Biotherapy

Jones and Bartlett Series in Oncology

2001 Oncology Nursing Drug Handbook, Wilkes/Ingwersen/Barton-Burke

American Cancer Society's Consumers Guide to Cancer Drugs, Wilkes/Ades/Krakoff

American Cancer Society's Patient Education Guide to Oncology Drugs, Wilkes/Ades/Krakoff

Biotherapy: A Comprehensive Overview, Second Edition, Rieger

Blood and Marrow Stem Cell Transplantation, Second Edition, Whedon

Cancer and HIV Clinical Nutrition Pocket Guide, Second Edition, Wilkes

Cancer Chemotherapy: A Nursing Process Approach, Second Edition, Barton-Burke/Wilkes/Ingwersen

Cancer Nursing: Principles and Practice, Fifth Edition, Yarbro, et al.

Cancer Nursing: Principles and Practice, Fourth Edition CD-ROM, Groenwald, et al

Cancer Symptom Management, Second Edition, Yarbro/Frogge/Goodman

Cancer Symptom Management, Patient Self-Care Guides, Second Edition, Yarbro/Frogge/Goodman.

Chemotherapy Care Plans Handbook, Second Edition, Barton-Burke/Wilkes/Ingwersen

A Clinical Guide to Cancer Nursing, Fourth Edition, Groenwald, et al.

A Clinical Guide to Stem Cell and Bone Marrow Transplantation, Shapiro, et al.

Clinical Handbook for Biotherapy, Rieger

Comprehensive Cancer Nursing Review, Fourth Edition, Groenwald, et al.

Contemporary Issues in Prostate Cancer: A Nursing Perspective, Held-Warmkessel

Fatigue in Cancer: A Multidimensional Approach, Winningham/Barton-Burke

Handbook of Oncology Nursing, Third Edition, Johnson/Gross

HIV Homecare Handbook, Daigle

HIV Nursing and Symptom Management, Ropka/Williams

Homecare Management of the Bone Marrow Transplant Patient, Third Edition, Kelley, et al.

The Love Knot: Ties that Bind Cancer Partners, Ross

Medication Errors: Causes, Prevention and Risk Management, Cohen

Memory Bank for Chemotherapy, Third Edition, Preston/Wilfinger

Oncology Nursing Review, Second Edition, Yarbro/Frogge/Goodman

Oncology Nursing Society's Instruments for Clinical Nursing Research, Second Edition, Frank-Stromborg

Physicians' Cancer Chemotherapy Drug Manual 2001, Chu

Pocket Guide to Breast Cancer, Hassey Dow

Pocket Guide to Prostate Cancer, Held-Warmkessel

Pocket Guide for Women and Cancer, Moore, et al.

Quality of Life: From Nursing and Patient Perspectives, King/Hinds

Radiation Therapy: Multidisciplinary Management of Patient Outcomes, Bruner

Women and Cancer: A Gynecologic Oncology Nursing Perspective, Second Edition, Moore-Higgs, et al.

Biotherapy

A Comprehensive Overview

Second Edition

Edited by

Paula Trahan Rieger, RN, MSN, CS, AOCN®, FAAN
Nurse Practitioner, Human Clinical Cancer Genetics
Department of Clinical Cancer Prevention
The University of Texas M.D. Anderson Cancer Center
Houston, Texas

JONES AND BARTLETT PUBLISHERS
Sudbury, Massachusetts
BOSTON   TORONTO   LONDON   SINGAPORE

To my father, Weldon Trahan, who instilled in me a love of science and learning, and my mother, Dolores Trahan, who taught me what it means to be a good person.

World Headquarters
Jones and Bartlett Publishers
40 Tall Pine Drive
Sudbury, MA 01776
978-443-5000
info@jbpub.com
www.jbpub.com

Jones and Bartlett Publishers Canada
2406 Nikanna Road
Mississauga, ON L5C 2W6
CANADA

Jones and Bartlett Publishers International
Barb House, Barb Mews
London W6 7PA
UK

PRODUCTION CREDITS

Acquisitions Editor: Penny Glynn
Editor: John Danielowich
Production Editor: Linda S. DeBruyn
Editorial/Production Assistant: Christine Tridente
V.P., Manufacturing and Inventory: Therese Bräuer

Typesetting: Modern Graphics, Inc.
Text Design: Modern Graphics, Inc.
Cover Design: Stephanie Torta
Printing and Binding: Malloy Lithographing

Library of Congress Cataloging-in-Publication Data

Biotherapy: a comprehensive overview / edited by Paula Trahan Rieger.—2nd ed.
   p. cm.—(Jones and Bartlett series in oncology)
Includes bibliographical references and index.
ISBN 0-7637-1428-3
1. Biological response modifiers—Therapeutic use.
2. Cancer—Immunotherapy. I. Rieger, Paula Trahan. II. Series.

RC271.B53 B57 2000
616.99′406—dc21

          00-062679
          CIP

Printed in the United States of America
04 03 02 01 00   10 9 8 7 6 5 4 3 2 1

The inclusion of information in the Quick Summary pages for professional and patient resources represents a selection of materials that were readily available at the time of publication of this handbook and is not meant to be all-inclusive. For complete information on resources that are available from a pharmaceutical company related to a given product, contact the product sales representative.

The selection and dosage of drugs presented in this book are in accord with standards accepted at the time of publication. The authors, editors, and publisher have made every effort to provide accurate information. However, research, clinical practice, and government regulations often change the accepted standard in this field. Before administering any drug, the reader is advised to check the manufacturer's product information sheet for the most up-to-date recommendations on dosage, precautions, and contraindications. This is especially important in the case of drugs that are new or seldom used.

CONTENTS

CHAPTER 7   **Hematopoietic Growth Factors   245**

Debra Wujcik, RN, MSN, AOCN®

CHAPTER 11   **Tumor Necrosis Factor   383**

Lynne Brophy, RN, MSN

CHAPTER 12   **The Retinoids   407**

Paula Trahan Rieger, RN, MSN, CS, AOCN®, FAAN
Fadlo R. Khuri, MD

CHAPTER 13   **Gene Therapy   431**

Yvette Payne, RN, MSN, MBA
Patricia Brusso, RN, MSN

PART III   **Nursing Management and Future Perspectives   459**

CHAPTER 14   **Patient Management   461**

Paula Trahan Rieger, RN, MSN, CS, AOCN®, FAAN

FOREWORD

We are in the midst of a revolution in the treatment of disease. In the area of classical drug development we have many new opportunities to target synthetic molecules at specific genetic or biochemical changes which lead to diseases such as cancer and cardiovascular disorders.

In parallel, a whole new area of therapeutics has developed, which takes advantage of our advancing knowledge about biological molecules produced in the human body that can have profound effects on disease. We have learned a great deal about molecules which carry out immune and inflammatory processes, and other molecules which regulate the proliferation and function of cells by binding to receptors on the cell surface. But these rapid advances could not be converted into clinically effective agents without major technical discoveries that have enabled scaled up production of biologicals. The two most important technological breakthroughs are:

- The discovery of the hybridoma technique for producing specific monoclonal antibodies in large quantities. This was reported in 1975 by Köhler and Milstein, who were awarded the Nobel Prize for their work.
- The discovery of restriction enzymes and other molecules which permit scientists to isolate genes and move them into new environments, where they can be expressed to produce "industrial quantities" of specific biological molecules.

In the mid-1980's the Food and Drug Administration approved the use of Interferon-α, and this was soon followed by approval of granulocyte colony stimulating factor and granulocyte-macrophage colony stimulating factor. By 1998 a number of monoclonal antibodies were approved for treatment. Among those are Rituximab, which binds to a specific antigen on B cells and is useful in lympho-proliferative diseases, and Herceptin which binds to the HER-2 receptor and is effective in breast cancer, especially in combination with chemotherapy. Thus, in the period of 25 years, an entirely new therapeutic field has been introduced into the armamentarium available for physicians treating patients.

The impact of these biologically based therapies is only beginning to be felt. It is safe to predict that their use will grow, as additional agents are discovered and produced in the quantities required to study them carefully.

In this textbook on biotherapy, Paula Trahan Rieger has gathered a group of skilled scientists, physicians and nurses who describe biologic agents and carefully explain their uses, and common side effects. Each chapter is thoroughly referenced. I believe the reader will find that the literature is critically and accurately summarized, so that most information needed by nurses who wish to thoroughly understand the biological basis and clinical indications for biotherapeutic treatments is available in the book. As stated in the title, it is truly "a comprehensive overview."

Finally, it is important to note that much of the research referenced in this textbook was carried out in collaboration with nurses. There are many areas that are fruitful for future investigation that are pointed out in the context of potential clinical applications for biological agents.

John Mendelsohn, M.D.
President,
The University of Texas
M. D. Anderson Cancer Center

xix

PREFACE

With the arrival of the millennium, we have seen the true integration of biotherapy as the fourth modality of cancer treatment. Since the publication of the first edition of this text in 1995, many changes have occurred which impact our world. Progress and discoveries in science and technology have continued at an astounding rate. The power of the World Wide Web has influenced our patients and consequently our practice. All major categories of biological agents have now received at least one regulatory approval, and additional indications are continually issued for those biological agents such as interferon-α and granulocyte colony-stimulating factor that received initial approval in the late 1980s or early 1990s.

The challenge for myself and the authors remained to synthesize an ever-expanding and rapidly changing field of knowledge into a text that is up-to-date, understandable, and clinically useful. Because most nurses now give biotherapy in their practice, the need for such a specialized and comprehensive text remained. Although articles on biotherapy are now common in the literature, and the subject is generally included in major source texts on cancer care, this book remains the only text of its kind. I have tried to integrate comments received from those who have used the text to improve upon this book, and continually strive to make it as clinically useful as possible.

This edition is targeted to both the oncology nurse who is a novice in biotherapy as well as the nurse with an expertise in this area. However, it is also a valuable text for nurses in other specialty fields that are now using biological agents to treat conditions such as hepatitis, autoimmune diseases, and multiple sclerosis. Additionally, other health care professionals, such as pharmacists, medical and surgical oncologists, and physicians' assistants will also find it useful as well as students in medical and nursing school.

Part I, **Biotherapy: Principles and Foundations,** now has four chapters. The first chapter provides an overview of the field of biotherapy, historical perspectives, technological developments, a framework to define and classify agents, and a brief overview of each category of agents and related approvals. Tables have been included that provide a quick overview of regulatory approvals for biological agents both within oncology (Table 1.6) and outside of oncology (Table 1.7). An expanded section has been added on biological agents with regulatory approval that do not fall under the major agent categories and includes immunomodulators. A section was also added in this chapter to cover cellular therapy. The chapter on the immune system has been updated to reflect new information, and a chapter was added on basic cell biology. All nurses must have a foundation in these concepts to understand the emerging therapies of the future. A chapter on optimizing the dose and schedule of biological agents provides a valuable perspective on the complex issue of selecting the proper dose.

Together, the chapters in Part I form a foundation for the information presented in Part II, **Major Categories of Biological Agents**. This section has undergone extensive revision to include new approvals and new avenues of clinical research. Chapters have been added on the retinoids, vaccines, and gene therapy. Because of the large volume of information on monoclonal antibodies, the information is now presented in two chapters—one focusing on hematological malignancies, and the other on applications in solid tumors. The authors selected are experts in their field. Each has provided an overview of the history of the development of each agent, the biological effects as they relate to the mechanism of action of each agent, the major clinical trials leading to an agent's approval, toxic effects, and areas of future research. Two new features have been added to these chapters. Clinical pearls, or tips, are presented that summarize key points a nurse should be aware of when administering an agent. Key references and resources are also cited to direct the reader to more comprehensive information or classic articles. Useful web sites have been integrated into these resources as well.

Part III, **Nursing Management and Future Perspectives** has also been expanded. A new chapter was added on the management of anorexia to provide more detailed information on this challenging toxic effect. A chapter was added to provide perspective from the patient's point of view regarding participation in clinical trials and receiving biological agents. The chapter on reimbursement issues was expanded to provide more information on disease management as it relates to the system of health care we currently work in. The future's chapter has been expanded to cover the emerging strategies in molecular medicine, which will assume an increasingly important role in the armamentarium to treat cancer. Health care in the year 2000 is increasingly focused on meeting needs of patients and families. A chapter on patient education remains and has been updated to reflect new technologies for teaching.

References are provided throughout the text to guide the reader in pursuing further information on clinical studies, biological actions of the major agents, and nursing care. Words included in the glossary are set in bold type throughout the text to assist the reader in developing the "new" vocabulary needed to understand this therapeutic modality. An appendix has been added to this addition to help the reader quickly locate key information. It includes examples of a clinical pathway for interleukin-2, and patient care plans. A new feature first used in the *Clinical Handbook for Biotherapy* (1999), the quick summary pages, is included in the appendix. These pages are designed to provide quick, easy-to-use information on the administration of regulatory-approved agents and associated resource materials. Information specific to drugs with regulatory approval was generated from the following resources: The World Wide Web; *The Physician's Desk Reference, 54th edition* (2000); and *Drug Facts and Comparison: Loose Leaf Drug Information Service* (2000).

This text represents the accumulated wisdom of the authors' many years of expertise in the field of biotherapy. Every attempt has been made to include the most up-to-date information, resources, and references. It is our hope that this text will provide you with a valuable resource that will expand your understanding of biotherapy as it is used in cancer management and will serve to enhance your practice.

Acknowledgments

The preparation of a text such as *Biotherapy: A Comprehensive Overview 2nd edition* requires significant commitment and time of those involved. One never achieves such a goal alone. There are many who contributed to this text and deserve acknowledgment.

First and foremost I would like to recognize and thank my husband Marty for his eternal support and assistance in helping me to achieve the goals I set. He helps to celebrate the successes and comfort me during the difficult times, and he built me the most beautiful office anyone could ask for. I thank Paula Shackelford, RN for the gift of her friendship and the many hours she spent helping to research key topics for this text, especially for the quick summary pages. I would like to pay special tribute to

Vickie Williams from Scientific Publications at the University of Texas M. D. Anderson Cancer Center for her innumerable hours of work in assuring the quality of this text through the standard of excellence she helped me to set. Her contribution has been invaluable. I would also like to recognize Suzan Stephens for secretarial assistance in revising manuscripts.

My sincere thanks to the many reviewers who assisted in assuring the quality of this text: Constance Johnson, RN (Chapter 1), Eric Wieder, PhD and Lisa St. John, PhD (Chapter 2), Michael Rosenblum (Chapter 4), John Thompson, MD (Chapter 5), James Lee Murray III, MD (Chapters 8 and 10), Christine Bennett, RN and Terese Knoop, RN (Chapter 13), Cynthia Hodges, RN and Bill Dana, PharmD (Chapter 14), Paula Shackelford, RN and Lee R. Berkowitz MD (Chapter 15), Paula R. Anderson, RN (Chapter 17), Faith Ottery, MD, PhD (Chapter 18), Louise Villejo (Chapter 20), Kris Hartigan, RN and Maggie O'Reilly, RN (Chapter 21), and Gordon Mills, MD, PhD (Chapter 22).

My most sincere appreciation and recognition are extended to the authors who participated in writing this text. They gave freely of their knowledge and spent the time requested of them to achieve the standard of excellence I hoped to attain in this text. They are to be commended. I recognize the many friends and colleagues who have inspired me over the years to be a better nurse and to strive for excellence in all that I do. And lastly, I would like to recognize the editorial staff at Jones and Bartlett, including Greg Vis, Penny Glynn, John Danielowich, Linda DeBruyn, and Christine Tridente; and Michael Granger at Modern Graphics for their contributions to this text.

The dedication of all involved has contributed to a 2nd edition that will ultimately benefit the patients for whom we, as oncology nurses, provide care.

CONTRIBUTORS

Lynne Brophy, RN, MSN (Chapter 11)
Consultant and Staff Nurse
Cincinnati Hematology Oncology
Cincinnati, OH

Charles K. Brown, MD, PhD (Chapter 10)
Biologic Therapy Fellow
University of Pittsburgh

Patricia Brusso, RN, MSN (Chapter 13)
At the time this chapter was written:
Senior Research Nurse
Head & Neck Surgical Oncology
The University of Texas M. D. Anderson
Cancer Center
Houston, TX

Linda Cuaron, RN, MN, AOCN®
(Chapters 5 & 18)
Senior Patient Care Consultant
Schering Oncology Biotech
Clinical Faculty
University of Washington
Seattle, WA

Grace E. Dean, RN, MSN (Chapter 17)
Research Specialist
Department of Nursing Research and Education
City of Hope National Medical Center
Duarte, CA

Alma Yvette DeJesus, RN, MSN, AOCN®
(Chapter 21)
Associate Director, Practice Outcomes
The University of Texas M. D. Anderson
Cancer Center
Houston, TX

Janet E. DiJulio, RN, MSN (Chapter 8)
Nurse Manager
Stanford University Hospital and Clinics
Palo Alto, CA

Danielle M. Gale, RN, ND, FNP, AOCN®
(Chapter 6)
Oncology Clinical Coordinator
Genentech BioOncology
San Francisco, CA

Marjorie Green, MD
Fellow – Medical Oncology
The University of Texas M. D. Anderson
Cancer Center
Houston, TX

Fadlo R. Khuri, MD (Chapter 12)
Assistant Professor of Medicine
Thoracic/Head and Neck Medical Oncology
The University of Texas M. D. Anderson
Cancer Center
Houston, TX

Krishna Komanduri, MD (Chapter 2)
Assistant Professor of Medicine
Section of Transplantation Immunology
Department of Blood and Marrow
Transplantation
The University of Texas M. D. Anderson
Cancer Center
Houston, TX

Donna M. Kinzler, RN, MSN, CRNP, OCN®
(Chapter 10)
Nurse Clinician
University of Pittsburgh Medical Center
Division of Surgical Oncology and Biologic
Therapy
Pittsburgh, PA

Christina A. Meyers, PhD, ABPP
(Chapter 19)
Associate Professor of Neuropsychology
The University of Texas M. D. Anderson
Cancer Center
Houston, TX

James Lee Murray III, MD (Chapter 9)
Professor of Medicine
Bioimmunotherapy and Breast Medical
Oncology
The University of Texas M. D. Anderson
Cancer Center
Houston, TX

Yvette Payne, RN, MSN, MBA (Chapter 13)
Senior Manager, Health Outcomes and Disease
Management
US Oncology
Houston, TX

**Paula Trahan Rieger, RN, MSN, CS,
AOCN®, FAAN** (Chapters 1, 4, 9, 12, 14, &
22)
Nurse Practitioner, Human Clinical Cancer
Genetics
Department of Clinical Cancer Prevention
The University of Texas M. D. Anderson
Cancer Center
Houston, TX

Kimberly A. Rumsey, RN, MSN, OCN®
(Chapter 20)
Family Nurse Practitioner-Private Practice
Tomball, TX

Brenda K. Shelton, RN, MS, CCRN, AOCN®
(Chapter 16)
Critical Care Clinical Nurse Specialist
The Johns Hopkins Oncology Center
Baltimore, MD

Scott Solomon, MD (Chapter 2)
Research Fellow, Hematology/Oncology
Stem Cell Allotransplantation Section
NHLBI, National Institutes of Health
Bethesda, MD

Patricia Sorokin, RN, BSN, OCN®
(Chapter 6)
Clinical Research Nurse
University of Illinois at Chicago
Section of Hematology/Oncology
Chicago, IL

Brian Stabler, PhD (Chapter 15)
Professor of Psychiatry and Pediatrics
School of Medicine
The University of North Carolina at Chapel Hill
Chapel Hill, NC

John Thompson, MD (Chapter 5)
Associate Professor of Medicine
University of Washington

Deborah L. Volker, RN, PhD, AOCN®
(Chapter 3)
Assistant Professor
School of Nursing
The University of Texas at Austin
Austin, TX

Debra Wujcik, RN, MSN, AOCN®
(Chapter 7)
Director, Clinical Trial Training and Outreach,
Vanderbilt-Ingram Cancer Center
Nashville, TN

PART I

Biotherapy:
Principles and Foundations

CHAPTER 1 | Biotherapy: An Overview

Paula Trahan Rieger, RN, MSN, CS, AOCN®, FAAN

As the field of biotherapy has evolved, it has generated, at varying times, feelings of excitement and frustration; however, scientific interest has remained undeterred. We now possess significant knowledge of the intricate workings of the immune system and how the immune system interacts with cancer cells; yet, we realize that there is much more to learn about biotherapy before we can maximize its therapeutic efficacy in the cancer setting (Rosenberg, 1999). This chapter provides a historical perspective of the field of biotherapy and the specific advances in technology that allowed for the mass production of biological proteins. The major categories of biological agents (e.g., the interferons, interleukins, hematopoietic growth factors, monoclonal antibodies, retinoids, vac-

cines, and tumor necrosis factor) and approvals to date will be covered in detail in subsequent chapters. The use of cellular therapy and immunomodulators, as more classic forms of immunotherapy, will be covered in detail in this chapter. Biotherapy represents the first attempt to target cancer therapies more specifically toward the cancerous cell. The understanding of cancer as a multifactorial disease that results from mutations in specific classes of genes controlling the cell's life cycle will ultimately lead to ever newer and more specific forms of cancer therapy in the future.

Historical Perspective

The use of **immunotherapy** as treatment for malignant disease can be traced back to the 19th century and even earlier (Hersh *et al.*, 1973; Oettgen and Old, 1991; Hall, 1997).

The author wishes to acknowledge the work of Patricia Jassak and Grace Dean, whose work on Chapters 1 and Chapter 9 (respectively) in the first edition of *Biotherapy: A Comprehensive Overview* formed the foundation of this chapter.

Immunotherapy, defined broadly, is a form of therapy that uses the immune system, its cells, and molecules that serve as messengers among cells involved in immune responses to battle disease. The beginning of immunotherapy is often traced to William Bradley Coley, a New York surgeon who noticed a connection between infection and the spontaneous regression of tumors in patients he had treated. The current use of cytokines is based on Dr. Coley's use of bacterial toxins to treat solid tumors. He used the toxins to induce an immune response that he hoped would activate the immune system to eliminate or reduce the tumor burden (Hall, 1997). Other early experiments in which tumor-specific immunity in the mouse was achieved by lymphocyte transfer laid the groundwork for the current use of cytotoxic T lymphocytes in conjunction with biological agents such as interleukin-2 (IL-2) (Oettgen and Old, 1991). Whereas the original vaccines were made from crude tumor preparations, today's vaccines contain purified cancer antigens. Modern investigations of monoclonal antibodies are refinements of early studies that used horse and rabbit antisera. A time line of the key events that occurred during the development of biotherapy is depicted in Table 1.1.

The quest to understand and control the relationship between the immune system and cancer is linked to three observations that have withstood the test of time: spontaneous remissions in patients with cancer, the increased incidence of cancer in immunosuppressed patients, and the presence of lymphoid infiltrates in solid tumors (Oettgen and Old, 1991). Oettgen and Old point out that although these observations are credible when viewed from an immunologic perspective, other explanations exist that are independent of immune system recognition and action. They postulate that these observations provide the impetus for continued scientific inquiry until it is clearly established that the human immune system is capable of recogni-

Table 1.1   Time line of key events in the development of biotherapy

Late 1800s to Mid-1900s
- Impure vaccines
- Coley's toxins
- Interferon discovered (1957)

1960s to Early 1970s
- Clinical trials of the use of bacterial agents to nonspecifically stimulate the immune system, examples, bacille Calmette-Guérin and *Corynebacterium parvum*
- Early immunotherapy trials
- Limitations of studies related to:
    Impure agents
    Variability in experimental procedures
    Incongruence between animal and human studies
    Lack of generalizable results

Late 1970s to Mid-1980s
- Major technological advances
- Increased understanding of immune system
- Advances in genetic engineering
- Continued advances in molecular biology
- Ability to mass produce biological proteins and antibodies
    Recombinant DNA technology
    Hybridoma technology
- Advances in laboratory methods and processes and computer systems
- Single-agent cytokine studies initiated
- Biological response modifier program initiated by the National Cancer Institute
- First biological agent (interferon-α) approved by the U.S. Food and Drug Administration

Late 1980s to Present
- Discovery and isolation of a variety of immune system products
- Numerous agents recombinantly produced for clinical trials
- Multisite clinical trials initiated; some ongoing
- Initiation of clinical trials of combination cytokine therapy
- Initiation of clinical trials of combination cytokine therapy plus chemotherapy
- Regulatory approval for all categories of biological agents

tion and surveillance of malignant cells. Thus, the therapeutic success of biotherapy is dependent on evolving insight into the physiologic mechanisms of the host-tumor relationship, host biology, and tumor biology (Creekmore *et al.*, 1991; Oldham, 1998a).

In 1894, Dr. Coley, a surgeon at New York's Memorial Hospital from 1891 to 1936, began studying the effects of bacterial products in patients with cancer. One of his first patients, a young woman less than 20 years old, had died of sarcoma, and the experience had intensely affected him. Following her death, he began a search of New York Hospital's records of prior cases of sarcoma to learn more about the rare disease. During the course of his research, he stumbled upon an unusual case of an immigrant treated at the hospital in 1885. The man had undergone 4 operations for cancer and had endured 4 recurrences of his tumor, a round-cell sarcoma. His last surgery was so extensive that surgeons were unable to close the wound, leaving a large, open area partially held together with sutures. His survival was believed to be hopeless.

Shortly after surgery, the patient had a raging case of erysipelas, a disease caused by *Streptococcus pyogenes*. In the 19th century, erysipelas was one of the most common postoperative infections, and it was often fatal. The man's first attack was severe, and a second attack followed two weeks later. Ultimately, to the astonishment of the hospital staff, the patient survived the infection; his wound healed, forming a healthy scar. He was discharged and disappeared from medical follow-up (Hall, 1997).

Seven years following his near-death experience, Dr. Coley tracked the patient to the tenements of New York. To everyone's astonishment, he was in good health and free of cancer. Dr. Coley reasoned that nature had provided a hint related to the patient's cure and that if an accidental case of erysipelas could cure a sarcoma, then an artificially induced epi-sode of the infection might produce the same result! In 1891, he initiated the American era of nonspecific immunotherapy by inoculating a patient with *S. pyogenes*, hoping to induce a case of erysipelas and produce an antitumor effect. Coley believed that a molecule, or "toxin," of some sort produced by the bacteria had a dramatic effect on the tumor.

In Coley's era, the accepted treatment for sarcomas was amputation, radiation therapy, or a combination of these. Until his death in 1936, Coley labored to prove his theory about the antitumor effect of toxins and that the use of toxins was as effective or even more effective than radiation therapy. To his credit, he had several patients who were long-term survivors of previously inoperable tumors (Coley, 1893; Coley, 1911).

Because his vision was a departure from popular thinking, Coley's work was widely criticized in his day despite numerous striking successes. Like many of the early immunotherapy trials, his work suffered from the lack of a standard formulation for his "toxins," the lack of standard doses and administration and treatment duration guidelines, and most troubling of all, a lack of replication of his results by others. Coley's toxin therapy continued to be used until 1975 and provided the rationale for the current investigations of cytokine therapy (Goodfield, 1984). However, with the advent of more predictable and comprehensive treatment options, that is, radiation therapy and, later, chemotherapy, the use of Coley's toxin therapy declined. Much of Coley's work was chronicled from his papers following his death by his daughter, Helen Coley Nauts (Nauts and McLaren, 1990). Oettgen and Old (1991) reported that only one clinical trial evaluated the use of Coley's toxin therapy in a rigorous scientific manner. In that trial, patients with non-Hodgkin's lymphoma were given chemotherapy alone or chemotherapy combined with Coley's toxins. At the first 5-year analysis, patients who received Coley's toxins demonstrated a higher rate of complete response, increased duration of response, and longer survival. However, as time passed, the differences between the two approaches diminished. Today, we might surmise that Coley's toxins caused the *in vivo* production of potent cytokines that led to antitumor responses, although no precise molecular or immunologic explanation for the results produced by the toxin therapy has been described (Oettgen and Old, 1991; Starnes, 1992).

Subsequent work in the field of biotherapy has used nonspecific stimulators of the immune system, such as **bacillus Calmette-Guérin (BCG)**, **methanol-extracted residue of BCG (MER-BCG)**, *Corynebacterium parvum*, and levamisole, in a variety of tumors. These agents appeared to be clinically effective only when used in patients with minimal tumor burden. Most studies failed to demonstrate any benefit from these agents when they were used alone in patients with a large tumor burden. In general, clinical outcomes were poor due to the use of impure agents and variability in experimental procedures. The variability in procedures led to results that were neither generalizable nor, when animal models were used, predictive of human response.

Biotechnology

In the 1980s, scientific advancement in the way biological agents were identified, isolated, produced, and used improved tumor responses to biotherapy and positioned it as a viable cancer-treatment modality. Advances in 4 areas were critical in establishing biotherapy as a promising treatment entity (Oldham and Smalley, 1983; Oldham, 1984; Gallucci, 1987; Oldham, 1998a; PhRMA, 1998):

- An increased understanding of the intricate complexities of the immune system

- Refinement of recombinant **deoxyribonucleic acid (DNA)** and hybridoma technology
- Laboratory success in establishing methods to produce large volumes of effector cells in culture
- Isolation and purification of new biological products aided by advances in computer hardware and software

The term "biotechnology" is used frequently and actually refers to 3 distinct types of technology: traditional biotechnology, gene technology, and reproduction technology. Traditional biotechnology uses living organisms or their parts to produce or modify chemical compounds. The process of fermentation, used for centuries to produce food and alcoholic beverages, is a type of traditional biotechnology. Gene technology or genetic engineering uses DNA properties to analyze and modify the genetic information. This methodology provides completely new avenues for the production of medications and other substances used in agriculture and food production. Lastly, reproduction technology refers to traditional breeding techniques, *in vitro* fertilization, and cloning of organisms. In reproduction biotechnology, the genetic information is not manipulated at all; hence, it should not be confused with gene technology. Biotechnology-derived medicines currently account for 5% of the value of the world market in medicines, and this percentage is expected to increase to greater than 15% by the year 2005 (PhRMA, 1999).

Clinical use of biological agents was limited until the advent of recombinant DNA technology. For recombinant technology to be successful, a system was needed that was able to support the large-scale production of cells that, because their DNA can be manipulated, could be made to express a desired protein. The bacterium *Escherichia coli* was developed as such an expression system, making a critical contribution to the evolution and expansion of the field of molecular biology. *E. coli* was a good choice for an expression system because it is relatively simple genetically, it grows rapidly, it is generally well characterized, and it has been extensively studied (Ramel *et al.*, 1983).

E. coli is made up of one large circular thread of chromosomal DNA and several smaller circular units of genetic material called plasmids. Because plasmids replicate independently of chromosomal DNA, they were quickly singled out as the target for genetic engineering. In recombinant DNA technology, special enzymes called restriction endonucleases are used to cut openings in the plasmid at specific locations and then fragments of DNA are inserted into the openings. Another enzyme, DNA ligase, is used to close the ends of the open plasmid to the ends of the DNA fragment.

The DNA fragment is derived in one of several ways (Ramel *et al.*, 1983). It can be chemically synthesized to code for the known amino acid sequence of a particular protein or excised from the chromosome of interest. Alternatively, complementary DNA may be synthesized (by using purified messenger RNA as a template) with the enzyme reverse transcriptase. The new plasmid created by this synthesis is called a **vector**, and it is introduced into the *E. coli* host, which in culture grows bacterial cells that produce the desired protein. **Cloning** refers to the selection of colonies for optimal growth in culture. Cloning enables the cells to produce an unlimited supply of the donor DNA. Figure 1.1 depicts this process schematically.

The *E. coli* expression system is somewhat restricted in that its natural structure does not include an enzyme system for adding sugar side chains to proteins (Ramel *et al.*, 1983). This is of little consequence when the substance to be cloned is not a glycoprotein. When the substance is a glycoprotein, however, its natural carbohydrate moiety will be missing. Clinical

trials must continue to address the importance of this variable. Other expression systems now in use, such as yeast, have the ability to bind glycosylating proteins.

The protein produced by this recombinant DNA technology is purified with the goal of 100% homogeneity and the highest possible product yield. Higher levels of homogeneity result in an unavoidable loss of product. Biological agents are examples of proteins produced by this process. The end result is the reliable mass production of pure amounts of natural body proteins. This methodology has led to the production of numerous biological products currently used in the treatment of such diseases as cancer, diabetes, cystic fibrosis, and hemophilia in addition to the production of vaccines.

A variety of expression systems may be used to produce biological proteins. Examples include yeast, mammalian cells (e.g., Chinese hamster ovary [CHO] cells), and transgenic animals. In the last case, the gene for a specific protein such as alpha-1 antitrypsin, which is used to fight emphysema, is injected into the fertilized egg of an animal such as a pig. The protein is then extracted from the transgenic pig's milk (Velander *et al.*, 1997; Wilmut, 1998). Increasingly, genetically modified mammalian cells are the preferred system for the production of recombinant therapeutic glycoproteins. Core genetic technologies are continually being refined and emerging strategies evaluated for their utility in optimizing recombinant-protein expression in genetically engineered mammalian cells. In addition, other applications of this technology include engineering of cell lines for drug screening and cell-base therapies and the construction of recombinant viruses for gene therapy (Fussenegger *et al.*, 1999; Wurm and Bernard, 1999).

The production of substances used in biological therapies must meet product quality control regulations and the good manufacturing product

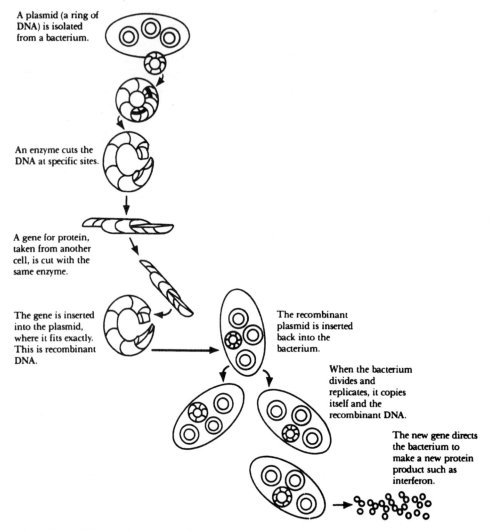

A plasmid (a ring of DNA) is isolated from a bacterium.

An enzyme cuts the DNA at specific sites.

A gene for protein, taken from another cell, is cut with the same enzyme.

The gene is inserted into the plasmid, where it fits exactly. This is recombinant DNA.

The recombinant plasmid is inserted back into the bacterium.

When the bacterium divides and replicates, it copies itself and the recombinant DNA.

The new gene directs the bacterium to make a new protein product such as interferon.

Figure 1.1   Recombinant DNA technology

Source: Schindler, L. 1988. *Understanding the Immune System.* NIH publication number 88-529. Bethesda, MD: U.S. Department of Health and Human Services, p. 29.

(GMP) guidelines. Evidence of the safety, efficacy, purity, and identity of a product must be presented to the Food and Drug Administration (FDA) before testing and when appropriate marketing approvals are granted. Recombinant products are designated by the placement of a lowercase "r" before the drug name.

Definition and Classification of Biotherapy

Biotherapy encompasses the use of agents derived from biological sources or of agents that affect biological responses (Oldham, 1998a). Primarily, these are products derived from the mammalian genome. In 1983, the National Cancer Institute, Division of Cancer Treatment Subcommittee on Biological Response Modifiers, defined **biological response modifiers (BRMs)** as "agents or approaches that modify the relationship between tumor and host by modifying the host's biological response to tumor cells with a resultant therapeutic effect" (Mihich and Fefer, 1983). This term distinguishes a class of agents composed of native and altered endogenous proteins that result in a specific desired cellular response. Most BRMs are either **lymphokines** or **cytokines** (Mazanet *et al.*, 1996).

The terms used to describe these agents and approaches have changed as scientific advances have increased our understanding of them. Historically, the term "immunotherapy" was used because the major focus of this therapeutic approach was modulation of the immune response. Although modulation of the immune response remains a major focus, the terms "biotherapy" or "biological therapy" have replaced "immunotherapy" because the scope of the field has widened. BRMs or more commonly biological agents—the agents used in this therapeutic modality—have pleiotropic effects, that is, they possess multiple actions. They are capable of producing immunological actions, other biological effects, or a combination of these activities. Biotherapy is generally used as a global term to refer to all of these activities.

No single classification system exists for biotherapy. It is also difficult to classify biological agents because they often perform multiple biological actions. Biological agents exert at least one of the following effects: they augment, modulate, or restore the host's immune response; they have direct cytotoxic or antiproliferative activity; or they produce other biological effects, for example, differentiation or maturation of cells or interference with tumor-cell metastasis or transformation (Clark and Longo,

1986; Borden and Sondel, 1990; Dutcher, 1992). In addition, they are used to increase the patient's ability to tolerate side effects of cytotoxic cancer treatment modalities and to target and bind to cancer cells and thereby induce more effective cytostatic or cytocidal antitumor activity (Oldham, 1998a). One system classifies the biotherapy of cancer into five broad categories based on the principal function of the agent or approach in the immune system (Mitchell, 1992). These categories are described in Table 1.2.

Clinical Development of Biological Agents

Identification, development, and testing of a biological agent requires that specific intricacies of physiologic and pharmacologic parameters be thoroughly investigated. This complete evaluation measures not only the agent's effectiveness but also takes into account the cellular immune response. Thus, the approach used in the clinical investigation of a biological agent is different from that used for a chemical agent.

The process of drug development begins with the discovery of the mechanisms involved in a specific disease. These discoveries are generated through research generated by government agencies, academic institutions, nonprofit foundations, and pharmaceutical companies. The disease mechanisms then become the targets of pharmaceutical interventions. Translational research brings the basic research into clinical practice, where the first phases of product development and initial human trials begin. Applied research, or the actual development and testing of medicines, is supported primarily by pharmaceutical companies and the government. It involves large-scale clinical trials, dosage testing, and research to determine information that should be included in product

Table 1.2   The effects of biotherapy on the immune system

Effect	Definition

Active	Stimulation of the host's intrinsic function
	• Nonspecific
	    Use of microbial or chemical agents to activate general host defense systems (e.g., bacillus Calmette-Guérin).
	• Specific
	    Use of vaccines to augment or induce host response to tumor cells or tumor-associated antigens. Immunization with purified antigen, immunodominant peptide (native or modified), "naked" DNA encoding the antigen, recombinant viruses encoding the antigen, or antigen-presenting cells pulsed with protein or peptide (or transfected with genes encoding the antigen).
	    Use of cytokine adjuvants such as IL-2 or IL-12 administered systemically or encoded by the immunizing vector.

Adoptive	Transfer of immune cells with antitumor properties to tumor-bearing host (e.g., lymphokine-activated killer cells or tumor-infiltrating lymphocytes). Transfer of cells sensitized *in vitro* to the specific antigen (bulk or cloned population). Transduction of effector cells (or stem cells) with genes encoding T-cell receptors that recognize specific antigens.
Restorative	Restoration of deficient immunologic subpopulations.
Passive	Transfer of antibodies or short-lived antitumor "factors."
Cytomodulatory	Agents that cause increased recognition of tumor-associated antigens and histocompatibility antigens on the surface of tumor cells.

Sources: Mitchell, M. 1992. Chemotherapy in combination with biomodulation: A 5-year experience with cyclophosphamide and interleukin-2. *Seminars in Oncology* 19(2 suppl 4): 80–87.

Rosenberg, S. 1999. A new era of cancer immunotherapy: Converting theory to performance. *CA: A Journal for Clinicians* 49(2): 70–73.

labeling (PhRMA, 1999). Figure 1.2 outlines the process of drug discovery.

Steps in the Drug Development Process

The FDA requires preclinical and clinical trial evaluation of all chemical and biological agents prior to their commercial approval (Johnson and Temple, 1985). The current process of drug development involves a very arduous, time-consuming, and costly set of procedures. The preclinical development of a new biological agent must encompass three major steps (Creekmore *et al.*, 1991; Siegel *et al.*, 1995;

Oldham, 1998b). The first step involves the identification, isolation, recombinant expression, and preclinical production of the new agent; determination of its physiologic role; and development of early therapeutic models. The vast majority of biological agents are species-specific. For this reason, the design of preclinical studies is especially important. The preclinical studies must carefully parallel the design of the proposed initial clinical trials, because results obtained with recombinant human biological agents administered to another species may not be transferable to the clinic (Mazanet, 1996). The second step focuses on the clinical development of the drug, including increased

The Process of Discovery

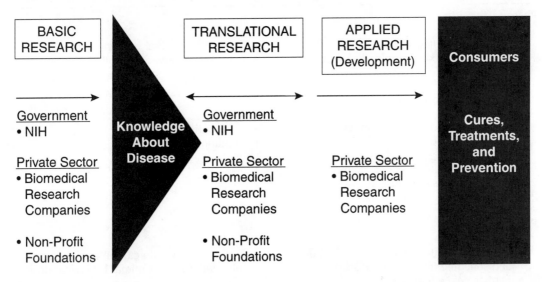

| BASIC RESEARCH | | TRANSLATIONAL RESEARCH | APPLIED RESEARCH (Development) | Consumers |

Figure 1.2 Drug development process

Reprinted with permission from Pharmaceutical Research and Manufacturers of America (PhRMA). 1998. *Biomedicine: Promises for Health.* Washington DC: Pharmaceutical Research and Manufacturers of America; and from Pharmaceutical Research and Manufacturers of America (PhRMA). 1999. *Pharmaceuticals Industry Profile 1999.* Washington DC: Pharmaceutical Research and Manufacturers of America.

production under the GMP guidelines and analysis of the preclinical toxicity profile, pharmacology studies, and application studies. In the third step, an investigational new drug (IND) application is completed and filed with the FDA. A phase I protocol accompanied by supporting preclinical toxicology and pharmacology studies is required for IND submission (Collins *et al.*, 1990). Once IND status is granted, the agent enters sequential clinical trials.

There are three main phases of clinical trials. The major characteristics of each phase and the specific objectives that must be addressed when evaluating biological agents are described in Table 1.3. When a company is ready to seek approval to market a biological product, a Product License Application (PLA) must be filed. This is comparable to the New Drug Applica-

tion filed for traditional pharmaceuticals. The PLA explains the process by which the product is manufactured and tested and includes the results of preclinical and clinical investigations using the products. In addition, historically, an Establishment License Application (ELA) was submitted to the FDA to obtain approval for the actual buildings where a biological product was to be manufactured, tested, or stored. The ELA and the PLA were generally submitted simultaneously. (Siegel *et al.*, 1995; Mazanet, 1996). The need for an ELA was eliminated by the FDA Modernization Act of 1997.

The Cost of Drug Development

The estimated pretax cost of drug development in the 1990s was $500 million, which included the cost of research failures as well as interest

Table 1.3   Objectives of clinical trials for biological and chemical agents (by phase) with specific objectives for biological agents

Objectives for Biological and Chemical Agents	Objectives Specific to Biological Agents Alone
Phase I	
Objectives:	*Objectives:*
• Define toxic effects	• Determine optimal biological dose
• Determine maximum tolerated dose and dose-limiting toxicity	• Correlate observed clinical responses with biological end points
• Use escalating doses	
• Determine pharmacokinetics	
Features:	*Features:*
• 3–6 patients/dose level (average)	• 5–15 patients/dose level
• Single-institution setting	• Immunologic monitoring
End Points:	
• Unacceptable toxic effects define maximum tolerated dose	
• Determination of dose schedules and toxicities	
Phase II	
Objectives:	*Objective:*
• Determine antitumor activity in given dose and schedule in a specific disease	• Dose and schedule can be at maximum tolerated dose or optimal biological dose
• Further define toxicity	
• Refine toxicity interventions/management	
Features:	
• Usually 30 patients at fixed dose	
• Multiple-institution setting	
End Points:	
• Substantial information obtained about drug's therapeutic activity related to best dose, route, and schedule of administration	
• Identification of tumor types for which treatment appears promising	
Phase III	
Objective:	*Objective:*
• Compare therapeutic efficacy	• In multiple disease states, no effective therapy exists; thus, most biological agents are approved for use after analysis of phase II data
Features:	
• Randomized study design	
• Large numbers of patients	
• Cooperative study groups	
End Point:	
• Comparison of new treatment and standard treatment	

over the entire period of the investment. The cost of drug development has increased since the 1970s for many reasons. A major factor has been the requirement by government regulatory agencies of an increase in the number of clinical trials and the number of study participants. In addition, it often takes an average of 15 years to develop a drug and bring it to market. Within this equation, pharmaceutical companies must balance projections about the potential market size and profitability of the drug as justification for the investment (Oldham, 1998b; PhRMA, 1999). Many biological agents are highly sought after, such as monoclonal antibodies that target only a subpopulation of cancer cells, thus limiting their market size. Market size may reach an unapproachable level given the current costs of drug development and the regulatory infrastructure in place.

Maximum Tolerated Dose Versus Optimal Biological Dose

The underlying hypothesis of cytotoxic drug research is that "more is better." Thus, a critical first step in evaluating a new drug is to determine the maximum tolerated dose (MTD). This step is also important for biological agents because the agent may exert the best antitumor effect at the MTD. The MTD, however, may not be the same as the optimal biological dose (OBD). Early clinical trials of biological agents demonstrated that immunologic effects occurred at doses lower than the identified MTD. This phenomenon led to the concept of the OBD (Herberman, 1985), which is defined as "that dose which, with a minimum of side effects, produces the optimal desired responses for the parameters deemed important with respect to a particular biological agent" (Creekmore et al., 1991; Mazanet, 1996). Further discussion of the importance of the OBD and dose response of biological agents can be found in Chapter 4.

Oldham (1985) identified 2 underlying differences between drugs and biological agents.

First, biological agents, unlike drugs, have pre-programmed mechanisms and receptors. Second, biological agents are derivatives of natural products found in mammalian or human genes. It is probably these differences that account for the variance between MTD and OBD. Whereas cytotoxic agents possess one clear clinical outcome, that is, the ability to maximize direct antitumor effects, biological agents are used both for their cytotoxic activity and for the pleiotropic, indirect immune effects they mediate to maximize tumor response.

To effectively evaluate the activity of a biological agent, clinical trials must routinely incorporate relevant measurements of bioavailability, pharmacokinetics, biological effects, and toxicity (Oldham, 1983; Mazanet et al., 1996). Other issues essential in clinical trials of biological agents include the characteristics of the study population, clinical monitoring of toxic effects (e.g., observation, grading of severity, and recording of duration), and the use of immunologic assays (Creekmore et al., 1991).

The Role of Nurses in the Development of Biological Agents

Nursing has consistently remained in the forefront in the clinical evaluation of biological agents. Many articles written in the 1970s and early 1980s addressed administration and monitoring issues related to BCG, C. parvum, and early trials of human interferon (IFN)-α. Numerous journal articles, book chapters, and pharmaceutical-company–sponsored series have described the involvement of nursing in identifying and managing the clinical toxic effects of biological agents. What is more, numbers of nurses are conducting clinical research to determine ways to manage symptoms related to biological agents. This research will doubtless have an effect on the well-being of the patient receiving biotherapy and the patient's family.

Biological Agents

Biotherapy differs from chemotherapy in several ways. The majority of biological agents in use clinically are cytokines, a broad class of protein cell regulators produced by the immune system. Cytokines have unique features:

- They have a low molecular weight and a polypeptide structure, and they are often **glycosylated**.
- They act at short range on cells that produce them or on nearby cells.
- They play a role in immune responses by functioning as a signaling system and thereby controlling growth, mobility, and differentiation of immune cells.
- They interact with high-affinity receptors on the surface of cells to alter protein synthesis.

These alterations cause deviations in cell behavior, such as directing the inhibition of growth, differentiation, or cytotoxicity; stimulating host defense cells; or disrupting the host/tumor relationship by acting on tumor vasculature and nutrient supply. Most cytokines are pleiotropic, that is, they possess multiple effects. The production or administration of one cytokine influences the production of others in a cascade effect. "Cytokine" is an umbrella term for this particular class of proteins. Cytokines produced by lymphocyte cells are known as lymphokines; cytokines produced by monocytes are known as **monokines**.

Clinical evaluation of biological agents in the 1980s enabled investigators to identify several principles of cytokine therapy (Table 1.4). The foundation for the development of these principles was the initial clinical experience with IFN and other cytokines. A brief discussion of the most important biological agents is provided here to familiarize the reader with each agent's investigational status and clinical

Table 1.4 Principles of cytokine therapy

- Simple dose-response relationship may not always occur (less may be better)
- Cytokine-responsive tumors may require longer periods to achieve therapeutic response
- Stable disease may become the acceptable outcome
- Common constellation of toxic effects; severity may vary by agent, dose, and other cumulative factors

uses (Table 1.5). In summary, biotherapy is a modality that capitalizes on the use of natural body proteins and their inherent ability to fight cancer.

Table 1.5 Categories of biological agents/approaches in clinical use

Cytokines
Interferons
Interleukins
Hematopoietic growth factors
Tumor necrosis factor
Monoclonal Antibodies
Differentiation Agents
Retinoids
Cellular Therapies
Lymphokine-activated killer cells
Tumor-infiltrating lymphocytes
Dendritic cells
T cells with chimeric receptors
T-cell receptor-activated cells
Immunostimulants
Nonspecific
Bacillus Calmette-Guérin
Levamisole
Specific
Specific vaccines
Gene Therapy

Interferons

Virologists in the 1940s noted that, under specific conditions, exposure to one virus protects against infection by other viruses. In 1957, Isaacs and Lindenmann isolated a protein substance whose presence appeared to interfere with viral activity in cells (Isaacs and Lindenmann, 1957). They called this substance interferon. Nearly a decade later, other properties of IFN were identified, including its antiproliferative capability. Because the difficulty of isolating and preparing the natural product precluded obtaining large amounts of the agent, clinical trials were limited until IFN was cloned, which then provided researchers access to large quantities in the 1980s (Pestka, 1983). Type I IFNs (IFN-α and IFN-β) are highly species specific.

Interestingly, IFN-α, in 1986, became the first biological agent to be approved by the FDA, thus it is often referred to as the prototypic biological agent. Initially, IFNs were described according to their cell of origin, then according to physical-chemical properties. Now they are classified according to their antigenic type (Fischer et al., 1993). Three major types of IFNs have been isolated, recombinantly produced, and approved by the FDA: IFN-α (Roferon®-A; Intron®-A), IFN-γ (Actimmune®), and IFN-β (Betaseron®; Avonex®). Additionally, there are two other types of IFN-α available: Alferon®, a purified natural human IFN produced from human leukocytes simulated by virus; and Infergen®, a recombinant nonnatural IFN produced by a compilation of genetic information from several subtypes of IFN-α. All three major types of IFN exhibit antiviral, immunomodulatory, and antiproliferative activity to varying degrees.

The FDA has approved IFN-α for use in the treatment of hairy cell leukemia, Kaposi's sarcoma related to AIDS, condyloma acuminata, hepatitis B, hepatitis C, lymphoma, melanoma, and chronic myelogenous leukemia, with specific doses and schedules established for each disease. Approvals differ by brand name.

IFN-β is approved for treatment of multiple sclerosis, and IFN-γ is approved for the treatment of infections associated with chronic granulomatous disease. Currently, the IFNs are approved for clinical use as single agents in specific disease states, but their optimal use may be in combination with chemotherapeutic agents or other biological agents. Their use in combination therapy and their indications in cancer other than regulatory approved uses may be determined only after continued clinical trials. See Chapter 5 for an in-depth discussion of the IFNs.

Interleukins

ILs can be produced by and can regulate many cell types. In 1986, the Sixth International Congress of Immunology decided that new cytokines would be named according to their biological properties but that on identification of the amino acid sequence, a sequential IL number would be assigned (Dinarello and Mier, 1987). Eighteen ILs have so far been identified and isolated as of July 2000 and are undergoing either preclinical or clinical evaluation. Only IL-2 and IL-11 have been approved by the FDA. IL-2 is indicated for treatment of metastatic renal cell cancer and metastatic melanoma. IL-11 has been approved for use in preventing severe thrombocytopenia and in decreasing the need for platelet transfusions following myelosuppressive therapy.

IL-2, discovered by Morgan and co-workers in 1976, is an excellent example of the impact of technology on scientific advancement. IL-2 was originally called T-cell growth factor (Morgan et al., 1976). It was entered into clinical trials in the early 1980s and was approved by the FDA in 1992, which is a speedy record for the development of an agent from the scientific laboratory to use in the clinical arena. The numerous, immune-mediated biological effects of IL-2 include the production of two cell subsets: lymphokine-activated killer cells and tumor-infiltrating lymphocytes. In preclinical models, the greatest antitumor response was achieved when the MTD of IL-2 was used. However, when the MTD of IL-2 was used in the clinical setting, there were severe, yet transient and reversible toxic effects (e.g., hypotension, capillary leak syndrome, and oliguria). Therefore, clinical trials continue to evaluate IL-2 alone at various doses, schedules, and routes of administration, especially regimens that can be administered in the ambulatory setting with less toxicity, to determine regimens that maintain clinical efficacy with less toxicity. The administration of IL-2 in combination with chemotherapeutic and other biotherapeutic agents also remains a major area of focus. An in-depth discussion of ILs can be found in Chapter 6.

Hematopoietic Growth Factors

Hematopoietic growth factors (HGFs) are a complex network of glycoprotein hormones responsible for the differentiation, proliferation, maturation, and functional activity of hematopoietic cells (Turner, 1992; Bociek and Armitage, 1996). These factors are classified as either lineage restricted (affecting only one cell type) or multilineage (affecting several different cell types) (Crosier and Clark, 1992). HGFs are primarily used as supportive therapy following chemotherapy or bone marrow transplantation. As of July 2000, 4 HGFs have been approved by the FDA: granulocyte colony-stimulating factor (G-CSF, filgrastim), granulocyte-macrophage CSF (GM-CSF, sargramostim), erythropoietin (EPO, epoetin alfa); and IL-11 (oprelvekin). Other HGFs such as IL-3 (multi-CSF), PIXY-321 (a combination of GM-CSF and IL-3), stem cell factor (ancestim), and macrophage CSF (M-CSF) are being investi-

gated in clinical trials. A detailed description of HGFs and their role in cancer therapy can be found in Chapter 7.

Monoclonal Antibodies

The use of antibodies as carriers to deliver drugs and toxins to tumor cells was proposed as early as the 1900s by Paul Ehrlich (1910). He termed these antibodies "magic bullets." In 1975, the development of hybridoma technology by Köhler and Milstein allowed for the production of large volumes of antibodies, called monoclonal antibodies (MABs), which are produced from a single clone of cells (Köhler and Milstein, 1975).

MABs have been investigated in clinical trials for use in cancer diagnosis and in cancer treatment (in both unconjugated and conjugated forms). In addition, they have been evaluated in bone marrow transplantation to prevent the development of graft-versus-host disease or to purge autologous marrow of lingering malignant cells prior to transplantation. MABs are used extensively by pathologists to classify leukemias and lymphomas and to aid in the differential diagnosis of tumors that look alike on routinely processed light microscope specimens.

Several MABs have now received regulatory approval both within and outside of oncology care. Orthoclone® OKT3 (muromonab-CD3), a murine MAB targeted to the CD3 receptor of human T cells, has regulatory approval for use in the treatment of acute allograft rejection in renal transplant patients. In 1997, Zenapax® (daclizumab) was approved as a prophylaxis for organ rejection through inhibition of IL-2–mediated activation of lymphocytes. OncoScint® CR/OV (satumomab pendetide) is approved for use in the detection of colorectal and ovarian cancer, and ProstaScint® (capromab pendetide) is approved for use in the detection of prostate cancer. Three MABs have now been approved for the treatment of cancer. In November 1997, Rituxan® (rituximab) was approved for use in the treatment of patients with non-Hodgkin's lymphoma, and in September 1998, Herceptin® (trastuzumab) was approved for use in the treatment of patients with metastatic breast cancer whose tumors express human epidermal growth factor receptor 2 (HER-2). In May 2000, Mylotarg™ (gemtuzumab ozogamicin) received regulatory approval for the treatment of patients aged 60 years or older with CD33-positive relapsed acute myeloid leukemia. More approvals can be expected as future investigations explore and refine this exciting area in cancer care. See Chapters 8 and 9 for detailed discussions of MABs.

Retinoids

The retinoids are a group of natural and synthetic analogues of vitamin A that perform a significant role in vision, growth and reproduction, epithelial-cell differentiation, and immune function. In chemoprevention research, retinoids are used to arrest or reverse the process of carcinogenesis to prevent cancer invasion and metastasis and to treat cancer (Singh and Lippman, 1998). The retinoids used in oncology clinical trials include all-*trans*-retinoic acid (*t*RA, tretinoin), 4-hydroxyphenyl all-*trans*-retinoic acid amide (4-HPR, fenretinide), 13-*cis*-retinoic acid (*c*RA, isotretinoin), and 9-*cis*-retinoic acid. As of July 2000, two retinoids have received regulatory approval. Tretinoin (Vesanoid®) has received regulatory approval for use in inducing remission in patients with acute promyelocytic leukemia, and bexarotene (Targretin®) is approved for the treatment of cutaneous manifestations of early and advanced cutaneous T-cell lymphoma. Several retinoid creams, Retin A® cream and Accutane®, have regulatory approval for the treatment of acne.

See Chapter 12 for a detailed discussion of retinoids.

Vaccines

The use of active-specific immunotherapy (ASI) to treat patients with cancer began in the early 1900s and was prompted by the success of vaccines against infectious disease. Current technological advances and improved understanding of the immune system and its response to cancer has fueled a rebirth of interest in the use of vaccines in cancer therapy. ASI is a method of reintroducing (the host already has the tumor) tumor-associated antigens (TAA) in a way that will be more **immunogenic** in the host. The specific goals of using cancer vaccines as a form of ASI are to overcome the immunosuppression produced by tumor-derived factors, stimulate specific immunity that will destroy tumor cells, and enhance the immunogenicity of TAAs. Nonspecific active immunotherapy (adjuvants) is used in conjunction with ASI to further augment immune responses.

TAAs are potentially immunogenic molecules. There are essentially 4 categories of TAAs: neoantigens, oncofetal antigens, tumor-specific antigens, and peptide antigens. Neoantigens are antigens that are not expressed by the normal cells from which cancer cells are derived but that are found in other normal tissues. Oncofetal antigens are antigens not expressed by any normal tissues but that are expressed on fetal tissues. Tumor-specific antigens are antigens that are not found in normal adult or fetal tissues. Peptide antigen systems are tumor antigens recognized by T cells that may also be found in normal progenitors.

There are 3 types of vaccines used in clinical trials: whole-cell autologous vaccines, whole-cell allogeneic vaccines, and purified TAA. As of July 2000, no vaccine has yet received regulatory approval for use in cancer care, although several are in phase III clinical trials. For a detailed discussion of vaccines, see Chapter 10.

Tumor Necrosis Factor

Tumor necrosis factor (TNF) was discovered in 1975 and was subsequently found to be the same molecule as cachectin (Tracey *et al.*, 1989). TNF is a protein that selectively targets and destroys malignant cells. Two distinct types of TNF have been isolated: TNF-α, which is produced primarily by activated macrophages, and TNF-β, also known as lymphotoxin, which is produced primarily by lymphocytes. Preclinical and clinical trials in which the efficacy of this agent has been evaluated have yielded only minimal therapeutic responses. The use of TNF as a regional perfusion in patients with melanoma has yielded promising results in recent clinical trials. However, the potential clinical impact of TNF depends on an increased understanding of its cellular mechanisms and tumor-cell resistance (Frei and Spriggs, 1989). A more detailed discussion of TNF and the nursing strategies for management of patients who receive TNF therapy can be found in Chapter 9.

Immunomodulators

Immunomodulators are substances capable of altering immune responses either through inhibition or suppression. Many of the agents used in early immunotherapy trials were nonspecific immunomodulators. They were used to stimulate the immune system in the hopes of having a beneficial effect against cancer cells. This section will discuss those immunomodulators that have received regulatory approval and will provide an overview of the clinical trials in which their utility in cancer has been investigated.

BACILLUS CALMETTE-GUÉRIN

The major public health problem in the late 1800s was tuberculosis. In 1908, two French scientists at the Pasteur Institute in France, León Calmette and Alphonse Guérin, discovered that the addition of a small aliquot of beef bile to the cultured medium of a highly virulent strain of bovine tubercle bacillus caused it to lose its pathogenic characteristics (Hanna *et al.*, 1992). After 13 years of culturing with 231 serial transplants, the tubercle bacillus was **attenuated** and could then be used for vaccination. In 1921, the first human was vaccinated with BCG as the isolated vaccine was designated (Weill-Hallé, 1980).

Old *et al.* (1959) demonstrated that BCG could prevent or delay the occurrence of sarcomas, carcinomas, and ascitic tumors in mice. This study and the work of others led to the clinical use of BCG in the treatment of cancer. Mathé and colleagues (Mathé *et al.*, 1969) were the first to use BCG as an adjuvant therapy in childhood acute lymphoblastic leukemia. The positive results of their study were the impetus for several hundred clinical trials investigating BCG in the treatment of a variety of cancers; some of these trials are still underway.

BCG is a microbial material made from an attenuated strain of a live virus, *Mycobacterium bovis*. It has been used for decades for immunization against tuberculosis and as a nonspecific immunopotentiating agent in cancer treatment. In the treatment of cancer, BCG acts as a nonspecific immunostimulatory agent. This effect is believed to be initiated not by a single mechanism but as the result of a cascade of immunologic events involving both humoral and cellular immunity. T cells, B cells, macrophages, and natural killer cells are all potentiated by a variety of lymphokines and cytokines induced as a result of BCG administration (Murahata and Mitchell, 1976; Mitchell and Murahata, 1979). The exact mechanism by which BCG causes tumor regression remains a mystery, but the local presence of BCG and development of a granuloma are believed to be important (Hanna *et al.*, 1972; Snodgrass and Hanna, 1973).

Mathé *et al.* (1969) used BCG as an adjuvant in the treatment of acute lymphoblastic leukemia. Intensive weekly multisite scarifications (Figure 1.3) with BCG were administered during both the induction and maintenance phases of chemotherapy. Improved survival over historical controls stimulated much interest in the area. Similar improvement in survival was demonstrated when a similar treatment schedule of BCG was used as therapy for acute myeloid leukemia (Freeman *et al.*, 1973). However, it had little effect on the duration of remission.

Morton *et al.* (1970) reported complete re-gression of cutaneous metastases of malignant melanoma in 5 of 8 patients treated with in-tralesional administration of BCG. Regression of noninjected adjacent nodules in the lym-phatic drainage area of the injected lesions was also noted in 2 of 8 patients. Minor effects were achieved at distant sites or for visceral disease.

Intracavity or intrapleural administration of BCG prior to surgery in patients with stage I or II lung cancer was described by McKneally *et al.* (1977). Two years after surgery, 93% of BCG-treated patients were disease-free com-pared with 67% of patients who were not treated with BCG. At the 4-year follow-up evaluation, it was determined that postoperative adminis-tration of BCG was effective only in stage I lung cancer. To date, however, no one has been able to reproduce the beneficial effect of

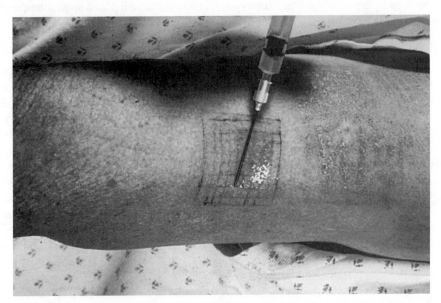

Figure 1.3 Scarification technique of bacillus Calmette-Guérin administration. A 5-cm × 5-cm area is anesthetized, then the skin is cleaned and allowed to dry. The vaccine preparation is then spread over the 5-cm × 5-cm area of skin. Straight lines (10 vertical and 10 horizontal) are scratched through the skin layers.

Source: Courtesy of The University of Texas M. D. Anderson Cancer Center, Houston, Texas.

intrapleural administration of BCG in the treatment of lung cancer.

BCG has been used successfully in the treatment of superficial bladder cancer (Herr, 1995). The majority of bladder cancers are superficial, which means the tumors are confined to the epithelium or lamina propria. Transurethral endoscopic resection is the standard initial treatment for these tumors. However, in most cases the disease ultimately recurs after this therapy. In a landmark study by Morales et al. (1976) 26 patients with superficial bladder cancer were treated with a combination of intravesical- and intradermal-administered BCG. This approach produced a dramatic reduction in the recurrence rate for up to 3 years after treatment. This study led to several prospective randomized trials that demonstrated that intravesical BCG was effective without concomitant intradermal BCG and that it prolonged the disease-free interval (Lamm et al., 1991; Herr et al., 1995).

In 1990, the FDA approved BCG for intravesical treatment of carcinoma in situ of the bladder. The treatment consists of induction and maintenance schedules. For the induction phase, 1 ampule of BCG (50 mg, 1 to 8 $\times$ 10^8 colony-forming units [TICE] or 81 mg, 1.05 $\times$ 10^9 $\pm$ 0.87 $\times$ 10^9 colony-forming units [ImmuCyst®/TheraCys®]) is suspended in 50 mL of saline. The solution is administered once per week for a minimum of 6 weeks intravesically and is retained in the bladder for 2 hours. While the BCG is retained, patients should lie 15 minutes each in the prone and supine positions and on each side. Urine voided for 6 hours after instillation should be diluted with an equal volume of household bleach and allowed to stand for 15 minutes before flushing. The maintenance phase consists of treatment once a month thereafter for up to 12 or 24 months, depending on the brand of BCG and the regimen used. Effectiveness is evaluated every 3 months by cystoscopy and urine cytology tests. This schedule remains empiric, and research

continues to evaluate different doses and schedules (Herr, 1995).

As with other biological agents, side effects of BCG depend on the dose, as well as the route, schedule, and even the timing of administration (Greenspan, 1986). When BCG is injected into a lesion, a local inflammatory reaction occurs within 4 hours. Within a week, tumor necrosis and ulceration develop and may require a few months to heal. Systemic side effects include a flu-like syndrome with fever, fatigue, myalgias, and possibly nausea and vomiting that may last several days. Side effects of scarification or intradermal BCG develop more gradually. An erythematous papule forms at the injection site but may heal in 1 or 2 days. Pruritis is common and occurs at the site of injection. As patients become sensitized to the treatment, however, the papules will ulcerate. Patients can expect permanent scarring and should be prepared for this.

When BCG is administered intravesically, the toxic effects are often localized, but there may be accompanying systemic symptoms. In a study by Hanna et al. (1992), more than half the patients who received intravesical BCG reported symptoms of bladder irritability such as dysuria, frequency, and hematuria. These symptoms can be managed with phenazopyridine, propantheline, and acetaminophen. A flu-like syndrome consisting of fever, chills, malaise, and myalgias occurred in one third of the patients, but fewer than 10% of them had severe symptoms. Systemic reactions usually last for 1 to 3 days after each intravesicular instillation (Kelly and Miaskowski, 1996; Skaugen, 1997; Swibold, 1999).

Two major complications may occur when BCG is administered: a hypersensitivity reaction or a disseminated BCG infection. Two cases of immediate hypersensitivity reaction to BCG have been reported that ultimately resulted in deaths (McKhaun et al., 1975). Presenting symptoms include fever, chills, hypotension, and oliguria (Groenwald *et al.*, 1987). Emergency equipment should be readily available when initiating BCG therapy in the event a hypersensitivity reaction occurs. Disseminated BCG infection presents with persistent fever, nausea, vomiting, fatigue, and weight loss and definitive antimicrobial treatment is typically used. Many clinicians recommend isoniazid.

BCG has clearly proven to be effective as a vaccine against tuberculosis and as primary treatment for bladder cancer (Alexandroff *et al.*, 1999). However, overtreatment, such as regimens that include injections into multiple sites, heavy doses, and frequently scheduled treatments, present probable cause for the numerous reports of negative results when BCG is used alone or in combination therapies (Greenspan, 1986). It is well recognized that smaller doses may be more effective when using biological agents (Hanna *et al.*, 1992). The most promising future use of BCG is as an adjuvant for tumor vaccines targeted toward a variety of cancers. Initial work by Berd *et al.* (1990) in the use of autologous tumor vaccines plus BCG in treating metastatic melanoma in addition to the early work of Hoover *et al.* (1985) using BCG postoperatively in the treatment of Dukes' stage B and C colorectal cancer produced encouraging results. Clinical trials continue to evaluate the efficacy of BCG as an adjuvant to vaccines in diseases such as melanoma (Yao *et al.*, 1999) and small-cell lung cancer (Grant *et al.*, 1999).

LEVAMISOLE

In the mid-1960s, levamisole, a broad-spectrum **anthelmintic** agent, was identified and found to have beneficial effects on the immune system. Investigators showed that levamisole potentiated the protective effect of a *Brucella* vaccine in mice. Although a tremendous amount of interest and research followed, it was short-lived. The overall conclusion from research conducted in the mid- to late-1970s was that leva-

misole restored depressed or anergic states to normal (DeBrabander *et al.*, 1992).

Levamisole has been effective in treating recurrent and chronic infections, postviral anergy, and rheumatic disorders by restoring to normal various functions of T lymphocytes and phagocytes. Levamisole has been evaluated in clinical trials of patients with cancer for over 20 years. In the 1990s, results from three major multicenter clinical trials revealed that levamisole is an effective adjuvant therapy for melanoma and colon carcinoma (Amery and Bruynseels, 1992). These new findings have stimulated renewed interest and research in the use of levamisole in treating cancer.

A **racemic** compound, tetramisole hydrochloride, was first introduced as an anthelmintic in 1966. It was soon discovered that the anthelmintic activity resided in the levorotatory isomer of levamisole. Today, levamisole is used as a broad-spectrum anthelmintic in the treatment of lungworm and gastrointestinal nematodes in animals and humans. It is administered as a single 5- to 40-mg/kg dose, depending on the parasite involved (Miller, 1980).

The mode of levamisole's action is still not completely understood, but several effects have been documented in *in vitro* and *ex vivo* experiments (Van Wauwe and Janssen, 1991; Amery and Bruynseels, 1992):

- Improvement of cell-mediated immune responses, particularly of macrophages and T cells
- Restoration of normal functioning of T lymphocytes and phagocytes, such as chemotaxis, random migration, adherence, intracellular killing, E rosette formation, and delayed skin hypersensitivity
- Synergization with mitogens and antigens in lymphocyte proliferation

Levamisole appears to have minimal effects on B lymphocytes and natural killer cells. Janik *et al.* (1993) conducted a phase I study that evaluated both the toxicity and immunobiological effects of levamisole alone and in combination with IFN-γ in patients with advanced cancer. In this study, the MTD was the same as the OBD (i.e., the dose that maximally stimulated biological effects). Patients were found to have elevated markers indicative of monocyte and T-cell stimulation.

Over the years, levamisole has undergone considerable study. As of July 2000, only 1 regulatory approval had been granted. Two significant trials of levamisole in combination with 5-fluorouracil (5-FU) in the treatment of colorectal cancer resulted in renewed interest in the use of levamisole as a biological agent and ultimately led to its regulatory approval in 1990. The first trial, a study by Laurie *et al.* (1989), involved 408 patients with resected Dukes' stage B_2 or C colorectal cancer. The trial consisted of 3 groups. One group received 150 mg levamisole orally for 3 consecutive days every 2 weeks for 1 year plus 5-FU 450 mg/m²/day by intravenous bolus for 5 days beginning at day 28 and then once a week for 1 year. The second group received levamisole only at 150 mg/day orally for 3 days every 2 weeks for 1 year. The third group received no postsurgery therapy. Levamisole plus 5-FU was superior in the treatment of patients with Dukes' stage C disease compared with no postsurgery treatment (5-year survival rates of 49% and 37%, respectively). There was also a difference in mean disease-free intervals (23 months versus 14 months, respectively) and tumor recurrence rate (41% versus 55%, respectively). Treatment with levamisole alone was only marginally beneficial. Another study by Moertel *et al.* (1990) used a similar treatment scheme but involved 1,296 comparable patients with matched controls. The combination of levamisole and 5-FU reduced the risk of recurrence by 41% and reduced the overall death rate by 33%. In the studies by Moertel *et al.* and Laurie *et al.*,

levamisole alone had no effect on either disease-free survival rate or overall survival rate.

As previously stated, levamisole was approved by the FDA in 1990 as an adjuvant treatment in combination with 5-FU following resection for Dukes' stage C colon cancer. The treatment consists of 150 mg of levamisole (50 mg every 8 hours) given orally for 3 consecutive days every 2 weeks for 1 year. It is recommended that treatment be initiated no earlier than 7 and no later than 30 days following resection.

The majority of randomized clinical trials have shown that no benefit is derived from combining levamisole and cytotoxic chemotherapy in the treatment of metastatic colon carcinoma (Bandealy *et al.*, 1998). In large-scale phase III trials, levamisole has also been evaluated alone and in combination with chemotherapy as adjuvant treatment or as treatment for advanced disease in patients with melanoma. Overall, no benefit has been demonstrated with either scheme. Although results from occasional trials have shown that levamisole has a beneficial effect against some cancers, overall randomized clinical trials evaluating levamisole as adjuvant therapy or as primary therapy in multiple malignancies, including head and neck cancers, breast cancer, bladder carcinoma, and ovarian cancer, have demonstrated no beneficial effects (Parkinson, 1995).

Levamisole is administered as an oral agent and is rapidly absorbed from the gastrointestinal tract. The results of a pharmacokinetic study of a single 50-mg dose revealed that the mean peak plasma level was reached within 1.5 to 2 hours. The drug is metabolized by the liver and excreted mainly by the kidneys (70% over 3 days) (Luyckx *et al.*, 1982). When compared with other biological agents, the side effects of levamisole as a single agent are relatively mild. Gastrointestinal problems (e.g., nausea, vomiting, and diarrhea) are the most common side effects and they occur in about 5% to 25% of patients. Flu-like symptoms, fatigue, headache, and dermatitis have also been reported. Granulocytopenia and agranulocytosis have been reported in as many as 10% of patients in some studies (Klefstrom *et al.*, 1985). However, when levamisole is combined with 5-FU, the side effects are slightly different. Moertel *et al.* (1990) reported nausea, vomiting, diarrhea, and stomatitis in more than half of the patients they studied, and nearly 25% had dermatitis and alopecia. Up to 14% of the patients had to discontinue combination therapy because of adverse reactions that included life-threatening exfoliative dermatitis, leukopenia, and sepsis.

Three conclusions regarding the effects of levamisole can be drawn from the results of the different experimental clinical trials: levamisole was more effective against slow-growing tumors than fast-growing ones, levamisole was more effective in preventing metastases than in shrinking established tumors, and levamisole has been most effective as an adjuvant following resection (DeBrabander *et al.*, 1992). Much can still be learned through this renewed interest in levamisole. Several concerns of paramount importance remain to be addressed, including the effect of levamisole plus 5-FU in treating Dukes' stage B colorectal carcinoma, the relative merits of preoperative and postoperative use of levamisole, the appropriate dosing of levamisole on chemotherapy treatment days, and the effects of levamisole on other types of tumors.

Cellular Therapy

In the mid-1980s, clinical trials evaluating the use of **adoptive cellular therapy** were initiated. Years of basic research and preclinical testing in animals led to human trials testing the utility of cellular therapy, primarily in conjunction with cytokines. The first-generation trials used natural killer cells stimulated *ex vivo* with IL-2. Once stimulated, these cells were called lymphokine-activated killer (LAK) cells and were administered in high numbers in conjunction with IL-2 infusions. Although success was seen in patients with renal cell cancer and melanoma, subsequent randomized clinical trials did not demonstrate any advantage of the combination regimen over IL-2 alone.

A second approach involved the use of lymphatic cells that had invaded the tumor. Once the tumor was surgically removed, the tumor-infiltrating lymphocytes (TILs) could be obtained, expanded *ex vivo* with IL-2, and reinfused in conjunction with high-dose IL-2. Clinical trials evaluating this combination, primarily in patients with renal cell cancer (Figlin *et al.*, 1999) and melanoma, found response rates ranging from approximately 10% to 60%. Although TIL cells (CD3+ cells) are more effective killers on a per cell basis than LAK cells, randomized trials have also failed to demonstrate that the addition of TILs to therapy with IL-2 increases the response rate. The combination of high-dose IL-2 and LAK or TIL cells was highly toxic and expensive, and the majority of patients did not experience sustained clinical responses.

Lessons were learned from these trials and provide clues that will help in the development of future approaches that will overcome or bypass immune defects in patients with cancer. Our increased understanding of the immune system has led to the evaluation of numerous new approaches. Table 1.6 provides an overview of emerging types of cellular therapy (Lum, 1999).

Summary

Biotherapy has been established, along with surgery, chemotherapy, and radiotherapy, as a treatment modality for cancer. Clearly, much has been learned about biotherapy in a very short period of time, but a vast amount of

Table 1.6   Cellular adoptive therapy

Cell Type	Description
Lymphokine-activated killer (LAK) cells	Natural killer cells are CD16$^+$. CD56$^+$ cells are responsible for tumor surveillance. When exposed to high concentrations of interleukin-2 (IL-2), they become LAK cells. Randomized clinical trials have not demonstrated a benefit from the addition of LAK to high-dose IL-2 regimens designed to treat patients with renal cell cancer and metastatic melanoma.
Tumor-infiltrating lymphocytes (TILs)	Lymphocytes derived from surgically removed tumor specimens. TILs are CD3$^+$ cells that display LAK activity. Cells are grown in culture with IL-2, and efficacy is believed to be linked to co-administration with IL-2. Primarily investigated in patients with renal cell cancer and melanoma. Randomized clinical trials have demonstrated no benefit from the addition of TIL to regimens using high-dose IL-2.
Activated T cells from tumor-draining lymph nodes	Lymph nodes that drain tumors contain sensitized, pre-effector T cells. When these cells are stimulated with anti-CD3 monoclonal antibodies (MABs) and cultured with IL-2, they assist in the generation of antigen-specific cytotoxic T lymphocytes. Preliminary clinical trials are underway in patients with renal cell cancer and melanoma. Results appear encouraging, yet further evaluation must occur.
Autolymphocyte therapy (ALT)	This approach uses the infusion of autologous peripheral blood mononuclear cells (PBMCs) produced by cultures containing extracts of autologous tumor and conditioned media. The conditioned media is derived from OKT3-stimulated (anti-CD3 MAB) PBMCs. Although preliminary studies in patients with renal cell cancer appeared promising, follow-up studies did not confirm significant differences compared with treatment with interferon.
T-cell receptor-activated T cells (TRAC)	This type of cell is produced by cross-linking the T-cell receptor with anti-CD3 MABs (OKT3), which results in T-cell proliferation, cytokine synthesis, and immune responses. TRACs are produced by OKT3- and IL-2-stimulated PBMCs and have LAK- and natural killer cell-like activity. In addition, they produce cytokines such as interferon, tumor necrosis factor, and granulocyte-macrophage colony-stimulating factor. They have the potential to serve as vehicles to deliver targeting antibodies or gene products. Clinical trials are preliminary.
New approach Anti-CD3/anti CD28 coactivated T cells (COACTS)	This type of cell is generated by cross-linking the T-cell receptor with anti-CD3, which triggers a signaling cascade that results in T-cell proliferation, cytokine synthesis, and immune responses. To produce optimal activation, the CD28 receptor on the T cells is stimulated with an anti-CD28 MAB. These interactions enhance proliferations and cytokine secretion. Early clinical trials have demonstrated modulation of the immune system. Future trials will evaluate COACTS in combination with chemotherapy and biological agents.

Table 1.6

Cell Type	Description
New approach Antigen-specific cytotoxic T lymphocytes (CTLs)	The development of CTLs targeted toward viruses or tumor-specific antigens. The generation of CTL directed toward *p21, ras, p53,* and HER-2/*neu* have been reported. The CTL would be produced by *in vitro* priming and then infused into patients.
New approach Dendritic cells (DCs)	A crucial component in the development of tumor-specific responses are "professional" antigen-presenting cells or DCs. These cells are capable of triggering powerful T-cell responses after encountering antigen. The *ex vivo* culture of DCs followed by peptide priming and then reinfusion or manipulation of cultured DCs to optimized vaccine strategies are being actively pursued. Infusion of primed DCs into patients will hopefully use the patient's own immune system as a "bioreactor" to sensitize and expand tumor-specific CTL.
New approach BiABs—combining the specificity of 2 MABs into 1 protein molecule	This approach combines MAB-targeting specificity with the cytotoxicity of T cells or other effector cells. BiABs are generated through a variety of sophisticated techniques to produce a molecule that binds to the T cell or other effector cell on 1 end and targets a tumor antigen on the other end. Clinical trials are actively investigating this approach. As the use of recombinant technology continues to expand, this will surely lead to the continued development of fusion proteins.
New approach T cells with chimeric receptors (T-bodies)	To produce long-lived, tumor-specific T cells, researchers have transduced T cells with genes containing chimeric receptors containing single-chain antibody fragments that target different tumor antigens. The term T-bodies describes T cells bearing the chimeric antibody receptor. Clinical trials are in progress.
New approach Infusion of genetically altered T cells	A form of gene therapy, this approach involves the infusion of T cells transduced with cytokine genes to deliver high concentrations of cytokines at the tumor site.
Adoptive immunotherapy in bone marrow transplant. Cellular therapy is used in an attempt to induce a graft-versus-leukemia (GVL) effect.	The types of cells used in approaches designed to induce GVL effect in clinical trials have been donor lymphocyte infusions; both low-dose and high-dose IL-2 therapy with reinfusion of LAK cells and the infusion of TRAC-2 following peripheral blood stem cell transplant transplantation in hematologic malignancies and solid tumors.

Source: Data from Lum, L. 1999. T cell-based immunotherapy for cancer: A virtual reality? *CA: A Journal for Clinicians* 49: 74–100.

information about these agents and their uses remains to be discovered, understood, and evaluated in preclinical and clinical trials. Tables 1.7 and 1.8 summarize the major biological agents with regulatory approval to date. These agents cannot be viewed as independent factors but rather as critical elements of a complex, intricate network that produces many positive and negative interactions. Although incomplete, our current understanding of biotherapy rests on the observations on page 32:

Table 1.7 Major biological agents with regulatory approval for oncology indications

Agent	Regulatory Approval
Interleukins (ILs)	
IL-2 (Proleukin®, Chiron Therapeutics)	Renal cell cancer, metastatic melanoma
Monoclonal antibodies	
Satumomab pendetide (OncoScint®, Cytogen)	Diagnostic imaging of colon and ovarian cancer
Capromab pendetide (ProstaScint®, Cytogen)	Diagnostic imaging of prostate cancer
Rituximab (Rituxan®, Genentech)	Treatment of relapsed or refractory low-grade or follicular CD20+ B-cell non-Hodgkin's lymphoma
Trastuzumab (Herceptin®, Genentech)	Treatment of patients with metastatic breast cancer whose tumors overexpress the HER-2 protein
Gemtuzumab ozogamicin (Mylotarg™, Wyeth-Ayerst)	Treatment of patients aged 60 years or older with CD33+ relapsed acute myeloid leukemia who are not considered candidates for cytotoxic chemotherapy
Hematopoietic Growth Factors	
GM-CSF (sargramostim; (Leukine®, Immunex, a subsidiary of American Home Products)	Acceleration of myeloid recovery in patients with non-Hodgkin's lymphoma; acute lymphoblastic leukemia; patients with Hodgkin's disease undergoing autologous BMT; BMT failure or engraftment delay; after induction chemotherapy in acute myelogenous leukemia in elderly patients; mobilization of peripheral stem cells for transplantation and following transplantation of autologous peripheral blood stem cells; and acceleration of myeloid recovery in patients undergoing allogeneic BMT from HLA-matched donors
G-CSF (filgrastim; Neupogen®, Amgen)	To decrease the incidence of infection in patients with nonmyeloid malignancies receiving myelosuppressive anticancer drugs; to reduce the duration of neutropenia and neutropenia-associated sequelae in patients with nonmyeloid malignancies who are receiving myeloablative chemotherapy followed by BMT; to mobilize peripheral stem cells for transplantation; to support treatment of patients with acute myeloid leukemia receiving induction or consolidation chemotherapy; and for the treatment of patients with severe chronic neutropenia

Table 1.7

Agent	Regulatory Approval
Procrit® (Ortho-Biotech)	Treatment of anemia in patients with chronic renal failure; anemia related to therapy with zidovudine in HIV-infected patients; and the treatment of anemia in cancer patients on chemotherapy and anemic patients undergoing elective noncardiac and nonvascular surgery to reduce the need for allogeneic blood transfusion
rhIL-11 (oprelvekin; Neumega®, Genetics Institute, a subsidiary of American Home Products)	Prevention of severe thrombocytopenia and reduction in the need for platelet transfusion following myelosuppressive chemotherapy in patients with nonmyeloid malignancies who are at high risk for severe thrombocytopenia
Retinoids	
All-*trans* retinoic acid (tretinoin; Vesanoid®, Roche Laboratories)	Induction of remission in patients with acute promyelocytic leukemia. All patients should receive standard consolidation and/or maintenance chemotherapy for acute promyelocytic leukemia after completion of induction therapy with tretinoin, unless otherwise contraindicated
Bexarotene (Targretin®, Ligand Pharmaceuticals)	Approved for the treatment of cutaneous manifestations of cutaneous T-cell lymphoma in patients who are refractory to at least 1 prior systemic therapy
Fusion Proteins	
DAB$_{389}$ IL-2 (denileukin difitox; ONTAK®, Ligand Pharmaceuticals)	Approved for the treatment of patients with persistent or recurrent CTCL whose malignant cells express the CD25 component of the IL-2 receptor. ONTAK® binds specifically to the IL-2 receptor and directs the cytocidal action of the diphtheria toxin to malignant CTCL cells inhibiting protein synthesis and causing cell death
Interferons (IFNs)	
IFN-α	
IFN-alfa-2a (Roferon-A®, Roche Lab)	Hairy-cell leukemia, AIDS-related Kaposi's sarcoma, chronic myelogenous leukemia, and chronic hepatitis C
IFN-alfa-2b (Intron-A®, Schering Corporation)	Hairy-cell leukemia, AIDS-related Kaposi's sarcoma, condyloma acuminata, chronic hepatitis C, and chronic hepatitis B; adjuvant therapy for melanoma (high risk for recurrence); and in conjunction with anthracycline-containing combination chemotherapy for the initial treatment of patients with clinically aggressive non-Hodgkin's lymphoma, a cancer of the lymphatic system

Source: Adapted with permission from Rieger, P. T. 1994. *Biotherapy.* In Otto, S. (ed). *Oncology Nursing,* 2nd ed. St. Louis, MO: Mosby, pp. 526–560.

BMT, bone marrow transplantation; CTCL, cutaneous T-cell lymphoma; G-CSF, granulocyte colony-stimulating factor; GM-CSF, granulocyte-macrophage colony-stimulating factor; HLA, human leukocyte antigen.

Table 1.8   Biological agents with regulatory approval for nononcology indications

Enzymes*

Tissue-type plasminogen activator (tPA),
converts plasminogen to plasmin, an
enzyme that helps break down the
blood clots

Alteplase (Activase®, Genentech, Inc.)	Approved for use in coronary artery and myocardial infarction; promotes thrombolysis of obstructing thrombus and limits infarct size in patients with acute myocardial infarction; used for lysis of acute pulmonary emboli
Reteplase (RETAVASE®, Centocor)	RETAVASE® is a potent fibrinolytic that is a variant of tPA. It is approved for the treatment of acute myocardial infarction to improve blood flow to the heart
Tenecteplase (TNKase, Genentech, Inc.)	Reduction of mortality associated with acute myocardial infarction

Glucocerebrosidase

Imiglucerase (Cerezyme®, Genzyme)	Indicated for long-term enzyme replacement therapy for patients diagnosed with Gaucher's disease type I

DNase

Dornase alfa (Pulmozyme®, Genentech, Inc.)	Approved for use in patients with cystic fibrosis to reduce the frequency of respiratory infection and to improve pulmonary function

Factor VIII

Antihemophilic factor (Recombinate®, Baxter; Kogenate®, Bayer; ReFacto, Genetics Institute)	Indicated for use in hemophilia A for prevention or control of bleeding episodes

Factor IX

Coagulation factor IX (BeneFix®, Genetics)	Indicated for use in the control and prevention of hemorrhagic episodes in patients with hemophilia B, including the peri-operative management of hemophilia B in patients undergoing surgery

Potent Specific Thrombin Inhibitor

Lepirudin (Refludan®, Hoechst Marion Roussel)	Indicated for anticoagulation in patients with heparin-induced thrombocytopenia and associated thromboembolic disease in order to prevent further complications

Hormones and Growth Factors

Erythropoietin

Epoetin alfa (Epogen®, Amgen)	For treatment of anemia in patients with chronic renal failure who are on dialysis; pediatric use approved 7/99

Human Growth Hormone

Somatrem (Protropin®, Genentech, Inc.)	Indicated for long-term treatment of children who have growth failure due to lack of adequate endogenous growth hormone

Table 1.8

Somatropin (Nutropin®, Genentech, Inc.)	Indicated for children with growth failure due to a lack of endogenous growth hormone secretion; also indicated for treating growth failure secondary to chronic renal failure up to the time of transplantation
Somatropin (Humatrope®, Eli Lilly)	Indicated for long-term treatment of children who have growth failure due to lack of adequate endogenous growth hormone
Somatropin (Genotropin™, Pharmacia and Upjohn)	Indicated for the long-term treatment of children who have growth failure due to an inadequate secretion of endogenous growth hormone
Somatropin (Serostim®, Serono)	Indicated for the treatment of AIDS wasting or cachexia
Human Insulin	
Recombinant human insulin (Humulin®, Eli Lilly)	Indicated for use as replacement therapy for the management of diabetes mellitus
Recombinant human insulin (Novolin®, Novo Nordisk)	Indicated for use as replacement therapy for the management of diabetes mellitus
Thyroid-Stimulating Hormone	
Thyrotropin alfa (Thyrogen®, Genzyme)	Indicated as an additional diagnostic tool in the follow-up of patients with a history of well-differentiated thyroid cancer
Follicle-Stimulating Hormone (Gonal-F®, Serono)	Used for the induction of ovulation and pregnancy in the anovulatory infertile patient in whom the cause of infertility is functional and not due to primary ovarian failure
Platelet-derived Growth Factor	
Becaplermin gel 0.01% (Regranex®, Chiron)	Indicated to promote healing in diabetic neuropathic foot ulcers
Interferons	
IFN-α	
IFN-α leukocyte (Alferon®, Purdue Fredric)	Approved for condyloma acuminata
IFN-alfa-N 1 (Wellferon®, Glaxo Wellcome Inc.)	Treatment of chronic hepatitis C
IFN-alfacon-1 (Infergen®, Amgen), a bioengineered, nonnaturally occurring type-I IFN	Treatment of chronic hepatitis C viral infection
IFN-β	
IFN-beta-1B (Betaseron®, Berlex Laboratories)	To reduce the frequency of clinical exacerbations that occur in multiple sclerosis
IFN-beta-1a (Avonex®, Biogen)	Treatment of relapsing forms of multiple sclerosis to slow the progression of physical disability and decrease the frequency of clinical exacerbations

(continued)

Table 1.8

Interferons (cont.)	
IFN-γ	
IFN-gamma 1b (Actimmune®, InterMune Pharmaceuticals Inc., marketer; Genentech Inc., manufacturer)	Approved for the treatment of chronic granulomatous disease; delaying the time to disease progression in patients with severe, malignant osteopetrosis
Vaccines	
Hepatitis B Vaccine (recombinant)	
Recombivax HB® (Merck & Co., Inc.), Energix® (Smith Kline Beecham), Comvax® (Merck & Co., Inc.)	Indicated for vaccination against hepatitis B
Recombinant OspA (Lyme disease) LYMErix® (Smith Kline Beecham)	Indicated for vaccination against Lyme disease
Monoclonal Antibodies	
Infliximab (Remicade®, Centocor, Inc.), an antitumor necrosis factor antibody	Treatment of moderately to severely active Crohn's disease in patients who have an inadequate response to conventional therapies
	For reduction of signs and symptoms of rheumatoid arthritis in patients who have had an inadequate response to methotrexate
Basiliximab (Simulect®, Novartis), Interleukin-2 receptor antibody	Prophylaxis for acute organ rejection in patients receiving renal transplantation when used as part of an immunosuppressive regimen that includes cyclosporine and corticosteroids
Muromonab-CD3 (Orthoclone® OKT3, Ortho Biotech), an anti-CD3 antibody	Treatment of rejection in organ transplants
Daclizumab (Zenapax®, Roche Laboratories), an anti-CD25 receptor antibody	Treatment of organ rejection, prophylaxis
Palivizumab (Synagis™, MedImmune, Inc.), a humanized monoclonal antibody produced by recombinant DNA technology, directed toward the respiratory syncytial virus	Prophylaxis of serious lower respiratory tract disease caused by respiratory syncytial virus in pediatric patients at high risk for respiratory syncytial virus disease
Abciximab (ReoPro®, Centocor) ReoPro®, is the Fab fragment of the chimeric human-murine monoclonal antibody 7E3. It binds to a receptor of human platelets and inhibits platelet aggregation	Approved for use as adjunctive therapy to prevent cardiac ischemic complications in a broad range of patients undergoing percutaneous coronary intervention as well as in unstable angina in patients not responding to conventional medical therapy when percutaneous coronary intervention is planned within 24 hours

Table 1.8

Fusion Proteins

Etanercept (ENBREL®, Immunex) Immunoadhesins are genetically engineered fusion proteins that combine certain structural features of antibodies with high-affinity cell-surface receptors. The resulting molecule can inhibit the activity of factors that normally bind to the receptors in the body. ENBREL® is a soluble receptor fusion protein and is the first product utilizing immunoadhesin technology to be approved by the U.S. Food and Drug Administration for medical use. ENBREL® consists of 2 soluble tumor necrosis factor receptors fused to the Fc fragment of a human immunoglobulin that acts by binding tumor necrosis factor. Tumor necrosis factor is one of the dominant cytokines or proteins that play an important role in the cascade of reactions that cause the inflammatory process of rheumatoid arthritis. ENBREL® competitively inhibits the binding of tumor necrosis factor molecules to the tumor necrosis factor receptor sites. The binding of ENBREL® to tumor necrosis factor renders the bound tumor necrosis factor biologically inactive and resulting in significant reduction in inflammatory activity

ENBREL® is approved to treat moderately to severely active rheumatoid arthritis in patients who have had an inadequate response to one or more disease-modifying antirheumatic drugs (DMARDS); approved May 1999 to treat moderately to severely active polyarticular-course juvenile rheumatoid arthritis in patients who have had an inadequate response to one or more DMARDs; approved June 2000 for reducing the signs and symptoms and delaying structural damage in patients with moderately to severely active rheumatoid arthritis

* Enzymes are proteins that act as a catalyst or inhibitor for biological reactions. The names of enzymes typically end in "ase," for example, "lipase."

- The majority of biological agents are produced by more than one type of cell.
- Each biological agent has its own distinct receptors but produces striking, overlapping biological effects.
- Most biological agents are pleiotropic, that is, they produce multiple effects.
- A single stimulus can induce responses from multiple cytokines.
- Biological agents interact within the cytokine network through a variety of actions, including stimulating production of other agents, modulating receptor sites, and enhancing or inhibiting the biological activity of other cytokines.

Significant achievement has occurred in a relatively short time in the use of biological agents to treat cancer. Before the full potential of these molecules may be realized, however, several challenges remain that must be addressed: toxicity, treatment cost, treatment guidelines, and issues related to dosing and scheduling. Technological changes are progressing at an unparalleled rate, so as they are discovered, new biological agents and approaches will continually be integrated into the management of patients with cancer and other diseases. The need for nurses who are knowledgeable in this area and who are able to direct the care of patients receiving biotherapy has never been greater.

References

Alexandroff, A., Jackson, A., O'Donnell, M., *et al.* 1999. BCG immunotherapy of bladder cancer: 20 years on. *Lancet* 353(165): 1689–1694.

Amery, W., and Bruynseels, J. 1992. Levamisole, the story and the lessons. *International Journal of Immunopharmacology* 143: 481–486.

Bandealy, M., Gonin, R., Loehrer, P., *et al.* 1998. Prospective randomized trial of 5-fluorouracil versus 5-fluorouracil plus levamisole in the treatment of metastatic colorectal cancer: A Hoosier Oncology Group trial. *Clinical Cancer Research* 4(4): 935–939.

Berd, D., Maguire, H., McCue, P., *et al.* 1990. Treatment of metastatic melanoma with an autologous tumor-cell vaccine: Clinical and immunologic results in 64 patients. *Journal of Clinical Oncology* 8(11): 1858–1867.

Bociek, R., and Armitage, J. 1996. Hematopoietic growth factors. *CA: A Journal for Clinicians* 46: 165–184.

Borden, E., and Sondel, P. 1990. Lymphokines and cytokines as cancer treatment: Immunotherapy realized. *Cancer* 65: 800–814.

Clark, J., and Longo, D. 1986. Biological response modifiers. *Mediguide to Oncology* 6(2): 1–4.

Coley, W. 1893. The treatment of malignant tumors by repeated inoculations of erysipelas: With a report of ten original cases. *American Journal of Medical Science* 105: 487.

Coley, W. 1911. A report of recent cases of inoperable sarcoma successfully treated with mixed toxins of erysipelas and *Bacillus prodigious*. *Surgical Gynecology and Obstetrics* 13: 174–190.

Collins, J., Grieshaber, C., and Chabner, B. 1990. Pharmacologically guided phase I clinical trials based upon preclinical drug development. *Journal of the National Cancer Institute* 80: 1321–1326.

Creekmore, S., Urba, W., and Longo, D. 1991. Principles of the clinical evaluation of biologic agents. In DeVita, V., Hellman, S., and Rosenberg, S. (eds). *Biological Therapy of Cancer*. Philadelphia, PA: W.B. Saunders Company, pp. 67–86.

Crosier, P., and Clark, S. 1992. Basic biology of the hematopoietic growth factors. *Seminars in Oncology* 19: 349–361.

DeBrabander, M., DeCree, J., Vandebroek, J., *et al.*

1992. Levamisole in the treatment of cancer: Anything new? (review). *Anticancer Research* 12: 177–188.

Dinarello, C., and Mier, J. 1987. Current concepts: Lymphokines. *New England Journal of Medicine* 317(15): 940–945.

Dutcher, J. 1992. Future directions in biological therapy of cancer. *Hospital Formulary* 27: 694–707.

Ehrlich, P. 1910. *Studies in Immunity*, 2nd edn. New York, NY: Wiley and Sons.

Figlin, R., Thompson, J., Bukowski, R., *et al.* 1999. Multicenter, randomized, phase III trial of CD8(+) tumor-infiltrating lymphocytes in combination with recombinant interleukin-2 in metastatic renal cell carcinoma. *Journal of Clinical Oncology* 17(8): 2521–2529.

Fischer, D., Knobf, M., and Durivage, H. 1993. *The Cancer Chemotherapy Handbook*, 4th edn. St. Louis, MO: Mosby-Year Book, Inc., pp. 217–246.

Freeman, C., Harris, R., Geary, C., *et al.* 1973. Active immunotherapy used alone for maintenance of patients with acute myeloid leukemia. *British Medical Journal* 4(892): 571–573.

Frei, E., and Spriggs, D. 1989. Tumor necrosis factor: Still a promising agent. *Journal of Clinical Oncology* 7(3): 291–294.

Fussenegger, M., Bailery, J., Hauser, H., *et al.* 1999. Genetic optimization of recombinant glycoprotein production by mammalian cells. *Trends in Biotechnology* 17(1): 35–42.

Gallucci, B. 1987. The immune system and cancer. *Oncology Nursing Forum* 14(6 suppl): 3–7.

Goodfield, J. 1984. Dr. Coley's toxins. *Science* 84: 68–73.

Grant, S., Kris, M., Houghton, A., *et al.* 1999. Long survival of patients with small cell lung cancer after adjuvant treatment with the anti-idiotypic antibody BEC2 plus bacillus Calmette-Guérin. *Clinical Cancer Research* 5(6): 1319–1323.

Greenspan, E. 1986. Is BCG an "orphan" drug suffering from chemotherapists' overkill? *Cancer Investigation* 4(1): 81–92.

Groenwald, S., Fisher, S., and McCalla, J. 1987.

Biological response modifiers. In Groenwald, S. (ed). *Cancer Nursing: Principles and Practice.* Boston, MA: Jones and Bartlett, pp. 385–404.

Hall, S. 1997. *A Commotion in the Blood: Life, Death, and the Immune System.* New York, NY: Henry Holt and Company.

Hanna, M., Jr., DeJar, R., Giunan, P., *et al.* 1992. Bacillus Calmette-Guérin (BCG) vaccine for tuberculosis: Antitumor effect in experimental animals and humans. *Vaccine Research* 1(2): 69–90.

Hanna, M., Snodgrass, M., Zbar, B., *et al.* 1972. Histopathology of tumor regression after intralesional injection of *Mycobacterium bovis*. IV. Development of immunity to tumor cells and to BCG. *Journal of the National Cancer Institute* 48: 245–257.

Herberman, R. 1985. Design of clinical trials with biological response modifiers. *Cancer Treatment Reports* 69: 1161–1164.

Herr, H. 1995. Instillation therapy for bladder cancer. In DeVita, V., Hellman, S., and Rosenberg, S. (eds). *Biological Therapy of Cancer* 2nd edn. Philadelphia, PA: W.B. Saunders Company, pp. 705–711.

Herr, H., Schwalb, D., Zhang, Z., *et al.* 1995. Intravesical bacillus Calmette-Guérin therapy prevents tumor progression and death from superficial bladder cancer: Ten-year follow-up of a prospective randomized trial. *Journal of Clinical Oncology* 13(6): 1404–1408.

Hersh, E., Gutterman, J., and Mavligit, G. 1973. *Immunotherapy of Cancer in Man: Scientific Basis and Current Status.* Springfield, IL: Charles C Thomas.

Hoover, H., Surdyke, M., Dangel, R., *et al.* 1985. Prospectively randomized trial of adjuvant active-specific immunotherapy for human colorectal cancer. *Cancer* 55: 1236–1243.

Isaacs, A., and Lindenmann, J. 1957. Virus interference. I. The interferon. *Proceedings of the Royal Society of London* (Series B): 259–267.

Janik, J., Kopp, W., Smith, J., *et al.* 1993. Dose-related immunologic effects of levamisole in patients with cancer. *Journal of Clinical Immunology* 11(1): 125–135.

Johnson, J., and Temple, R. 1985. Food and Drug Administration requirements for approval of anticancer drugs. *Cancer Treatment Reports* 69: 1155–1159.

Kelly, L., and Miaskowski, C. 1996. An overview of bladder cancer: Treatment and nursing implications. *Oncology Nursing Forum* 23(3): 459–470.

Klefstrom, P., Holsti, P., Grohn, P., *et al.* 1985. Levamisole in the treatment of stage II breast cancer. *Cancer* 55: 2753–2757.

Köhler, G., and Milstein, C. 1975. Continuous cultures of fused cells secreting antibody of predefined specificity. *Nature* 256: 495–496.

Lamm, D., DeHaven, J., Shriver, J., *et al.* 1991. Prospective randomized comparison of intravesical and percutaneous bacillus Calmette-Guérin versus intravesical bacillus Calmette-Guérin in superficial bladder cancer. *Journal of Urology* 145: 738–740.

Laurie, J., Moertel, C., Fleming, T., *et al.* 1989. Surgical adjuvant therapy of large bowel carcinoma: An evaluation of levamisole and the combination of levamisole and fluorouracil. *Journal of Clinical Oncology* 7: 1447–1456.

Lum, L. 1999. T cell-based immunotherapy for cancer: A virtual reality? *CA: A Journal for Clinicians* 49(2): 74–100.

Luyckx, M., Rousseau, F., Cazin, M., *et al.* 1982. Pharmacokinetics of levamisole in healthy subjects and cancer patients. *European Journal of Drug Metabolism and Pharmacokinetics* 7(4): 247–254.

Mathé, G., Amiel, J., Schwarzenberg, L., *et al.* 1969. Active immunotherapy for acute lymphocytic leukemia. *Lancet* 1: 697–699.

Mazanet, R., Morstyn, G., and Foote, M. 1996. Development of biological agents. In Schilsky, R., Milano, G., and Ratain, M. (eds). *Principles of Antineoplastic Drug Development and Pharma-*

cology. New York, NY: Marcel Dekker, Inc., pp. 55–73.

McKhaun, C., Hendrickson, C., and Spitler, L. 1975. Immunotherapy of melanoma with BCG: Two fatalities following intralesional injection. *Cancer* 35: 514–520.

McKneally, M., Maver, C., and Kausal, H. 1977. Intrapleural BCG stimulation in lung cancer. *Lancet* 1: 593.

Mihich, E., and Fefer, A. (eds). 1983. Biological response modifiers: Subcommittee report. *National Cancer Institute Monograph.* Washington, D.C.: National Cancer Institute, p. 63.

Miller, M. 1980. Use of levamisole in parasitic infections. *Drugs* 20: 122–130.

Mitchell, M. 1992. Chemotherapy in combination with biomodulation: A 5-year experience with cyclophosphamide and interleukin-2. *Seminars in Oncology* 19(2 suppl 14): 80–87.

Mitchell, M., and Murahata, R. 1979. Modulation of immunity by bacillus Calmette-Guérin (BCG). *Pharmacological Therapeutics* 4: 329–353.

Moertel, C., Fleming, T., MacDonald, J., *et al.* 1990. Levamisole and fluorouracil for adjuvant therapy of resected colon carcinoma. *New England Journal of Medicine* 322: 352–358.

Morales, A., Eidinger, D., and Bruce, A. 1976. Intracavity bacillus Calmette-Guérin in the treatment of bladder tumors. *Journal of Urology* 116: 180–183.

Morgan, D., Ruscetti, F., and Gallo, R. 1976. Selective in vitro growth of T lymphocytes from normal human bone marrow. *Science* 193: 1007–1008.

Morton, D., Eilber, F., Malmgren, R., *et al.* 1970. Immunological factors which influence response to immunotherapy in malignant melanoma. *Surgery* 68: 158.

Murahata, R., and Mitchell, M. 1976. Modulation of the immune response by BCG: A review. *The Yale Journal of Biology and Medicine* 49: 283–291.

Nauts, H., and McLaren, J. 1990. Coley's toxins—

The first century. *Advances in Experimental Medicine and Biology* 267: 483–500.

Oettgen, H., and Old, L. 1991. The history of cancer immunotherapy. In DeVita, V., Hellman, S., and Rosenberg, S. (eds). *Biological Therapy of Cancer*. Philadelphia, PA: W.B. Saunders Company, pp. 87–119.

Old, L., Clarke, D., and Benacerrat, B. 1959. Effect of bacillus Calmette-Guérin infection on transplanted tumors in the mouse. *Nature* 184: 231.

Oldham, R. 1983. Biologicals: New horizons in pharmaceutical development. *Journal of Biological Response Modifiers* 2: 199–206.

Oldham, R. 1984. Biologicals and biological response modifiers: Fourth treatment modality of cancer treatment. *Cancer Treatment Reports* 68(1): 221–232.

Oldham, R. 1985. Biologicals and biological response modifiers: Design of clinical trials. *Journal of Biological Response Modifiers* 4: 117–128.

Oldham, R. 1998a. Cancer biotherapy: General principles. In Oldham, R. (ed). *Principles of Cancer Biotherapy*, 3rd edn. Dordrecht, Netherlands: Kluwer Academic Press, pp. 1–15.

Oldham, R. 1998b. Developmental therapeutics and the design of clinical trials. In Oldham, R. (ed). *Principles of Cancer Biotherapy*, 3rd edn. Dordrecht, Netherlands: Kluwer Academic Press, pp. 39–50.

Oldham, R., and Smalley, R. 1983. Immunotherapy: The old and the new. *Journal of Biological Response Modifiers* 2: 1–37.

Parkinson, D. 1995. Levamisole. In DeVita, V., Hellman, S., and Rosenberg, S. (eds). *Biological Therapy of Cancer*, 2nd edn. Philadelphia, PA: W.B. Saunders Company, pp. 795–801.

Pestka, S. 1983. The purification and manufacture of human interferons. *Scientific American* 249(2): 37–43.

Pharmaceutical Research and Manufacturers of America (PhRMA). 1998. *Biomedicine: Promises for Health*. Washington, DC: Pharmaceutical Research and Manufacturers of America.

Pharmaceutical Research and Manufacturers of America (PhRMA). 1999. *Pharmaceutical Industry Profile 1999*. Washington, DC: Pharmaceutical Research and Manufacturers of America.

Ramel, A., McGregor, W., and Dziewanowska, Z. 1983. Methods of preparation. In Sikora, K. (ed). *Interferon and Cancer*. New York, NY: Plenum Press, pp. 17–32.

Rosenberg, S. 1999. A new era of cancer immunotherapy: Converting theory to performance. *CA: A Journal for Clinicians* 49(2): 70–73.

Siegel, J., Gerrard, T., Savagnaro, J.A., *et al.* 1995. Development of biological therapeutics for oncologic use. In DeVita, V., Hellman, S., Rosenberg, S. (eds). *Biologic Therapy of Cancer*, 2nd edn. Philadelphia, PA: J.B. Lippincott, pp. 879–890.

Singh, D., and Lippman, S. 1998. Cancer chemoprevention—Part I: Retinoids and carotenoids and other classic antioxidants. *Oncology* 12(11): 1643–1658.

Skaugen, P. 1997. Bacillus Calmette-Guérin therapy for bladder carcinoma *in situ*: Use in a clinical setting. *Urologic Nursing* 17(2): 69–71.

Snodgrass, M., and Hanna, M., Jr. 1973. Ultrastructural studies of histiocyte-tumor cell interactions during tumor regression after intralesional injection of *Mycobacterium bovis*. *Cancer Research* 33: 701–716.

Starnes, C. 1992. Coley's toxins in perspective. *Nature* 357: 11–12.

Swibold, L. 1999. Maintenance therapy with bacillus Calmette-Guérin in patients with superficial bladder cancer. *Urology Nursing* 19(1): 38–41.

Tracey, K., Vlassara, H., and Cerami, A. 1989. Cachectin/tumor necrosis factor. *Lancet* 1: 1122–1126.

Turner, S. 1992. Colony-stimulating factors: An understandable approach. *Pharmacy and Therapeutics* 17: 1423–1428.

Van Wauwe, J., and Janssen, P. 1991. On the biochemical mode of action of levamisole: An update. *International Journal of Immunopharmacology* 13(1): 3–9.

Velander, W., Lubon, H., and Drohan, W. 1997. Transgenic livestock as drug factories. *Scientific American* 276(1): 70–74.

Weill-Hallé, B. 1980. Routes and methods of administration: Oral vaccination. In Rosenberg, S. (ed). *BCG Vaccine: Tuberculosis-Cancer.* Littleton, MA: P.S.G. Publishing Co., Inc., pp. 165–170.

Wilmut, I. 1998. Cloning for medicine. *Scientific American* 279(6): 58–63.

Wurm, F., and Bernard, A. 1999. Large-scale transient expression in mammalian cells for recombinant protein production. *Current Opinions in Biotechnology* 10(20): 156–159.

Yao, T., Meyers, M., and Livingston, P. 1999. Immunization of melanoma patients with BEC2-keyhole limpet hemocyanin plus BCG intradermally followed by intravenous booster immunizations with BEC2 to induce anti-GD3 ganglioside antibodies. *Clinical Cancer Research* 5(1): 77–81.

Resources and Key References

Print Material

DeVita, V., Jr., Hellman, S., and Rosenberg, S. (eds). 1995. *Biologic Therapy of Cancer*, 2nd edn. Philadelphia, PA: Lippincott Publishers.

Hall, S. 1997. *A Commotion in the Blood: Life, Death and the Immune System*. New York, NY: Henry Holt and Company.

Herberman, R., and Ignoffo, R. (eds). 1996. *Biotherapy in Cancer: Continuing Education for Oncology Nurses*. Richmond, CA: Berlex Laboratories.

Kelly, L., and Miaskowski, C. 1996. An overview of bladder cancer: Treatment and nursing implications. *Oncology Nursing Forum* 23(3): 459–470.

Mire-Sluis, A.R., and Thorpe, R. 1998. *Cytokines*. San Diego, CA: Academic Press.

Oldham, R. (ed). 1998. *Principles of Cancer Biotherapy*, 3rd edn. Boston, MA: Kluwer Academic Publishers.

Rieger, P. (guest ed). 1996. Biotherapy: Present accomplishments and future projections. *Seminars in Oncology Nursing* 12(2): 81–171.

Rieger, P. 1998. Nursing implications of biotherapy.

In Itano, J., and Taoka, K. (eds). *ONS Core Curriculum for Oncology Nursing*, 3rd edn. Philadelphia, PA: W.B. Saunders Company.

Rosenberg, S.A. (ed). 2000. *Principles and Practice of the Biological Therapy of Cancer*, 3rd edn. Philadelphia, PA: Lippincott, Williams & Wilkins.

Thomson, A.W. 1998. *The Cytokine Handbook*, 3rd edn. San Diego, CA: Academic Press.

Tomaszewski, J., DeLaPena, L., Molenda, J., *et al.* 1995. Programmed instruction. Biotherapy: Overview of biotherapy. *Cancer Nursing* 18(5): 397–415.

Walsh, G. (ed) (In press). *Biopharmaceuticals: Biochemistry and Biotechnology*. New York, NY: Wiley-Liss.

Wilmut, I. 1998. Cloning for medicine. *Scientific American* 279(6): 58–63.

Web Sites

For a listing of biopharmaceuticals by company: *http://www.biopharma.com/products.html*

For a listing of approvals for biological agents: *http://www.fda.gov/cber*

CHAPTER 2 | The Immune System

Scott Solomon, MD

Krishna Komanduri, MD

The roots of modern biotherapy for cancer may be traced to 1774, when a French physician attempted to treat a patient with inoperable breast cancer by injecting pus into her leg, inducing inflammation and an eventual disappearance of the cancer. Despite the substantial evolution of biotherapy since its beginnings in the 18th century, clinical trials with new biotherapeutic agents have often outpaced our understanding of precise mechanisms of action. Since the early 1960s when it became clear for the first time that thymus-derived lymphocytes played a role in immunity, remarkable strides have been made in understanding the cells and proteins that mediate protective immune responses. An increasingly clearer understanding of the regulatory pathways of the immune response, as well as the advent of modern biotechnology have formed the basis for novel

interventions that we can classify as **biotherapy**. Biotherapy connotes the administration of products that (1) are coded by the mammalian genome, (2) modify the expression of mammalian genes, or (3) stimulate the immune system. This chapter outlines some basic concepts about the human immune response that provide the intellectual basis for modern biotherapy.

Overview of the Immune System

The immune system is a complex, dynamic system made up of a number of different physical barriers, cell types, and blood-borne proteins that protect us from a hostile environment. There are two types of immunity: innate and adaptive. **Innate immunity**, also called nonspecific or natural immunity, is the first line of defense against pathogenic organisms. Innate immunity is present prior to exposure to infectious organisms and it is not enhanced by such exposures; it is seen clinically as the inflammatory response. **Adaptive immunity**, also known as specific or acquired immunity, is characterized by specific recognition of foreign determinants and a memory response. This allows the immune system to increase in magnitude its responsive and defensive capabilities with each successive exposure to infectious organisms. For a comparison of innate and adaptive immunity, see Table 2.1.

Foreign substances that induce a specific immune response are called **antigens**. Specific immune responses, seen in adaptive immunity, are normally stimulated when an individual is exposed to a foreign antigen. This process is called **immunization**, and the immunity is termed active immunity. Specific immunity can also be conferred upon an individual by transferring cells or serum from a specifically immu-

nized individual. This **adoptive transfer** of immune response between individuals is called passive immunity.

Specific immune responses are classified as humoral or cell mediated, depending on the components of the immune system that mediate the response (Figure 2.1). **Humoral immunity** is characterized by its ability to be adoptively transferred in the cell-free portion of blood. It is mediated by molecules called **antibodies** that specifically recognize and eliminate circulating antigens. **Cell-mediated immunity**, as the name implies, can only be passively transferred with cells from an immunized individual. The cells responsible for specific antigen recognition are called **lymphocytes**. One of the most remarkable features of the immune system is its ability to distinguish between self antigens and foreign antigens. Immunologic unresponsiveness to self is called **tolerance**. The induction of tolerance is an important acquired process that takes place during the development of cell-mediated immunity.

Table 2.1   Innate and adaptive immunity

System	Hallmarks	Features and Functions
Innate immunity	Primary line of defense Nonspecific No memory	Mechanical barriers Intact skin Mucous membranes Chemical barriers Inflammatory response Fever Phagocytic cells Soluble factors Protects against pathogens

Adaptive immunity	Secondary line of defense
	Specific
	Memory
		Lymphocytes
		  T cells: Provide cell-mediated immunity
		    Primarily protects against intracellular organisms, immune surveillance, responsible for rejection of transplanted organs, and modulation of immune response
		  B cells: Provide humoral immunity
		    Primarily protects against viruses and bacteria

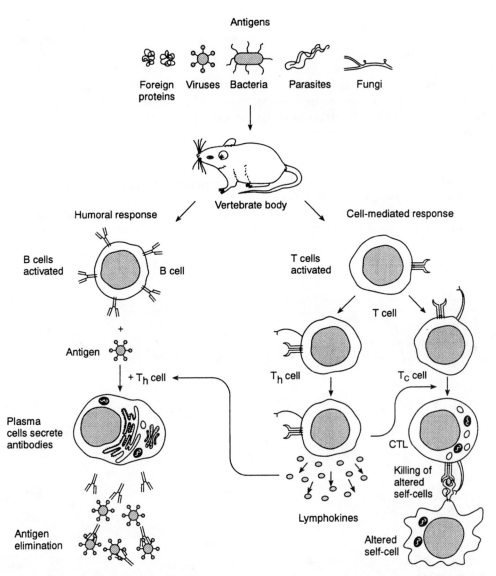

Figure 2.1   Humoral and cell-mediated responses in the immune system. The B lymphocyte is central to the humoral immune response. Interaction of B lymphocytes with antigen (in the presence of appropriate signals provided by T helper [T$_h$] cells) leads to their differentiation into antibody-secreting plasma cells. The secreted antibodies may circulate in the body, bind to target antigens, and facilitate their clearance from the body. The cell-mediated immune response is coordinated by T$_h$ cells that secrete cytokines and aid in the destruction of self-cells by cytotoxic T lymphocytes (CTLs). CTLs recognize self-cells that have been altered in some way (e.g., by viral infection or by malignant transformation).

Source: IMMUNOLOGY by Janis Kirby. Copyright © 1992 by W. H. Freeman and Company. Reprinted with permission.

Innate Immunity

The body's first lines of defense against a foreign invader (e.g., microbes) are mechanical barriers such as intact skin and mucous membranes. If these defenses fail, the innate immune system provides a quick response to limit the colonization of the microbe. The innate immune system has several major components, including **complement** proteins, professional **phagocytes**, and **natural killer (NK) cells**. When an individual's mechanical barriers are breached, an acute inflammatory response follows that includes the physiological processes of capillary dilation, exudation of fluid and plasma protein into the tissues, and accumulation of neutrophils at the site of infection. These responses are manifested clinically as the 5 cardinal signs of inflammation: heat, redness, swelling, pain, and loss of function. The invading organism is then killed through the destructive effects of phagocytosis or soluble chemical factors (Figure 2.2).

Complement System

The complement system consists of about 20 plasma proteins, including multiple proteolytic

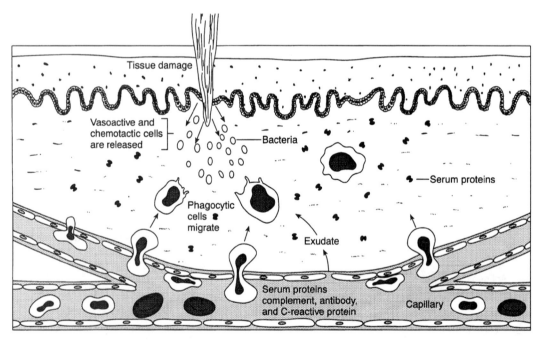

Figure 2.2   The inflammatory response. A bacterial infection or other injury induces tissue damage associated with the release of proteins including vasoactive and chemotactic factors. These proteins lead to the cardinal signs of inflammation, including redness (*rubor*), heat (*calor*), swelling, pain (*dolor*); and loss of function. These findings are caused by increased capillary permeability, influx of macrophages and other white blood cells, and the production of cytokines by the infiltrating leukocytes. Bacterial clearance is enhanced by the antimicrobial properties of the secreted cytokines and by direct phagocytosis by macrophages.

Source: IMMUNOLOGY by Janis Kirby. Copyright © 1992 by W. H. Freeman and Company. Reprinted with permission.

enzymes, that become sequentially activated in a highly regulated multistep process reminiscent of the coagulation cascade. This proteolytic cascade allows for tremendous amplification. The end product of complement activation is the membrane-attack complex, which inserts a donut-shaped channel into the membrane, causing cell lysis. The complement cascade can be activated through 2 separate but interconnected mechanisms. The classical pathway activates the complement cascade only where antibody has bound specific antigens and thus serves as an important effector mechanism for specific humoral immunity. The alternative pathway allows for activation of the complement cascade on microbial surfaces in the absence of antibody. The complement cascade thus acts as a bridge between the specific antibody response (part of the adaptive immune system) and the nonspecific inflammatory response.

When inactive complement proteins are activated, small polypeptides are released. These small "split products" are nonspecific activators of inflammation and act as chemotactic agents, which attract white blood cells to the area; opsonins, which enhance clearance by phagocytic cells; and anaphylactoid agents, which induce the release of histamine, a mediator of increased capillary permeability and edema. These functions are vital for clearance of micro-organisms from the host. Individuals who have a congenital deficiency of one of the complement proteins are at higher risk for some infections.

Phagocytic Cells

GRANULOCYTES

Neutrophils or polymorphonuclear leukocytes are important, early cellular mediators of the inflammatory process. They are also critical to the body's response to acute infections. Neutrophils are the most numerous of all the leukocytes, accounting for approximately 50% to 70% of circulating white blood cells. Neutrophils respond rapidly to chemotactic signals, migrating from the bloodstream into the tissue where they play an important role in acute inflammation and natural immunity. They avidly phagocytose opsonized pathogens and cellular debris. **Eosinophils** are phagocytes, and they are important effector cells in immune reactions to antigens that induce high levels of **immunoglobulin** (Ig)E antibodies, such as parasites. An increase in the circulating eosinophil count is also a hallmark of acute and chronic allergic responses to environmental antigens as well as hypersensitivity reactions to medications. **Basophils** are the circulating counterparts of tissue mast cells. On their surface, they have high-affinity receptors for IgE that, when stimulated, cause these cells to release mediators such as histamine, which are also important in allergic reactions.

MONOCYTES AND MACROPHAGES

The **mononuclear phagocyte system** is made up of cells that have a common lineage and can take several morphologic forms. In the peripheral blood, they are termed **monocytes**. They contain finely granular cytoplasm consisting of lysosomes and phagocytic vacuoles. Once they settle in tissues, they complete maturation and are called **macrophages** or **histiocytes**. Macrophages are found in all tissues, and some have special names reflecting their specific location, for example, alveolar macrophages in the lung, Kupffer cells in the liver, and microglia in the central nervous system. These cells are present late in the inflammatory process and in chronic infections, and they are very effective in removing cellular debris. Macrophages also produce **cytokines**, a group of proteins that signal other immune cells and are responsible for many of the systemic effects of inflammation, such as fever. Macrophages also play a vital role in adaptive immune responses where they are involved in processing antigens and presenting them to antigen-specific T lymphocytes.

Natural Killer Cells

NK cells are large lymphocytes that possess membrane-bound granules that contain hydrolytic enzymes. They constitute about 15% of the circulating lymphocytes. These large granular lymphocytes can spontaneously destroy malignant cell lines in culture. Functionally, NK cells can recognize and destroy target cells without having prior exposure. It has recently been shown that NK cells express a family of proteins called killer-cell Ig-like receptors or **killer-cell inhibitory receptors (KIRs)**, which recognize the **class I** proteins that are part of the **major histocompatibility complex (MHC)**. Class I MHC proteins are expressed on most cells. A more detailed discussion of the MHC follows. When an NK cell encounters

a cell expressing a class I protein, the result is KIR triggering, which inhibits the NK cell from killing the target. Cells lacking class I proteins (e.g., invading bacteria cells) are unable to trigger KIRs and are thus susceptible to attack (see Figure 2.3). NK cells can destroy cells by direct contact and release of **perforins**, molecules that form donut-shaped pores in the target cell's membrane. NK cells can also destroy targets by **antibody-dependent cell-mediated cytotoxicity (ADCC)**. In ADCC, NK cells bind antibodies to their surfaces. When these antibodies bind to cell-surface antigens, cytotoxic enzymes are released, resulting in cell destruction.

Adaptive Immunity

The innate and adaptive immune systems are intimately linked. The innate immune system plays a crucial role in alerting the adaptive

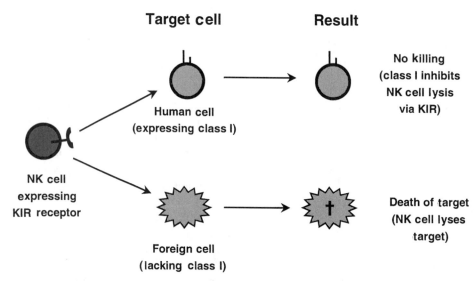

Figure 2.3   Natural killer cell-mediated lysis and inhibition by KIRs. Natural killer (NK) cells express killer-cell inhibiting receptors (KIRs) that are triggered by the binding of KIRs to class I MHC molecules found on the surface of most human cells. NK cells nonselectively kill target cells they encounter that do not express class I MHC molecules (e.g., invading bacteria). When an NK cell encounters a self-cell (expressing class I MHC on its surface), the KIR is triggered, and NK-mediated killing is inhibited, preventing damage to host tissues.

immune system to danger. In return, the adaptive immune response helps amplify the protective mechanisms of innate immunity while at the same time focusing these mechanisms to the sites of antigen entry.

The major cellular effector of the adaptive immune system is the lymphocyte. There are two major classes of lymphocytes: B lymphocytes and T lymphocytes. Some general distinctions can be drawn concerning these two subsets of lymphocytes. For the most part, antibodies produced by B lymphocytes recognize extracellular antigens, whereas T lymphocytes recognize intracellular antigens presented at the surface of cells. Furthermore, antibodies generally recognize intact proteins, whereas T cells recognize only antigenic protein fragments presented in the context of molecules encoded by MHC molecules.

The key features of the adaptive immune response are its diversity, specificity, and memory. The immune system has an amazing capacity to respond specifically to a vast number of foreign antigens. To achieve this, the immune system maintains lymphocytes with a large number of antigenic specificities, estimated to be at least 10^7. The clonal selection principle states that this amazingly diverse lymphocyte repertoire is present in the individual prior to and independent of antigenic stimulation. Subsequently, antigenic stimulation of one of these lymphocyte clones leads to proliferation and differentiation of these cells. The secondary immune response is more pronounced and occurs more quickly than a primary immune response because of the rapid expansion of antigen-specific lymphocytes following priming with antigen. This property of specific immunity is called immunologic memory.

Major Histocompatibility Complex and Antigen Presentation

T cells can only recognize antigenic peptides when they are presented in the context of an appropriate MHC molecule on the surface of a cell. Cells that bear MHC molecules are said to present antigen to the T cell. For foreign proteins to be recognized, the cell must first process them into smaller peptide fragments, associate them with an MHC molecule, and display them on the cell surface. The presence or absence of MHC molecules that can bind and present antigenic peptides to T cells determines the immune response to a foreign protein. The MHC complex refers to a region of highly polymorphic genes. Many different alleles exist within a population, and these alleles differ in their ability to present different antigenic determinants of proteins.

The MHC locus was first studied to determine its relationship to transplantation of tissue. "Transplantation antigens" were initially defined using models of skin or tumor allografts in genetically nonidentical mice. Antigens that mediated rejection of allografts were termed histocompatibility antigens. The strongest of these antigens, termed H2 in mice, was named the major histocompatibility complex. The MHC complex in man is designated the **human leukocyte antigen (HLA) complex** and is located on the short arm of chromosome 6. The HLA antigens were originally defined serologically. The first 3 genes identified, *HLA-A, HLA-B,* and *HLA-C,* make up the class I HLA locus. The next 3 genes identified, which map to a similar region of the chromosome (HLA-D), are called *HLA-DR, HLA-DQ,* and *HLA-DP.* These three genes make up the class II HLA locus.

These two major MHC loci, class I and class II, represent two distinct functional subsets, and any given T cell recognizes foreign proteins bound to only one specific type. In general, class II MHC molecules bind peptides derived from extracellular proteins, whereas endogenously synthesized proteins are associated with class I MHC molecules. As will be discussed in detail in a later section of this chapter, a subset of T cells bearing the surface marker

CD4 are called **CD4$^+$ T cells**. Most of these T cells are cytokine-producing **T helper (T$_h$)** cells and only recognize peptide in association with class II MHC molecules. In contrast, **CD8$^+$ T cells**, most of which are **cytotoxic T lymphocytes (CTLs)**, only recognize peptide in association with class I MHC molecules. This condition is termed **MHC restriction** of the T-cell response, and it is a direct consequence of the way in which T cells mature and are selected in the **thymus**.

Class I MHC molecules are present on most nucleated cells, where they present endogenously synthesized peptides to CTLs. For a CTL to recognize a tumor cell or virus-infected cell as foreign, the antigen must be associated with a class I MHC molecule. Considering that a virus can infect any cell in the body and that the CTL is responsible for killing cells infected with viruses, it makes sense that class I MHC molecules are ubiquitous. Class I MHC molecules are absent in sperm and in trophoblasts. Some cells of the body (e.g., liver cells, fibroblasts, and neurons) express very low levels of these genes. Cytokines such as tumor necrosis factor (TNF) and interferons (IFNs) can upregulate the expression of these genes, increasing the numbers of class I MHC molecules on the surfaces of these cells.

Unlike class I MHC molecules, which are expressed on almost every type of cell in the body, class II MHC molecules are expressed exclusively on cells of the immune system, most notably macrophages, dendritic cells (DCs), and activated B lymphocytes. These cells are called **antigen-presenting cells (APC)** because of their importance in the presentation of class II MHC molecules and target antigens to T$_h$ cells.

T Cells and Thymic Education

The T cell is so named because the vast majority of these lymphocytes are thought to be derived from the thymus, an organ in the anterior mediastinum above the heart. As uncontroversial as this simple statement now seems, it was not until the early 1960s that Jacques Miller demonstrated that the thymus was an important source of lymphocytes and, therefore, central to the development of effective immune responses. Subsequent experiments demonstrated that lymphocytes produced in the thymus were essential for protection against opportunistic infection and for the rejection of allogeneic skin grafts. It was first assumed that a homogeneous population of small lymphocytes was capable of initiating cell-mediated and humoral immune response (i.e., responses mediated by circulating antibodies). However, further work established that these responses were dependent on distinct cellular subsets, with the thymus-derived T-cell subset essential for the production of antibody by cells later termed B cells. Because the thymus is quite prominent in childhood and decreases in size with age, it was long assumed that the thymus was only active in the preadolescent years of life. Instead, it has recently been demonstrated that the thymus continues to function throughout life to produce a steady supply of new T cells, albeit at a lower level with advancing age.

A quick introduction to the development of T cells in the thymus serves to illustrate several important features of T cells (an overview of stages of human thymocyte development is presented in Figure 2.4). **Hematopoietic stem cells**, the most primitive of all blood cells, probably migrate from the bone marrow to form the most immature **thymocytes**. These thymocytes initially lack expression of CD4 and CD8, the two markers that define the most significant peripheral T-cell subsets. Thymocytes then progress through intermediates, including a cell that expresses both CD4 and CD8 (the double-positive thymocyte). These cells increase their expression of the **T-cell receptor (TCR)** as they mature to single-positive thymocytes, the immediate precursors of peripheral lymphocytes. The TCR is the surface protein that

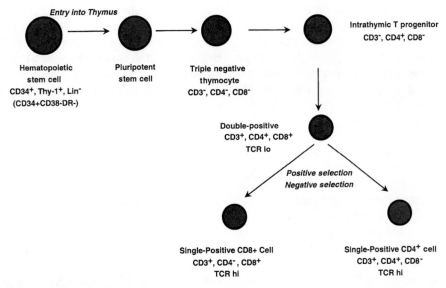

Figure 2.4 Stages of human thymocyte maturation. T lymphocytes, the most important effector cells in the human immune response, develop in the thymus, hence the term thymocyte. Hematopoietic stem cells migrate from the bone marrow and enter the thymus where they give rise to several successive immature stages of development, which are identified by the expression of cluster definition (CD) antigens, denoted below each stage. The majority of thymocytes are double-positive and express CD4 and CD8. These cells then undergo positive and negative selection, and around 1% of thymocytes complete maturation as CD4+ or CD8+ cells that act as helper or cytotoxic cells, respectively, after leaving the thymus. T cells that are ineffective or self-reactive do not survive positive and negative selection. TCR, T-cell receptor. Thy−1+, cells expressing the Thy−1 surfaceantigen, described initially on thymocytes (hence Thy). Lin−, cells lacking markers defining maturation in various lineages.

enables each T cell to recognize a unique target and that initiates effector functions of the T cell (either destroying the target directly for CTLs or orchestrating the immune response for T_h cells). The random rearrangement of a number of different genes, including the variable, joining, and diversity genes at the TCR gene locus, allows for a virtually infinite variety of different T-cell receptors to be expressed on the surface of developing thymocytes.

Although this potential diversity is what allows us to respond to a host of pathogens in our environment, many of the T cells thus produced will have ineffective TCRs or have receptors capable of damaging our own tissues,

leading to **autoimmunity**. Autoimmunity mediated by T cells is thought to underlie the devastating consequences of such human diseases as rheumatoid arthritis, childhood-onset diabetes mellitus, and multiple sclerosis, among others. To produce a healthy and diverse (but safe) TCR repertoire, the processes of positive and negative selection occur in maturing T cells. Together, these processes have been termed thymic education, because the product is a functional T-cell repertoire that is best able to respond to a variety of pathogens but is less likely to induce autoimmune disease.

As double-positive thymocytes mature, they downregulate either CD4 or CD8 and continue to express the other of these proteins, serving as a marker of their function in the peripheral lymphoid system. During this maturation process, thymocytes also sequentially undergo positive and negative selection. In positive selection, only thymocytes bearing TCRs capable of binding appropriately to the correct MHC molecule (class I for CD8$^+$ cells and class II for CD4$^+$ cells) are allowed to survive. The others undergo death by **apoptosis**, a form of cellular suicide important in the regulation of developmental processes. In this manner, the immune system eliminates ineffective T cells before they are exported from the thymus. T cells surviving this step are then screened for their ability to bind proteins present in our own bodies (self-antigens), a process called negative selection. Cells that are likely to provoke autoimmune reactions die, a process that has been termed central tolerance, because cells that survive this step are likely to "tolerate" (i.e., not attack) their host. Because cancer cells are derived from host tissues, this step explains why we may often be unable to eliminate them unless they develop new antigens on their surfaces that can be recognized by T cells that survive negative selection.

Cells that pass positive and negative selection (perhaps only 1% of double-positive thymocytes) then migrate out of the thymus into the blood and other peripheral lymphoid tissues, including **lymph nodes**. At this time, prior to seeing their target antigen for the first time, newly produced T cells are considered **naive T cells** and can be identified by the expression of the surface marker CD45RA and other proteins. Once they encounter their target antigen for the first time, they proliferate and differentiate into **memory cells** or **effector cells** that express the marker CD45RO rather than its isoform CD45RA. These cells can persist for decades in the blood and lymph nodes, forming a basis for immunity that is nearly lifelong. Whereas negative selection eliminates the vast majority of T cells capable of initiating autoimmune reactions, the immune system also may limit the extent of immune activation through **peripheral tolerance**. Peripheral tolerance consists of mechanisms by which activated T cells naturally undergo a death that is termed activation-induced cell death to prevent beneficial immune reactions from becoming harmful to surrounding tissues and to reduce the pool of memory T cells to levels sufficient to sustain immunological memory.

Antigen-Presenting Cells

The two properties that allow a cell to function as an APC are its ability to process endocytosed proteins into smaller peptides and the expression of class II MHC molecules. After APCs internalize extracellular antigens, intracellular proteolysis produces multiple peptide fragments that can bind to MHC. Only short peptide chains (8 to 20 amino acids in length) can be presented to T cells because of the size of the MHC binding cleft. This requirement explains why T cells recognize linear but not conformal determinants of proteins. Furthermore, polysaccharide and lipid antigens are not recognized by T cells, which is a result of their inability to associate with MHC molecules. The best-defined APCs are DCs, macrophages, and activated B lymphocytes. In addition, other cell types can be induced to express class II MHC molecules and present antigen to T$_h$ cells by the cytokine IFN-γ, facilitating potent upregulation of the immune response.

The functional activation of T cells requires more than binding of MHC-conjugated antigen to the TCR. In addition to expressing MHC molecules, an efficient APC must also provide important costimulatory signals required for T-cell activation (described below). Macrophages and B cells, once activated by the immune response, efficiently express both MHC and costimulatory molecules. Once activated, these APCs provide the appropriate signals to activate T lymphocytes. DCs perform similar functions but appear to be unique in their powerful ability to stimulate naive T cells and thus initiate immune responses to novel antigens.

DENDRITIC CELLS

DCs are specialized APCs that reside in all lymphoid and most nonlymphoid tissues, including a subset in the skin known as Langerhans cells. DCs are extremely efficient APCs compared with macrophages, and they play a critical role in the initiation and regulation of immune responses. DCs are believed to play an important role in surveillance at sites of antigen entry, as well as in activation of naive T cells during primary immune responses.

DC progenitors are derived from bone marrow, and they subsequently seed most nonlymphoid tissues, where they exist in an immature stage. Immature DCs are effective scavengers with an increased capacity for antigen capture and processing but have low T-cell stimulatory capability. Inflammatory mediators promote DC maturation and migration out of nonlymphoid tissues into the blood or afferent lymph. These migratory cells reach secondary lymphoid organs where they home to the T-cell areas and undergo a dramatic phenotypic change. Mature DCs lose the ability to capture antigen and acquire an increased capacity to stimulate T cells. They achieve this through upregulation of MHC, expression of costimulatory signals, and secretion of specialized cytokines such as interleukin (IL)-12. Mature DCs therefore present to naive T cells antigen that has been captured at the level of peripheral tissues and so can be viewed as the sentinels of the immune system.

Important recent advances have included the development of techniques for culture of DCs from progenitors and the capacity to generate DCs with distinct functions *in vitro*. There is increasing evidence for distinct developmental pathways that generate different DC subsets both *in vitro* and *in vivo*. Recently, a lymphoid DC was described that appears to represent a unique DC subset. After production in the bone marrow, this DC directly seeds the thymus, where it appears to be involved in the induction of central T-cell tolerance rather than T-cell activation. Future studies of various DC subsets will most certainly increase our understanding of immune function.

Helper and Cytotoxic T Lymphocytes

As discussed previously, the T-lymphocyte population can be further divided into two major subpopulations that can be distinguished by the cell-surface markers CD4 and CD8. The CD4-expressing T cells are also called T_h cells. Their major function is to orchestrate the immune response. In response to antigenic stimulation, T_h cells secrete protein hormones called cytokines, which function to promote the proliferation and differentiation of T cells, B cells, and macrophages. The T_h cells also induce the generation of CTLs. In addition, these cytokines can recruit and activate inflammatory leukocytes, providing an important link between specific T-cell immunity and the nonspecific inflammatory response. T_h cells can only recognize antigen when presented in the context of a class II MHC molecule and are thus called class II-restricted cells. $CD4^+$ T cells also express the protein CD154, which is the ligand for the CD40 receptor present on DCs and other APCs. Activation of T_h cells allows them to interact with DCs, a process that has been termed "licensing," inducing licensed DCs to better present antigens to naive T cells. CD154-CD40 interactions are also important in activating B cells to better secrete antibodies in the humoral response, further demonstrating the importance of T_h cells in coordinating complex immune responses. It is important to note that CD4 is a co-receptor for the human immunodeficiency virus (HIV-1, thus, HIV-mediated killing of CD4$^+$ lymphocytes is central to the immunodeficiency of the acquired immunodeficiency syndrome (AIDS).

CTLs express the cell-surface marker CD8 and recognize only those antigens that are associated with class I MHC molecules, that is, that are class I MHC-restricted. CTLs recognize and bind to cells expressing foreign antigens (e.g., viral and tumor-associated antigens) bound to class I MHC molecules. Once bound, they release a variety of mediators that induce cell killing. Studies of experimental viral infection in animals, such as murine infections with viruses including lymphocytic choriomeningitis virus and influenza, have established the crucial role of the CD8$^+$ CTL as the most important cell in protective immune responses. Recent studies of human viral infections such as HIV and cytomegalovirus (CMV), a major pathogen in subjects with HIV infection and those undergoing bone marrow transplantation, have demonstrated similar results. Further studies have demonstrated in both animal models and human subjects that CTL responses to individual pathogens are unlikely to be sustained over time unless the CD4$^+$ T$_h$ response to the same virus is preserved.

Other, less well understood lymphocyte subsets may exist, including suppressor T cells, which may express CD8 and may have a role in limiting immune activation and in transplantation tolerance. A better understanding of T-cell subsets has been facilitated by the use of sophisticated **flow cytometry**, a technique that allows precise definition of the multiple surface markers that can be used to distinguish cells. Flow cytometric evaluation of T cells has recently defined a far greater diversity of T-cell subsets than has been previously suggested by expression of CD4 and CD8 alone. Further characterization of the role of such subsets in

performing regulatory roles in the immune system will likely be crucial to our understanding of tumor immunology and other fields.

T lymphocytes are responsible for many important clinical immune reactions such as delayed-type hypersensitivity reactions, graft rejection, graft-versus-host disease, and contact skin sensitivity.

T-Cell Receptor Complex

As previously stated, T lymphocytes specifically recognize antigenic peptides in a MHC-restricted fashion via a specialized receptor complex, the TCR. The TCR is a heterodimer composed of two polypeptide chains, α and β, which are covalently linked to each other by disulfide bonds. Each chain is composed of variable and constant regions, structurally related to Ig. Another less-common type of TCR that is found on a small subset of T cells is composed of γ and δ chains. These γδ T cells may arise through extrathymic development and may play a role in immune responses on mucosal surfaces such as the gut. The αβ TCR heterodimer enables T cells to recognize antigen-MHC complexes, but cellular signaling is dependent on an associated protein complex, CD3. When antigen binds to the TCR, the associated CD3 transduces an activation signal to the T cell. Antibodies directed against CD3 proteins can stimulate T-cell responses identical to antigen-induced responses. Other antigens, termed **superantigens**, are capable of activating large subsets of T cells bearing certain variable-region (or Vβ) genes. An example of a superantigen-mediated disease is toxic shock syndrome, which is mediated by a toxin secreted by the bacterium *Staphylococcus aureus*.

CD4 and CD8 Receptors

The CD4 and CD8 receptors are important cell-surface molecules on T cells that extend beyond their ability to define functional subsets. CD4 and CD8 also help to facilitate the MHC-restricted interactions of T_h cells with APCs, as well as interactions of CTLs with their appropriate target cell (i.e., virally infected cells). These proteins have at least two important functions. Most important, they act as cell-cell adhesion molecules, anchoring the TCR to the appropriate MHC molecule (i.e., class II for $CD4^+$ T cells and class I for $CD8^+$ T cells). Secondly, $CD4^+$ and $CD8^+$ molecules also possess cell-signaling ability and are believed to facilitate T-cell activation.

Costimulation

Engagement of the TCR by antigen is necessary but not sufficient to promote T-cell proliferation and differentiation into helper and effector lymphocytes. The two-signal hypothesis, first articulated by Peter Bretscher and Melvin Cohn in 1970, states that the signal produced by the TCR ("signal one") must be accompanied by a second signal to induce T-cell activation. The molecules that provide this second signal were identified much later and act to provide what has been termed **costimulation**. The most important providers of a costimulatory signal are APCs, which provide this signal at the same time that they present antigens to responding T cells. When T cells encounter antigen but do not receive an appropriate costimulatory signal, a state of T-cell unresponsiveness, or **anergy**, ensues; in some cases, however, this anergic state can be overcome by signals induced by the cytokine IL-2.

Although a large number of costimulatory proteins have been described, the most important molecule appears to be **B7**. B7 actually represents a family of proteins consisting of at least two related molecules: B7-1 (CD80) and B7-2 (CD86). **CD28**, expressed on resting and activated T lymphocytes, is a receptor for both of these molecules. Costimulation through B7-

CD28 results in high-level IL-2 production, an essential survival stimulus for activated T cells. Another receptor for CD80 and CD86 is the CTLA-4 receptor. In contrast to CD28, this receptor may serve to slow down or limit activation of the T cell and may play a role in preventing harmful overexpansion of an immune response.

As discussed previously, activation of $CD4^+$ T cells leads to interaction of the $CD4^+$ T-cell-surface protein CD154 also known as CD40 ligand (CD40L) with its receptor CD40 on the surface of DCs and activated B cells. CD154-CD40 interactions have pronounced immunostimulatory effects, enhancing T-cell activation through upregulation of B7-1 and B7-2 expression on DCs and induction of IL-12 secretion. CD154-CD40 interactions also enhance B-cell activation and are essential to promoting T-cell-dependent antibody responses. Some of the important interactions between an APC and a $CD4^+$ T cell are illustrated in Figure 2.5.

Helper T-Cell Subsets

$CD4^+$ T_h lymphocytes are crucial to the initiation of specific immunity, both cell-mediated and humoral. In response to antigenic stimulation and appropriate costimulation, T_h cells secrete cytokines that function to orchestrate the immune response. Once activated, T_h cells proliferate through an autocrine response to IL-2 in order to build up a clone of T_h cells with the same TCR specificity. Further stimulation results in the secretion of other cytokines, such as IFN-γ, TNF, IL-4, IL-5, and IL-10.

In general, a single T_h cell does not secrete every cytokine. Although not a perfect rule, T_h cells tend to secrete subsets of cytokines that are frequently categorized into two different groups: T_h1 cytokines, including IL-2, IFN-γ, and TNF; and T_h2 cytokines, including IL-4, IL-5, and IL-10. These T_h subsets perform very different functions. The T_h1 cytokine profile is

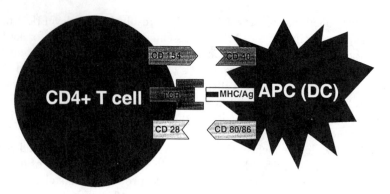

Figure 2.5 Major interactions between antigen-presenting cells (APCs) and T lymphocytes. Three major interactions between a dendrite cell (DC) and a CD4+ T lymphocyte are depicted: (1) the triggering of CD40 on the surface of the DC, leading to its activation or "licensing" by CD154 expressed by the T cell; (2) the interaction of the T-cell receptor (TCR) with a major histocompatibility complex/antigen (MHC/Ag) complex presented by the DC; and (3) costimulation, mediated by the binding of CD80 and CD86 (a.k.a. the B7 proteins) to CD28, an interaction necessary to fully activate the T cell.

well suited to help defend the body against viral or bacterial invasion because these cytokines instruct the innate and adaptive immune responses to produce cells and antibodies that are effective against these organisms. The T_h2 cytokines, on the other hand, lead to IgE and IgA antibody production and are ideally suited for defense against parasitic and mucosal infections. An overview of peripheral human T-cell subsets is presented in Figure 2.6.

Mechanisms of Cytotoxic T-Lymphocyte Killing

CTLs express CD8, are class I MHC-restricted, and require direct cell-cell contact for cell killing. Because almost every cell in the body expresses class I MHC antigens, almost every cell can be killed by a CTL; in contrast, cell killing by NK cells is inhibited by class I expression. CTLs are important effector cells in 3 noteworthy settings: viral infection, allograft rejection, and tumor rejection.

Cell killing by CTLs is directed by cytokines secreted by T_h1 cells. In response to cytokines such as IL-2 and antigen stimulation, the resting CTL is stimulated to proliferate and differentiate. After target-cell contact, the CTL possesses several weapons for effective cell killing. The first involves the production of a protein called perforin, that, like the membrane-attack complex of the complement system, inserts a donut-shaped channel into the membrane, causing cell lysis. In addition, CTLs can secrete a cell toxin called granzyme B, which kills target cells by apoptosis. Another major mechanism of CTL-mediated killing involves a cell-surface protein on CTLs called Fas ligand that can bind to the Fas receptor protein (CD95) on target cells, triggering apoptotic cell death. Other downstream mediators of the apoptotic pathway are the caspases. A better definition of the apoptotic cascade is likely to be important in the design of immunomodulatory drugs that could potentiate CTL killing as well as an understanding of tumor escape mechanisms.

T-Cell Receptor Diversity

For a viral or tumor antigen to be recognized and effectively cleared by the immune system, a preexisting T cell with a receptor capable of

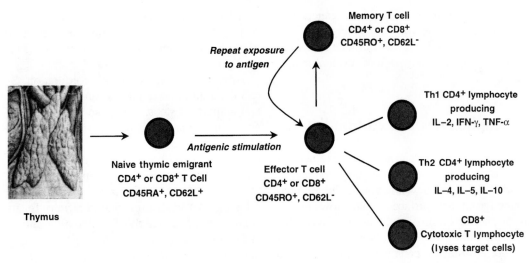

Figure 2.6 Phenotypes of peripheral human T cells. When CD4$^+$ or CD8$^+$ T cells first leave the thymus, they are referred to as naive until their initial encounter with their cognate antigen. Following antigenic stimulation, a single cell expands into a pool of effectors, some of which die; others contract to form a memory T-cell subset that can regain effector activity with repeated stimulation. Effector cells include the cytotoxic T lymphoctye as well as functional subsets of T$_h$ cells, including the T$_h$1 and T$_h$2 subsets characterized by their cytokine secretion profiles.

recognizing the target antigen must be activated and expanded to initiate the immune response. If no T cells capable of recognizing the target antigens exist, no response will be generated. Therefore, maintaining sufficient diversity to deal with evolving pathogens (and tumor antigens) is an important part of T-cell homeostasis.

There are approximately 10^{12} T cells in an average human. Diversity among $\alpha\beta$ T cells, which constitute the majority of the T cells in our bodies, is generated by recombining the 42 variable and 61 joining segments in the α locus and the 47 variable, 2 diversity, and 13 joining segments in the β locus. The number of theoretical combinations with this number of different gene segments is approximately 10^{15} different TCRs. In reality, far fewer T cells bearing different TCRs actually exist in an individual. Recent quantitative analysis has demonstrated that approximately 2 to 3 $\times$ 10^7 different TCR-bearing $\alpha\beta$ T cells exist in the naive T-cell

compartment. Although the memory T-cell compartment consists of nearly the same number of T cells as the naive compartment in most adults, it only contains 100,000 to 200,000 different TCRs. Whereas persistent input from the thymus may help keep this diversity relatively broad in some individuals, other consequences may damage the repertoire and severely limit this diversity. For example, HIV-1-infected subjects may experience HIV-mediated killing of T cells that may substantially limit TCR diversity, leading to vulnerability to many opportunistic infections. Cytotoxic chemotherapy and steroids are widely used classes of drugs that also destroy T cells and may substantially diminish the T-cell repertoire that is capable of responding to viral and tumor antigens.

Currently, there is great interest in combining antitumor cytotoxic therapies with immunologic interventions as treatment for cancer. It will be important to design biotherapeutic approaches that maximally inhibit cancer cell growth while preserving the diversity of the TCR repertoire to allow the immune system to participate in the destruction of residual malignant cells.

B Lymphocytes and Antibodies

Antibodies, or **Igs**, are synthesized exclusively by plasma cells derived from B lymphocytes. Resting B lymphocytes express membrane-bound Igs on their surface, which allows recognition and activation of antigen-specific B cells. Following antigenic stimulation, B cells differentiate into **plasma cells**, which function is to secrete antibodies into the circulation. All the daughter cells derived from a single B cell will produce the same antibody; therefore, the name **monoclonal antibody** is given to the Ig secreted from a particular clone of B cells.

B-Cell Activation

Resting B cells are activated to proliferate and secrete antibody by antigenic stimulation of their cell-surface receptor, membrane-bound Ig. Effective B-cell signaling also requires crosslinking of membrane-bound Ig on the surface of the cell. This can be achieved through closely spaced antigens or an antigen with multiple similar epitopes. The requirement for receptor cross-linking can be significantly decreased when complement proteins are bound (opsonized) to pathogens.

In addition to antigen recognition, B-cell activation requires a costimulatory signal, usually provided by a T_h cell. The most important costimulatory signal involves direct cell-cell contact between the 2 cells and is likely to include the interaction of CD154 on the T cell with CD40 on the B cell. After antigen stimulation, the B cell internalizes the antigen and presents it along with a class II MHC molecule to the T cell. This T-cell/B-cell interaction causes secretion of various cytokines by the T cell, resulting in proliferation and maturation of B cells (Figure 2.7).

After B-cell activation and proliferation, B-cell maturation takes place. This involves several important steps. First, isotype switching occurs in which the B cell decides what class of Ig it will make. The choice of antibody class is driven by exposure to various cytokines. Second, affinity maturation takes place in which membrane-bound Ig undergoes mutation and selection that leads to increased affinity for its cognate antigen. Lastly, B cells differentiate and commit to being either an antigen-secreting plasma cell or a long-lived memory B cell.

Immunoglobulins

All antibodies have a common core structure of 2 identical light chains and 2 identical heavy chains. One light chain is attached to each heavy chain, and the 2 heavy chains are attached to each other. All antibody light chains fall into one of two classes: κ or λ. The heavy chains take their name from the Ig class or **isotype**. There are 5 main isotypes of immunoglobulins: IgA, IgD, IgE, IgG, and IgM, and the heavy chains are thus denoted α, δ, ε, γ, and μ, respectively. All heavy chains may be expressed in two molecular forms, a secretory form and a membrane-bound form that contains additional hydrophobic amino acid residues at the carboxyl terminal.

Igs are considered bifunctional proteins. A highly variable region at one end serves as the antigen-binding site, whereas the constant region on the other end serves as the effector end of the molecule. In an intact Ig molecule, 3 hypervariable regions in each light chain and 3 hypervariable regions in each heavy chain are brought together in 3-dimensional space to form the antigen-binding surface. Because each

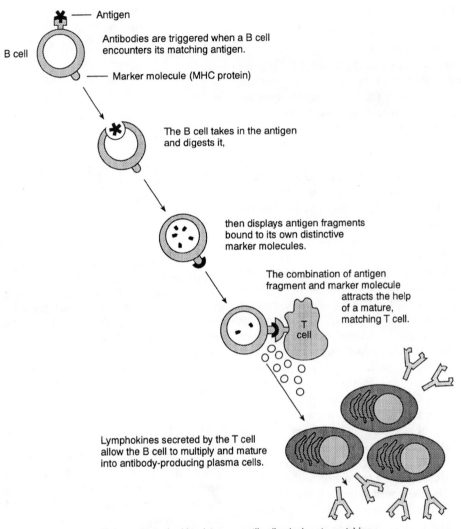

Antigen

Antibodies are triggered when a B cell encounters its matching antigen.

B cell

Marker molecule (MHC protein)

The B cell takes in the antigen and digests it,

then displays antigen fragments bound to its own distinctive marker molecules.

The combination of antigen fragment and marker molecule attracts the help of a mature, matching T cell.

T cell

Lymphokines secreted by the T cell allow the B cell to multiply and mature into antibody-producing plasma cells.

Released into the bloodstream, antibodies lock onto matching antigens. These antigen-antibody complexes are soon eliminated, either by the complement cascade or by the liver and the spleen.

Figure 2.7   Activation of B lymphocytes to produce antibodies. Surface immunoglobulin receptors on B cells bind their cognate antigens, which are then processed by the cell and presented to T helper cells. Surface protein interactions (including the association of CD154 on the T cell with CD40 on the B cell) and cytokine signals delivered by the T cell help transform the B cell into an antibody-secreting plasma cell. Secreted antibodies may freely circulate, binding antigens and targeting antibody-coated targets for elimination by phagocytes and by the complement cascade. MHC, major histocompatibility complex.

Source: Schindler, L. 1992. *Understanding the Immune System.* NIH publication no. 92-3229. Bethesda, MD: U.S. Department of Health and Human Services, June 1992, p. 12.

monomer of an Ig has 2 heavy and 2 light chains, an Ig can bind 2 antigenic sites.

ANTIBODY CLASSES

Of all the Ig classes, IgG is present in the highest concentration in the plasma. It is the principal antibody secreted in the secondary immune response, and it is responsible for most specific antibody reactions in the adult. It is also the antibody passed from the maternal blood to the fetus and is responsible for enhancing neonatal immunity. The constant region of IgG contains the **Fc** receptor-binding site, which allows binding of antibody to neutrophils, macrophages, and NK cells. Furthermore, 2 of the 4 subclasses of IgG are able to activate complement proteins.

IgM is the first class of Igs to be formed when naive B cells are activated. It is a large pentameric molecule, composed of 5 separate Ig molecules. IgM is produced early during an infection, where it is extremely efficient at both neutralizing circulating pathogens and activating complement proteins (see Figure 2.8). IgA is the main antibody class that guards the mucosal surfaces of the body, preventing antigens from gaining access to the systemic circulation. Comprised of a dimer, IgA is very good at agglutinating pathogens, allowing them to be cleared in the mucus. IgA is also secreted into breast milk, providing protection to the nursing infant. IgE, the fourth class of Igs, plays an important role in allergic reactions and in immunity against parasites. It is a monomeric Ig that attaches to high-affinity receptors on mast cells and basophils, which when activated cause cellular degranulation. Not much is known about IgD, which is present in small amounts in the circulation and is involved in the regulation of Ig synthesis.

Distribution of Lymphoid Cells

It is tempting and potentially misleading to think of the immune system as an organ that

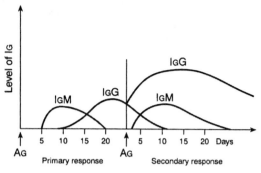

Primary and secondary immune responses

Figure 2.8 Primary and secondary humoral immune responses. The kinetics of the immunoglobulin M (IgM) and immunoglobulin G (IgG) responses are depicted following primary and secondary antigenic stimulation, as occurs following immunization or repeated viral infections. There is a decreased latency and greater magnitude of the secondary immune response, resulting from expansion of increasingly specific B cells.

Source: Reprinted with permission from Galluci, B. 1987. The immune system and cancer. *Oncology Nursing Forum* 14 (suppl 6): 3–12.

may be sampled easily (e.g., by drawing peripheral blood). It is important to realize that the majority of cells in the immune system actually reside in tissue compartments contained in the primary lymphoid and secondary lymphoid organs.

The organs capable of producing cells of the immune system (e.g., the APCs or lymphocytes) have been termed the primary lymphoid or hematopoietic tissues. These organs include the bone marrow and the thymus. In birds, these organs also include the Bursa of Fabricius, a specialized organ capable of generating B lymphocytes. The name reflects the cell's "bursal" origin. Following their "central" production, cells of the immune system (e.g., lymphocytes) express homing receptors, specialized adhesion molecules expressed on their surfaces that allow them to "home" (or locate) and bind to entry areas of secondary lymphoid tissues. For example, as mature thymocytes exit the thymus and become naive lymphocytes in the periphery, they express CD62L, also known as L-selectin. CD62L expression enables the naive lymphocyte to bind to lymph nodes, where most lymphocytes in the body reside. Lymph nodes are encapsulated organs in drainage areas where antigens from the skin and other organs may be concentrated and processed by APCs. The presence of memory lymphocytes in lymph nodes enables these APCs to stimulate an effector response more efficiently than would be possible if most lymphocytes were circulating freely. Other specialized lymphoid tissues include the **mucosa-associated lymphoid tissues** (**MALT**), a group of tissues that includes the bronchus-associated lymphoid tissues (BALT) and the gut-associated lymphoid tissues (GALT).

Once a naive lymphocyte becomes activated following presentation of its cognate antigen by an APC (e.g., a Langerhans cell in the skin or a macrophage in a lymph node), it proliferates, giving rise to many daughter cells with similar specificities. Until relatively recently, it was believed that the frequency of an individual antigen-specific response could never rise much above 1 in 1,000 lymphocytes. It is now known that such responses in both CD4$^+$ and CD8$^+$ lymphocytes may rise to much higher levels in both acute and chronic infections. For example, in experimentally infected mice, a single clone of antigen-specific CD8$^+$ T cells can expand to nearly 50% of the total number of peripheral CD8$^+$ T cells. In human subjects infected with the chronic viral pathogen CMV, CMV-specific responses in the CD4$^+$ T-cell compartment greater than 10% of peripheral CD4$^+$ T cells have been reported. Although in most cases these acute responses ultimately decrease (following apoptotic death of many of the effectors), it is likely that long-lived memory cells reside in lymph nodes and similar tissues waiting for a repeat exposure to antigen. Only about 1% of total lymphocytes freely circulate at any given time. The remainder may move, or traffic, between the blood and lymphoid organs like the lymph nodes or the spleen, a process termed lymphocyte recirculation.

Cancer and the Immune System

Tumor Biology

Cancer is characterized by unregulated cell growth and division, and underlying this abnormal cellular state are genetic changes. **Carcinogenesis** is a multistep process, whereby increasing numbers of genetic changes or mutations accumulate as the tumor progresses. The normal cellular genes that are mutated in cancer are generally grouped into two categories. The first group of genes, the **proto-oncogenes**, promote cell growth and tumor spread (metastasis). The second group of genes, the **tumor-suppressor genes**, protect us against cancer-causing mutations.

Oncogenes were first recognized in experimental virology, where viral genes were shown to have the ability to transform cells in culture. Transformation is the process by which a cellular phenotype is altered in culture, so that it takes on the appearance of a tumor cell. It was subsequently discovered that viral oncogenes have normal cellular equivalents or proto-oncogenes. The initiating event in cell growth and division is termed cell signaling. The signal, which could be a growth factor, hormone, cytokine, or antigen, initiates a complex series of actions at the cell surface as well as in the cytoplasm and nucleus. Proto-oncogenes are involved in coding for the proteins that act as growth factors, growth factor receptors, and signaling complexes at the membrane; second messengers in the cytoplasm; and regulators of gene expression. Proto-oncogenes also control the highly regulated processes of the cell cycle, that is, the sequencing and coordination of the cell through the G_0, G_1, S, G_2, and M phases.

The existence of tumor-suppressor genes was first hypothesized from epidemiologic data. Knudson developed a mathematical model to explain the difference in age at onset of unilateral and bilateral (familial) retinoblastoma (Rb). He suggested that individuals with familial disease were born with one defective gene of the pair of maternal and paternal genes, alleles, which control Rb development. As the presence of at least one functioning gene inhibits the growth of the tumor, tumor formation requires the loss of both alleles. Therefore, the loss of both alleles occurs at an earlier age in bilateral disease. Unilateral disease occurs later in life, given the requirement for acquired mutations in both alleles. The responsible tumor-suppressor gene, *Rb,* appears to be very important in the process of regulating cell-cycle progression. Great progress has also been made in identifying tumor-suppressor genes associated with other diseases, such as Wilms' tumor, von Recklinghausen's neurofibromatosis, and familial adenomatous polyposis. Tumor-suppressor genes have a variety of actions, including suppression of cellular transcription factors, DNA replication, and gene transcription.

One tumor-suppressor gene, *p53*, deserves special mention. Mutations at the *p53* locus occur in almost all malignancies, including cancers of the colon, breast, liver, and lung. Indeed, alterations in the expression of *p53* are found more commonly in neoplasia than abnormalities of any other known tumor-suppressor genes or proto-oncogene. A master regulator of cell-cycle progression, *p53* plays an important role in protecting the cell from cancer-causing mutations. When *p53* senses that mutations have occurred in cellular genes, it will either halt cell proliferation until these mutations can be repaired or, if irreversible genetic damage has occurred, the cell is destroyed through apoptosis. Transgenic mice carrying a mutant

p53 gene develop many types of cancer, including a high incidence of sarcomas. Furthermore, patients with the **Li-Fraumeni syndrome**, who have inherited *p53* mutations, develop a broad spectrum of cancers, including osteosarcomas, breast cancer, soft-tissue sarcoma, and leukemias, some of which may appear at a very early age. Statistical analyses have demonstrated that 50% of these individuals will develop a malignancy before the age of 30, with this proportion rising to 90% by age 70.

Mutations in cellular genes often lead to altered protein expression. Expression of mutant proteins in tumor cells may lead to the production and expression of unique tumor-specific antigens. The expression of such antigens might theoretically lead to enhanced potential of tumor recognition by the cellular immune response. The identification and characterization of such tumor antigens has served as a focus of considerable interest among those developing immunotherapeutic approaches for cancers.

Immune Surveillance

As stated above, powerful defense mechanisms exist within the cell to protect it from cancer-causing mutations. Whether the immune system plays a role in protecting us from the majority of human cancers remains speculative. In the 1950s, the concept of **immune surveillance** was popularized. This hypothesis suggests that in most individuals, occult, early-stage cancers are likely to be controlled and destroyed by the immune system. Unfortunately, direct testing of this hypothesis has proved difficult because, by definition, the development of occult, early-stage cancers that may be controlled by the immune system may not be quantitated. There is good evidence that the incidence of cancer is increased in people who are immunosuppressed, either by chemotherapy or in the setting of HIV-1 infection. Specific cancers such as lymphomas, leukemias, and virus-associated cancers clearly occur more commonly in these patients; however, a similar increase is not seen for many other human malignancies. Furthermore, most of the tumors arising in immunodeficient mice and other animal models are derived from the abnormal immune system (e.g., lymphoma) rather than from solid organs such as the breast or lung.

To summarize, evidence to date has not demonstrated a conclusive role of the immune system in protection against most human tumors. However, under appropriate circumstances, it is likely that tumors may express antigens that make them potentially susceptible to immune attack. The ability to manipulate the immune system to recognize tumor cells that were once invisible forms the basis of current immunotherapeutic approaches to treating cancer.

Immune Responses to Tumors

Much of the early work in tumor immunology was performed in inbred strains of mice. In these animal models, tumor antigens are also called tumor transplantation antigens, reflecting the experimental design used to test these ideas. In these experiments, nonviable tumor cells obtained from another animal of the same inbred line were injected as a tumor-cell vaccine. After rechallenging the animal with live tumor cells, the mice did not always develop tumors. In contrast, control animals without prior exposure to the tumor-cell vaccine were unable to reject the live tumor cells and thus developed malignancies. Manipulation of antigens, APCs, cytokines, and costimulatory pathways has been done effectively to prevent or delay tumor recurrence in similar animal models.

In humans, there are several lines of evidence arguing for an immune response to established tumors. The first comes from the study of tumor histopathology. When examined under the microscope, some tumors have marked inflammatory infiltrates, consisting of lymphocytes and macrophages, suggesting that the tumor has stimulated an immune response in the individual. In some cancers (e.g., medullary carcinoma of the breast), the presence of a mononuclear infiltrate portends a more favorable prognosis. Secondly, immune responses to some malignancies can be inferred by the clinical observation of waxing and waning in tumor size. This phenomenon has been most frequently described in melanoma, where malignant lesions may be easily visible on the skin. In some cases of melanoma, lesions have been noted to disappear from one area whereas others appeared simultaneously at distant sites, providing putative evidence for immune surveillance. Spontaneous regression of a diagnosed malignancy is an extremely rare event but has been well documented in various cancers such as carcinoma of the kidney, melanoma, neuroblastoma, and choriocarcinoma. In allogeneic human stem-cell transplantation, relapse rates have been found to vary inversely to the degree of genetic relatedness of the donor and recipient. Furthermore, donor lymphocyte infusions alone have induced remissions in subjects who have relapsed following allogeneic transplantation. These data provide compelling evidence that immunologic recognition of residual cancer cells by donor T cells may eradicate residual cancer cells (the graft-versus-malignancy effect).

Tumor antigens elicit both humoral and cell-mediated immune responses *in vivo*, and almost every immunologic effector mechanism tested has been shown to kill tumor cells *in vitro*. It is probable that the most protective responses to tumors are cellular responses, which are similar to those generated against viruses. The most important cells in these reactions are cytotoxic T cells, NK cells, and APCs.

Cell-Mediated Cytotoxicity

CTLs can recognize and destroy malignant cells by the same mechanisms they use to recognize and destroy cells infected with viruses. The cytotoxic TCR attaches to the tumor antigen, which is complexed with a class I MHC antigen. The direct contact and binding results in the release of enzymes and lysis of the tumor cell within a few minutes. As with many other specific cytotoxic T-cell reactions, T_h activation is likely to be necessary. T_h cells are activated by the presentation of tumor antigens linked to class II MHC on macrophages or DCs. In addition to facilitating cytotoxic T-cell reactions, activation of T_h cells can also result in nonspecific cytotoxicity. These cells release cytokines, which activate macrophages in the area of the tumor. The activated macrophages release lytic enzymes, proteases, and reactive oxygen intermediates that destroy the tumor cells. NK cells are also responsible for the killing of tumor cells, but unlike CTLs, NK cells destroy their targets in an MHC-unrestricted manner and do not require prior exposure to a tumor antigen to induce a cytotoxic response. In another type of cytotoxicity, antibody-dependent cytotoxicity, antibodies bound to an NK cell or a macrophage may cross-link the cytotoxic and tumor cells. This binding creates changes in the cell membrane of the macrophage or NK cell, causing release of lytic granules and death of the tumor cell.

Antitumor Antibodies

In animal experiments, the injection of tumor cells has resulted in the production of antitumor antibodies. The binding of these antibodies to macrophages can lead to tumor-cell lysis, as described above in antibody-dependent cytotoxicity. Antitumor antibodies can also act as an opsonin, allowing phagocytosis by macrophages to occur more readily as well as resulting in activation of the complement system. Paradoxically, it has been shown in some animal models that the production of antibodies to tumors can interfere with cell-mediated, antitumor immune responses. In humans, there is

no compelling evidence that the presence of antitumor antibodies blocks tumor growth.

Clinical evidence with rituximab, a monoclonal antibody directed against the B-lymphocyte marker CD20, has resulted in surprising efficacy for many patients with lymphoma previously resistant to cytotoxic therapies. The mechanism of action of such antibodies may include increased clearance by the immune system following antibody binding or, alternatively, induction of apoptosis in target cells facilitated by antibody binding. It is likely that the success of such therapies is highly individualized and dependent on both the binding properties of the antibody used as well as properties of the cellular target antigen and its cellular function.

Cytokines as Cancer Therapy

Several cytokines are known to have an antitumor effect; they may act alone or in concert with other cytokines. IFN, TNFs, and IL-2 are some of the well-known cytokines with cytotoxic or antiproliferative effects. For instance, IFN-γ activates NK cells, thereby increasing NK cytotoxicity. Furthermore, IFNs are antiproliferative agents and can increase the expression of MHC antigens, which are necessary for T-cell activation. Macrophages, NK cells, and T_h cells secrete TNF, which can directly lyse tumor cells and can act in a synergistic fashion with IFN. The cloning of cytokine genes and their commercial production has led to an explosion of knowledge about these powerful cell regulators and to their exploitation for therapeutic purposes. Both IL-2 and IFN-γ have been demonstrated to have therapeutic efficacy in a variety of human cancers, including renal cell carcinoma, melanoma, and various hematopoietic tumors. Other cytokines, such as **granulocyte-macrophage colony-stimulating factor** and IL-3 may facilitate the activation or culturing of DCs for immunotherapy. Still other cytokines, such as **granulocyte colony-stimulating factor** have been used to speed recovery of neutrophil counts following chemotherapy and also to aid in the mobilization and harvesting of hematopoietic stem cells for transplantation.

Tumor Escape Mechanisms

By the time an individual has been diagnosed with malignancy, cancer cells have obviously evaded recognition or, at the very least, have evaded complete destruction by the immune system. A major focus of tumor immunology is to understand the mechanisms by which this happens. One mechanism utilized by cancer cells involves hiding from the immune system through selective loss of immunogenic antigens or downregulation of MHC molecules. Alternatively, tumors can promote immunologic tolerance by presenting antigens to the immune system without the appropriate costimulatory signals. Furthermore, tumor cell products may produce local or systemic immunosuppression by the production of immunoregulatory cytokines. One example of this is transforming growth factor (TGF)-β, which is secreted in large quantities by many tumors. TGF-β antagonizes many activities of the immune system, including lymphocyte activation and proliferation, in addition to its direct effect of promoting tumor metastatic potential. Some tumors may also express proteins such as the recently identified FLIP protein, an inhibitor of apoptosis. Because one major pathway for CTL activity is induction of apoptosis in target cells, it is likely that this renders such cells much more resistant to CTL-mediated killing. It has also been demonstrated that some human cancers (as recently shown for melanoma) may elicit T-cell responses in human subjects that are atypical in their cellular phenotype, resulting in high-frequency responses that are ineffective at killing. How tumors may preferentially elicit expansion of these T-cell subsets (e.g., T cells lacking $\alpha\beta$ TCRs) is unknown, although such mechanisms might limit the expansion of other, more productive T-cell immune responses. The protean mechanisms used by tumor cells to escape cell-mediated killing remains a significant barrier to the development of effective immunotherapy strategies.

Summary

The immune system is a complex, integrated network of cells, physical barriers, and blood-borne molecules that defend the body against pathogenic organisms. Immune responses are classified as innate and adaptive. Innate immunity provides the first defense against an invading organism. It is present prior to infectious exposure and thus allows for rapid response. It consists of nonspecific defenses such as physical barriers and the powerful inflammatory response. Complementing innate immunity, the adaptive immune response has several distinctive features. The hallmarks of the adaptive response are specificity and memory. Adaptive immunity is induced by exposure to a foreign substance, is exquisitely specific for distinct macromolecules, and is characterized by an increasingly strong response with each successive exposure. It also encompasses central and peripheral mechanisms to induce tolerance to self-antigens, preventing potentially catastrophic autoimmune responses. Lymphocytes are the primary effector of the adaptive immune system and include the antibody-producing B cells as well as distinct T-cell subsets that mediate cytotoxic and regulatory functions.

The Ig receptor on B cells and the TCR are responsible for the specificity of the adaptive immune system. Whereas B cells recognize intact proteins, T cells recognize antigenic peptides presented in the context of appropriate MHC molecules. For CD4$^+$ T$_h$ cells, peptides are presented in the context of class II MHC molecules by professional APCs. CD8$^+$ CTLs, on the other hand, recognize peptide complexed to class I MHC molecules. Cytokines are powerful mediators released during the inflammatory response as well as in specific immune reactions. Although considered separately for classification purposes, there is significant interaction between the innate and adaptive immune responses, and both are typically required to effect a sufficient response to eliminate pathogens.

Although the importance of immune surveillance in the healthy individual remains uncertain, there is considerable experimental evidence demonstrating the capacity of the immune system to recognize and destroy tumors under controlled circumstances. However, this potential is often overshadowed by the amazing ability of cancer cells to evade the immune response. Under appropriate conditions, however, the immune system can recognize tumor-associated antigens in a fashion analogous to the immune response to viruses. The challenge for current research is to learn how to manipulate the immune system so that effective anti-tumor responses can be achieved. A more complete understanding of the immune response coupled with rapid advances in technology has led to some exciting new strategies for tumor immunotherapy. Various avenues are being explored, including therapy with recombinant cytokines, directed antibody-based approaches, adoptive cellular therapy, and tumor vaccines. We must learn how to specifically activate the immune response and preserve T-cell diversity while limiting the toxicities and autoimmunity we presently associate with activation of the immune response. We must also better understand the mechanisms by which tumor cells are able to evade recognition and killing by the immune system. As we are better able to achieve creative solutions to these basic challenges, increasingly more effective biotherapeutic approaches to the treatment of malig-

nancies and other illnesses will continue to emerge, providing new hope for future patients.

Key References

Abbas, A., Lichtman, H., and Pober, J. (eds). 2000. *Cellular and Molecular Immunology,* 4th edn. Philadelphia, PA: W.B. Saunders Company.

Abbas, A., Murphy, K., and Sher, A. 1996. Functional diversity of helper T lymphocytes. *Nature* 383: 787–793.

Ahmed, R., and Gray, D. 1996. Immunological memory and protective immunity: Understanding their relation. *Science* 272(5258): 54–60.

Altman, J., Moss, P., Goulder, P., *et al.* 1996. Phenotypic analysis of antigen-specific T lymphocytes. *Science* 274: 94–96.

Arstila, T., Casrouge, A., Baron, V., *et al.* 1999. A direct estimate of the human αβ T cell receptor diversity. *Science* 286(5441): 958–961.

Austyn, J. 1998. Dendritic cells. *Current Opinion in Hematology* 5(1): 3–15.

Austyn, J., and Wood, K. (eds). 1994. *Principles of Cellular and Molecular Immunology.* Oxford, UK: Oxford University Press.

Bretscher, P. 1992. The two-signal model of lymphocyte activation twenty-one years later. *Immunology Today* 13: 74–79.

Burnet, F. 1967. Immunological aspects of malignant disease. *Lancet* 1(7501): 1171–1174.

Burnet, F. 1991. The Nobel Lectures in Immunology. The Nobel Prize for Physiology or Medicine, 1960. Immunologic recognition of self. *Scandinavian Journal of Immunology* 33(1): 3–13.

DeLisle Dupré. 1774. *Traite du Vice Cancereux.* Paris: Couturier Fils.

Douek, D., McFarland, R.D., Keiser, P., *et al.* 1998. Changes in thymic function with age and during the treatment of HIV infection. *Nature* 396(6712): 690–695.

Froelich, C., Dixit,V., and Yang, X. 1998. Lymphocyte granule-mediated apoptosis: Matters of viral mimicry and deadly proteases. *Immunology Today* 19(1): 30–36.

Gallucci, B. 1987. The immune system and cancer. *Oncology Nursing Forum* 14(suppl 6): 3–12.

Goldrath, A., and Bevan, M., 1999. Selecting and maintaining a diverse T-cell repertoire. *Nature* 402(6759): 255–262.

Kalams, S., and Walker, B. 1998. The critical need for CD4 help in maintaining effective cytotoxic T lymphocyte responses. *Journal of Experimental Medicine* 188(12): 2199–2204.

Komanduri, K., and McCune, J. 2000. Development and reconstitution of T lymphoid immunity. In Pantaleo, G., and Walker, B. (eds). *Retroviral Immunology*, Totawa, NJ: Humana Press.

Lewis, S. 1994. The mechanism of V(D)J joining: Lessons from molecular, immunological, and comparative analyses. *Advances in Immunology* 56(1): 27–150.

Lum, L. 1987. The kinetics of immune reconstitution after human marrow transplantation. *Blood* 69(2): 369–380.

Mackey, M., Gunn, J., Maliszewsky, C., *et al.* 1998. Dendritic cells require maturation via CD40 to generate protective antitumor immunity. *Journal of Immunology* 161(5): 2094–2098.

Marrack, P., and Kappler, J. 1997. Positive selection of thymocytes bearing $\alpha\beta$ T cell receptors. *Current Opinion in Immunology* 9(2): 250–255.

Miller, J., and Mitchell, G. 1967. The thymus and the precursors of antigen reactive cells. *Nature* 216(5116): 659–663.

Miller, J.F.A.P. 1961. Immunological function of the thymus. *Lancet* 2: 748–749.

Oettgen, H., and Old, L. 1991. The history of cancer immunotherapy. In DeVita, V., Hellman, S., and Rosenberg, S. (eds). *Biologic Therapy of Cancer.* Philadelphia, PA: J.B. Lippincott, pp. 87–119.

Poulin, J. F., Viswanathan, M., Harris, J.M., *et al.* 1999. Direct evidence for thymic function in adult humans. *Journal of Experimental Medicine* 190(4): 479–486.

Riddell, S., and Greenberg, P. 1995. Principles for adoptive T cell therapy of human viral diseases. *Annual Review of Immunology* 13(16): 545–586.

Ridge, J., Di Rosa, F., and Matzinger, P. 1998. A conditioned dendritic cell can be a temporal bridge between a CD4$^+$ T-helper and a T-killer cell. *Nature* 393(6684): 474–478.

Roitt, I., Brostoff, J., and Male, D. (eds). 1998. *Immunology*, 5th edn. Philadelphia, PA: Mosby.

Romagnani, S. 1997. The Th1/Th2 paradigm. *Immunology Today* 18(6): 263–266.

Schindler, L. 1992. *The Immune System: How it Works*. U.S. Department of Health and Human Services. Bethesda, MD: National Institutes of Health (NIH) Publication #92-3229.

Sprent, J. 1994. T and B memory cells. *Cell* 76(2): 315–322.

Sprent, J., and Tough, D. 1994. Lymphocyte lifespan and memory. *Science* 265(5177): 1395–1400.

Tonegawa, S. 1983. Somatic generation of antibody diversity. *Nature* 302(5909): 575–581.

von Boehmer, H., and Rajewsky, K. 1997. Lymphocyte development: Essential features. *Current Opinion in Immunology* 9(2): 213–215.

Zinkernagel, R., and Hengartner, H. 1997. Antiviral immunity. *Immunology Today* 18(6): 258–260.

CHAPTER 3 | Normal Cell Biology and the Biology of Cancer

Deborah L. Volker, RN, PhD, AOCN®

Cancer is a genetic disease. Over the past 20 years, tremendous advances have been made in our understanding of how genes regulate normal cell structure and cell function and how genetic aberrations influence the evolution of malignancies. The field of biotherapy uses knowledge of the molecular basis of cancer and host interactions with the disease to develop new therapies to treat cancer. The purpose of this chapter is to review normal cell biology and explore the genetic basis of cancer pathogenesis.

Normal Cell Biology

The basis of modern medicine is the axiomatic assumption that the cell is the fundamental unit of life. The human body contains about 100 trillion cells of different types. Each group of cells performs a specialized function and hence has a specific structure to support that function (Thibodeau and Patton, 1999). For example, B lymphocytes have a system that produces antibodies, whereas nerve cells contain structures that transmit neural impulses. The study of cell structure and function is fundamental to understanding the basis of disease and the clinical opportunities to prevent, detect, and successfully treat disease. This section explores the structure of cells and how cells function to support life activities.

Structural and Functional Elements

Human cells are composed of 3 core elements: the plasma membrane, the cytoplasm, and the nucleus. The **plasma membrane** (also known as the cell membrane) composes the outer boundary or envelope of the cell. In addition to providing the "scaffolding" or support for the cell, the plasma membrane regulates the movement of substances in and out of the cell. The plasma membrane is a double phospholipid structure interspersed with protein, carbohydrate, and cholesterol molecules (Seely *et al.*, 1996). The proteins facilitate movement of substances through the membrane by functioning as carriers, channels, receptors, enzymes, or even "markers" that assist in the recognition of cells and organelles (Thibodeau and Patton, 1999).

Cytoplasm is a fluid substance within the cell. **Organelles** are literally "little organs" that

are suspended within the cytoplasm and that vary greatly in number and type based on their specific cellular function. The **nucleus**, typically the largest organelle, is located at the center of the cell. Surrounded by a nuclear membrane or envelope, the nucleus contains **deoxyribonucleic acid** (**DNA**) molecules that guide protein synthesis within the cell. Figure 3.1 and Table 3.1 summarize some key cell structures and their functions.

Cell Metabolism

Cell metabolism refers to the chemical reactions that occur within a cell, including (1) catabolic

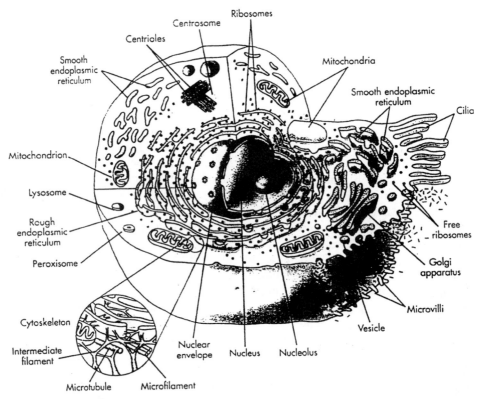

Figure 3.1   Typical or composite cell

Source: Reprinted with permission from Thibodeau, G., and Patton, K. 1999. *Anatomy & Physiology,* 4th edn. St. Louis, MO: Mosby, Inc., p. 76.

Table 3.1   Some major cell structures and their functions

Cell Structure	Functions
Membranous	
Plasma membrane	Serves as the boundary of the cell, maintaining its integrity; protein molecules embedded in the plasma membrane perform various functions (for example, they serve as markers that identify cells of each individual, as receptor molecules for certain hormones and other molecules, and as transport mechanisms)
Endoplasmic reticulum (ER)	Ribosomes attached to rough ER synthesize proteins that leave cells via the Golgi complex; smooth ER synthesizes lipids incorporated in cell membranes, steroid hormones, and certain carbohydrates used to form glycoproteins
Golgi apparatus	Synthesizes carbohydrate, combines it with protein, and packages the product as globules of glycoprotein
Lysosomes	A cell's "digestive system"
Peroxisomes	Contain enzymes that detoxify harmful substances
Mitochondria	Catabolism; adenosine triphosphate synthesis; a cell's "power plants"
Nucleus	Houses the genetic code, which in turn dictates protein synthesis, thereby playing an essential role in other cell activities, namely, cell transport, metabolism, and growth
Nonmembranous	
Ribosomes	Site of protein synthesis; a cell's "protein factories"
Cytoskeleton	Acts as a framework to support the cell and its organelles; functions in cell movement; forms cell extensions (microvilli, cilia, flagella)
Cilia and flagella	Hairlike cell extensions that serve to move substances over the cell surface (cilia) or propel sperm cells (flagella)
Nucleolus	Plays an essential role in the formation of ribosomes

Source: Reprinted with permission from Thibodeau, G., and Patton, K. (1999). *Anatomy & Physiology,* 4th edn. St. Louis, MO: Mosby, Inc., p. 77.

processes that break down larger molecules, such as nutrients, into smaller molecules; and (2) anabolic processes that build larger molecules from smaller ones. Cellular respiration, the conversion of glucose molecules into carbon dioxide and water, is a key catabolic process. Glycolysis, the citric acid cycle, and the electron transport system all constitute cellular respiration and result in the release of energy via heat production or energy stored in adenosine triphosphate (ATP). ATP is used by the cell to fuel virtually all cellular metabolic activities.

Protein synthesis is a prototype anabolic process. DNA controls the synthesis of proteins within a cell. These proteins may take the form of enzymes that regulate biochemical reactions or form the structural components of both cellular and extracellular materials. Because DNA controls protein synthesis, it directs all cellular activities and, thus, all structural, functional, and growth characteristics of a human being from the time of conception to full maturity and beyond.

DNA is a large, complex, double-helix molecule that is comprised of many smaller molecules (nucleotides) linked together in a recurrent sequence (Figure 3.2). Nucleotides are compounds formed by phosphoric acid, a sugar (deoxyribose), and a nitrogenous base. DNA is composed of 4 types of nucleotides

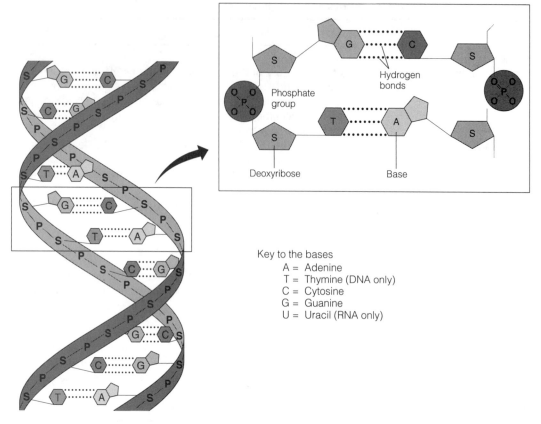

Figure 3.2   Watson-Crick model of the DNA molecule. The DNA structure illustrated here is based on that published by James Watson and Francis Crick in 1953. Note that each side of the DNA molecule consists of alternating sugar and phosphate groups. Each sugar group is united to the sugar group opposite it by a pair of nitrogenous bases (adenine-thymine or cytosine-guanine). The sequence of these pairs constitutes a genetic code that determines the structure and function of the cell.

Source: Reprinted with permission from Thibodeau, G., and Patton, K. 1999. *Anatomy & Physiology,* 4th edn. St. Louis, MO: Mosby, Inc., p. 107.

characterized by the presence of one of four nitrogenous bases: cytosine, guanine, adenine, and thymine. Sugar and phosphoric acid form the sides or "backbone" of the DNA molecule; the nitrogenous bases join together in pairs to form the linkages that resemble steps on a twisted ladder or staircase. Adenosine only links to thymine and guanine only to cytosine.

The sequence of the paired bases varies from one DNA molecule to the next.

Chromosomes are structural units that contain the DNA molecules and other associated proteins. **Genes** are sections of DNA and are the core units of heredity. Genes are comprised of long chains of base pairs; each gene may contain a chain of as many as 1,000 pairs of nucleotides (Thibodeaux and Patton, 1999). In humans, the genome (total genetic information carried by a cell) consists of at least 100,000 genes distributed among 23 chromosomes. Each somatic cell is diploid, that is, it contains 2 copies of the genome, resulting in 23 pairs or 46 chromosomes. Each gene encodes or contains the manufacturing instructions and capability to produce a given protein.

Gene expression, a term used to refer to the process of protein synthesis, was often called the "central dogma" of molecular biology and genetics (Lea and Jenkins, 1997; Rieger, 1997). Because errors in gene expression can precipitate a wide variety of disease entities, an understanding of this process is guiding the development of treatment approaches designed to correct or repair such errors. Protein synthesis is a 2-step process: it involves **transcription** and **translation.** In essence, transcription is the process of making a copy of the information within the DNA that is required to make a protein. Transcription occurs within the cell nucleus and is much like the process of photocopying or "transcribing" an original document. A section of DNA separates and pairs with ribonucleic acid (RNA) nucleotides (already present in the nucleus) to form messenger RNA (mRNA). The newly formed mRNA contains a copy of the instructions necessary to produce a protein. The mRNA then moves out into the cytoplasm to begin the second step of protein synthesis, translation. During translation, cytoplasmic ribosomes are attracted to the mRNA and use transfer RNA, ribosomal RNA, and enzymes to produce sequenced chains of amino acids that form proteins.

Cell Proliferation and Regulation

Cell proliferation via cell growth and reproduction is the essence of the cell life cycle. Genetic controls guide cell growth and ensure that the genome is passed on from a cell to its progeny.

When errors in gene expression occur, resulting in genetic mutations, alterations in the growth, reproduction, and death of cells may arise. These alterations are key factors in the pathogenesis of numerous illnesses, including cancer, viral infections, autoimmune diseases, neurodegenerative disorders, and acquired immune deficiency syndrome or AIDS (Kliche and Hoffken, 1999).

CELL LIFE CYCLE

Cell proliferation is a multistep process. Typically, human cells proliferate, grow to a preprogrammed size and extent, become mature, and eventually die. Figure 3.3 summarizes key points in the normal cell life cycle. In essence, the cell life cycle is comprised of a series of systematic events that are precisely regulated by 2 kinds of molecular controls: (1) a cascade of cyclin (cell-cycle proteins), cyclin-dependent kinases (CDKs), and CDK inhibitors; and (2) a series of checkpoints that monitor the molecular activities of each phase and delay progression to subsequent phases if problems arise (Cotran *et al.,* 1999). The key purpose of checkpoints is to avoid accumulation of genetic mistakes during cell division (Bartek *et al.,* 1999).

The G_0 phase is a quiescent period in which cells are either "resting" in a nonreproductive mode or have terminally differentiated and cannot undergo any further division. A quiescent cell can be stimulated to move from the G_0 to the G_1 phase, which is a preparatory mode in which cells reside prior to the S phase, where DNA replication occurs. Factors that influence transition to G_1 include mitogens, nutrients, and growth factors (Kasten, 1997).

As illustrated in Figure 3.3, transition from the G_1 to the S phase is marked by a transition or "restriction" point. This checkpoint in the cell life cycle is designed to block movement to the S phase if the cell has incurred DNA damage. The restriction point is critical because

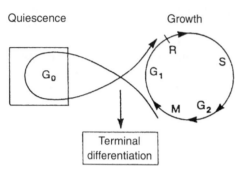

Figure 3.3   The cell life cycle. When a cell is not synthesizing DNA (S phase) or completing mitosis (M phase), it is commonly described as being in a G (gap) phase. Normal cells are capable of resting in a nondividing state, called G_0. They can begin one or more cycles of cell division when there is a need to maintain or replace tissue, and they stop dividing when the necessary growth is complete. In G_1, protein and RNA synthesis are active. If conditions are permissive for subsequent cell division, cells pass through the R (restriction) point and quickly move into the S (synthetic) period, when new DNA is synthesized. Another gap (G_2) follows when the newly duplicated chromosomes condense. In the M period, the chromosomes divide into 2 sets, the cell forms 2 nuclei, and then divides into 2 daughter cells. When normal cells differentiate, typically with a gain in the properties required for organ or tissue functions, they generally lose the capacity to continue cell division.

Source: Reprinted with permission from Fingert, H., Campisi, J., and Pardee, A. 1997. Cell proliferation and differentiation. In Holland, J., Frei, E., Bast, R., Kufe, D., Morton, D., and Weichselbaum , R. (eds). *Cancer Medicine,* 4th ed. Baltimore, MD: Williams and Wilkins, p. 4.

it can prevent damaged or mutated cells from propagating. The *p53* gene plays an important role in this process because it integrates a variety of intracellular messages and either allows the cell to repair the DNA or causes cell death (Prives and Hall, 1999). Thus, *p53* plays a crucial gatekeeping function at this checkpoint.

The S phase of the cell cycle focuses on DNA replication. Although the S phase only lasts a few hours, all 3 billion bases of the human genome must be accurately copied within this time frame (Kasten, 1997). Biochemical regulation of the S phase is not completely understood, but it appears that DNA replication occurs at multiple sites in the genome simultaneously and is controlled by a variety of enzymes. Each time the DNA strand is copied, however, there is a risk that some of the genetic material at each end of the chromosomes will be lost. **Telomeres** are structures comprised of small bits of DNA that form the ends of chromosomes. Telomeres ensure that chromosomes replicate completely and that degradation of the chromosome ends is prevented (Cotran *et al.,* 1999). Over time, however, as the cell continues to proliferate, the telomeres progressively shorten. Eventually, the cell loses its ability to replicate. Hence, Fossel (1998) described the telomere as the "clock of replicative senescence" but noted that this clock can be reset or turned back by the presence of an enzyme, **telomerase**. Simply put, telomerase slows the erosion rate of telomere bases.

Once DNA synthesis is complete, the cell transitions to the G_2 phase. In G_2, the cell undergoes cyclin-mediated activities to create molecules and organelles in preparation for the M phase, the reproductive phase of cell division. Another key checkpoint occurs in G_2: assessment of the newly formed DNA for any errors prior to beginning mitosis. *p53* may also play a key role at this checkpoint (Levine, 1997). Checkpoints also occur within mitosis to assess for error or weakness within the mitotic process (Dirks and Rutka, 1997). Table 3.2 summarizes the key events of cell mitosis.

Once mitosis is complete, the cell may either cycle out of the active proliferation process to the G_0 (quiescent) phase or it may cycle back to the G_1 phase and continue dividing. Examples

Table 3.2   The major events of mitosis

Prophase	Metaphase	Anaphase	Telophase
1. Chromosomes shorten and thicken (from coiling of DNA molecules that compose them); each chromosome consists of 2 chromatids attached at centromere 2. Centrioles move to opposite poles of cell: spindle fibers appear and begin to orient between opposing poles 3. Nucleoli and nuclear membrane disappear	1. Chromosomes align across equator of spindle fibers: each pair of chromatids attached to spindle fiber at its centromere	1. Each centromere splits, thereby detaching two chromatids that compose each chromosome from each other 2. Sister chromatids (now called chromosomes) move to opposite poles; there are now twice as many chromosomes as there were before mitosis started	1. Changes occurring during telophase essentially reverse of those taking place during prophase; new chromosomes start elongating (DNA molecules start uncoiling) 2. Nuclear envelope reappears, enclosing each new set of chromosomes 3. Spindle fibers disappear

Centrioles

Nucleus

Spindle fibers

Chromatids

Centromere

Sister chromatids

Nuclear envelope

Source: Reprinted with permission from Thibodeau, G., and Patton, K. (1999). *Anatomy & Physiology*, 4th edn. St. Louis, MO: Mosby, Inc., p. 114.

of cells that continuously divide include hematopoietic stem cells and epithelial cells of the mucosal lining of the gastrointestinal tract and other organs. Kidney, liver, and smooth muscle cells are more likely to be quiescent and to replicate at a much lower level (Cotran *et al.*, 1999).

CELL GROWTH AND DIFFERENTIATION

Once a new cell is formed, growth and **differentiation** are activated by external stimuli or signals at the cell-membrane surface. Such stimuli may include growth factors, stressors, **cytokine** receptors, and antigen receptors (Zanke, 1998). Growth factors are proteins that bind to the cell-surface membrane and activate **signal transduction**, the process of transmitting information (signals) received on the cell surface to the cell's inner structures and nucleus. Signal transduction is a communication process by which information is relayed through a variety of intracellular components, much like a "telephone tree" of callers passes on information from one individual to another. In any event, the end response can be cell proliferation, cell death, or a host of other activities. Some of the growth factors that stimulate signal transduction are epidermal growth factor, platelet-derived growth factor, and granulocyte-macrophage colony-stimulating factor. Signal transduction also can be initiated by a wide variety of other external stimuli such as insulin, epinephrine, angiotensin, and serotonin (Hannun, 1997). In sum, cell responses are unique based on the stimulus received.

Cell growth is also affected by stressors such as heat, radiation, or exposure to biological agents such as interleukin-1 or tumor necrosis factor (Zanke, 1998). In this instance, signaling pathways are involved in either coordinating the cell's efforts to repair damage incurred by the stressor or to initiate cell death.

The action of cytokine receptors is another mediator of cell proliferation and differentiation. Cytokine receptors likely include both extracellular and intracellular structures and modulate the effects of hematopoietic, neural, and embryonal development via interleukins, interferons, and colony-stimulating factors (Zanke, 1998). Not surprisingly, cell signal-transduction processes are an essential communication tool for cytokine-receptor activity.

Cell-surface antigen receptors play a key role in the function and proliferation of B and T lymphocytes. Antigen receptors use signal transduction to stimulate T and B lymphocytes, resulting in genetically modulated cytokine production and other activity (Zanke, 1998).

APOPTOSIS

In order to maintain normal homeostasis, the human body must have an orderly means to eliminate aging or defective cells. **Apoptosis** is the genetically controlled process of cell death. It is also termed "programmed cell death" and "cell suicide." Apoptosis can occur in the following circumstances (Cotran *et al.*, 1999):

• During cell development
• As a homeostatic mechanism to maintain cell populations in tissues
• As a defense mechanism such as in immune reactions
• When cells are damaged by disease or noxious agents
• During the aging process

Consistent with all other events that control cellular developmental processes, apoptosis is a genetically controlled series of molecular events initiated by a variety of stimuli. Although described as "the highly orchestrated form of cell death in which cells neatly commit suicide by chopping themselves into membrane-packaged bits" (Miller and Marx, 1998), the term apoptosis literally means "falling off" as in the falling of leaves from a tree (Nakano, 1997).

Apoptosis may be triggered by a variety of stimuli, including (1) the lack of a necessary growth factor; (2) internal signals indicating harmful changes such as errors in DNA replication; and (3) specific, injurious external agents (Cotran *et al.*, 1999). Signaling pathways play a key role in activation of apoptosis. Such pathways can be triggered by the activity of "death sensors" on their cell-surface membranes. These sensors are members of the tumor necrosis factor receptor gene family and guide a type of immune-modulated apoptosis, including deleting activated T lymphocytes at the completion of an immune response, killing cancer or viral cells by cytotoxic T cells and natural killer cells, and killing inflammatory cells (Ashkenazi and Dixit, 1998). Signaling pathways for apoptosis may also be stimulated when conflicting or paradoxical signals for growth are received, such as when a proliferative gene (proto-oncogene) such as *c-myc* tries to stimulate growth in the absence of a necessary growth factor (Slingerland and Tannock, 1998). Numerous other intracellular events can trigger signaling pathways.

Regardless of the trigger, apoptosis is controlled and integrated within the cell by 2 types of activities: one guided by a series of adapter proteins and the other guided by proteins generated by the *Bcl-2* family of genes (Cotran *et al.*, 1999). The *Bcl-2* genes are characterized as arbiters or the "rheostat" of cell survival in that some members of the family block cell death by inhibiting necessary enzyme activity, whereas other types of *Bcl-2* genes promote apoptosis by disrupting action of the adaptor proteins (Adams and Cory, 1998).

Once the cell is destined for death, a proteolytic cascade of enzymes, termed caspases, oversee the process of cell destruction. Morphologically distinct from the processes of cell lysis or necrosis, features of apoptosis include cell shrinkage, chromatin condensation, and formation of smaller, membrane-bound apoptotic bodies (Figure 3.4). Subsequently, the apoptotic bodies are phagocytized by surrounding cells.

Given that apoptosis is a genetically controlled process, mutations can either cause hyperactivation, resulting in premature cell death, or suppress apoptosis, leading to a type of cell immortality (Schmitt and Lowe, 1999). Any number of diseases may arise due to abnormalities in the process of cell death. For example, cancer and autoimmune disorders may result from insufficient apoptotic activity; conversely, too much apoptosis may contribute to stroke damage and neurodegeneration in patients with Alzheimer's disease (Miller and Marx, 1998). Clearly, treatments that alter the threshold or timing of apoptosis have the potential to change the course of such diseases (Kliche and Hoffken, 1999).

Cancer Biology

Cancer is the term used to refer to a group of malignant diseases characterized by a series of

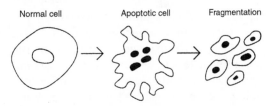

Figure 3.4 Schematic diagram to illustrate the morphological appearance of an apoptotic cell. Note condensation of chromatin to form apoptotic bodies and blebbing of the cell membrane. Fragmentation of the cell into membrane-bound fragments occurs subsequently.

Source: Reprinted with permission from Slingerland, J., and Tannock, I. 1998. Cell proliferation and cell death. In Tannock, I., and Hill, R. (eds). *The Basic Science of Oncology,* 3rd edn. New York, NY: McGraw Hill, p. 141.

cellular, genetic changes that result in cell proliferation. Most cancers arise from a single transformed cell that gives rise to increasingly malignant progeny. Although the different types of cancer vary considerably in terms of natural history, pathology, and response to treatment, all cancers have 2 unifying attributes: (1) the propensity for unchecked local cell growth (tumor formation) and invasion into adjacent tissue and (2) the propensity to **metastasize** or spread to distant sites and form secondary tumors.

The Molecular Basis of Cancer

Cancer is a multistep process that occurs due to cumulative alterations in a cell's genes. Nearly all cancers contain malignant cells that have acquired chromosomal abnormalities (Le Beau, 1997). Hence, an overview of the molecular basis of cancer must begin with an examination of the genetic features of malignancy. Figure 3.5 illustrates the key points in the genetic evolution of cancer. In essence, a potential cancerous change is thought to occur when a normal cell suffers some type of DNA damage that does not destroy the cell. Such damage seems to target any of the cell's growth-regulating genes, including proto-oncogenes (growth promoters), **tumor suppressor genes** (growth inhibitors), DNA repair genes, or the apoptosis genes (regulators of cell death) (Cotran et al., 1999). Once a faulty clone emerges, other host factors combine to enhance tumor progression and tumor-cell genetic diversity.

However, genetic changes alone do not tell the entire story of cancer pathogenesis or **carcinogenesis**. Numerous mechanisms precipitate and influence the growth of an abnormal clone of cells. The etiologic factors that cause damage to DNA or give rise to carcinogenesis can be chemical, physical, viral, or hormonal. These factors and processes are well described elsewhere (Ruddon, 1995; Hall, 1997; Henderson

et al., 1997; Poeschla and Wong-Stall, 1997; Yuspa and Shields, 1997; Goss and Tye, 1998; Okey et al., 1998; Yarbro, 2000).

ONCOGENES AND PROTO-ONCOGENES

As emphasized in the section of this chapter titled "Normal Cell Biology," a wide variety of genes regulate the development, division, and death of cells. Proto-oncogenes are normal genes that serve as cell-growth promoters. They encode protein products that respond to external signals, resulting in gene expression, DNA synthesis, cytoskeleton membrane changes, cell-to-cell contacts, and cell metabolism (Benchimol and Minden, 1998). An analogy to traffic lights is useful for describing genes that influence cell growth and differentiation. Accordingly, a proto-oncogene is the green light signaling for cell growth processes to proceed. However, this green light does not stay on indefinitely; it turns off when normal cell growth processes are completed.

Oncogenes are mutated or "activated" versions of proto-oncogenes. Oncogenes may arise as a result of: (1) changes in gene structure, which then cause production of abnormal proteins; or (2) changes in the regulation of gene expression, resulting in overproduction of normal growth proteins (Cotran et al., 1999). To extend the traffic light analogy, oncogenes cause problems, as the green traffic light stays on too long, allowing for unregulated growth processes that exceed normal bounds. Specifically, oncogenic protein products disrupt the signal-transduction process and the cell life cycle. Recall that signal transduction begins with a stimulus such as a growth factor. One way in which oncogenic proteins promote abnormal cell growth is by overproduction of growth factor receptors on the cell-membrane surface. These mutant receptors will provide continuous or excessive growth signals to the cell. This problem is compounded when other mutations send abnormal messages to other

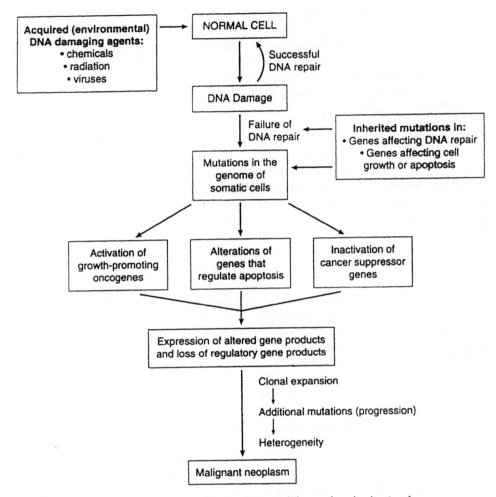

Figure 3.5   Flow chart depicting a simplified scheme of the molecular basis of cancer

Source: Reprinted with permission from Cotran, R., Kumar, V., and Collins, T. 1999. *Robbins Pathologic Basis of Disease,* 6th edn. Philadelphia, PA: W. B. Saunders Company, p. 278.

transmission points within the signal-transduction communication pathway.

Oncogenic proteins can also affect nuclear activities, including faulty encoding of nuclear transcription factors and activators, sustained transcription of critical target genes, and potential malignant transformation of the cell (Cotran *et al.,* 1999). Oncogenes may impact cycle activity by disrupting the activity of cyclins and

CDKs. When genetic mutations cause overexpression of the cyclins and CDKs, activity at critical checkpoints in the cell cycle is disregulated (Slingerland and Tannock, 1998). Hence, damaged DNA may escape scrutiny, and the cell will continue through each phase of the cell cycle unscathed. The end result of these oncogenic changes is uncontrolled cell division.

Most oncogenes arise somatically, that is,

they are "acquired" and not "inherited" genetic changes. A few notable exceptions do occur in germ cells and are associated with familial or inherited predisposition to cancer. Examples of proto-oncogenes that can become oncogenic include the *Ras* genes (among the most frequently detected oncogenes in human cancers) (Hannun, 1997), the *Ret* genes (associated with inherited cancer syndromes such as multiple endocrine neoplasia and familial medullary thyroid cancer), the HER-2/*neu* oncogene (associated with breast and ovarian cancers), and *c-myc* (associated with Burkitt's lymphoma, lung cancer, and neuroblastoma) (Perkins and Stern, 1997; Benchimol and Minden, 1998; Cotran *et al.*, 1999; Ross and Fletcher, 1999).

TUMOR SUPPRESSOR GENES

Tumor suppressor genes limit cell growth and are active in suppressing the development of cancer. Unlike oncogenes, they serve as "red traffic lights" and restrain genetic molecular processes that support cell proliferation. Also unlike oncogenes, tumor suppressor genes figure much more predominantly in inherited cancers but are also prevalent in acquired cancers (Benchimol and Minden, 1998).

The *p53* gene plays a key role in normal cell function by regulating cell response to DNA damage. A gatekeeper of sorts, *p53* regulates transition between various phases of the cell life cycle and plays a key role in apoptosis. Levels of *p53* are activated by DNA damage secondary to irradiation, hypoxia and chemicals. Normally, the *p53* gene stops cell proliferation via activation of other gene products, allowing DNA damage to be repaired (Prives and Hall, 1999). If the damage cannot be repaired, *p53* guides the cell toward destruction via apoptosis. Thus, *p53* has earned the name "guardian of the genome" (Cotran *et al.*, 1999). When mutated, *p53* restraint on cell proliferation is lost, allowing for faulty DNA to be repli-

cated within the cell cycle and malignant changes to ensue. More than one half of all human cancers contains mutations of the *p53* gene; indeed, *p53* gene mutations are among the most frequent abonormalities in human cancer (Prives and Hall, 1999). Cancers associated with *p53* mutations include melanoma; colorectal cancer; and cancers of the lung, breast, testes, bladder, and prostate (Levine, 1997).

Examples of other tumor suppressor genes associated with hereditary cancers include *BRCA1* (familial breast and ovarian cancer), *p16* (melanoma and glioblastoma), *RB1* (retinoblastoma), and *APC* (familial polyposis) (Squire *et al.*, 1998; Fahraeus *et al.*, 1999).

DNA-REPAIR GENES

Despite almost continual exposure to environmental agents that damage DNA, human cells have an amazing ability to repair such damage and prevent mutations. This process is supported by proto-oncogenes, tumor suppressor genes, and DNA-repair genes. Defective DNA-repair genes are not oncogenic per se, but do allow mutations in other genes to occur during cell division. The *hMSH2, hMLH1, hPMS1,* and *hPMS2* genes are examples of DNA-repair genes implicated in hereditary nonpolyposis colon carcinoma. Inherited mutations in these genes cause errors in "proofreading" the accuracy of DNA replication, thus allowing mutations to occur (Cotran *et al.*, 1999). The *p53* gene may also serve a DNA-repair function in other inherited cancers, such as xeroderma pigmentosum (Benchimol and Minden, 1998).

APOPTOSIS GENES

The apoptosis genes are the fourth category of genes associated with carcinogenesis. Much like the other types of genes, the genes that modulate apoptosis can be overexpressed and lead to a malignancy. The *Bcl-2* group of genes is implicated in such a scenario. Overexpression of *Bcl-2* protects lymphocytes from apoptosis.

The *Bcl-2* oncogene is found in most follicular lymphomas and in some cases of chronic lymphocytic lymphoma and diffuse large-cell lymphoma (Adams and Cory, 1998). Similarly, the *c-myc* oncogene may collaborate with *Bcl-2* to delay apoptosis in lymphoid malignancies.

In sum, the study of the genetic basis of cancer is leading to exciting breakthroughs in diagnosis, prognosis, and treatment of disease. Recent discoveries regarding the HER-2/*neu* oncogene serve as an example. Overexpression of this growth factor receptor gene has been associated with 10% to 34% of certain breast cancers (Ross and Fletcher, 1999). Investigation is underway to examine associations between HER-2/*neu* abnormalities, estrogen receptor status, and response to hormone therapy, chemotherapy, adjuvant treatments, and monoclonal antibody therapy (Ross and Fletcher, 1999).

Characteristics of Cancer Cells

STRUCTURAL CHANGES

Microscopic studies of cancer cells reveal a number of structural features that distinguish them from normal cells. Morphologically, cancer cells demonstrate the property of **pleomorphism**, that is, they tend to be more variable in size and shape than the cells in surrounding tissue. The nucleus in a cancer cell tends to be larger than in normal cells, as evidenced by a high nucleus-to-cytoplasm ratio. The nucleus of cancer cells is also **hyperchromatic** (chromatin are more pronounced when stained) and pleomorphic (variable in size and shape), and contains large nucleoli. Cancer cells typically contain unusual numbers of chromosomes (**aneuploidy**) and have abnormal chromosome arrangements, including translocations, deletions, and amplifications.

BIOCHEMICAL CHANGES

Given the genetic changes in cancer cells, variations in cell metabolism and biochemical products are notable. In particular, numerous changes occur at the cell membrane, including production of surface enzymes that aid in cellular invasion and metastasis, loss of glycoproteins that normally promote cell-to-cell adhesion and organization, and loss of cell-surface antigens that normally label the cell as "self." As noted previously, oncogenic mutations may produce abnormal growth factor receptors on the cell membrane. These receptors can activate signal transduction without exposure to a growth factor and may persist in delivering growth signals to the cell (Gribbon and Loescher, 2000). Normal versions of growth factor receptors may be overexpressed, which may cause the tumor cell to be highly sensitive to otherwise normal amounts of growth factor. This property could account for the aggressive growth of certain cancers (Cotran *et al.*, 1999).

Other biochemical changes may be evident. For example, certain types of cancer cells may produce new tumor-associated antigens (refer to the discussion of tumor antigens in Chapter 2). Normal cells use aerobic glycolysis for cell metabolism, whereas cancer cells use higher rates of anaerobic glycolysis. Hence, cancer cells are less dependent on oxygen and are more likely to survive despite poor oxygenation. Cancer cells may also abnormally produce hormones or hormone-like substances, procoagulant materials, growth factors, and catecholamines, causing disorders termed paraneoplastic syndromes. For example, hypercalcemia can be termed a paraneoplastic syndrome when it is caused by a cancer cell's production of a substance that mimics the effect of the parathyroid hormone.

CELL KINETIC CHANGES

Studies of cancer cell kinetics reveal that malignant cells grow unrestrained. Both the genetic and biochemical properties reviewed previously promote autonomous growth that does not respond to normal checks and balances for cell growth. Normally, cell proliferation is limited by the principle of contact inhibition, which occurs when cells stop dividing when they come in contact with each other. Cancer cells ignore this constraint and also lose the properties of adhesion and cell-to-cell recognition, the normal tendency of cells to stick together. Collectively, these features promote metastasis. Loss of contact inhibition and adhesion result from increased production of degradative enzymes that promote both invasion and metastasis.

Cancer cells also demonstrate an increased **mitotic index**, the proportion of cells in a given tissue that are in mitosis at any given time. This increase is indicative of the high proliferative activity of some cancers but is not diagnostic of cancer per se. Many normal tissues also have a higher mitotic index because of their proliferative functions (e.g., bone marrow or gastrointestinal mucosa). Another hallmark of cancer is the presence of abnormal cell differentiation, or the inability to mature completely. The lack of differentiation occurs in all malignant cells but ranges along a continuum from a fairly well-differentiated cell type to a poorly differentiated cell type.

Cancer cells tend to live longer than normal cells. Typically, cells undergo a limited number of divisions, with telomeres mediating that process. As the telomeres shorten with each sequence of DNA replication, the life of the cell shortens. Once the telomere reaches a certain threshold point, the cell stops dividing and begins the aging process with apoptosis as the end point. Telomerase is the enzyme that activates the telomeric DNA prior to each cell division. Telomerase is present in embryonic cells, germ cells, and certain mature cells (such as lymphocytes) but is inactive in most mature somatic cells (Slingerland and Tannock, 1998). However, telomerase is activated in many types of cancers. Although the connection between expression of telomerase and malignant transformation is unclear, use of drugs that block telomerase and allow the cells to die presents an exciting therapeutic potential (Fossel, 1998; Greider, 1999).

The immune system also plays a key role in regulating cancer cell growth. Refer to the discussion of immune surveillance and responses to cancer cells in Chapter 2.

GROWTH CHARACTERISTICS

Many variables influence the length of time it takes for a mass of malignant cells to become clinically detectable. In general, superficial tumors can be clinically detected once they contain about 1 billion cells and are 1 gram in weight (Slingerland and Tannock, 1998). Because of anatomic considerations, more deeply situated tumors tend to be larger upon clinical detection. A tumor's growth rate is directly linked to its **growth fraction,** the proportion of cells in active proliferation. Similar to the concept of mitotic index, the growth fraction varies widely in both normal tissues and in cancer cells. Another way to characterize tumor growth is to measure the **tumor-volume-doubling** time. This refers to the time within which the total cancer cell population doubles. Depending on the tissue type, a tumor's growth trajectory will cause variance in the rate at which cells die or break away from the original tumor mass and the vascularity of the tumor. The growth of cancers that arise from hormone-dependent tissue (e.g., cancers of the breast, prostate, and endometrium) also may be influenced by the presence or absence of high hormone levels. Proliferation of some of these tumors may be slowed if the stimulating hormone is reduced. In general, tumors increase in size because the rate of cell production exceeds the rate of cell death.

The Biology of Tumor Growth: Invasion and Spread of Disease

Once a group of malignant cells is established, continued growth and spread depend on several processes. Figure 3.6 illustrates the sequence of steps that constitute the formation of metastases. **Metastasis** refers to the spread of a malignancy beyond the primary tumor to distant sites. Metastatic disease is the primary cause of treatment difficulties and death. If tumors remained localized, surgery could substantially increase cancer cure rates. Unfortunately, by the time people with solid tumors first present to a physician for treatment, about 70% already have micrometastases (Rosenberg, 1997).

ANGIOGENESIS

Tumors that are 1 to 2 mm in diameter can survive by obtaining necessary nutrients through the normal vasculature in surrounding

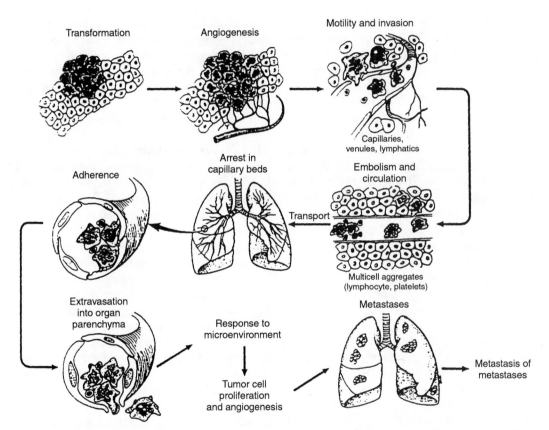

Figure 3.6 Pathogenesis of cancer metastasis. To produce metastases, tumor cells must detach from the primary tumor, invade the extracellular matrix, enter the circulation, survive in the circulation to arrest in the capillary bed, adhere to subendothelial basement membrane, gain entrance into the organ parenchyma, respond to paracrine growth factors, proliferate and induce angiogenesis, and evade host defenses. The pathogenesis of metastasis is therefore complex and consists of multiple sequential, selective, and interdependent steps whose outcome depends on the interaction of tumor cells with homeostatic factors.

Source: Reprinted with permission from Fidler, I. 1997. Molecular biology of cancer: Invasion and metastasis. In DeVita, V., Hellman, S., and Rosenberg, S. (eds). *Cancer: Principles and Practice of Oncology,* 5th edn. Philadelphia, PA: Lippincott-Raven Publishers, p. 136.

tissue (Dedhar *et al.*, 1998). Tumor **angiogenesis** (also termed neovascularization) refers to the tumor's ability to stimulate rapid proliferation of new blood vessels from the host. This process permits rapid growth of tumor cells and increases the risk for metastasis. However, growth beyond that size requires the generation of new supporting vasculature for the tumor.

Angiogenesis is induced by multiple growth factors and enzymes released by both tumor cells and host cells, including endothelial cells, epithelial cells, mesothelial cells, and leukocytes (Fidler, 1997). Oncogenes play a key role in activating angiogenesis. Numerous tumor-associated angiogenic factors have been identified; vascular endothelial growth factor and basic fibroblast growth factor are among the most important. These factors can be detected in body fluid. Studies investigating a potential prognostic role for such measurements as tumor markers are ongoing (Nguyen, 1997; Pluda, 1997). Additionally, an understanding of the action of angiogenic factors has important implications for cancer treatment. Promising clinical studies of pharmaceutical angiogenesis inhibitors such as interferons, platelet-derived-growth factors, retinoids, and other chemotherapeutic agents are now underway (Gradishar, 1997).

INVASION

Invasion refers to the spread of a tumor into adjacent tissues. Three processes promote invasion: (1) mechanical pressure exerted by the rapidly growing cells, (2) migration of individual cells due to decreased tumor-cell adhesiveness and increased motility, and (3) release of destructive enzymes that degrade host tissue (Fidler, 1997). Tumor cells are thus able to penetrate the basement membrane of the tissue of origin, move through the interstitial cellular matrix, and penetrate the basement membrane of a nearby blood vessel or lymphatic channel. This process gives the tumor cell access to circulation throughout the body.

The propensity for a primary tumor to form metastases is directly linked to the genetic instability of the tumor cells. As tumor cells grow and divide, they become increasingly heterogeneous in genetic composition, invasiveness, growth rate, hormonal responsiveness, metastatic potential, and susceptibility to antineoplastic therapy (Cotran, *et al.*, 1999). Figure 3.7 illustrates tumor **heterogeneity** in primary tumors and metastases. Cancer cells are inherently genetically unstable. As they divide, random spontaneous mutations occur. The tumor thus becomes increasingly resistant to both host immune-modulated destruction and the toxic effects of chemotherapy. Additionally, heterogeneity seems to render the tumor more adept at invasion and formation of metastases.

METASTATIC SPREAD

Once tumor cells or emboli escape the host tumor, they may circulate via blood vessels, the lymphatic system, or both. Dissemination via the lymphatic system may lead to lymph node metastasis. Emboli may lodge in the first node encountered or may move through several nodes before lodging in a more distant node. This is known as "skip metastasis."

Most metastases disseminate via blood capillaries and veins. Fortunately, the majority of cells that break away from the primary tumor and enter the circulation are quickly destroyed by immune defenses (Fidler, 1997). However, once in circulation, tumor cells tend to aggregate and form emboli. The emboli interact with platelets and fibrin, which may help to form a protective sheath that counteracts the destructive effects of immune system surveillance. The emboli then adhere to the blood vessel endothelial linings of distant organs and extravasate into adjacent tissue. Penetration of the vascular endothelium follows an enzymatic process similar to that of tumor cell escape from the host tissue described above. A series of adhesion molecules facilitate the process. In particular,

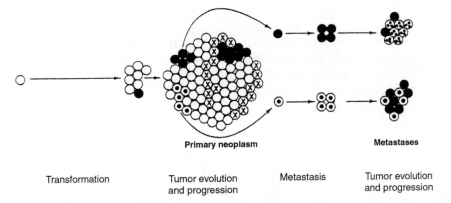

Primary neoplasm   **Metastases**

Transformation   Tumor evolution   Metastasis   Tumor evolution
                      and progression   and progression

Figure 3.7.   The origin of biological heterogeneity in primary neoplasms and metastases. Biological heterogeneity in tumors that are unicellular in origin is due to genetic and epigenetic instability. By the time of diagnosis, most neoplasms consist of multiple subpopulations of cells with different properties. Metastases can have a clonal origin and different metastases can originate from different progenitor cells. Even in clonal metastases, biological diversification gives rise to heterogeneous lesions.

Source: Reprinted with permission from Fidler, I. 1997. Molecular biology of cancer: Invasion and metastasis. In DeVita, V., Hellman, S., and Rosenberg, S. *Cancer: Principles and Practice of Oncology,* 5th edn. Philadelphia, PA: Lippincott-Raven Publishers, p. 142.

variant or mutated forms of the adhesion molecule CD44 (expressed by normal T lymphocytes) may play a key role in the metastatic spread of colon cancer and other cancers (Cotran *et al.*, 1999). Subsequent proliferation of these newly implanted tumor cell emboli gives rise to the metastatic site.

The question of why certain tumor types predictably metastasize to certain distant organs while avoiding others remains under scrutiny. Clearly, the rate of blood flow, organ vascularity, and the number of tumor cells that disseminate and reach an organ are not determining factors (Fidler, 1997). The formation of regional metastases may be linked to anatomical patterns of lymphatic drainage and venous circulation. But the formation of distant metastases is guided by other factors. The "seed and soil" theory of metastasis proposes that only certain metastatic cancer cells (seed) will grow in specific target organs (soil). Three types of mechanisms may influence this process: (1)

tumor cell production of adhesion molecules that prefer only certain target tissues, (2) production of chemical signals by distant organs to attract tumor cells, and (3) production of inhibitor substances by organs that are not typically sites for metastatic growth of a particular tumor (Cotran *et al.,* 1999).

Conclusion

In summary, the evolution of cancer is a complex, multistep process encompassing a wide variety of factors that interact to both suppress and support dissemination of cancer. Discovery of the molecular genetic basis of these factors is now the platform for developing exciting new diagnostic and treatment alternatives. Both the lay and scientific communities are continually bombarded with news releases covering exciting breakthroughs in genetic discoveries that enhance our understanding of cancer and many other diseases. Understandably, patients and families eagerly review such information through print, audiovisual, and Internet sources and bring questions to their health care providers. Nurses must couple an understanding of the molecular basis of cancer with an awareness of clinical discoveries and advances in care to provide competent, up-to-date teaching and guidance for patients and families.

References

Adams, J., and Cory, S. 1998. The Bcl-2 protein family: Arbiters of cell survival. *Science* 281: 1322–1326.

Ashkenazi, A., and Dixit, V. 1998. Death receptors: Signaling and modulation. *Science* 281: 1305–1308.

Bartek, J., Lukas, J., and Bartkova, J. 1999. Perspective: Defects in cell cycle control and cancer. *Journal of Pathology* 187(1): 95–99.

Benchimol, S., and Minden, M. 1998. Viruses, oncogenes, and tumor suppressor genes. In Tannock, I., and Hill, R. (eds). *The Basic Science of Oncology,* 3rd edn. New York, NY: McGraw Hill, pp. 79–105.

Cotran, R., Kumar, V., and Collins, T. 1999. *Robbins Pathologic Basis of Disease,* 6th edn. Philadelphia, PA: W. B. Saunders Company.

Dedhar, S., Hannigan, G., Rak, J., and Kerbel, R. 1998. The extracellular environment and cancer. In Tannock, I., and Hill, R. (eds). *The Basic Science of Oncology,* 3rd edn. New York, NY: McGraw Hill, pp. 197–218.

Dirks, P., and Rutka, J. 1997. Current concepts in neuro-oncology: The cell cycle—A review. *Neurosurgery* 40(5): 1000–1015.

Fahraeus, R., Fischer, P., Krausz, E., and Lane, D. 1999. New approaches to cancer therapies. *Journal of Pathology* 187(1): 138–146.

Fidler, I. 1997. Molecular biology of cancer: Invasion and metastasis. In DeVita, V., Hellman, S., and Rosenberg, S. (eds). *Cancer: Principles and Practice of Oncology,* 5th edn. Philadelphia, PA: Lippincott-Raven Publishers, pp. 135–150.

Fingert, H., Campisi, J., and Pardee, A. 1997. Cell proliferation and differentiation. In Holland, J., Frei, E., Bast, R., Kufe, D., Morton, D., and Weichselbaum, R. (eds). *Cancer Medicine,* 4th edn. Baltimore, MD: Williams and Wilkins, p. 4.

Fossel, M. 1998. Telomerase and the aging cell. *Journal of the American Medical Association* 279: 1732–1735.

Goss, P., and Tye, L. 1998. Hormones and cancer. In Tannock, I., and Hill, R. (eds). *The Basic Science of Oncology,* 3rd edn. New York, NY: McGraw Hill, pp. 263–294.

Gradishar, W. 1997. An overview of clinical trials involving inhibitors of angiogenesis and their mechanism of action. *Investigational New Drugs* 15(1): 49–59.

Greider, C. 1999. Telomerase activation: One step on the road to cancer? *Trends in Genetics* 15(3): 109–112.

Gribbon, J. and Loescher, L. 2000. Biology of cancer. In Yarbro, C., Frogge, M., Goodman, M., and Groenwald, S.(eds). *Cancer Nursing: Principles and Practice,* 4th edn. Subury, MA: Jones and Bartlett, pp. 17–34.

Hall, E. 1997. Etiology of cancer: Physical factors. In DeVita, V., Hellman, S., and Rosenberg, S. (eds). *Cancer: Principles and Practice of Oncology,* 5th edn. Philadelphia, PA: Lippincott-Raven Publishers, pp. 203–218.

Hannun, Y. 1997. Signal transduction in cancer. In Holland, J., Frei, E., Bast, R., Kufe, D., Morton, D., and Weichselbaum, R. (eds). *Cancer Medicine,* 4th edn. Baltimore, MD: Williams and Wilkins, pp. 65–83.

Henderson, B., Bernstein, L., and Ross, R. 1997. Etiology of cancer: Hormonal factors. In DeVita, V., Hellman, S., and Rosenberg, S. (eds). *Cancer: Principles and Practice of Oncology,* 5th edn. Philadelphia, PA: Lippincott-Raven Publishers, pp. 219–229.

Kasten, M. 1997. Molecular biology of cancer: The cell cycle. In DeVita, V., Hellman, S., and Rosenberg, S. (eds). *Cancer: Principles and Practice of*

Oncology, 5th edn. Philadelphia, PA: Lippincott-Raven Publishers, pp. 121–134.

Kliche, K., and Hoffken, K. 1999. The role of apoptosis in hematologic malignancies and modulation of apoptosis as a new therapeutic approach. *Journal of Cancer Research and Clinical Oncology* 125(3–4): 226–231.

Le Beau, M. 1997. Molecular biology of cancer: Cytogenetics. In DeVita, S., Hellman, S., and Rosenberg, S. (eds). *Cancer: Principles and Practice of Oncology,* 5th edn. Philadelphia, PA: Lippincott-Raven Publishers, pp. 103–119.

Lea, D., and Jenkins, J. 1997. Cancer genetics for nurses: Part I. The genetic basis of cancer. *Oncology Nursing Updates* 4(5): 1–11.

Levine, A. 1997. p53, the cellular gatekeeper for growth and division. *Cell* 88: 323–331.

Miller, L., and Marx, J. 1998. Apoptosis. *Science* 281: 1301.

Nakano, R. 1997. Apoptosis: Gene-directed death. *Hormone Research* 48(suppl 3): 2–4.

Nguyen, M. 1997. Angiogenic factors as tumor markers. *Investigational New Drugs* 15(1): 29–37.

Okey, A., Harper, P., Grant, D., and Hill, R. 1998. Chemical and radiation carcinogenesis. In Tannock, I., and Hill, R. (eds). *The Basic Science of Oncology,* 3rd edn. New York, NY: McGraw Hill, pp. 166–196.

Perkins, A., and Stern, D. 1997. Molecular biology of cancer: Oncogenes. In DeVita, V., Hellman, S., and Rosenberg, S. (eds). *Cancer: Principles and Practice of Oncology,* 5th edn. Philadelphia, PA: Lippincott-Raven Publishers, pp. 79–102.

Pluda, J. 1997. Tumor-associated angiogenesis: Mechanisms, clinical implications, and therapeutic strategies. *Seminars in Oncology* 24(2): 203–218.

Poeschla, E., and Wong-Staal, F. (1997). Etiology of cancer: Viruses. In DeVita, V., Hellman, S., and Rosenberg, S. (eds). *Cancer: Principles and Practice of Oncology,* 5th edn. Philadelphia, PA: Lippincott-Raven Publishers, pp. 153–184.

Prives, C., and Hall, P. 1999. The *p53* pathway. *Journal of Pathology* 187(1): 112–126.

Rieger, P. 1997. Emerging strategies in the management of cancer. *Oncology Nursing Forum* 24(4): 728–737.

Rosenberg, S. 1997. Principles of cancer management: Surgical oncology. In DeVita, V., Hellman, S., and Rosenberg, S. (eds). *Cancer: Principles and Practice of Oncology,* 5th edn. Philadelphia, PA: Lippincott-Raven Publishers, pp. 295–306.

Ross, J., and Fletcher, J. 1999. The *HER-2/neu* oncogene: Prognostic factor, predictive factor and target for therapy. *Seminars in Cancer Biology* 9(2): 125–138.

Ruddon, R. (1995). *Cancer Biology,* 3rd edn. New York, NY: Oxford University Press.

Schmitt, C., and Lowe, S. 1999. Apoptosis and therapy. *Journal of Pathology* 187(1): 127–137.

Seeley, R., Stephens, T., and Tate, P. 1996. *Essentials of Anatomy & Physiology,* 2nd edn. St. Louis, MO: Mosby Year-Book.

Slingerland, J., and Tannock, I. 1998. Cell proliferation and cell death. In Tannock, I., and Hill, R. (eds). *The Basic Science of Oncology,* 3rd edn. New York, NY: McGraw Hill, pp. 134–165.

Squire, J., Whitmore, G., and Philips, R. 1998. Genetic basis of cancer. In Tannock, I., and Hill, R. (eds). *The Basic Science of Oncology,* 3rd edn. New York, NY: McGraw Hill, pp. 48–78.

Thibodeau, G., and Patton, K. 1999. *Anatomy & Physiology,* 4th edn. St. Louis, MO: Mosby, Inc.

Yarbro, J. 2000. Carcinogenesis. In Yarbro, C., Frogge, M., Goodman, M., and Groenwald, S., (eds). *Cancer Nursing: Principles and Practice,* 5th edn. Subury, MA: Jones and Bartlett, pp. 48–59.

Yuspa, S., and Shields, P. 1997. Etiology of cancer: Chemical factors. In DeVita, V., Hellman, S., and Rosenberg, S. (eds). *Cancer: Principles and Practice of Oncology,* 5th edn. Philadelphia, PA: Lippincott-Raven Publishers, pp. 185–202.

Zanke, B. (1998). Growth factors and intracellular signaling. In Tannock, I., and Hill, R. (eds). *The Basic Science of Oncology,* 3rd edn. New York, NY: McGraw Hill, pp. 106–133.

Resources and Key References

Print Materials

Bronchud, M. H. (ed.). 2000. *Principles of Molecular Oncology*. Totowa, NJ: Humana Press.

Gonick, L., and Wheeler, M. 1991. *Cartoon Guide to Genetics*. New York, NY: Harper Perennial.

Lea, D., Jenkins, J., and Francomano, C. 1998. *Genetics in Clinical Practice: New Directions for Nursing and Health Care*. Sudbury, MA: Jones and Bartlett.

Lewin, B. 2000. *Genes VII*. New York, NY: Oxford University Press.

Ouellette, F. 1999. Internet resources for the clinical geneticist. *Clinical Genetics* 56(3): 179–185.

Web Sites

Cancer Genetics Network. National network of centers specializing in the study of inherited predisposition to cancer. *http://www-dccps.ims.nci.nih.gov/CGN*

CancerNet. The National Cancer Institute's cancer information web site: *http://cancernet.nci.nih.gov*

Genomic and Genetic Data. Site for the National Human Genome Research Institute: *http://www.nhgri.nih.gov/Data*

National Center for Biotechnology Information. Resource for molecular biology information: *http://www.ncbi.nlm.nih.gov*

National Human Genome Research Institute. Heads the human genome project: *http://www.nhgri.nih.gov*

CHAPTER 4 | Optimizing the Dose and Schedule of Biological Agents

Paula Trahan Rieger, RN, MSN, CS, AOCN®, FAAN

Developments in biological approaches to cancer treatment continue to progress rapidly, and regulatory approvals in each major category of biological agents have now occurred. However, the optimal dose, route of administration, and schedule are still not known for the majority of biological agents and will most likely differ for each disease treated. Questions continue to be raised as to what constitutes optimal dosing and how it should be achieved in clinical trials. In fact, several terms are used to describe optimal dosing for biological agents: **optimal biological dose (OBD)**, optimal immunomodulatory dose, biologically optimal dose, biologically active dose, optimal biological response modifier dose, and maximum tolerated dose (MTD). The aim of this chapter is to define optimal biological dosing and to address issues regarding the dosing of biological agents and

the combination of these agents with other types of therapy. A description of the basic concepts of pharmacokinetics and pharmacodynamics as they relate to dosing provides a foundation for understanding concerns related to dosing. Methods of evaluating biological effects and analysis of end points (therapeutic outcomes) in the treatment of cancer serve as clinical examples to highlight these end points.

Drug Development

The process of developing a new drug is both time consuming and costly. The development of biological agents for therapeutic use in the Unites States is regulated by the Center for Biologics Evaluation and Research (CBER), an arm of the Food and Drug Administration

(**FDA**) (Siegel *et al.*, 1995). The role of this center is to ". . . protect and enhance the public health through regulation of biological and related products including blood, vaccines, and biological therapeutics according to statutory authorities. The regulation of these products is founded on science and law to ensure their purity, potency, safety, efficacy, and availability." The FDA Modernization Act of 1997 (FDAMA), signed into law on November 21, 1997, amended the Food, Drug and Cosmetic Act and the Public Health Service Act to modernize the regulation of food, medical products, and cosmetics. Initiatives within FDAMA included measures to modernize the regulation of biological products by bringing them into harmony with regulations of drugs. Specific changes included eliminating the need for establishment of license applications, streamlining the approval processes for manufacturing changes, and reducing the need for environmental assessment as part of a product application. Another important component of the FDAMA was the establishment of parameters for distributing sound and balanced information about "off-label uses" for marketed drugs, biologics, and medical devices (CBER, 1999).

In general, the development of biological agents is similar to that of chemotherapeutic agents but biological agents follow a different path. Both endeavors initially begin with the discovery of a new agent. For chemotherapeutic agents, the next step is extraction or synthetic formulation. For biological agents, the next step is finding the gene or determination of the DNA sequence that codes for the biological protein. With hybridomas, this phase involves selecting the hybridoma that produces the desired monoclonal antibody. Biological activities and mechanism of action, both *in vitro* and *in vivo*, are documented, and then animal studies are done to evaluate the toxicity of the agent. A limiting factor in the preclinical investigation of the physiological effects of biological agents is that the majority of these agents are strongly species specific. Increasingly, many of the preclinical developmental studies with biologicals occur in nonhuman primates. The production of transgenic and knockout mice may prove useful in resolving this problem (Mazanet *et al.*, 1996). During development, preclinical toxicology studies must also be done. The goal of this preclinical safety evaluation is to recommend a safe starting dose and dose-escalation scheme for use with humans. Other goals of this study are to identify potential target organs, toxic effects, appropriate parameters to monitor in the clinical setting, and potential mechanisms of action of the drug (Siegel *et al.*, 1995).

At this point, if an agent has demonstrated clinical usefulness, the company or academic center developing the drug will file an investigational new drug application (**INDA**). Barriers to this process include, but are not limited to, the cost, the expertise, and the development resources involved in bringing a new drug to market. A new program by the National Cancer Institute (NCI), Rapid Access to Intervention Development (RAID), is designed to address these barriers. Through RAID, the NCI makes its resources available to the investigating institution on a competitive basis so that preclinical drug development and INDA filing are done by the researchers who originated the potential therapy (Anonymous, 1998).

Once declared an investigational new drug, the new agent is entered into clinical trials for evaluation in humans. The purposes of phase I trials are to establish the MTD and to recommend an administration schedule. The MTD is the highest dose at which side effects are tolerable. Increasingly, phase I trials of biological agents are designed to also evaluate the biological effects of the drug. A 2-tiered phase I trial is often conducted: the phase Ia study seeks to determine the MTD and the phase Ib study seeks to determine the optimal dose for achieving the desired biological effect or effects (Creekmore *et al.*, 1991; Oldham, 1998).

In phase II trials, therapeutic activity with respect to a given disease is tested. In phase III trials, the agent's usefulness is compared with the standard therapy for that particular disease. At this point, if the agent appears promising, a new drug application is made to the FDA. Dosage, route, schedule, toxicity, and indications for the agent are then specified (Oldham, 1998).

There are many problems inherent to this system. The majority of advances in biotherapy have been made through empirical discoveries rather than findings based on rational principles (Creekmore *et al.*, 1991). The time it takes to move a drug through the approval process is often as long as 8 to 10 years, and the costs can run as high as $80 million to $100 million. Only companies with substantial resources are able to persevere through the lengthy and expensive approval process (Oldham, 1998). Although improvements have been made, the current system is often not sufficiently flexible to optimize the development of biological agents.

Optimal Biological Dosing

It has been demonstrated in studies with animal models that there may be a wide disparity between the MTD and the OBD of biological agents. The OBD is defined as the minimum dose at which biological activity is maximally stimulated (Creekmore *et al.*, 1991). Parameters deemed important for treating a particular disease with biological agents must be determined so that the desired response can be assessed. Within the current framework of drug development, several crucial issues unique to biological agents are not addressed: the diversity and selectivity of these agents, the **cytokine cascade**,

the existence of physiological mechanisms of action and receptors for biological agents (because they are natural products), and the measurement of biological effects within the context of clinical trials (Creekmore *et al.*, 1991; Talmadge, 1992).

Diversity and Selectivity

Biological agents are both diverse and selective. Owing to their **pleiotropic** nature, many have more than one mechanism of action (Balkwill, 1997; Kelso, 1998). Which mechanism of action can yield the desired antitumor effect when a biological agent is given as treatment for a particular disease is often unknown. For example, the key antitumor action of interferon (IFN)-α may be its immunomodulatory effects or its antiproliferative effects. The approach to dosing is very different depending on which effect is to be maximally stimulated (Mihich, 1987; Creekmore *et al.*, 1991). The relationship of dosing to antitumor activity is not the same for biological agents as it is for chemotherapeutic agents. Moreover, biological agents are generally much more selective than are chemotherapeutic agents. Many function as receptor-mediated molecules, that is, select cells bear receptors for a given agent. Monoclonal antibodies are an excellent example of a group of agents with high selectivity (Oldham, 1998).

The Cytokine Cascade

The biology of the immune system is complex. This system contains a multitude of cells that communicate with each other through secretion of a variety of cytokines, or biological proteins, that act as messengers (see Chapter 2). The term "cytokine cascade" is used to describe the network of interactions that occur through mutual cytokine induction; through transmodulation of cell surface receptors; and by

synergistic, additive, or **antagonistic** interactions that affect the function of a target cell (Balkwill, 1997; Kelso, 1998). Assessment of a cytokine's action is often done *in vitro* or in animal models. It is difficult to determine whether these activities will also be seen when the agent is given *in vivo*. The ultimate response of a cell may be determined by the number of different messages it receives concurrently at its surface (Sporn and Roberts, 1988). When a cytokine is administered exogenously, it is not always known which other cytokines may be stimulated *in vivo* as a result of the cytokine cascade.

Toxicity of Natural Products

The toxicity of biological agents may need to be viewed differently from that of chemotherapeutic agents. Because biological agents are natural proteins, we would expect them to have a less acute or milder cumulative toxic effect. To a certain extent, this is true, because when administration of biological agents is stopped, side effects generally resolve very quickly. This characteristic may be related to the fact that both receptors and physiological mechanisms for these natural proteins are already in place (Oldham, 1998).

Measurement of Biological Effects in Clinical Trials

The issue of evaluating biological effects within the context of clinical trials is gaining increasing attention. How does the administration of a biological agent affect a patient's normal cytokine cascade? What is the agent's predominant antitumor effect? What is the rationale for using a certain biological agent to treat a particular disease based on the underlying pathophysiology of the disease? The answers to these questions are essential to maximizing the use of biological agents in the management of can-

cer. The majority of clinical trials to date have attempted immunological monitoring using data obtained from analysis of peripheral blood, partly because of the ease of obtaining specimens. One might question the relevance of this information, because the primary target of therapy and likely the most important site of immunological effects is the tumor site. Data obtained from the peripheral blood might provide no conclusions at all about the effects obtained at the tumor site. Indeed, most studies utilizing immunological monitoring have failed to demonstrate a correlation between any observed changes in peripheral blood cells and an antitumor effect. New approaches to immunological monitoring are being developed, and studies utilizing this technique are being tailored to the specific treatment being tested in an attempt to obtain relevant and more meaningful data that will hopefully guide the development of effective regimens (Kopp and Holmlund, 1996).

Drug Activity and Dosing

In essence, the end effect of a drug depends on its ultimate concentration at the site of action. A medication must proceed through 3 specific phases of drug action as it passes through the body: the pharmaceutical phase, the pharmacokinetic phase, and the pharmacodynamic phase.

The concepts of pharmacokinetics, pharmacodynamics and measurement of response can be used to understand biological dosing issues and to evaluate the aforementioned issues in more detail.

Pharmaceutical Phase

During the pharmaceutical phase, the medication enters the body in one form (as an orally administered tablet, capsule, or elixir) and changes into another form to be utilized. Because few biological agents are given orally, this phase is often not relevant in biotherapy.

Most biological agents are given either by subcutaneous or intramuscular injection and absorbed rapidly into the bloodstream or intravenously, which deposits the agent directly into the bloodstream.

Pharmacokinetic Phase

Pharmacokinetics can be defined simply as what the body does to the drug (Benet *et al.*, 1996; Kuhn, 1998). The pharmacokinetic phase encompasses an agent's absorption, distribution to the site of action, biotransformation, and clearance (see Figure 4.1). This phase may be affected by such factors as body weight, age, disease state, immune factors, psychological factors, environment, and timing of the dose (chronobiology).

Once a drug is administered, it must then be absorbed so that it can make its way into the systemic circulation. **Absorption** is the rate at which the drug leaves the site of administration and the extent to which this occurs. Absorption involves the passage of the drug across the surface of cell membranes. Once the drug enters the blood it can circulate either independently or while bound to plasma proteins. Factors affecting absorption include bioavailability, solubility, drug pH, concentration, circulation, and route (see Table 4.1).

Once absorption occurs, the drug must then make its way to the site of action. This process is termed **distribution.** For most biological agents, the site of action is receptors on target cells. Factors affecting distribution are blood flow and drug properties such as solubility and

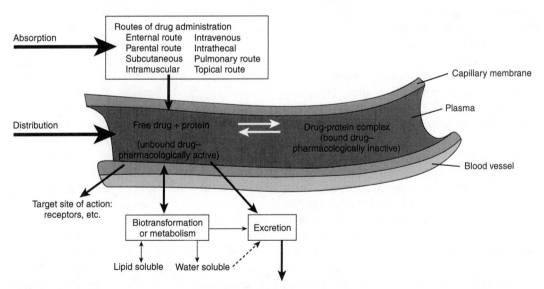

Figure 4.1 Schema of pharmacokinetic phase of drug action, showing absorption, distribution, biotransformation, and excretion of drugs. Note that only free drug is capable of movement for absorption, distribution to the target site of action, biotransformation, and excretion; the drug-protein complex represents bound drugs; and because the molecule is large, it is trapped in the blood vessel and serves as a storage site for the drug.

Source: Reprinted with permission from McKenry, L., and Salerno, E. 1998. *Mosby's Pharmacology in Nursing,* 20th edn. St. Louis: Mosby, Figure 3.3, p. 32.

Table 4.1 Factors affecting drug absorption

Factor	Definition
Bioavailability	The percentage of drug that is absorbed. Dosage forms of a drug from different manufacturers may differ in their bioavailability.
Solubility	The ability of a medication to dissolve and form a solution.
Concentration	The relative content of a component (strength or potency). The more concentrated a drug, the more rapidly it will be absorbed.
Circulation	The amount of blood flow available to carry the drug to the site of action.
Route	Method by which medication can be introduced into the body. Possible routes are: oral, via mucous membranes, via inhalation, and parenteral. Places the drug near the absorbing surface for absorption into the vascular system.

binding ability. Drugs generally bind to plasma proteins or physiological receptors after which an equilibrium is reached between the concentration of drug in the blood and in plasma and target receptors or in certain tissue reservoirs such as fat cells. **Plasma concentration** is the amount of both free and bound drug in the plasma. The maximal effect of a drug usually occurs when the peak level of drug concentration at the target site is reached.

Biotransformation, or metabolism, refers to the enzymatic alteration of the drug. Generally occurring in the liver, biotransformation can be affected by factors such as genetics, preexisting liver disease, or the concomitant administration of other drugs.

Lastly, drugs are excreted through the liver and kidneys in either altered (as metabolites) or natural form. The whole-body **clearance** rate of a drug is a measure of the speed at which the drug leaves the system. The rate of clearance will impact the frequency of administration. For example, a drug with a low clearance rate requires less frequent administration than a drug with a high clearance rate (Benet *et al.*, 1996; Kuhn, 1998). The ability to relate these concepts to the clinical evaluation of biological agents is important. For example, in phase I trials, pharmacologic studies relate the concentration of drug in the circulation to the concen-

tration needed at the site of action to obtain the desired biological effect. These studies represent a way to quantify the relationship between dose and the effect of a drug.

The results of a pharmacologic study can be plotted on a pharmacology curve (Figure 4.2). In this case, the **area under the curve** defines the exposure of the target cell to the drug and is a function of the concentration of the drug and time. Half-life is defined as the time it takes for the concentration of drug in the blood to decrease by 50% (Benet *et al.*, 1996).

The pharmacokinetic profiles of IFN-α and granulocyte macrophage-colony-stimulating factor (GM-CSF), determined during the original phase I trials, serve to illustrate these concepts. Note Figure 4.3, which depicts intramuscular administration of IFN. The pharmacology curve for intramuscular administration of IFN shows a slow and gradual absorption from the muscle into the bloodstream with a gradual decline over the course of 1 to 2 days. Escalation of the IFN dose shows higher levels of the drug initially, with a slower clearance time. Peak serum concentrations are generally achieved 4 to 6 hours after injection, with maximum-observed serum concentrations increasing with dose (Gutterman *et al.*, 1982).

The pharmacology curves of colony-stimulating factors are similar to those seen with IFN.

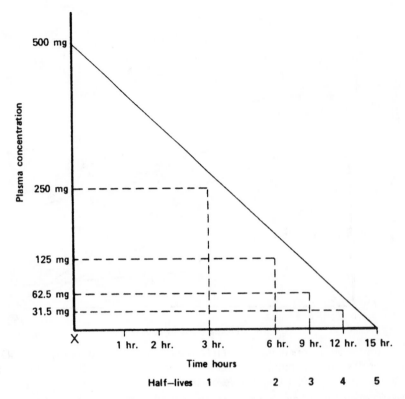

Figure 4.2   Linear medication curve shows the biological half-life of a medication. A dose of 500 mg of the drug, which has a half-life of 3 hours, is given at point X. At 3 hours, 250 mg are excreted; at 6 hours, an additional 125 mg are excreted; at 9 hours, an additional 62.5 mg are excreted. This continues for approximately 5 half-lives.

Source: Reprinted with permission from publisher F. A. Davis. Kuhn, M. 1998. Pharmaceutical, pharmacokinetic, and pharmacodynamic phases of drug action. In Kuhn, M. (ed). *Pharmacotherapeutics: A Nursing Approach*, 4th edn. Philadelphia, PA: F. A. Davis, Figure 4.6, p. 43.

For GM-CSF administered intravenously, the serum concentration is very high initially but falls rapidly over several hours (Figure 4.4A). When GM-CSF is given subcutaneously, a more gradual absorption occurs, with the peak serum concentration occurring after approximately 2 to 4 hours, depending on the dose (Figure 4.4B–D) (Cebon *et al.*, 1988; Morstyn *et al.*, 1989).

Pharmacologic studies in phase I trials are clinically important because the results are used to determine the appropriate route, dose, and schedule for administration of a drug. The concentration of drug needed at the site of action usually correlates with the dose that yields this concentration in the blood. This information can also be correlated clinically with side effects. Peak concentrations of drugs often relate to the peak occurrence of side effects. Again, IFN serves as an excellent model. Fever and chills generally occur 2 to 4 hours after injection, which correlates with the beginning of a

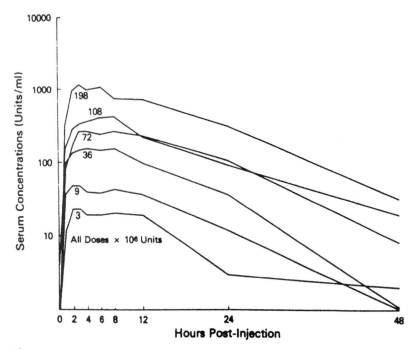

Figure 4.3 The mean serum concentrations of IFN as measured by the bioassay with MDBK (bovine kidney) cells as target cells. The numbers of patients measured at 3, 9, 36, 72, 108, and 198 million units are 16, 16, 16, 16, 14, and 5, respectively.

Source: Reprinted with permission from *Annals of Internal Medicine* and the authors Gutterman, J., Fine, S., and Quesado, J. 1982. Recombinant leukocyte A interferon: Pharmacokinetics, single-dose tolerance, and biologic effects in cancer patients. *Annals of Internal Medicine* 96: 549–555. Figure 2, p. 551.

peak concentration in the blood. When drugs are given intravenously, side effects generally occur much more quickly.

Many cytokines have a short half-life and are given daily or every other day by subcutaneous injection or continuous infusion. Agents that have a longer half-life, such as thrombopoietin and trastuzumab, are likely to be dosed on a different schedule. Thrombopoietin has an elimination half-life approaching 30 hours, which is longer than that of other hematopoietic growth factors, and it also has prolonged biological action. These factors must be taken into consideration when designing dose schedules for thrombopoietin (Kaushansky, 1998). Trastuzumab (Herceptin®), a monoclonal antibody

targeted toward the HER-2 receptor, has a half-life measured in days: 1.7 days at the 10-mg-dose level and up to 12 days at the 500-mg-dose level. Trastuzumab is administered as a loading dose and is followed by weekly maintenance doses (Genentech, Inc., 1998).

Other less commonly used routes of administration include intraperitoneal infusion and inhalation, both of which facilitate high, site-specific concentrations of drug. For example, natural interleukin-2 (IL-2) has been administered by inhalation for the treatment of pulmonary malignancies refractory to conventional therapy. A phase I study by Lorenz and colleagues (1996) evaluated the toxicity, pharmacokinetics, and biological effects of inhalation.

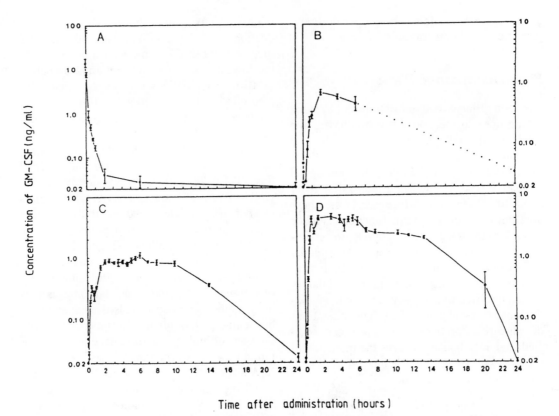

Figure 4.4 Pharmacokinetics of human GM-CSF in humans: (A) 0.3 mcg/kg administered intravenously, (B) 1 mcg/kg administered subcutaneously, (C) 3 mcg/kg administered subcutaneously, and (D) 10 mcg/kg administered subcutaneously. Serum levels are expressed as means of triplicate determinations ± standard deviation. GM-CSF was injected at time 0.

Source: Reprinted with permission from *Blood* and the authors Cebon, J., Dempsey, P., Fox, R., *et al.* 1988. Pharmacokinetics of human granulocyte-macrophage colony-stimulating factor using a sensitive immunoassay. *Blood* 72(4): 1340–1347. Figure 6, p. 1344.

The adverse effects observed with this approach were different from those observed with systemic administration and were limited primarily to pulmonary toxicity. A dose-dependent expansion of pulmonary immunocompetent cells was observed, with little systemic biological effect detectable. The investigators concluded that aerosolized natural IL-2 merited further investigation as a site-specific treatment for malignant and inflammatory lung disease. Huland and colleagues (2000) have reviewed the clinical experiences of over 300 patients receiving inhaled IL-2 therapy for the treatment of pulmonary metastases. They concluded that the route is efficacious and has low toxicity.

The primary pharmacokinetic factors affecting the concentration of drug in the blood and therefore the patient's response include the rate and amount of drug absorbed, the distribution of the drug to the site of action, biotransformation of the drug, and clearance or elimination of the drug from the body. These are key principles in determining the proper dose and schedule for administration of a drug.

Pharmacodynamic Phase

The term **pharmacodynamics** refers to what a drug does to the body. It encompasses the biochemical and physiological effects and mechanisms of action of the drug (Ross, 1996; McKenry and Salerno, 1998). Most biological agents are receptor-mediated molecules. After interaction with cell-surface receptors, these molecules stimulate certain functions, induce secondary messengers, or suppress select immune functions. IFN can be used as a model to illustrate this point. It has several biological actions: antiviral effects, immunomodulatory and antiproliferative activity, oncogene regulation, and metabolic and phenotypic alterations of cell-surface proteins. IFN is receptor mediated, and once bound it causes the induction of secondary messengers inside the cell (Balkwill, 1989; Pfeffer et al., 1998).

INTERFERON

If the biological actions of IFN were to be assessed, what response parameters would be measured? Useful parameters evaluated in early trials assessing biological effects included the activation of natural killer cells (NK); β_2-microglobulin production, which relates to the induction of major histocompatibility complex antigens; and neopterin production, which relates to the activation of macrophages (Borden et al., 1987; Aulitzky et al., 1989; Huber and Herold, 1989).

In a classic study, Aulitzky et al. (1989) evaluated the effects of IFN-γ on biological responses in 16 patients with renal cell cancer and observed a bell-shaped response curve. As the concentration of drug increased, responses also increased to a certain point. Past a certain dose, however, responses began to decrease or

plateau. An evaluation of β_2-microglobulin induction at IFN-γ doses of 10, 100, and 500 mcg once weekly is depicted in Figure 4.5. At the lowest dose, there was minimal induction of β_2-microglobulin levels. A significant increase in levels was seen at the 100-mcg dose, but levels were not greatly increased at the 500-mcg-dose level, although toxic effects were significantly more severe. This illustrates how the MTD may differ from the biologically optimal dose. The MTD (500 mcg) was not the dose at which maximal biological activity was obtained (100 mcg), as determined by the aforementioned parameters. A similar pattern was observed with neopterin levels (Figure 4.6). In the next phase of the study, Aulitzky and colleagues treated patients at the biologically optimal dose of 100-mcg IFN-γ, and found that some patients did respond to this dose. This is an example of how clinical trials might be designed to evaluate the issue of biologically optimal dosing in conjunction with determination of MTD.

A key to determining the OBD is identifying which biological effects contribute to the antitumor effect. With most biological agents, it is difficult to say which biological property is responsible for the primary antitumor effect in a given disease. With IFNs, OBD may differ for different types of tumors. For example, hairy-cell leukemia responds to very low doses of IFN-α (Huber et al., 1987). For the treatment of renal cell cancer and chronic myelogenous leukemia (Guilhot and Lacotte-Thierry, 1998), moderate doses of IFN-α are needed, whereas for treatment of Kaposi's sarcoma, much higher doses of IFN-α are required to produce clinical response.

HEMATOPOIETIC GROWTH FACTORS

The evaluation of hematopoietic growth factors, specifically GM-CSF and granulocyte colony-stimulating factor (G-CSF, filgrastim) serve as additional clinical examples. Hematopoietic growth factors are involved in the matu-

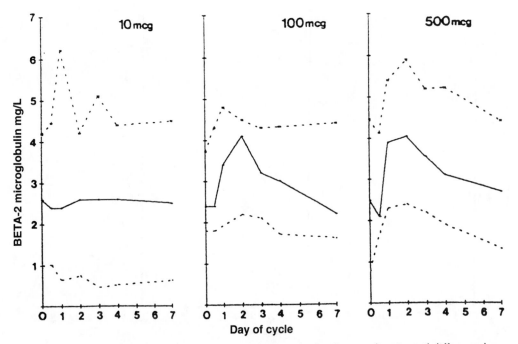

Figure 4.5 Kinetics of β_2-microglobulin serum levels after the first application of different dose levels of IFN-γ. Median values and range of all determinations performed in 16 patients with renal cell carcinoma are demonstrated.

Source: Reprinted with permission from the *Journal of Clinical Oncology* and the authors Aulitzky, W., Gastl, G., Aulitzky, W., *et al.* 1989. Successful treatment of metastatic renal cell carcinoma with a biologically active dose of recombinant interferon-gamma. *Journal of Clinical Oncology* 7(12): 1875–1884. Figure 1, p. 1878.

ration and differentiation of hematopoietic cells. They are also able to enhance the function of these cells (Metcalf, 1990). For example, GM-CSF can enhance the function of neutrophils and macrophages. Key functions of neutrophils in the body include the ability to move to an area of inflammation or infection and to phagocytize foreign bodies (Wiernik, 1989).

A simple way to evaluate the biological effects of hematopoietic growth factors is examination of peripheral blood cell counts. In early phase I trials with GM-CSF, analysis of the white blood cell count demonstrated increasing numbers of white blood cells as the dose was increased, with a rapid decline in counts once therapy was discontinued (Vadhan-Raj *et al.*, 1988) (Figure 4.7). Lower doses, at which there are minimal toxic effects, may be adequate to stimulate the desired number of white blood cells.

As discussed previously, the endogenous normal cellular cytokine cascade appears to be delicately balanced. The therapeutic use of a biological agent may occasionally produce unintended biological effects. During early clinical trials, a controversial point surrounding the use of GM-CSF was that neutrophils appeared to not "function" properly. Work by Peters *et al.* (1988) evaluated the function of neutrophils by measuring their margination, phagocytosis, peroxide production, and migration in patients receiving GM-CSF. Evaluation of these

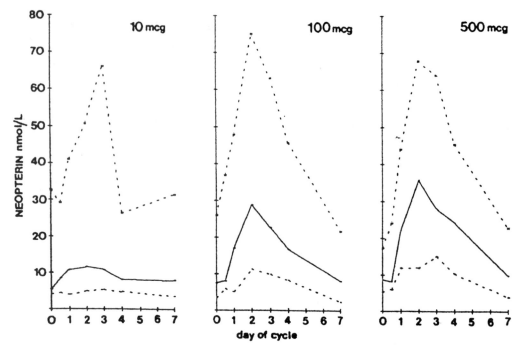

Figure 4.6 Kinetics of neopterin serum levels after the first application of different dose levels of IFN-γ. Median values and range of all determinations performed in 16 patients with renal cell carcinoma are demonstrated.

Source: Reprinted with permission from *Journal of Clinical Oncology* and the authors Aulitzky, W., Gastl, G., Aulitzky, W., *et al.* 1989. Successful treatment of metastatic renal cell carcinoma with a biologically active dose of recombinant interferon-gamma. *Journal of Clinical Oncology* 7(12): 1875–1884. Figure 1, p. 1878.

functions demonstrated that margination, phagocytosis, and peroxide production levels were similar both before and after therapy, whereas neutrophil migration was decreased. Neutrophils tended to stay in the bloodstream because of the concentration gradient that resulted from GM-CSF administration. It is uncertain whether decreased neutrophil migration has a negative clinical effect.

G-CSF also produces a dose-dependent increase in the total circulating neutrophil pool by 2 major mechanisms: cytokinetics (the mobilization of mature neutrophils into the blood) and accelerated granulopoiesis. Figure 4.8 demonstrates how G-CSF causes a dose-dependent

acceleration in precursor maturation time, that is, the higher doses result in a shortened time frame for maturation of neutrophils. To date, no MTD has been established for G-CSF. Each indication has a recommended starting dose that can be titrated to obtain the desired biological effect, that is, absolute neutrophil count (Campbell, 1998; Roskos *et al.*, 1998).

LEVAMISOLE
Clinical studies evaluating levamisole provide another relevant example of OBD. Although levamisole was approved in 1990 for use in standard adjuvant therapy for patients with Dukes' stage C colon cancer, little is known

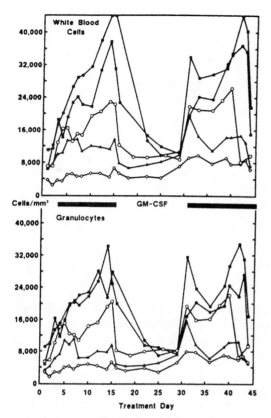

Figure 4.7 White blood cell counts and absolute granulocyte counts (neutrophils and bands) in patients with solid tumors treated with recombinant human granulocyte-macrophage colony-stimulating factor (rhGM-CSF). rhGM-CSF was administered by intravenous bolus injection on day 1, followed by continuous intravenous infusion (solid bar) on days 2 through 14. After a 2-week rest period, a second 2-week cycle by intravenous continuous infusion was repeated. Each of the five patients traced here received rhGM-CSF at a dose of 30 (◇–◇), 60 (▲–▲), 120 (○–○), 120 (●–●), or 250 (■–■) mcg/ m² of body surface area.

Source: Reprinted with permission from *Blood* and the authors. Vadhan Raj, S., Buescher, S., Le Maistre, A., *et al.* 1988. Stimulation of hematopoiesis in patients with bone marrow failure and in patients with malignancy by recombinant human granulocyte-macrophage colony-stimulating factor. *Blood* 72(1): 134–141. Figure 1, p. 136.

about its optimal dose and schedule or the mechanism by which it exerts its antitumor effects (Janik *et al.*, 1993). A phase I study by Janik and colleagues evaluated levamisole alone and in combination with IFN-γ in treating patients with advanced cancers. Patients were divided into 2 groups: those with advanced disease in whom standard therapy had failed and those with either renal cancer or melanoma who received adjuvant therapy. The main objective of the trial was to determine the MTD and immunomodulatory activity of levamisole alone and in combination with IFN-γ. Immunologic monitoring involved measurement of neopterin levels, flow cytometric **immunophenotyping**, and NK cell assays. In both groups, it appeared that a threshold dose of 5.0 mg/kg of levamisole was needed to induce levels of both neopterin and soluble IL-2 receptor (sIL-2R). Expression of monocyte surface markers associated with activation increased in response to treatment with levamisole alone at this dose level, but multiple doses were needed to induce this effect. These data suggest that monocytes were activated *in vivo*. Increased levels of sIL-2R suggest that T cells were activated by levamisole with subsequent secretion of IFN-γ. Monocytes may then have been stimulated by IFN-γ to make neopterin. Natural killer cell activity was not reproducibly elevated above baseline, regardless of levamisole dose.

Therefore, in this study, the MTD of levamisole alone and in combination with IFN-γ was 5.0 mg/kg, which was also the optimal immunomodulatory dose. The reported dose of levamisole when used as adjuvant therapy in other cancers is below the MTD (Moertel *et al.*, 1990; Quirt *et al.*, 1991) and also below the OBD, according to calculations by Janik and colleagues (Janik *et al.*, 1993). These data argue for additional trials evaluating higher doses of levamisole with alternate schedules. These trials should include both immunologic and clinical end points. A study published by Reid *et*

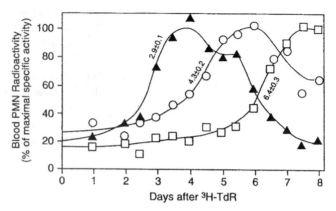

Figure 4.8   Filgrastim (G-CSF) causes a dose-dependent acceleration of precursor maturation time. Solid triangles, 300 mcg; open circles, 30 mcg; open squares, no drug.

Source: Reprinted with permission from Valle, J., and Scarffe, H. 1998. *Filgrastim in Clinical Practice,* 2nd edn. New York: Marcel Dekker, Inc., Figure 1, p. 377.

al. (1998) evaluated high-dose levamisole in combination with 5-fluorouracil (5-FU) in patients with advanced cancer. The goal of the study was to determine the MTD and activity of levamisole in conjunction with 5-FU. This study concluded that levamisole may be administered safely with 5-FU at doses 4 to 5 times greater than those presently given in conventional regimens. They recommended a dose of 75 mg/m² 3 times daily for levamisole in combination with 5-FU for 5 days for future studies (Reid *et al.*, 1998).

INTERLEUKIN-6

In recent years, evaluation of the biological effects of cytokines has become more sophisticated. A study published on the immunomodulatory and hematopoietic effects of recombinant human (rh)IL-6 illustrates this point (Nieken *et al.*, 1999). IL-6 is a pleiotropic cytokine synthesized under inflammatory conditions by numerous cell types. In this study, the researchers investigated the immunomodulatory effects of low-dose subcutaneous rhIL-6 in patients with metastatic renal cell carcinoma or malignant

melanoma. Prior to their study, clinical trials concerning the immunomodulatory impact of rhIL-6 had produced contradictory data. In this study by Nieken *et al.* (1999), patients received 150 mcg of rhIL-6 once daily for 42 consecutive days. Immunologic data was adjusted to correct for concurrent hemodilution resulting from rhIL-6 administration. To better determine the range of its biological effects, the following parameters were measured: total and differential white blood cell counts; quantitative determination of immunoglobulins G, A, and M; serum levels of GM-CSF, IL-1β, tumor necrosis factor (TNF), and IL-6; and flow cytometric analysis for phenotypic analysis of peripheral blood mononuclear cells. Nieken *et al.* found no consistent changes in total and differential white blood cell counts. The lymphocyte subset was not altered, nor did it express specific cell activation markers such as CD25 and HLA-DR. Levels of IgA, IgG, and IgM remained unaffected. Levels of secondary cytokines such as IL-1β, TNF, and GM-CSF remained below detection limits before, during, and after the rhIL-6 administration. The investigators surmised that their data differed from other clinical data on rhIL-6 due to divergent dosage regimens, routes of administration, or a combination of these factors. They concluded from their data that the immunomodulatory impact of rhIL-6 at low doses is limited and does not support a role for this agent as single treatment in cell-mediated tumor regression in patients with disseminated renal cell cancer and metastatic melanoma.

LOW-DOSE VERSUS HIGH-DOSE THERAPY

An intense area of investigation surrounding the use of cytokines in patients with cancer is the investigation of low-dose therapy. Because of the toxicity associated with higher doses of cytokines such as IFN-α and IL-2, researchers have attempted to determine whether clinical efficacy can be maintained with lower doses. In 1993, Mäas and associates reviewed the issue of high-dose versus low-dose IL-2 (Mäas *et al.*, 1993). In many trials, IL-2 has been used like a chemotherapeutic agent (i.e., at the MTD). Therapy at this dose level appears to best stimulate nonspecific antitumor activity (lymphokine-activated killer [LAK] cell activity). Therapy with low doses of IL-2, however, preferentially stimulates a specific antitumor immune response. Many studies have evaluated the immunological effects of IL-2 administration both in animal models and in patients with cancer. High-dose IL-2 causes an increase in the number of lymphocytes in the peripheral blood and induces LAK-cell activity. In addition, cytokines such as IFN-γ, IL-1, IL-6, and TNF are released. If LAK-cell cytotoxicity is the predominant antitumor mechanism, then IL-2 therapy should be effective against a wide range of different tumors. To date, however, IL-2 therapy has been found to be effective primarily in patients with melanoma and renal cell cancer, tumors known to be very immunogenic. These facts may suggest the involvement of a specific antitumor reaction. Mäas and colleagues argued for the use of low IL-2 doses which give optimal stimulation of a specific immune reaction, particularly the intratumoral application of low doses of IL-2, which does not induce toxic effects (Mäas *et al.*, 1993). A more recent report by Lissoni (1997) presents a review of the literature regarding the immunomodulatory activity and clinical efficacy of low-dose recombinant IL-2. Although the threshold is somewhat controversial, low-dose therapy is defined as doses ranging from less than 1 MIU/m^2/day to 6 MIU/day. Numerous studies have now evaluated the immunomodulatory effects of low-dose IL-2 by measuring cytokine production and immune cell numbers and activity. In addition to its biological role as the main growth factor for T cells, the anticancer action of IL-2 is likely caused by the activation of NK cells and by their evolution into LAK cells. Data have demonstrated that sequential injections of low-dose IL-2 seem to induce a preferential increase in activated NK cells and eosinophils. This author postulates that not only is low-dose IL-2 less toxic than high-dose IL-2, but low-dose IL-2 is the most physiologically immunotherapeutic strategy to activate the anticancer immune response *in vivo*. In addition, abnormally low levels of IL-2 are found in blood samples from cancer patients and appear to correlate with poor prognosis and lower survival. Because of the important physiologic role of IL-2 in antitumor immune responses, these reduced endogenous levels of IL-2 may be considered one of the most important immune alterations associated with cancer and may be responsible, at least in part, for cancer progression. Therefore, the exogenous injection of IL-2 would represent not only an effective immunotherapy for cancer but also the best replacement therapy to correct one of the main pathological mechanisms responsible for cancer-related immunosuppression. From this author's perspective, the end point of clinical trials of IL-2 therapy should be the determination of the lowest dosage of IL-2 necessary to activate an effective *in vivo* anticancer immune response (Lissoni, 1997).

In 1995, the FDA approved high doses of IFN-α2b as adjuvant therapy for treatment of patients with melanoma who were at high risk for recurrence. IFN-α2b significantly prolonged both relapse-free survival and overall survival. Several other studies have attempted to replicate these results with lower-dose regimens that have less-toxic effects (Grob *et al.*, 1998; Pehamberger *et al.*, 1998; Ascierto *et al.*, 1999). Whereas data from these studies have demonstrated an improvement in relapse-free survival compared with observation only, no demonstrable effect on overall survival has been demonstrated. The majority of patients in these trials were categorized as being at intermediate risk for disease recurrence. The mechanism of action of IFN when used as adjuvant therapy for melanoma has yet to be elucidated, and may be due to direct antitumor effects, altered antitumor immune responses, or induction of tumor antigens that mark tumors for immune elimination. As future trials are designed and efforts are made to determine the optimal dose for IFN in the adjuvant setting, it will be increasingly important to understand the influence of IFN-α on immune responses in melanoma to determine the OBD (Kirkwood, 1998).

In summary, the optimal dose for many biological agents remains uncertain. Continuation of research that incorporates measurement of biological effects into clinical trials will provide the answer. Currently, with some biological agents, cost considerations have begun to impact dosing. With many of the hematopoietic growth factors, for example, doses are rounded up or down to approximate the nearest vial size so that drug is not wasted or so that it is not necessary to access a new vial for a small amount of drug to achieve the calculated per m^2 dose. An editorial by Ratain (1998) questioned the use of body surface area (BSA) as a basis for dosing of anticancer agents. BSA may not be the best tool to use to estimate dosing based on pharmacologic principles. Body size does not necessarily correlate with organ size and function. It has been suggested that lean body mass may be a better measure to use in determining dose, although it also does not take into account other important factors that determine drug clearance such as genetically determined polymorphisms in drug-metabolizing activity and reduced drug clearance caused by the effects of age or the malignancy itself (Ratain, 1998). This author calls for a new paradigm for determining dose levels that would simplify regimens and potentially eliminate BSA-based dosing when there has been no correlation between BSA and drug clearance.

Scheduling

Dose is not the only important factor to consider in achieving maximal biological effects. Scheduling may also have an impact. A study by Vadhan-Raj *et al.* (1992) evaluated the scheduling of GM-CSF after chemotherapy in patients with sarcoma to determine a schedule that would best abrogate myelosuppression. In the initial schedule, chemotherapy with cyclophosphamide, doxorubicin, and dacarbazine (CyADIC) was given on days 1 through 5 and GM-CSF was administered on days 8 through 21 by continuous intravenous infusion following the second cycle of chemotherapy (Figure 4.9). Although the rate of neutrophil recovery was enhanced, severe neutropenia was not eliminated. A modified schedule was then initiated to allow earlier administration of GM-CSF. The CyADIC treatment was compressed from 5 to 3 days, and GM-CSF was infused immediately

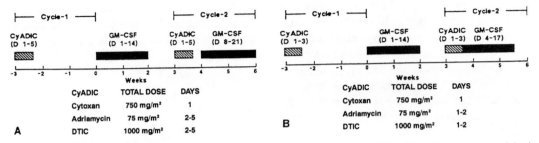

Figure 4.9   Schema of the initial therapeutic schedule of CyADIC and GM-CSF (A) and the modified therapeutic schedule (B) Abbreviations: CyADIC, cytoxan (cyclophosphamide), Adriamycin (doxorubicin), and DTIC (dacarbazine); GM-CSF, granulocyte-macrophage colony-stimulating factor; M-CSF, macrophage-colony stimulating factor.

Source: Reprinted with permission from the authors. Vadhan-Raj, S., Brormeyer, H., Hittleman, W., *et al.* 1992. Abrogating chemotherapy-induced myelosuppression by recombinant granulocyte-macrophage colony-stimulating factor in patients with sarcoma: Protection at the progenitor cell level. *Journal of Clinical Oncology* 10(8): 1266–1277. Figure 1, p. 1268.

following the completion of the second cycle of chemotherapy. On the modified schedule, GM-CSF significantly reduced both the degree and the duration of neutropenia and incidence of mucositis, and it allowed for higher doses of chemotherapy in 17 patients. These findings suggest that the timing of administration of growth factors and chemotherapy has a great impact on the degree of myeloprotection. This clinical study illustrates the point that optimal dose may not be the only factor important in obtaining the desired biological effect.

In an effort to continue to optimize dosing regimens, a study was done to determine whether administration of a single high dose of epoetin alfa was as effective as repeated administration of lower doses given by the subcutaneous route (Cheung *et al.*, 1998). In a randomized, placebo-controlled study, these researchers evaluated the traditional 3 times per week dosing schedule of 150 IU/kg versus 600 IU/kg given once weekly for 4 weeks. Other groups received single doses ranging from 300 IU/kg to 2,400 IU/kg. Data from these studies clearly demonstrated that the pharmacologic response of epoetin alfa is a function of both the dose and dosing regimen. After single subcutaneous doses ranging from 300 IU/kg to 2,400 IU/kg, serum erythropoietin concentrations rapidly increased then declined to endogenous erythropoietin levels by day 15. The mean percentage of reticulocytes increased then declined to baseline values by day 22. In contrast, 150 IU/kg administered 3 times a week was able to maintain serum erythropoietin concentrations and mean percentage of reticulocytes above the respective predose levels continuously through day 22. The 600 IU/kg once per week dosing regimen maintained serum erythropoietin levels at about the predose endogenous erythropoietin level for 5 to 8 days in a dosing week, and this regimen was also able to sustain the mean percentage of reticulocytes above the predose level through day 22. The investigators concluded that repeated subcutaneous administration (either 3 times weekly or higher doses weekly) was more effective in stimulating a reticulocyte response than large single doses of the same total amount of epoetin alfa.

Another area not often considered that may impact scheduling of drugs and ultimately determination of dose, is chronotherapy. Circadian variation in drug metabolism and tissue sensitivity to drugs impacts their activity and toxicity. A growing body of data suggests that response to therapy may be improved and toxicity may be reduced by administering antineoplastic agents at carefully selected times of the day. A proponent of this theory, William J. Hrushesky, noted that data exist that support the predictable and exploitable nonlinear dynamic relationship between dose and effect that occurs each day (Hrushesky, 1991; Hrushesky, 1995). He contends that researchers must explore the ways in which clinical research can determine when to treat and must wrestle with the question of the stability of circadian time structure in chronically ill cancer patients. Few studies have evaluated this concept in conjunction with the administration of biological agents. Levi *et al.* (1991) provided an overview of chronotherapy and biological agents. They noted that immune defenses are organized along both 24-hour and yearly time scales. Two circadian systems have been isolated in man, which can be desynchronized: the circulation of T-, B-, and NK-lymphocyte subsets in peripheral blood and the density of epitope molecules at their surface. They hypothesize that the temporally optimized delivery of biological agents may be guided by immunologic rhythms. They also reviewed several small-scale preliminary studies that yielded dose intensities 2 to 4 times higher than those usually recommended when IFN was given at specific times of the day, specifically the evening. Iacobelli *et al.* (1995) presented results from a phase I trial of IFN-α administered at a circadian-rhythmn-modulated rate to evaluate MTDs and toxicity. The IFN-α was administered as a 7-day continuous intravenous infusion with maximum delivery between 6 P.M. and 3 A.M. A programmable-in-time infusion pump was used. They reported that compared with standard subcutaneous and intramuscular injection, this circadian schedule allowed delivery of high doses of IFN with acceptable toxicity. Based on empiric evidence, nurses often recommend that biologics such as

IFN be given in the evening to lessen side effects. As of yet, chronobiology and the administration of biologics remains a largely unexplored area.

Biotherapy in Combination Therapy Regimens

As success was achieved with the use of biological agents in the treatment of cancer, the next logical step in assessing these agents was evaluation of their combination with other biological agents or with other therapies (chemotherapy or radiation therapy) to improve their therapeutic indices. Issues such as the rationale for selecting a certain combination and the dose and schedule to be used remain important. This section will review and analyze the rationale for combining biotherapy with chemotherapy, review historical work that has evaluated the proposed benefits of combination therapies, and highlight several clinical examples of combination therapies. The toxicities associated with these combinations will also be discussed.

Goals of Combination Therapy

The ultimate goal of cancer therapy is patient survival. The first principle in reaching this goal is that the patient must first achieve a complete response. When the patient has maintained a complete response over a defined period of time (usually 5 years), he or she can then be considered cured. The question then is how available therapies can be better utilized to achieve cure.

One approach is the use of combination therapies with the intent of increasing response rates. Two agents would ideally provide better results than one. Generally, when agents are combined, it is because they have demonstrated synergistic and not just additive effects. A useful illustration of the difference between synergistic and additive effects is as follows: with additive effects,

$$1 + 1 = 2,$$

whereas with synergy,

$$1 + 1 = 4.$$

To design an effective combination regimen, several issues, including dosing, scheduling, and rationale, must be addressed. An ideal combination would have less severe toxicity than either agent alone; thus, one of the primary goals of combining agents is to achieve non-overlapping toxicity.

Although certain of the biological agents that are used singly have been observed to induce responses, only a small percentage of patients receiving these single agents have achieved long-standing remission or cure. The major opportunity for success may rest on rational combinations of biological agents. Because of their redundant and pleiotropic nature, combinations of cytokines may be synergistic or antagonistic; amplification or limitation of a response may also occur through the cytokine cascade when one cytokine induces the synthesis of another (Kelso, 1989). Determination of effective combinations through *in vitro* work or animal models should serve as the foundation for designing effective combinations.

Combinations of Biological Agents

A variety of combinations of biological agents have now been tested clinically. A brief overview of key studies of these combinations is given here; more thorough overviews are provided in other chapters. Refer to Atkins *et al.* (1995) for a thorough review of biotherapy combined with cytokines. Combinations of different IFNs, IFN and IL-2, IFN or IL-2 with monoclonal antibodies, and TNF with IFN or IL-2 are representative of the major combina-

tions that have undergone investigation (Mulé and Rosenberg, 1989; Gilewski and Golomb, 1990; Mulé and Rosenberg, 1991). In addition, the investigation of combinations of hematopoietic growth factors has also been an area of intense research (Valle and Scarffe, 1998).

Numerous clinical trials have evaluated the combination of IFN and IL-2 in patients with advanced malignancies. The rationale for combining IFN and IL-2 is based on their differing mechanisms of action: IL-2 acts primarily as an immunomodulatory agent, whereas IFN has antiproliferative effects. However, IFN may also serve to augment the expression of histocompatibility antigens on tumor cells, making them more susceptible to IL-2-sensitized lymphocytes (Figlin, 1992). Even though potent synergism is seen *in vitro* with this combination, its mechanism is as yet undetermined. To date, most responses to this combination are seen in patients with renal cell cancer or melanoma. A recent review by Bukowski (1999) summarized the results of clinical trials evaluating this combination in renal cancer. Over 1,400 patients have received IFN-α therapy in combination with several differing IL-2 regimens (e.g., subcutaneous administration, continuous intravenous infusion, and intravenous bolus infusion). Overall, the response rate was approximately 20%, with about 3% to 5% of patients achieving a durable, complete remission. Randomized trials have also evaluated this combination (Henriksson *et al.*, 1998; Negrier *et al.*, 1998) and found higher response with the combination but in association with more significant toxicity. Event-free survival was increased in the Negrier study, but not overall survival. Based on the sum results of the work completed to date, it appears that the combination of IFN-α and IL-2 may increase response rates in renal cancer, but improvement in overall survival is not yet clear. In metastatic melanoma, a number of phase II trials have evaluated the combination of IFN-α and IL-2 (Keilholz *et al.*, 1997). The combined data from the studies yields an average response rate of 22% (range, 10% to 41%), demonstrating no significant clinical benefit. A randomized trial evaluating the difference between single-agent IL-2 and the combination of IFN-α and IL-2 was terminated because of low response rates in both arms (Sparano *et al.*, 1993). In this area, the current focus of therapy is on the use of biochemotherapy.

Another area of exploration involves combinations of monoclonal antibodies and other biological agents. The proposed rationale for using monoclonal antibodies and IL-2 lies with the antibody's reaction with target cells and mediation of tumor destruction through binding complement or via effector cells by **antibody-dependent cell-mediated cytotoxicity**. In short, IL-2 would be used to stimulate LAK effector cells (Mulé and Rosenberg, 1991). With IFNs, upregulation of tumor-associated antigens or major histocompatibility antigens on tumor cells may serve to improve targeting of antibodies to tumor cells.

Clinical trials evaluating these combinations remain an active area of investigation. Early trials investigating the combination of IL-2 and monoclonal antibodies in patients with neuroblastoma concluded that the approach may be more effective in patients with minimal residual disease. Additional phase II studies and future phase III trials will be necessary to fully determine the efficacy of this combination (Sondel and Hank, 1997). Other trials have evaluated the ability of IFN-α to upregulate tumor-associated antigens. A report by Macey *et al.* (1997) summarized the results of using IFN-α to upregulate tumor-associated glycoprotein 72 (TAG-72) on tumors. To determine whether recombinant IFN-α (rIFN-α) could enhance TAG-72 expression *in vivo* in patients, 15 women with breast cancer were randomized to receive daily injections of rIFN-α (3 $\times$ 10^6 units/m^2 for 14 days) beginning on day 1 (group 1, 7 patients) or on day 6 (group 2, 8 patients). On day 3, all patients received a 10 to 20 mCi

tracer dose of ^{131}I-CC49, a high-affinity murine monoclonal antibody reactive against TAG-72, followed by a therapeutic dose of 60 to 75 mCi/m^2 of ^{131}I-CC49 on day 6. Treatment with rIFN-α was found to enhance TAG-72 expression in tumors from patients receiving rIFN-α (group 1) by 46 $\pm$ 19% ($p < .05$) compared with only 1.3 $\pm$ 0.95% in patients not initially receiving IFN (group 2). The uptake of CC49 in tumors was also significantly increased in rIFN-α-treated patients. One partial and two minor tumor responses were seen. In summary, rIFN-α treatment altered the pharmacokinetics and tumor uptake of ^{131}I-CC49 in patients at the expense of increased toxicity. This study demonstrates how monitoring of biological effects can determine the additive benefit of combination therapies. Although these data are encouraging, further study of the combination of IFN-α and monoclonal antibodies remains necessary.

The availability of recombinant hematopoietic growth factors has made possible the study of both the physiology of the cytokines and their pharmacodynamic effects when used alone and in combination with other hematopoietic growth factors. Numerous studies have investigated the *in vitro* and *in vivo* combination of white blood cell growth factors (single-lineage factors) plus multilineage growth factors and white blood cell growth factors plus erythropoietin. The majority of clinical studies to date are limited to phase I/II safety and toxicity-defining studies. Prospective, randomized trials will be needed to determine whether the coadministration of hematopoietic growth factors leads to a more rapid rescue of hematopoietic activity after myelosuppressive treatment or bone marrow transplantation. The *ex vivo* expansion of progenitor cells is also a major focus of research. Figure 4.10 demonstrates preclinical studies evaluating the coadministration of stem cell factor and G-CSF. A significant increase in peripheral blood nucleated cells was seen. Clinical trials in patients are currently being

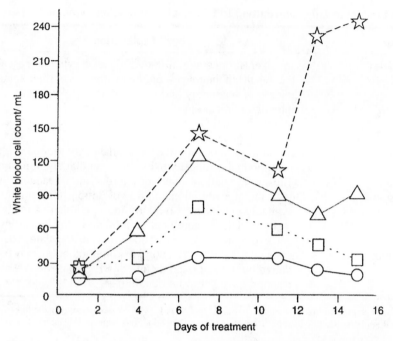

Figure 4.10   The changes in peripheral blood nucleated cell count in mice during treatment with recombinant rodent stem cell factor (rrSCF) (100 μg/kg/day) either alone or in combination with filgrastim (G-CSF) at doses between 0.1 and 2.5 μg/kg/day. Circles = rrSCF; squares = rrSCF + filgrastim 0.1 μg/kg/day; triangles = rrSCF + filgrastim 1 μg/kg/day; stars = rrSCF + filgrastim 25 μg/kg/day.

Source: Reprinted with permission from Mazanet, R., Morstyn, G., and Foote, M. 1998. *Filgrastim in Clinical Practice*, 2nd edn. New York: Marcel Dekker, Inc., Figure 2, p. 53.

done to evaluate the use of this combination for improving the yield of stem cell harvests for transplantation (Valle and Scarffe, 1998).

Investigation of the many possible combinations of biological agents continues. As predicted by Kelso (1989), it is unlikely that all possible combinations of the 20-plus known cytokines will be tested. It is crucial, therefore, that *in vitro* and animal model data be used to guide the rational combination of these agents. When clinical successes are seen, prospective randomized trials must then be used to delineate the full benefit. Atkins *et al.* (1995) discussed some of the potential factors that may contribute to the failure of combination cytokine thera-

pies that appear so promising in preclinical study. Table 4.2 outlines these issues.

Biological Agents and Chemotherapy

RATIONALE

Studies of the combination of biotherapy and chemotherapy became an active area of investigation in the late 1980s (Mitchell, 1988). The interaction of cytokines and cytotoxic drugs may occur on several levels (Figure 4.11) (Kreuser, 1992; Kreuser *et al.*, 1995). The rationales for using the biotherapy/chemotherapy combination approach are that (1) the two

Table 4.2   Factors potentially contributing to failure of combination cytokine therapy

Factor	Explanation
Cytokine cascades	Many agents, once administered, trigger a cytokine cascade *in vivo* that results in the release of other cytokines or their antagonists. The release of secondary and even tertiary cytokines may impact the intended clinical effect as well as toxicity. More subtle dosing and scheduling may be required to achieve the desired therapeutic goal and biological effect.
Overlapping mechanisms of action	The antitumor mechanism of any single agent remains obscure. It is possible that distinct cytokines have similar antitumor mechanisms. Thus, combinations may not improve the therapeutic index.
Scheduling issues	Due to the almost unlimited array of options for combining the available cytokines, it remains an incredible challenge to design rational trials for combination therapies. Preclinical investigation and exploration in animal models may not translate to use in humans.
Genetic limitations	Each patient's ability to respond to immunotherapy may be genetically determined. Factors predictive of which patients are most likely to respond have yet to be determined.

Source: Adapted with permission from Atkins, M., Tréhu, E., and Mier, J. 1995. Combination cytokine therapy. In DeVita, V., Hellman, S., and Rosenberg, S. (eds). *Biologic Therapy of Cancer,* 2nd edn. Philadelphia, PA: Lippincott, pp. 443–460.

therapies have different mechanisms of action, in essence resulting in a two-pronged attack on the tumor; (2) the combination facilitates modulation of the pharmacokinetics or action of the chemotherapeutic agent on key enzymes, alteration of drug-resistance mechanisms, and alteration of cell-cycle kinetics; and (3) the two therapies have nonoverlapping toxicities. Further rationales include modifications in the permeability of the vascular system that allow increased accumulation of chemotherapeutic drugs at the tumor site, reduction of the tumor burden, use of one modality as maintenance therapy, and use of one modality to improve patient tolerance of cytotoxic agents (Parmiani and Rivoltini, 1991; Krueser, 1992; Pazdur, 1992; Baselga and Mendelsohn, 1995).

It is useful to explore in more depth the concept of differing mechanisms of action. Chemotherapy targets rapidly dividing cells and through various mechanisms causes cell death. Biological agents or cytokines, which are some-times termed "biomodulators," modulate biological responses through various actions, including (1) augmenting the patient's antitumor response (e.g., stimulation of effector cells or increased production of cytokines), (2) decreasing suppressor mechanisms, (3) increasing the patient's immunological defenses, (4) increasing the patient's ability to tolerate damage by cytotoxic modalities, (5) changing membrane characteristics of the tumor cell to make it more susceptible to killing by chemotherapeutic agents, (6) preventing or reversing transformation, or (7) decreasing the ability of tumor cells to metastasize (Kreuser, 1992; Baselga and Mendelsohn, 1995; Kreuser *et al.*, 1995).

The term "biomodulation" may also be used in another context. When agents are combined, one agent can cause the biochemical modulation of another. A definition of this type of modulation would be the enhancement of the antitumor activity of an effector agent by a second agent (Schmoll *et al.*, 1992). With

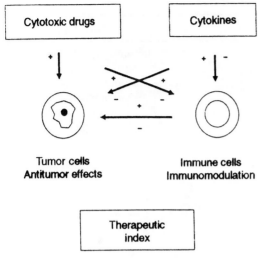

Figure 4.11 Interaction of cytokines and cytotoxic drugs.

Source: Reprinted with permission from *Seminars in Oncology* and the authors Kreuser, E., Wadler, S., Theil, E., *et al.* 1992. Interactions between cytokines and cytotoxic drugs: Putative molecular mechanisms in experimental hematology and oncology. *Seminars in Oncology* 19(2 Suppl 4): 1–7. Figure 1, p. 3.

biochemical modulation, the modulator manipulates the metabolic pathway of a cytotoxic drug to increase the efficacy or selective protection of normal tissue or both. Cytokines can also serve as biochemical modulators, with multiple levels of interaction between chemotherapy and cytokines possible. Targets of modulation include specific enzymes of drug metabolism, receptors for adhesion or growth, cell-cycle phases, gene expression, and the immune system (Table 4.3) (Kreuser, 1992).

DOSING

Dosing has already been reviewed. Although the hope is that combining agents will decrease the amount that is needed of each, this may not be the case. Again, the desired biological effect must be identified so that the proper dose can be administered.

SCHEDULING

To avoid one agent negating the effects of the other or to obtain maximum benefit, scheduling issues are of utmost importance when combining chemotherapy with biotherapy. *In vitro* studies can be used as a guide to determine whether biotherapy should be given before, during, or after chemotherapy. A primary question that must be answered in determining sequence is whether the chemotherapy agent being used is immunosuppressive. Typically, chemotherapy is given before biotherapy, proposedly because this sequence reduces the tumor burden; allows for recovery from the immunosuppressive effects of chemotherapy; eliminates suppressor influences (such as CD8$^+$ cells); and alters the tumor cell membranes, which may lead to exposure of antigens, thereby increasing the susceptibility of tumor cells to lysis by immune cells. Table 4.4 illustrates the relative immunosuppressive activity of various chemotherapeutic agents (Gilewski and Golomb, 1990). It is interesting to note that not all chemotherapy agents are immunosuppressive, and the immunosuppressive effects of those that are are dose dependent.

CLINICAL EXAMPLES

IFN-α again serves as a clinical example to illustrate the principles of combination therapy. Many *in vitro* studies using both tumor cell lines and animal tumor models have analyzed the activity of IFN-α in combination with other cytotoxic agents. Preclinical data have identified a variety of chemotherapeutic agents that are positively modulated by IFN (Table 4.5) including at least one from every class of chemotherapeutic drugs: alkylating agents, mitotic spindle inhibitors, anthracyclines, heavy metals, antibiotics, antimetabolites, and steroids (Wadler and Schwartz, 1992). This broad spectrum of activity suggests at least two possible mechanisms. Either IFN-α possesses a single fundamental action that affects nearly every

Table 4.3 Cytotoxic drug-cytokine interactions: levels of mechanisms

Tumor Cells	Host Cells
Cellular modulation	Immunomodulation
Enzymes	Natural killer cells
Topoisomerase	Monocytes
Thymidylate synthase	Macrophages
Thymidine kinase	Cytotoxic T lymphocytes
Pyrimidine phosphorylase	Pharmacologic modulation
DNA	Liver cells
Gene expression	
Receptors	
Adhesion receptors	
Growth factor receptors	
Cytokine receptors	
Cell-cycle phase	
G_0/G_1 arrest	
G_0/G_1 recruitment	
Effects on tumor-cell vasculature	

Source: Reprinted with permission from *Seminars in Oncology* and the authors. Kreuser, E., Wadler, S., and Thiel, E. 1992. Interactions between cytokines and cytotoxic drugs: Putative molecular mechanisms in experimental hematology and oncology. *Seminars in Oncology* 19(2 suppl 4): 1–7. Table 3, p. 3.

Table 4.4 Immunosuppressive activity of chemotherapeutic agents

Class of Agent	Demonstrated Activity	Minor Activity
Alkylating agents	Cyclophosphamide Nitrosoureas	Busulfan, dimethyl busulfan, dacarbazine
Antibiotics	Daunorubicin	Bleomycin, doxorubicin, mithramycin
Folic acid antagonists	Methotrexate	
Purine analogs	6-Mercaptopurine Azathioprine	
Pyrimidine analogs	5-FU, Cytarabine	
Vinca alkaloids	Vincristine Vinblastine	

Source: Reprinted with permission from *Seminars in Oncology* and the authors. Gilewski, T., and Golomb, H. 1990. Design of combination biotherapy studies: Future goals and challenges. *Seminars in Oncology* 17(1 suppl 1): 3–10. Table 1, p. 4.

aspect of cell growth and replication or it acts at multiple levels, with different actions predominating in different cell types. In all likelihood, the predominant mechanism of action depends on the cytotoxic drug used (Wadler and Schwartz, 1992).

One of the most exciting areas to initially emerge in the study of combination therapy was the evaluation of the combination of IFN-α with 5-FU. *In vitro* studies have demonstrated that synergy was both dose- and schedule-dependent and was seen only when IFN-α was given

Table 4.5 Cytotoxic drugs with activity modulated by IFNs

Cisplatin	Cyclophosphamide
Doxorubicin	Fluorouracil
Melphalan	Methotrexate
Mitomycin	Mechlorethamine
Vinblastine	Vincristine
Dactinomycin	ACNU
Carmustine	Bleomycin
Cytarabine	Difluoromethylornithine
Neocarzinostatin	(DFMO)
Prednisone	Peplomycin
	Thioguanine

Source: Reprinted with permission from *Seminars in Oncology* and the authors. Wadler, S., and Schwartz, E. 1992. Principles in the biomodulation of cytotoxic drugs by interferons. *Seminars in Oncology* 19(2 suppl 3): 45–48. Table 2, p. 47.

before or concurrently with 5-FU (Sznol and Longo, 1993). Proposed explanations for this synergy include the ability of IFN-α to increase plasma levels of active metabolites of 5-FU, decrease resistance to 5-FU by inhibiting overexpression of thymidylate synthase, alter the cell cycle to enhance antiproliferative effects, activate the patient's immunological defense mechanisms, and induce direct but separate antiproliferative effects (Meadows *et al.*, 1991; Kreuser, 1992; Schuller *et al.*, 1992; Wadler, 1992; Wadler and Schwartz, 1992). Initial studies by Wadler *et al.* (1989) showed a 76% rate of response to this combination in patients with colon cancer. Even though most responses were only partial remissions, the study generated tremendous excitement and follow-up studies in other types of cancer. Further clinical evaluation of this combination by Wadler and other investigators (Wadler and Wiernick, 1990; Kemeny and Younes, 1992; Pazdur, 1992; Pazdur *et al.*, 1992) demonstrated efficacy in a lower percentage of patients (see Chapter 5). Ultimately, the optimism was followed by disappointment. Nine phase III randomized trials that included over 1,700 patients failed to dem-

onstrate any improvement in response, and many trials concluded a substantial increase in toxicity. In conclusion, the combination that initially yielded such excitement has not fulfilled original expectations (Kjaer, 1996). The use of subcutaneous rhIL-2, IFN-α, and 5-FU has been investigated in patients with renal cancer. Preliminary data have been published from 1 randomized trial, but no definitive conclusions have yet been made as to the benefits of the combination in renal cell cancer (Bukowski, 1999). A review by Hernber *et al.* (1999) reported the results of a meta-analysis comprising all available randomized trials comparing regimens with or without IFN-α in metastatic melanoma and renal cell carcinoma. This included trials with biological agents, chemotherapy, biological agents plus chemotherapy, and IFN. The analysis showed that regimens including IFN-α improved response rates compared with regimens without IFN-α, and in metastatic melanoma, a trend toward prolonged survival was noted. The authors recommend that future randomized trials both in metastatic melanoma and advanced renal cell carcinoma should evaluate not only response rate but also overall survival as primary end points to allow the evaluation of the total benefit of immunotherapy in advanced disease. Many authors contend that with biological treatment, instead of recording only the responses, one should take into account disease stabilization and survival.

The combination of IL-2 and chemotherapy has also been evaluated extensively. The use of low-dose cyclophosphamide to eliminate suppressor influences prior to administration of IL-2 was evaluated by Mitchell (1992). A 26% rate of response to this combination was reported in patients with melanoma (Mitchell, 1992). The median survival period of responders in the study was 18 months compared with the historical overall survival duration of 12 months in melanoma patients with recurrent disease. Although these data did not conclusively prove that the combination regimen resulted in greater longevity, there was a strong suggestion to that effect. However, one clear and important finding from the study was that patients do not need to achieve a complete remission to have an increased lifespan and good quality of life. Although the overall response rate of 26% was not better than traditional response rates to chemotherapy with dacarbazine, nitrosoureas, vindesine/vinblastine, or cisplatin alone, the suggestion of improved survival and relative lack of toxicity certainly warrants further exploration.

A large number of experiments have evaluated the combination of chemotherapy and IL-2 in animal models. In most cases, these combinations are effective only if the host immune system is intact and if the tumor is sensitive to IL-2 (i.e., immunogenic). Possible explanations for the beneficial effect of adding chemotherapy to treatment with IL-2 include modulation of the immune system as noted in the example above, alteration of the tumor-cell membrane to increase immunogenicity, and debulking of the tumor. To date, many different combinations of chemotherapy with IL-2 or IL-2 and IFN-α have been tested in the clinical setting. Impressive results have been seen in trials using combination biotherapy and chemotherapy (i.e., biochemotherapy). Beginning in early 1990, several investigators began to examine the efficacy of combination chemotherapy regimens used in conjunction with combination biotherapy for the treatment of melanoma. Initial protocols developed by Legha (1997) used a sequential regimen of cisplatin, vinblastine, and dacarbazine in combination with biotherapy using recombinant IL-2 and recombinant IFN-α. The regimen ultimately evolved to a concurrent regimen of all 5 drugs and was termed concurrent biochemotherapy. Between the 2 regimens, Legha and associates reported 114 evaluable patients with a 21% complete response rate and 39% partial

response rate, yielding an overall response rate of 60% (Legha et al., 1997). The response rates were essentially the same for sequential and concurrent biochemotherapy; however, the latter had less toxicity. Although no immunological monitoring has been reported for this regimen, this study does illustrate the important implications of scheduling on toxicity. The average response rate for combination chemotherapy regimens alone is approximately 30%, thus biochemotherapy appears to be superior to combination chemotherapy. Several other investigators have reported similar results using different chemotherapy regimens (Legha, 1997). To determine whether biological therapy definitely enhances the effects of chemotherapy, randomized phase III trials are ongoing (Sznol and Longo, 1993; Legha et al., 1997; McDermott et al., 2000).

Biotherapy may also be used as maintenance therapy after chemotherapy. In one of the first clinical trials reporting the use of IFN-α as maintenance therapy, Mandelli et al. (1990) evaluated its utility in patients with multiple myeloma and found improved duration of response that translated into overall improved survival in the group that received IFN. This statistically significant advantage was seen only in patients who had achieved an objective response to induction chemotherapy. Rationale for the use of IFN-α as maintenance therapy includes its ability to reduce the capacity for self-renewal in myeloma cells, its modulation of oncogene expression, and its antiproliferative activity (Cooper, 1991). A review of the use of IFN in the treatment of myeloma (Gisslinger, 1997) evaluated data from 8 trials comprising 929 patients randomized for IFN treatment or watchful waiting following chemotherapy for multiple myeloma. IFN maintenance treatment prolonged the average relapse-free survival by 7 months and prolonged the average overall survival by 5 months. Younger patients, patients with good performance status, and patients with lower tumor burden seem to benefit most from the addition of IFN to chemotherapy or from IFN as maintenance therapy. This author concluded that IFN has a minor beneficial effect on response rates, progression-free survival, and overall survival in the above-mentioned patient group and might be applied when high-dose chemotherapy with transplantation is not feasible. IFN has been shown to be effective for maintenance therapy in patients with lower tumor burden who have responded to induction therapy.

IFN has also been actively investigated as maintenance therapy and as an addition to combination chemotherapy in non-Hodgkin's lymphoma. Randomized trials in the use of IFN both in combination approaches and as maintenance has demonstrated a longer duration of response and time to progression (or treatment failure) (Baselga and Mendelsohn, 1995). Arrantz et al. (1998) reported that adding IFN alfa-2b to induction chemotherapy in low-grade NHL did not induce a higher response rate, but it significantly increased the duration of the responses. The investigators found significant differences in progression-free survival that favored the patients who received chemotherapy plus IFN, but not in overall survival. To date, no additional benefit has been seen from the administration of IFN for maintenance. Research continues in this area.

The introduction of hematopoietic growth factors to combination regimens was an attempt to use biological agents to significantly reduce the toxicity associated with chemotherapy. In general, the effectiveness of chemotherapy in treating most tumors is limited by two major problems: drug resistance and the toxic effects of the drug in normal tissues. Although hematopoietic growth factors represent a major breakthrough in treating the problem of chemotherapy-induced myelosuppression, several problems remain. Although these agents are highly effective in ameliorating myelosuppres-

sion, increased doses of chemotherapy may lead to other organ toxicities upon which hematopoietic growth factors have no protective effect or in which myelosuppression may not be the dose-limiting toxic effect of a chemotherapeutic agent. Also, whether more dose-intensive chemotherapy will lead to improved response and prolonged overall survival has not yet been determined. Large-scale studies are needed to prove that dose-intensive therapies with hematopoietic growth factor support can be administered with acceptable toxicity and costs (Demetri and Griffin, 1990; Canelos and Demetri, 1993). At the 1999 meeting of the American Society of Clinical Oncology, five studies on the use of high-dose chemotherapy and bone marrow transplantation were presented. The presentation at a plenary session sparked controversy because only one study from a South African team of researchers showed any benefit with the use of the high-dose therapy. The other four studies revealed no survival difference between women given standard therapy for breast cancer and those given high doses of drugs followed by bone marrow or stem cell transplant. Discussion during and after the plenary session offered no additional insight regarding the use of high-dose therapy (Stadtmauer et al., 1999). The South African team, led by Dr. Bezwoda, later admitted to scientific misconduct by using a different control regimen than that described in the abstract (Horton, 2000).

FURTHER ISSUES REGARDING COMBINATIONS OF BIOTHERAPY AND CHEMOTHERAPY

Although exciting results have emerged from the use of combination chemotherapy and biotherapy, many issues are yet to be addressed. It is disappointing that randomized trials are often not confirmatory of initial results. Often, agents are combined solely because each has shown clinical activity in treating a given disease. A clinical trial, however, should be based on firm, preclinical rationale rather than an empirical approach. Elucidation of the mechanisms of action of biological agents and chemotherapeutic agents as well as an understanding of mechanisms of synergism are musts in applying a rational approach to combination therapy. Refinement of dose, schedule, and route of administration will then be facilitated. Early work with the use of animal models focused mostly on evaluating schedules, sequencing and doses rather than on understanding the mechanisms of synergism (Parmiani and Rivoltini, 1991). The need for more predictive preclinical models remains critical. Until these are available, however, the design of combination trials must rely partly on reasonable evaluation of preclinical data and partly on empiricism (Sznol and Longo, 1993). If heightened responses are seen, evaluation of remission rates and durability of response must be assessed through large-scale randomized trials. Future directions include targeting therapy by using monoclonal antibodies with biotherapy, chemotherapy, or radioisotopes attached and introducing new hematopoietic growth factors or combinations of growth factors that can further abrogate chemotherapy-induced suppression of bone marrow. A better understanding of cancer biology, the use of chemotherapy plus target-specific biological agents, bioactive peptides, or organic molecules with well-defined mechanisms of action and nonoverlapping toxicities hold promise for clinical investigation in the future (Baselga and Mendelsohn, 1995). Exciting possibilities remain for the combination of very different modalities that will ultimately lead to improved patient responses, cure rates, and survival rates.

BIOTHERAPY AND RADIATION THERAPY

Evaluation of combinations of radiation therapy and biotherapy, and the rationale for doing so, remains at an early stage (Hallahan et al., 1990;

Devine et al., 1991; Hallahan et al., 1993). An active area of study involves the use of monoclonal antibodies conjugated to radioisotopes to selectively deliver radiation to the tumor site. This form of therapy, known as radioimmunotherapy, has demonstrated clinical success most specifically in the hematologic malignancies and will be discussed in more detail in Chapter 8.

TOXICITY

Toxicity remains an important issue when considering combination therapy. In theory, the use of combinations of biotherapy and chemotherapy would capitalize on the fact that these agents have essentially nonoverlapping toxic effects. Toxicities are often additive with biological agents, unless lower doses are utilized. The most common side effects of biological agents (constitutional symptoms, fatigue, anorexia, changes in mental status, reversible changes in laboratory values, and allergic reactions) differ significantly from those of chemotherapy (bone marrow suppression with resultant anemia, thrombocytopenia, neutropenia, nausea and vomiting, mucositis, and alopecia). Nurses caring for patients receiving combination therapies should be aware of the expected toxic effects of individual agents and should also assess for unexpected adverse reactions. Such unexpected adverse effects seen with combinations of IFN-α and 5-FU include increased incidence and severity of mucositis, diarrhea, neurotoxicity (dependent on patient age and degree of liver involvement), and prolonged granulocytopenia (Kemeny and Younes, 1992; Pazdur, 1992). With combinations of IFN-α and IL-2, the major treatment-limiting toxic effects were neurologic (e.g., confusion), gastrointestinal (e.g., nausea and vomiting), and fatigue (Rosenberg et al., 1989; Figlin, 1992). Many of the biochemotherapy regimens for melanoma have substantial toxicity and require administration in the inpatient setting and intensive nursing care (Legha *et al.*, 1997).

Outcomes of Therapy

The final factor to consider with respect to dosing in biotherapy is determination of the outcome of therapy. An essential component of determining the appropriate dose of a drug is determining how long therapy should be administered. This decision ultimately hinges on measurement of a clinical response. As we gain sophistication in the use of biological agents and as successes are seen in various disorders, questions of when to stop therapy will arise. In some diseases, achieving a complete response is the desired goal, whereas in other situations, it may be argued that stabilizing disease with improved quality of life is an appropriate goal (Mitchell, 1992). Typically, the time period required to achieve responses with biological agents is longer than that required with chemotherapy; hence, caution must be exercised to avoid halting therapy prematurely.

For many diseases, technology has changed the way response to therapy is evaluated. Patients with chronic myelogenous leukemia provide an interesting illustration of technology's role in changing the definition of response and ultimately of cure in certain diseases. Traditionally, hematologic remission (normalization of peripheral blood counts) has been used as the benchmark for evaluating response. Cytogenetic analysis now provides a more precise determination of when therapy should be discontinued. The use of **cytogenetics** (the study of cytology in relation to **genetics**) to measure response in patients with this disease facilitated a more accurate determination of complete response.

Cytogenetics specifically looks at the behavior of **chromosomes** during **mitosis** and **meio-**sis (Heim and Mitelman, 1987). Bone marrow smears of the majority of patients with chronic myelogenous leukemia exhibit the **Philadelphia chromosome**, a shortened chromosome number 22, as a marker for this disease. The classic Philadelphia chromosome results from a **translocation** between chromosomes 9 and 22, which results in the production of a new protein (Kurzrock *et al.*, 1988). Because of this translocation, the *ABL* gene is transferred from its normal location on chromosome 9 and placed next to the disrupted proximal end of the *BCR* gene on chromosome 22. A chimeric gene, *BCR-ABL*, is produced and codes for the new protein. IFN-α, which is used to treat patients with chronic myelogenous leukemia, has demonstrated the ability to suppress the Philadelphia chromosome in some patients (Talpaz *et al.*, 1991). The degree of disappearance of the Philadelphia chromosome from the bone marrow is now used to determine response.

Technology has progressed even further with the introduction of molecular analysis. This technique, which involves the use of molecular probes that can identify the altered gene produced in the translocation, can be used to monitor therapies even more precisely. Molecular analysis provides for the evaluation of both dividing and nondividing cells and detects minute amounts of the Philadelphia chromosome in patients (Yoffe, 1987). For example, a patient who shows a complete disappearance of the Philadelphia chromosome by cytogenetic analysis may still exhibit a small amount of disease with this new technique. Indeed, many studies have suggested that most if not all patients with chronic myelogenous leukemia who are in IFN-α-induced cytogenetic remission remain positive for BCR-ABL transcripts when analyzed by the reverse transcriptase polymerase chain reaction (PCR) technique. A study by Kurzrock and colleagues examined 18 patients who had been in cytogenetic remission for over one year

(Kurzrock *et al.*, 1998). Ten of 18 patients demonstrated reverse-transcription PCR negativity for BCR-ABL transcripts. Research is attempting to correlate PCR positivity and PCR negativity with potential for relapse. The results of this study together with other experience and data from patients who received bone marrow suggest that serial PCR studies of IFN-α-treated patients with CML in long-term cytogenetic remission should be performed to ascertain whether persistent negativity is relevant to outcome and useful in determining a time point at which discontinuation of IFN therapy is reasonable (Kurzrock *et al.*, 1998). PCR technology is also used to assess response in indolent lymphoma. From the available literature, it seems that the achievement of a molecular complete response (PCR negativity for *bcl-2*) is a desirable objective. Patients who achieve a persistently negative PCR state seldom relapse. Whereas IFN has been shown to increase the length of remission in patients with advanced indolent lymphomas, the question of whether it is capable of increasing the molecular complete-response rate as measured by PCR remains unknown (Cabanillas, 1997).

Efforts have also begun to focus on how to best predict which patients will respond to therapy. Keilholz and colleagues (1998) reported on the European Organization for Research and Treatment of Cancer Melanoma Cooperative Group experience with IL-2. This group activated the first prospectively randomized phase III trial in 1993 to evaluate the individual components of chemoimmunotherapy regimens for their impact on response, response duration, and survival in melanoma patients. They reported analysis of survival data from previous nonrandomized studies. This first analysis of data from twelve institutions revealed that serum lactate dehydrogenase and the presence of high tumor burden were the most important prognostic factors for survival. A database of over 600 melanoma patients was analyzed to address the question of what factors are prognostic for response and survival. The authors concluded that serum lactate dehydrogenase, metastatic site, and performance status are useful stratification factors for randomized trials in metastatic melanoma. This important information, which has provided factors that will ultimately serve as prognostic indicators, will certainly guide the selection of patients that may benefit the most from high-dose, aggressive combination therapies.

Studies have also evaluated the goal of predicting response in the use of hematopoietic growth factors. Adamson and Ludwig (1999) reported that changes in levels of serum transferrin receptor protein, hemoglobin, ferritin, and reticulocyte count following a short course of epoetin alfa therapy were useful markers for predicting later hematopoietic response to epoetin alfa. Data have suggested that low baseline erythropoietin levels, in association with an increase of greater than 0.5 g/dL in hemoglobin or greater than or equal to a 25% increase in circulating levels of transferrin receptor protein after 2 weeks of epoetin alfa therapy are highly predictive of a response ($\geq$ 2 g/dL increase in hemoglobin). These authors contend that progress has clearly been made in the development of predictive models that can identify those patients most likely to respond to epoetin alfa by monitoring several specific hematological parameters at baseline and early in therapy.

Although cure is generally the desired goal, with many biological agents, only partial or minor responses are seen. In a small percentage of these patients, however, disease may remain stable or quiescent for long periods of time. If stabilization of disease and improved quality of life were valued as a desired therapeutic goal, then less sophisticated means of determining response could be used to evaluate response (Pyrhönen, 1992). Measurement of quality of life, an increasingly active focus in oncology research, can also be used to evaluate the outcome of therapy in conjunction with more traditional diagnostic tests when quality of life is included as a component of outcome.

Future Directions

The issue of attaining the OBD is complex, and at this point there are more questions than answers. Determination of the OBD often appears insurmountable because of the complexity of biological proteins. Indeed, an OBD must be determined not only for each agent but also for each disease that agent may be used for.

Parameters crucial to immune function must be identified and measured so that pertinent mechanisms of response for a given disease can be identified (Osband and Ross, 1990). With IFN-α, pinpointing whether the antiproliferative effect or the immunomodulatory effect is most dominant will determine optimum dose. Doses are generally much higher when antiproliferative effects are desired. Basic knowledge about the pathophysiology of the disease, tumor antigenicity, the pleiotropic mechanisms of host defenses, the mode of action of a BRM, and the dynamic status of these defenses must be improved so that therapy may be more selectively applied. Furthermore, "each sick patient is immunologically deficient in his or her own way" (Osband and Ross, 1990), and if factors predictive of response were identified, they could be used to target therapy to individual patients most likely to respond. The administration of high-dose IL-2 and biochemotherapy regimens to patients has demonstrated that durable and clinically meaningful antitumor responses can be mediated in select patients with advanced cancer. These successes have helped to establish the principle that immunologic manipulation can lead to the regression of bulky tumor deposits. The continued need for development of laboratory techniques that can measure the impact of biotherapy on immune and other pertinent responses will ultimately lead to an improved understanding of the factors that lead to successful therapy in patients and will open the door for newer, improved therapies (Rosenberg, 1997).

An ideal phase I biotherapy study would thus include determining an agent's bioavailability, pharmacokinetic properties, biological response, and toxicity, all in the context of escalating doses and with a dose-response curve to be assessed for each property (Osband and Ross, 1990; Oldham, 1998). Creekmore and colleagues suggested the development of a two-tiered phase I trial: phase Ia to determine MTD and phase Ib to determine the optimal dose for achieving the desired biological effect or effects (Creekmore et al., 1991). As previously discussed, the desired biological response and MTD of a biological agent may occur at different doses. This now occurs in many current phase I and phase II trials and should ultimately lead to a more scientifically based development of therapeutic regimens.

In the development of biological agents, patient selection, dose escalation, measurement of biological effect, determination of optimal dose, and route of administration will need to be assessed differently than for chemotherapeutic agents. The question of the amount of tumor burden as it relates to patient selection remains an issue. Because certain kinds of biological agents may work only in a specific patient population, more selectivity in patient eligibility may be required. Such selectivity is now required, to a certain extent, for studies involving monoclonal antibodies, and it may need to be instituted for other biological agents as well. Determining the underlying pathophysiology of a disease will allow for the more rational selection of an agent or combination of agents for use in treating the disease. Dose-escalation studies are traditionally conducted with successive groups of patients receiving higher doses. For biological agents, however, dose escalation may need to occur for each patient. With natural body proteins, toxic effects are not expected to be as severe as with chemotherapy drugs. For studies with a given patient, we should be able to increase doses without the fear of excess toxicity. The dose and route of administration should be determined by pharmacokinetics, as well as by biological effects. The desired antitumor effect to be stimulated should also be considered. One may argue, for example, that a serum concentration may not even be necessary to have a biological effect (Kelso, 1989); perhaps it is more important that secondary messengers be set in motion by the biological agent. These same principles apply for the rational design of combination therapies. Although exciting results are beginning to emerge from clinical studies, a great deal remains to be learned about designing effective combinations. Determination of underlying mechanisms of action will provide the cornerstone for designing these combinations.

Determining when to stop therapy can be viewed from two sides. To cure a patient, obtaining a complete remission must be the ultimate goal. Biotherapy is often regarded as less than desirable, because few complete remissions are obtained with biological agents. However, could stable disease be viewed as a desirable end point? In cases where the course of disease is slowed or quiescent, is this not a potentially valuable goal? With diseases in which biotherapy has shown efficacy, technology is beginning to provide the capability to more precisely measure responses. With these advances, the selection of end points for determining the clinical usefulness of biological agents may need to be reevaluated.

Biotherapy is now well recognized as the fourth modality of cancer care; however, the ultimate role of biotherapy in the treatment of many diseases remains uncertain. Determination of the appropriate dose and schedule in treating a given disease and determination of

rational combination therapies lie at the core of this challenge.

References

Adamson, J., and Ludwig, H. 1999. Predicting the hematopoietic response to recombinant human erythropoietin (epoetin alfa) in the treatment of the anemia of cancer. *Oncology (Karger)* 56: 46–53.

Anonymous. 1998. NCI offers expertise to aid preclinical drug development. *Cancer Letter* April 24: 4–7.

Arranz, R., Garcia-Alfonso, P., and Sobrino, P. 1998. Role of interferon alfa-2b in the induction and maintenance treatment of low-grade non-Hodgkin's lymphoma: Results from a prospective, multicenter trial with double randomization. *Journal of Clinical Oncology* 16(4): 1538–1546.

Ascierto, P., Palmieri G., Parasole, R., *et al.* 1999. 3-year treatment with recombinant interferon-α as adjuvant therapy of cutaneous malignant melanoma. *International Journal of Molecular Medicine* 3(3): 303–306.

Atkins, M., Tréhu, E., and Mier, J. 1995. Combination cytokine therapy. In DeVita, V., Hellman, S., and Rosenberg, S. (eds). *Biologic Therapy of Cancer*, 2nd edn. Philadelphia, PA: Lippincott, pp. 443–460.

Aulitzky, W., Gastl, G., Aulitzky, W., *et al.* 1989. Successful treatment of metastatic renal cell carcinoma with a biologically active dose of recombinant interferon-gamma. *Journal of Clinical Oncology* 7(12): 1875–1884.

Balkwill, F. 1989. Interferons. In Balkwill, F. (ed). *Cytokines in Cancer Therapy*. Oxford: Oxford University Press, pp. 8–53.

Balkwill, F. 1997. Cytokine amplification and inhibition of immune and inflammatory responses. *Viral Hepatology* 4 (suppl 2): 6–15.

Baselga, J., and Mendelsohn, J. 1995. Interaction of biologic agents with chemotherapy. In DeVita, V., Hellman, S., and Rosenberg, S. (eds). *Biologic*

Therapy of Cancer, 2nd edn. Philadelphia, PA: Lippincott, pp. 863–875.

Benet, L., Kroetz D., and Sheiner L. 1996. Pharmacokinetics: The dynamics of drug absorption, distribution, and elimination. In Hardman, J., and Limbird, L. (eds). *Goodman & Gilman's The Pharmacological Basis of Therapeutics*, 9th edn. New York, NY: McGraw-Hill Health Professions Division, pp. 3–28.

Borden, E., Paulnock, D., Spear, G., *et al.* 1987. Biological response modification in man: Measurement of interferon-induced proteins. In Baron, S., Dianzani, F., Stanton, G., and Fleischmann, W. (eds). *The Interferon System: A Current Review to 1987*. Austin, TX: The University of Texas Press, pp. 423–429.

Bukowski, R. 1999. Immunotherapy in renal cell carcinoma. *Oncology* 13(6): 801–809.

Cabanillas, F. 1997. Can we cure indolent lymphomas? *Clinical Cancer Research* 3(12 pt 2): 2655–2659.

Campbell, J. 1998. Practical aspects of filgrastim (r-metHuG-CSF) administration. In Morstyn G., Dexter T., and Foote, M. (eds). *Filgrastim (r-metHuG-CSF) in Clinical Practice*, 2nd edn. New York, NY: Marcel Dekker, Inc. pp. 603–613.

Canellos, G., and Demetri, G. 1993. Myelosuppression and "conventional" chemotherapy: What price, what benefit? *Journal of Clinical Oncology* 11(1): 1–2.

Cebon, J., Dempsey, P., Fox, R., *et al.* 1988. Pharmacokinetics of human granulocyte-macrophage colony-stimulating factor using a sensitive immunoassay. *Blood* 72(4): 1340–1347.

Center for Biologics Evaluation and Research (CBER). 1999. Available at *http://www.fda.gov/cber/inside/mission.htm.*

Cheung, W., Goon, B., Guilfoyle, M., and Wacholtz, M. 1998. Pharmacokinetics and pharmacodynamics of recombinant human erythropoietin after single and multiple subcutaneous doses to healthy subjects. *Clinical Pharmacology and Therapeutics* 64(4): 412–423.

Cooper, R. 1991. A review of the clinical studies of

alpha-interferon in the management of multiple myeloma. *Seminars in Oncology* 18(5 suppl 7): 18–29.

Creekmore, S., Longo, D., and Urba, W. 1991. Principles of the clinical evaluation of biologic agents. In DeVita, V., Hellman, S., and Rosenberg, S. (eds). *Biologic Therapy of Cancer*. Philadelphia, PA: J.B. Lippincott Co., pp. 67–86.

Demetri, G., and Griffin, J. 1990. Hematopoietic growth factors and high-dose chemotherapy: Will grams succeed where milligrams fail? *Journal of Clinical Oncology* 8(5): 761–764.

Devine, S., Vokes, E., and Weichselbaum, R. 1991. Chemotherapeutic and biological radiation enhancement. *Current Opinion in Oncology* 3: 1087–1095.

Figlin, R., Bellegrun, A., Moldawer, N., *et al.* 1992. Concomitant administration of recombinant human interleukin-2 and recombinant interferon alfa-2a: An active outpatient regimen in metastatic renal cell carcinoma. *Journal of Clinical Oncology* 10(3): 414–421.

Genentech, Inc. 1998. Herceptin® (trastuzumab) package insert. South San Francisco, CA: Genentech, Inc.

Gilewski, T., and Golomb, H. 1990. Design of combination biotherapy studies: Future goals and challenges. *Seminars in Oncology* 17(1 suppl 1): 3–10.

Gisslinger, H. 1997. Interferon alpha in the therapy of multiple myeloma. *Leukemia* 11(suppl 5): S52–S56.

Grob, J., Dreno, B., de la Salmonière, P., *et al.* 1998. Randomized trial of interferon alfa-2a therapy in resected primary melanoma thicker than 1.5 mm without clinically detectable node metastases. *Lancet* 351: 1905–1910.

Guillhot, F., and Lacotte-Thierry, L. 1998. Interferon-alpha: Mechanisms of action in chronic myelogenous leukemia in chronic phase. *Hematology Cell Therapy* 40(5): 237–239.

Gutterman, J., Fine, S., Quesada, J., *et al.* 1982. Recombinant leukocyte A interferon: Pharmacokinetics, single-dose tolerance, and biological effects in cancer patients. *Annals of Internal Medicine* 96: 549–555.

Hallahan, D., Beckett, M., Kuff, D., *et al.* 1990. The interaction between recombinant human tumor necrosis factor and radiation in 13 human tumor cell lines. *International Journal of Radiation, Oncology, Biology, Physics* 19: 69–74.

Hallahan, D., Haimovitz-Friedman, A., Kute, D., *et al.* 1993. The role of cytokines in radiation oncology. In DeVita, V., Hellman, S., and Rosenberg, S. (eds). *Important Advances in Oncology.* Philadelphia, PA: J.B. Lippincott Co., pp. 71–81.

Heim, S., and Mitelman, F. 1987. *Cancer Cytogenetics.* New York, NY: Alan R. Liss, Inc.

Henriksson, R., Nilsson, S., Colleen, S., *et al.* 1998. Survival in renal cell carcinoma—Randomized evaluation of tamoxifen vs interleukin 2, α-interferon (leukocyte) and tamoxifen. *British Journal of Cancer* 77: 1311–1317.

Hernberg, M., Pyrhönon, S., and Muhonen, T. 1999. Regimens with or without interferon-α as treatment for metastatic melanoma and renal cell carcinoma: An overview of randomized trials. *Journal of Immunotherapy* 22(2): 145–154.

Horton, R. 2000. After Bezwoda. *Lancet* 355(9208): 942–943.

Hrushesky, W. 1991. Temporally optimizable delivery systems—sine qua non for molecular medicine. Preface. *Annals of the New York Academy of Science* 618: xi–xvii.

Hrushesky, W. 1995. Cancer chronotherapy: Is there a right time in the day to treat? *Journal of Infusion Chemotherapy* 5(1): 38–43.

Huber C., Aulitzky W., Tilg H., *et al.* 1987. Studies on the optimal dose and the mode of action of alpha-interferon in the treatment of hairy cell leukemia. *Leukemia* 1(4): 355–357.

Huber, C., and Herold, M. 1989. The importance of patient monitoring in clinical cytokine trials: Use of serum markers to define biologically active doses. *Cancer Surveys* 8(4): 809–815.

Huland, E., Heinzer, H., Huland, H., *et al.* 2000. Overview of interleukin-2 inhalation therapy. *Cancer Journal of Scientific American* 6(suppl 1): 5104–5112.

Iacobelli, S., Garufi, C., Irtelli, L., *et al.* 1995. A phase I study of recombinant interferon-alpha administered as a seven-day continuous venous infusion at circadian-rhythm modulated rate in patients with cancer. *Journal of Clinical Oncology* 18(1): 27–31.

Janik, J., Kopp, W., Smith II, J., *et al.* 1993. Dose-related immunologic effects of levamisole in patients with cancer. *Journal of Clinical Oncology* 11(1): 125–135.

Kaushansky, K. 1998. Thrombopoietin. *New England Journal of Medicine* 339: 746–754.

Keilholz, U., Conradt, C., Legha, S., *et al.* 1998. Results of interleukin-2-based treatment in advanced melanoma: A case record-based analysis of 631 patients. *Journal of Clinical Oncology* 16(9): 2921–2929.

Keilholz, U., Stoter, G., Punt, C., *et al.* 1997. Recombinant interleukin-2-based treatments for advanced melanoma: The experience of the European Organization for Research and Treatment of Cancer Melanoma Cooperative Group. *The Cancer Journal for Scientific American* 3(suppl 1): S22–S28.

Kelso, A. 1998. Cytokines: Principles and prospects. *Immunology and Cell Biology* 76(4): 300–317.

Kemeny, N., and Younes, A. (1992) Alfa-2a interferon and 5-fluorouracil for advanced colorectal carcinoma: The Memorial Sloan-Kettering experience. *Seminars in Oncology* 19(2 suppl 3): 171–175.

Kirkwood, J. 1998. Adjuvant IFN-α2 therapy of melanoma. *The Lancet* 351: 1901–1903.

Kjaer, M. 1996. Combining 5-fluorouracil with interferon-α in the treatment of advanced colorectal cancer: Optimism followed by disappointment. *Anti-Cancer Drugs* 7: 35–42.

Kopp, W., and Holmlund, J. 1996. Cytokines and immunological monitoring. In Pinedo, H., Longo, D., and Chabner, B. (eds). *Cancer Chemotherapy and Biological Response Modifiers Annual 16.* London: Elsevier Science B.V., pp. 189–238.

Kreuser, E., Wadler, S., and Thiel, E. 1992. Interactions between cytokines and cytotoxic drugs: Putative molecular mechanisms in experimental hematology and oncology. *Seminars in Oncology* 19(2 suppl 4): 1–7.

Kreuser, E., Wadler, S., and Thiel, E. 1995. Biochemical modulation of cytotoxic drugs by cytokines: Molecular mechanisms in experimental oncology. *Recent Results in Cancer Research* 139: 371–382.

Kuhn, M. 1998. Pharmaceutical, pharmakokinetic, and pharmacodynamic phases of drug action. In Kuhn, M. (ed). *Pharmacotherapeutics: A Nursing Process Approach*, 4th edn. Philadelphia, PA: F. A. Davis Co., pp. 36–51.

Kurzrock, R., Estrov, Z., Kantarjian, H., *et al.* 1998. Conversion of interferon-induced, long-term cytogenetic remissions in chronic myelogenous leukemia to polymerase chain reaction negativity. *Journal of Clinical Oncology* 16(4): 1526–1531.

Kurzrock, R., Gutterman, J., and Talpaz, M. 1988. The molecular genetics of Philadelphia chromosome-positive leukemias. *New England Journal of Medicine* 319: 990–998.

Legha, S., Ring, S., Eton, O., *et al.* 1997. Development and results of biochemotherapy in metastatic melanoma: The University of Texas M.D. Anderson Cancer Center experience. *The Cancer Journal for Scientific American* 3(suppl 1): S9–S15.

Levi, F., Canon, C., Dipalma, M., *et al.* 1991. When should the immune clock be reset? From circadian pharmacodynamics to temporally optimized drug delivery. *Annals of the New York Academy of Sciences* 618: 312–329.

Lissoni, P. 1997. Effects of low-dose recombinant interleukin-2 in human malignancies. *The Cancer Journal for Scientific American* 3(suppl 1): S115–S120.

Lorenz, J., Wilhelm, K., Kessler, M., *et al.* 1996. Phase I trial of inhaled natural interleukin 2 for treatment of pulmonary malignancy: Toxicity, pharmacokinetics, and biological effects. *Clinical Cancer Research* 2: 1115–1122.

Mäas, R., Dullens, H., and Otter, W. 1993. Interleukin-2 in cancer treatment: Disappointing or (still) promising? A review. *Cancer Immunology and Immunotherapy* 36: 141–148.

Macey, D., Grant, E., Kasi, L., *et al.* 1997. *Clinical Cancer Research* 3(9): 1547–1555.

Mandelli, F., Avvisati, G., Madori, S., *et al.* 1990. Maintenance treatment with recombinant interferon alfa-2b in patients with multiple myeloma responding to conventional induction chemotherapy. *New England Journal of Medicine* 322(20): 1430–1434.

Mazanet, R., Morstyn, G., and Foote, M. 1996. Development of biological agents. In Schilsky, R., Milano, G., and Ratain, M. (eds). *Principles of Antineoplastic Drug Development and Pharmacology*. New York, NY: Marcel Dekker, Inc., pp. 55–73.

McDermott, D.F., Mier, J.W., Lawrence, D.P., *et al.* 2000. A phase II pilot trial of concurrent biochemotherapy with cisplatin, vinblastine, dacarbazine, interleukin-2, and interferon-alpha 2b in patients with metastatic melanoma. *Clinical Cancer Research* 6(6): 2201–2208.

McKenry, L., and Salerno, E. 1998. Principles of drug action. In McKenry, L., and Salerno, E. (eds). *Mosby's Pharmacology in Nursing*, 20th edn. St. Louis, MO: Mosby, pp. 29–47.

Meadows, L., Walther, P., and Ozer, H. 1991. Alpha-interferon and 5-fluorouracil: Possible mechanisms of antitumor action. *Seminars in Oncology* 18(5 suppl 7): 71–76.

Metcalf, D. 1990. The colony-stimulating factors: Discovery, development and clinical applications. *Cancer* 5(10): 2185–2195.

Mihich, E. 1987. Modulation of antitumor immune responses. *Cancer Detection and Prevention Supplement* 1: 399–407.

Mitchell, M. 1988. Combining chemotherapy with biological response modifiers in treatment of cancer. *Journal of the National Cancer Institute* 80: 1445–1450.

Mitchell, M. 1992. Chemotherapy in combination with biomodulation: A 5-year experience with cyclophosphamide and interleukin-2. *Seminars in Oncology* 19(2 suppl 4): 80–87.

Moertel, C., Fleming, T., MacDonald, J., *et al.* 1990. Levamisole and fluorouracil for adjuvant therapy of resected colon carcinoma. *New England Journal of Medicine* 322: 352–358.

Morstyn, G., Lieschke, G., Sheridan, W., *et al.* 1989. Pharmacology of the colony-stimulating factors. *Trends in Pharmacological Sciences* 10: 154–159.

Mulé, J., and Rosenberg, S., 1989. Immunotherapy with lymphokine combinations. In DeVita, V., Hellman, S., and Rosenberg, S. (eds). *Important Advances in Oncology*. Philadelphia, PA: J.B. Lippincott Co., pp. 99–126.

Mulé, J., and Rosenberg, S. 1991. Combination cytokine therapy: Experimental and clinical trials. In DeVita, V., Hellman, S., and Rosenberg, S. (eds). *Biologic Therapy of Cancer*. Philadelphia, PA: J.B. Lippincott Co., pp. 393–416.

Negrier, S., Escudier, B., Lasset, C., *et al.* 1998. Recombinant human interleukin-2, recombinant interferon alfa-2a, or both in metastatic renal cell carcinoma. *New England Journal of Medicine* 338: 1272–1278.

Nieken, J., Mulder, N., Pietens, J., *et al.* 1999. The modulatory impact of recombinant human interleukin-6 on the immune system of cancer patients. *Journal of Immunotherapy* 22(4): 363–370.

Oldham, R. 1998. Developmental therapeutics and the design of clinical trials. In Oldham, R. (ed). *Principles of Cancer Biotherapy*, 3rd ed. Dordrecht, Netherlands: Kluwer Academic Press, pp. 39–50.

Osband, M., and Ross, S. 1990. Problems in the investigational study and clinical use of cancer immunotherapy. *Immunology Today* 11: 193–195.

Parmiani, G., and Rivoltini, L. 1991. Biologic agents as modifiers of chemotherapeutic effects. *Current Opinion in Oncology* 3: 1078–1086.

Pazdur, R. 1992. Combination of fluorouracil and interferon: Mechanisms of interaction and clinical studies. In Holdstein, A., and Garaci, E. (eds).

Combination Therapies. New York, NY: Plenum Publishing Corp., pp. 73–78.

Pazdur, R., Moore, D., and Bready, B. 1992. Modulation of fluorouracil with recombinant alfa interferon: M.D. Anderson clinical trial. *Seminars in Oncology* 19(2 suppl 3): 176–179.

Pehamberger, H., Soyer, P., Steiner, A., *et al.* 1998. Adjuvant interferon alfa-2a treatment in resected primary stage II cutaneous melanoma. *Journal of Clinical Oncology* 16(4): 1425–1429.

Peters, W., Stuart, A., Affronti, M., *et al.* 1988. Neutrophil migration is defective during recombinant human granulocyte-macrophage colony-stimulating factor infusion after autologous bone marrow transplantation in humans. *Blood* 72: 1310–1315.

Pfeffer, L., Dinarello, C., Herberman, R., *et al.* 1998. Biological properties of recombinant α-interferons: 40th anniversary of the discovery of interferons. *Cancer Research* 58: 2489–2499.

Pyrhönen, S., Kouri, M., Holsti, L., *et al.* 1992. Disease stabilization by leukocyte alpha interferon and survival of patients with metastatic melanoma. *Oncology* 49: 22–26.

Quirt, J., Shelley, W., Pater, J., *et al.* 1991. Improved survival in patients with poor-prognosis malignant melanoma treated with adjuvant levamisole: A phase III study by the National Cancer Institute of Canada clinical trials group. *Journal of Clinical Oncology* 9: 729–735.

Ratain, M. 1998. Body-surface area as a basis for dosing of anticancer agents: Science, myth, or habit? Editorial. *Journal of Clinical Oncology* 16(7): 2297–2298.

Reid, J., Kovach, J., O'Connell, M., *et al.* 1998. Clinical and pharmacokinetic studies of high-dose levamisole in combination with 5-fluorouracil in patients with advanced cancer. *Cancer Chemotherapy and Pharmacology* 41(6): 477–484.

Rosenberg, S. 1997. Keynote address: Perspectives on the use of interleukin-2 in cancer treatment. *The Cancer Journal of Scientific American* 3(suppl 1): S2–S6.

Rosenberg, S., Lotze, M., Yang, J., *et al.* 1989. Combination therapy with interleukin-2 and alpha-interferon for the treatment of patients with advanced cancer. *Journal of Clinical Oncology* 7(12): 1863–1874.

Roskos, L., Cheung, E., Vincent, M., *et al.* 1998. Pharmacology of filgrastim (r-metHuG-CSF). In Morstyn, G., Dexter, T., and Foote, M. (eds). *Filgrastim (r-metHuG-CSF) in Clinical Practice*, 2nd edn. New York, NY: Marcel Dekker, Inc., pp. 51–71.

Ross, E. 1996. Pharmacodynamics: Mechanisms of drug action and the relationship between drug concentration and effect. In Hardman, J., and Limbird, L. (eds). *Goodman & Gilman's The Pharmacological Basis of Therapeutics*, 9th edn. New York, NY: McGraw-Hill Health Professions Division, pp. 29–42.

Schmoll, H., Hiddemann, W., Rustum, Y., *et al.* 1992. Introduction: The emerging role for biomodulation of antineoplastic agents. *Seminars in Oncology* 19(2 suppl 3): 1–3.

Schuller, J., Czejka, M., Schernthaner, G., *et al.* 1992. Influence of interferon alfa-2b with or without folinic acid on pharmacokinetics of fluorouracil. *Seminars in Oncology* 19(2 suppl 3): 93–97.

Siegel, J., Gerrard, T., Cavagnaro, J., *et al.* 1995. In DeVita, V., Hellman, S., and Rosenberg, S. (eds). *Biologic Therapy of Cancer,* 2nd edn. Philadelphia, PA: W.B. Saunders, pp. 879–890.

Sondel, P., and Hank, J. 1997. Combination therapy with interleukin-2 and antitumor monoclonal antibodies. *The Cancer Journal for Scientific American* 3(suppl 1): S121–S127.

Sparano, J., Fisher, R., Sunderland, M., *et al.* 1993. Randomized phase III trial of treatment with high-dose interleukin-2 either alone or in combination with interferon-alfa-2a in patients with advanced melanoma.

Sporn, M., and Roberts, A. 1988. Peptide growth factors are multifunctional. *Nature* 332: 217–219.

Stadtmauer, E., O'Neill, A., Goldstein, P., *et al.* 1999. Phase III randomized trial of high-dose chemotherapy (HDC) and stem cell support (SCT) show no difference in overall survival or severe toxicity compared to maintenance chemotherapy with cyclophosphamide, methotrexate and 5-fluorouracil (CMF) for women with metastatic breast cancer who are responding to conventional induction chemotherapy: The "Philadephia" intergroup study (PBT-1). *Proceedings of the American Society of Clinical Oncology* 18: 1a, abstract 1.

Sznol, M., and Longo, D. 1993. Chemotherapy drug interactions with biological agents. *Seminars in Oncology* 20(1): 80–93.

Talmadge, J. 1992. Development of immunotherapeutic strategies for the treatment of malignant neoplasms. *Biotherapy* 4(3): 215–236.

Talpaz M., Kantarjian H., Kurzrock R., *et al.* 1991. Interferon-alpha produces sustained cytogenetic responses in chronic myelogenous leukemia. *Annals of Internal Medicine* 114: 532–538.

Vadhan-Raj, S., Broxmeyer, H., Hittelman, W., *et al.* 1992. Abrogating chemotherapy-induced myelosuppression by recombinant granulocyte-macrophage colony-stimulating factor in patients with sarcoma: Protection at the progenitor cell level. *Journal of Clinical Oncology* 10(8): 1266–1277.

Vadhan-Raj, S., Buescher, S., LeMaistre, A., *et al.* 1988. Stimulation of hematopoiesis in patients with bone marrow failure and in patients with malignancy by recombinant human granulocyte-macrophage colony-stimulating factor. *Blood* 72(1): 134–141.

Valle, J., and Scarffe, H. 1998. Use of combinations of cytokines with filgrastim (r-metHuG-CSF). In Morstyn G., Dexter T., and Foote, M. (eds). *Filgrastim (r-metHuG-CSF) in Clinical Practice*, 2nd ed. New York, NY: Marcel Dekker, Inc. pp. 371–396.

Wadler, S., and Schwartz, E. 1990. Atineoplastic activity of the combination of interferon and cytotoxic agents against experimental and human malignancies: A review. *Cancer Research* 50: 3473–3486.

Wadler, S. 1992. Antineoplastic activity of the combination of 5-fluorouracil and interferon:

Preclinical and clinical results. *Seminars in Oncology* 19(2 suppl 4): 38–40.

Wadler, S., and Schwartz, E. 1992. Principles in the biomodulation of cytotoxic drugs by interferons. *Seminars in Oncology* 19(2 suppl 3): 45–48.

Wadler, S., Schwartz E., Goldman, M., *et al.* 1989. Fluorouracil and recombinant alfa-2a-interferon: An active regimen against advanced colorectal carcinoma. *Journal of Clinical Oncology* 7(12): 1769–1775.

Wadler, S., and Wiernik, P. 1990. Clinical update on the role of fluorouracil and recombinant interferon alfa-2a in the treatment of colorectal carcinoma. *Seminars in Oncology* 17: 16–21.

Wiernik, P. 1989. Neutrophil function in infection. *Mediguide to Infectious Diseases* 9(1): 1–8.

Yoffe, G., Blick, M., Kantarjian, H., *et al.* 1987. Molecular analysis of interferon-induced suppression of Philadelphia chromosome in patients with chronic myeloid leukemia. *Blood* 69(3): 961–963.

PART II

Major Categories of Biological Agents

CHAPTER 5 | The Interferons

Linda Cuaron, RN, MN, AOCN®

John Thompson, MD

It has been known since the early 1930s that cells infected with **viruses** are capable of protecting other cells from viral infection. Isaacs and Lindemann (1957) discovered the protein that partially explains this phenomenon and named it interferon (IFN) because of its ability to "interfere" with viral replication. Within a few years, the **antiproliferative** and **immuno-modulatory** cellular effects of this molecule had been identified. There are 5 major species of IFN: alpha (α), beta (β), gamma (γ), omega (ω), and tau (τ) (Roberts, 1996; Viscomi, 1997). IFN-ω and IFN-τ are in the early stages of study and not yet approved for therapeutic use in

The authors wish to thank and acknowledge Nancy Moldawer and Robert Figlin, MD, whose work from the first edition of *Biotherapy: A Comprehensive Overview* served as a foundation for this chapter.

humans. Cantell and co-workers (1975) developed techniques for purifying IFN-α from donated human blood. This method proved to be costly as well as time- and resource-consuming and resulted in an impure product. However, it provided the opportunity to test this molecule as an antitumor agent. The development of **recombinant DNA** technology in 1980 and the birth of the biotechnology industry led to the production of highly purified IFN molecules. In 1981, the first human trials with recombinant IFN-α began. Since then, research has led to Food and Drug Administration (FDA) approval of IFN-α as treatment for nine different diseases and approval of IFN-β and IFN-γ as treatment for one disease each (see Table 5.1).

In 1986, just a few years after its introduction as an anticancer agent, the first IFN-α was approved by the FDA for its significant role in

Table 5.1 Type I and type II interferons in clinical use

Species	Subtype	Trade Name	Manufacturer	FDA Approved Indications
Alpha (α)	Recombinant alpha (IFN-alfa-2a)	Roferon-A®	Hoffmann-LaRoche	Hairy-cell leukemia AIDS-related Kaposi's sarcoma Chronic myelogenous leukemia Chronic hepatitis C
	Recombinant alpha (IFN-alfa-2b)	Intron-A®	Schering-Plough	High-risk melanoma Non-Hodgkin's lymphoma Hairy-cell leukemia AIDS-related Kaposi's sarcoma Condylomata acuminata Chronic hepatitis C Chronic hepatitis B (adult and pediatric)
	Lymphoblastoid (IFN-alfa N1)	Wellferon®	Glaxo-Wellcome	Not commercially available in the United States
	Human leukocyte-derived (IFN-alfa N3)	Alferon®	Purdue Frederick	Condylomata acuminata
	Recombinant consensus (IFN-Con₁)	Infergen®	Amgen	Chronic hepatitis C
Beta (β)	Recombinant beta-1a (IFN-beta-1a)	Avonex®	Biogen	Multiple sclerosis
	Recombinant beta-1b (IFN-beta-1b)	Betaseron®	Chiron/Berlex	Multiple sclerosis
Gamma (γ)	Interferon gamma-1b (IFN-gamma-1b)	Actimmune®	Intermune	Chronic granulomatous disease

the treatment of hairy cell leukemia (HCL). Shortly thereafter, in 1989, IFN-α received its second FDA approval for the treatment of acquired immunodeficiency syndrome (AIDS)-related Kaposi's sarcoma (KS). Additional oncology indications for IFN-α include melanoma, non-Hodgkin's lymphoma (NHL), and chronic myelogenous leukemia (CML). In viral diseases, IFN-α has clinical application for the treatment of hepatitis B, hepatitis C, and condylomata acuminata. Chronic granulomatous disease (CGD) is an inherited abnormality of certain cells of the immune system that "ingest" bacteria and kill them (phagocytic cells). The abnormality results in chronic infection by certain types of bacteria that result in severe, recurrent infections of the skin, lymph nodes, liver, lungs, and bone. Because treatment with IFN-γ led to a 70% reduction of serious infections in patients with this disease (Gallin *et al.*, 1991), this agent was approved in 1990.

In 1993, IFN-β was approved for the treatment of relapsing-remitting (RR)-multiple sclerosis (MS). IFN therapy provides the first hope for an effective treatment for MS since the disease was first described in 1868 (Rolak, 1996). Because of the research efforts of many people and groups such as the Multiple Sclerosis Collaborative Research Group, MS is now considered a treatable disease (Aranson, 1999).

The IFNs have been referred to as the "prototype" biological agents and have undergone intensive molecular, preclinical, and investigational scrutiny. IFN therapy has an established role in the treatment of several advanced malignancies. Numerous phase II and phase III trials have demonstrated its efficacy as a single agent. Additional studies have shown its ability to induce responses in refractory neoplasms and to modify chromosomal disorders in CML. Studies that utilize IFN as a component of combination therapies have demonstrated that IFN can modulate the activity of cytotoxic, biological, and differentiating agents. The **antiangiogenic** effect of IFN-α has led to its use in several malignant and nonmalignant diseases.

This chapter will focus on the FDA-approved indications for IFN-α, IFN-β, and IFN-γ. The biological properties and mechanisms of action of IFN will be described. Additionally, an overview of the studies that suggest potential uses for IFNs and possible future applications will be discussed.

Biological Activity

The IFN family comprises a very complex set of proteins and glycoproteins. Because of this heterogeneity, it is not surprising that several attempts have been made to classify these agents. One approach to classifying IFNs is the **phylogenetic** system. To date, two types and five species of IFNs have been described: type I, which includes IFN-α, -β, -ω, and -τ, and type II, which includes IFN-γ. IFN-ω and IFN-τ are the newest additions (Roberts, 1996; Qin *et al.*, 1997; Soos, 1997; Viscomi, 1997).

Type I IFNs differ from the type II IFN in structure and interaction with cell-surface receptors (Viscomi, 1997). Type I IFNs are more effective in inducing an antiviral state in cells, whereas the type II IFN is associated more with the proper functioning of the immune system (Durelli *et al.*, 1995). Additionally, type I IFNs share a common ligand binding site and induce common biological effects. These proteins are usually defined by the cell that produces them. Both IFN-α and IFN-ω are derived from **leukocytes**, and IFN-β is derived from **fibroblasts**. IFN-τ is derived from **trophoblasts** and is being investigated in the treatment of MS (Roberts, 1996). Type II IFN-γ is secreted by CD8[+] T cells and some CD4[+] T cells. These cells secrete IFN-γ only when activated by interleukin (IL)-2 and IL-12 (Oppenheim *et al.*, 1997).

Antiviral Effects

The IFNs have very high antiviral-specific activity and are protective against both DNA and RNA viruses (Samuels, 1988). When a cell is infected with a virus, it synthesizes and releases IFN into the extracellular space. IFN then binds to receptors on other cells and is internalized. The IFN-induced cells then produce several enzymes that can regulate the process of viral protein synthesis. The best studied of these enzymes are **2'-5'-oligoadenylate synthetase** and a **protein kinase**. Indirectly, the IFNs may mediate antiviral effects by stimulating cytotoxic T lymphocytes (CTLs) to lyse virally infected cells.

In general, **CD8+ cytotoxic T cells** and **CD4+ T-helper 1 (T$_h$1) cells** are the primary components of cell-mediated host defense once virus has entered the cell and become latent. Activated T$_h$1 cells produce several secondary **cytokines,** including IL-2, IFN-γ, and tumor necrosis factor (TNF). IFNs act to induce an antiviral state in the uninfected cells. The secondary cytokine IL-2 contributes to the activation of CTL precursors, with both IL-2 and IFN activating the **natural killer (NK) cells** (Abbas et al., 1991; Oppenheim et al., 1997).

Intercellular Protein Changes

The anticancer activity of IFN-α probably results from a number of different mechanisms, including induction of intracellular proteins, enhancement of immune **effector** cells, and changes in cell-surface structures. The signaling pathways that are activated by IFNs directly activate a recently characterized class of enzymes known as Janus kinases (JAKs), which are associated with the catalytic activity in the cytoplasm of cytokines that are necessary to transmit intracellular signals. The term "Janus" was taken from the name of the Roman god who had 2 faces and refers to the fact that JAKs have 2 active binding sites (Durelli et al., 1995; Williams and Haque, 1997).

Binding of IFNs to their receptors results in signal transmission from the cell surface to the nucleus. This is followed by induction of several IFN-stimulated genes (ISGs). This action is mediated by a group of proteins known as signal transducers and activators of transcription (STAT). The function of these proteins is signal **transduction** from the cell surface to the nucleus and activation of **transcription**. At least seven types of STATs have been identified and cloned. STAT1 and STAT2 have been identified as part of an ISG complex. Some of the effects of ISG induction include the release of arachidonic acid and production of proteins. It is thought that these actions may be implicated in some of the side effects that patients experience with IFN therapy (Leonard and O'Shea, 1998; Yong et al., 1998).

Together, these proteins form the JAK-STAT pathway, a signaling cascade that is showing that significant cross talk exists between cytokine, hormone, and growth-factor signaling systems (Haque and Williams, 1998).

Antiproliferative Effects

IFN-α has an antiproliferative effect on many malignant tumor cells. Inhibition of hematologic tumors by IFN-α has been observed in Burkitt's lymphoma, lymphocytic lymphoma, acute myelogenous leukemia (AML), CML, chronic lymphocytic leukemia (CLL), and multiple myeloma (MM) (Rodriguez et al., 1998; Salmon et al., 1998; Faderl et al., 1999; Huang et al., 1999). Other studies have suggested that IFN-α has a greater inhibitory effect on cells of **hematopoietic** origin than either IFN-β or IFN-γ. Research has demonstrated that nondividing tumor cells (cells in **cell-cycle** phases G_0 and G_1) appear to have increased sensitivity to the antiproliferative activity of human IFN (Creasey et al., 1980; Qin et al., 1997). There is also a direct antiproliferative effect, which is supported by studies of transplanted human tumors in immunodeficient nude mice in which the immunomodulatory effects of IFN were minimal. Dose-dependent growth inhibition was observed in these models, but it lasted only for the duration of IFN exposure (Yoshitake *et al.*, 1976; Balkwill *et al.,* 1982).

Additional contributions to the understanding of the regulation of antiproliferation involve the role of transcription factors that mediate IFN signaling. Protein **phosphorylation** is an important action of the JAK-STAT pathway. The JAK-STAT pathway consists of a cascade of specific protein-to-protein interactions. These proteins culminate in protein DNA engagement and specific transcriptional regulation, resulting in antiviral activity, cell-growth control, and **apoptosis** (Williams and Haque, 1997). One of the specific mediators of IFN-induced antiproliferation is protein kinase R, a dsRNA-activated kinase that may work by suppressing the expression of c-*myc* (Kaempfer, 1998). The **myc protein** is a transcription factor that contributes to regulation of cell division by binding to DNA in the control region of the gene. Myc behaves as an **oncogene** (a cancer-causing gene) whenever it becomes stuck in hyperactive form (Clark and Russell, 1997). It is now believed that in many cases, the neoplastic transformation of normal cells to malignant cells is regulated by the expression of cellular oncogenes. Thus, another mechanism whereby IFN may exert its antitumor activity is by its effects on oncogene expression.

Immunomodulatory Effects

The anticancer effects of IFN have been attributed to several of its immunomodulatory activities, but the most relevant appears to be its effects on NK cells and **macrophages.** The **pleiotropic** effects of IFN-α on the immune system are well established. IFN-α activates pathways that may induce, inhibit, or modify the effects of several cytokines, including IFN-γ, IL-1, IL-2, IL-6, IL-8, and TNF-α (see Figure 5.1). Side effects may be induced by the stimulatory or inhibitory effects of IFN-α on the production or activation of other cytokines or **chemokines** (Taylor and Grossberg, 1998). The effects of IFN-α on NK cells and the augmentation of the cytotoxic activity have been extensively reviewed. Brief exposure (1 to 2 hours) of NK cells to IFN-α results in a significant increase in the ability of NK cells to kill NK-sensitive tumor target cells. The ability of IFN-α to modulate NK cell activity is thought to be caused by several factors, including accelerated kinetics, recycling (by lysing multiple targets), IL-2–dependent growth, mediation of antibody-dependent cellular cytotoxicity, and the release of various cytokines that might broaden the immunomodulatory effects (Herberman, 1997).

In part, the immunomodulatory effects of type I IFNs stem from activation of macrophages, T and B lymphocytes, and large granular lymphocytes with NK activity. Type I IFNs also regulate the differentiation and function of monocytes and macrophages. This results in an increase in the tumoricidal and bacteriocidal activity of macrophages. Macrophages that have been activated by IFN *in vitro* show morphologic changes that are characteristic of maturation, including enlargement, pseudopod formation and vacuolization, and increased expression of receptors for the **Fc** portion of immunoglobulins. Upregulation of the macrophage **Fc receptor** promotes increased phagocytosis of immune complexes and enhanced **lytic** ability. For the most part, macrophage activation is the result of increased gene transcription. The genes activate the functional capacities of the macrophage that are not present in the resting monocyte. IFN-γ is a potent macrophage activator as well. Although the properties of an activated macrophage have

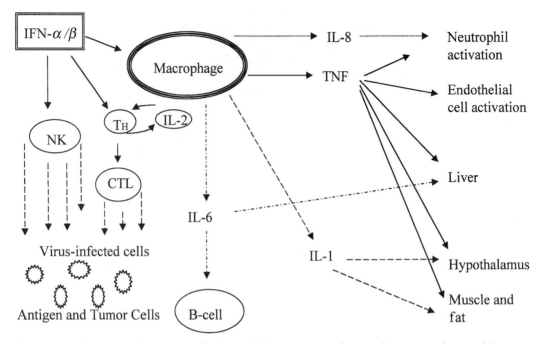

Figure 5.1   Type I interferon cascade. Type I IFNs activate pathways that may induce, inhibit, or modify the effects of several cytokines. This figure demonstrates a few of the pleiotropic effects of type I IFNs. CTL, cytotoxic T lymphocyte; IFN, interferon; IL, interleukin; NK, natural killer cells; TH, T helper; TNF, tumor necrosis factor.

Source: Adapted courtesy of Sidney Grossberg, MD, and Jerry Taylor, PhD, Medical College of Wisconsin.

been well described, it is not yet clear which specific activities are induced by the different types of IFNs. Furthermore, there may be variation in the specific activities of the subtypes within each species of IFN (Bordens *et al.*, 1997; Pestka, 1997a; Pestka, 1997b; Taylor and Grossberg, 1998).

Some of the side effects associated with type I IFNs are the result of the activation of macrophages and CD4+ T cells. As our understanding of the molecular aspects of type I IFNs increases, the complexity of the interactions and induction of cytokines leads to a theoretical basis for describing some of the side effects that occur when IFNs are used therapeutically.

Research has increased our understanding of the IFN cascade as well as other actions of the

activated macrophage. The activated macrophage, by definition, is able to perform specific activities that the resting macrophage cannot, such as killing microorganisms, killing tumor cells, stimulating acute inflammation, and becoming a more efficient **antigen presenting cell (APC)**. Additionally, the products of the activated macrophage (e.g., cytokines and growth factors) are able to effect the process of angiogenesis (Abbas *et al.*, 1991).

Macrophage activation occurs as the result of new or increased gene transcription. IFN-α can induce the expression of ISG-15, which can stimulate IFN-γ production. IFN-γ can stimulate the activity of the inducible nitric oxide synthetase (iNOS) enzyme. This enzyme produces the free-radical gas nitric oxide, which is toxic and may play a role in some IFN-associated side effects. IFN-γ can also induce the macrophage to release a substance known as "tissue factor," which can initiate the extrinsic clotting cascade (Abbas *et al.*, 1991; Taylor and Grossberg, 1998).

Activated macrophages also contribute to an acute inflammatory process through the secretion of mediators such as prostaglandins, platelet-activating factor, and **leukotrienes**. Certain T-cell-derived cytokines stimulate the macrophage to secrete secondary cytokines. Together with IFN-γ, which is secreted by the activated T lymphocyte in the presence of type I IFN, the macrophage is stimulated to release secondary cytokines such as TNF, IL-1, IL-6, and IL-8. Activated macrophages also secrete a substance known as fibroblast growth factor. This leads to endothelial cell migration and proliferation and results in the formation of new blood vessels or angiogenesis (Abbas *et al.*, 1991).

IL-8 is an inflammatory chemokine. Together with TNF, it stimulates the migration or chemotaxis of **neutrophils** from the vascular space to the endothelial space. TNF causes the endothelial cells to secrete IL-8 and the monocyte chemotactic protein-1. This results in a type of neutropenia that differs from chemotherapy-induced neutropenia and is attributed in part to the increased mobility of leukocytes. IL-8 and monocyte chemotactic protein-1 act preferentially on leukocytes that are bound to endothelial cells. TNF is known to stimulate endothelial cells to express endothelial leukocyte adhesion molecule-1 (ELAM-1). ELAM-1 selectively binds neutrophils, and as the level of ELAM-1 declines, the levels of intercellular adhesion molecule-1 and vascular cell adhesion molecule-1 increase (Abbas *et al.*, 1991). Because there has not been a cytotoxic effect on progenitor cells, the neutropenia seen with IFN therapy is primarily one of storage or redistribution of the neutrophils outside the vascular space. Once neutrophils enter the tissues, they live only a short while (one to two days). Dose reduction or temporary discontinuation usually results in a fairly rapid return to baseline levels as new neutrophils mature and enter the periphery.

IL-6 was first thought to be an IFN (IFN-β₂). Early work characterized IL-6 as both a hepatocyte-stimulating factor and a B-cell growth factor. As a hepatocyte-stimulating factor, IL-6 impacts the liver by inducing the synthesis of acute-phase proteins such as C-reactive protein, fibrinogen, and C3, while also inhibiting the synthesis of albumin and prealbumin. IL-1 and TNF also act synergistically with some of these acute-phase proteins. This may account, in part, for the increase in liver enzyme release that is seen in some patients receiving IFN therapy. When healthy volunteers were injected with IL-6 they showed decreased levels of thyroid-stimulatory hormone and thyroid hormone T3. They also experienced headache, tachycardia, chills, and fever (Abbas *et al.*, 1991; Oppenheim *et al.*, 1997; Taylor and Grossberg, 1998).

TNF is an inflammatory cytokine, and it contributes to neutrophil chemotaxis by causing vascular endothelial cells to become adhesive. It is also an endogenous pyrogen and acts on cells in the temperature-regulating regions of the brain to induce fever. It is similar to IL-1 in this activity.

IFN-inducible protein-10 (IP-10) can be stimulated by both IFN-α and IFN-γ. Some of the activities of IP-10 include inhibition of bone marrow colony formation, enhancement of T-cell adhesion to endothelial cells, and inhibition of angiogenesis. IP-10 is a chemokine that is structurally similar to the IL-8 family (Taylor and Grossberg, 1998).

Antiangiogenesis

Angiogenesis or neovascularization is now known to play a significant role in tumor metastasis. In addition to enabling the metastatic spread of tumor cells, the process of angiogenesis is also believed to reduce the tumor's accessibility to chemotherapeutic drugs (Folkman, 1995). Endogenous IFN is one of many negative regulators of angiogenesis. Fibroblast growth factor is an endogenous angiogenic factor. As illustrated in Figure 5.2, the switch to neovascularization, which results in tumor growth and spread, requires both the upregulation of an angiogenic factor and downregulation of inhibitors of blood vessel growth. Many endogenous angiogenic factors as well as the negative regulators (inhibitors) of angiogenesis have been identified (Table 5.2).

In addition to slowing endothelial migration, as described earlier in this chapter, the mechanism by which IFN-α inhibits angiogenesis involves inhibiting mRNA and protein production of two known angiogenic factors: basic fibroblast growth factor and IL-8 (Singh and Fidler, 1996).

IFN-α has shown success as an anticancer agent for diseases that overexpress basic fibroblast growth factors such as giant-cell tumor of the mandible or bladder cancer (Dinney et al., 1998; Dickerman, 1999; Kaban et al., 1999). Furthermore, the combination of retinoic acid and IFN-α have demonstrated dramatic decreases in angiogenesis and tumor growth in head and neck squamous-cell carcinoma (Lingen et al., 1998). Similarly, IFN-α has also demonstrated efficacy in the treatment of hemangiomas (Folkman, 1995). Control or regulation of angiogenesis will be an important component of new anticancer treatment models.

Clinical Experience: Interferon-α

Hematologic Malignancies and Lymphomas

HAIRY-CELL LEUKEMIA
HCL is a rare, chronic, lymphoproliferative disorder. Characteristic clinical features include splenomegaly, pancytopenia, and the presence of distinctive irregular projections on lymphoid

Table 5.2   Endogenous angiogenic and anti-angiogenic factors

Endogenous Angiogenic Factors	Endogenous Negative Regulators of Angiogenesis
Fibroblast growth factors, basic (bFGF) and acidic (aFGF)	Interferon-α
	Platelet factor-4
Angiogenin	Thrombospondin-1
Transforming growth factors α and β	Tissue inhibitors of metalloproteinases (TIMP-2)
Tumor necrosis factor α	Prolactin
Vascular endothelial growth factor	Angiostatin
Platelet-derived endothelial-cell growth factor	Placental proliferin-related protein
Granulocyte colony-stimulating factor	
Placental growth factor	bFGF soluble receptor*
Interleukin-8	Transforming growth factor β†
Hepatocyte growth factor	
Proliferin	

* bFGF soluble receptor has not been tested *in vivo*.
† Transforming growth factor β has not been shown to inhibit angiogenesis.

Source: Adapted from Folkman, J. 1995. Clinical applications of research on angiogenesis. *Seminars in Medicine of the Beth Israel Hospital*, Boston 333(26): 1757–1762.

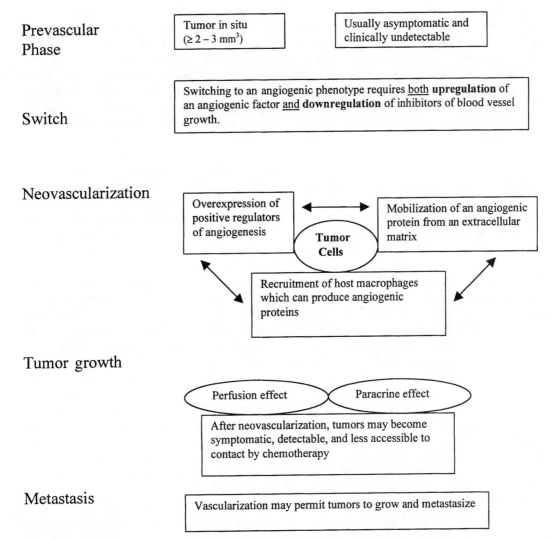

Prevascular Phase

> Tumor in situ ($\geq 2 - 3$ mm^3)

> Usually asymptomatic and clinically undetectable

Switch

> Switching to an angiogenic phenotype requires <u>both</u> **upregulation** of an angiogenic factor <u>and</u> **downregulation** of inhibitors of blood vessel growth.

Neovascularization

> Overexpression of positive regulators of angiogenesis

> Tumor Cells

> Mobilization of an angiogenic protein from an extracellular matrix

> Recruitment of host macrophages which can produce angiogenic proteins

Tumor growth

> Perfusion effect   Paracrine effect

> After neovascularization, tumors may become symptomatic, detectable, and less accessible to contact by chemotherapy

Metastasis

> Vascularization may permit tumors to grow and metastasize

Figure 5.2   Angiogenesis in neoplastic disease. Tumors may persist for years before neovascularization occurs. Neovascularization involves a switch that changes the local equilibrium between positive and negative regulators of microvessel growth factors. Upregulation of an angiogenic factor alone is not enough to signal neovascularization. Down-regulation of negative regulators or inhibitors of vessel growth is also necessary. Perfusion augments tumor growth because in crowded tissue, perfusion is more efficient than diffusion in allowing inward passage of nutrients and outward passage of catabolites. The paracrine effect comes from the production of growth factors by endothelial cells.

Source: Adapted from Folkman, J. 1995. Clinical applications of research on angiogenesis. *Seminars in Medicine of the Beth Israel Hospital,* Boston 333(26): 1757–1762.

cells in the bone marrow, peripheral blood, and reticuloendothelial system. The cytopenias seen in HCL are multifactorial and related to abnormal progenitor stem cells, deficiency in hematopoietic growth factors, and hypersplenism. Indications for therapeutic intervention because of cytopenias include a hemoglobin level less than 10 g/dL, an absolute neutrophil count equal to or less than 1×10^9/L, and a platelet count equal to or less than 100×10^9/L (Diesseroth et al., 1997).

HCL was initially described in 1958, and for 25 years, splenectomy was the mainstay of treatment. Splenectomy resulted in improvement in peripheral blood cytopenias in approximately 50% of patients; however, because splenectomy does not address the underlying bone marrow disease, the majority of patients with HCL treated with splenectomy relapse with progressive cytopenias.

In 1984, IFN was introduced as a treatment for HCL by Quesada et al. (1984). In general, low-dose IFN-α therapy (2×10^6 mU/m^2 every day with IFN-alfa-2b or 3×10^6 mU 3 times a week with IFN-alfa-2a) leads to a high overall response rate with normalization of peripheral blood cell counts. In subsequent studies, high response rates have been noted in patients who underwent splenectomy or who were previously untreated, but a complete response (CR) was seen in only 5% to 11% of cases (Diesseroth et al., 1997). The FDA approved IFN-α for treatment of HCL in 1986.

One of the largest multicenter trials of IFN-α for the treatment of progressive HCL included 212 patients. Objective responses (complete, partial, and minor) were recorded in 89% of the study group and were characterized by a marked reduction in infections as well as in the need for transfusions (Thompson and Fefer, 1987). CR, defined as a normal complete blood cell count and less than 5% hairy cells in the marrow, was achieved in 4% of the subjects. Partial response (PR), defined as normal complete blood cell count, was attained in 74% of subjects. Minor responses (normalization of subnormal hematocrit, granulocyte, or platelet counts) were seen in 11% of subjects. Overall, the results of this study indicated that IFN-α was well tolerated, produced durable responses, and improved quality of life in a high percentage of patients with progressive HCL.

Initial therapy for HCL with IFN-α doses of 3×10^6 units 3 times a week is associated with chills and flu-like symptoms early in the course of therapy. With continued therapy, however, **tachyphylaxis** to the acute toxic effects of IFN usually develops. The major chronic toxic effect associated with this dose and schedule of IFN is fatigue. Lower doses of IFN are associated with minimal or undetectable side effects and yet may be effective in maintaining remissions induced by higher doses (Thompson et al., 1989). Many patients with HCL have been treated with IFN continuously for over 10 years with persistent remission of their leukemia.

Although early results yielded mostly PRs, the survival rates have greatly improved, and the estimated survival of patients treated with IFN-α is 85% to 90% at 5 years. Retrospective analysis of patients who experience long-term response to IFN-α therapy has led to identification of specific histological factors that are seen in patients who have a durable sustained response to treatment. One of these factors is use of the hairy-cell index (HCI). The HCI is defined as the percent of cellularity times the percent of hairy cells divided by 100 (% cellularity $\times$ % hairy cells/100). An HCI of less than 0.50 at the time of diagnosis and an HCI of less than 0.10 at the end of IFN-α therapy is a characteristic of patients who have a durable sustained response to treatment. Another parameter shared by long-term responders was treatment for more than 18 months ($p = .003$) (Zinzani et al., 1997). Combination therapy with hydroxyurea (HU), cytarabine (Ara-C), and IFN-α in a group of 361 patients was compared with the combination of HU and IFN-α in 360 patients. After 3 years, the survival rate was 85.7% for the group that received the Ara-C with HU plus IFN-α and 79.1% for the HU plus IFN-α only group. The rate of hematological response (HR) was also higher in the Ara-C–treated group ($p = .003$) (Guilhot et al., 1997). The toxicities were all higher in the Ara-C–treated group, with the greatest increase seen in hematologic toxicity, gastrointestinal toxicity, weight loss, and skin rash, all of which are expected toxicities with this chemotherapy.

The combination of HU and IFN-α in the treatment of leukemia cell lines has been shown to be more effective than IFN-α alone. This may occur because of the following mechanism. The IFN-α antitumor effect occurs through binding of IFN-α to specific cell-surface receptors. HU is a DNA synthesis inhibitor that promotes a dose- and time-dependent increase in receptor binding affinity. HU may cause the DNA synthesis to proceed more slowly. Because it has been demonstrated that nondividing cells are more sensitive to IFN-α, the addition of a drug that causes DNA synthesis to slow down may provide another explanation for why IFN efficacy is improved with the addition of HU (Tamura et al., 1997).

The treatment of HCL with IFN-α has recently been challenged by the development of newer drugs. Pentostatin (Nipent®) or 2'-deoxycoformycin exerts its biological activity by inhibiting the enzyme adenosine deaminase and was reported by Spiers et al. (1984) to have clinical activity in HCL. Subsequent trials of this drug have demonstrated that it yields a higher percentage of CRs than IFN-α with excellent durability of response. Pentostatin has also been demonstrated to be non-cross-resistant with IFN-α and to be effective in HCL patients who are unresponsive to IFN. Other studies have evaluated a regimen of alternating cycles of pentostatin and IFN-α (Habermann et al., 1990; Martin et al., 1990). Because of

evidence that IFN-α and pentostatin are clinically non-cross-resistant and that patients who do not respond to IFN-α may respond to pentostatin, Martin et al. (1990) studied their use in combination. The rate of improvement in peripheral blood cell counts was comparable with that of single-agent pentostatin (Johnston et al., 1988) and was more rapid than IFN-α alone (Quesada et al., 1984; Foon et al., 1986; Golomb et al., 1987). In contrast to other reports, no patient who received the combination achieved a pathologic CR. This may have been due in part to the study's frequent sampling of bone marrow, allowing detection of minimal residual disease. Pentostatin is now approved by the FDA for use as treatment of IFN-α–refractory HCL (*Physician's Desk Reference*, 2000).

Cladribine (Leustatin®) or 2-CdA is another drug evaluated in the treatment of HCL. This drug is a chlorinated purine nucleoside that is resistant to degradation by adenosine deaminase. Once administered, a resultant accumulation of 2-CdA nucleotides occurs in cells with high levels of deoxycytidine kinase and low levels of 5'-nucleotidase activity (e.g., lymphocytes and monocytes). Within the cell, 2-CdA is metabolized into a triphosphate derivative that ultimately causes cell death. In initial investigations with 2-CdA in 12 patients with HCL, there was a marked response (11 CRs and 1 PR with one 7-day course of treatment) (Piro et al., 1990). Subsequent studies confirmed the efficacy of this agent in the treatment of HCL (Estey et al., 1992; Tallman et al., 1992). In 1993, the FDA approved 2-CdA for the treatment of HCL (*Physician's Desk Reference*, 2000).

Zaja et al. (1997) compared the outcome of patients with HCL who were treated with IFN-α with those treated with 2-CdA. Thirty-four patients were enrolled, with 26 receiving 3 mU of IFN-α every other day for 3 months. 2-CdA (0.1 mg/kg each day for 7 days for 1 or 2 cycles) was given as first-line therapy for 8 patients and as second-line therapy for 14 patients resistant to (2 cases) or relapsed after (12 cases) IFN-α. The CR rate was 19% for IFN-α treatment versus 75% for 2-CdA as first-line therapy and versus 86% for 2-CdA as second-line therapy. The PR rate was 58% with IFN-α treatment versus 25% for 2-CdA as first-line therapy and versus 14% for 2-CdA as second-line therapy. Treatment-associated toxicities were evaluated, and both drugs were determined to be safe. The main side effect of IFN-α was flu-like syndrome, whereas 2-CdA induced a hematological toxicity described as initial neutropenia and a long-lasting lymphocytopenia. Only 1 patient developed a major infectious complication (pneumonia), which occurred 3 months after treatment.

Further evaluation of the durability of response to treatment with 2-CdA alone was evaluated in a study by Lauria et al. (1997). Forty patients were followed for a median duration of 48 months (range 30 to 66 months). These patients were treated with 0.1 mg/kg of 2-CdA each day for 7 days. Thirty (75%) patients had CRs, and 10 (25%) had PRs. Among the patients with CRs, one each experienced a relapse at 12, 24, 26, 30, and 36 months after treatment as determined by the HCI; 2 of them were re-treated. Twelve of the original complete responders were still disease-free after 5 years. Eight of the 10 partial responders progressed after 8 to 36 months and were re-treated with 0.15 mg/kg each day for 5 days. Four of these patients attained a CR, three a better PR, and 1 patient died of infection complications. Notably, 1 patient each died after 24 and 37 months because of a second neoplasm. The primary treatment-related toxicity was neutropenia, with the risk of infection being greater in those who started therapy with fewer than 1.0×10^9/L neutrophils.

The purine antagonist 2-CdA has become the most commonly used systemic treatment for patients newly diagnosed with HCL because clinical trials in large numbers of patients have shown a 50% to 60% chance of achieving a durable CR after a single 7-day course of therapy. However, 2-CdA is associated with severe, if temporary, immunosuppression and an attendant risk of infection. For patients who relapse after 2-CdA or for whom 2-CdA is contraindicated because of risk for infection, IFN-α represents an effective alternative treatment strategy.

CHRONIC MYELOGENOUS LEUKEMIA

CML is a hematopoietic stem cell disease of clonal expansion. This malignant clonal disorder results in decreases in myeloid cells, erythroid cells, and platelets in peripheral blood. It also results in distinct myeloid hyperplasia in the bone marrow. CML usually has a biphasic or triphasic course. After an initial chronic phase, there is progression to a blastic phase. For 75% to 80% of patients, this transformation occurs after an intermediate or accelerated phase. The natural history of CML is usually typified by progression from a benign chronic phase to blastic crisis in 3 to 5 years. Survival after the development of blast transformation is usually very short (2 to 4 months). The criteria for chronic and blastic phases have been well defined, but the criteria for the accelerated phase is less well defined. The typical symptoms at presentation are fatigue, anorexia, and weight loss, but in 40% to 50% of cases, patients are asymptomatic, and diagnosis is based solely on abnormal blood counts (Cortes et al., 1998; Sawyers, 1999). Remissions in CML are currently evaluated at several levels: hematologic, cytogenetic, and molecular. Hematologic remissions alone are not sufficient to prevent progression of the disease to a terminal stage. Consequently, current therapeutic goals include the eradication of the malignant clone (the Philadelphia [Ph] chromosome) and the restoration of normal hematopoiesis (Kurzrock et al., 1998).

Most patients diagnosed with CML possess the cytogenic abnormality of oncogene translocation known as the Ph chromosome. The Ph chromosome is characterized by a translocation between chromosomes 9 and 22 that juxtaposes the c-*abl* oncogene from chromosome 9 with the breakpoint cluster region (bcr) on chromosome 22. This results in the abnormal bcr-abl transcripts, which generate a bcr-abl tyrosine kinase gene product. This abnormal tyrosine kinase protein is thought to be responsible for cell proliferation, tranformation of immature hematopoietic cells, and suppression of apoptosis, which are the typical pathogenic features of CML (Enright and McGlave, 1997).

The traditional treatment approach for patients in the chronic phase has been therapy with HU alone or busulfan. HU is a cell-cycle–specific inhibitor of DNA synthesis. Busulfan is an alkylating agent. HU and busulfan achieve hematologic control in 50% to 80% of patients. These agents have little or no effect on disease progression, and cytogenetic remissions are rare. Patients who are treated with these drugs will ultimately experience tranformation to blastic phase, and after a median three to six years, they will die from complications of the disease. Median duration of survival and median duration of chronic phase are longer with HU than with busulfan, and exposure to HU before the transplant is associated with better posttransplant outcome (Faderl *et al.*, 1999).

Use of **p value** (or **alpha level**) in the statistical evaluation of IFN-α in the treatment of CML was first reported by Talpaz *et al.* (1986). This and other early studies of IFN-α for CML (Talpaz *et al.*, 1987) were the first, except for studies of the effect of IFN-α as a pretreatment to allogeneic stem cell transplant, to demonstrate that a single agent was capable of inducing a cytogenetic remission. Another early study conducted at The University of Texas M. D. Anderson Cancer Center (Houston, TX) with 274 patients in early chronic-phase CML showed promising results (Faderl *et al.*, 1999). IFN-α was given daily at a dose of 5 mU/m^2 or the maximum tolerated lower dose. Hematologic CRs were seen in 80% of the patients, and cytogenetic responses were seen in 58% of the patients. Of the cytogenetic responses, 26% were CRs and 38% were major responses.

Three other trials confirmed higher response rates with higher doses of IFN. They also demonstrated a statistically significant survival benefit that showed survival rates were associated with cytogenic response (Alimena *et al.*, 1988; Ozer *et al.*, 1993; Mahon *et al.*, 1996).

Since the introduction of IFN-α for the treatment of CML, there have been many randomized clinical trials that have looked at the impact of the addition of IFN-α to a treatment regimen or comparisons of IFN-α with chemotherapy (Kantarjian *et al.*, 1996). The Chronic Myeloid Leukemia Trialists' Collaborative Group (Oxford, UK) collaborated in a worldwide review of all such clinical trials. Data were compiled from seven trials that represented 1,554 patients with CML, most of whom were Ph-chromosome positive. For these patients, combination-agent regimens that contained IFN-α produced a statistically significant improvement in survival when compared with single-agent studies using HU ($p = .001$) or busulfan ($p = .00007$). Five-year survival rates were 57% with IFN-α and 42% with chemotherapy. These rates may be conservative, because some of the patients in the studies were not in early chronic phase (Chronic Myeloid Leukemia Trialists' Collaborative Group, 1997).

O'Brien *et al.* (1999) designed a chemoimmunotherapy regimen that consisted of homoharringtonine (HHT), which is a novel plant alkaloid, and IFN-α. HHT has been shown to effectively produce hematologic CR in 72% of treated patients with late chronic-phase CML. It also produced 31% cytogenetic remission in this patient group. This study compared patients who received 6 courses of HHT plus maintenance with IFN-α at a target dose of 5 mU/m^2 every day. The IFN-α dose was adjusted to maintain hematologic CR, so the actual median dose delivered to the treatment group was 2.4 mU/m^2. The treatment arm was compared with a cohort of historical controls who received IFN-α alone. This study demonstrated that 66% of patients who received a combination of HHT and IFN-α achieved cytogenetic response and that 61% of patients who received IFN-α alone (historical controls) achieved cytogenetic response (statistical significance was not cited). The authors concluded that induction therapy with HHT followed by maintenance with IFN-α resulted in achievement of hematologic and cytogenetic response with decreased side effects, particularly gastrointestinal side effects and myalgias, although neurotoxicity and fatigue were comparable in both groups. The authors recommended that future studies examine the efficacy of combinations of HHT, IFN-α, and low-dose Ara-C.

There are other chemotherapy agents and investigational approaches to note. Decitabine is a cytidine analogue that has been shown to produce responses in 53% of patients with accelerated-phase CML and 25% with blastic-phase CML. Clinical trials are currently evaluating the use of decitabine in combination with busulfan and cyclophosphamide as preparatory agents for allogeneic transplantation. Another approach is the use of antisense oligonucleotides. These are short DNA sequences modified to bind specific RNA sequences within the cell, thereby prohibiting the translation of the RNA message into functional proteins. The targets for the antisense sequence include bcr-abl, Ras, PI-3-kinase, c-myb, and c-myc. This strategy is also being used *ex vivo* as an element of purging of autologous cells for bone marrow transplantation (BMT). Tyrosine kinase inhibitors are also being studied for their growth-inhibiting effect on CML cell lines. Clinical trials with bcr-abl–specific tyrosine kinase in-

hibitors are underway. Lastly, the role of adoptive immunotherapy is the focus of considerable research. In one study, CML progenitor cells were incubated with granulocyte-macrophage colony-stimulating factor, IL-4, and TNF. This process stimulated the *in vitro* formation of dendritic cells, which are leukemic APCs. The dendritic cells are strong inducers of T-cell responses, and it is hoped that identification of leukemia-specific antigens and stimulation of leukemia-specific T-cell responses will open the door to other approaches, such as immune gene therapy and peptide vaccination (Faderl et al., 1999).

Questions remain about the effectiveness of IFN-α as a post-BMT measure and its efficacy in regimens treating patients with late chronic-phase CML. Higano and fellow researchers (1997) from the Fred Hutchinson Cancer Research Center (Seattle, WA) reported on 14 patients who had a cytogenetic relapse of CML after BMT (12 related donors and 2 syngeneic donors). Daily IFN-α was administered at doses of 1 to 3 mU/m^2 based on initial blood counts. The dose was reduced after a stable cytogenetic remission was achieved with a median time to achieve this remission of 7.5 months (range 1.2 to 12 months). Twelve patients achieved a cytogenetic CR on at least one occasion, and 10 of them remain on IFN. Of these 10, 6 remain in continuous cytogenetic remission for 10+ to 54+ months. Two patients had no response to IFN, and 1 of them relapsed early (day 36) and progressed to blast crisis. The reappearance of the Ph chromosome in the early months after BMT may not be a sign of relapse. Higano et al. (1997) observed this in 4 of 14 patients who were not eligible for the study described above. These 4 patients showed evidence of the Ph chromosome while on cyclosporine therapy for immunosuppression. Signs of the Ph chromosome disappeared after the therapy was stopped. Emergence of the Ph chromosome six months or more after transplant is often predictive of onset of clinical relapse within two years' time. It has also been reported that this chromosome produces hematologic control in the majority of patients treated (Higano *et al.*, 1992; Higano *et al.*, 1993).

Patients diagnosed early in chronic-phase CML and treated with IFN-α have shown hematologic CR of 70% to 80%, with cytogenetic CRs of 5% to 32%. Those who have a cytogenetic response experience a survival benefit, with 80% of these patients alive and in remission after eight years (Sacchi *et al.*, 1997). The benefit to patients with late chronic-phase CML is unclear. Researchers at M. D. Anderson Cancer Center studied the efficacy of IFN-α regimens in 137 patients who were Ph-chromosome positive and in late chronic phase (diagnosis of more than 12 months). In the study, IFN-α regimens induced an overall hematologic CR of 57% and a cytogenetic response rate of 15% (8% with major response and 2% with CR). Regimens that combined IFN-α and low-dose Ara-C were associated with higher hematologic CR. Cytogenetic response rates were associated with an estimated 3-year improvement in survival. Although only the hematologic CR reached statistical significance, the results show promise for further studies that examine the efficacy of IFN-α–based and Ara-C–based therapies and clearly point to the importance of earlier treatment, that is, during early chronic-phase (Sacchi *et al.*, 1997).

CML is a complex disease. The role of therapies for patients newly diagnosed with the disease has been condensed into an algorithm by Faderl *et al.* (1999), as seen in Figure 5.3. As demonstrated in this algorithm, patients who are in late chronic phase of transformed stages of CML should either be enrolled in investigational protocols or should undergo BMT if a donor is available. Patients in early chronic phase should be offered matched sibling transplants if a donor is available and if treatment-related morbidity and mortality (TRMM) is ex-

pected to be less than 20%. This would include younger patients with matched-related donors. For patients with expected TRMM between 20% to 40%, a trial of IFN-α is indicated. This group would include older patients with matched-related donors and younger patients with molecularly matched unrelated donors. If the expected TRMM is greater than 40%, it may be advisable to defer stem cell grafting until clear signs of disease acceleration appear. Patients who fall into this group would include older individuals who will receive a matched-unrelated donor transplant or transplant with molecular mismatches. For these patients, IFN-α–based therapies or other investigational modalities may be preferable. Additionally, for patients who are total nonresponders to initial therapy as well as those who lose their initial hematologic or cytogenetic response, investigational therapies such as autografting, matched-unrelated donor transplants, and new agents (either alone or in combination) are recommended. Table 5.3 outlines guidelines for therapy with IFN-α in patients with CML (Talpaz *et al.*, 1997; Faderl *et al.*, 1999).

IFN-α continues to be an effective therapy for many patients with CML, with evidence of both hematologic and cytogenetic remissions. There are, however, complexities in determining the optimal therapy based on the phase of the disease (chronic phase versus accelerated phase versus blast phase), the role of the Ph chromosome, the age and performance status of the patient, and availability of an appropriate bone marrow donor.

B-Cell Malignancies

MULTIPLE MYELOMA

MM is a plasma-cell dyscrasia that results from the clonal proliferation of plasma cells. MM accounts for about 10% of all hematologic malignancies in the United States, is considered a disease of older adults (over 50 years of age;

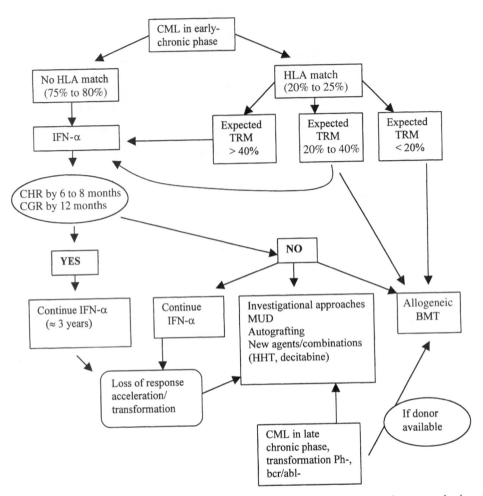

Figure 5.3 Suggested treatment algorithm for newly diagnosed chronic myelogenous leukemia patients (CML). Patients with CML in late chronic phase of transformed stages should either be enrolled in investigational protocols or undergo allogeneic bone marrow transplant (BMT) if a donor can be found. Patients in early chronic phase should be offered matched-sibling transplants if a donor is available and treatment-related morbidity and mortality is expected to be less than 20%, (e.g., in younger patients with matched related donors). For patients with expected mortality between 20% and 40% (e.g., older patients with matched related donors and younger patients with a molecularly matched unrelated donor [MUD]), a trial of IFN-α is indicated. If expected mortality exceeds 40% (e.g., MUD transplant in older patients or transplant with molecular mismatches), it may be advisable to defer stem cell grafting until clear signs of disease acceleration appear. In such patients interferon (IFN)-α–based therapies or other investigational modalities may be preferable. Likewise, in those who never respond to initial therapy and those who lose their initial hematologic or cytogenetic response, investigational therapies, including autografting, MUD transplants, and new agents (either alone or in combination) should be tried.

CGR, cytogenetic response; CHR, complete hematologic response; HHT, homoharringtonine; HLA, human lymphocyte antigen; TRM, transplant-related mortality.

Source: Adapted from Faderl *et al.* 1999. Chronic myelogenous leukemia: Update on biology and treatment. *Oncology* 13(2): 169–181.

Table 5.3   Guidelines of chronic myelogenous leukemia with interferon-α

Initiating therapy
- Start cytoreduction with hydroxyurea (1 to 5 g/day) to decrease WBC count to 10 to 20 × 10^9 before starting IFN-α therapy.
- Initiate IFN-α at lower dose and increase gradually (3 mμ/day for 3 to 7 days, then 5 mU/day for 3 to 7 days, then 5 mμ/m^2 or maximum tolerated dose).
- Older patients are more sensitive to side effects of IFN-α and may not tolerate full doses.
- Premedicate with acetaminophen to lessen fever and chills.
- Inject doses at bedtime.
- Common chronic side effects include a triad of fatigue, depression, and insomnia. Low doses of tricyclic antidepressants, e.g., amitriptyline 2.5 to 50 mg at bedtime may be of benefit. Neuropsychiatric consultation can be helpful in some cases.

Dosage adjustments
- Do not reduce the dose of IFN-α if WBC count is low, unless WBC count is <2 × 10^9 or platelet count is <50 × 10^9.
- For grade 3 and 4 toxicities, withhold dose until toxicity lessens or resolves and restart at 50% of dose. For grade 2 persistent toxicities, reduce dose by 25%.
- Withhold IFN-α during moderate acute intercurrent illness.

Monitoring
- Monitor complete blood counts weekly until stable, then twice monthly.
- Aim for a WBC count between 2 and 4 x 10^9 and platelet count >50 × 10^9.
- Monitor cytogenetic response on bone marrow aspirates every 3 months during the first year, then every 4 to 6 months.
- Perform I-FISH on peripheral blood samples every 3 months until Ph-positive cells are <10%.
- Perform H-FISH on bone marrow when Ph-positive cells are <10%.
- Monitor for unusual complications, e.g., T4, TSH for thyroid abnormalities.

Severe bone pain when WBC >20 × 10^9
- Hold IFN-α.
- Give hydroxyurea to decrease WBC count.
- Give steroids (solumedrol 50 mg by mouth, bid until pain resolves then taper over 1 week, or give narcotics (dilaudid 2 mg by mouth every 3 hours as needed with NSAID until pains resolve).
- Restart IFN-α after pain resolves for 1 week and WBC count is <5 × 10^9, continue giving hydroxyurea for approximately 1 month.

bid, twice a day; IFN, interferon; H-FISH, hypermetaphase fluorescence *in situ* hybridization; I-FISH, interphase fluorescence *in situ* hybridization; NSAID, nonsteroidal anti-inflammatory drug; Ph, Phildelphia chromosome; T4, levothyroxine; TSH, thyroid-stimulating hormone; WBC, white blood cell.

Source: Adapted from Faderl *et al.* 1999. Chronic myelogenous leukemia: Update on biology and treatment. *Oncology* 13(2): 1999. 169–181; Talpaz *et al.* 1997. The M. D. Anderson Cancer Center experience with interferon-alpha therapy in chronic myelogenous leukemia. *Ballieres Clin Haematol* 10(2): 291–305.

median age 70 for men, 68 for women), and occurs in African-Americans twice as frequently as in whites. Advances in the understanding of the biology of MM indicate that this disease is a multistep tranformation process that probably involves a series of molecular events, including gene mutation, oncogene activation, and growth-factor dysregulation. Additionally, a number of studies have indicated that IL-6 is a major cytokine regulator in the growth and survival of myeloma cells (Huang *et al.*, 1999).

Although MM, a disease characterized by uncontrolled proliferation of malignant plasma cells, responds initially to a variety of chemotherapeutic agents, once it becomes refractory to first-line therapies, further responses and prolonged survival are difficult to achieve. As a single agent, recombinant IFN-α continues to demonstrate response rates of 10% to 20% in previously treated patients with MM and 50% in previously untreated patients (Costanzi *et al.*, 1985; Quesada *et al.*, 1986a;). This response rate is clearly inferior to that of conventional chemotherapy (Huang *et al.*, 1999).

Whereas little progress has been made over the last 2 decades in clinical studies of MM, recent studies suggest that dose intensification requiring stem cell rescue has demonstrated higher CR rates. In 1 reported case-controlled study of 116 patients with MM, the treatment group received "total therapy" consisting of an induction regimen followed by autologous transplant, with a maintenance period (after hematologic recovery) of IFN-α until disease recurrence or progression. This group was compared with matched historic controls who received standard therapy with melphalan and prednisone. The "total therapy" regimen resulted in CR in 40% of the intent-to-treat group. Median duration of event-free survival was 49 months, and overall survival was 62+ months. Abnormalities of chromosomes 11q and 13 were negative prognostic indicators. Attainment of a CR within 6 months after induction therapy was associated with a favorable prognosis (Barlogie *et al.*, 1997).

Data from a 1990 study by Mandelli *et al.* (1990) demonstrated that the addition of IFN-α as maintenance therapy after 12 months of chemotherapy had a positive impact on response and survival durations. In this study, response duration and median survival duration were significantly longer in the group that re- ceived IFN-α maintenance therapy. The treated group in this study showed an advantage of 12 to 13 months over the control group in response duration and survival duration respectively.

Subsequently, IFN-α was found to prolong the duration of response in patients with MM treated with the vincristine, doxorubicin, and dexamethasone (VAD) regimen. The treatment group consisted of those patients recruited after 1990 ($n = 33$) who received VAD followed by 5 mU IFN-α subcutaneously 3 times a week for a maximum of 2 years. They were compared with patients treated between 1985 and 1990 with VAD alone ($n = 31$). Time to response and rate of objective response were similar for both groups; however, the survival analysis differed. A longer median progression-free period was noted for the VAD plus IFN group compared with the IFN-alone group (39.6 months versus 12 months, respectively). The overall survival duration was also longer for the VAD plus IFN group compared with the IFN-alone group (65+ months versus 24 months, respectively) (Kars *et al.*, 1997).

In a 1998 report of the Southwest Oncology Group (SWOG) study 9028, Salmon *et al.* described the results of treatment with IFN-α plus prednisone (IFN-α/P) for remission maintenance in patients with MM. Of the 233 patients who were treated with VAD or VAD plus verapamil and quinine, 89 patients became eligible for the study after achieving remission. Early in the trial, the data-monitoring committee closed the arm that contained VAD plus verapamil and quinine because there were nine deaths in that arm in comparison with only one death on the VAD-alone arm. Maintenance therapy consisted of two arms. Patients on the IFN-α–alone arm received IFN-α 3 mU subcutaneously 3 times a week. Patients on the IFN-α/P arm received IFN-α at the same schedule plus 50 mg prednisone as a single dose 3 times a week the morning after IFN-α administration. Protocol guidelines permitted a 50% reduction in IFN dose for patients who experienced significant toxicity, but after resolution of toxicity, the dose was escalated if feasible. Results were statistically significant in favor of the IFN-α/P arm. This group had improved, progression-free survival duration (median 19 months versus 9 months; $p = .008$).

A preliminary report from Byrne *et al.* (1998) showed that adjuvant IFN-α could improve remission rates for MM following allogeneic BMT. Although this form of therapy may be curative in some patients with MM, relapse is the major cause of treatment failure. This study reports on 5 of 14 evaluable patients who were undergoing allogeneic sibling-donor BMT or peripheral blood stem cell transplant. At a median time of 126 days posttransplant, those patients who met the criteria were started on IFN-α at a dosage of 3 mU 3 times a week with the potential of reducing it to 2 times per week if there was exacerbation of graft-versus-host disease or development of significant thrombocytopenia ($<50 \times 10^9$/L). Treatment continued until achievement of CR or until disease progression. Cyclosporin therapy was tapered from day 50 or longer posttransplant and had to be discontinued for at least 1 month prior to starting IFN-α therapy. Durable CRs were achieved between 8 and 36 weeks after initiating therapy with IFN-α. None of the patients who achieved CR following IFN-α therapy had relapsed when these data were reported.

Overall, it appears that IFN-α has activity in patients with MM; however, IFN-α as monotherapy appears to be less active than chemotherapy regimens. There appears to be promise in the utilization of IFN-α in combination with certain chemotherapy regimens or following BMT as a form of maintenance treatment. Utilization of results from these studies requires careful attention to the specific regimens because there can be significant differences between protocols apart from the addition of IFN-α.

NON-HODGKIN'S LYMPHOMA

Clinically, most cases of NHL can be categorized into 2 major groups: low grade and high grade. The low-grade or indolent NHLs are usually not curable and have a long natural history with a median survival duration of 8 to 10 years. High-grade or aggressive NHL tends to progress quickly and can become fatal within a few months if not treated (Shipp, 1997).

Based on consistent demonstration of its activity against lymphomas in phase I trials, especially in the indolent (low-grade) lymphomas, several phase II studies of IFN-α were undertaken to define more precisely the rate and duration of response to this agent in patients with lymphomas. Early studies used both crude-natural and recombinant forms of IFN-α. Antitumor responses were reported in 33% to 50% of patients with early indolent lymphoma, whereas patients with intermediate-grade NHL tended to have fewer objective responses (Wagstaff *et al* , 1986; Price *et al.*, 1991; Smalley *et al.*, 1992). It was not until 1982 that IFN-α was studied in combination with standard chemotherapy. McLaughlin *et al.* (1993) reported on a study with 127 patients with stage IV, low-grade lymphoma. Prior to treatment with cyclophosphamide, doxorubicin, vincristine, prednisone, and bleomycin (CHOP-Bleo), 51 patients were pretreated with 3 mU of IFN-α given intramuscularly every day for 8 weeks. Excluded from this group were patients with high-risk features such as bulky adenopathy, mediastinal or pleural disease, cytopenias, or visceral displacement. All patients were treated with CHOP-Bleo for 9 to 18 months. Those patients who attained CR were treated with IFN-α at 3 mU intramuscularly 3 times a week for 24 months as maintenance therapy.

There was a significant improvement in relapse-free survival for patients who received maintenance therapy with IFN-α after achieving a CR with CHOP-Bleo. The overall response rate for the entire treatment program was

73% CR and 23% PR, with a median follow-up of 59 months. At 5 years, the relapse-free survival rate was 47%, and for those who had attained a CR, it was 60%. When compared with historical controls treated with CHOP-Bleo during the period between 1972 and 1982, these data represent statistical significance for overall relapse-free survival ($p = .01$) and for relapse-free survival in the CR group ($p = .01$). The authors noted that the problem of tolerance of IFN was surprising, given the low dose that was utilized. Some of the side effects that were underemphasized at that time included nasal congestion, the occasional severity of the fatigue/involution/depression syndrome, and impotence. The authors call for a better means to ameliorate IFN toxicity and maximize the potential for benefit from maintenance therapy with IFN-α. In this study, IFN-α also demonstrated activity in NHL as a single agent in patients who received induction therapy. After 8 weeks of induction, 29% of patients experienced major response, and 33% experienced minor response.

The efficacy of maintenance therapy with IFN-α in clinically aggressive low-grade or intermediate-grade NHL was studied by Smalley et al. (1992). A four-drug cytotoxic regimen of cyclophosphamide, vincristine, prednisone, and doxorubicin (COPA) was chosen on the basis of its efficacy in an Eastern Cooperative Oncology Group (ECOG) study of patients who had advanced NHL with unfavorable histologic features. In a pilot feasibility study, it had been demonstrated that adding IFN-α to this regimen was feasible, but the schedule had to be altered so that treatment was given every 28 days rather than every 21 days. The rationale was to avoid additive myelotoxicity and a desire to avoid simultaneous administration of prednisone and IFN-α. Patients received 8 to 10 cycles of therapy every 4 weeks. The treatment consisted of cyclophosphamide, vincristine, and doxorubicin on day 1 and prednisone on days 1 through

5 for both groups. The experimental group also received IFN-α on days 22 through 26 of each 28-day cycle.

IFN-alfa-2b was approved by the FDA in 1997 for use with CHOP-like regimens in patients with advanced low-grade follicular NHL. The approval was based on research by the French cooperative group, Groupe d'Etude des Lymphomes Folliculaires (GELF). The pivotal trial compared CHVP alone against CHVP plus IFN-α. The CHVP regimen used in the trial consisted of cyclophosphamide 600 mg/m^2, doxorubicin 25 mg/m^2, and teniposide 60 mg/m^2 (all on day 1) and prednisone 40 mg (for 5 days). CHVP is somewhat less intensive than the American CHOP regimen, which consists of cyclophosphamide 750 mg/m^2, doxorubicin 50 mg/m^2, and vincristine 1.4 mg/m^2 (maximum 2.0 mg) and 5 days of prednisone 100 mg.

The pivotal GELF study by Solal-Celigny et al. (1997) involved 242 patients with advanced follicular lymphoma. Chemotherapy with CHVP was administered once a month for 6 months. Patients who responded by month 6 or who had stable disease continued with chemotherapy once every other month for an additional 12 months or until disease progression. In addition to and during CHVP therapy, the experimental group received IFN-α 5 mU subcutaneously 3 times per week for 18 months. The FDA-approved usage of IFN-alfa-2b is 5 mU 3 times a week to be administered with an **anthracycline**-containing chemotherapy regimen. It is important to note that the doses of CHVP are lower than those of CHOP and that concurrent use of IFN-α with full-dose CHOP therapy has not been studied. It is recommended that, if concurrent use of IFN-α is desired with the CHOP regimen, the initial anthracycline and cyclophosphamide doses should be decreased by 25%.

The median progression-free survival for the CHVP plus IFN-α group was 2.9 years compared with 1.5 years for the group that received

CHVP alone ($p = .0002$). A follow-up report from May 1996 showed that median survival duration had not been reached for the CHVP plus IFN-α group, whereas the CHVP-alone group had reached a median survival duration of 5.6 years ($p = .0084$) (Solal-Celigny et al., 1998). Risk factors for overall survival, using Cox's stepwise regression model, included number of extranodal sites ($p = .004$), treatment with CHVP plus IFN-α ($p = .011$), performance status ($p = .02$), and age ($p = .04$). Adverse events with World Health Organization (WHO) grade 3 or 4 disease were more frequent in the IFN-α–treated group and included asthenia (10% versus 3%, respectively), neutropenia (34% versus 6%, respectively), and elevation in liver enzymes (4% versus 0%, respectively). The increase in neutropenia in the IFN-treated group did not result in an increase in the incidence of neutropenic infections.

Quality of life was also measured using the Q-Twist (quality time without symptoms or toxicity) analysis. In cancer treatment, it is usually expected that there will be a period of time in which toxicity will be increased (the treatment-related period). By plotting data derived from Cox regression analysis using a Kaplan-Meier curve, a survival plot is developed that reflects the gain of time free from symptoms of the cancer or from side effects of the treatment regimen. The quality-adjusted years gained may then be calculated. The Q-Twist analysis used in the GELF study demonstrated that the IFN-α group had more time without symptoms of disease progression or treatment-related toxicity and a significantly prolonged quality-adjusted survival duration ($p < .05$).

IFN-α has demonstrated efficacy in patients with follicular lymphoma when added to an anthracycline-containing chemotherapy regimen. A course of maintenance therapy following an anthracycline-containing regimen such as CHOP appears to prolong remissions in patients with indolent lymphomas (Shipp, 1997).

Quality-of-life studies also support the use of IFN-α as approved by the FDA.

T-Cell Malignancies

Cutaneous T-cell lymphomas (CTCLs) such as mycosis fungoides, Sézary syndrome, and reticulum-cell sarcoma of the skin are NHLs characterized by a malignant proliferation of mature T_h lymphocytes. CTCLs consist of neoplasms that home to the skin and to the T-cell zones of lymphoid tissue but rarely involve the bone marrow. Effective therapies include topical mechlorethamine hydrochloride (nitrogen mustard, NM) or bischoloethyl-nitrosourea (BCNU), psoralen plus ultraviolet (PUVA) therapy, local external-beam irradiation, total-skin electron beam therapy, and IFN-α (Mostow et al., 1993; Kuzel et al., 1995; Wilson et al., 1997).

Topical chemotherapy with the alkylating agents NM or BCNU can result in CR in 64% to 92% of patients with early-stage (T1 or T2) disease. Median survival duration for these patients was 8 years; however, 7 of 8 patients have a relapse within 3 years unless treated with maintenance therapy. PUVA kills CTCLs. It also interferes with antigen presentation and cytokine production in the skin. This therapy is effective for patients with patches or thin plaques but is unlikely to produce a CR in patients with thicker plaques or tumors (Zackheim, 1994).

Systemic therapies initially included cytotoxic chemotherapy regimens but their efficacy in the treatment of CTCL was limited. Practice has since been changed to include immune-modulating therapies such as IFNs, monoclonal antibodies, or investigational agents combined with photopheresis. Several phase II clinical trials of IFN-α have been performed (Bunn et al., 1984; Covelli et al., 1987; Olsen et al., 1987). The response rate in these early studies was variable: about 79% of previously untreated patients responded to IFN therapy, whereas the response rates in pretreated patients ranged between 45% and 70%. The average duration of response was about 9 months in previously treated patients.

Bunn *et al.* (1989) evaluated recombinant IFN-α at a dose of 50 mU/m^2 3 times a week in patients with CTCL who were previously untreated. Nine of 20 patients responded (2 CRs and 7 PRs). Responses in both cutaneous and extracutaneous sites were reported. These results were similar to those found by other investigators (Olsen *et al.*, 1989) who treated patients with skin involvement only with either 3 mU IFN daily or in escalating doses of 3 to 36 mU IFN daily for 10 weeks. Three patients had a CR, and 10 had a PR. From these results, the authors concluded that there is a dose-response relationship.

The maximum tolerated dose of IFN-α given in combination with PUVA therapy is reported to be 12 mU/m^2 (Springer *et al.*, 1991). CRs were achieved in some patients who were refractory to PUVA therapy at IFN-α doses of 3 to 6 mU. Kuzel *et al.* (1995) reported on the effectiveness of IFN-α in combination with phototherapy; in this treatment scheme, IFN-α is considered to be a "PUVA booster."

Solid Tumors

In solid tumors, the objective response rates from treatment with single-agent IFN-α have not been as high as those for the hematologic malignancies and lymphomas. Despite this, IFN-α has significant activity in solid tumors, often when combined with cytotoxic chemotherapy or biological or differentiating agents.

ACQUIRED IMMUNODEFICIENCY SYNDROME-RELATED KAPOSI'S SARCOMA

KS, once a rare malignancy of the skin, is now the most frequent malignancy in men with AIDS (Scandinavian Study Group, 1997). Prognosis is poor for those with progressive disease, with a median survival duration of less than 6 months. There are several therapies now available for palliation. Radiation therapy is a choice for those with a limited number of lesions. Severe or progressive KS has been treated with chemotherapy regimens such as bleomycin and vincristine (BV), doxorubicin plus BV (DBV), or liposomal daunorubicin. Fewer than 10% achieve CR but 50% to 80% will have a PR. IFN-α has been useful in patients with predominantly mucocutaneous disease. It is most effective in patients with limited lymphadenopathy, no history of opportunistic infections, absence of B symptoms (e.g., fever, night sweats, cachexia, and diarrhea), and an intact immune system (CD4 count greater than 200/mm^3) (Morris and Valley, 1996).

Prior to the recognition of the human immunodeficiency virus 1 (HIV-1) as the causative agent of AIDS, several studies were conducted in groups of homosexual men with KS. These studies were based on evidence that IFN-α had a therapeutic effect in viral diseases. Krown and colleagues (1983) reported the earliest phase I trial of recombinant IFN-α in AIDS-related KS. Five of 12 patients had major objective responses to IFN-α (3 CR and 2 PR). These data have been confirmed in larger groups of patients treated with IFN-alfa-2a (Krown *et al.*, 1984; Krown *et al.*, 1986a; Krown *et al.*, 1986b; Real *et al.*, 1986) and IFN-alfa-2b (Groopman *et al.*, 1984; Mitsuyasu *et al.*, 1984; Volberding and Mitsuyasu, 1985). Objective response rates approaching 30% were reported when IFN-α was administered in high doses (>20 mU/m^2) (Abrams and Volberding, 1987). It appears that high (10 to 36 mU) and very high (> 36 mU) doses daily have been associated with better response rates than lower doses (Goldstein and Laszlo, 1986). Retrospective analyses have identified positive prognostic indicators, including higher CD4 count, skin test reactivity to recall antigens, or greater proliferative responses to mitogens and bacterial antigens (Miles *et al.*, 1997).

The combination of azidothymidine (AZT) and IFN-α has been observed to have a synergistic antiretroviral effect both *in vivo* and *in vitro* (Hartshorn *et al.*, 1987). Early pilot studies based on this combination have reported tumor response rates between 33% and 63%. In addition to tumor response, *in vivo* antiviral effects have been reported (Fischl *et al.*, 1988; Mullen *et al.*, 1988; Krown *et al.*, 1989). In studies in which IFN-α was given at doses ranging from 4.5 to 18 mU in combination with AZT at either 100 or 200 mg every 4 hours, tumors regressed at every dose level, with higher doses producing more responses (Hartshorn *et al.*, 1987). Tumor remissions were seen with much lower doses of IFN-α in the combination regimen than were acquired with IFN alone. Responses occurred in patients with prior opportunistic infections and other poor prognostic features. Myelotoxicity and hepatotoxicity were the dose-limiting side effects of this combination.

IFN-α is an important investigational agent in patients with HIV infection without KS. The well-documented efficacy of IFN-α against AIDS-related KS led to its approval by the FDA as therapy for that condition. The recent success seen with protease inhibitors and the subsequent elevation of CD4 counts in patients with AIDS will probably contribute to reconsideration of the types of therapy available to those who were previously severely immunocompromised. The therapeutic effect of IFN-α seems to be dose-related and is greatest at high doses (>20 mU/m^2) (Abrams and Volberding, 1987), higher daily doses (10 to 36 mU), and very high doses (>36 mU daily). Some studies are currently looking at the combination of protease inhibitors and lower-dose IFN-α (Miles *et al.*, 1997).

Although no clear-cut immunologic improvement has been observed in AIDS patients treated with IFN-α, in a study by Mitsuyasu (1988), opportunistic infections were less frequently diagnosed and survival was improved in a subset of treated patients. Systemic cytotoxic chemotherapy is still the primary treatment choice for patients with visceral KS or widespread KS.

GASTROINTESTINAL MALIGNANCIES

Although IFN-α has shown therapeutic activity in several hematologic malignancies, its performance as a single agent as treatment for adenocarcinomas and other solid tumors has been disappointing. Colon carcinoma is a solid tumor with a low rate of response to all agents, including IFN; however, 5-fluorouracil (5-FU) may induce a relatively brief PR in 15% to 20% of patients. Preclinical studies suggest that the coadministration of IFN-α and 5-FU elevates the serum level of the chemotherapeutic agent from 1.5-fold to 64-fold (Grem *et al.*, 1990; Lindley *et al.*, 1990). Recombinant IFN-α has been shown to enhance the cytotoxic effect of 5-FU *in vitro*. In a pilot clinical trial conducted by Wadler and colleagues; the combination induced a PR in 63% of the patients (Wadler *et al.*, 1984; Wadler and Wiernik, 1990). To confirm these findings, a phase II clinical trial (Wadler *et al.*, 1991) was conducted by the ECOG in 1989. The treatment regimen consisted of 5-FU (750 mg/m^2 each day for 5 days) by continuous infusion followed by weekly outpatient bolus therapy and IFN-α (9 mU) subcutaneously 3 times a week beginning on day 1. The objective response rate was 42%, including 1 clinical CR and 14 PRs. Doses were modified for gastrointestinal, hematologic, and neurologic toxic effects and for fatigue.

A phase II trial evaluated the effects of the addition of IFN-α to systemic 5-FU and leucovorin in patients with colorectal cancer and liver metastasis (Patt *et al.*, 1997). Patients were selected if they were refractory to previous 5-FU–based treatment. Percutaneous catheters and internal pumps were installed for the intrahepatic instillation. IFN-α at a dose of 5 mU/ m^2 was infused over 6 hours followed by 1,500 mg/m^2 of 5-FU over 18 hours. The criteria for CR included complete disappearance of all disease as observed by computed tomography (CT) scanning and normalization of carcinoembryonic antigen (CEA) levels. Responses were evaluable in 45 of 48 patients. Three (6.6%) patients had a CR, and 12 (26.6%) had a PR (greater than 50% reduction of all tumor nodules by CT scan). The median response duration was 7 months. Interestingly, a steroid (dexamethasone) was administered at either 10 mg intravenously or 8 mg by mouth as premedication prior to IFN instillation.

In phase II clinical trials of recombinant IFN-α plus 5-FU in advanced colorectal carcinoma, the combination had a greater therapeutic effect than would be expected for 5-FU alone (Huberman *et al.*, 1990; Kemeny *et al.*, 1990; Pazdur *et al.*, 1990; Wadler and Wiernik, 1990; Wadler *et al.*, 1991). To better understand the efficacy and safety of this combination, an international multicenter randomized trial in 234 patients was conducted and reported by York *et al.* (1993). Patients with advanced colorectal carcinoma were randomized to receive 5-FU alone at a dose of 750 mg/m^2 daily for 5 days by continuous infusion, followed by a weekly dose of the same 5-FU schedule plus 9 mU IFN-α 3 times a week. The overall response rates (CR and PR) were 20% in the group that received 5-FU alone and 25% in the group that received the combination treatment. Although mild nausea, vomiting, diarrhea, and stomatitis were common side effects in both groups, fever and fatigue were more common in the patients who received IFN. In this randomized study, the combination of 5-FU and IFN-α had activity similar to that of 5-FU alone with no prolongation of the duration of remission or survival.

In another phase III trial, 496 patients with advanced colorectal cancer were randomized to receive either 5-FU plus IFN-α or 5-FU plus leucovorin (Kocha, 1993). The overall response rates were 21% in the 5-FU plus IFN-α group and 18% in the 5-FU plus leucovorin group, indicating that these 2 regimens yield more or less equal periods of response and survival. Severe diarrhea, nausea and vomiting, and stomatitis were more common in the leucovorin arm; whereas fatigue, somnolence, and fever were more frequent in the IFN-α arm. The combination of 5-FU and IFN-α, therefore, appears comparable with either high-dose 5-FU or 5-FU plus leucovorin, but none of the 3 treatments has clear-cut superiority.

Although studies have demonstrated that the combination of IFN-α and 5-FU can enhance the cytotoxicity of the chemotherapeutic agent, the value of using the combination at standard doses remains under question. Dose intensification of 5-FU is hindered by the rapid onset of mucosal toxic effects such as diarrhea and stomatitis and the secondary toxicity of myelosuppression. 5-FU–induced diarrhea may be caused by the alteration in balance between the host flora and normal leukocytes in the bowel. Following mucosal damage, a release of inflammatory cytokines occurs and may lead to malabsorption of water and decreased bowel transit time. Studies have shown that granulocyte colony-stimulating factor (G-CSF) can accelerate the migration and survival of neutrophils in mucosal tissue, resulting in healing of ulcers in a patient with idiopathic neutropenia and reduction of oral ulceration and gingivitis in patients with cyclic neutropenia (Wadler *et al.*, 1998). Given these results, and in an effort to reduce the severity of toxicity in a dose-escalation study, Wadler *et al.* (1998) designed a clinical trial of weekly intensive therapy with 5-FU on two different schedules in combination with IFN-α and G-CSF in patients with advanced solid tumors (ECOG P-Z991). The complex study schema incorporated four treatment arms. In arms A and B, patients received 5-FU as a 5-day continuous infusion plus IFN-α and

G-CSF. Patients in arms C and D received 2.6 to 3.4 g/m² of 5-FU as a 24-hour, high-dose infusion along with IFN-α and G-CSF. In all arms, IFN-α was administered subcutaneously 3 times a week at doses ranging between 3 and 9 mU. IFN-α was administered immediately before 5-FU on the days 5-FU was administered. In all arms G-CSF was administered at 5 mcg/kg subcutaneously. In arms A and B, G-CSF was given 24 hours after the initial 5-FU infusion was completed, stopped 48 hours before each weekly dose of 5-FU, and restarted 24 hours after completion of each weekly dose. Another goal of arms A and C was to demonstrate the safety and tolerability of combining IFN-α with G-CSF.

Although the questions asked by this study were related to dose escalation and tolerability of a novel combination of therapeutic agents, there were 4 PRs: 2 patients with colon cancer, 1 patient with prostate cancer, and 1 patient with endometrial carcinoma. The study demonstrated that IFN-α and G-CSF could be administered simultaneously without causing any additional side effects. Specifically, there did not appear to be an increase in the symptoms commonly associated with IFN-α (e.g., flu-like symptoms and fatigue) nor an increase in common symptoms associated with G-CSF (e.g., bone pain and dyspnea). Other studies have reported profound myelosuppression when 5-FU and G-CSF were combined, which has resulted in a consensus that there should be at least 24 hours between administration of G-CSF and the start of 5-FU. In this study, however, G-CSF was administered approximately 6 hours after the 5-FU was completed, which allowed for 5 rather than 4 doses between schedules and treatment and resulted in only infrequent myelosuppression. The authors conclude that weekly intensive therapy with 5-FU, IFN-α, and G-CSF is feasible. G-CSF had its greatest impact on reducing neutropenia, but it remains unclear whether it significantly decreases the mucosal toxicities of this regimen. Recommendations were made for use of this combination in a phase II trial (Wadler et al., 1998).

The role of IFN-α in the treatment of colorectal cancer remains under investigation. IFN-α may be useful in combination with cytotoxic chemotherapy, but research in this area is still in its early stages.

BLADDER CANCER

Bladder cancer is the second most common urological malignancy in the United States, occurring as the fourth most frequent malignancy in men and tenth most frequent for women. The majority of these tumors (90%) are transitional cell carcinomas (TCC), which are usually superficial and limited to the mucosal lining of the bladder. TCC often presents with superficial tumors that are treated with transurethral resection and intravesicular chemotherapy or immunotherapy. After initial treatment, most of these TCCs will recur, and 20% will progress to invade the muscle or become metastatic. This suggests the need for prophylactic or adjuvant therapy after surgery. Carcinoma in situ (CIS) is a superficial bladder tumor that lies within the confines of the urothelial lining. It has a higher histological grade and carries a greater potential for deeper invasion than TCC.

Bacille de Calmette-Guérin (BCG) is a potent, nonspecific, immunomodulatory drug. Intravesicular instillation of BCG for the treatment of TCC and CIS of the bladder has demonstrated average response rates of 40% to 70% (Glashan, 1990; Zhang et al., 1997). Intravesical chemotherapy has shown far less success, with response rates of 0% to 36% for thiotepa, 10% to 23% for doxorubicin, and 2% to 39% for mitomycin C (Glashan, 1990). Chemotherapy administered intravesically can result in bladder irritation as well as systemic toxicities.

BCG has been the mainstay of therapy for superficial bladder cancer, but it has been associated with significant complications, including cystitis, dysuria, hematuria, pneumonitis, and BCG sepsis (Stricker *et al.*, 1996). Standard BCG immunotherapy consists of 6 weekly treatments and a maintenance regimen of 3 weekly treatments every 6 months for 3 years. Although the response rates have been good, there is a relapse rate of 20% to 40% (Belldegrun *et al.*, 1998). Recognition of the antiproliferative effects of IFN-α in human bladder cancer cell lines led to the study of IFN-α as therapy for this disease. Early phase I and phase II trials demonstrated a potential for efficacy without dose-limiting systemic or local toxicity.

In a prospective, randomized trial, Glashan *et al.* (1990) treated 87 patients with CIS of the bladder. Fifty-four percent of these patients had received previous treatment with chemotherapy or BCG. Two different dose levels of IFN-alfa-2b (10 mU [$n = 38$] or 100 mU [$n = 47$]) were administered intravesically every week for 12 weeks and then monthly for 1 year. Therapy was administered within 1 month of a documented positive cytology. The IFN-alfa-2b was reconstituted in 30 mL of sterile water and instilled directly into the bladder via catheterization. Patients had been instructed to take nothing by mouth for 8 hours prior to the procedure to minimize premature voiding, because the IFN-alfa-2b was to be retained for 2 hours. They were asked to rotate positions every 15 minutes to ensure contact for the entire mucosal surface. Current practice has eliminated the rotation of positions, and patients are free to leave after instillation of the IFN-alfa-2b, although they are asked to restrain from voiding for 2 hours. Responses were seen in both the low- and high-dose arms, with a statistically significant difference of 43% versus 5% ($p \leq .0001$) in favor of the high-dose treatment. Patients with a lower tumor stage had a more favorable response. Prior treatment with either chemotherapy or BCG did not affect the ability of a patient to respond to IFN-alfa-2b, suggesting a lack of

cross-resistance and providing a rationale for future research using combination therapy. Some of the mechanisms thought to be responsible for the therapeutic effects of IFN on bladder cancer include inhibition of tumor proliferation, induction of differentiation, upregulation of NK cells, and enhanced expression of tumor-associated antigens (Molto *et al.*, 1995; Zhang *et al.*, 1997).

In an effort to determine the mechanism by which intravesicular administration of IFN-α exerts its anticancer effects, the NK cell activity of peripheral blood mononuclear cells (PBMNCs) was studied in two groups of previously untreated patients with superficial bladder cancer. Seventeen patients (all men) received weekly intravesicular therapy with 50 mU IFN-α for 3 months. Twelve patients (10 men and 2 women) received mitomycin C at 30 mg each week for 3 months; these patients served as the control group. Additionally, 48 healthy, age- and sex-matched subjects were selected as healthy controls. All patients were studied prior to surgical resection of the tumor and at months 2, 3, and 6. Results showed that treatment with IFN-α significantly enhanced the NK cell activity of PBMNCs in those patients who remained free of recurrence after 1 year of follow-up. The authors suggested that the therapeutic effects of intravesicular IFN-α are not due to an expansion of NK cells in the PBMNCs cells but rather to an activation of effector cells. They also acknowledge that cyclic use of IFN-α might further enhance the therapeutic effects (Molto *et al.*, 1995).

In vitro and *in vivo* studies have been developed to examine the mechanism and efficacy of combining 2 immunomodulatory agents: BCG and IFN-α. It was found that BCG and IFN-α had an additive antiproliferative effect on selected human bladder cancer cells. Further studies showed that those cell lines that were less sensitive to BCG were highly sensitive to IFN-α. The authors suggest that the enhanced cytolytic and antiproliferative effects seen with the combination of these agents may be caused by the induction of cytokines. This may result in increased clinical benefit (Zhang *et al.,* 1997).

The use of BCG and IFN-α in combination has shown promise in a phase I study of 12 patients with superficial bladder cancer (Stricker *et al.,* 1996). Patients were randomized to receive low-dose BCG (60 mg) plus IFN-α (10 to 100 mU). BCG and IFN-α were mixed in 50 mL of sterile water and instilled into the bladder once a week for 6 weeks. Because this was a feasibility study without maintenance therapy, the long-term responses cannot be predicted. At 12 months posttreatment, however, the results have been promising. Further, the study demonstrated that coadministration of BCG plus IFN-α is safe and well tolerated (Stricker *et al.,* 1996). The role of IFN-α intravesicular therapy in superficial bladder cancer is recommended for patients who relapse after treatment with BCG or who cannot tolerate the side effects of BCG.

RENAL CELL CARCINOMA

Renal cell carcinoma (RCC) is the most common malignancy of the kidney and affects nearly 20,000 Americans per year. The most common histologic types of RCC are clear-cell cancer (75%) followed by papillary tumors (15%). Malignancies of the collecting duct and medulla and sarcomatoid tumors account for the remaining 10% of RCCs. Only half of the patients who present with local disease are cured by surgery, and those with metastatic disease have a median survival duration of approximately 10 months. Neither chemotherapy nor radiation therapy has a significant role in the treatment of metastatic RCC. It has been discovered that most renal cell tumors express P-glycoprotein, which sets up multidrug resistance by pumping the chemotherapeutic agent out of the tumor cell. Mutations in the von Hippel Lindau (*VHL*) gene have been identified in patients with clear-cell carcinoma. Mutant forms of vascular endothelial growth factor, a protein that is regulated by the *VHL* gene, are found in clear-cell forms of renal tumors. Some renal tumors express the proto-oncogene c-*met*, which is a gene that codes for a protein that functions as a hepatocyte growth-factor receptor (Bukowski, 1999).

For a long time, patients with metastatic RCC have been treated with a variety of investigational protocols. The majority of these protocols have involved the use of biological agents. In 1983, the University of California Los Angeles (Dekernion *et al.,* 1983) and M. D. Anderson (Quesada *et al.,* 1983) reported independently on the regression of metastatic RCC with partially purified human leukocyte IFN. Objective responses (complete and partial) occurred in 16.5% and 26% of patients, respectively. Numerous phase II trials have confirmed a reproducible objective response rate of 15% to 20%. Responses are independent of the type of IFN-α used and correlate positively with prior nephrectomy, good performance status, a long disease-free interval, and lung as the predominant site of metastasis. The median duration of response is 6 to 10 months, with few durable CRs. Minasian *et al.* (1988) from the Memorial Sloan-Kettering Cancer Center (New York, NY) reported on a large, single-institution experience with IFN-α in 159 patients with metastatic RCC. The overall response rate was 10% (2 CRs and 14 PRs). The median response duration was 12.2 months, and the median survival duration was 11.4 months. Only 3% of patients were alive at 5 years. Although the response rate of 10% is lower than that reported elsewhere, it is within the range of the overall clinical experience with IFN-α. This report demonstrated the need for continued investigation to find more effective therapies for advanced RCC and supports the studies in which IFN-α is combined with new agents.

In a 1999 review of several studies that included 1,500 patients who had been treated with IFN-α, tumor regression occurred in 12% to 15% of patients (Bukowski, 1999). CRs were seen in 2% to 5% of patients and were more commonly seen in patients with pulmonary metastasis.

In an attempt to improve the therapeutic index of IFN therapy in patients with RCC, there has been great interest in the combination of IL-2 and IFN-α. The mechanisms of action of these two biological agents are different but may result in therapeutic synergy. IL-2 acts almost exclusively as an immune modulator, whereas IFN-α has a direct antiproliferative effect. Additionally, the IFN may increase the immunogenic response of tumor cells by enhancing their histocompatibility and tumor-associated antigens, which results in greater sensitivity to IL-2–sensitized lymphocytes (Figlin *et al.*, 1992).

In experimental murine models, the combination of IL-2 and IFN-α has greater antitumor effect than either agent alone (Cameron *et al.*, 1988). Many phase I trials have studied different administration schedules (intravenous bolus versus continuous infusion) and different doses of both IL-2 and IFN-α. These studies reported that this combination of cytokines had antitumor activity.

In a phase II study of IL-2 and IFN-α for patients with metastatic RCC the course of treatment involved 4 weeks of therapy followed by 2 weeks of rest. IL-2 was administered as a continuous intravenous infusion for 4 days of each treatment week and IFN-alfa-2a was administered intramuscularly or subcutaneously on days 1 and 4 of each treatment week. Although there were no CRs with this regimen; 9 of 30 patients had PR and 4 of 30 had stable disease. Patients received a median of 3 courses of therapy (range, 1 to 6).

Since both agents are associated with toxicities, it is interesting to note the types and frequency of side effects as well as the common strategies for ameliorating the toxicities. Nausea and vomiting (5), fatigue (4), neurologic symptoms (5), arrhythmia (2), diarrhea (2), pulmonary problems (1), and granulocytopenia (1) were severe enough in 16 patients to result in modification or discontinuation of therapy. All patients developed an erythematous, pruritic maculopapular rash that began early in treatment and resolved and did not return after completion of cycle one. Clinically significant capillary leak syndrome was not seen. Hypotension requiring vasopressors did not occur although 23% of patients required parenteral fluids between cycles for postural hypotension. There was one death from cardiac arrest that occurred 12 days after therapy was discontinued for gastrointestinal toxicity. Some of the supportive care measures included acetaminophen PRN for fever, premedication for IFN-α with indomethacin, meperidine 50 mg by mouth 30 minutes after IFN-α and PRN to control rigors, and diphenhydramine 25 mg to 50 mg by mouth for rash and pruritus. Volume depletion and postural hypotension were managed with parenteral fluid administration (Figlin *et al.*, 1992).

A 1999 review of numerous studies that included a sum total of 1,400 patients who received IFN-α and recombinant human IL-2 reported an overall response rate of 20%, with 3% to 5% of patients experiencing CRs. These results were independent of the schedule of IL-2 and were equivocal regardless of whether the route of administration was subcutaneous, continuous intravenous, or bolus intravenous (Bukowski, 1999).

In a randomized trial, IFN-alfa-2a has been administered as adjuvant therapy to patients at risk for relapse of their kidney cancer (Porzolt, 1992). Results have demonstrated no differences in survival duration or time to treatment failure in patients who did not receive IFN-alfa-2a compared with those patients who did.

The role of IFN-α in the treatment of RCC is still under investigation. When tested in randomized trials, the overall survival of the patient receiving IFN-α appears improved to a limited degree. Immune dysregulation may decrease the effects of biotherapy in patients with RCC. Patients with single metastatic sites are treated surgically, and those with an adequate performance status are candidates for cytokine therapy or clinical trials (Bukowski, 1999).

METASTATIC MELANOMA

The incidence of melanoma is rising faster than that of any other cancer except for lung cancer in women. For example, the lifetime risk of developing melanoma in the United States in 1935 was 1 in 1,500. It is estimated that this risk will reach 1 in 75 in the year 2000. Increased recreational exposure to **ultraviolet light** and increased awareness leading to early detection are thought to be important contributors to the increased incidence of melanoma. Although most new patients with melanoma are diagnosed early, the outlook is dismal if the disease is left unchecked until later stages. The median survival period for patients with stage IV melanoma who go untreated is 5 to 6 months, with fewer than 20% surviving 1 year (Balch et al., 1993).

Kirkwood et al. (1996) reported on the results of the ECOG trial that evaluated high-dose, single-agent IFN-alfa-2b as adjuvant therapy in patients with high-risk, resected, cutaneous melanoma. Individuals with deep primary lesions have a high incidence of relapse and a mortality rate of 50% to 90%. This was a randomized, controlled study of 280 patients with stage IIB or III melanoma. One group was randomized to observation for 1 year. The experimental group received 1 month of induction therapy (20 mU/m^2 intravenously 5 times a week) followed by maintenance therapy (10 mU/m^2 subcutaneously 3 times a week) for 48 weeks. Both overall and relapse-free results favored the treatment arm. The median 5-year overall survival rate for those treated with IFN-

alfa-2b compared with those in the observation arm was 37% versus 26%, respectively ($p = .047$). The median increment in disease-free survival (DFS) was 1 year in the observation arm versus 1.7 years in the IFN-alfa-2b treated arm ($p = .005$). The increments of median overall survival duration was from 2.8 to 3.8 years, which represents a 42% improvement in relapse-free survival over nontreatment or the "watch and wait" approach. Retrospective subset analysis was performed and seemed to demonstrate that the most significant benefit was in patients with nodal metastases. However, those with nodal metastases made up 89% of the treatment arm, and there were only 31 patients (11%) in the subset of those with negative lymph nodes; these factors prevent any meaningful conclusions (Balch and Buzaid, 1996).

The impact of therapy on survival has been sustained over the median 7-year follow-up (reported in 1996), with the greatest reduction in deaths occurring early during active treatment. Dosing delays or reductions were necessary at least once for 50% of the patients during the induction phase and for 48% during the maintenance phase. Side effects were significant but tolerable, with constitutional (flu-like), hematologic, and neurologic toxicities noted most frequently. Sixty-seven percent of the patients had severe (WHO grade 3) toxicity at some point during the year of treatment, and 12 (9%) patients had life-threatening toxicity (5 constitutional and seven neurological). Two treatment-related deaths attributed to hepatotoxicity were reported. In both cases, there was suggestion of antecedent liver disease, and the biochemical testing of liver function, as specified by the protocol, had been omitted. Notification of the importance of monitoring regular liver function tests occurred, and no further deaths due to hepatotoxicity have been reported in the subsequent five years of this study. Optimal treatment for any patient depends on the tumor burden and personal preferences regarding toxicity and disease relapse (Cole *et al.*, 1996). Quality-of-life analysis was completed for this study using the Q-Twist analysis, and the results concluded that the clinical benefits of high-dose IFN-alfa-2b are similar to those for standard chemotherapeutic adjuvant regimens for breast and colorectal cancer.

Several groups have looked at IFN-α regimens as treatment for earlier-stage melanoma. A randomized prospective trial with high-risk stage I and II melanoma was conducted in 262 patients following complete resection of their lesions (Creagan *et al.*, 1995). Patients were randomized to a treatment group designed to receive intramuscular injections of 20 mU IFN-alfa-2a 3 times a week for 12 weeks or to an observation group. Routine lymph node dissections were not performed unless clinically palpable nodes were noted. Almost half of the patients in the treatment arm had a primary lesion 1.7 to 3.5 mm in thickness. The 5-year survival rate for patients with lesions in this range is 69%, compared with the 93% 5-year survival rate for thinner lesions. The median disease-free survival duration for the treatment arm was 2.4 years versus 2.0 years for the observation arm ($p = .24$). Recurrence rates were similar in both arms (59% in the treatment arm versus 65% in the observation arm; $p = .37$). Subset analysis demonstrated no therapeutic advantage for patients with stage I disease. Median survival was 6.6 years for the treatment group and 5.0 years for the observation group ($p = .40$). The stage II group showed some improvement (overall survival 4.1 years for the treatment group versus 2.7 years for the control group), but the treatment effect only achieved statistical significance in an adjusted analysis. The authors conclude that the magnitude of the treatment effect seems promising but recommend a randomized trial to ensure that this finding is not due to chance from subset analysis. Severe flu-like toxicity was seen in 44% of patients, and 45% experienced a worsening of

their performance status. This may be due to the lack of supportive medications because patients were only scheduled to take acetaminophen prior to their first treatment.

Pehamberger *et al.* (1998) conducted a study of patients with primary cutaneous melanoma with lesions 1.5 mm or deeper. The choice of patients with stage II melanoma was based on results of the Creagan study (Creagan *et al.*, 1995), which showed that IFN-α could possibly improve DFS for this group of patients. Patients were randomized to receive IFN-alfa-2a daily at a dose of 3 mU subcutaneously for 3 weeks followed by 1 year at 3 mU subcutaneously 3 times a week. Elective lymph node dissection was not performed. The end point of this study was DFS; no data are shown for overall survival. A prolongation of DFS was seen in the treatment arm. Thirty-seven of 154 patients (24%) on the treatment arm developed metastases versus 57 of 157 (36%) in the observation arm ($p = .02$).

The French Cooperative Group on Melanoma conducted a trial of 499 patients with stage IIA or IIB melanoma (Grob *et al.*, 1998). This patient group is considered at high risk for recurrence because 55% of patients with stage IIA melanoma (Breslow thickness 1.5 to 4 mm) and 75% of patients with stage IIB melanoma (Breslow thickness greater than 4 mm) are expected to experience relapse within five years after surgical resection. Thirty percent of patients with stage IIA and 50% with stage IIB are expected to die in the same time interval. The end point of the study was DFS, although it also reported on overall survival. The researchers performed an 18-month study of IFN-alfa-2a following surgery with patients who had primary cutaneous melanoma. The treatment arm received IFN-alfa-2a at 3 mU subcutaneously 3 times a week. Patients did not receive elective lymph node dissection or sentinel-node dissection. The efficacy analysis showed that the patients in the treatment arm had a significant increase in relapse-free interval. In the treatment arm, 100 of 244 (40%) patients relapsed versus 119 of 245 (48%) in the control arm ($p = .035$). With respect to overall survival rate, 59 of 244 (24%) patients in the treatment arm died versus 76 of 245 (31%) in the observation arm ($p = .59$). Although these results do not represent statistical significance, they do demonstrate a trend (Grob *et al.*, 1998).

In summarizing the use of biotherapy for melanoma over the past 40 years, Kirkwood (1998) identified several factors that need to be considered in the assessment of therapies for melanoma. The chief prognostic variable is stage of disease, which is defined by presence or absence of lymph node or distant metastases and Breslow depth in patients without metastases. Although elective lymph node dissection has not demonstrated a significant therapeutic effect on survival, the need to identify lymph node metastases more precisely has important implications in assessing patient risk for relapse (Essner, 1997). Sentinel lymph node mapping and selective lymphadenectomy directed by isotopic lymphoscintigraphy and blue-dye lymphography are described elsewhere in this section and have been useful in accurate staging of melanoma. The refinement of the therapies for treatment of melanoma will benefit from consistency in staging of the disease. Kirkwood drew the following conclusions regarding trials of adjuvant IFN-α for patients who had undergone resection of their melanoma but were at high risk and intermediate risk for relapse:

- Relapse-free interval is prolonged with low doses of IFN-α given for 12 to 18 months.
- The inhibition of relapse by low doses of IFN-α occurs gradually and is lost over time after discontinuation of therapy.

These conclusions are in contrast with results of the use of high-dose IFN-alfa-2b, which has shown an impact on overall survival (Kirkwood *et al.*, 1996). Kirkwood suggests that regimens with low doses of IFN-α given for longer periods of time and higher doses for shorter periods should be evaluated (see Table 5.4).

Because lymph node metastases decrease the 5-year survival rate of patients with melanoma by 40% compared with patients with no metastasis, the shift has been to move forward to develop accurate staging and early identification and treatment of melanoma. The staging of disease is dependent on factors such as vertical thickness of the lesion and presence of histologically positive lymph nodes. Intraoperative lymphatic mapping and sentinel-node biopsy has changed the way nodal metastases are identified. Injection of isosulfan blue dye at the site of a cutaneous lesion during surgical resection leaves a visible blue color on the sentinel node in the draining nodal basin. If the node is negative, there is a strong likelihood ($\approx$95%) that all the nodes are negative and that there is no metastatic spread, so the patient is spared a total lymphadenectomy. Another technique, radiolymphoscintigraphy, utilizes a combination of isosulfan blue dye and technetium injected at the site of the melanoma. A gamma nuclear probe can then track the lymphatic flow to the draining lymphatic basin (Reintgen *et al.*, 1995). This is especially useful in the head and neck area and in ambiguous areas of lymphatic drainage. The Melanoma Sunbelt Trial is currently utilizing these techniques to accurately stage patients who have thinner lesions and to test the efficacy of treatment with IFN-alfa-2b in earlier-stage disease.

Along with the development of IFN-α for adjuvant therapy of high-risk melanoma patients, trials of melanoma vaccines are underway at several research centers. It is hypothesized that melanoma vaccines will amplify host T-cell and/or humoral immunity to melanoma-specific or melanoma-associated antigens. Specific strategies being evaluated include combinations of IFN-α and vaccines

Table 5.4   Trials of adjuvant IFN-alfa-2 for resected high-risk and intermediate-risk melanoma

Cooperative Group (PI)	Eligibility	n	Treatment Agent/Dosage/Duration	Impact on DFS	Impact on OS	Median F/U
T3-4/node (+) (AJCC Stage IIB/III)						
ECOG 1684	T4, N1	287	IFN-alfa-2b 20 mU/m²/d IV × 1 mo, 10 mU/m²/SC TIW for 11 mo	(+)	(+)	~7 years
NCCTG 837052	T3-4, N1	262	IFN-alfa-2a 20 mU/m²/d IM TIW × 3 mo	(−)	(−)	~7 years
ECOG 1690 (Kirkwood)	T4, N1	642	IFN-alfa-2b 20 mU/m²/IV × 1 mo vs 3 mU/d SC TIW × 2 yr	(?)	(?)	Masked
WHO 16	N1, N2	444	IFN-alfa-2a 3 mU/d SC TIW × 2 yr	(−)	(−)	3.3 years
EORTC 18871 (Kleeberg)	T3-4, N1	800	IFN-alfa-2a 1 mU/d SC × 1 yr vs IFN-γ 0.2 mg/d SC × 1 yr	(−)	(−)	
EORTC 18952 (Eggermont)	T4, N1	1,000	IFN-alfa-2b 10 mU/d/SC x 1 mo, then IFN-alfa-2b 10 mU/d SC	(?)	(?)	In progress
ECOG 1694/SWOG 9512	T4, N1	851	IFN-alfa-2b 20 mU/m²/d IV × 1 mo, 10 mU/m² SC TIW × 11 mo vs GM-2-KLH/QS-21 vaccine			Ongoing in U.S.
T3/node (−) (AJCC Stage II)						
ECOG 1697 (Agarawala/ Kirkwood)	T3, N0	1,420	IFN-alfa-2b 20 mU/m²/d IV × 1 mo			Planned
Austrian	T3, N0	311	IFN-alfa-2a 3 mU/d SC × 3 wk, then TIW × 11 mo	(+)	(?)	3 years
French (Grob)	T3, N0, IIA	499	IFN-alfa-2a 3 mU SC TIW × 18 mo	(+)	(−)	5 years

d, day; DFS, disease-free survival; ECOG, Eastern Cooperative Oncology Group; EORTC, European Organization for Research and Treatment of Cancer; IFN, interferon; IM, intramuscularly; IV, intravenously; Median F/U, median follow-up; mo, month; mU, million units; NCCTG, North Central Cancer Treatment Group; OS, overall survival; SC, subcutaneous; TIW, three times a week; vs, versus; WHO, World Health Organization; wk, week; (+), statistically significant outcome; (−), no statistically significant outcome; (?), analysis not yet reported; SWOG, Southwest Oncology Group; yr, year

Source: Adapted from Kirkwood, J. 1998. Adjuvant IFNα2 therapy of melanoma. *The Lancet* 351(June 27): 1902.

composed of gangliosides, peptides, proteins, or tumor-cell preparations (see Chapter 10).

Once melanoma metastasizes to distant sites, the prognosis becomes poor; median survival duration in such cases is 6 months. Several regimens have been evaluated for this group of patients, with most containing cytotoxic chemotherapy and immunomodulating agents such as IFN-α, IL-2, or both.

Thompson et al. (1997) reported on an outpatient protocol with monthly cycles of intravenously administered carmustine, dacarbazine, cisplatin, and tamoxifen plus IL-2 and IFN-α self-administered as subcutaneous injections. The overall response rate with this regimen was 43% (13% CR and 30% PR). Toxicities were manageable, with nausea and vomiting being the most common. The goal of this study was to evaluate the feasibility of providing an outpatient regimen of chemoimmunotherapy that could be delivered with less toxicity and at a lower cost. The results of this study were promising, and the 43% overall response rate was considered equivalent to trials that used bolus intravenous IL-2 and IFN-α, which produced significantly higher levels of toxicity.

Rosenberg et al. (1999) compared the responses of 102 patients who were randomized to receive either cisplatin, dacarbazine, and tamoxifen alone or followed by IL-2 and IFN-α. Of the group randomized to receive chemotherapy alone, 14 (27%) patients had a response (4 CRs and 10 PRs). Of the patients randomized to receive chemoimmunotherapy, there were 22 (44%) objective responses (3 CRs and 19 PRs). The duration of the PRs, however, was short. There was a trend toward survival in the chemotherapy-alone arm; however, treatment-related toxicities were greater in the patients who received chemoimmunotherapy. These study results were confirmed in a report by Margolin et al. (1999) of a phase II SWOG study. Patients were treated with the same agents but at different schedules, and only one objective response was observed in the 25 patients treated. Based on these results, neither study supports the use of these regimens as standard therapy for metastatic melanoma.

Richards et al. (1999) reported on a 6-week protocol that involved patients with brain metastasis. Patients received cisplatin, dacarbazine, and carmustine plus IFN-α and IL-2. The purpose of this study was to test the therapeutic potential of the combination, clarify the toxicities of the regimen, and further evaluate immunological changes. Eighty-three of the 84 patients studied were evaluable, and 46 (55%) patients had an objective response (12 CRs and 34 PRs). The time to disease progression was 7 months, and the median survival duration from study entry was 12.2 months. Patients were hospitalized for this regimen. Some patients (10%) experienced survival beyond 4 years, suggesting that in some cases, there may be a long-term benefit to this therapy.

CARCINOID TUMORS

Carcinoid tumors are neuroendocrine in nature and have been found in individuals 10 to 93 years of age. The most frequent site of occurrence for carcinoid tumors of clinical significance is the jejunoileum of the small intestine. Symptoms are vague with periodic abdominal pain and intermittent bowel obstruction. Many of those with carcinoid tumors will develop malignant carcinoid syndrome. The features of carcinoid syndrome include flushing attacks (unpleasant feeling of warmth, erythema of the face and neck, itching, and palpitations), diarrhea, cardiac manifestations (due to fibrous deposits on the heart), and asthma-like symptoms (Jensen and Norton, 1997). Carcinoid tumors of the intestinal tract are thought to arise from cells in the base of the intestinal crypts. Confirmation of diagnosis is made by tumor markers such as chromogranin

A, which is a glycoprotein that is stored and released from neuroendocrine cells (Oberg, 1999).

The mechanism by which IFN-α acts against tumor growth in carcinoid tumors has been theorized as follows. It is known that IFN-α exerts an antiproliferative effect. A rapid induction of cyclin-dependent kinase inhibitors precedes the arrest of the G_0-G_1 phase of the cell cycle and prolongs the S_1 phase of the cell cycle (Sangfelt et al., 1999). Additionally, it has been demonstrated that the levels of circulating 5H1AA hormone in patients with carcinoid tumors is significantly reduced within one month of starting IFN-α therapy. If IFN-α is administered into the feeding artery of an area of metastasis, the tumor-cell count and expression of RNA for chromagranin A are reduced. This results in reduction in protein and hormone synthesis. Oberg and Alm (1997) recognized that expression of the *neu* oncogene protein is reduced after IFN-α treatment. These mechanisms are thought to contribute to the control of hormone synthesis and abrogation of tumor growth for extended periods of time, although cure of the disease is unlikely at this time.

Treatment with IFN-α of more than 350 patients with neuroendocrine tumors resulted in a 44% biochemical response and 11% tumor response rate, with a small number of select patients surviving for more than 80 months (Oberg, 1996a). Side effects for these patients included mainly flu-like syndrome and low-grade chronic fatigue syndrome. Combination of IFN-α and octreotide improved the biochemical response rate and improved the tolerability of the IFN-α but did not demonstrate a significant antitumor effect.

Medical treatment is based on chemotherapy, somatostatin analogues, and IFN-α. Streptozotocin plus 5-FU or doxorubicin are considered first-line therapy for the majority of endocrine pancreatic tumors. Somatostatin analogues and IFN-α are considered first-line for classical midgut carcinoid tumors (Oberg, 1996b).

SQUAMOUS CARCINOMAS OF THE SKIN OR CERVIX

Several preclinical and clinical studies provide a rationale for evaluating the combination 13-cis-retinoic acid (isotretinoin) and IFN-α. Preclincial data indicate that the 2 drugs have different mechanisms of action (Lotan et al., 1990; Pitha, 1990) and show enhanced activity when used in combination in a variety of human hematologic and solid tumor cell lines (Frey et al., 1991; Higuchi et al., 1991; Peck and Bollag, 1991). Data on the use of each agent alone suggest that each, when used systemically at high doses, produces response rates of 40% to 50% (less than 15% CRs) in locally advanced skin cancer. IFN-α and isotretinoin are synergistic in their antiproliferative effect. Some of the mechanisms that may contribute to this synergy include changes in gene expression that are mediated by nuclear and cell-surface receptors, inhibition of angiogenesis, or promotion of apoptosis (Look et al., 1998).

In the first phase II trial of systemic therapy in metastatic squamous-cell carcinoma of the skin, Lippman and colleagues reported on the combination of isotretinoin and IFN-α (Lippman et al., 1992a). This carcinoma is extremely common. Although 90% of patients are cured by local therapy, the remaining 10%, which represent tens of thousands of cases, often suffer severe disfigurement with cosmetic deformities as a result of their treatment. The purpose of the trial by Lippman was to evaluate whether a high rate of CRs could be achieved by using a combination of these two agents in patients in whom local therapy had failed or who had regional metastasis, distant metastasis, or both. Ultimately, 7 patients had CRs and 12 had PRs.

The combination of isotretinoin and IFN-α has also been reported by Lippman et al. (1992b) to be effective in the treatment of squamous-cell carcinoma of the cervix. Twenty-six patients with locally advanced bulky disease received daily oral isotretinoin (1 mg/kg) and subcutaneous IFN-α (6 mU). Thirteen (50%) patients achieved major responses (1 CR and 12 PRs). Side effects were mild. Studies of the long-term response rates, response durations, and survival durations are ongoing, and further study is needed before defining this regimen's role in squamous-cell carcinoma of the cervix.

In 1998, the Gynecologic Oncology Group reported on a phase II trial of 37 patients with unresectable squamous-cell carcinoma of the cervix. Patients were scheduled to receive a 4-week course of oral isotretinoin at 1 mg/kg a day with 6 mU IFN-α administered subcutaneously. Thirty-four patients were actually evaluable for toxicity, and 26 were evaluable for response. Most of the patients had received prior chemotherapy (23) and radiation therapy (25). The overall response rate was 3.8%. The authors state that in this pretreated population, the schedule and doses evaluated had minimal activity against the disease but cite other research that suggests that regimens with moderate activity in previously untreated patients perform less well in patients who have been previously treated (Look *et al.*, 1998).

Nononcologic Indications for Interferon-α Therapy

HEPATITIS B VIRUS

Many types of hepatitis viruses have been identified, but the development of chronic disease is associated with hepatitis B, C, and D viruses. Hepatitis D does not exist independently, only as a coinfection with hepatitis B virus (HBV). The causative agent of hepatitis C, the hepatitis C virus (HCV), was identified in 1989. Prior to 1989, most cases of hepatitis C were called hepatitis non-A, non-B. It is now thought that up to 90% of patients diagnosed with non-A, non-B were actually infected with HCV.

Five percent to 10% of patients infected with HBV will develop chronic viral hepatitis. Premature death will come to 15% to 25% of those affected, with about 22% of the deaths resulting from hepatocellular carcinoma (HCC). The mechanism by which HBV contributes to HCC is thought to be a direct carcinogenic effect through interaction with oncogenes, growth factors, or tumor suppressor genes (Di Bisceglie, 1997). Chronic viral hepatitis is the primary cause of serious liver disease in the world and is now the major reason for liver transplantation in adults. It has the potential to cause cirrhosis and HCC (Hoofnagle, 1997a). HCC incidence varies from country to country and region to region. In Italy, Spain, and Japan between 50% and 75% of cases of HCC are connected to hepatitis C infection. In the United States, the hepatitis-related incidence of HCC is about 30% (Di Bisceglie, 1997).

Several multicenter clinical trials have demonstrated that IFN-α has significant activity in the treatment of chronic hepatitis B (Coppens *et al.*, 1989; Fattovich *et al.*, 1989; Saracco *et al.*, 1989; Perrillo *et al.*, 1990). Approximately 30% to 50% of patients with chronic hepatitis B infection respond to IFN-α therapy. Remissions of chronic hepatitis B following IFN therapy are reported to be of long duration and are often associated with loss of viral hepatitis B surface antigen (Korenman *et al.*, 1991). Several studies have indicated that treatment of chronic hepatitis B with a sufficient dose of IFN-α (30 to 35 mU/week divided into daily or 3 times a week doses) for at least 6 months slows progression of disease and can result in long-term remission. Evaluation of IFN-alfa-2b in children (aged 1 to 17 years) with hepatitis B infection demonstrated results similar to adult trials, with response rates of 24% to 32%. The dosing schedule for children is 3 mU/m² 3 times a week subcutaneously for 1 week followed by 6 mU/m² 3 times a week (maximum 10 mU 3 times a week) for 15 to 23 weeks (Schering Plough Product Information, 1998).

HEPATITIS C VIRUS

Between 60% and 100% of patients infected with HCV will develop chronic hepatitis (Colquhoun, 1996; Woo et al., 1997). Transmission of HCV is most often via the parenteral route. The most frequently identified risk factors for acquiring hepatitis C include receipt of a blood transfusion (prior to June 1992), needle-sharing or intravenous-drug use, hemodialysis, body piercings, or tattoos placed under nonsterile conditions or with nonsterile ink. Health care workers have a risk of contracting HCV ranging from 0% to 6%. One report showed that members of a liver transplant team had a 5.3% prevalence of infection compared with 0.5% among other health care workers (Colquhoun, 1996). Sexual transmission of HCV is low (5%) in monogamous couples, but the risk increases with multiple sexual partners, co-infection with HIV, or a sexually transmitted disease. Perinatal transmission is also in the low area of 5% to 6%, and breast-feeding does not appear to increase the risk of transmission of HCV in infants of mothers with hepatitis C (Dienstag, 1997).

The conceptual development of research and treatment patterns for hepatitis C has been and continues to be an evolutionary process. The natural history of HCV is not yet fully understood. Compounding the difficulty of treating these viruses is the presence of at least 6 **genotypes** of hepatitis C with differing characteristics and response to treatment profiles. This century saw the spread of hepatitis C in the United States associated with genotypes 2 and 1b. Most recently, genotypes 1a and 3a have appeared, with 3a most frequently found in the intravenous-drug-user population. The clinical implications reflect the tenacity of the genotype, with type 1 viruses more difficult to eradicate than type 2 or 3 (Simmonds, 1997). HCV has the ability to mutate rapidly and exist simultaneously as a series of "quasi-species" that are related but immunologically distinct. This provides a mechanism for the virus to escape the host immune response and may be one of the reasons behind the persistence of chronic infection in some patients (Alter and Mose, 1994; Alter, 1995; Alter, 1997; Hoofnagle, 1997a; Hoofnagle and Di Bisceglie, 1997b; Purcell, 1997; Seef, 1997).

Development of new laboratory tests that actually measure the HCV RNA include reverse transcription-**polymerase chain reaction (RT-PCR)** and branch-chain DNA (bDNA®; Chiron Laboratories, Emeryville, CA) testing. Serologic tests are also in the developmental stage. Additionally, a test that identifies the genotype of the virus has been developed. These advances have given practitioners the tools to establish, monitor, and modify a treatment pattern based on individual response. There is variation in the sensitivity and reliability of quantitative tests for HCV RNA. The range extends from detection of a lower limit of 200,000 viral particles per milliliter of serum by using bDNA to more sensitive RT-PCR kits that are able to detect 1,000 viral particles per milliliter of blood, such as the Roche Monitor® assay (Hoffman-LaRoche, Nutley, NJ). There are specialized laboratories that can reliably measure as few as 100 viral particles per milliliter of blood (Superquant®; National Genetics Institute, Los Angeles, CA). There are kits available that yield a sensitivity of 100 viral copies/per milliliter of serum (Amplicor®; Hoffman-La Roche, Nutley, NJ) reported by Gretch (1997) in his reference laboratory. Prior to the development of highly sensitive RT-PCR, surrogate markers such as liver enzymes (alanine aminotransferase [ALT], formerly known as SGPT; aspartate aminotransferase [AST], formerly known as SGOT; or a combination of these) were used as indicators of biochemical response. These tests do not correlate with virological status. One study reported that more than 30% of patients with chronic hepatitis C had normal liver enzymes (Conry-Cantilena et al., 1996).

IFN-α has demonstrated efficacy in the treatment of infection with HBV and HCV. The dosage of IFN-α used to treat hepatitis B is higher (5 mU daily or 10 mU 3 times a week, depending on the schedule), but the duration of therapy is less (Perrillo *et al.*, 1990). Side effects seen with lower doses are minor and usually do not require dose modification. Tachyphylaxis or tolerance develops after the first or second injection, and most side effects diminish over the next few weeks. The most common and predictable side effects include flu-like syndrome; neuropsychiatric changes such as apathy, irritability, insomnia, and mood or cognitive changes; gastrointestinal changes such as diarrhea, nausea, and abdominal pain; and cutaneous reactions such as pruritus or alopecia. Changes in laboratory values include a decrease in granulocytes, platelets, and red blood cells and an increase in serum triglyceride, serum ALT, serum AST, and proteinuria. Most of these changes are transient and resolve after completion of therapy but require careful monitoring and adherence to dose modification guidelines that are available from the pharmaceutical company that makes the particular type of IFN being used (see Table 5.1). Overall, fatal and life-threatening adverse events are rare at the doses used to treat hepatitis. A large multicenter study that looked at adverse events in 11,241 patients with either hepatitis B or hepatitis C reported 5 (0.04%) deaths as a result of therapy with IFN. All 5 developed liver failure or sepsis. Other life-threatening events occurred in eight (0.07%) patients and included severe depression with suicide attempt and bone marrow suppression (granulocytes < 500/μL; platelet counts < 25,000 μL). Other serious but not life-threatening adverse events occurred in 131 (1.2%) of the 11,241 patients and included symptomatic thyroid disease (n = 71), diabetes mellitus (n = 10), psychosis (n = 10), seizures (n = 4), and peripheral neuropathy (n = 3) (Dusheiko, 1997).

The treatment of hepatitis C has evolved rapidly since the development of molecular assays. The overall pattern seen as a result of research with IFN-α is that increasing the duration of treatment increased the end-of-treatment response and sustained response (measured by absence of virus 6 months after completion of therapy). Responses were greatly improved with the approval of combination therapy (Rebetron™, Schering Corporation, Kenilworth, NJ) with ribavirin (Rebetrol®) and IFN-alfa-2b for hepatitis C.

Initial studies showed efficacy in the treatment of hepatitis C when patients were treated with IFN-α for 6 months. Unfortunately, approximately half of the patients who showed an end-of-treatment response relapsed within 6 months. Subsequent studies demonstrated that higher rates of sustained response could be achieved by increasing the duration of therapy to 12 months or longer (Chemello *et al.*, 1995; Reichard *et al.*, 1995; Lindsay *et al.*, 1996; Manesis *et al.*, 1997). Carithers and Emerson (1997) conducted a rigorous meta-analysis of IFN-α trials and also confirmed that there was a clear-cut increase in sustained response in patients who were treated for 12 to 24 months when compared with those treated for 6 months. A "good treatment profile" included having an early stage of liver fibrosis. Those patients whose profile included the early stage of liver fibrosis, nongenotype 1b, and low baseline virologic load achieved the best responses.

In 1997, recombinant IFN-alfacon-1 (Infergen®) also gained approval as a treatment of chronic infection with HCV, marking the first time a nonnaturally occurring IFN had been approved by the FDA for clinical use. IFN-alfacon-1 was derived by scanning the sequences of several natural IFN subtypes. This synthetic IFN was created using codons for the most frequent amino acids in 8 of the different known type I IFNs. IFN-alfacon-1 has 20 amino acid differences from IFN-alfa-2a and approximately 30% identity with IFN-β (Dhib-Jalbut et al., 1996). Other changes were made for purposes of completing the molecular construction. The end product was a 19,434-dalton synthetic IFN that shares many of the properties of type I IFNs, including antiviral, antiproliferative, NK cell activation and gene induction activity. One difference between IFN-alfacon-1 and natural IFN-α is the way the drug is dosed. IFN-alfacon-1 is dosed in micrograms, and IFN-α is dosed in the international million units (mU). IFN-alfacon-1 has gained FDA approval for treatment of chronic HCV infection in patients 18 years or older with compensated liver disease (Pfeffer, 1997; Amgen, Thousand Oaks, CA).

Preclinical trials with IFN-alfacon-1 have produced results that demonstrate a higher affinity for an array of IFN type I receptors. In a study examining the treatment of experimental tumors with, the *IFN-alfacon*-1 gene, there was successful transfection of the cancer-producing cells, causing the cells to lose their oncogenic potential by causing phenotypic reversion. Other characteristics of the transformed cancer cells included a decrease in growth rate and an increase in the major histocompatibility II surface markers. This response was similar to that seen following treatment with exogenous consensus IFN or IFN-α (Blatt *et al.*, 1996). Dhib-Jalbut *et al.* (1996) compared IFN-alfacon-1 and IFN-β to see whether the immunomodulatory effects were similar. They found that IFN-alfacon-1 possesses immunomodulatory properties similar to other type I IFNs, including enhancement of human lymphocyte antigen (HLA) class I expression, inhibition of IFN-γ-enhanced HLA class II expression, and an antiproliferative effect on mitogen-driven lymphoproliferation.

A phase III research study compared the effects of IFN-alfacon-1 with IFN-alfa-2b (Tong *et al.*, 1997) in the treatment of HBV. IFN-

alfacon-1 was administered at doses of 3 or 9 mcg and was compared with 3 mU of IFN-alfa-2b, which was also given subcutaneously 3 times weekly for 24 weeks followed by 24 weeks of observation. Biochemical responses (a surrogate for improved liver histology) measured by serum ALT and virological responses (or eradication of the virus) measured by RT-PCR were monitored. Sustained biochemical responses at the end of the 24-week, posttreatment observation period did not achieve statistical difference. Normalization of ALT was seen in 6.5% of the patients treated with 3 mcg IFN-alfacon-1, 20.3% of the patients treated with 9 mcg IFN-alfacon-1, and 6% of the patients treated with 3 mU IFN-alfa-2b. Virological responses at the end of the treatment period were seen in 6.5% of the patients treated with 3 mcg IFN-alfacon-1, 34.9% of the patients treated with 9 mcg IFN-alfacon-1, and 27.1% of the patients treated with 3 mU IFN-alfa-2b. Sustained virologic responses diminished over the 24-week observation period. Results showed that 2.6% of the patients treated with 3 mcg IFN-alfacon-1, 12.1% of the patients treated with 9 mcg IFN-alfacon-1, and 11.3% of the patients treated with 3 mU IFN-alfa-2b had nondetectable levels of HCV RNA, as assessed by the most sensitive RT-PCR test. The adverse events reported in more than 94% of the patients receiving IFN-alfacon-1 at any dose level were similar to those seen with IFN-α and included flu-like syndrome, fatigue, headache, arthralgia, and myalgia. Forty-five of the 697 patients who were evaluated in the safety evaluation group were withdrawn from the study. Of this group, 46.7% were withdrawn for psychiatric adverse events such as nervousness and depression. Only 3 of the 13 patients who were treated on the 3 mcg IFN-alfacon-1 regimen were withdrawn for psychiatric reasons, which suggests that the psychiatric adverse event was dose-related.

HEPATITIS C COMBINATION THERAPY

Combination therapy with the nucleoside analogue ribavirin (Rebetol®) plus IFN-alfa-2b (packaged together as Rebetron™) has shown increased efficacy over therapy with IFN-α therapy alone. Ribavirin is a synthetic nucleoside analogue that has shown activity in some viruses. As a single-agent therapy for treatment of hepatitis C it has reduced the level of liver enzymes but has not reduced the level of the HCV. A pivotal trial compared the efficacy of IFN-alfa-2b alone with that of IFN-alfa-2b plus ribavirin in 345 patients with chronic hepatitis C who had previously shown an initial response to any type of IFN but had subsequently relapsed (Davis *et al.*, 1998). Patients were randomly assigned and stratified according to the presence of cirrhosis, high serum HCV RNA levels, and HCV genotype 1 (factors known to reduce response to IFN) to maintain equal representation in both groups. The group receiving the combination-agent therapy received IFN-alfa-2b at 3 mU 3 times a week subcutaneously and ribavirin in daily divided doses of 1,000 mg (if 165 pounds or less in weight) or 1,200 mg (if more than 165 pounds in weight). The control group received IFN-alfa-2b at 3 mU 3 times a week plus placebo. The two end points for this study were disappearance of HCV RNA from serum and histologic improvement at the end of the 6-month follow-up period. Patients were treated for 24 weeks, at which time the end-of-treatment response was reported. Sustained virologic remission, the more significant end point, was measured 6 months after the completion of therapy. A complete sustained response was defined as having no detectable virus by highly sensitive (100 copies/mL) RT-PCR at 6 months after completion of therapy.

Ribavirin accumulates in red blood cells and results in an intravascular hemolysis, which was demonstrated as a mean decline in hemoglobin of 14.4 ± 1.2 to 12.4 ± 1.4 g/dL during the first month of treatment. This condition was followed by a reticulocytosis, which was mirrored by a stabilization of hemoglobin after which patients returned to near-baseline values. Both groups experienced a decline in white blood cell count (35% in the combination-agent group and 23% in the monotherapy group) and neutrophil count (33% in the combination-agent group and 28% in the monotherapy group). Platelet count decreased in both groups but significant thrombocytopenia was less in the combination therapy group (7%) than in the monotherapy group (15%). The side effects of the combination-agent therapy were similar to those seen with IFN-α alone, except for nausea (35% versus 20%, respectively), dyspnea (14% versus 6%, respectively), and rash (13% versus 6%, respectively). There were no serious or life-threatening complications with combination-agent therapy; however, one woman, with a history of alcohol and substance abuse, committed suicide 3 months after treatment was stopped. She had not reported depression during her treatment.

When the end points of this study were evaluated at 6 months after completion of therapy, 49% of those receiving combination therapy had a sustained virological response (undetectable levels of HCV RNA) compared with 5% of patients who received IFN-alfa-2b alone. For the second end point, 47% of those patients who received combination therapy achieved a sustained biochemical response (normalization of ALT levels) compared with 5% in the monotherapy group. Further analysis demonstrated that for those patients with a lower viral load (HCV RNA $< 2 \times 10^6$/mL) and having a genotype other than 1, a 100% sustained virological response was seen. For the difficult-to-treat patients (HCV RNA $> 2 \times 10^6$ and genotype 1), the sustained response rate was 25% for those treated with combination-agent therapy compared with 0% for the IFN-alfa-2b–alone group. These results led to the approval of Rebetron™ combination therapy for patients with hepatitis C who had relapsed following a course of IFN therapy.

Two additional studies evaluated the role of combination therapy as initial treatment for chronic hepatitis C. McHutchinson *et al.* (1998) evaluated 912 patients in a large multicenter trial. The baseline characteristics of the patients studied were similar, with 72% of the patients exhibiting genotype 1. Patients were randomly assigned to IFN-alfa-2b plus placebo or IFN-alfa-2b combination with ribavirin. In the combination regimen, ribavirin was dosed at 1,000 to 1,200 mg a day depending on body weight, and IFN-alfa-2b was given at 3 mU 3 times a week. There were two arms in this study: a comparison of monotherapy versus combination therapy at 24 weeks or the same comparison at 48 weeks. Adverse events were graded as mild, moderate, severe, or life threatening and were based on the WHO toxicity model. For severe adverse events (other than anemia), the IFN-alfa-2b was reduced to 1.5 mU 3 times a week, and the ribavirin was reduced to 600 mg a day until resolution of the event. If the patient's hemoglobin fell to 10 g/dL, the ribavirin was reduced to 600 mg a day and discontinued if the hemoglobin level fell below 8.5 g/dL.

Anemia, as measured by hemoglobin reduction to less than 10 g/dL, occurred in 8% of patients treated with combination therapy. Dose reduction of the ribavirin resulted in hemoglobin increases of 1 to 1.5 g/dL. White blood cell counts decreased in all groups, but the mean value remained within normal limits. The mean platelet counts remained above 100×10^3 in 95% of all patients. Other side effects that were more common with combination therapy than IFN-alfa-2b alone were dyspnea, pruritus, rash, nausea, insomnia, and anorexia.

Higher sustained virological response (SVR) rates were seen in the group treated with combination therapy for 48 weeks. The combination therapy for 24 weeks yielded a 31% SVR, and 48 weeks of therapy yielded a 38% SVR. For patients treated with monotherapy for 24 weeks, the SVR was 6%; for those treated for 48 weeks it was 13%. Those patients with genotype 1 received greater benefit from 48 weeks of combination-agent therapy (28% SVR) than from monotherapy (7%). No significant differences were seen in the genotype 2 or 3 groups when treated for 48 weeks as compared with those treated for 24 weeks.

Poynard *et al.* (1998) reported on a randomized, placebo-controlled study of 832 patients comparing safety and efficacy of combination-agent therapy for 24 or 48 weeks versus IFN-α plus placebo for 48 weeks. The primary end point for this study was loss of detectable HCV RNA (serum HCV RNA < 100 copies/mL at week 24 after treatment). The genotypes represented in this study reflected the demographics of European patients with hepatitis C, with 57% having genotype 1, 35% genotype 2 or 3, and 8% another genotype.

In this study, patients treated with combination-agent therapy began showing a decrease in hemoglobin at week 1, and they stabilized by week 4. Duration of therapy did not increase the need for dose reduction. White blood cell count decreased in both groups but remained within the normal range. Platelet counts decreased in both groups but were greater in the monotherapy group. Other side effects for combination therapy were similar to those seen with IFN-α. Dyspnea, pharyngitis, pruritus, rash, nausea, anorexia, and insomnia were reported more frequently with the combination group but were not dose-limiting.

Primary end points were measured at 6 months after completion of therapy. The SVR rates were 43% for those receiving 48 weeks of

Rebetron™ combination therapy, 35% for those receiving 24 weeks of Rebetron™ combination therapy, and 19% for those receiving 48 weeks of IFN-alfa-2b monotherapy. The similarities in treatment response and side effect profile in all three studies led to guidelines for treatment monitoring and dose reduction schedules that provide for safe and effective delivery of this therapy.

In the oncology setting, hepatitis C may be a concomitant illness in persons with cancers such as acute leukemia. The presence of HCV is common in this population, with some acquiring HCV before developing leukemia. There have been no prospective studies of the long-term impact of HCV on long-term survivors of leukemia. Another issue that remains to be clarified is the etiology of abnormal liver biochemical tests in leukemia patients with HCV who are receiving chemotherapy and whether drug dose modification guidelines for HCV-related liver abnormalities should be developed (Ribas *et al.*, 1997).

Toxicity Profile of Interferon-α

The toxicity profile of IFN-α is dependent on the dose, the route of administration, and the treatment schedule. The occurrence of side effects in patients receiving IFN can be predictable, and these side effects have often been categorized according to their frequency (Table 5.5). The majority of side effects associated with IFN are constitutional. They include fatigue, fever, chills, myalgias, headache, and anorexia. This constellation of side effects is often referred to as flu-like symptoms. They are reported almost universally following initial administration of treatment. The appearance of subsequent tachyphylaxis or tolerance depends on the dose, the route, and the schedule of administration.

Table 5.5   Side effect profile of type 1 interferons

	Frequent	Less Frequent
Acute	Fever	Nausea
	Chills	Vomiting
	Malaise	Diarrhea
	Headache	
	Anorexia	
Chronic	Fatigue	Mild neutropenia
	Weight loss	Elevated liver enzymes
	Alopecia (mild)	Thrombocytopenia
		Central nervous system
		Depression
		Confusion
		Mental slowing
		Retinal changes
		Proteinuria
		Hypertriglyceridemia

Fever and Flu-like Syndrome

The endogenous pyrogens, IL-1 and TNF, along with prostaglandin E2, exert effects that raise the temperature set point in the hypothalamus, the body's thermoregulatory center. The physical response to this temporary change in temperature set point is to generate heat with normal heat-promoting mechanisms such as shivering and vasoconstriction. A period of temperature elevation often occurs 1 to 4 hours after receiving IFN-α and can persist for 2 to 4 hours. This is often followed by a period of diaphoresis, as the body attempts to decrease the temperature. Corticosteroids can inhibit the transcription of IL-1, TNF, and nearly all cytokines (Dinarello, 1997). Because of the immunosuppressive effect of steroids, they are not recommended for management of these side effects because the full scope of the desired immunomodulatory therapeutic effects of IFN are not known. There are some therapeutic regimens that combine the use of steroids with IFN for their anticancer or antiautoimmune effect; however, steroids should not be routinely used to decrease the side effects of IFN.

Temperature elevations following administration of high-dose IFN may reach 104°F, usually 2 to 6 hours after administration, depending on the route of administration. Patient education and prophylactic premedication is critical for this usually benign but very uncomfortable side effect. If not properly controlled, patients may experience chest pain and dyspnea. Adverse cardiovascular events may be associated with rigors due in part to the vasoconstriction that occurs and the increased demand for oxygen by the myocardial tissue during the chilling phase.

Fatigue

Fatigue is the most frequently observed side effect of IFN-α treatment, occurring in up to 70% of patients. The fatigue experienced with this therapy is usually dose-related and most frequently seen in doses of 10 mU/m^2 or greater (Dalakas *et al.,* 1998). Compounding the problem of fatigue for patients with the conditions for which IFN is utilized as therapy is the high incidence of fatigue reported before undergoing treatment (e.g., fatigue associated with cancer, hepatitis B, hepatitis C, and MS).

In the patient receiving IFN, fatigue can be associated with depression, anemia, hypoglycemia, hypovolemia, or thyroid abnormality. It can also be related to alterations in levels of electrolytes or nutritional status (Dean *et al.,* 1995; Nail and Winningham, 1995). The induction of proinflammatory cytokines is a possible mechanism of neuromuscular pathology that could be experienced as fatigue (Dalakas *et al.,* 1998). Other physical stressors that can contribute to fatigue in the cancer patient include chronic pain, anorexia/cachexia, infection/fever, anemia, and dyspnea (Aistars, 1987). Dehydration can be a factor in the ongoing pres-

ence of fatigue. Although there is little in the literature specifically related to the role and impact of either intravenous or oral hydration for the patient receiving IFN therapy, anecdotal and personal experience have supported this concept. Biochemical processes also support the need for water in the generation of energy. Adenosine triphosphate (ATP) has been termed "the universal currency" of free energy in biological systems. The generation of ATP as described by the Kreb's cycle requires two molecules of water for each molecule of ATP to be formed (Stryer, 1981).

Assessment of factors that contribute to fatigue should be ongoing for the patient receiving IFN therapy. Baseline thyroid assessment and periodic repeat testing during treatment is important. Fatigue can be greatly reduced by correcting the thyroid condition. Other key laboratory tests to monitor and correct include electrolyte, hemoglobin, and serum glucose levels. Depression and anxiety should be assessed and intervention should be provided. There may be an additive effect of depression on fatigue due to disturbances in sleep.

A study of an intervention for IFN-induced fatigue is being conducted at the University of Washington Cancer Center. Melanoma patients are participating in a study to test the effect of physical activity and methylphenidate (Ritalin®). Patients take 20 mg of sustained-release methylphenidate every day and are asked to exercise 3 to 4 days per week for 15 to 30 minutes at a pace that is comfortable for them. They are asked to choose an aerobic activity that they enjoy, such as walking. This pilot study also shows promise and is expected to provide the basis for a multicenter study after its completion. The principal investigator for this study has also developed a tool, the Schwartz Cancer Fatigue Scale (Schwartz, 1998), which will also aid in further research evaluating interventions for fatigue.

Dean *et al.* (1995) reported on perceived

causes of fatigue in patients receiving IFN-α. They identified psychological issues such as bad news, fears, depression, nervousness, poor mental outlook, stress, and worrying. Symptom issues included fever, flu-like symptoms, lack of appetite, nausea, pain, and shortness of breath. Other factors cited by patients included long hospital visits, traveling, work, cancer treatments, anemia, arthritis, and little sleep. Patients were also asked what helped provide relief from fatigue, and they cited interventions that fell into five categories: distraction, energy conservation, expending energy, medical treatment, and other. Under distraction, they cited daydreaming, laughter, meditation, prayer, reading, soft music, soaking in the tub, watching television, and writing. Energy conservation techniques included avoiding exertion, getting extra sleep or a quick nap, resting or sitting quietly, slowing down, relaxing, or planning activities. Under expending energy, they listed exercise, swimming, and walking. Medical treatments that helped to relieve fatigue included blood transfusions and pain control. Under the "other" category, they listed consuming food and ice water.

It is valuable to see the scope of interventions that have been found to be helpful for patients receiving IFN therapy. The development of research that looks specifically at the issues of IFN-related fatigue is also an important step toward helping patients receive the prescribed doses of IFN and also improve the patients' quality of life. A more detailed discussion of fatigue is provided in Chapter 17.

Anorexia

Anorexia is commonly reported, and weight loss may occur with prolonged treatment. The occurrence of nausea, vomiting, or diarrhea is usually related to dose, but these effects tend to be mild and self-limiting. The generation of secondary cytokines such as TNF-α may play a role in the development of anorexia. In addition to being an inflammatory cytokine, TNF-α is also known as a cachectin, which is responsible for increased muscle catabolism and lipolysis (Oppenheim *et al.*, 1991). A more thorough description of nutritional issues with biotherapy is addressed in Chapter 18.

Myalgia and Arthralgia

Prostaglandins are implicated in the sensitization of nerve endings to bradykinin, a pain substance. Nonsteroidal anti-inflammatory drugs (NSAIDs) may block the synthesis of prostaglandins and thereby decrease the inflammatory response; however, the use of NSAIDs in patients must be individualized because of possible side effects such as the blocking of thromboxane, which leads to increased bleeding time. Nonacetylated NSAIDs may be useful in situations where risk for bleeding is a concern.

Hematological Effects

The hematological effects of IFN-α therapy include leukopenia, anemia, and thrombocytopenia. The white blood cell counts are usually lowered by 40% to 60%, but they usually rebound rapidly to normal after discontinuation of therapy. Infectious sequelae do not increase in IFN-α–induced leukopenia, and granulocytopenia is rarely dose-limiting. Anemia is generally seen with chronic therapy but is rarely severe. Mild thrombocytopenia has been reported in 5% to 50% of patients but generally is not clinically significant. Patients previously treated with chemotherapy, radiation therapy, or both may be more susceptible to the hematological side effects of IFN-α. The pathophysiological mechanisms that may underlie the hormonal, neurologic, endocrine, and hypothalamic systems that are involved in the generation of side effects are described in the literature (Borden and Parkinson, 1998; Dalakas *et al.*,

1998; Jones *et al.*, 1998; Moldawer and Sattler, 1998; Plata-Salaman, 1998).

Neurological Effects

It is impossible to anticipate all the possible side effects that may be associated with a drug during development and implementation of a clinical trial. Reporting of adverse drug reactions (ADR) after a drug has been approved, as required by the FDA, provides valuable information about side effects that may not have surfaced during the research treatment period. Drug manufacturers are required by law to submit ADR reports received by any means from health professionals and consumers. As a result of post-marketing ADRs, psychiatric disorders associated with IFN-α therapy have been recognized more frequently. A review of these ADR reports revealed that approximately 4% of the adverse event reports involved psychiatric disturbance. The increased incidence of psychiatric disturbance in IFN-α–treated patients when compared to randomized control groups suggests a causal relationship between IFN-α and mood disorders (Weiss, 1998). Studies evaluating low-dose IFN-α showed mild neurologic dysfunction without psychiatric symptoms or neuropsychological impairment; however, a small number of patients did experience action tremor (Caraceni *et al.*, 1998).

Researchers have now begun to describe possible mechanisms whereby IFN-α, secondary cytokines, or both act directly on the brain to induce alterations in mood and cognition. Although major depressive disorder is not a common or frequently seen outcome, careful routine assessment for depression is indicated for patients receiving IFN-α therapy (Licinio *et al.*, 1998; Valentine *et al.*, 1998).

The most frequent neurological side effects of IFN-α therapy are alteration in mental status such as slowed thinking, difficulty concentrating, and problems with memory. With higher doses, more significant toxicity such as somnolence, lethargy, and confusion may occur. Several mechanisms have been proposed to explain the phenomenon of neurological toxicity. First, IFN-α administration alters the secretion of neuroendocrine hormones. Cortisol levels are increased, as are levels of ACTH and β-endorphin. Second, IFNs appear to share a structural similarity to ACTH and β-endorphin as well as common signaling pathways with these hormones. Third, IFNs can induce the production of cytokines such as TNF and IL-1. These cytokines cross the blood-brain barrier and mimic the neurological changes seen with septic shock. Management of neurological toxicities includes obtaining a baseline neurological assessment, which would include sensory and motor function, gait, range of motion, cranial nerve function, and reflexes (Bender *et al.*, 1996).

IFN-α administered at high doses has the ability to induce **anhedonia**, fatigue, disrupted sleep, and altered cognitive function. This constellation of side effects has been termed "sickness behavior" (Musselman *et al.*, 1999). Researchers at Emory University School of Medicine are evaluating the effect of prophylactic pretreatment with the selective serotonin re-uptake inhibitor (SSRI) antidepressant paroxetine (Paxil®) for patients who are to receive high-dose IFN-alfa-2b as adjuvant therapy for melanoma. Miller *et al.* (1999) reported the interim results of a randomized, blinded, placebo-controlled study. Patients on the treatment arm were pretreated for two weeks prior to starting induction therapy and continued with the antidepressant with increases in dosage as needed. Eighteen patients have completed the study and the researchers report interim results. Of the 9 patients who received placebo, 7 (78%) met the criteria for major depression and 4 discontinued therapy. Of the 9 patients on the treatment arm, only 2 (22%) developed depression and only one patient discontinued therapy. The investigators conclude that paroxetine pretreatment may be an important clinical intervention to block the development of "sickness behavior" and depression in patients receiving high-dose IFN-α therapy.

Although the exact etiology of IFN-α neurotoxicity has not been firmly established, the interaction with the opioid receptor has been studied in a report by Valentine *et al.* (1995). Their pilot study reports on the use of the μ-opioid receptor antagonist naloxone in outpatients with CML or essential thrombocytopenia who were experiencing neurobehavioral side effects. Naloxone was selected because it has a long duration of action and can be administered orally. Nine patients (8 women and one man) were identified and treated. Two patients had near-complete resolution of neurotoxic symptoms that were sustained over time and still effective when the IFN-α dose was increased in one patient. Five patients had partial relief but either could not escalate their dose of IFN-α or required an increase in naloxone to obtain or maintain relief. Two patients had severe side effects to the naloxone that resolved when it was discontinued.

Capuron and Ravaud (1999) reported on the use of a self-rating scale for depression for prediction of the depressive effects of IFN-α. They evaluated the mood of patients before the initiation of treatment with high-dose IFN for melanoma using the Montgomery-Asberg Depression Rating Scale (MADRS). They excluded patients who had prior history of psychiatric problems from this study. They evaluated patients before initiation of treatment and at the end of the fourth week of treatment. They found that the MADRS scores significantly predicted the intensity of the patient's depressive symptoms at week 4. A self-rating scale such as the MADRS may be useful for identifying those patients at greater risk for development of depression and in need of antidepressant therapy.

Retinal Changes

Retinal complications have been reported primarily in patients with viral hepatitis. The most common manifestation has been the appearance of mild to moderate ischemic retinopathy manifested as cotton-wool spots and hemorrhages similar to those seen in diabetic retinopathy (Kawano *et al.*, 1996). Although the long-term effects of retinal complications may vary among individual patients, the potential risk makes this an important pretreatment topic for patient education. Middle-aged patients (>55 years of age) with hypercholesterolemia may be at greatest risk for this complication (Manesis *et al.*, 1998).

Hypertriglyceridemia

Elevations in triglyceride level have been seen in patients treated with IFN for more than 12 months. A recent study suggests that hypertriglyceridemia is a minor problem and that gemfibrozil might be an appropriate treatment (Sgarabotto *et al.*, 1997).

Autoimmune Effects

Other issues that are of concern involve the possibility of cytokine-induced exacerbation of underlying diseases or immune dysregulation. Over the period of time that the different types of IFN-α have been studied in humans, there have been case reports of exacerbation of autoantibodies or autoimmune diseases, such as thyroiditis, systemic lupus erythematosus, and insulin-dependent diabetes. Others have seen the development of diseases involved with cell-mediated immune functions such as inflammatory dermatological diseases, nephritis, pneumonitis, and colitis (Vial and Descotes, 1995; Deutsch *et al.*, 1997). These are rare side effects seen with IFN-α. Recently, Schwid *et al.* (1997) reported on a group of 200 women with MS who were being treated with IFN-beta-1b. Two women in this group developed autoimmune hyperthyroidism. Hyperthyroidism has been reported in as many as 4.9% of patients with MS. There have not been many reports of autoimmune disorders attributed to IFN-β or IFN-γ; this may be because clinical experience is far greater with IFN-α.

Cutaneous Effects

Patients given IFN at high doses may experience hypotension, tachycardia, skin rashes, and peripheral neuropathies. Urticaria and rash can be a clinical manifestation of immunological and inflammatory mechanisms. Certainly the cause of rash must be carefully evaluated and other factors such as foods, drugs, heat, cold, pressure, and sun exposure should be considered. Treatment with histamine blockers (e.g., H1 and H2), if started early, may ameliorate the urticaria and rash (Asnis and Gaspari, 1995; Presser, 1997). Instruction on skin care should be given, such as avoiding hot baths or showers, maintaining well-moisturized skin, and avoiding soaps and lotions with drying properties. Topical steroids may be used for localized rashes but long-term use is discouraged.

Renal and Hepatic Effects

The most common renal toxic effect is mild proteinuria, but nephrotic syndrome and acute renal insufficiency have been reported. Transaminase elevation, usually mild, has occurred more often in the presence of pretreatment hepatic abnormalities and is dose-related.

Antibody Development

Some patients treated with IFN-α develop neutralizing antibodies to the IFN preparation. The development of these antibodies depends on which IFN-α preparation is used and which assay system is employed (Figlin et al., 1988; Antonelli et al., 1991). McKenna and Oberg (1997) reviewed 10 different studies to determine the influence of neutralizing antibodies on response to IFN-α therapy. Sixty-three percent of the patients who developed antibodies became resistant to therapy or relapsed, compared with 13% of the patients who did not develop antibodies. Meaningful comparisons are only obtained with studies in which IFN is given by the same route and according to the same treatment schedule to patients with the same underlying disease (Itri et al., 1987). Data are available from three hepatitis studies that compare patients with chronic viral hepatitis. In these studies, antibodies developed more frequently in patients treated with IFN-alfa-2a than with IFN-alfa-2b ($p = .0001$) (McKenna and Oberg, 1997). Several studies have looked for the development of neutralizing and nonneutralizing antibodies for the purpose of determining whether there is any significant impact on outcome of treatment. Oberg and Alm (1997) reported on the significance of antibodies in patients with solid tumors. They reported that in studies with patients with malignant carcinoid tumors treated with various types of IFN, 8 (28%) of 28 developed high-titer neutralizing antibodies with IFN-alfa-2a, 9 (4%) of 204 with IFN-alfa-2b, and 0 of 45 (0%) with natural IFN. A significant number of patients lost the antitumor effect during development of neutralizing antibodies at high titers. The authors suggest that human leukocyte IFN can be used as a rescue (Oberg and Alm, 1997).

Psychosocial Issues During Therapy

In addition to the physiological issues that a patient receiving biotherapy faces, there are psychosocial issues that impact the patient's ability to cope with the process. Some of these factors include any previous treatment with biotherapy, the efficacy of that therapy, control of previous treatment-related symptoms, and the competence and supportiveness of health care providers. The ability to assimilate new information and the degree to which the normal adult developmental process have been impacted will also influence the patient's ability to cope and adapt.

Levinson's model of adult developmental levels provides a framework for helping caregivers understand the issues and priorities their patients may be facing. When a person is in his or her 20s, they are entering the adult world, and it is a time full of potential and pressure. Some of these individuals are likely to have concerns about reproductive issues. The third decade of life is usually a time of transition and settling down. The patient may be very concerned with interruption of career advancement, and fatigue and flu-like symptoms may be perceived as overwhelming. In midlife or middle adulthood, there may be a sense of loss related to one's youth. Alopecia and side effects that affect performance may be more difficult for patients in this age group. At age 50, people are typically involved in leadership positions in work and in family and community relationships. Therapy-related side effects may result in loss of role function and may also impede travel and leisure plans. Late adulthood, the period when individuals are preparing for retirement, may also find patients dealing with other chronic illnesses. Conversely, the previously healthy older adult may feel robbed of an enjoyable retirement and may have difficulties with side effects such as depression (Hogan, 1991).

When the nurse employs coaching and educational strategies to help the patient move from the unknown to the familiar, the patient learns to effectively cope and adapt to the illness and treatment and to reclaim personal control. It has also been noted that fostering hope is an important role for the nurse and that it may positively impact the coping response. However, the ability to be hopeful requires energy, which implies that patients must have their physical symptoms fully addressed, and the caregiver must foster self-care activities that will further decrease symptoms such as fatigue and anorexia (Hogan, 1991).

Nursing Issues

Kiley and Gale (1998) emphasize the importance of pretreatment assessment before initiation of therapy with IFN-α for high-risk melanoma. A thorough medication, nutrition, medical, and psychological history is essential. In particular, assessment of cardiovascular or pulmonary disease, diabetes, a thyroid disorder, or a previous psychiatric disorder should be undertaken. A nursing management plan should be outlined based on establishing a nursing diagnosis, defining outcomes that will support the patient in maintaining activities of daily living and quality of life. Donnelly (1998) describes the importance of nurses being well versed in the expected side effects of IFN-α. She states that patients who know what to expect are usually better able to manage the side effects of therapy. Family and other caregivers should be included in the educational process.

Nurses should distinguish between short-term and longer-term side effects so that patients can be guided through the treatment process. Compliance with IFN-α therapy is critical if the patient is to achieve the benefits of therapy. The role of the nurse in understanding the spectrum of side effects and helping the patient to find relief for these side effects is challenging. Successful accomplishment of this goal can transform the care of the patient and offer the best chance for extending the life of the patient.

Clinical Experience: Interferon-β

IFN-β is produced primarily by fibroblasts and epithelial cells. Its biological effects are similar to those of IFN-α and may be summarized as antiviral, immunomodulatory, and antiproliferative (Riechmann, 1997). The use of IFN-β in the treatment of cancer remains investigational.

Multiple Sclerosis

MS is a neurological disease that affects 300,000 people in the United States and over 1 million people worldwide (Reder, 1997). IFN-β therapy has represented the first hope for an effective treatment since the disease was first described in 1868 (Rudick and Ransohoff, 1995; Rolak, 1996). Central nervous system (CNS) demyelination occurs in patients with MS, resulting in chronic disability that follows periods of relapse and remission. Extensive research has failed to identify the cause of MS, but an immunological basis is strongly suggested (Yong et al., 1998). The disease also has an autoimmune element and there is a proposed defect in the suppresser T-cell subset (Pfeffer, 1997).

Oligodendrocytes are involved in the formation of myelin in the CNS. Oligodendrocytes or the myelin they form are the targets in MS. It has been postulated that damage to these cells and tissue in MS is either cell mediated, antibody mediated, or cytokine mediated (Genc et al., 1997; Vartanian, 1997). Vartanian and colleagues (1997) found that IFN-γ induces the degeneration and ultimate death of cultured oligodendrocytes. Genc and colleagues (1997) found that during MS exacerbations, the cytokines produced by T_h1 cells are elevated. Subsequent blood-derived immune cells are activated, causing damage to the oligodendroglia. This supports the idea that inflammatory cytokines such as IFN-γ contribute to the exacerbation of MS.

The IFN-beta-1b (Betaseron®) pilot study (Knobler et al., 1993) was designed to evaluate the relationship between the dose and side effects, the route of administration, and the clinical safety of IFN-β for patients with MS. Thirty patients aged 18 to 50 years were randomized into 5 groups by dose. The doses ranged from 0 (placebo) to 16 mU. Two well-established rating scales of neurologic impairment were used. The Kurtzke Expanded Disability Status Scale (EDSS) has a range from 0 (normal) to 10 (death) (Kurtzke, 1983). The Scripps Neurologic Rating Scale (NRS) attempts to quantify impairment based on the traditional neurological examination. Scores were used to define neurological disability and exacerbation severity of MS. A dose-related therapeutic trend at six months after initiation of treatment suggested a reduction of the exacerabation rate. The fewest exacerbations were seen with patients treated with 16 mU of IFN-beta-1b. Although the number of patients studied was too small to achieve statistical significance, this study opened the door to further research. Further, this study identified the subcutaneous route of administration as an effective route of administration (Knobler et al., 1993).

A pivotal, multicenter study of IFN-beta-1b was reported by the IFN-β Multiple Sclerosis Study Group (1993). The study involved 372 men and women age 18 to 50 years with RR-MS who were randomized into 1 of 3 arms: the placebo group, those receiving 1.6 mU every other day, and those receiving 8 mU every other day. Two performance scores (Kurtzke EDSS and Scripps NRS) were used to assess neurological status. Magnetic resonance imaging (MRI) was incorporated into the study as a screening tool to determine a pattern of lesions and to provide follow-up studies that could compare any change in the pattern of lesion burden and to further evaluate the effects of the treatment. Again, the fewest exacerbations were seen at the higher dose. These results achieved statistical significance that was maintained throughout the 5 years of the study.

Several studies have confirmed the efficacy of IFN-beta-1a (Avonex®) for the treatment of RR-MS (Jacobs *et al.*, 1995; Munschauer and Kinkel, 1997; Munschauer and Stuart, 1997; Rudick *et al.*, 1997; Rudick *et al.*, 1999). A phase III trial by the Multiple Sclerosis Collaborative Research Group confirmed that 6 mU (30 mcg) of IFN-beta-1a administered by weekly intramuscular injections could be effective in delaying the onset of sustained disability in patients with RR-MS (Jacobs *et al.*, 1995). The Prevention of Relapses and Disability by IFN-beta-1a Subcutaneously in Multiple Sclerosis Study Group (1998) reported on a double-blind, placebo-controlled study designed to describe clinical benefit and optimum dose of IFN-β. They utilized IFN-beta-1a at doses of 22 mcg or 44 mcg or placebo 3 times a week for 2 years. The relapse rate at 1 to 2 years was significantly lower for both doses of IFN-β than for placebo. The mean number of relapses per patient was 1.82 for the 22-mcg group and 1.73 for the 44-mcg group. The proportion of relapse-free patients was significantly increased ($p < .05$), and the time to first relapse was prolonged by 3 months for the 22-mcg group and by 5 months for the 44-mcg group. Early treatment is favored for patients with RR-MS because MRI studies indicate that these patients frequently have evidence of CNS inflammation before onset of clinical symptoms (Munschauer and Stuart, 1997).

Safety data for adverse reactions to IFN-beta-1b and IFN-beta-1a report a high incidence of depression. The other side effects noted were similar for both drugs, with the exception of injection-site reaction. In placebo-controlled studies, IFN-beta-1a was associated with a 4% incidence of injection-site reaction (placebo = 0%) at the 30-mcg dose given once a week intramuscularly. By contrast, IFN-beta-1b was associated with an 85% incidence of injection-site reaction (placebo = 37%) and 2% necrosis at the 8-mU dose given 3 times a week subcutaneously. In the prescribing information and approval studies, the use of IFN-beta-1a yielded a 37% reduction in the risk of accumulating disability at the end of 2 years of treatment with 38% of patients who were exacerbation-free versus placebo 26% ($p = .10$). Treatment with IFN-beta-1b resulted in a 31% reduction in the annual exacerbation rate at the end of 2 years of treatment with 25% of patients exacerbation-free versus placebo 16% ($p = .094$) (Boothman, 1997; Calabresi *et al.*, 1997).

Side Effect Management

Medications that have been used for both MS-associated side effects or for amelioration of type I IFN therapy side effects include:

- For fatigue, methylphenidate or fluoxetine (Prozac®)
- For depression, amitriptyline (Elavil®), fluoxetine, and sertraline (Zoloft®)
- For pain, amitriptyline (Elavil®)
- For bladder dysfunction, amitriptyline and oxybutinin (Ditropan®)
- For muscle spasm, clonazepam (Klonopin®)

Bladder dysfunction and muscle spasm are manifestations of MS but are not IFN side effects. It is important to premedicate patients with MS prior to administration of IFN to help ameliorate the side effects of fever, fatigue, and flu-like symptoms. Worsening of MS symptoms has been associated with transient increases in core body temperature. Regular use of acetaminophen and NSAIDs is useful in this situation (Knobler, 1997). Approximately 55% of the patients who receive IFN therapy experience these flu-like symptoms, but the symptoms usually diminish over time, and by the sixth week of therapy, many do not experience these side effects at all (Rolak, 1996).

Much of the information gained in the study of IFN-α has helped to shape the current understanding of the role of IFN in the treatment and etiology of MS (Kastrukoff and Oger, 1997). One of the key points detailed in this article that summarizes the clinical trials of IFN for treatment of relapsing MS is the importance of having a placebo-controlled group in the experimental design, because exacerbation rates rise and fall even when the patient is not receiving therapy. It also appears that patients with RR-MS responded more favorably to IFN-α than patients with relapsing-progressive MS. A natural IFN preparation was used in some of the studies but had the disadvantage of potential contamination. Finally, the appearance of certain predictable side effects has the potential to unblind a study.

The IFN-β Multiple Sclerosis Study Group states that the following four components are integral to the outcome measures of a well-designed study to evaluate the use of IFN-α and IFN-β in MS. The 2 "physician-oriented" outcomes are (1) the physiological measurement of disease such as MRI and (2) the agreement on clinical end points such as relapse rate. The two "patient-oriented" outcomes are (1) relevant aspects of health status, such as disability, and (2) health-related quality of life (Hobart and Thompson, 1997). These are important features to remember as research continues to provide information about this complex disease state. Side effect management for patients with MS being treated with IFN-β is an important aspect of health-related quality of life. Patients with MS may also experience side effects as a result of decreased nerve impulse conduction or the release of inflammatory cytokines in the CNS. The use of the Kurtzke EDSS has helped to define more clearly the "patient-oriented" outcomes related to health status and disability (Rudick et al., 1997). Advances in "physician-oriented" measurement

of response to therapy or progression of disease have occurred. Changes in lesions or degree of cerebral atrophy identified by gadolinium-enhanced MRI are important markers of disease progression (Aranson, 1999; Simon et al., 1999). Additionally, studies have demonstrated that cerebral spinal fluid white blood cell counts are positively correlated with both clinical and MRI-measured disease activity (Rudick et al., 1999).

Clinical Experience: Interferon-γ

IFN-γ shares many properties with IFN-α and IFN-β but has many differences as well. It shows greater antiproliferative activity than the other IFNs but is more likely to result in myelosuppression. Hypotension is also a more common toxic effect of IFN-γ (at higher doses) than the type I IFNs. IFN-γ appears to be a more potent immune stimulator of monocytes and class II HLA activity than IFN-α or IFN-β.

Recombinant human IFN-γ can be administered intravenously, intramuscularly, or subcutaneously. It has also been prepared as an aerosol and in this form, induces the activation of the alveolar macrophage in a nonsystemic fashion. It has been administered intralesionally in cutaneous leishmaniasis (Murray, 1996). Typically, single daily doses of 50 to 100 mcg/m² have induced systemic immunomodulatory and antimicrobial effects.

IFN-gamma-1b (Actimmune®) is an approved immunomodulatory agent for the treatment of CGD, a rare disorder that is characterized by either a diminished or absent neutrophil oxidative function. The efficacy of neutrophils is dependent on the rapid and carefully controlled generation of toxic oxygen compounds, which are lethal to most pathogenic organisms. The complex enzyme that is responsible for this oxidative function, NADPH oxidase, is composed of 4 separate protein subunits. Each of these proteins is critical to oxidase function. These proteins are encoded by a series of unrelated genes which are each located on a different chromosome. Mutations in any 1 of the 4 genes can result in impairment or loss of oxidase activity. Three of the proteins are inherited in an autosomal recessive manner, and one is transmitted in an X-linked manner.

CGD is characterized by life-threatening infections that are typically caused by organisms such as *Staphylococcus aureus, Escherichia coli, Pseudomonas cepacia*, and *Aspergillus fumigatus*. These infections most often affect the skin, lung, lymph glands, liver, bones, and intestinal tract. The basic defect is a malfunction of the polymorphonuclear (PMN) leukocytes (Ahlin *et al.*, 1997).

A recent dose-comparison study of IFN-gamma-1b evaluated the differences in functional responses of neutrophils in patients with CGD at 50 and 100 mcg/m^2 administered for 2 consecutive days (Ahlin *et al.*, 1997). The drugs were administered subcutaneously in a double-blind manner. Four patients received the higher dose, and 5 received the lower dose. Reported side effects for those receiving the 100 mcg/m^2 dose were headache, muscle pain, and a severe-grade fever lasting 2 to 7 hours. Four of the patients receiving 50 mcg/m^2 and 1 receiving 100 mcg/m^2 reported headache and fever of minor or moderate grade lasting 2 hours. Three of the patients (2 in the high-dose group and 1 in the low-dose group) did not report any adverse reactions. The variables being measured included the factors that are directly dependent on the pathogenesis of CGD, such as expression of FcγRI, a receptor for immunoglobulin on neutrophils that is important for PMN phagocytosis. They also examined the PMN aspergillicidal capacity. This study suggested a dose-dependent effect with a maximal effect on day 3 after the 100 mcg/

m^2 dose. This may be a very important finding, because fungal infections have been reported to be a major cause of death for patients with CGD (Ahlin *et al.*, 1997).

CGD is a disease for which long-term administration of IFN therapy may be indicated. In a phase IV study, Bemiller and colleagues (1995) investigated the safety and effectiveness of long-term IFN-gamma-1b in patients with CGD. Prior to this study, there were no data to describe whether the clinical effectiveness of IFN-gamma-1b would wane over time or whether there was no late or cumulative toxicity. Thirty patients, ranging in age from 0.8 months to 34.7 years, were enrolled in the study. Three quarters of these patients had previously or were currently receiving IFN-gamma-1b in phase III therapeutic or compassionate-use studies at Scripps Research Institute (San Diego, CA).

In this study, results were positive when compared with historical controls. The placebo arm of the published phase III study that was used as the control averaged 1.10 serious infections per patient year for 30 of 65 patients (46%) with an average of 48 days in the hospital. The patients in this study had an average of 0.13 serious infections per patient year, with 3 patients having serious infections requiring an average of 23 days in the hospital. The 3 patients who experienced serious infections had X-linked CGD; for reasons that are yet unknown, this group tends to have a more severe clinical course.

Adverse events were mild to moderate and included fever (23%), diarrhea (13%), and flu-like syndrome (13%). In 9 patients, treatment was temporarily held or the dose was reduced because of adverse events (abnormal liver function tests in 2 patients; neutropenia in 3 patients; and hallucinations, headache with joint stiffness, rule-out sepsis, and chills with fever in 1 patient each). Patients were able to resume therapy with complete resolution of side effects in all but 3 cases. There was 1 case of an adolescent male developing psychotic depression that did not improve following withdrawal of therapy. There was one patient who had elevated thyroid-stimulating hormone levels during therapy, an abnormality that has been reported in treatment with type one IFN but has not been reported before in patients with CGD receiving IFN-γ. In both the postpubertal and adult groups, there was no decrement in sexual function historically or in measured sex hormone levels. Three of three adolescents (aged 15 to 17 years) experienced Tanner stage 4 or 5 development and had normal testosterone or estrogen levels for their age. Two postpubertal women reported normal menses, and one patient fathered a normal child while on this study. Steady growth and development was observed in 23 of 30 patients who were not yet of adult age and who were actively growing. Although children with CGD tend to be shorter than their peers, the majority in this study remained within 10 percentile points of their baseline height. Only one of the 9 infants experienced neutropenia ($<1,000$ cells/mm^3); however, infants and children require careful monitoring for this side effect, as do all patients. The authors concluded that when IFN-gamma-1b is used for infection prophylaxis in patients with CGD, it does not appear to delay growth and maturation nor does it seem to cause any worrisome trends or clues that would lead us to expect to see late toxicities associated with this treatment. Additionally, even after 2½ years of continuous treatment, IFN-gamma-1b has measurable benefit in reducing the frequency and severity of serious infections.

The role of biotherapy apart from the treatment of disease has been described in a study of IFN-γ in the critical care setting. Dries (1996) reported on the results of a randomized, double-blind, placebo-controlled trial with 416 hospitalized patients who were being treated for severe trauma. Subjects received treatment with IFN-gamma-1b at 100 mcg subcutaneously for 21 days or placebo in addition to standard antibiotic therapy. Sixty-five percent of the patients in the experimental arm completed therapy. Deaths during treatment were comparable, with fatalities reported for 17 (8%) of the placebo-treated patients and 18 (9%) of the IFN-treated patients. Major infections were seen in 83 (40%) of the placebo-controlled group and in 89 (43%) of the IFN-gamma-1b–treated group. Infection-related death occurred in 18 (9%) patients in the placebo-treated group and in 7 (3%) of the IFN-gamma-1b–treated group (statistical significance not reported). The researcher noted that a disproportionate number of major infections (29%) and deaths (47%) occurred at one study center. Other notable issues include the difficulty in assessing immunological competence and interpreting immunological data in injured patients. This continues to be an area that will benefit from further research.

Other areas that may also show benefit for prophylaxis with IFN-γ include replacement therapy for patients with persistent T-cell defect, patients with CD4 cell deficiency, and patients receiving immunosuppressive therapy. Short-term prophylactic IFN-γ therapy for those known to be at risk for infection include burn or trauma patients, postchemotherapy or post-BMT patients, or those with debilitating illness who require hospitalization in intensive care units. Adjuvant therapy with IFN-γ may be a consideration for treatment of infections that require toxic or long-term antibiotic therapy such as leprosy, progressive leishmaniasis, atypical and drug-resistant tuberculosis, and systemic or focal fungal infections (Murray, 1996).

Regulatory Approvals

IFN-α was first approved by the FDA in 1986 for its significant role in the treatment of HCL.

Since then, two other types of IFN (β and γ) have been approved. In all, IFN has been approved for treatment of a total of 11 different diseases (see Table 5.1). There are seven commercially available and FDA-approved IFNs available in the United States. IFN-alfa-2a has been approved for treatment of CML, HCL, AIDS-related KS, and chronic hepatitis C. IFN-alfa-2b has received FDA approval for the treatment of high-risk melanoma, follicular NHL, HCL, AIDS-related KS, condylomata acuminata, chronic HBV (adult and pediatric), and chronic hepatitis C (alone or in combination with ribavirin). IFN-alfa-N3 (Alferon®) has received FDA approval for the treatment of condylomata acuminata. IFN-alfacon-1 has received FDA approval for the treatment of hepatitis C. Both IFN-beta-1a and IFN-beta-1b have received FDA approval for use in the treatment of RR-MS. IFN-gamma-1b has FDA approval for treatment of CGD. There are many diseases for which IFNs are being evaluated either as a single agent or in combination with other agents. As research culminates and data mature, we are likely to see the list of approvals continue to grow.

Summary

IFN-α was the first pure human protein found to be effective in the treatment of cancer. When this molecule was introduced into the clinical arena over 20 years ago, it was hailed as a wonder drug and "magic bullet" by the media. For patients, the medical community, and the drug industry, that announcement was the beginning of an arduous period of watching and waiting for clinical results to come forth. Today, IFN has clearly demonstrated its usefulness in inducing regressions in both hematologic malignancies and solid tumors. Some of its antitumor effects have been dramatic, others only partial or relatively brief in duration.

Treatment with IFN-α has been shown to be effective in inducing regression in several malignancies. They are the first human therapeutic proteins to show a survival benefit in cancer patients. They also have the ability to interact synergistically with other anticancer drugs. The strategies of the future will likely include gene modulation or complementary effects with other modalities such as chemotherapy or immunomodulatory agents. An influx of information on the immunomodulatory processes, genetic identity, and the signaling pathways involved in IFN-related therapies is upon us. Molecular technology will provide greater sophistication in targeting and controlling secondary cytokines that contribute to side effects. Additional strategies for side effect reduction will be critical and are likely to come from the area of biochemical or molecular research.

The majority of IFN research in cancer treatment has dealt with invasive, advanced cancer. Between 1992 and 1994, approximately 1,500 manuscripts related to the treatment of advanced cancer were published, whereas only a few dealt with the role of IFN in early disease (Tanneberger and Hrelia, 1996). Identification of appropriate end points and markers of response to treatment with IFN is one of the greatest impediments to the study of cancer and other disease states.

The most important future direction for research on IFNs and possibly their greatest value will be in prolonging the disease-free interval and, ultimately, survival. Numerous studies have demonstrated improvement in these areas. The hope remains that as biotherapy with IFN becomes applied to earlier-stage disease, greater gains in survival and disease-free intervals may be sustained. The challenge remains in reducing the patient's experience of side effects. Several approaches have been described in the nursing literature and provide a strong basis to pursue further research in this area (Dean *et al.*, 1995; Skalla, 1996; Donnelly, 1998; Kiley and Gale, 1998). Nursing research can make a substantial contribution to the success of therapy with IFN in terms of the management and support of the patient receiving IFN, but this needs the strength of empirical study to make a true impact.

References

Abbas, A., Lichtman, A., and Pober, J. 1991. Cytokines. In *Cellular and Molecular Immunology*. Abbas, A., Lichtman, A., and Pober, J. (eds). Philadelphia, PA: W.B. Saunders Company, pp. 226–242.

Abrams, D., and Volberding, P. 1987. Alpha interferon of AIDS-associated Kaposi's sarcoma. *Seminars in Oncology* 14(2 suppl 2): 42–47.

Ahlin, A., Elinder, G., Palmblad, J., *et al.* 1997. Dose-dependent enhancements by interferon-γ on functional responses of neutrophils from chronic granulomatous disease patients. *Blood* 89(9): 3396–3401.

Aistars, J. 1987. Fatigue in the cancer patient: A conceptual approach to a clinical problem. *Oncology Nursing Forum* 14(6): 25–30.

Alimena, G., Morra, E., Lazzarino, M., *et al.* 1988. Interferon alpha-2b as therapy of Ph-positive chronic myelogenous leukemia: A study of 82 patients treated with intermittent or daily administration. *Blood* 72(2): 642–647.

Alter, H. 1995. To C or not to C: These are the questions. *Blood* 85(7): 1681–1695.

Alter, M. 1997. Epidemiology of hepatitis C. *Hepatology* 26(3 suppl 1): 62S–65S.

Alter, M., and Mase, E. 1994. The epidemiology of viral hepatitis in the United States. *Gastroenterology Clinics of North America* 21: 437–455.

Antonelli, G., Currenti, M., Turriziani, O., *et al.* 1991. Neutralizing antibodies to interferon alpha: Relative frequency in patients treated with different interferon preparations. *Journal of Infectious Diseases* 163(4): 882–885.

Aranson, B. 1999. Immunologic therapy of multiple sclerosis. *Annual Review of Medicine* 50: 291–302.

Asnis, L., and Gaspari, A. 1995. Cutaneous reactions to recombinant cytokine therapy. *Journal of the American Academy of Dermatology* 33(3): 393–410.

Balch, C., and Buzaid, A. 1996. Finally, a successful adjuvant therapy for high-risk melanoma (Editorial). *Journal of Clinical Oncology* 14(1): 1–3.

Balkwill, F., Moodie, E., Freedman, V., *et al.* 1982. Human interferon inhibits the growth of established human breast tumors in the nude mouse. *International Journal of Cancer* 30(3): 231–253.

Barlogie, B., Jagannath, S., Vesole, D., *et al.* 1997. Superiority of tandem autologous transplantation over standard therapy for previously untreated multiple myeloma. *Blood* 89(3): 789–793.

Belldegrun, A., Franklin, J., O'Donnell, M., *et al.* 1998. Superficial bladder cancer: The role of interferon-α. *The Journal of Urology* 159: 1793–1801.

Bemiller, L., Roberts, D., Starko, K., *et al.* 1995. Safety and effectiveness of long-term interferon gamma therapy in patients with chronic granulomatous disease. *Blood Cells, Molecules, and Diseases* 21(24 December 31): 239–247.

Bender, C., Monti, E., and Kerr, M. 1996. Potential mechanisms of interferon neurotoxicity. *Cancer Practice* 4(1): 35–39.

Blatt, L., Davis, J., Klein, S., *et al.* 1996. The biologic activity of molecular characterization of a novel synthetic interferon-alpha species, consensus interferon. *Journal of Interferon and Cytokine Research* 16: 489–499.

Boothman, B. 1997. Interferon beta: The current position. *British Journal of Hospital Medicine* 57(6): 277–280.

Borden, E., Hogan, T., and Voelkel, J. 1982. Comparative antiproliferative activity in vitro of natural interferons alpha and beta for diploid and transformed human cells. *Cancer Research* 42: 4948–4953.

Borden, E., and Parkinson, D. 1998. A perspective

on the clinical effectiveness and tolerance of interferon-a. *Seminars in Oncology* 25(1 suppl): 3–8.

Bordens, R., Grossberg, S., Trotta, P., *et al.* 1997. Molecular and biologic characterization of recombinant interferon-a2b. *Seminars in Oncology* 24(9 suppl): S941–S951.

Bukowski, R. 1999. Immunotherapy in renal cell carcinoma. *Oncology* 13(6): 801–810.

Bunn, P., Foon, K., Ihde, D., *et al.* 1984. Recombinant leukocyte A interferon: An active agent in advanced cutaneous T-cell lymphomas. *Annals of Internal Medicine* 101(4): 484–487.

Bunn, P., Ihde, D., Foon, K., *et al.* 1989. The role of recombinant interferon alpha-2a in the therapy of cutaneous T-cell lymphomas. *Cancer* 57(8): 1689–1695.

Byrne, J., Carter, G., Bienz, N., *et al.* 1998. Adjuvant a-interferon improves complete remission rates following allogeneic transplantation for multiple myeloma. *Bone Marrow Transplantation* 22: 639–643.

Calabresi, P., Stone, L., Bash, C., *et al.* 1997. Interferon beta results in immediate reduction of contrast-enhanced MRI lesions in multiple sclerosis patients followed by weekly MRI. *Neurology* 48(5): 1446–1448.

Cameron, R., McIntosh, J., and Rosenberg, S. 1988. Synergistic antitumor effects of combination immunotherapy with recombinant interleukin-2 and recombinant hybrid alpha-interferon in the treatment of established hepatic metastases. *Cancer Research* 8(6): 1637–1649.

Cantell, K., Hervonen, S., Cavalletto, L., *et al.* 1975. Human leukocyte interferon production, purification and animal experiments. In Waymouth, C. (ed). *In Vitro*. Baltimore: Baltimore Tissue Culture Association, pp. 35–38.

Capuron, L., and Ravaud, A. 1999. Prediction of the depressive effects of interferon alfa therapy by the patient's initial affective state. *The New England Journal of Medicine,* April 29: 1370.

Caraceni, A., Gangeri, L., Martini, C., *et al.* 1998. Neurotoxicity of interferon-alpha I melanoma

therapy: Results from a randomized controlled trial. *Cancer* 83(3): 482–489.

Carithers, R., and Emerson, S. 1997. Therapy of hepatitis C: Meta-analysis of interferon alfa-2b trials. *Hepatology* 26(3 suppl 1): 85S–88S.

Chemello, L., Bonetti, P., Cavalletto L., *et al.* 1995. Randomized trial comparing three different regimens of alpha-2a-interferon in chronic hepatitis C. *Hepatology* 22(3): 700–706.

Chronic Myeloid Leukemia Trialists Group. 1997. Interferon alfa versus chemotherapy for chronic myeloid leukemia: A meta-analysis of seven randomized trials. *Journal of the National Cancer Institute* 89(21): 1616–1620.

Clark, D., and Russell, L. (eds). 1997. *Molecular Biology Made Simple and Fun*. Vienna, IL: Cache River Press.

Cole, B., Gelber, R., Kirkwood J., *et al.* 1996. Quality-of-life-adjusted survival analysis of interferon alfa-2b adjuvant treatment of high-risk resected cutaneous melanoma: An Eastern Cooperative Oncology Group study. *Journal of Clinical Oncology* 14: 2666–2673.

Colquhoun, S. 1996. Hepatitis C: A clinical update. *Archives of Surgery* 131(January): 18–23.

Conry-Cantilena, C., VanRaden, M., Gibble, J., *et al.* 1996. Routes of infection, viremia, and liver disease in blood donors found to have hepatitis C virus infection. *The New England Journal of Medicine* 334: 1691–1696.

Coppens, J., Cornu, C., Lens, E., *et al.* 1989. Prospective trial of recombinant leukocyte interferon in chronic hepatitis B: A 10-month follow-up study. *Liver* 9(5): 307–313.

Cortes, J., Talpaz, M., O'Brien, S., *et al.* 1998. Suppression of cytogenetic clonal evolution with interferon alfa therapy in patients with Philadelphia chromosome-positive chronic myelogenous leukemia. *Journal of Clinical Oncology* 16(10): 3279–3285.

Costanzi, J., Cooper, M., Scarffe, J., *et al.* 1985. Phase II study of recombinant alpha-2 interferon in resistant multiple myeloma. *Journal of Clinical Oncology* 3(5): 654–659.

Covelli, A., Cavalieri, R., *et al.* 1987. Recombinant leukocyte A interferon (IFN-ra) as initial therapy in mycosis fungoides and Sezary syndrome. *Proceedings of the American Society of Clinical Oncology* 6(189): abstract.

Creagan, E., Dalton, R., Ahmann, D., *et al.* 1995. Randomized surgical adjuvant clinical trial of recombinant interferon alfa-2a in selected patients with malignant melanoma. *Journal of Clinical Oncology* 13(11): 2776–2783.

Creasey, A., Bartholomew, J., and Merigan, T. 1980. Role of G_0–G_1 arrest in the inhibition of tumor cell growth by interferon. *Proceedings of the National Academy of Sciences USA* 77(3): 1471–1475.

Dalakas, M., Mock, V., Hawkins M., *et al.* 1998. Fatigue: Definitions, mechanisms, and paradigms for study. *Seminars in Oncology* 25(1 suppl): 48–53.

Davis, G., Esteben-Mur, R., Rustgi, V., *et al.* 1998. Interferon alfa-2b alone or in combination with ribavirin for the treatment of relapse of chronic hepatitis C. *The New England Journal of Medicine* 339(21): 1493–1499.

Dean, G., Spears, L., Ferrell, B., *et al.* 1995. Fatigue in patients with cancer receiving interferon alpha. *Cancer Practice* 3(3): 164–172.

Deisseroth, A., Kantarjian, H., *et al.* 1997. *Chronic Leukemia.* Phildelphia, PA: Lippincott-Raven.

Dekernion, J., Sarna, G., Figlin, R., *et al.* 1983. Treatment of renal cell carcinoma with human leukocyte (alpha) interferon. *The Journal of Urology* 130: 1063–1066.

Denz, H., Lechleitner, M., Marth, C., *et al.* 1985. Effect of human recombinant alpha-2a and gamma interferon on the growth of human cell lines from solid tumors and hematologic malignancies. *Journal of Interferon Research* 5(1): 147–157.

Deutsch, M., Dourakis, S., Manesis, E., *et al.* 1997. Thyroid abnormalities in chronic viral hepatitis and their relationship to interferon alfa therapy. *Hepatology* 26: 206–210.

DeWit, R. 1992. AIDS-associated Kaposi's sarcoma and the mechanisms of interferon alpha's activity: A riddle within a puzzle. *Journal of Internal Medicine* 231: 321–325.

Dhib-Jalbut, S., Jiang, H., Xia, Q., *et al.* 1996. Comparative effects of interferon-consensus1, interferon-a2a, and interferon-b1b on HLA expression and lymphoproliferation: A preclinical model for treatment of multiple sclerosis. *Journal of Interferon and Cytokine Research* 16: 195–200.

Di Bisceglie, A. 1997. Hepatitis C and hepatocellular carcinoma. *Hepatology* 26 (3 suppl 1): 34S–38S.

Dickerman, J. 1999. Interferon and giant cell tumors. *Pediatrics* 103(6): 1282–1283.

Dienstag, J. 1997. Sexual and perinatal transmission of hepatitis C. *Hepatology* 26(3 suppl 1): 66S–70S.

Dinarello, C. 1997. Induction of interleukin-1 and interleukin-1 receptor antagonist. *Seminars in Oncology* 24(9 suppl): S981–S993.

Dinney, C., Bielenberg, D., Perrotte, P., *et al.* 1998. Inhibition of basic fibroblast growth factor expression, angiogenesis, and growth of human bladder carcinoma in mice by systemic interferon-a administration. *Cancer Research* 58: 808–814.

Donnelly, S. 1998. Patient management strategies of interferon alfa-2b as adjuvant therapy of high-risk melanoma. *Oncology Nursing Forum* 25(5): 921–927.

Dries, D. 1996. Interferon gamma in trauma-related infections. *Intensive Care Medicine* 22(suppl): S462–S467.

Durelli, L., Bongioanni, M., Cavallo, R., *et al.* 1995. Interferon alpha treatment of relapsing-remitting multiple sclerosis: Long-term study of the correlations between clinical and magnetic resonance imaging results and effects on the immune function. *Multiple Sclerosis* 1(suppl 1): S32–S37.

Dusheiko, G. 1997. Side effects of alpha interferon in chronic hepatitis C. *Hepatology* 26(3 suppl 1): 112S–121S.

Enright, H., and McGlave, P. 1997. Biology and treatment of chronic myelogenous leukemia. *Oncology* 11: 1295–1306.

Essner, R. 1997. The role of lymphoscintigraphy and sentinel node mapping in assessing patient risk in melanoma. *Seminars in Oncology* 24(1 suppl 4): S4–S8.

Estey, E., Kurzrock, R., Kantarjian, H., et al. 1992. Treatment of hairy cell leukemia with 2-chloro-deoxyadenosine (2-CdA). *Blood* 79: 882–887.

Faderl, S., Kantarjian, H., and Talpaz, M. 1999. Chronic myelogenous leukemia: Update on biology and treatment. *Oncology* 13(2): 169–181.

Fattovich, B., Brollo, L., Boscaro, S., et al. 1989. Long-term effect of low-dose recombinant interferon therapy in patients with chronic hepatitis B. *Journal of Hepatology* 9(3): 331–337.

Figlin, R., Belldegrun, A., Moldawer, J., et al. 1992. Concomitant administration of recombinant human interleukin-2 and recombinant interferon alfa-2a: An active outpatient regimen in metastatic renal cell carcinoma. *Journal of Clinical Oncology* 10(3): 414–421.

Figlin, R., Dekernion, J., Mukamel, E., et al. 1988. Recombinant interferon alfa-2a in metastatic renal cell carcinoma: Assessment of antitumor activity and anti-interferon antibody formation. *Journal of Clinical Oncology* 6(10): 1604–1610.

Fischl, M., Reese, J., et al. 1988. Phase I study of interferon-alpha and AZT in patients with AIDS-related Kaposi's sarcoma. *Fourth International Conference on AIDS* 1(253): abstract.

Folkman, M. 1995. Clinical applications of research on angiogenesis. *The New England Journal of Medicine* 333(26): 1757–1763.

Foon, K., Maluish, A., Abrams, P., et al. 1986. Recombinant leukocyte A interferon therapy for advanced hairy cell leukemia. *American Journal of Medicine* 80(3): 351–356.

Frey, J., Peck, R., and Bollag, W. 1991. Antiproliferative activity of retinoids, interferon alpha and their combination in five human transformed cell lines. *Cancer Letters* 57(3): 223–227.

Gallin, J., Malech, H., et al. 1991. A controlled trial of recombinant human interferon gamma to prevent infection in chronic granumomations dis-ease. *The New England Journal of Medicine* 324: 509–516.

Genc, K., Dona, D., and Reder, A. 1997. Increased CD8[(+)] B cells in active multiple sclerosis and reversal by interferon beta-1b therapy. *Journal of Clinical Investigation* 99(11): 2664–2667.

Glashan, R. 1990. A randomized controlled study of intravesical a-2b-interferon in carcinoma in situ of the bladder. *Journal of Urology* 144(September): 658–661.

Goldstein, D., and Laszlo, J. 1986. Interferon therapy in cancer: From imaginon to interferon. *Cancer Research* 38(1): 259–278.

Golomb, H., Fefer, A., Golde, D., et al. 1987. Sequential evaluation of alpha-2b interferon treatment in 128 patients with hairy cell leukemia. *Seminars in Oncology* 14(1): 13–17.

Grem, L., Allegra, C., et al. 1990. Phase I study of interferon alfa-2a (IFN-A), 5-fluorouracil (5-FU) and high-dose leucovorin (LV) in metastatic gastrointestinal cancer. *Proceedings of the American Society of Clinical Oncology* 9: 70 (abstract).

Gretch, D. 1997. Diagnostic tests for hepatitis C. *Hepatology* 26(suppl 1): 43S–47S.

Grob, J., Dreno, B., de la Salmoniere, P., et al. 1998. Randomised trial of interferon a-2a as adjuvant therapy in resected primary melanoma thicker than 1.5 mm without clinically detectable node metastases. *The Lancet* 351: 1905–1910.

Groopman, J., Gottleib, M., Goodman, J., et al. 1984. Recombinant alpha-2 interferon therapy for Kaposi's sarcoma associated with the acquired immunodeficiency syndrome. *Annals of Internal Medicine* 100(5): 671–676.

Guilhot, F., Chastang, C., Michallet, M., et al. 1997. Interferon alfa-2b combined with cytarabine versus interferon alone in chronic myelogenous leukemia. *The New England Journal of Medicine* 337(4): 223–229.

Habermann, T., Cassileth, P., et al. 1990. A phase II trial for the evaluation of alpha-2a interferon (Roferon-A) (Alpha-IFN) followed by 2'-deoxycoformycin (pentostatin) (dCF) in the therapy of hairy cell leukemia (HCL) in previously splenectomized patients. *Blood* 76(suppl 1): 277a.

Haque, S., and Williams, B. 1998. Signal transduction in the interferon system. *Seminars in Oncology* 25(1 suppl): 14–22.

Hartshorn, M., Vogt, M., Chou, T., *et al.* 1987. Synergistic inhibition of human immunodeficiency virus in vitro by azidothymidine and recombinant alpha A-interferon. *Antimicrobiology Agents in Chemotherapy* 31(2): 168–172.

Herberman, R. 1997. Effect of alpha-interferon on immune function. *Seminars in Oncology* 24(3 suppl 9): S978–S980.

Higano, C., Chielens, D., Raskind, W., *et al.* 1997. Use of α--2a-interferon to treat cytogenetic relapse of chronic myeloid leukemia after marrow transplantation. *Blood* 90(7 October 1): 2549–2554.

Higano, C., Raskind, W., and Singer, J. 1992. Use of α-interferon for the treatment of relapse of chronic myelogenous leukemia in chronic phase after allogeneic bone marrow tranplantation. *Blood* 80(6): 1437–1442.

Higano, C., Raskind, W., and Singer, J. 1993. Use of interferon alfa-2a to treat hematologic relapse of chronic myelogenous leukemia after bone marrow transplantation. *Acta Haematologica* 89(suppl 1): 8–14.

Higuchi, T., Hannigan, G., Malkin, D., *et al.* 1991. Enhancement by retinoic acid and dibutyryl cyclic adenosine 3'-5'-monophosphate of the differentiation and gene expression of human neuroblastoma cells induced by interferon. *Cancer Research* 51(15): 3958–3964.

Hobart, J., and Thompson, A. 1997. Clinical trials of multiple sclerosis. In Reder, A. (ed). *Interferon Therapy of Multiple Sclerosis.* New York, NY: Marcel Dekker, Inc., pp. 499–508.

Hogan, C. 1991. Coping with biotherapy: Physiological and psychosocial concerns. *Oncology Nursing Forum* 18(1 suppl 1): 19–23.

Hoofnagle, J. 1997a. Hepatitis C: The clinical spectrum of the disease. *Hepatology* 26(suppl 1): 15S–20S.

Hoofnagle, J., and Di Bisceglie, A. 1997b. The treatment of chronic viral hepatitis. *The New England Journal of Medicine* 336(5): 347–356.

Huang, Y.W., Hamilton, A., Arnuk, O., *et al.* 1999. Current drug therapy for multiple myeloma. *Drugs* 57(4): 485–506.

Huberman, M., Bering, H., *et al.* 1990. 5-fluorouracil (5FU) plus recombinant alpha interferon (Roferon A) in advanced colorectal cancer. *Proceedings of the American Society of Clinical Oncology* 9: 116 (abstract).

Isaacs, A., and Lindemann, J. 1957. Virus interference I. The interferon. *Proceedings from the Royal Society Service* B147: 258–267.

Itri, L., Campion, M., Dervin, R.A., *et al.* 1987. Incidence and clinical significance of neutralizing antibodies in patients receiving recombinant interferon alfa-2a by intramuscular injection. *Cancer* 59(3): 668–674.

Jacobs, L., Cookfair, D., Rudick, R., *et al.* 1995. A phase III trial of intramuscular recombinant interferon beta as treatment for exacerbating-remitting multiple sclerosis: Design and conduct of study and baseline characteristics of patients. Multiple Sclerosis Collaborative Research Group. *Multiple Sclerosis* 1(2): 118–135.

Jensen, R., and Norton, J. 1997. Carcinoid Tumors. In DeVita, V., Hellman, S., and Rosenberg, S. (eds). *Cancer: Principles and Practice of Oncology,* 5th edn. Philadelphia, PA: Lippincott-Raven, pp. 1704–1723.

Johnston, J., Eisenhauer, E., Corbett, W., *et al.* 1988. Efficacy of 2'deoxycoformycin in hairy cell leukemia: A study of the National Cancer Institute of Canada Clinical Trials Group. *Journal of the National Cancer Institute* 80: 765–769.

Jones, T., Wadler, S., Hupart, K., *et al.* 1998. Endocrine-mediated mechanism of fatigue during treatment with interferon-alfa. *Seminars in Oncology* 25(1 suppl 1): 54–63.

Kaban, L., Mulliken, J., Ezekowitz, R., *et al.* 1999. Antiangiogenic therapy of a recurrent giant cell tumor of the mandible with interferon alfa-2a. *Pediatrics* 103(6): 1145–1149.

Kaempfer, R. 1998. Cytokine and interferon research in Israel. *Cytokine and Growth Factor Reviews* 9(2): 99–108.

Kantarjian, H., Deisseroth, A., Kurzrock, R., *et al.* 1993. Chronic myelogenous leukemia: A concise update. *Blood* 82(3): 691–703.

Kantarjian, H., Keating, M., *et al.* 1992. Treatment of advanced stages of Philadelphia chromosome positive chronic myelogenous leukemia with alpha interferon and low dose cytosine arabinoside. *Proceedings of the American Society of Clinical Oncology* 11: 260 (abstract).

Kantarjian, H., O'Brien, S., Anderlini, P., *et al.* 1996. Treatment of chronic myelogenous leukemia: Current status and investigational options. *Blood* 87(8): 3069–3081.

Kars, A., Celik, I., Kansu, E., *et al.* 1997. Maintenance therapy with alpha-interferon following first-line VAD in multiple myeloma. *European Journal of Haematology* 59(2): 100–104.

Kastrukoff, L., and Oger, J. 1997. Interferon-α in the treatment of multiple sclerosis. In Reder, A. (ed). *Interferon Therapy of Multiple Sclerosis*. New York, NY: Marcel Dekker, Inc., pp. 287–306.

Kawano, T., Shigehira, M., Uto, H., *et al.* 1996. Retinal complications during interferon therapy for chronic hepatitis C. *American Journal of Gastroenterology* 91(2): 309–313.

Kelly, C. 1996. The role of interferons in the treatment of multiple sclerosis. *Journal of Neuroscience Nursing* 28(2): 114–120.

Kemeny, N., Kelsen, D., *et al.* 1990. Combination 5-fluorouracil and recombinant alpha-interferon in advanced colorectal carcinoma: Activity but significant toxicity. *Proceedings of the American Society of Clinical Oncology* 9: 109 (abstract).

Kiley, K., and Gale, D. 1998. Nursing management of patients with malignant melanoma receiving adjuvant alpha interferon-2b. *Clinical Journal of Oncology Nursing* 2(1): 11–16.

Kirkwood, J. 1998. Adjuvant IFNalpha2 therapy of melanoma. *The Lancet* 351(June 27): 1901–1903.

Kirkwood, J., Strawderman, M., Ernstoff, M., *et al.* 1996. Interferon alfa-2b adjuvant therapy of high-risk resected cutaneous melanoma: The Eastern Cooperative Oncology Group Trial EST 1684. *Journal of Clinical Oncology* 14(1): 7–17.

Knobler, R. 1997. Interferon B-1b (Betaseron) treatment of multiple sclerosis. In Reder, A. (ed). *Interferon Therapy of Multiple Sclerosis*. New York, NY: Marcel Dekker, Inc., pp. 353–413.

Knobler, R., Greenstein, J., Johnson, K., *et al.* 1993. Systemic recombinant human interferon-beta treatment of relapsing-remitting multiple sclerosis: Pilot study analysis and six-year follow up. *Journal of Interferon Research* 13: 333–340.

Kocha, W. 1993. 5-fluorouracil (5-FU) plus interferon alfa-2a (Roferon-A) versus 5-fluorouracil plus leucovorin (LV) in metastatic colorectal cancer—Results of a multicenter, multinational phase III study. *Proceedings of the American Society of Clinical Oncology* 12: 562 (abstract).

Korenman, J., Baker, B., Waggoner, J., *et al.* 1991. Long-term remission of chronic hepatitis B after alpha interferon therapy. *Annals of Internal Medicine* 114(8): 629–634.

Kosmidis, P., Bacoyiannis, C., Fountzilas, G., *et al.* 1997. 5-fluorouracil, interferon-alpha-2b and cisplatin (FAP) for advanced urothelial cancer. A phase II study. *Annals of Oncology* 8: 373–378.

Krown, S., Bundow, D., *et al.* 1989. Interferon alpha + AZT in AIDS-associated Kaposi's sarcoma: Final results of a phase I trial. *V. International Conference. AIDS WBP* 374: abstract.

Krown, S., Gold, J., *et al.* 1986a. Interferon alfa-2a + vinblastine (VLB) in AIDS-associated Kaposi's sarcoma: Therapeutic activity, toxicity, and effects on HTLV-III/LAV viremia. *Journal of Interferon Research* 6(3 suppl 1): abstract.

Krown, S., Real, F., *et al.* 1986b. Therapeutic trials of interferon alfa-2a (IFNa2a) in AIDS-related Kaposi's sarcoma (KS/AIDS). *Proceeding, International Conference on AIDS, Paris, France, June 23–25, 1986, Communication* 88: 35 (abstract).

Krown, S., Real, F., Cunningham-Rundles, S., *et al.* 1983. Preliminary observations on the effect of recombinant leukocyte A interferon in homosexual men with Kaposi's sarcoma. *The New England Journal of Medicine* 308(18): 1071–1076.

Krown, S., Real, F., Krim, M., *et al.* 1984. Recombinant leukocyte A interferon in Kaposi's sarcoma. *Annals of the New York Academy of Sciences* 437: 431–437.

Kurtzke, J. 1983. Rating neurologic impairment in multiple sclerosis: An expanded disability status scale (EDSS). *Neurology* 33(11): 1444–1452.

Kurzrock, R., Estrov, Z., Kantarjian, H., *et al.* 1998. Conversion of interferon-induced, long-term cytogenetic remissions in chronic myelogenous leukemia to polymerase chain reaction negativity. *Journal of Clinical Oncology* 16(4): 1526–1531.

Kuzel, T., Roenigk, H., Samuelson, E., *et al.* 1995. Effectiveness of interferon alfa-2a combined with phototherapy for mycosis fungoides and the Sezary syndrome. *Journal of Clinical Oncology* 13(1): 257–263.

Lai, M.Y., Kao, J.H., Yang, P., *et al.* 1996. Long-term efficacy of ribavirin plus interferon alfa in the treatment of chronic hepatitis C. *Gastroenterology* 111: 1307–1312.

Lauria, F., Rondelli, D., Zinzani, P., *et al.* 1997. Long-lasting complete remission in patients with hairy cell leukemia treated with 2-CdA: A 5-year survey. *Leukemia* 11: 629–632.

Lee, W. 1997. Therapy of hepatitis C: Interferon alfa-2a trials. *Hepatology* 26(3 suppl 1): 89S–93S.

Leonard, W., and O'Shea, J. 1998. JAKS and STATS; Biological implications. *Annual Review of Immunology* 16: 293–322.

Licinio, J., Kling, M., and Hauser, P. 1998. Cytokines and brain function: Relevance to interferon-α-induced mood and cognitive changes. *Seminars in Oncology* 25(1 suppl): 30–38.

Lindley, C., Bernard, S., *et al.* 1990. Interferon-alpha increases 5-fluorouracil (5FU) plasma levels 64-fold within one hour: Results of a phase I study. *Journal of Interferon Research* 10(132 suppl): (abstract).

Lindsay, K., Davis, G., Schiff, E., *et al.* 1996. Response to higher doses of interferon alfa-2b in patients with chronic hepatitis C: A randomized multicenter trial. *Hepatology* 24(5): 1034–1040.

Lingen, M., Polverini, P., and Bouck, N. 1998. Retinoic acid and interferon alpha act synergistically as antiangiogenic and antitumor agents against human head and neck squamous cell carcinoma. *Cancer Research* 58: 5551–5558.

Link, H. 1998. The cytokine storm in multiple sclerosis. *Multiple Sclerosis* 4(1): 12–15.

Lippman, S., Kavanagh, J., Paredes-Espinoza, M., *et al.* 1992a. 13-Cis-retinoic acid plus interferon alpha-2a: Highly active systemic therapy for squamous cell carcinoma of the cervix. *Journal of the National Cancer Institute* 84(4): 241–245.

Lippman, S., Parkinson, D., Itri, L., *et al.* 1992b. 13-Cis-retinoic acid and interferon alpha-2a: Effective combination therapy for advanced squamous cell carcinoma of the skin. *Journal of National Cancer Institute* 84(4): 235–241.

Look, K., Blessing, J., Nelson, B., *et al.* 1998. A phase II trial of isotretinoin and alpha interferon in patients with recurrent squamous cell carcinoma of the cervix. *American Journal of Clinical Oncology* 21(6): 591–596.

Lotan, R., Francis, G., Freeman, C., *et al.* 1990. Differentiation therapy. *Cancer Research* 50(11): 3453–3464.

Mahon, F., Faberes, C., Montastruc, M., *et al.* 1996. High response rate using recombinant alpha interferon in patients with newly diagnosed chronic myeloid leukemia: Analysis of predictive factors. *Bone Marrow Transplant* 7(suppl 3): S33–S37.

Makawer, D., Wadler, S., Haynes, S., *et al.* 1997. Interferon induces thymidine phosphorylase/platelet-derived endothelial cell growth factor expression *in vivo*. *Clinical Cancer Research* 3: 923–929.

Mandelli, F., Avvisati, G., Amadori, S., *et al.* 1990. Maintenance treatment with recombinant interferon alpha-2b in patients with multiple myeloma responding to conventional induction chemotherapy. *The New England Journal of Medicine* 322(20): 1430–1434.

Manesis, E., Moschos, M., Brouzas, D., *et al.* 1998. Neurovisual impairment: A frequent complication of alpha-interferon treatment in chronic viral hepatitis. *Hepatology* 27(5): 1421–1427.

Manesis, E., Papaioannou, C., Gioustozi, A., *et al.* 1997. Biochemical and virological outcome of patients with chronic hepatitis C treated with interferon alfa-2b for 6 or 12 months: A 4-year follow-up of 211 patients. *Hepatology* 26: 734–739.

Margolin, K., Doroshow, J., Akman, S., *et al.* 1992. Phase II trial of cisplatin and alpha-interferon in advanced malignant melanoma. *Journal of Clinical Oncology* 10(10): 1574–1578.

Margolin, K., Liu, P., Unger, J., *et al.* 1999. Phase II trial of biochemotherapy with interferon alpha, dacarbazine, cisplatin and tamoxifen in metastatic melanoma: A Southwest Oncology Group trial. *Journal of Cancer Research in Clinical Oncology* 125: 292–296.

Martin, A., Nerenstone, S., Urba, W., *et al.* 1990. Treatment of hairy cell leukemia with alternating cycles of pentostatin and recombinant leukocyte A interferon: Results of a phase II study. *Journal of Clinical Oncology* 8(4): 721–730.

McGlave, P. 1997. Biology and treatment of chronic myelogenous leukemia. *Oncology* 11(9): 1295–1300.

McHutchison, J., Gordon, S., Schiff, E., *et al.* 1998. Interferon alfa-2b alone or in combination with ribavirin as initial treatment for chronic hepatitis C. *The New England Journal of Medicine* 339(21): 1485–1492.

McKenna, R., and Oberg, K. 1997. Antibodies to interferon-alpha in treated cancer patients: Incidence and significance. *Journal of Interferon and Cytokine Research* 17: 141–143.

McLaughlin, P., Cabanillas, F., Hagemeister, F., *et al.* 1993. CHOP-Bleo plus interferon for stage IV low-grade lymphoma. *Annals of Oncology* 4: 205–211.

Miles, S., Mitsuyasu, R., Aboulafia, D., *et al.* 1997. AIDS-related malignancies. In DeVita, V., Hellman, S., and Rosenberg, S. (eds). *Cancer: Principles and Practice of Oncology* 5th edn. Philadelphia, PA: Lipincott-Raven, pp. 2445–2467.

Miller, A., Musselman, D., Penna, S., *et al.* 1999. Pretreatment with the antidepressant paroxetine prevents cytokine-induced depression during IFN-alpha therapy for malignant melanoma. (Psychoneuroimmunology Research Society, 1999). *Neuroimmunomodulation* 6: 237 (abstract).

Minasian, L., Motzer, R., Gluck, L., *et al.* 1993. Interferon alfa-2a in advanced renal cell carcinoma: Treatment results and survival in 159 patients with long-term follow-up. *Journal of Clinical Oncology* 11(7): 1368–1375.

Mitsuyasu, R. 1988. The role of alpha interferon in the biotherapy of hematologic malignancies and AIDS-related Kaposi's sarcoma. *Oncology Nursing Forum* 15(6 suppl): 7–12.

Mitsuyasu, R., and Groopman, J. 1984. Biology and therapy of Kaposi's sarcoma. *Seminars in Oncology* 11(1): 53–59.

Moldawer, L., and Sattler, F. 1998. Human immunodeficiency virus-associated wasting and mechanisms of cachexia associated with inflammation. *Seminars in Oncology* 25(1 suppl): 73–81.

Molina, P., Burzstein, S., and Abumrad, N. 1995. Theories and assumptions on energy expenditure: Determinations in the clinical setting. *Critical Care Clinics* 11(3): 587–601.

Molto, L., Alvarez-Mon, M., Carballido, J., *et al.* 1995. Use of intracavitary interferon-alfa-2b in the prophylactic treatment of patients with superficial bladder cancer. *Cancer* 75(11): 2720–2726.

Morris, A., and Valley, A. 1996. Overview of the management of AIDS-related Kaposi's sarcoma. *Annals of Pharmacotherapy* 30(10): 1150–1163.

Morton, D., and Barth, A. 1996. Vaccine therapy for malignant melanoma. *California Cancer Journal for Clinicians* 46: 225–244.

Mostow, E., Neckel, S., Oberhelman, L., *et al.* 1993. Complete remissions in psoralen and UV-A (PUVA)-refractory mycosis fungoides-type cutaneous T-cell lymphoma with combined interferon alfa and PUVA. *Archives of Dermatology* 129: 747–752.

Mullen, M., Spicehandler, D., *et al.* 1988. Phase I study of combination zidovudine (AZT) and interferon alfa-2b in patients with AIDS. *Proceedings of the American Society of Clinical Oncology* 7: 1 (abstract).

Munschauer, F., and Kinkel, R. 1997. Managing side effects of interferon-beta in patients with relapsing-remitting multiple sclerosis. *Clinical Therapeutics* 19(5): 883–893.

Munschauer, F., and Stuart, W. 1997. Rationale for early treatment with interferon beta-1a in relapsing-remitting multiple sclerosis. *Clinical Therapeutics* 19(5): 868–882.

Murray, H. 1996. Current and future clinical applications of interferon-gamma in host antimicrobial defense. *Intensive Care Medicine* 22(suppl): S456–S461.

Musselman, D., Lawson, D., Penna, S., *et al.* 1999. Paroxetine pretreatment reduces interferon-alpha induced depression. *Biologic Psychiatry* 45(suppl): 110S (abstract).

Nail, L., and Winningham, M. 1995. Fatigue and weakness in cancer patients: The symptom experience. *Seminars in Oncology Nursing* 11(4): 272–278.

O'Brien, S., Kantarjian, H., Koller, C., *et al.* 1999. Sequential homoharringtonine and interferon-alpha in the treatment of early chronic phase chronic myelogenous leukemia. *Blood* 93(12): 4149–4153.

Oberg, K. 1996a. Interferon-alpha versus somatostatin or the combination of both in gastro-enteropancreatic tumors. *Digestion* 57(suppl 1): S81–83.

Oberg, K. 1996b. Neuroendocrine gastrointestinal tumors. *Annals of Oncology* 7(5): 453–463.

Oberg, K. 1998a. Advances in chemotherapy and biotherapy of endocrine tumors. *Current Opinion in Oncology* 10(1): 58–65.

Oberg, K. 1998b. Carcinoid tumors: Current concepts in diagnosis and treatment. *Oncologist* 3(5): 339–345.

Oberg, K. 1999. Neuroendocrine gastrointestinal tumors—a condensed overview of diagnosis and treatment. *Annals of Oncology* 10(suppl 2): S3–8.

Oberg, K., and Alm, G. 1997. The incidence and clinical significance of antibodies to interferon-a in patients with solid tumors. *Biotherapy* 10: 1–5.

Oberg, K., Norheim, I., and Alm, G. 1989. Treatment of malignant carcinoid tumors: A randomized controlled study of steptozocin plus 5-FU and human leukocyte interferon. *European Journal of Cancer and Clinical Oncology* 25(10): 1475–1479.

Oberg, K., Norheim, I., Lind, E., *et al.* 1986. Treatment of malignant carcinoid tumors with human leucocyte interferon: Long-term results. *Cancer Treatment Reports* 70(11): 1297–1304.

Olsen, E., Rosen, S., Vollmer, R., *et al.* 1989. Interferon alpha-2a in the treatment of cutaneous T-cell lymphoma. *Journal of the American Academy of Dermatology* 20: 395–407.

Olsen, E., Vollmer, R., *et al.* 1987. Interferon alfa-2a in the treatment of cutaneous T-cell lymphoma. *Proceedings of the American Society of Clinical Oncology* 6: 189 (abstract).

Oppenheim, J., Ruscett, F., and Faltynek, C. 1997. Cytokines. In Stites, D., Terr, A., and Parslow, T. (eds). *Medical Immunology* 9th edn. Stamford, CT: Appleton & Lange, pp. 146–168.

Ozer, H., George, S., Schifer, G., *et al.* 1993. Prolonged subcutaneous administration of recombinant alfa-2b interferon in patients with previously untreated Philadelphia chromosome-positive chronic-phase chronic myelogenous leukemia: Effect on remission duration and survival. *Blood* 82(10): 2975–2984.

Patt, Y., Hogue, A., Lozano, R., *et al.* 1997. Phase II trial of hepatic arterial infusion of fluorouracil and recombinant human interferon alfa-2b for liver metastases of colorectal cancer refractory to systemic fluorouracil and leucovorin. *Journal of Clinical Oncology* 15(4): 1432–1438.

Pazdur, R., Ajani, J., Patt, Y., *et al.* 1990. Phase II study of fluorouracil and recombinant interferon alfa-2a in previously untreated advanced colorectal carcinoma. *Journal of Clinical Oncology* 8(12): 2027–2031.

Peck, R., and Bollag, W. 1991. Potentiation of retinoid-induced differentiation of HL-60 and U937 cell lines by cytokines. *European Journal of Cytokines* 27(1): 53–57.

Pehamberger, H., Soyer, H., Steiner, A., *et al.* 1998. Adjuvant interferon alfa-2a treatment in resected primary stage II cutaneous melanoma. *Journal of Clinical Oncology* 16(4): 1425–1429.

Perrillo, R., Schiff, E., Davis, G., *et al.* 1990. A randomized controlled trial of interferon alfa-2b alone and after prednisone withdrawal for the treatment of chronic hepatitis B. *The New England Journal of Medicine* 323(5): 295–301.

Pestka, S. 1997a. The interferon receptors. *Seminars in Oncology* 24(9 suppl): S918–S940.

Pestka, S. 1997b. The human interferon-alpha species and hybrid proteins. *Seminars in Oncology* 24(9 suppl): S94–S917.

Pfeffer, L. 1997. Biologic activities of natural and synthetic type I interferons. *Seminars in Oncology* 24(9 suppl): S963–S969.

Physician's Desk Reference, 51st edn. 2000. Montvale, NJ: Medical Economics Data.

Piper, B., Rieger, P., Brophy, L., *et al.* 1989. Recent advances in the management of biotherapy-related side effects: Fatigue. *Oncology Nursing Forum* 16(6 suppl): 27–34.

Piro, L., Carrerra, C., Carson, L., *et al.* 1990. Lasting remissions in hairy-cell leukemia induced by a single infusion of 2–chlorodeoxyademosine. *The New England Journal of Medicine* 332(16): 1117.

Pitha, P. 1990. Interferons: A new class of tumor suppressor genes? *Cancer Cells* 2(7): 215–216.

Plata-Salaman, C. 1998. Cytokines and anorexia: A brief overview. *Seminars in Oncology* 25(1 suppl): 64–72.

Porzolt, F. 1992. Adjuvant therapy of renal cell cancer (RCC) with interferon alfa-2a. *Proceedings of American Society of Clinical Oncology* 11: 202 (abstract).

Poynard, T., Leroy, V., Cohard, M., *et al.* 1996. Meta-analysis of interferon randomized trials in the treatment of viral hepatitis C: Effects of dose and duration. *Hepatology* 24: 778–789.

Poynard, T., Marcellin, P., Lee, S., *et al.* 1998. Randomized trial of interferon-alfa-2b plus ribavirin for 48 weeks or for 24 weeks versus interferon-alfa-2b plus placebo for 48 weeks for treatment of chronic infection with hepatitis C virus. *The Lancet* 352: 1426–1432.

Presser, R. 1997. Urticaria: A nurse practitioner's approach. *Journal of the American Academy of Nurse Practitioners* 9(9): 437–443.

Price, C., Rohatiner, A., Stewart, W., *et al.* 1991. Interferon-alfa-2b in the treatment of follicular lymphoma: Preliminary results of a trial in progress. *Annals of Oncology* 2(suppl 2): 141–145.

PRISMS. 1998. Randomised double-blind placebo-controlled study of interferon beta-1b in relapsing/remitting multiple sclerosis. PRISMS (Prevention of Relapses and Disability by Interferon beta-1a Subcutaneously in Multiple Sclerosis) Study Group. *The Lancet* 352(9139): 1498–1504.

Purcell, R. 1997. The hepatitis C virus: Overview. *Hepatology* 26(3 suppl 1): 11S–14S.

Qin, X.Q., Runkel, L., Deck, C., *et al.* 1997. Interferon-beta induces S phase accumulation selectively in human transformed cells. *Journal of Interferon and Cytokine Research* 17: 355–367.

Quesada, J., Swanson, D., Trindada, A., *et al.* 1983. Renal cell carcinoma: Antitumor effects of leukocyte interferon. *Cancer Research* 43(2): 940–947.

Quesada, J., Reuben, J., Manning, J., *et al.* 1984. Alpha interferon for induction of remission in hairy-cell leukemia. *The New England Journal of Medicine* 310(1): 15–18.

Quesada, J., Alexanian, R., Hawkins, M., *et al.* 1986a. Treatment of multiple myeloma with recombinant alpha interferon. *Blood* 67(2): 275–278.

Quesada, J., Hersh, E., Manning, J., *et al.* 1986b. Treatment of hairy cell leukemia with recombinant alpha interferon. *Blood* 68(2): 493–497.

Quesada, J., Talpaz, M., Rios, A., *et al.* 1986c. Clinical toxicity of interferons in cancer patients: A review. *Journal of Clinical Oncology* 4(2): 234–243.

Real, F., Oettgen, H., and Krown, S. 1986. Kaposi's sarcoma and the acquired immunodeficiency syndrome: Treatment with high and low doses of recombinant leukocyte A interferon. *Journal of Clinical Oncology* 4(4): 544–551.

Reder, A. (ed). 1997. *Interferon Therapy of Multiple Sclerosis.* Chicago, IL: Marcel Dekker, Inc.

Reichard, O., Glaumann, H., Fryden, A., *et al.* 1995. Two-year biochemical, virological and histological follow-up in patients with chronic hepatitis C responding in a sustained fashion to interferon alfa-2b treatment. *Hepatology* 21: 918–922.

Reintgen, D., Altertini, J., *et al.* 1995. The accurate staging and modern day treatment of malignant melanoma. *Cancer Research Therapy and Control* 4: 183–197.

Reintgen, D., and Conrad, A. 1997. Detection of occult melanoma cells in sentinel lymph nodes and blood. *Seminars in Oncology* 24(1 suppl 4): S4–S11.

Ribas, A., Butturini, A., Locascuilli, A., *et al.* 1997. How important is hepatitis C virus (HCV)-infection in persons with acute leukemia? *Leukemia Research* 21(8): 785–788.

Richards, J., Gale, D., Mehta, N., *et al.* 1999. Combination of chemotherapy with interleukin-2 and interferon alfa for the treatment of metastatic melanoma. *Journal of Clinical Oncology* 17(2): 651–657.

Riechmann, P. 1997. The effects of interferon-beta on cytokines and immune responses. In Reder, A. (ed). *Interferon Therapy of Multiple Sclerosis.* New York, NY: Marcel Dekker, Inc., pp. 161–191.

Roberts, M. 1996. Interferon-τ and pregnancy. *Journal of Interferon and Cytokine Research* 16: 271–273.

Rodriguez, J., Cortes, J., Smith, T., *et al.* 1998. Determinants of prognosis in late chronic-phase chronic myelogenous leukemia. *Journal of Clinical Oncology* 16(12): 3782–3787.

Rolak, L. 1996. The diagnosis of multiple sclerosis. *Neurology Clinics* 14(1): 27–43.

Rook, A., and Heald, P. 1995. The immunopathogenesis of cutaneous T-cell lymphoma. *Hematology/ Oncology Clinics of North America* 9(5): 997–1010.

Rosenberg, S., Yang, J., Schwartzentruber, D., *et al.* 1999. Prospective randomized trial of the treatment of patients with metastatic melanoma using chemotherapy with cisplatin, dacarbazine, and tamoxifen alone or in combination with interleukin-2 and interferon alfa-2b. *Journal of Clinical Oncology* 17(3): 968–975.

Rudick, R., and Ransohoff, R. 1995. Biologic effects of interferons: Relevance to multiple sclerosis. *Multiple Sclerosis* 1(suppl 1): S12–S16.

Rudick, R., Cookfair, D., Simonian, N., *et al.* 1999. Cerebrospinal fluid abnormalities in a phase III trial of Avonex (IFNbeta-1a) for relapsing multiple sclerosis. The Multiple Sclerosis Collaborative Research Group. *Journal of Neuroimmunology* 93(1–2): 8–14.

Rudick, R., Goodkin, D., Jacob, L., *et al.* 1997. Impact of interferon beta-1a on neurologic disability in relapsing multiple sclerosis. The Multiple Sclerosis Collaborative Research Group. *Neurology* 49(2): 358–363.

Sacchi, S., Kantarjian, H., O'Brien, S., *et al.* 1997. Long-term follow-up results of alpha-interferon-based regimens in patients with late chronic phase chronic myelogenous leukemia. *Leukemia* 11: 1610–1616.

Salmon, S., Crowley, J., Balcerzak, S., *et al.* 1998. Interferon versus interferon plus prednisone remission maintenance therapy for multiple myeloma: A Southwest Oncology Group Study. *Journal of Clinical Oncology* 16(3): 890–896.

Samuels, C. 1988. Mechanisms of the antiviral action of interferons. *Progress in Nucleic Acid Research and Molecular Biology* 35: 27–72.

Sangfelt, O., Erickson, S., Castro, J., *et al.* 1999. Molecular mechanisms underlying interferon-alpha induced G_0/G_1 arrest: CKI-mediated regulation of GI CDK-complexes and activation of pocket proteins. *Oncogene* 18(18): 2798–2810.

Saracco, G., Mazella, G., Rossina, F., *et al.* 1989. A controlled trial of human lymphoblastoid interferon in chronic hepatitis B in Italy. *Hepatology* 10(3): 336–341.

Sawyers, C. 1999. Chronic myeloid leukemia. *The New England Journal of Medicine* 340(17): 1330–1340.

Scandinavian Study Group. 1997. Kaposi's sarcoma and its management in AIDS patients: Recommendations from a Scandinavian Study Group. *Scandinavian Journal of Infectious Diseases* 29(1): 3–12.

Schwartz, A. 1998. The Schwartz Cancer Fatigue Scale: Testing reliability and validity. *Oncology Nursing Forum* 25(4): 711–717.

Schwid, S., Goodman, A., and Mattson, D. 1997. Autoimmune hyperthyroidism in patients with multiple sclerosis treated with interferon beta-1b. *Archives of Neurology* 54: 1169–1170.

Seef, L. 1997. Natural history of hepatitis C. *Hepatology* 26(3 suppl 1): 21S–28S.

Sgarabotto, D., Vianello, F., Stefani, P., *et al.* 1997. Hypertriglyceridemia during long-term interferon-alpha therapy in a series of hematologic patients. *Journal of Interferon and Cytokine Research* 17: 241–244.

Sharrack, B., and Hughes, R. 1996. Clinical scales for multiple sclerosis. *Journal of Neuroscience* 135(1): 1–9.

Shipp, M. 1997. Can we improve upon the international index? *Annals of Oncology* 8(suppl 1): 43–47.

Simmonds, P. 1997. Clinical relevance of hepatitis C virus genotypes. *Gut* 40: 291–293.

Simon, J., Jacobs, L., Campion, M., *et al.* 1999. A longitudinal study of brain atrophy in relapsing multiple sclerosis. The Multiple Sclerosis Collaborative Research Group. *Neurology* 53(1): 139–148.

Singh, R., and Fidler, I. 1996. *Current Topics in Microbiology and Immunology.* Berlin: Springer-Verlag.

Skalla, K. 1996. The interferons. *Seminars in Oncology Nursing* 12(2): 97–105.

Smalley, R., Anderson, J., Hawkins, M., *et al.* 1992. Interferon alfa combined with cytotoxic chemotherapy for patients with non-Hodgkin's lymphoma. *The New England Journal of Medicine* 327(November 5): 1336–1341.

Solal-Celigny, P., LePage, B., Brousse, N., *et al.* 1993. Recombinant interferon alfa-2b combined with a regimen containing doxorubicin in patients with advanced follicular lymphoma. *The New England Journal of Medicine* 329(22): 1608–1614.

Solal-Celigny, P., Lepage, E., *et al.* 1997. A doxorubicin-containing regimen with or without interferon alpha 2b (IFN a2B) in advanced follicular lymphomas. Final analysis of survival, toxicity and quality of life of the GELF trial. *Blood* 38(10 suppl 1).

Solal-Celigny, P., Lepage, E., Brousse, N., *et al.* 1998. Doxorubicin-containing regimen with or without interferon alfa-2b for advanced follicular lymphomas: Final analysis of survival and toxicity in the Groupe d'Etude des Lymphomes Folliculaires 86 trial. *Journal of Clinical Oncology* 16(7): 2332–2338.

Soos, J., Schiffenbauer, T., *et al.* 1997. Interferon-τ: A potential treatment for inflammatory central nervous system disease. In Reder, A. (ed). *Interferon Therapy of Multiple Sclerosis.* New York, NY: Marcel Dekker, Inc.

Spiers, A., Parekh, S., and Bishop, M. 1984. Hairy cell leukemia: Induction of complete remission with pentostatin (2′ deoxycoformycin). *Journal of Clinical Oncology* 2(12): 1336–1342.

Springer, E., Kuzel, T., Rosen, S., and Roenigk, H. 1991. International symposium on cutaneous T-cell lymphoma. *Journal of the American Academy of Dermatology* 24: 136–138.

Statement, N. I. O. H. C. D. C. P. 1997. National Institutes of Health Consensus Development Conference Panel Statement: Managment of hepatitis C. *Hepatology* 26(3 suppl): 2S–10S.

Stedmans Medical Dictionary, 26th edn. 1995. Baltimore, MD: Williams & Wilkins.

Stricker, P., Pryor, K., Nicholson, T., *et al.* 1996. Bacillus Calmette-Guérin plus intravesical interferon alpha-2b in patients with superficial bladder cancer. *Urology* 48: 957–962.

Strohmaier, W. 1999. New treatment modalities—

The urologist's view. *Anticancer Research* 19: 1605–1610.

Stryer, L. 1981. *Biochemistry*. San Francisco, CA: W. H. Freeman and Co.

Tallman, M., Hakimian, D., Variakojis, D., *et al.* 1992. A single cycle of 2-chlorodeoxyadenosine results in complete remission in the majority of patients with hairy cell leukemia. *Blood* 80: 2203–2209.

Talpaz, M., Kantarjian, H., McCredie, K., *et al.* 1986. Hematologic remission and cytogenetic improvement induced by recombinant human interferon alpha in chronic myelogenous leukemia. *The New England Journal of Medicine* 314(17): 1065–1069.

Talpaz, M., Kantarjian, H., McCredie, K., *et al.* 1987. Clinical investigation of human alpha interferon in chronic myelogenous leukemia. *Blood* 69(5): 1280–1288.

Talpaz, M., Kantarjian, H., O'Brien, S., *et al.* 1997. The M. D. Anderson Cancer Center experience with interferon-alpha therapy in chronic myelogenous leukaemia. *Baillieres Clin Haematol* 10(2): 291–305.

Tamura, T., Matsuzaki, M., Harada, H., *et al.* 1997. Upregulation of interferon-a receptor expression in hydroxyurea-treated leukemia cell lines. *Journal of Investigative Medicine* 45(4): 160–167.

Taylor, J., and Grossberg, S. 1998. The effects of interferon-alpha on the production and action of other cytokines. *Seminars in Oncology* 25(1 suppl): 23–29.

Thompson, J., and Fefer, A. 1987. Interferon in the treatment of hairy cell leukemia. *Cancer* 59(suppl 3): 605–609.

Thompson, J., Gold, P., and Fefer, A., *et al.* 1997. Outpatient chemoimmunotherapy for the treatment of metastatic melanoma. *Seminars in Oncology* 24(1 suppl 4): S44–S48.

Thompson, J., Kidd, P., and Rubin, E. 1989. Very low dose alpha-2b interferon for the treatment of hairy cell leukemia. *Blood* 73(6): 1440–1443.

Tong, M., Reddy, K., Lee, W., *et al.* 1997. Treatment of chronic hepatitis C with consensus interferon: A multicenter, randomized controlled trial. *Hepatology* 26(3): 747–754.

Valentine, A., Meyers, C., Kling, M., *et al.* 1998. Mood and cognitive side effects of interferon-alpha therapy. *Seminars in Oncology* 25(1 suppl): 39–47.

Valentine, A., Meyers, C., and Talpaz, M. 1995. Treatment of neurotoxic side effects of interferon-alpha with naltrexone. *Cancer Investigation* 13(6): 561–566.

Vartanian, T. 1997. Interferons and the central nervous system glia. In Reder, A. (ed). *Interferon Therapy of Multiple Sclerosis*. New York, NY: Marcel Dekker, Inc., pp. 95–113.

Vial, T., and Descotes, J. 1995. Immune-mediated side-effects of cytokines in humans. *Toxicology* 105: 31–57.

Viscomi, G. 1997. Structure-activity of type I interferons. *Biotherapy* 10(1): 59–86.

Volberding, P., and Mitsuyasu, R. 1985. Recombinant interferon alpha in the treatment of acquired immunodeficiency syndrome-related Kaposi's sarcoma. *Seminars in Oncology* 12(4): 2–6.

Wadler, S., and Wiernik, P. 1990. Clinical update on the role of fluorouracil and recombinant interferon alpha-2a in the treatment of colorectal carcinoma. *Seminars in Oncology* 17(suppl): 516–521.

Wadler, S., Atkins, M., Karp, D., *et al.* 1998. Clinical trial of weekly intensive therapy with 5-fluorouracil on two different schedules combined with interferon alpha-2a and filgrastim in patients with advanced solid tumors: Eastern Cooperative Oncology Group Study P-Z991. *The Cancer Journal for Scientific American* 4(4): 261–268.

Wadler, S., Lembersky, B., Atkins, M., *et al.* 1991. Phase II trial of fluorouracil and recombinant interferon alfa-2a in patients with advanced colorectal carcinoma: An Eastern Cooperative Oncology Group study. *Journal of Clinical Oncology* 9(10): 1806–1810.

Wadler, S., Schwartz, E., Goldman, M., *et al.* 1989. 5-Fluorouracil and recombinant alpha-2a interferon: An active regimen against advanced colorectal cancer. *Journal of Clinical Oncology* 7: 1769–1775.

Wadler, S., Wagstaff, J., Loyonds, P., *et al.* 1986. A phase II study of human rDNA alpha-2 interferon in patients with low grade non-Hodgkin's lymphoma. *Cancer Chemotherapy and Pharmacology Journal* 18(1): 54–58.

Weiss, K. 1998. Safety profile of interferon-alpha therapy. *Seminars in Oncology* 25(1 suppl): 9–13.

Williams, B., and Haque, S. 1997. Interacting pathways of interferon signaling. *Seminars in Oncology* 24(9 suppl): S970–S977.

Wilson, L., Kacinski, B., Edelson, R., *et al.* 1997. Cutaneous T-cell lymphomas. In DeVita, V., Hellman, S., and Rosenberg, S. (eds). *Cancer Principles and Practice of Oncology*, 5th edn. Philadelphia, PA: Lippincott-Raven, pp. 2220–2232.

Yong, V., Chabot, S., Stuve, O., *et al.* 1998. Interferon beta in the treatment of multiple sclerosis: Mechanisms of action. *Neurology* 51(3): 682–689.

York, M., Greco, R., *et al.* 1993. A randomized phase III trial comparing 5-FU with or without interferon alfa-2a for advanced colorectal cancer. *Proceedings of the American Society of Clinical Oncology* 12: 590 (abstract).

Yoshitake, Y., Kishida, T., *et al.* 1976. Antitumor effects of interferon on transplanted tumors in congenitally athymic nude mice. *Giken Journal* 19: 125–127.

Zackheim, H. 1994. Topical carmustine (BCNU) for patch/plaque mycosis fungoides. *Seminars in Dermatology* 13(3): 202–206.

Zaja, F., Fanin, R., Silvestri, F., *et al.* 1997. Retrospective analysis of 34 cases of hairy cell leukemia treated with interferon-alpha and/or 2-chlorodeoxyadenosine. *Haematologica* 82: 468–470.

Zhang, Y., Khoo, H., and Esuvaranathan, K. 1997. Effects of bacillus Calmette-Guérin and interferon-alpha-2b on human bladder cancer in vitro. *International Journal of Cancer* 71: 851–857.

Zinzani, P., Lauria, F., Salvucci, M., *et al.* 1997. Hairy-cell leukemia and alpha-interferon treatment: Long-term responders. *Haematologica* 82: 152–155.

Clinical Pearls

1. Most patients will experience flu-like symptoms upon initiation of therapy. The intensity and duration is related to the dose, route, and schedule of administration. Acetaminophen, given pretreatment and repeated in 4 hours should be used to lessen flu-like symptoms. If this is ineffective, nonsteroidal anti-inflammatory drugs (NSAIDs) may be helpful. Over time, patients usually develop a tolerance to these side effects, which is termed tachyphylaxis.

2. Fever may be preceded by chills and rigors. If rigors are unusually severe, meperidine is effective for symptom control.

3. With intravenous administration, especially during acute flu-like symptoms, nausea and vomiting may be seen more frequently. Premedication with antiemetics may be helpful.

4. It is important that patients maintain adequate hydration because significant fluid loss can occur following defervescense or with nausea/vomiting or decreased oral intake.

5. Depression can occur in patients receiving interferon (IFN). Premedication may be valuable for patients receiving high-dose therapy with IFN-α. Use of an objective assessment tool will also aid in assessing the need for and efficacy of antidepressants.

6. Selective serotonin re-uptake inhibitors are effect antidepressants in patients receiving IFN. Dosages may need to be augmented or increased if therapy duration exceeds 6 months.

7. Depression may be exacerbated if the patient is inactive or experiencing insomnia. Social and emotional support is important in helping the patient cope with issues such as change in health, role, activity level, etc.

8. Insomnia or intermittent wakefulness may occur in patients receiving IFN. Use of medications such as temazepam, zolpidem tartrate, or trazadone hydrochloride may aid in restoring sleep patterns. Sleep hygiene measures such as setting patterns prior to sleep and ensuring a quiet, darkened room with enough warm blankets if needed will be helpful. Change injection time to earlier in the day if patient experiences period of hyperexcitability after administration of IFN.

9. Fatigue is often a multifactorial problem. With onset of significant fatigue, patient should be evaluated for thyroid abnormality. Other factors to consider include electrolyte imbalance, anemia, dehydration, malnutrition due to inadequate intake, hypoglycemia, insomnia, depression, and inactivity. Any abnormality needs to be corrected immediately. Maintaining a moderate level of activity, such as walking for 15 minutes per day, may help reduce the severity of fatigue and should be encouraged prophylactically. The use of a stimulant such as methylphenidate hydrochloride coupled with an exercise program may help decrease the severity of fatigue.

10. The need for monitoring a patient following his or her initial dose of IFN should be guided by clinical judgment and the patient's underlying medical condition.

11. Patients should be monitored closely over the duration of therapy for chronic side effects such as fatigue, anorexia, and mental status changes. Working closely with the patient and family to design a plan of care that manages these side effects is essential.

12. Patient and/or family education to learn medication self-administration should be instituted as soon as possible.

13. Because of the manufacturing process, the strength and type of IFN may vary for different IFN formulations. A change in brands may require a change in dosage. Therefore, physicians are cautioned not to change from one IFN product to another without considering these factors.

Related Web Sites

http://www.nlm.nih.gov. National Library of Medicine/National Institute of Health

www.centerwatch.com. Center Watch—search for information on clinical trials by geographic location

www.actis.org. AIDS Clinical Trials Information Service

http://cancernet.nci.nih.gov. National Cancer Institute. Search for clinical trial abstract information using the PDQ (Physician Data Query)

www.cdc.gov. Centers for Disease Control and Prevention

http://www.nih.gov. National Institute of Health

http://www.pharminfo.com/phrmlink.html #pharmco. Pharmaceutical manufacturer Web sites

http://www.cansearch.org/canserch/canserch.htm. Internet cancer resources

http://www.oncolink.upenn.edu/. Information updated daily on cancer treatment and research advances

http://www.meds.com/. Medical information and education in oncology, Medline, literature searches, Daily Oncology News Digest, Cancer Forums, reports from medical meetings

http://www.cancercare.org. Links for specific diagnoses, financial assistance, patient resources, financial assistance, resources for minorities

www.roche.com. Manufacturer of Roferon®-A

www.sp-research.com. Manufacturer of Intron-A®

www.amgen.com. Manufacturer of Infergen®

www.interferonsciences.com. Manufacturer of Alferon® N

www.biogen.com. Manufacturer of Avonex®

www.berlex.com. Manufacturer of Betaseron®

http://skincancer.cool.net.au/. Skin cancer information

www.melanoma.com. Melanoma resource site

http://www.nmss.org. National multiple sclerosis

www.oncology.com. Online oncology resource with numerous links, drug and disease information, support programs, news, free registration

http://www.cancercare.org. Links for specific diagnoses, financial assistance, patient resources, financial assistance, resources for minorities

http://www.oncolink.upenn.edu/. Information updated daily on cancer treatment and research advances

http://www.aad.org. American Academy of Dermatology, links for skin cancer screenings, CME programs, therapies

http://www.peel.edu.on.ca/~applewd/cybercafe/previouslessons. Information and lesson plans for skin cancer education and screening

www.cancerfacts.com. Online site for information on oncology treatment-related issues

http://www.jacksonwalter.com/hcv/comboguide .htm Side effect management tips for hepatitis patients

Key References

Balch, C., Buzaid, A., Atkins, M., *et al.* 2000. A new American Joint Committee on Cancer staging system for cutaneous melanoma. *Cancer* 88(6): 1484–1490.

Belldegrun, A., Franklin, J., O'Donnell, M. A., *et al.* 1998. Superficial bladder cancer: The role of interferon-α. *The Journal of Urology* 159: 1793–1801.

Birkel, A., Caldwell, L., Stafford-Fox, V., *et al.* 2000. Combination interferon alfa-2b/ribavirin therapy for the treatment of hepatitis C: Nursing implications. *Gastroenterology Nursing* 23(2): 55–62.

Borden, E., and Parkinson D. 1998. A perspective on the clinical effectiveness and tolerance of interferon-alpha. *Seminars in Oncology* 25(1 suppl): 3–8.

Bukowski, R. M. 2000. Cytokine combinations: Therapeutic use in patients with advanced renal cell carcinoma. *Seminars in Oncology* 27(2): 204–212.

Buzzaid, A., Meyers, M., and Agarawala, S. (1998). Adjuvant high-dose interferon-α therapy in melanoma—Practical guidelines. *Cancer Therapeutics* 1(3): 178–183.

Chronic Myeloid Leukemia Trialists' Collaborative

Group. 1997. Interferon alfa versus chemotherapy for chronic myeloid leukemia: A meta-analysis of seven randomized trials. *Journal of the National Cancer Institute* 89(21): 1616–1620.

Costello, K., and Conway, K. 1997. Nursing management of MS patients receiving interferon beta-1b therapy. *Rehabilitation-Nursing* 22(2): 62–66, 81, 112.

Dalakas, M., Mock, V., and Hawkins, M. J. 1998. Fatigue: Definitions, mechansims, and paradigms for study. *Seminars in Oncology* 25(1 suppl): 48–53.

Dean, G., Spears, L., Ferrell, B. R., *et al.* 1995. Fatigue in patients with cancer receiving interferon alpha. *Cancer Practice* 3(3): 164–172.

Donnelly, S. 1998. Patient management strategies of interferon alfa-2b as adjuvant therapy of high-risk melanoma. *Oncology Nursing Forum* 25(5): 921–927.

Faderl, S., Kantarjian, H., and Talpaz, M. 1999. Chronic myelogenous leukemia: Update on biology and treatment. *Oncology* 13(2): 169–181.

Herberman, R. B. 1997. Effect of alpha-interferon on immune function. *Seminars in Oncology* 24(3 suppl 9): S9-78–S9-80.

Jones, T. H., Wadler, S., and Hupart, K. H. 1998. Endocrine-mediated mechanism of fatigue during treatment with interferon-alfa. *Seminars in Oncology* 25(1 suppl 1): 54–63.

Kelly, C. L. 1996. The role of interferons in the treatment of multiple sclerosis. *Journal of Neuroscience Nursing* **28**(2): 114–120.

Kiley, K., and Gale, D. 1998. Nursing management of patients with malignant melanoma receiving adjuvant alpha interferon-2b. *Clinical Journal of Oncology Nursing* 2(1): 11–16.

Leonard, W.J. and Lin, J.X. 2000. Cytokine receptor signaling pathways. *Journal of Allergy and Clinical Immunology* 105(5): 877–888.

Licinio, J., Kling, M., and Hauser, D. 1998. Cytokines and brain function: Relevance to interferon-alpha-induced mood and cognitive changes. *Seminars in Oncology* 25(1 suppl): 30–38.

Malkower, D., and Wadler, S. 1999. Interferons as biomodulators of fluoropyrimidines in the treatment of colorectal cancer. *Seminars in Oncology* 26(6): 663–667

Pfeffer, L. 1997. Biologic activities of natural and synthetic type I interferons. *Seminars in Oncology* 24(9 suppl): S963–S969.

Plata-Salaman, C. (1998). Cytokines and anorexia: A brief overview. *Seminars in Oncology* 25(1 suppl): 64–72.

Poynard, T., McHutchison, J., and Goodman, Z. et al. 2000. Is an "a la carte" combination interferon alfa-2b plus ribavirin regimen possible for the first line treatment in patients with chronic hepatitis C? *Hepatology* 31(1): 211–218.

Quesada, J., Talpaz, M., Rios, A., *et al.* 1986. Clinical toxicity of interferons in cancer patients: A review. *Journal of Clinical Oncology* 4(2): 234–243.

Rieger, P. T. 1995. Interferon alpha: A clinical update. *Cancer Practice* 3(6): 356–365.

Skalla, K. (1996). The interferons. *Seminars in Oncology Nursing* 12(2): 97–105.

Stafford-Fox, V., and Guindon, K. M. 2000. Cutaneous reactions associated with alpha interferon therapy. *Clinical Journal of Oncology Nursing* 4(4): 164–168.

Taylor, J. L., and Grossberg, S. 1998. The effects of interferon-a on the production and action of other cytokines. *Seminars in Oncology* 25(1 suppl): 23–29.

Trask, P., Esper, P., Riba, M., *et al.* 2000. Psychiatric side-effects of interferon therapy: Prevalence, proposed mechanisms, and future directions. *Journal of Clinical Oncology* 18(11): 2316–2326

Valentine, A., Meyers, C., Kling, M. A., et al. 1998. Mood and cognitive side effects of interferon-alpha therapy. *Seminars in Oncology* 25(1 suppl): 39–47.

CHAPTER 6 | The Interleukins

Danielle M. Gale, RN, ND, FNP, AOCN®

Patricia Sorokin, RN, BSN, OCN®

The interleukins (ILs) are a family of cytokines that represent a major communication network in living organisms (Aulitzky *et al.*, 1994). ILs are proteins that exist as natural components of the human immune system. They are produced by monocytes, endothelial cells, astrocytes/glial cells, fibroblasts, bone marrow stromal cells, and thymocytes as well as lymphocytes. The term "interleukin" was originally used to define substances produced by leukocytes that had activity on other leukocytes (Holcombe, 1994). However, this early definition fails to adequately describe the production and range of activities now attributed to the family of ILs.

The primary function of ILs is the **immuno-**

A special note of recognition to Eileen Sharp, RN, BSN, OCN®, author of the original chapter on interleukins in the first edition of *Biotherapy: A Comprehensive Overview.*

modulation and **immunoregulation** of leukocytes; however, most ILs have **pleiotropic** functions, that is, they are capable of inducing multiple biological activities in a variety of target cells. As a result of the many ILs described in early research, each had several names which described a different function. In an effort to standardize the nomenclature, ILs are now designated by the order in which they are approved (i.e., IL-1, IL-2, IL-3, etc.).

To qualify as an IL, a cytokine must have a documented unique amino acid sequence and functional activity involving leukocytes. The evidence is evaluated by the Nomenclature and Standardization Committee of the International Cytokine Society and the Union of Immunological Societies that make a recommendation to the World Health Organization (Oppenheim, 1998). There is no ranking in terms of importance or specific activity. Table 6.1 summarizes the biological activities of all 18 ILs described through July 2000 (Holcombe, 1994; Cohen and Cohen, 1996; Kluth and Rees, 1996; Nielsen *et al.*, 1996; Tsuji-Takayama *et al.*, 1997; Muir-Sluis, 1998; Thompson, 1998).

The activities of the ILs are receptor mediated. ILs activate target cells by binding to receptor sites present on the cell-surface membranes. The binding of the IL to the membrane receptor signals the interior of the cell to alter the cell's activation level or functional capacity. In many cases, IL receptors are expressed specifically by cells in the immune system after antigen exposure. Many ILs share the same receptor-site subunits. This sharing of subunits is one of the mechanisms by which functional redundancy of cytokine activity occurs, suggesting the sharing of a common signal transduction pathway as well (Hibi *et al.*, 1996). Examples of this include the gp130 subunit, which is shared by the receptors for IL-6 and IL-11; the β subunit, which is shared by granulocyte-macrophage colony-stimulating factor (GM-CSF), IL-3, and IL-5; and the cytokines IL-4 and IL-13, which share a common subunit for signal transduction (Yin *et al.*, 1993; Zurawski *et al.*, 1993; Hibi *et al.*, 1996). The sharing

Table 6.1   Biological activities of interleukins

Interleukin (IL)	Biological Activities
IL-1	Activates resting T cells
	Mediates inflammation
	Activates endothelial cells and macrophages
	Functions as a cofactor for hematopoietic growth factors
	Induces sleep, fever, ACTH release, acute-phase response
	Enhances activity of NK cells
	Chemotactically attracts neutrophils and macrophages
	Stimulates the synthesis of lymphokines
IL-2	Induces the synthesis and secretion of lymphokines
	Induces proliferation of antigen-primed T cells
	Functions as a cofactor for growth and differentiation of B cells
	Augments LAK activity
	Enhances NK activity
IL-3	Supports the growth of pluripotent bone marrow stem cells
	Acts as a growth factor for mast cells
	Stimulates histamine secretion
IL-4	Acts as a growth factor for activated B cells
	Induces MHC class II antigens on B cells
	Acts as a growth factor for resting T cells
	Enhances cytolytic activity of cytotoxic T cells
	Acts as a growth factor for mast cells
	Promotes growth of melanoma TILs
	Induces class switch to IgE and IgG$_1$
	Increases phagocytic activity of macrophages
IL-5	Induces B-cell proliferation and differentiation
	Induces eosinophil growth and differentiation
	Acts with IL-4 to stimulate IgE production

Table 6.1

Interleukin (IL)	Biological Activities
IL-6	Increases secretion of antibodies by plasma cells
	Co-stimulates T-cell activation with IL-1
	Aids in differentiation of myeloid stem cells
	Induces B-cell differentiation into plasma cells
IL-7	Supports the growth of B-cell precursors
	Stimulates the growth of thymocytes
	Increases the expression of IL-2 and IL-2R by resting T cells
IL-8	Chemotactically attracts neutrophils
	Induces adherence of neutrophils to vascular endothelial cells and aids migration to tissues
IL-9	Acts as a mitogen to induce T-helper cell growth
	Acts as a growth factor for mast cells
IL-10	Suppresses cytokine production by T-helper 1 subset
	Stimulates cytotoxic T-cell growth
IL-11	Enhances early hematopoietic progenitor cells
	Enhances megakaryocytopoiesis with IL-3
	Inhibits lipoprotein lipase activity
IL-12	Activates NK-mediated cytotoxicity
	Facilitates cytotoxic T-cell responses, LAK cells
	Enhances survival and proliferation of stem cells
	Enhances production of IFN-γ in infection
	Plays a key role in the differentiation of the T-helper cell system
IL-13	Inhibits the production of macrophage-derived cytokines, end effect is anti-inflammatory effects on monocytes and macrophages
	Induces B-cell proliferation and differentiation (similar actions to IL-4)
	Decreases production of IL-1β and increases production of anti-inflammatory factor IL-1 receptor antagonist
	Inhibits the procoagulant effects of tumor necrosis factor and IL-1
	Reduces production of nitric oxide and reactive oxygen species
IL-14	Induces B-cell proliferation and expands some B-cell populations
	No reported activity on T cells
	Augments proliferation of B-cell non-Hodgkin's lymphoma cell lines *in vitro*
IL-15	Stimulates proliferation of T lymphocytes
	Stimulates both CTL and LAK activity as well as NK cells
IL-16	Initiates T-cell–mediated inflammatory process associated with atopic asthmatic phenotype
IL-17	Induces other cytokine production including IL-6 and IL-8
	Induces protein tyrosine kinase-mediated signaling
IL-18	Stimulates T cells to produce IFN-γ
	Induces protein tyrosine-kinase–mediated signaling

ACTH, adrenocorticotropin hormone; CTL, cytotoxic T lymphocyte; IFN-γ, interferon-gamma; Ig, immunoglobulin; IL, interleukin; LAK, lymphokine-activated killer; MHC, major histocompatibility complex; NK, natural killer; TIL, tumor-infiltrating lymphocyte.

of receptors by various cytokines and growth factors has been called the cytokine receptor superfamily and helps to explain the pleiotropic and often redundant actions of ILs (Ihle *et al.*, 1994).

Various ILs may produce autocrine, paracrine, or endocrine actions within the body. **Autocrine** action refers to the binding and activation of the same cell that produced the IL. **Paracrine** action describes the binding and activation of nearby cells. **Endocrine** action occurs when ILs are secreted and bind to distant cells in the body (Vassilopoulou-Sellin, 1994; Kuby, 1997). Primarily, ILs affect local or regional cells rather than distant cells as in endocrine action. The complex balance between cellular activation and immunoregulation is orchestrated by the secretion of ILs and the resultant effects of the immune system on cells. Actions produced by the ILs may by redundant, synergistic, or antagonistic. **Redundant** actions are similar actions that may be produced by different ILs. **Synergistic** activity occurs when more than one IL is essential to produce activity in a particular target cell. **Antagonistic** effects occur when an IL inhibits the target-cell activity induced by another cytokine (Kuby, 1997; Vilček, 1998).

This chapter focuses on IL-1, IL-2, IL-4, IL-6, IL-10, and IL-12 and includes information about their biological activities, clinical trials and regulatory approvals for these agents, side effects of IL therapy and future applications for ILs. Specific information about IL-3 and IL-11 may be found in Chapter 7.

Interleukin-1

IL-1, originally known as "lymphocyte-activating factor" and "endogenous pyrogen" and first described by Gery *et al.* (1972), is a glycoprotein molecule primarily secreted by activated macrophages in the body. IL-1 is also produced by a variety of other cells, including B and T lymphocytes, neutrophils, natural killer (NK) cells, fibroblasts, endothelial cells, smooth-muscle cells, and vascular tissues in response to trauma, infection, or exposure to antigens (Kuby, 1997). Two forms of the IL-1 molecule, α and β, have been identified. The two forms are related but are products of separate genes and have different amino acid sequences; however, both bind to the same cell-surface receptors and therefore share biological activities (Dinarello and Wolff, 1993; Nikolic-Paterson *et al.*, 1996).

Biological Actions

The biological actions of IL-1 are numerous and include immunomodulation, promotion of hematopoiesis, mediation of inflammation, and mediation of disease in the body. Other activities of IL-1 include promoting bone resorption, stimulating fibroblasts, and conferring radioprotective effects on normal tissues. These actions may benefit the human body by conveying protective or healing properties following inflammation and injury or may negatively affect the body through their pathogenetic role (Dinarello and Wolff, 1993; Dinarello, 1998a).

IMMUNOMODULATION
The immunomodulatory functions of IL-1 include the activation of T cells, NK cells, polymorphonuclear cells, and monocytes. IL-1 also enhances B-cell growth and antibody production. IL-1 has direct antiproliferative activity against certain human cell lines and several murine tumors, and it enhances the antitumor effects of monocytes and NK cells and induces the secretion of secondary cytokines that may possess antitumor activities (Curti and Smith, 1995). Tumor necrosis factor (TNF) and IL-1 may act synergistically to enhance TNF cytotoxicity (Spriggs, 1991).

PROMOTION OF HEMATOPOIESIS

Preclinical and *in vitro* studies have demonstrated that IL-1 induces the production of hematopoietic growth factors such as GM-CSF, macrophage colony-stimulating factor, and IL-6. IL-1 acts synergistically with these colony-stimulating factors (CSFs) to promote the proliferation and differentiation of hematopoietic progenitor cells *in vitro* (Moore, 1991). Preclinical studies have shown that IL-1 can accelerate the recovery of granulocytes and platelets if given after chemotherapy or radiation therapy and can be myeloprotective if given before (Futami *et al.*, 1990).

MEDIATION OF INFLAMMATION

IL-1 is an important mediator of the inflammatory response and can be detected in the circulatory system within a few hours after the onset of infection or trauma (Kluth and Rees, 1996). IL-1 induces fever, sleep, acute-phase protein synthesis, and production of adrenocorticotropic hormone, cortisol, and insulin. IL-1 induces local inflammation via its effects on hematopoietic cells, fibroblasts, vascular endothelial cells, and secondary cytokine production. During inflammatory reactions, IL-1 induces neutrophils to travel from the bone marrow through the peripheral circulatory system and then to extravasate through capillary walls to extravascular spaces and tissue sites. Both neutrophils and monocytes are activated by and chemotactically attracted to IL-1, which induces an increase in phagocytic cells during an inflammatory response (Kluth and Rees, 1996; Kuby, 1997). IL-1 also induces endocrine effects on liver hepatocytes to produce acute-phase proteins, including fibrinogen, C-reactive protein, and haptoglobin, which contribute to host defense during an inflammatory response (Kuby, 1997).

MEDIATION OF DISEASE

IL-1 appears also to have a role as a mediator of diseases in the human body. In septic shock, IL-1 induces the synthesis and production of platelet-activating factor, prostaglandins, and nitric oxide. In laboratory animals, these mediator molecules act as potent vasodilators and produce hypotension and shock. TNF, which produces similar effects, also stimulates the production of IL-1 (Dinarello and Wolff, 1993). IL-1 may also play a role in autoimmune disorders such as insulin-dependent diabetes mellitus (Mandrup-Poulsen *et al.*, 1989), which is characterized by the destruction of beta cells in the islets of Langerhans. *In vitro* incubation of human and animal islet cells with IL-1 induces beta cell death. Therefore, the destruction of beta cells in patients with insulin-dependent diabetes may be caused by IL-1 that has been produced as a result of an autoimmune process within the islet cells (Dinarello and Wolff, 1993).

IL-1 may also play a role in the pathogenesis of such inflammatory diseases as rheumatoid arthritis and inflammatory bowel disease (IBD). In patients with rheumatoid arthritis, IL-1 can be detected in the synovial fluid and lining. In animals, intra-articular injections of IL-1 induce leukocyte infiltration and cartilage degeneration. These findings have led to postulation of a role for IL-1 in the pathophysiology of rheumatoid arthritis (Dinarello and Wolff, 1993). In IBD (ulcerative colitis and Crohn's disease), the lesions contain activated neutrophils and macrophages. In these bowel lesions, concentrations of IL-1 and IL-8 (an inflammatory cytokine whose production is stimulated by IL-1) in tissue are high. In animals, blocking the effects of IL-1 with an IL-1–receptor antagonist (IL-1Ra) reduces the severity of IBD (Dinarello and Wolff, 1993). This evidence links IL-1 to the pathophysiology of IBD.

The role of IL-1 as a direct or an indirect growth factor for both acute myelogenous leukemia (AML) and chronic myelogenous leukemia also is being investigated as a result of observations that IL-1β messenger RNA (mRNA) can be detected in cells from patients with AML (Rambaldi *et al.*, 1991) or in chronic granulocytic leukemia cells of the juvenile type (Bagby *et al.*, 1988). The mechanism of action by which IL-1 may stimulate myelogenous leukemia cells is similar to the action by which IL-1 stimulates the production of CSFs and serves as a cofactor for the proliferation of stem cells (Dinarello and Wolff, 1993).

Based on increased IL-1 concentrations in plasma and evidence of IL-1 gene expression in affected tissues, the pathogenetic contributory role of IL-1 is being investigated to determine its role in other diseases or conditions. These conditions include atherosclerosis, psoriasis, asthma, osteoporosis, periodontal disease, transplant rejection, graft-versus-host disease, sleep disturbances, alcoholic hepatitis, and premature labor secondary to uterine infection (Dinarello and Wolff, 1993; Colatta *et al.*, 1998; Dinarello, 1998b).

Clinical Trials

Theoretically, the potential for therapeutic application of the biological actions of IL-1 is significant because of its beneficial and harmful effects in the body. Thus, there is interest in the development of both **agonists** and **antagonists** of this cytokine. IL-1 may be useful in the treatment of cancer because of its ability to activate effector cells, induce production or activity of secondary cytokines, protect cells from radiation-induced injury, restore bone marrow damaged by chemotherapy, and confer anti-infection properties. Antagonists of IL-1 may be useful in reducing the production or action of IL-1 in other diseases (Starnes, 1991; Patarca and Fletcher, 1997).

Clinical trials continue to study the toxic and hematologic effects of IL-1 in patients with advanced malignant disease. In one of the first phase I studies, intravenous (IV) IL-1 was administered over 15 minutes every day for 7 days to patients with advanced malignancies. The maximum tolerated dose (MTD) of IL-1 was determined to be 0.3 mcg/kg. Dose-limiting toxic effects included hypotension, confusion, renal insufficiency, myocardial infarction, and severe abdominal pain. Observed hematologic effects may have potential benefit. Therapy with IL-1 induced a significant dose-related increase in the total white blood cell count. Platelet counts temporarily decreased during IL-1 therapy, but there was a significant increase in the platelet count 1 to 2 weeks after therapy. Bone marrow cellularity also increased during therapy (Smith *et al.*, 1992).

Other studies have shown IL-1 to accelerate the recovery of platelets after high-dose carboplatin therapy (Smith *et al.*, 1993; Vadhan-Raj *et al.*, 1994). Early studies evaluating IL-1β postchemotherapy with 5-fluorouracil (5-FU) demonstrated fewer days of neutropenia in patients receiving 5-FU plus IL-1β than in those patients receiving 5-FU alone. This difference, however, did not achieve statistical significance. The data did show that IL-1β had stimulatory effects in human hematopoiesis. Hypotension was a dose-limiting factor in this study (Crown *et al.*, 1991).

Studies evaluating the use of IL-1β following bone marrow transplant (BMT) have shown some promise. Neumunaitis *et al.* (1994) reported on a phase one trial of patients undergoing BMT who received IL-1β at 3 dose levels (0.01, 0.02, and 0.05 mcg/kg) by a 30-minute IV infusion once a day beginning on the day of the bone marrow infusion and continuing for a total of 5 doses. A total of 17 patients were entered on the trial, and their results were compared with those of 74 consecutive historical control subjects who did not receive CSFs. The number of days required to reach an absolute neutrophil count greater than 500 mL in patients who received recombinant human (rh)IL-1β was less than in the control group; however, the results did not reach statistical significance

(25 days versus 34 days; $p = .02$). This appeared to correlate with a reduced incidence of infection between days 0 and 28 after bone marrow infusion (12% versus 23%; $p = .049$). Survival was improved in the patients who received treatment but was not statistically significant (30% versus 20%: $p = .04$). Common toxicities included fever, chills, and hypotension, with 30% of patients requiring therapy for hypotension with either normal saline or dopamine.

A phase I/II clinical trial of 40 patients with Hodgkin's disease (n = 9) and non-Hodgkin's lymphoma (NHL) (n = 31) found that patients treated with IL-1α following autologous BMT achieved neutrophil recovery (absolute neutrophil count > 500 mL) significantly earlier (median 12 days versus 27 days; $p < .0001$) with earlier engraftment leading to earlier hospital discharge and reduced costs (Weisdorf *et al.*, 1994). The dose-limiting toxicity was hypotension.

Actual tumor responses to IL-1-containing regimens have been uncommon. Redman *et al.* (1994) found no response in 19 patients with metastatic renal cancer treated with IL-1β in a phase II trial. There was evidence of a biological effect in the form of leukocytosis, thrombocytosis, and increased IL-6 and IL-2 levels. Minor but objective tumor responses were seen in only 2 of 18 patients with recurrent ovarian cancer treated with IL-1α before their first dose of carboplatin (Verschraegen *et al.*, 1996). The MTD was 3 mcg/m²/day. The dose-limiting effects seen at 10 mcg/m²/day were fever, chills, hypotension, and fluid retention. Dosik *et al.* (1996) reported a 30% response rate in a phase I clinical trial of 9 patients with metastatic melanoma (MM) who received cisplatin followed by IL-1α. The first 8 patients received 0.08 mcg/m², and the second dosing level began at 0.2 mcg/m². The use of IL-1 resulted in decreases in carcinoembryonic antigen levels in 3 of 22 patients when the drug was given along with a cancer vaccine in treatment of patients with metastatic colon cancer (Woodlock *et al.*, 1996). In general, the use of IL-1 alone appears to have little antitumor activity against melanoma, renal cell carcinomas, or other malignancies. Beneficial hematopoietic effects, including megakaryocytopoietic effects, are modest and do not warrant exposure to the toxicity necessary to achieve them given the availability of other less-toxic hematopoietic growth factors. However, IL-1 seems to endow certain progenitor cells with responsiveness to other hematopoietic cytokines, including CSFs and IL-3. One potential application of IL-1 is to help expand bone marrow *ex vivo* following stem cell harvest, which could allow further chemotherapy dose escalations in chemotherapy-sensitive tumors (Veltri and Smith, 1996). Toxic effects such as fever, flu-like symptoms, and dose-limiting hypotension can be severe yet manageable, and IL-1 can be given safely to patients with cancer.

Because IL-1 is involved in the pathophysiology of several disease states, strategies to reduce the production or action of IL-1 have been investigated. Medications such as corticosteroids, nonsteroidal anti-inflammatory drugs, and cytokines such as IL-4 or IL-10 may reduce IL-1 production. Inhibition of IL-1–converting enzymes may decrease IL-1 processing and release from cells. More attention has been devoted to neutralizing IL-1 by using anti–IL-1 antibodies and soluble IL-1 receptors. Another strategy to decrease the action of IL-1 is the use of IL-1Ra to compete with and bind to the IL-1 receptor sites on the target cells (Figure 6.1). This naturally occurring protein was first described in 1985 and subsequently expressed in recombinant form (Eisenberg *et al.*, 1990; Dinarello, 1991; Dinarello, 1998a; Dinarello, 1998b). Administration of IL-1Ra has been shown to reduce mortality among patients with septic shock syndrome (Fisher and Zheng, 1996). However, in two phase III trials of IL-1Ra in treatment of septic shock syndrome,

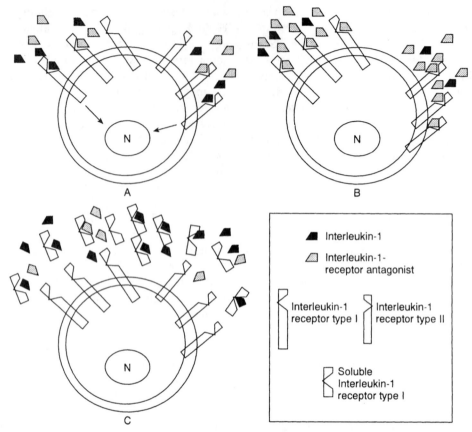

Figure 6.1   Interactions between interleukin (IL)-1, IL-1-receptor antagonist (IL-1Ra), and IL-1-receptor (IL-1R). Panel A depicts a cell with the 2 types of IL-1Rs. The 2 types have similar extracellular structures, and both bind IL-1 (α or β) and IL-1Ra. Normally, there is partial occupancy by IL-1R and partial occupancy by IL-1Ra. In this cell, IL-1 is still able to trigger a response, as indicated by the arrows directed toward the nucleus (N). The cell in panel B is exposed to a large excess of IL-1Ra, so all the IL-1Rs are occupied by the receptor antagonist. No stimulation occurs under these conditions, because IL-1 cannot bind to the IL-1Rs. The cell in panel C is exposed to soluble type I receptors and IL-1. The soluble type I receptors bind to IL-1, so IL-1 cannot bind to and activate its cell-surface receptors.

Source: Reprinted with permission from Dinarello, C., and Wolff, S. 1993. The role of interleukin-1 in disease. *The New England Journal of Medicine* 328(2): 106–113. Copyright 1993 Massachusetts Medical Society. All rights reserved.

retrospective analysis revealed decreased mortality in patient subgroups, particularly during the first 7 days after entry into the trials. The results suggested that factors other than IL-1 contributed to the cause of death in patients with septic shock. In the trial reported by Opal *et al.* (1997), a 72-hour continuous IV infusion of rhIL-1Ra failed to demonstrate a statistically significant reduction in mortality when compared with standard therapy in this multicenter clinical trial. If rhIL-1Ra treatment has any therapeutic activity in severe sepsis, the incremental benefits are small and will be difficult to demonstrate in a patient population as defined by this clinical trial. IL-1Ra is being used to suppress IL-1 production in glomerulonephritis, which slows disease progression in animal studies. In studies of rheumatoid arthritis, IL-1Ra has a demonstrated benefit when combined with conventional immunosuppressive treatment (Nikolic-Paterson *et al.*, 1996). Investigation of the blocking of IL-1 receptors with IL-1Ra continues to help increase the understanding of IL-1 as a mediator of human disease.

Regulatory Approval

As of July 2000, clinical trials of IL-1 were ongoing, but the drug had not received Food and Drug Administration (FDA) approval.

Side Effects

The most common adverse reactions observed in patients who received IL-1 include constitutional side effects (e.g., fever, chills, headache, and myalgias) and gastrointestinal side effects (e.g., nausea and vomiting). The majority of patients experienced chills followed by a monophasic elevation in body temperature. Chills were successfully treated by administering an IV and covering the patient with warm blankets. Nausea and vomiting, which occurred soon after therapy, was common but not severe in nature (grade 2 or less). When IL-1 was administered by subcutaneous (SC) injection, patients experienced significant local pain, erythema, and swelling (Laughlin *et al.*, 1993). Less common side effects of IL-1 include somnolence, abdominal pain, dyspnea, and peripheral vein phlebitis (Smith *et al.*, 1992). Hypotension has been the dose-limiting toxicity in the clinical trial setting (Dinarello, 1998a).

Future Directions

Future applications and clinical trials evaluating IL-1 will involve the areas of immunomodulation, inflammation, hematopoiesis, autoimmune disorders, wound healing, and radioprotection. Thus far, the direct administration of IL-1 appears to have modest benefit in treating patients with cancer, but its effect has been impacted by its formidable toxicity. Clinical testing of IL-1 in combination with chemotherapy and with biotherapy continues. As an antitumor agent, it has demonstrated some effect in MM and colon cancer.

IL-1 has shown considerable activity as a hematopoietic agent. Its combination with other growth factors is just beginning and may produce the best hematopoietic effects. Perhaps combinations will allow for lower doses of IL-1 and will demonstrate positive effects without the severe toxicities seen thus far. Reducing the production or activity of IL-1 may be a useful strategy for the treatment of patients who have acute or chronic inflammatory or autoimmune disorders. This is an active area of investigation (Dinarello, 1998a).

Interleukin-2

IL-2 is a lymphokine first described in 1976 as a T-cell growth factor (Morgan *et al.*, 1976). Produced primarily by activated T-helper (T_h) cells, IL-2 is a messenger regulatory molecule that has profound immunomodulatory effects in the body. The regulation of IL-2 production is dependent on the activation of T cells by antigens. This production and release of IL-2 requires two signals. First, the T_h cell must recognize an antigen in conjunction with the major histocompatibility complex antigens expressed on an antigen-presenting cell. Second, the T_h cell interacts with IL-1 produced by the antigen-presenting cell. Once activated, T_h cells begin to produce and secrete IL-2 and express IL-2 receptors. Autocrine activity is displayed by IL-2 as it binds to and activates the same cell line by which it was secreted (Malek and Gutgsell, 1993; Smith, 1993; Thorpe, 1998).

Biological Actions

The biological actions of IL-2 are critical for generation of an immune response. The specific actions of IL-2 are numerous and complex (Thorpe, 1998). In addition to its primary role in the proliferation of all T-cell subpopulations, IL-2 promotes the activation of cytotoxic T cells, NK cells, and monocytes (Boldt and Ellis, 1993). The activation of peripheral blood lymphocytes into **lymphokine-activated killer (LAK) cells** is induced by IL-2 (Grimm, 1993). B-cell growth and antibody production are supported by IL-2 and by the secretion of secondary cytokines (IL-4, IL-5, and IL-6) induced by IL-2 that serve as B-cell growth and differentiation factors. Through the activation of target cells, IL-2 also induces the release of other cytokines such as interferon (IFN)-γ, GM-CSF, and TNF. In addition, IL-2 shares some of the activities of other molecules such as IL-4, IL-7, and IL-15 (Thorpe, 1998). IL-2 also enhances expression of the IL-2 receptor (IL-2R) on T-cell surfaces (Rubin, 1993; Lewko et al., 1998; Barth and Mulé, 2000).

The activation of target cells by IL-2 is accomplished by the binding of the IL-2 protein molecule to IL-2R located on the target cell-surface membrane. IL-2R is composed of 3 separate chains: the α chain, the β chain, and the γ chain, as shown in Figure 6.2. When all 3 chains are expressed simultaneously, a high-affinity heterotrimeric receptor is formed. If cells display heterodimers such as the β chain and the γ chain, or the α and the γ chain, an intermediate-affinity receptor is formed. The α chain of the IL-2R, classified as the CD25 surface marker, binds IL-2 with relatively low af-finity. Cells that display only the α chain do not generate a signal when IL-2 binds. Resting T cells do not express high-affinity IL-2Rs; however, when T cells are exposed to antigens, low concentrations of IL-2 will saturate high-affinity IL-2Rs, and antigen-specific T-cell pro-liferation will occur. Withdrawal of the antigen leads to reduction of the high-affinity IL-2Rs and of T-cell clonal expansion despite the pres-ence of IL-2 (Smith, 1993; Gaffen et al., 1998; Thorpe, 1998). These findings have been ap-plied in the laboratory to increase proliferation of cytotoxic T cells for use in cancer clinical trials.

Clinical Trials

Early studies demonstrated that native IL-2 alone or in combination with LAK cells caused tumor regression in animal models. Production of the recombinant form of IL-2 began when the DNA sequence coding for IL-2 was identified. Although the recombinant form of IL-2 differs slightly from its native form, the two have simi-lar functional and biological activities (Dudjak, 1993). The recombinant form differs primarily in that the protein is not glycosylated and the amino acid serine is substituted for cysteine at amino acid position 125. rhIL-2 has no direct cytostatic or cytotoxic effects on tumor cells. The therapeutic effect is mediated by its ability to modulate immune reactions in patients (Ro-senberg, 1997). Large-scale clinical trials using IL-2 were begun in 1984, and rhIL-2 has been used in clinical trials to treat a variety of human malignancies. Used either as a single agent or in conjunction with LAK cells, **tumor-infil-trating lymphocytes (TILs)**, other biological agents, or chemotherapy, IL-2 has induced re-sponses against some tumors, especially renal cell carcinoma and malignant melanoma (Ro-senberg et al., 1989; Atkins and Mier, 1993; Dillman et al., 1993; Rosenberg et al., 1994; Thorpe, 1998).

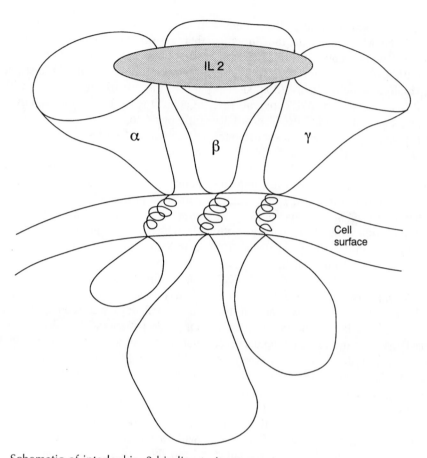

Figure 6.2   Schematic of interleukin–2 binding to its receptor

Source: Reprinted with permission from Smith, K. 1993. Lowest dose interleukin-2 immunotherapy. *Blood* 81(6): 1414–1423.

In May 1992, the FDA licensed IL-2 for use in the treatment of adult patients with metastatic renal cell carcinoma (MRCC). That approval was based on an evaluation of 255 patients treated with single-agent IL-2 at a dosage of 600,000 IU/kg of body weight administered every 8 hours by 15-minute IV bolus infusion for a total of 14 doses. After 9 days of rest, the schedule was repeated. Objective responses were observed in 37 patients (15%), with 9 complete responses (CRs) and 28 partial responses (PRs). Responses were noted in metastases to the lung, liver, lymph node, soft tissue,

and renal bed. The median duration of the objective responses was 23.2 months (Cetus Corporation, 1992).

In an update of the original 255 patients, a median survival duration of 16.3 months was noted and the median response duration for all objective responders was 54 months (Fisher *et al.*, 2000). The median duration of response for complete responders has not been reached but the range is 3 to 131 months, and approximately 10% to 20% of patients are estimated to be alive 5 to 10 years after treatment (Fisher *et al.*, 2000). An additional study by Rosenberg *et al.* (1994) of long-term survival of 283 patients with MRCC and MM treated in the Surgery Branch at the National Cancer Institute between September 1985 and December 1992 with single-agent, high-dose bolus IL-2 (720,000 IU/kg every 8 hours) revealed a 20% overall response rate for patients with MRCC (9% CR and 11% PR) and a 17% overall response rate for patients with MM (7% CR and 10% PR). CRs were more durable, with only 5 of the 24 patients with CRs recurring and 19 in complete regression for 46 to 137 months. These results suggest that single-agent IL-2 has activity in MM. Long-term follow-up in 266 patients with MM treated with high-dose IL-2 revealed a 17% overall response rate, with a median response duration of 6.5 months (Atkins, 1997). The CR rate was 6%, with 69% of the patients in remission for longer than 5 years without further treatment. This data led to the granting of a marketing license by the FDA on January 12, 1998 for the use of IL-2 in the treatment of MM (Chiron Corporation, 1998). At the described dose and schedule of administration, close patient monitoring was needed because many patients suffered severe side effects that often necessitated intensive care. The most acute side effects involved the cardiovascular, pulmonary, and renal systems or were related to vascular leak syndrome (Rosenberg *et al.*, 1989). Recent trends in IL-2 treatment have involved lower doses of the drug and have resulted in substantially less toxicity (Figlin, 1997).

Since its approval by the FDA, IL-2 continues to be studied in clinical trials in an effort to define its activity using different doses, routes, schedules, and combination regimens that produce fewer toxic effects while maintaining efficacy. IL-2 has been administered by a variety of traditional routes, including IV (bolus versus continuous infusion), SC, intra-arterial, intra-lymphatic, and intraperitoneal routes. Huland *et al.* (1999) reported on their experience using IL-2 via inhalation routes. They concluded from their results that inhaled IL-2 effectively prevents the progress of pulmonary metastases in 70% of patients. Local administration of IL-2 allows the use of higher doses with the hope of achieving the full potential of cytokines with little or no toxicity.

Numerous studies are using IL-2 alone at various doses, routes, and schedules. Use of low-dose IL-2 regimens has enabled a greater number of patients to receive therapy and has permitted prolonged exposure to IL-2. Sleijfer *et al.* (1992) reported on one of the first phase II studies of IL-2 administered SC to outpatients with MRCC. IL-2 was administered SC in a 5-day/week cycle for 6 consecutive weeks. During the first 5-day cycle, the dose was 18 million IU/day. In subsequent weeks, the daily dose for the first 2 days was reduced to 9 million/IU. Of the 26 patients whose disease could be evaluated for response, 2 achieved a CR and 4 achieved a PR (overall response rate, 23%). These results suggest that IL-2 has activity against MRCC when administered by low-dose, SC injection. The observed response rate was similar to that of high-dose IL-2 administered with or without LAK cells.

In the initial report of a study comparing high-dose IL-2 (720,000 IU/kg/dose IV every 8 hours for 15 doses) and low-dose IL-2 (72,000 IU/kg/dose IV every 8 hours for 15 doses) for treatment of 125 patients with MRCC, response rates were similar in the 2 groups (15% overall response rate in the low-dose group versus 20% overall response rate in the high-dose group) with substantially fewer complications, reduced admissions to the intensive care unit, and reduced use of vasopressor support in the low-dose group (Yang *et al.*, 1994). Later, a third arm was added to the study using SC injections of IL-2 (week 1, 250,000 IU/kg/day for 5 days; weeks 2 to 6, 125,000 IU/kg/day). In the 2-arm comparison of high-dose versus low-dose IV rhIL-2, 116 and 112 patients, respectively, were randomized, and the median follow-up was 52 months. Low-dose rhIL-2 induced significantly less hypotension, thrombocytopenia, malaise, pulmonary toxicity, and neurotoxicity than high-dose rhIL-2. The initial overall response rate (PR plus CR) was 19% with high-dose rhIL-2 and 10% with low-dose rhIL-2. Responses to high-dose rhIL-2 tended to be more durable. With 54 to 56 patients randomized per arm in the 3-arm comparison, the high-dose IV, low-dose IV, and SC outpatient rhIL-2 regimens have produced response rates of 16%, 4%, and 11%, respectively. SC rhIL-2 therapy was infrequently associated with grade 3 or 4 toxicity (similar to low-dose IV rhIL-2 therapy). Survival data remain incomplete, with a median 27-month follow-up in the 3-arm trial. Further accrual and follow-up will be necessary to properly compare the impact of these regimens on patient survival. The optimal IL-2 regimen for treating MRCC remains unknown (Yang and Rosenberg, 1997).

The evaluation of outpatient low-dose SC IL-2 remains an area of intense investigation. An overall response rate of 19% (n = 9) was seen in a group of 47 patients with MRCC treated with SC IL-2 (Vogelzang et al., 1993). In a group of 50 patients with MRCC treated with SC IL-2 at 18 IU/m^2/day for 2 days followed by 6 IU/m^2/day 5 days a week for 6 weeks, Lissoni et al. (1994) found an overall response rate of 28%. In both series, the lower doses were well tolerated with fewer systemic side effects than have been associated with higher-dose IV regimes (see Table 6.2).

Dutcher et al. (1997) reviewed long-term follow-up from three phase II studies conducted by the Cytokine Working Group from 1989 to 1995 of patients with MRCC treated with IL-2 and found similar response rates among high-dose IV IL-2 alone (17%), high-dose IL-2/IFN-α (11%), SC IL-2/IFN-α (7%), and IL-2/IFN-α plus 5-FU/IFN-α (16%). However, high-dose IV IL-2 alone produced a 7% CR rate compared

with 0%, 4%, and 4% rates (respectively) in the other groups, with the median duration of response again much longer in the high-dose group (53 months versus 7, 12, and 9 months, respectively). For more information regarding combination therapy with IL-2/IFN-α with or without chemotherapy agents for the treatment of MRCC, refer to the review by Bukowski (1999).

IL-2 has also been combined with adoptive cellular therapy using LAK cells or TILs. LAK cells are generated from peripheral blood lymphocytes after exposure to IL-2. These activated lymphocytes are capable of lysing a variety of tumor cell lines. Early reports of IL-2 given together with LAK cells seemed to indicate a higher incidence of complete responders in these patients over patients historically treated with IL-2 alone (Rosenberg et al., 1989). However, in a prospective randomized clinical trial comparing IL-2 with LAK cells to IL-2 without LAK cells, the overall survival difference between the groups did not reach statistical significance (Rosenberg et al., 1993). In 1997, Gold et al., reported on 123 patients who received continuous infusion IL-2 (18 to 22 IU/m^2/day on days 1 through 5 and 6 to 8 IU/m^2/day on days 10 through 19) of which the first 76 patients also received LAK cells. They found an overall response rate of 19% (7.3% CR and 11.4% PR), with no statistically significant difference in response rates or survival compared with patients who received LAK cells. Overall, the results of IL-2 plus LAK therapy are similar to the results of IL-2 alone or IL-2 combined with IFN-α (Bukowski, 1997).

TILs are expanded and activated lymphocytes obtained from tumor specimens. In theory, TILs have specific activity against the tumor from which they were derived, which contrasts with LAK cells, which have broader cytolytic activity (Itoh and Balch, 1993). Trials utilizing IL-2 plus TILs have focused primarily on patients with renal cell carcinoma and melanoma and have demonstrated some objective responses (Rosenberg *et al.*, 1988; Dillman *et al.*, 1991; Oldham *et al.*, 1991; Rayman *et al.*, 1994). At the National Cancer Institute, the results of a clinical trial in which 84 patients with MM were treated with TILs plus IL-2 found a 34% response rate, including patients that had previously failed treatment with IL-2 alone (Rosenberg, 1997). The availability of TILs associated with tumor regression is a valuable tool for identifying human tumor regression antigens. TILs have been used to clone the gene that encodes for the antigens recognized by the TILs. This has facilitated the identification of specific melanoma-associated antigens and may allow for the generation of immune cells with far greater specificity and hence new possibilities for adoptive immunotherapy (Rosenberg, 1997).

Figlin *et al.* (1997) performed a series of trials of IL-2 plus TIL therapy in 62 patients with renal cell carcinoma. Patients were treated with cytokines before nephrectomy, and a preparation of cytokine-primed TILs or CD8+ TILs was isolated for infusion into patients. Of the 62 patients enrolled, 55 were treated with TILs and IL-2 and were evaluable for toxicity, response, and survival. Overall, 5 patients (9.1%) achieved a CR and 14 (25.5%) achieved a PR. The responses were durable, with a median duration of 14 months (range, 0.8+ to 64+ months). The actuarial survival was 65% at 1 year and 43% at 2 years from the time of nephrectomy, with an overall median survival duration for all patients of 22 months (range, 2 to 70+ months). At the time the study was reported, the median survival duration for the responding patients had not yet been reached, but the range was 2 to 63+ months. From these results, the investigators concluded that immunotherapy with radical nephrectomy, TILs, and IL-2 provides substantial clinical benefit in the majority of patients. In 1999, Figlin *et al.* reported the results of a randomized clinical trial

of nephrectomy and CD8+ TILs plus IL-2 versus nephrectomy and IL-2 alone. Of the 178 patients enrolled, only 160 were randomized and treated. In the TIL-therapy arm, 40% of patients were unable to receive TILs because of an insufficient number of viable cells. Of those treated, the objective response rates were 9.9% in the TIL plus IL-2 postnephrectomy arm versus 11.4% in the IL-2 alone arm. The technical difficulties experienced in this trial impeded its original goal of resolving whether cellular therapy with TILs provides any clinical benefit. Additional randomized trials are needed to evaluate the potential benefits of **adoptive cellular therapy** combined with IL-2. The toxic reactions experienced by patients who receive IL-2 plus LAK cells or TILs are mainly dependent on the dose and schedule of IL-2 (Brogley and Sharp, 1990).

IL-2 has been combined with chemotherapeutic agents as treatment for a variety of malignancies in an attempt to produce synergistic antitumor effects. The sequencing of the 2 therapies may affect their efficacy and toxicity patterns. If chemotherapy is administered first, it may prime the immune system or decrease the tumor burden. If IL-2 and chemotherapy are administered concurrently, synergistic actions may include chemotherapy-induced damage to the tumor cell membrane or IL-2-induced intratumoral capillary leak. Among theoretical reasons for administering IL-2 prior to chemotherapy is to allow IL-2 immunomodulation without immunosuppression and alteration of tumor cells by IL-2 or secondary cytokines, which would render the tumor cells more susceptible to the cytotoxic effects of chemotherapy (Sznol and Longo, 1993).

Combination regimens of IL-2 plus chemotherapy have been studied in a variety of malignancies, including melanoma, renal cell carcinoma, gastrointestinal malignancies, non-small-cell lung cancer, and head and neck cancer. Generally, these drug combinations have

Table 6.2   Interleukin-2 dosing schedule examples

Interleukin-2 Dose	Administration Route	Care Setting
High Dose		
600,000 IU/kg Q 8 hours	Intravenous bolus	Inpatient intensive care (potential)
Intermediate Dose		
18 million IU/m²/day	Intravenous continuous infusion	Inpatient General Oncology Unit
Low Dose		
18 million IU/day	Subcutaneous	Outpatient

response rates equivalent to those achieved with chemotherapy alone. However, combination therapy using agents with proven activity against melanoma has generated more promising results with potential additive activity. Richards *et al.* (1992) reported a phase II study using carmustine, cisplatin, dacarbazine, IL-2, and IFN-α for treatment of melanoma. Among 36 patients who completed one treatment cycle, there was one CR, 23 PRs, and one minor response (overall response rate, 69%). The median duration of response was 7 months, and the median survival duration was 11.5 months. A follow-up study was designed to further evaluate the therapeutic potential, clarify the toxicities, and explore associated immunologic changes.

Richards *et al.* (1999) reported on 84 patients with melanoma who were treated on a 6-week protocol using cisplatin, dacarbazine, carmustine, and INF-α and IL-2. The biological agents were administered both before and after the combination cytotoxic chemotherapy. The overall response rate was 55% (12 CRs and 34 PRs). The median survival duration was 12.2 months from the time of study entry. A small percentage of patients appeared to derive long-term benefit. The authors concluded that a randomized trial of chemoimmunotherapy versus chemotherapy should be performed to es-

tablish the value of chemoimmunotherapy for melanoma.

Other investigators have studied the effects of IL-2 plus chemotherapy for MM. In 1993, Khayat *et al.* (1993) reported a 54% overall response rate in a series of 39 patients with MM treated with cisplatin followed by IL-2 and INF-α. Legha *et al.* (1993) studied the effects of IL-2, IFN-α, and chemotherapy with cisplatin, vinblastine, and dacarbazine and achieved response rates superior to those achieved with either biotherapy or chemotherapy alone. Legha and colleagues (Legha *et al.*, 1993; Legha and Buzaid, 1993) examined the sequence of administration of biotherapy plus chemotherapy and observed response rates ranging from 47% (arm with biotherapy administered first) to 73% (arm with chemotherapy administered first). More recently, Legha *et al.* (1998) reported on concurrent biochemotherapy combinations to treat patients with MM. In a series of 53 patients, an overall 64% response rate was reported with 21% CRs and 43% PRs, with durable CRs in about 10% of patients. Randomized phase III clinical trials evaluating this approach are currently underway (Flaherty, 2000). The toxic effects of these treatments are significant and include myelosuppression, fatigue, fevers, chills, nausea, vomiting, and capillary-leak syndrome and have required inpatient hospitalization. The authors conclude that concurrent biochemotherapy for patients with advanced melanoma is capable of producing high CR and overall response rates and did result in durable CRs in a small number of patients. Toxicity, though severe, was manageable in a routine inpatient hospital setting. An unexpected side effect from these biochemotherapy combinations has been vitiligo, a depigmentation of the skin. Richards *et al.* (1992) found that 77% of patients who developed vitiligo also had responses to therapy. In an effort to decrease toxicities, lower-dose combinations given on an outpatient basis are being tried. Thompson *et al.* (1997) reported on a series of 32 patients treated with chemotherapy (cisplatin, dacarbazine, carmustine, and tamoxifen) plus self-administered SC IL-2 and IFN-α. The response rate was 43%, and toxicity was tolerable, with only 7% of patients requiring hospitalization for management. The long-term durability of this outpatient regimen is still unknown. Rosenberg *et al.* (1999) reported on a prospective randomized trial in which patients with MM were treated with chemotherapy alone or in combination with IL-2 and IFN-α. In this study, 102 patients with MM were prospectively randomized to receive chemotherapy with tamoxifen, cisplatin, and dacarbazine or the same regimen followed by IFN-alfa-2b and IL-2. Responses were evaluated at a median follow-up of 42 months. In the 52 patients randomized to receive chemotherapy alone, there were 14 objective responses compared with 22 objective responses in the chemoimmunotherapy group. In both groups, the duration of PRs was often short, and treatment toxicity was greater in patients receiving chemoimmunotherapy. The authors concluded that the addition of immunotherapy to chemotherapy increased toxicity but did not increase survival. They recommended that chemoimmunotherapy regimens be given only in the setting of well-designed, prospective, randomized protocols showing the benefit of this treatment strategy.

The role of IL-2 in hematological malignancies has yet to be defined. Numerous clinical studies have begun to evaluate the use of IL-2 as salvage therapy or following BMT. IL-2 has been evaluated in patients with AML both for treatment of relapsed-refractory AML and as a means of preventing relapse in patients achieving a second CR. In a pilot trial, Meloni *et al.* (1997) treated 24 AML patients with advanced disease and low blastosis. Patients received 5 days of continuous-infusion IL-2 with daily dose escalations (8 to 18 MIU/m^2/day). At the completion of the induction cycles, 54% of patients had achieved a CR, and 2 patients demonstrated stable disease. The positive results of this trial led to a large, cooperative, prospective, randomized phase III study initiated in 1992 by Meloni and colleagues. In their study, 264 patients who had previously been treated for AML received mitoxantrone, etoposide, and cytarabine. Of these, 55% (n = 146) achieved a second CR. Of this group, 32 patients who were not eligible for BMT were randomized to receive no treatment or IL-2. Because of low recruitment, the investigators were unable to obtain a sufficient number of patients for a statistically meaningful comparison. However, a trend toward improved survival was observed in the patients on maintenance IL-2 (Meloni *et al.*, 1997). A large, randomized, controlled phase III cooperative group study is now being conducted to further investigate this approach. As of July 2000, results were yet to be reported.

In other trials with small numbers of patients with various hematological malignancies, including NHL, some patients with refractory malignancies have responded to IL-2 with or without IL-activated lymphocytes (Fefer, 1997). The use of IL-2 following allogeneic BMT has been based on the principle that a donor lymphocyte-mediated, graft-versus-leukemia effect can be induced without exacerbation of graft-versus-host disease (Fefer, 1997). Initial studies in which IL-2 was infused immediately after BMT for hematologic malignancies resulted in severe toxicity but did not delay engraftment (Mazumder, 1997). When IL-2 is administered after neutrophil engraftment, it is well tolerated, and immunologic changes, including increased NK activity, IL-2R expression, and cytokine production, have been documented (Higuchi *et al.*, 1991). In a clinical trial involving patients with lymphoma who received IL-2 with or without LAK cells after autologous BMT, the probability of relapse was 23%, and the probability of survival was 71%, which is far superior to the outcomes of historical control patients (Fefer *et al.*, 1997).

Several investigators have demonstrated that the incubation of autologous bone marrow with IL-2 results in significant antitumor results (Verma *et al.*, 1994; Meehan *et al.*, 1995; Margolin, 2000). These studies also included patients with breast cancer, but follow-up was too short to determine the impact of this treatment on relapse and survival in patients with breast cancer. Randomized clinical trials are currently under way to better determine the role of IL-2 following BMT in both solid tumors and hematologic malignancies.

Regulatory Approval

In May 1992, the FDA approved aldesleukin, a form of human IL-2 produced by recombinant DNA technology, for the treatment of MRCC in adults 18 years of age or older. On January 12, 1998, the FDA granted a marketing license for IL-2 for the treatment of patients with MM. Aldesleukin is manufactured by the Chiron Corporation under the trade name Proleukin® (Chiron Corporation, 1998). The recommended treatment for both diseases is high-dose therapy consisting of two 5-day cycles of aldesleukin at 600,000 IU/kg administered every 8 hours as a 15-minute IV bolus infusion for a total of 14 doses. The cycles are separated by a 9-day rest period. Because adverse effects at this dosage level are frequent, often serious, and sometime fatal, it is recommended that patients have normal cardiac, pulmonary, hepatic, and central nervous system function prior to initiation of therapy.

Side Effects

The side effect profile for patients who receive IL-2 therapy differs depending on the dose, route, and schedule of IL-2 given. In general, high-dose IL-2 therapy produces more severe toxic effects. Analysis of 775 consecutive patients treated with high-dose IL-2 between May 1989 and January 1997 revealed no treatment-related deaths compared with initial studies in which there was a 3% mortality rate (Rosenberg, 1997). This drop in mortality rate was felt to be attributable to more care-appropriate management skills and better patient selection. Factors such as patient performance status, major organ function, age, duration of therapy, and tumor burden also can affect the onset, duration, and severity of side effects. Prior to IL-2 therapy, patients should be thoroughly screened to determine their ability to tolerate this treatment. The side effects of IL-2 have the potential to involve nearly every major organ system (Sandstrom, 1996; Rieger, 1997; Wheeler, 1997; Sundin and Wolin, 1998). Protracted therapy with IL-2 may produce more toxic effects. Side effects generally begin shortly after the initiation of therapy and intensify over time. Once therapy has been completed, most side effects resolve within a few days. Irreversible or permanent side effects from IL-2 therapy are rare.

A major side effect experienced by patients who receive IL-2 therapy is the flu-like syndrome. Patients may experience chills or rigors followed by fevers. Other constitutional symptoms include myalgias, arthralgias, malaise, headache, and nasal stuffiness. The onset of these symptoms is usually 4 to 6 hours after initiation of therapy (see Chapter 16). Fatigue is also a significant side effect in patients who receive IL-2 therapy (Piper *et al.*, 1989; Rust and Rosenzweig, 1997). IL-2 triggers the release of cytokines such as IL-1, IL-6, and IFN-γ from target cells, and that release may induce these symptoms (Sergi, 1991; Rieger, 1992; Weidmann *et al.*, 1992; Bukowski, 1997).

Potential cardiovascular side effects related to IL-2 therapy include tachycardia, hypotension, arrhythmias, edema, and weight gain. In part, these toxic effects result from dose-related fluid imbalances caused by a vascular leak syndrome. Release of cytokines such as IL-1, TNF, and IFN-γ may affect the permeability of vascular walls, decrease systemic vascular resistance, and allow fluids to leak from the vascular bed to the interstitial spaces (Mier, 1993b; Schwartzentruber, 1997).

Potential pulmonary side effects include dyspnea and pulmonary congestion. These side effects may occur as a result of interstitial pulmonary edema related to increased vascular permeability, the migration of activated T cells to the lungs, or the release of secondary cytokines in the lungs (Sergi, 1991; Berthiaume *et al.*, 1995). In extreme cases, patients who receive high-dose IL-2 therapy may develop adult respiratory distress syndrome, which can progress to severe respiratory failure requiring intubation (Farrell, 1992; Gaynor and Fisher, 1993; White *et al.*, 1994). Patients with poor pulmonary reserve should be screened carefully prior to receiving IL-2 therapy and should be monitored closely during therapy.

Renal dysfunction, another potential side effect of IL-2 therapy, is manifested by decreased urine output and increased serum creatinine and blood urea nitrogen levels. Contributing factors include hypoperfusion of the kidneys and direct effects of IL-2 on the kidneys (Guleria *et al.*, 1994). Patients with MRCC who have under-

gone prior nephrectomy or who have impaired renal function prior to IL-2 therapy should be monitored closely.

Liver function may also be temporarily impaired during IL-2 therapy. Signs of this include elevated liver enzymes (which are reflective of liver function) and jaundice. The reversible cholestasis that occurs may be a result of the direct effects of IL-2 or indirect effects of secondary cytokines such as TNF or IL-6 (Fisher *et al.*, 1989; Rieger, 1992). Patients who have metastatic disease in the liver should be monitored closely.

Skin changes associated with IL-2 therapy are common. Patients may experience a diffuse erythematous rash, intense pruritus, and dry skin with desquamation. The palms of the hands and the soles of the feet may peel. Results of histologic examinations of skin biopsy samples have been inconclusive (Rieger, 1992; Wolkenstein *et al.*, 1993). Patients who receive SC IL-2 have experienced local inflammatory responses at injection sites (Atzpodien *et al.*, 1991; Hossan and Rieger, 1997). Inflammation may begin 4 to 6 hours after injection and may persist for up to 5 days. The injection site may be painful, erythematous, and indurated. SC nodules may also develop at injection sites. These nodules are usually small and painless but may take several months to resolve.

Gastrointestinal toxic effects are commonly experienced by patients who receive IL-2 therapy. Nausea, vomiting, diarrhea, anorexia, and mucositis are symptoms experienced by the majority of patients at all dose levels of IL-2 and may be severe. Nausea, vomiting, and diarrhea commonly occur within several hours after IV bolus IL-2 or SC IL-2. With continuous infusion IL-2, these side effects may occur intermittently. Anorexia can be a severe side effect of long-term or repeated IL-2 therapy and may result in significant weight loss. The gastrointestinal side effects generally resolve rapidly on completion of therapy.

Neurological changes may also occur in patients who receive therapy with IL-2 (Sparber and Biller-Sparber, 1993; Forman, 1994; Lerner *et al.*, 1999). Lethargy, confusion, sleep disturbances, decreased concentration, mood swings, and depression may occur. Severe neurological changes may represent a dose-limiting toxic effect with high-dose IL-2 therapy.

Hematological changes during IL-2 therapy, including mild anemia, leukopenia, and thrombocytopenia, are possible (Paciucci *et al.*, 1990; Oleksowicz *et al.*, 1991). With prolonged or repeated courses of IL-2, eosinophilia is common (Silberstein *et al.*, 1989). After IL-2 has been discontinued, a marked rebound of lymphocytosis occurs as activated lymphocytes circulate in the peripheral bloodstream (Thompson *et al.*, 1988; Boldt and Ellis, 1993).

Impaired neutrophil function with resultant decreased chemotaxis is associated with IL-2 therapy. Therefore, patients with a pre-existing infection should be treated with antibiotics prior to receiving IL-2 therapy. Consideration should also be given to the use of prophylactic antibiotics in patients with indwelling central lines or long-term venous access devices (Hartman *et al.*, 1989; Bock *et al.*, 1990; Snydman *et al.*, 1990; Klempner and Snydman, 1993; Pockaj *et al.*, 1993).

An increased incidence of reactions to both ionic and nonionic radiographic computed tomography contrast media has been reported in patients who have received therapy with IL-2. Symptoms have included fever, chills, nausea, vomiting, hypotension, leukocytosis, skin rash, and elevation in serum creatinine (Oldham and Brogley, 1990; Zukiwski *et al.*, 1990; Abi-aad *et al.*, 1991; Fishman *et al.*, 1991; Choyke *et al.*, 1992). Because the risk of contrast media reactions may be greater early after IL-2 therapy, the use of contrast agents should be avoided during this time (Shulman *et al.*, 1993).

Nursing Considerations

Nursing considerations specific to IL-2 include measures to manage capillary leak syndrome such as strict monitoring of fluid balance, judicious use of IV fluids, need for vasopressor support for hypotension, and monitoring of cardiac and pulmonary functions (Gale, 1997). Table 6.3 summarizes guidelines for nursing management of capillary leak syndrome (Seipp, 1997). The SC nodules, pain, and skin irritation associated with SC administration of IL-2 can be of concern for patients and their families.

Table 6.3 Guidelines for nursing management of capillary leak syndrome

- Monitor blood pressure before and after IL-2 doses.
- Assess clinical symptoms of hypotension, dizziness, light-headedness, and fainting.
- Report persistent hypotension < 90 mm Hg that does not respond to 2 L normal saline solution (0.9%) IV boluses; begin dopamine and transfer to ICU.
- Auscultate for breath sounds.
- Monitor O_2 saturation.
- Monitor heart rate; assess with ECG; report significant tachycardia or arrhythmias.
- Monitor urine output (strict intake and output recording); Foley catheter may be needed to monitor hourly output.
- Monitor daily weight.
- Monitor electrolytes, blood urea nitrogen, creatinine, liver enzymes; replace ↓ magnesium, ↓ phosphorus, ↓ potassium.
- Initiate diuretics when hypotension is controlled and creatinine is stable.
- Help patient adjust physical activity to conserve energy.
- Report significant changes to physician.

ECG, electrocardiogram; ICU, intensive care unit; IL, interleukin; IV, intravenous.

Source: Reprinted with permission from Seipp, C. 1997. Capillary leak syndrome: Nursing considerations. *Biotherapy: Considerations for Nurses* 2(2): 12.

Administration of a cold pack prior to injection may prevent some discomfort, and application of warm compresses for 20 minutes 4 times a day to painful nodules may be helpful. Patient education should stress the importance of rotating the injection site, bringing prefilled syringes to room temperature, and proper injection into the SC tissue, as improper intradermal injection can lead to severe skin reactions (Hossan and Rieger, 1997). The use of clinical pathways may maximize available resources and ensure consistent patient outcomes. An example of a clinical pathway utilized in the inpatient setting at Lutheran General Hospital (Park Ridge, IL) is provided in Appendix A.

Future Directions

Research of the use of IL-2 for a wide variety of malignancies continues. Studies of renal cancer and melanoma are focusing on outpatient SC administration or infusion by using an ambulatory pump to decrease costs and toxicity while maintaining clinical response (Hossan and Rieger, 1997). The ability to identify tumor-specific antigens in a wide variety of malignancies, including melanoma, breast cancer, colon cancer, and lymphomas, may enhance development of disease-specific vaccine therapy (Rosenberg, 1997). Inhaled IL-2 in patients with pulmonary MRCC showed promise in preventing progression of disease without systemic toxicities in 70% of patients (Huland et al., 1999). As stated by Atkins (1997), ". . . the challenge for the next decade will be to devise therapies to improve outcomes for a majority not minority of patients; it is likely IL-2 will play a pivitol role in these therapies." The use of IL-2 to incubate bone marrow collections and expand and activate T cells is still being studied (Fefer, 1997). It has also been suggested that the addition of IL-2 may prolong responses not only to BMT but postchemotherapy in patients with lymphomas, leukemias, myelomas,

breast cancer, and colon cancer. Studies are ongoing, and long-term results are not yet known.

IL-2 has been investigated extensively in the treatment of patients with human immunodeficiency virus (HIV) infections and acquired immunodeficiency syndrome (AIDS) (Schwartz and Merigan, 1990; Schwartz et al., 1991; Smith, 1993). The goal of such therapy is to increase the numbers of lymphocytes as well as their functional capacity. Studies have demonstrated that a temporary increase in T-cell numbers can be achieved with 2 to 3 weeks of low-dose IL-2 therapy. The full impact of this therapy and the potential risks of promoting HIV transcription or viral entry into healthy activated cells has yet to be determined. Research will continue to elucidate the regulatory network of cytokines that affect virtually every step of the virus life cycle, from cell entry to budding of new progeny virions, both proinflammatory cytokines and anti-inflammatory cytokines. The role of IL-2, as exemplified by the potent enhancing effect on the number of circulating CD4+ T lymphocytes, will continue to be investigated as a means of immune reconstitution (Poli, 1999) or to decrease the incidence of AIDS-related malignancies such as lymphoma (Khatri et al., 1997).

Because of its profound effects as an immunostimulant, IL-2 is being tested as a proactive anti-infection agent (Smith, 1993). Low doses of IL-2 administered to patients with lepromatous leprosy led to a significant reduction in the bacterial load in those patients. With this observation, consideration is being given to the use of IL-2 for treating bacterial, fungal, viral, and parasitic infections and for preventing infections in burn patients (Smith, 1993).

Another area of interest is the reduction of IL-2–induced toxic effects, especially hypotension and the vascular leak syndrome. Because these hemodynamic effects of IL-2 are related to secondary cytokines such as TNF and IL-1, strategies are being employed to use other agents to interfere with the secretion of these cytokines. Pentoxifylline, an agent that suppresses TNF synthesis, has been shown to reduce IL-2 toxicity in mice while preserving antitumor efficacy (Edwards *et al.*, 1992). Preliminary studies also indicate that the presence of pentoxifylline does not inhibit human LAK cytotoxicity (Thompson *et al.*, 1993). Clinical trials continue to investigate pentoxifylline for its usefulness in delivering higher doses of IL-2 without severe toxic effects. Other agents being considered for use with IL-2 include dexamethasone, anti-TNF antibodies, soluble TNF receptors, platelet-activating factor antagonists, and IL-1-Ras (Mier, 1993a). Initial studies of dexamethasone have shown blockage of all IL-2 effects (Vetto *et al.*, 1987). It has yet to be determined what effect these agents may have on the potential antineoplastic activity of IL-2. Although there is interest in decreasing IL-2 toxicity so that higher doses of it may be given, there is also interest in delivering low doses of IL-2 that bind to high-affinity IL-2Rs and signal the target cell without triggering secondary cytokine production (Smith, 1993).

Future investigations of IL-2 will involve combination regimens that include other cytokines, activated lymphocytes, vaccines, and chemotherapeutic agents for a variety of malignancies and other diseases. Doses, routes of administration, and schedules will be altered to attempt to achieve greater efficacy with less toxic effects. As more complex therapies are delivered to outpatients, IL-2 therapy will be applied in that setting (Smith, 1997).

Interleukin-4

In 1982, IL-4 was initially described as a B-cell growth factor and as an IgG$_1$-enhancing factor (Howard *et al.*, 1982). IL-4 is a cytokine produced primarily by activated T$_h$ cells and mast cells (Puri and Siegel, 1993). Antigens, antigen-presenting cells, or antibodies in conjunction with the T cells induce production of IL-4. It exerts its functional activity by binding to receptors on the cell-surface membranes of target cells (Paul, 1991; Chomarat *et al.*, 1998; Muir-Sluis, 1998).

Biological Actions

Like most cytokines, IL-4 displays pleiotropic functions. It exerts different effects on resting and activated B cells by binding to a receptor that consists of 2 or possibly 3 chains. The biochemical and signaling events that occur when IL-4 binds to its receptor remain poorly understood (Muir-Sluis, 1998). IL-4 stimulates the growth of resting B cells by increasing cell numbers and by enhancing the expression of class II major histocompatibility antigens. Following antigen activation, IL-4 serves as a B-cell growth factor by stimulating the B cell to replicate its DNA. IL-4 also promotes the differentiation of antibody-stimulated B cells, and it is therefore known as a B-cell growth and differentiation factor. As a "switch factor," IL-4 is a major regulator of Ig isotope expression, inducing IgE and IgG$_1$ production (Feldmann and Male, 1989; Oppenheim *et al.*, 1991; Chomarat *et al.*, 1998).

IL-4 also induces T-cell growth, enhances production of IL-2 (Paul, 1991), and increases the expression of the IL-2R to increase T-cell stimulation by IL-2 (Lewko *et al.*, 1998). The proliferation and differentiation of cytotoxic T cells are enhanced by IL-4. *In vitro*, the combination of IL-2 and IL-4 has synergistic effects on the growth and lytic activity of cytotoxic T cells but may inhibit LAK activity, although induction of LAK activity may be mediated by IL-4. When lymphocytes are exposed to suboptimal doses of IL-2, IL-4 may stimulate LAK activity (Higuchi *et al.*, 1989). In addition, IL-4 promotes the growth of TILs that exert a cytotoxic effect on human melanoma (Kawakami *et al.*, 1988; Lotze *et al.*, 1992). IL-4 also acts synergistically with IL-2 to enhance the expansion of activated CD4+ cells while inhibiting nonspecific cytotoxicity (Tso *et al.*, 1992). In sum, IL-4 has a variety of effects on cytotoxic cells, depending on the phenotype of the cells, the presence of other cytokines, and the state of activation of the cells (Muir-Sluis, 1998).

In addition to stimulating B and T cells, IL-4 also activates granulocytes, macrophages, megakaryocytes, thymocytes, and mast cells. IL-4 enhances the growth of hematopoietic progenitor cells in the presence of granulocyte colony-stimulating factor (G-CSF), IL-6, and IL-11 but inhibits colony formation in the presence of GM-CSF, macrophage colony-stimulating factor, or IL-3 (Muir-Sluis, 1998). Increased antitumor activity is stimulated in macrophages by IL-4, yet it downregulates other aspects of the function of macrophages such as production of superoxide (Jansen *et al.*, 1990; Dawson 1991; Puri and Siegel, 1993). IL-4 has been shown to inhibit the growth of macrophages, yet it induces differentiation of monocytes to macrophages (Jansen *et al.*, 1990).

Clinical Trials

Numerous phase I clinical trials have been conducted using IL-4. It has been administered alone and in combination with IL-2 by IV bolus injection, continuous IV infusion, or SC injection. In a phase I study by Atkins *et al.* (1992), the MTD was determined to be 10 mcg/kg/dose when administered by IV bolus every 8 hours on days 1 to 5 and days 15 to 19. No tumor responses were observed. When administered by daily SC injection, dose-limiting toxicity was reached at a dose of 5 mcg/kg/day (Gilleece *et al.*, 1992). Sosman *et al.* (1994) used escalating doses of IL-4 up to 360 mcg/m^2/day administered by continuous IV infusion for 7 days and found this to be the MTD. No significant

responses were seen in this trial. A phase I clinical trial of 19 patients with advanced cancer found that the MTD was 400 mcg/m^2/day, and 2 patients with NHL showed a transient response (Prendiville *et al.*, 1993).

IL-4 has also undergone study in phase II trials, primarily for the treatment of renal cell carcinoma and melanoma. In a phase II study of patients with MRCC and MM, the MTD was found to be 600 mcg/m^2 after 3 of 27 patients treated at 800 mcg developed cardiac toxicities. There were no responses in the patients with MRCC, and only 1 patient with MM responded. Several phase II studies of MRCC patients treated with IL-4 or a single agent confirmed a lack of response, with only 1 minor response of 18 patients treated by Stadler *et al.* (1995) and 1 response in 50 patients treated by Whitehead *et al.* (1995). A phase II trial of rIL-4 administered at a dose of 5 mcg/kg/day for 28 days followed by a second course after a 7-day rest was reported by Whitehead *et al.* (1998). Of 34 eligible patients with MM who had received no prior therapy for metastatic disease, there was 1 CR and 2 patients with stable disease. In a phase II trial of patients with chronic lymphocytic leukemia and indolent NHL treated with IL-4 as a single agent, 4 of 17 eligible patients had reductions in adenopathy, but none qualified as a response (Venkatraj *et al.*, 1997). Single-agent IL-4 did show a 9% response rate and a survival advantage (median survival duration, 372 days) in patients with advanced non-small-cell lung cancer with doses of 1, 2, 4, and 8 mcg/kg 3 times a week for 6 months (Modiano, 1997). A study published in 1998 by Vokes *et al.* found that a small number of patients with advanced or recurrent non-small-cell lung cancer achieved a PR (1 in 55 evaluable patients) or stabilization of disease (8 in 55 evaluable patients) at a dosage of 1.0 mcg/kg administered by SC injection 3 times per week. Only 1 patient in the group receiving a lower dose of IL-4 (0.25 mcg/kg) achieved stabilization of disease. Because the therapy was well tolerated and there was a trend toward stabilization of disease at the higher dose, the investigators recommended further study of IL-4 in lung cancer either alone or in combination with other therapies.

Based on the premise that IL-4 may activate cytotoxic effector cells most effectively following IL-2, phase I studies have also incorporated the use of continuous IV infusion of IL-4 followed by IL-2. Several phase I trials with IL-4 either followed by IL-2 or with IL-2 given simultaneously with IL-4 have demonstrated that the combination is tolerable, with toxicities similar to the profile of IL-2 alone. In one trial, only 2 of 39 patients with refractory malignancies had a response (Olencki et al., 1996), and in another study, 1 of 17 had a minor response (Sosman et al., 1994). In both studies there was evidence of immune stimulation such as increases in percentages of CD56+ lymphocytes and CD3+ and CD4+ lymphocyte subsets (Sosman et al., 1994; Olencki et al., 1996).

Phase II trials have been conducted using TILs whose proliferation has been increased *in vitro* by IL-2 and IL-4 administration. The TILs were administered in conjunction with IL-2 to patients with MRCC. Although a few tumor responses were observed, the response rate was not greater than that noted with IL-2 alone. The toxic effects were those expected with IL-2 plus TIL therapy (Puri and Siegel, 1993).

Regulatory Approval

As of July 2000, IL-4 continues to be studied in clinical trials and has not yet been approved by the FDA.

Side Effects

The most common side effects observed in patients receiving single-agent IL-4 are fever, nasal congestion, headache, nausea/vomiting, diarrhea, anorexia, fatigue, capillary-leak syndrome, weight gain, and dyspnea. Asymptomatic elevations in liver function tests have also occurred but were transient. In a review of 73 patients with advanced malignancies who were treated with either single-agent IL-4 or combination therapy with IL-2 and IL-4, Rubin and Lotze (1992) reported that 12 of 84 courses of therapy were associated with the development of gastroduodenal erosion or ulceration. Transfusions were required in 3 of these courses, and no treatment-related deaths occurred. Upper-gastrointestinal bleeding without evidence of local tumor involvement has also been seen by other investigators (Margolin et al., 1994; Stadler et al., 1995). Several studies have reported cardiac abnormalities including biopsy-proven myocarditis in 1 patient (Trehu et al., 1993), cardiac ischemia with pericarditis in 1 patient, arrhythmias in 2 others (Margolin et al., 1994), and an asymptomatic 14% decrease in cardiac ejection fraction in 1 patient (Stadler et al., 1995). In studies evaluating the administration of IL-2 plus IL-4-stimulated TIL cells, the side effect profile is similar to that observed with IL-2 alone. The safety and tolerability of *Escherichia coli*-derived rhIL-4 have been evaluated in phase I and phase II studies in human patients with a variety of malignancies. Clinical trials have demonstrated that SC administration of rhIL-4 is safe and well tolerated at doses as high as 5 mcg/kg/day and as high as 10 mcg/kg when administered 3 times a week (Leach et al., 1997).

Future Directions

Although IL-4 appears to demonstrate antitumor activity in animal models, it has yet to produce useful antitumor responses in humans. The role of IL-4 in the activation of cytolytic T cells and TILs continues to be studied in an attempt to develop clinical applications for this cytokine. Additional strategies include the transduction of the *IL-4* gene into immune cells for localized secretion of IL-4. In a phase I trial conducted at the Pittsburgh Cancer Center, Pittsburgh, PA, this approach was evaluated in patients with advanced malignancies. The patients were vaccinated with irradiated autologous tumor cells together with *IL-4*–transduced irradiated autologous fibroblasts (Suminami *et al.*, 1995). Following vaccination, mRNA for the *IL-4* gene was detected in tissue biopsies of the vaccinated sites. Cytokine gene therapy is a potentially powerful antineoplastic strategy. It provides paracrine cytokine secretion in the region of putative tumor antigen that maximizes antitumor immune responses and minimizes systemic toxicity. A wealth of animal experimentation has demonstrated the effectiveness of cytokine gene therapy in a variety of tumor models. Enough evidence has mounted so that human cytokine gene therapy trials are under way throughout the United States and elsewhere (D'Angelica and Fong, 1998).

Another possible application for IL-4 lies in its ability to induce class switch in Ig production to IgE and IgG$_1$. Control of Ig synthesis could prevent or minimize IgE-mediated allergic conditions. Strategies to neutralize IL-4, block the production of IL-4, or inhibit the activity of IL-4 may be explored. The inhibitory effects of IL-4 on the production of cytokines provides a strong rationale for its use in chronic inflammatory diseases such as rheumatoid arthritis.

Interleukin-6

The various activities of IL-6 were originally described by many investigators who initially thought they each had found a new cytokine. Weissenbach *et al.* (1979) first called "IL-6 IFN-β2". Teranishi *et al.* (1982) described a new factor that induced the differentiation of B cells to antibody-producing plasma cells. Haegeman *et al.* (1986) called it an IL-1–induc-

ible 26-kDa protein. The advent of molecular cloning revealed that all these activities were encoded by the same gene and hence were actually one and the same cytokine, now known as IL-6 (Kammuller, 1995). IL-6 is an endogenous cytokine involved in numerous physiological processes that are predominantly related to host defense maintenance (i.e., inflammation, immunity, and hematopoiesis). T lymphocytes, monocytes, fibroblasts, endothelial cells, and keratinocytes all produce IL-6 (Veldhuis *et al.*, 1996). A variety of peptide factors, including IL-1, TNF, IL-2, IFN-β, and platelet-derived growth factor, also induce IL-6 production (Hirano, 1998).

Biological Actions

It is known at present that IL-6 plays a pivotal role in the body's defenses through induction of the immune response as well as in the stimulation of hematopoiesis (Herodin *et al.*, 1992). The overproduction of IL-6 either experimentally or in human disease is associated with various levels of disease, so IL-6 antagonists may play a role in the suppression of certain disease states such as multiple myeloma, Alzheimer's disease, or multiple sclerosis (MS) (Scholz, 1996). Myeloma cell growth in culture appears to be regulated in an autocrine fashion by IL-6 (Richards, 1998). Known actions of IL-6 include inducing megakaryocyte maturation, causing B-cell differentiation to antibody-producing cells, T-cell growth and maturation, differentiation of myeloid leukemic cells into macrophages, development of osteoclasts, and inducting acute-phase protein synthesis in hepatocytes. In fact, one of the primary roles of IL-6 *in vivo* is that it serves as the major cytokine in initiating the hepatic acute-phase response. IL-6 also appears to be active in neurological systems that are integrated into the acute inflammatory response and causes neural differentiation of a specialized laboratory cell line (chromaffin cell line PC 12) (Hibi *et al.*, 1996; Richards, 1998).

The activities of IL-6 are mediated through the human IL-6R complex, consisting of a binding molecule termed IL-6Rα and a signal transducer, gp130 (Hibi *et al.*, 1996). As previously discussed, other cytokines, such as IL-11, also share the signal transducer gp130, making this receptor part of the cytokine-receptor super-family (Yin *et al.*, 1993). Once the receptor and the ligand are bound, signaling pathways that target certain genes are induced.

Of particular importance to clinical use of this cytokine is the stimulatory actions of IL-6 on hematopoiesis, especially its effect on the thrombocytopoietic system and its impact on regulatory activities of the cellular and humoral immune function, possibly leading to antitumor effects (Veldhuis *et al.*, 1996). IL-6 may have an antitumor effect in chronic lymphocytic leukemia (Aderka *et al.*, 1993) and other tumors such as renal cell carcinoma, breast cancer, sarcomas, and melanoma (Sandoz Pharmaceuticals, 1991; Veldhuis *et al.*, 1996).

Clinical Trials

Early studies of rhIL-6 administration in rodents and animals have shown its ability to stimulate the production of platelets and significantly lessen the degree of thrombocytopenia induced from radiation therapy (Herodin *et al.*, 1992). In addition, IL-6 has been found to accelerate recovery from myelosuppression induced by cytotoxic chemotherapy or following BMT in murine models (Lotem *et al.*, 1989). Castell *et al.* (1989) have shown that in addition to its hematologic effects, IL-6 is a major stimulator of the acute-phase response.

The ability of IL-6 to stimulate platelet production and its impact on regulatory activities of cellular and humoral immune function (e.g., activation of T lymphocytes, differentiation of cytotoxic T lymphocytes, activation of NK cells, and maturation of B lymphocytes into antibody-producing cells) have led investigators to study its antineoplastic activities in animals. Mulé *et al.* (1990) demonstrated that rhIL-6 caused inhibition of experimental hepatic and pulmonary metastases by syngeneic methylcholanthrene-induced sarcomas in mice. The antitumor activities of IL-6 are thought to be caused by stimulation of immune and host defense systems.

Initial phase I/II clinical trials in humans with rIL-6 given before chemotherapy have demonstrated significant increases in platelet counts. Doses up to 20 mcg/kg given either intravenously or subcutaneously were well tolerated, with flu-like syndrome being the most common side effect. Dose-limiting toxicity was seen at 30 mcg/kg and consisted of neurotoxicity in one study and cardiac dysrhythmia and severe hepatotoxicity in another (Veldhuis *et al.*, 1996). Fay *et al.* (1994) reported on concomitant administration of IL-6 and GM-CSF given after autologous BMT for the treatment of breast cancer. The combination seemed to be well tolerated, and preliminary results indicated that the combination may result in rapid recovery of the bone marrow after marrow-ablative therapy and autologous BMT for breast cancer. Lestingi *et al.* (1994) found that administration of rhIL-6 following a total of 53 cycles of chemotherapy in patients with MM was generally safe and well tolerated. Platelet nadirs were similar to those of historical controls with chemotherapy alone. However, only 1 patient of 19 had a platelet nadir lower than 20,000/mL versus 10% of historical controls, who had a nadir of 20,000/mL or less. Constitutional symptoms were common and included fevers, chills, rigors, fatigue, and anorexia. rhIL-6 was stopped in one patient for intolerable fatigue and another for depression/suicidal ideation. Grade 3 neutropenia was observed in 11 of 53 cycles, but no infectious episodes were noted. Hematocrit nadirs lower than 25% were noted in 18 of 53 cycles. A response rate of 30% in this study compared with historical response rates of 40% to 50% for chemotherapy alone demonstrated no benefit in survival for patients receiving chemotherapy followed by rhIL-6. Additional studies of rhIL-6 postchemotherapy reported no effect on platelet nadir but a tendency toward faster recovery of platelets (Veldhuis *et al.*, 1996). A phase III trial of IL-6 plus G-CSF versus placebo following high-dose cytoxan and doxorubicin in patients with advanced breast cancer found no impact on platelet transfusion events and a second-cycle platelet nadir in the treatment group (Hamm *et al.*, 1997). Shen *et al.* (1997) reported that a combination of IL-6 and G-CSF compared with G-CSF alone appeared to enhance absolute neutrophil count and platelet recovery following chemotherapy with ifosfamide, cytoxan, and etoposide in children with recurrent solid tumors. In sum, although numerous clinical trials have evaluated its utility in diminishing thrombocytopenia following chemotherapy or BMT, the effects of IL-6 appear to be modest at most, and the side effects likely limit its clinical application in this setting (Maslak and Nimer, 1998; Hochster *et al.*, 1999).

The role of rIL-6 as an antitumor agent has yet to be fully explored. Patients with renal cell carcinoma and melanoma treated with IL-6 alone exhibited low response rates (8% and 14%, respectively) (Veldhuis *et al.*, 1996). Because IL-6 and IL-6R play a major role in autocrine/paracrine growth regulation of myeloma cells are the central mediators for bone destruction and other systemic manifestations of multiple myeloma, modulation of the IL-6/IL-6R cytokine loop represents a rational therapeutic approach for treatment of this disease. Chen *et al.* (1997) updated and reviewed the studies of the agents that targeted IL-6/IL-6R modulation and the results of selected clinical trials. Thus far, clinical trials show largely lim-

ited benefits to these agents but they remain an area of interest. Given tumor-cell heterogeneity and the complexity of the interconnected cytokine network *in vivo*, these authors suggest that future emphasis should be on the strategy of combination treatment that would modulate this cytokine loop at multiple sites. Further advances in delineating IL-6 and related cytokine signal transduction pathways also suggest other targets for therapeutic intervention.

Regulatory Approval

As of July 2000, IL-6 continues to be studied in clinical trials and has not yet been approved by the FDA.

Side Effects

The side effects associated with IL-6 are similar to those of other ILs and include flu-like symptoms, fevers, chills, fatigue, myalgias, anorexia, mild nausea, and vomiting. Transient elevations in liver transaminase, alkaline phosphatase, and bilirubin were also seen and were dose-limiting in some patients. Thrombocytosis and anemia were observed as well. The etiology of the anemia seen with IL-6 has been found to be dilutional in nature. It occurs rapidly after the administration of IL-6 and resolves soon after IL-6 is completed. It does not appear to cause a direct inhibition of erythroid precursor maturation or an ongoing hemolytic process. Transfusions of packed red blood cells may be required if patients are symptomatic. Thrombocytosis was directly related to the administration of IL-6; however, no adverse experiences have been shown to be related to its development. Neurological symptoms were experienced by some patients, including confusion, dizziness, mood and sleep disturbances, headache, parsthesias, and vision changes. Lestingi *et al.* (1994) reported that one patient was removed from the study for depression/suicidal ideation.

Cardiovascular toxicities reported by Sandoz Pharmaceutical (1991) from data on file were mild to moderate in severity and included hypertension, bradycardia, atrial fibrillation, dizziness, and pedal edema. More serious cardiac toxicities included cardiac ischemia in one patient, cardiac tamponade in another patient, and hypotension in one patient requiring vasopressor support for 7 hours after the first dose of IL-6 given at 30 mcg/kg as a 1-hour infusion. For this patient, the remainder of the treatment course was given on time, and the patient did not experience a recurrence of hypotension (Sandoz Pharmaceutical, 1991).

A variety of respiratory side effects resulting from IL-6 treatment have been reported, including abnormal breath sounds, cough, dyspnea, nasal congestion, pharyngitis, pleuritic pain, tachypnea, and thick mucous. These toxicities were mild to moderate in severity and did not necessitate interruption in treatment for most patients. Erythema and pain at the injection site were the most common dermatologic side effects seen by patients receiving SC IL-6. Rotation of injection sites and avoidance of reinjection at reddened sites did not result in skin reactions severe enough to require interruption of therapy. Other mild dermatologic reactions included facial flushing, burning eyes, palate petechiae, pruritus, rash, and cyanosis of the lips, nailbeds, and periorbit (Sandoz Pharmaceutical, 1991).

Nursing Considerations

Nursing considerations include administration issues such as dose and route. At present, the optimal dose and method for administering IL-6 have yet to be determined. Clinical trials have demonstrated it is safe to administer IL-6 by the IV route and by SC injection. Doses in clinical trials have ranged from 0.3 to 30 mcg/kg/day. Schedules for administration of IL-6 have varied. The most common method of administration has been SC injections given by the patient or a caregiver in the home. IL-6 is reconstituted with sterile nonbacteriostatic water and should be used within 24 hours of reconstitution or discarded. Because of the possibility of erythema at the injection site, it is important to instruct patients on site rotation in order to ensure safe home therapy. Patients were instructed to inject themselves at bedtime in the hope they would sleep through the worst of the side effects and be able to conduct their usual activities during the day.

Future Directions

Phase II/III trials studying IL-6 alone and in combination with other growth factors are needed to focus on its ability to reduce thrombocytopenia following chemotherapy and its possible antitumor effects (Veldhuis *et al.*, 1996; Hirano, 1998; Richards, 1998). Overproduction of IL-6 is associated with various diseases such as plasmocytoma, myeloma, and some autoimmune disorders (Scholz, 1996). Thus, an IL-6 antagonist may be beneficial in treating these types of disease.

Interleukin-10

IL-10 was originally named "cytokine synthesis inhibitory factor" because of its ability to inhibit cytokine production by activated T_{h1} cells. It was also termed "macrophage deactivating factor" owing to its ability to inhibit activation of cells of the macrophage monocyte and dendritic lineage. IL-10, like other ILs, has multiple biological activities and affects monocytes, macrophages, T cells, B cells, NK cells, neutrophils, endothelial cells, and peripheral blood mononuclear cells (PBMCs).

Biological Actions

The specific actions of IL-10 include inhibition of cytokine synthesis and proliferation of T cells activated in the presence of antigen-presenting cells. This effect is due mostly to its downregulatory effects on the function of antigen-presenting cells. IL-10 inhibits the production of proinflammatory cytokines such as IL-1, IL-2, TNF-α, IFN-γ, and IL-6 through inhibitory action on T_{h1} cells and macrophages (Fiorentino et al., 1991; Beutler et al., 1995; Kucharzik et al., 1995; de Waal Malefyt and Moore, 1998). IL-10 has been shown to enhance proliferation of activated human B lymphocytes and to induce them to secrete large amounts of Igs (Burdin et al., 1993). IL-10 is produced by T_{h0}, T_{h1}, and T_{h2} cell clones; B cells; keratinocytes (mouse); and monocytes and macrophages (de Waal Malefyt et al., 1991; DeVita et al., 1995).

Physiological Activities

INFLAMMATORY BOWEL DISEASE
Active IBD is characterized by increased monocyte secretion of proinflammatory cytokines. Immunoregulatory cytokines such as IL-10, IL-4, and IL-13 are capable of inhibiting the proinflammatory cytokine response of activated monocytes (Kucharzik et al., 1997). The pathogenesis of ulcerative colitis and Crohn's disease may be associated with decreased production of IL-10 and IL-4 cytokines, which are capable of suppressing macrophage and T-cell function. IL-4 mRNA expression has been found to be decreased in intestinal tissue from patients with Crohn's disease, whereas IL-10 mRNA expression is decreased in a majority of patients with ulcerative colitis, suggesting that these diseases have a different immunopathogenesis (Nielsen

et al., 1996). IL-6 is a proinflammatory cytokine and is most likely the main cytokine factor responsible for induction of hepatic acute-phase proteins in Crohn's disease (Niederau et al., 1997). In an in vitro study, PBMCs were isolated from 27 patients with Crohn's disease, 27 patients with ulcerative colitis, and 16 healthy controls and were stimulated with pokeweed mitogen after treatment with IL-13, IL-4, and IL-10, and secretion of IL-1β, TNF-α, and IL-6 was assessed using sandwich enzyme-linked immunosystems. These researchers found that IL-10 was able to downregulate all pro-inflammatory cytokines in active IBD as well as in the controls (Kucharzik et al., 1996). Serum IL-10 levels were assessed in another study of 44 patients with ulcerative colitis, 40 patients with Crohn's disease, and in 30 healthy controls. IL-10 serum levels were increased in patients with active Crohn's disease and active ulcerative colitis compared with the control group. Only patients with active disease presented with significantly increased IL-10 serum levels, whereas patients with inactive disease did not show any significant increase. This finding may suggest that IL-10 acts as a naturally occurring damper of the acute inflammatory process of IBD (Kucharzik et al., 1995). In vitro and in vivo studies of IL-10 have shown it to downregulate the enhanced secretion as well as mRNA levels of proinflammatory cytokines by mononuclear phagocytes in patients with IBD. In vivo topical application of IL-10 induces the downregulation of pro-inflammatory cytokine secretion both systemically and locally (Schreiber et al., 1995).

HUMAN IMMUNODEFICIENCY VIRUS
In HIV infection, there is a progressive deterioration of cell-mediated immune responses as cytokine production and regulation become increasingly dysregulated (Blazevic et al., 1996). IL-10 is a cytokine that is overexpressed in HIV-infected individuals (Dereuddre-Bosquet

et al., 1997). Studies have demonstrated that IL-10 is expressed and produced spontaneously in PBMCs of those infected with HIV. IL-10 mRNA was detected in both T lymphocytes and monocytes and macrophages isolated from the peripheral blood of HIV-infected patients. It has also been shown that IL-10 inhibits the replication of the virus in infected monocytes and PBMCs in a dose-dependent manner (Masood *et al.*, 1994). The inhibitory effect of IL-10 on HIV replication in maturing monocytes is thought to be mediated mainly by the inhibition of cellular gene expression and the inhibition of maturation of monocytes into macrophages. This would result in the downregulation of HIV mRNA (Naif *et al.*, 1996). Study results show that HIV-specific T-cell antigens induce production of IL-10 in infected individuals. This increase in IL-10 may have a role in the immunosuppression of T cells often found in this virus infection (Blazevic *et al.*, 1996). Preclinical results of *in vitro* studies suggest that IL-10 can interfere with HIV replication in monocyte-derived macrophages (Koostra *et al.*, 1994). At present, results from a series of studies suggest that IL-10 may inhibit HIV replication or production at early stages of infection but may be detrimental in advanced stages of the disease when immune responses are compromised (de Waal Malefyt and Moore, 1998).

RHEUMATOID ARTHRITIS

Rheumatoid arthritis is an autoimmune disease with inflammatory manifestations in the peripheral synovial joints, which are infiltrated by activated T cells, macrophages, and plasma cells (Feldmann *et al.*, 1994). IL-10 has been found to have an inhibitory effect on synovial cells and is an important immunoregulatory component of the cytokine network in rheumatoid arthritis (Kawakami *et al.*, 1997). Biopsies from patients with rheumatoid arthritis and osteoarthritis suggest that IL-10 is spontaneously produced in both of these types of arthritis; in

rheumatoid arthritis, IL-10 is responsible for regulating monocyte and, in some cases, T-cell cytokine production (Katsikes *et al.*, 1994). Although IL-10 is present in the inflamed joints of patients with rheumatoid arthritis, its level of expression may not be sufficient for down-modulation of immune activation (Bucht *et al.*, 1996). Data indicate that endogenously produced IL-10 functions as an immunoregulatory molecule in rheumatoid synovium. Importantly, exogenous IL-10 has potent anti-inflammatory effects on synovial fluid mononuclear cells, suggesting that IL-10 may be useful in the treatment of patients with rheumatoid arthritis (Isomaki *et al.*, 1996).

SYSTEMIC LUPUS ERYTHEMATOSUS

In systemic lupus erythematosus (SLE), IL-10 is produced in large amounts by B lymphocytes and monocytes and is responsible for auto-antibody production (Emilie *et al.*, 1997). It has been previously reported that the production of IL-6 is often enhanced in SLE. Because the production of both IL-6 and IFN-α is regulated by IL-10, the enhancement of the production of these cytokines could reflect a defect in either IL-10 production or responsiveness. However, spontaneous production of IL-10 was enhanced in cultures of B cells and monocytes from patients with lupus compared with normal controls. These findings imply an abnormality in IL-10–mediated suppression in patients with SLE and that there may be an intrinsic defect in IL-10–induced suppression of cytokine synthesis. This could explain the increased levels of IL-10 and IL-6 found in this condition (Mongan *et al.*, 1997). Increased IL-10 production by non-T cells in SLE might exert an inhibitory effect on T_{h1} CD4$^+$ T cells, which would explain the decreased T-cell functions observed in these patients. The potential therapeutic use of monoclonal antibodies to IL-10 in patients with SLE seems to be gathering strength, whereas in rheumatoid arthritis, IL-10 is used as a therapeutic intervention (Alcocer-Varela *et al.*, 1996).

PSORIASIS

In a study comparing cytokine patterns of active and lesion-free skin in patients with psoriasis, it was found that lesional skin had an increased expression of mRNA for IL-2, IFN-γ, and lymphotoxin concurrent with a lack of the cytokines IL-4, IL-5, and IL-10 (Uyemura and Nickoloff, 1993). Cloned epidermal cells from psoriatic lesions produced IFN-γ, with only a minority producing IL-4. These same cells produced little or no IL-10 but high amounts of IL-2. Biopsies from psoriatic lesions confirmed production from mRNA of IFN-γ but not of IL-4 or IL-10 (Schlaak *et al.*, 1994). It has also been found that blister fluid from psoriatic lesions have significantly less IL-10 than fluids from noninvolved psoriatic skin and normal controls (Mussi *et al.*, 1994). When exogenously added to cultured psoriatic skin lesions, IL-10 has been shown to inhibit dendritic-cell function (Mitra *et al.*, 1995).

MULTIPLE SCLEROSIS

Low serum IL-10 levels have been found in patients with MS, regardless of clinical activity (Salmaggi *et al.*, 1996). Studies have observed that monocytes from these patients produce a significant amount of IL-10 when induced by IFN-β. Secretion of TNF-α and IL-6 was induced *in vitro* in PBMCs of these patients and in normal controls. When IL-10 was added to the cultures, TNF-α and IL-6 secretions were inhibited in both groups. Based on this result, it was suggested that IL-10 may block secretion of pro-inflammatory cytokines *in vivo* in patients with MS (Porrini *et al.*, 1995). Other studies have found that IFN-β induces upregulation of IL-10, which may have a therapeutic effect in relapsing-remitting MS (Rudick *et al.*, 1996).

Regulatory Approval

As of July 2000, IL-10 had not been approved by the FDA.

Nursing Considerations

Initial clinical investigation of IL-10 administered as a single IV or SC injection found very mild adverse effects. These included injection-site reactions, headaches, and myalgias (Huhn *et al.*, 1996). Many of these side effects can be effectively relieved with acetaminophen or ibuprofen. Moderate reductions in platelet counts associated with multiple-dose administration of IL-10 have been observed in patients with rheumatoid arthritis and Crohn's disease and healthy volunteers. Platelet counts did return to normal when the IL-10 was discontinued A trial is currently underway to investigate the mechanism of IL-10-induced thrombocytopenia in health volunteers.

Future Directions

IL-10 plays a major regulatory role in the course of inflammatory responses by downregulating the synthesis of cytokines and cell-mediated immunity and upregulating humoral immune responses. The evaluation of IL-10 in clinical trials for management of autoimmune and infectious disease is currently in progress. Many phase I/II studies have been completed; few, however, have been published. The therapeutic role of IL-10 will continue to be explored in a variety of laboratory and clinical settings (Opal *et al.*, 1998; Sands, 1999). Challenges to developing such new therapeutic strategies include not only identifying novel agents and defining their effects *in vivo* (Huhn *et al.*, 1999) but also improving the definition of clinical end points and efficacy at the biological level.

Interleukin-12

IL-12 is a cytokine with potent immunoregulatory and antitumor activity. IL-12 was discovered independently by Genetics Institute, Cambridge, MA; Wistar Institute, Philadelphia, PA; and Hoffmann-La Roche, Nutley, NJ. It was originally given the names "natural killer cell stimulatory factor" and "cytokine lymphocyte maturation factor" based on its stimulatory effects on these cytolytic lymphokine populations (Atkins *et al.*, 1997). This cytokine provides an important link between natural resistance (mediated by NK cells) and adaptive immune responses (mediated by T cells). IL-12 is unusual compared with other cytokines because it is a heterodimer composed of 2 subunits that represent unrelated gene products (Chizzonite *et al.*, 1998). Monocytes appear to be the major source of IL-12 in activated PBMC suspensions *in vitro* (D'Andrea *et al.*, 1992). Epstein-Barr virus–transformed B cells and other APCs (antigen-presenting cells) also appear to produce IL-12 (Kobayashi *et al.*, 1989; Cassatella *et al.*, 1995; Chizzonite *et al.*, 1998; Storkus *et al.*, 1998).

Biological Actions

Once produced, IL-12 allows continued proliferation of activated T and NK cells (Gately *et al.*, 1991; Bertagnolli *et al.*, 1992; Perussia *et al.*, 1992). IL-12 is able to activate spontaneously cytotoxic human NK/LAK cells to become cytolytic. IL-12 is also a potent inducer of IFN-γ release from both T lymphocytes and NK cells, while inducing much lower amounts of other inflammatory cytokines (Mier *et al.*, 1988; Naume *et al.*, 1992). IL-12 promotes T_{h1} cell development while inhibiting T_{h2} cell development. T_{h1} cells produce IL-2 and IFN and stimulate cell-mediated immunity; T_{h2} cells produce IL-4, IL-5, and IL-10 (Mossman *et al.*,

1986; Germann *et al.*, 1993; Scott, 1993). It is also thought that IL-12 may mediate humoral immunity by enhancing production of antigen-specific murine IgG_2a antibodies *in vivo* and altering isotope profiles of primary and secondary antibody responses (Metzger *et al.*, 1995). The IL-12 receptor has 2 known subunits now classified as IL-12Rβ_1 and IL-12Rβ_2. Coexpression of these two subunits leads to the formation of a functional high-affinity IL-12 receptor complex (Chizzonite *et al.*, 1998).

Clinical Trials

The clinical evaluation of IL-12 as treatment for patients with cancer remains in its early stages. One of the earliest clinical trials involved patients with metastatic cancer who were refractory to standard therapy. The study was a randomized, multicenter, phase I, dose-escalation trial. In this study, IL-12 was administered by bolus IV injection initially as a single test dose, then daily for 5 days every 3 weeks, for 6 maximum 5-day cycles. Forty patients were treated (the majority had MRCC or MM at doses ranging from 3 to 1,000 ng/kg. The MTD on this regimen was determined to be 500 ng/kg. A total of 14 patients were treated at this dose level (Atkins *et al.*, 1997), and the dose and schedule were essentially well tolerated by all 14 patients treated in the dose-escalation and safety studies. Biological effects included dose-dependent increases in circulating IFN-γ, which exhibited attenuation with subsequent cycles, increases in serum neopterin levels (a measure of immune activation), and no detectable levels of TNF-α.

A phase II trial of IL-12 administration at 500 ng/kg using the same schedule as the phase I trials but without the single test dose was initiated in MRCC in 4 institutions. Unfortunately, this trial had to be closed because of unexpected severe toxicity. Of the 17 patients treated, 12 were hospitalized, and 2 of the 12 died. In contrast to the phase I study, most patients in the phase II study experienced serious adverse events during the first cycle with some patients unable to tolerate more than 2 successive doses of the IL-12. The clinical study was halted immediately, and no patient entered a second cycle. The adverse events involved multiple organ systems and were associated with constitutional, cardiac, renal, hematopoietic, hepatic, neurologic, and gastrointestinal toxicities. Extensive analysis confirmed that a single injection of IL-12 1 week before starting the consecutive daily treatment with IL-12 has a profound and unexpected abrogating effect on toxicity (Atkins *et al.*, 1997; Leonard *et al.*, 1997). Due to this unique, schedule-dependent phenomenon, careful attention to dose and especially schedule has been required to ensure safe and effective clinical development of this highly promising cytokine. Additional clinical studies of IL-12 have been conducted, and several hundred subjects have been safely treated (Genetics Institute, Inc., unpublished data).

Another pilot study was initiated at a single center with 10 previously treated patients who had progressive MM. Patients received IL-12 at a dosage of 0.5 mcg/kg by SC injection for 2 identical 28-day cycles. Injections were administered on days 1, 8, and 15 of each cycle. If the patients had evidence of response or disease stabilization, the treatment was continued for 2 additional cycles. Toxicity consisted mainly of flu-like symptoms, transient increases in transaminases (6 of 10 patients), and triglyceridemia (8 of 10 patients). Peak serum levels of IL-12 were reached 8 to 12 hours after the first injection in all patients. No serum IL-12 was detected in 6 of 9 evaluable patients after the last injection of the second cycle, and no antibody response to rhIL-12 could be detected in any of the patients. Tumor shrinkage, not reaching PR or CR, was exhibited as regression of SC nodules in 2 of 3 patients. Tumor regression was detected after the first cycle of treatment and maintained in spite of progression at different sites. Based on the results of this study, the investigators concluded that SC rhIL-12 is well tolerated and has potential antitumor activity. Further trials may investigate the safety and tolerability of IL-12 at a dose of 0.75 mcg/kg SC. It is possible that this dosage can be administered without reaching the dose-limiting liver toxicity and leukopenias observed at higher doses and would translate into an improved therapeutic benefit (Bajetta *et al.*, 1998). Patients with renal cell carcinoma have also been treated with a similar regimen at dose levels of 0.1, 0.5, and 1.0 mcg/kg in cohorts of 3 to 6 subjects. On the basis of the toxicity profile, a second scheme (up-titration) was undertaken in which rhIL-12 was escalated for each patient from week 1 to week 2 to a target dose given from week 3 and continuing thereafter. Target dose levels in this scheme were 0.5, 0.75, 1.0, 1.25, and 1.5 mcg/kg. The MTD for the fixed-dose scheme was 1.0 mcg/kg with dose-limiting toxicities of increased liver transaminases, pulmonary toxicity, and leukopenia. With the up-titration scheme, the MTD was 1.5 mcg/kg. Of 50 evaluable patients treated, 1 had a CR, 34 had stable disease, and 14 showed progression of disease. The authors concluded that rhIL-12 was well tolerated by SC injection. Phase II trials have been initiated in patients with renal cell carcinoma and melanoma (Motzer *et al.*, 1998).

Regulatory Approval

As of July 2000, IL-12 had not been approved by the FDA. Golab and Zagozdon (1999) have outlined the clinical trials of IL-12 that have been conducted and the side effects noted.

Side Effects

Based on the phase I/II trials conducted in patients with metastatic disease, the potential side effects of IL-12 are flu-like symptoms; skin problems, and cardiac, gastrointestinal, hematologic; liver, metabolic, renal, and respiratory toxicities. Most side effects of IL-12 were proportional in frequency and severity to the dose level administered. The side effects described here are based on the MTD unless otherwise noted (Atkins *et al.*, 1997; Leonard *et al.*, 1997; Bajetta *et al.*, 1998).

Flu-like symptoms included fever (usually occurring 8 to 12 hours after the IV administration and 12 to 24 hours after SC administration), chills, fatigue, headache, and myalgias. These conditions were universal at all dose levels. The cardiac conditions included orthostasis with dehydration, which was observed in 1 patient but was not thought to be related to the IL-12. Among the gastrointestinal toxicities noted, nausea and vomiting were rare; however, stomatitis has been reported, appears to be dose-dependent, and usually resolves within 3 days. Gastrointestinal bleeding was observed but was not thought to be directly related to the IL-12. No mucositis was documented. One patient was admitted for abdominal pain and anemia and died following rapid onset of shock. The death was felt to be secondary to sepsis, presumably from necrotic intra-abdominal tumor, and was classified as "possibly related to the IL-12." Anemia, neutropenia, and thrombocytopenia were the hematologic toxicities noted and appeared to be independent of dose. Absolute neutrophil count nadir occurred around day 5 of each cycle without cumulative toxicity, and full recovery occurred by day 15. Lymphocytopenia occurred in a majority of patients at all dose levels and resolved without rebound of lymphocytosis. Hypertransaminasemia as well as increases in alkaline phosphatase, bilirubin, and lactate dehydrogenase levels were dose-dependent. Hypoalbuminemia was also documented. Levels usually returned to baseline in 7 to 10 days. Hyperglycemia and increases in triglyceride levels were observed frequently. BUN and creatinine levels were not found to be elevated. A slight decrease in CO_2 diffusion was noted (grade 1). In 10% of patients who received IL-12 by SC administration, SC induration occurred at the site of the injection. Skin rashes were rare.

Nursing Considerations

It is important to note that fevers have a delayed onset with IL-12. When IL-12 is administered intravenously, the fevers may occur 8 to 12 hours after administration. The fever may be incompletely suppressed with nonsteroidal anti-inflammatory drugs. Fevers may occur 12 to 24 hours after SC administration and may wane in a median 3 days. When IL-12 is administered SC, fever is usually easily treated with acetaminophen. To monitor for potential gastrointestinal bleeding, patients should have a rectal examination to assess for blood in the stool.

Future Directions

IL-12 is an experimental agent that continues to be studied and should not be considered a treatment option. Several studies in the area of oncology are ongoing and the data has yet to be analyzed. New clinical trials are being developed to determine the therapeutic role of IL-12 in several diseases, including melanoma.

Summary

The ILs play a pivotal role in maintaining the complex balance of the human immune system. ILs provide a communication link among a wide variety of cells within the body, including T cells, B cells, macrophages, hematopoietic cells, and antigen-producing cells. Knowledge of the roles and functions of the ILs continues to grow, with new ILs identified almost yearly. Further clinical study will continue to elucidate the role of ILs in the pathophysiology of disease and in the treatment of cancer and other diseases. Many opportunities are available for nurses in the study of new ILs and the discovery of new applications for existing ILs.

References

Abi-aad, A., Figlin, R., Belldegrun, A., et al. 1991. Metastatic renal cell cancer: Interleukin-2 toxicity induced by contrast agent injections. *Journal of Immunotherapy* 10: 292–295.

Aderka, D., Manor, Y., Novick, D., et al. 1993. Interleukin-6 inhibits the proliferation of B-chronic lymphocytic leukemia cells that is induced by the tumor necrosis factor-α or -β. *Blood* 81(8): 2076–2084.

Alcocer-Varela, J., Llorente, L., and Alarcon-Segovia, D. 1996. Immunoregulatory circuits and potential treatment of connective tissue diseases. *Journal of International Archives of Allergy and Immunology* 111: 348–354.

Atkins, M. 1997. Interleukin-2 in metastatic melanoma: Establishing a role. *The Cancer Journal from Scientific American* 3(suppl 1): S35–S36.

Atkins, M., and Mier, J. (eds). 1993. *Therapeutic Application of Interleukin-2.* New York, NY: Marcel Dekker, pp. 3–476.

Atkins, M., Robertson, M., Gordon, M., et al. 1997. Phase I evaluation of intravenous recombinant human interleukin-12 in patients with advanced malignancies. *Journal of Clinical Cancer Research* 3: 409–417.

Atkins, M., Vachino, G., Tilg, H., et al. 1992. Phase I evaluation of thrice-daily intravenous bolus interleukin-4 in patients with refractory malig-

nancy. *Journal of Clinical Oncology* 10(11): 1802–1809.

Atzpodien, J., Poliwoda, H., and Kirchner, H. 1991. Alpha-interferon and interleukin-2 in renal cell carcinoma: Studies in non-hospitalized patients. *Seminars in Oncology* 18(5 suppl 7): 108–112.

Aulitzky, W., Schuler, M., Peschel, C., et al. 1994. Interleukins: Clinical pharmacology and therapeutic use. *Drugs* 48(5): 667–677.

Bagby, G., Dinarello, C., Neerhout, R., et al. 1988. Interleukin-1 dependent paracrine granulopoiesis in chronic granulocytic leukemia of the juvenile type. *Journal of Clinical Investigations* 82: 1430–1436.

Bajetta, E., Del Vecchio, M., Mortarini, R., et al. 1998. Pilot study of subcutaneous recombinant human interleukin-12 in metastatic melanoma. *Journal of Clinical Cancer Research* 1(4): 75–85.

Barth, R.J., Jr., and Mulé, J.J. 2000. Interleukin-2: Preclinical trials. In Rosenberg, S.A. (ed). *Principles and Practice of Biologic Therapy of Cancer.* 3rd edn. Philadelphia, PA: Lippincott, Williams & Wilkins, pp. 19–31.

Bertagnolli, M., Lin, B-Y., Young, D., et al. 1992. IL-12 augments antigen-dependent proliferation of activated T lymphoctyes. *Journal of Immunology* 149: 3778–3783.

Berthiaume, Y., Boiteau, P., Fick, G., et al. 1995. Pulmonary edema during IL-2 therapy: Combined effect of increased permeability and hydrostatic pressure. *American Journal of Respiratory Critical Care Medicine* 152: 329–335.

Blazevic, V., Heino, M., Lagerstedt, A., et al. 1996. Interleukin-10 gene expression induced by HIV-1 Tat and Rev in the cells of HIV-1 infected individuals. *Journal of Acquired Immune Deficiency Syndrome Human Retrovirology* 13(3): 208–214.

Bock, S., Lee, R., Fisher, B., et al. 1990. A prospective randomized trial evaluating prophylactic antibiotics to prevent triple-lumen catheter-related sepsis in patients treated with immunotherapy. *Journal of Clinical Oncology* 8(1): 161–169.

Boldt, D., and Ellis, T. 1993. Biological effects of

interleukin-2 administration on the immune system. In Atkins, M., and Mier, J. (eds). *Therapeutic Applications of Interleukin-2.* New York, NY: Marcel Dekker, pp. 73–91.

Brogley, J., and Sharp, E. 1990. Nursing care of patients receiving activated lymphocytes. *Oncology Nursing Forum* 17(2): 187–193.

Bucht, A., Larsson, P., Weisbrot, L., *et al.* 1996. Expression of interferon-gamma, IL-10, IL-12 and transforming growth factor-beta mRNA in synovial fluid cells from patients in the early and late phases of rheumatoid arthritis. *Journal of Clinical Experimental Immunology* 103: 357–367.

Bukowski, R. 1997. Natural history and therapy of metastatic renal cell carcinoma: The role of interleukin-2. *Cancer* 80(7): 1198–1220.

Bukowski, R. 1999. Immunotherapy in renal cell carcinoma. *Oncology* 13(6): 801–809.

Bukowski, R., Rayman, P., Gibson, V., *et al.* 1992. Treatment of human metastatic renal cell carcinoma with IL-2/IL-4-grown tumor-infiltrating lymphocytes (TIL) and rIL-2. *Proceedings of the Annual Meeting of the American Association of Cancer Research* 33: A1941, p. 325.

Burdin, N., Peronne, C., Banchereau, J., *et al.* 1993. Epstein-Barr virus transformation induces B lymphocytes to produce human interleukin-10. *Journal of Experimental Medicine* 177: 295–304.

Cassatella, M., Meda, L., Gasperini, S., *et al.* 1995. Interleukin-12 production by human polymorphonuclear leukocytes. *European Journal of Immunology* 25: 1–5.

Castell, J., Gomez-Lechon, M., David, M., *et al.* 1989. Interleukin-6 is a major regulator of acute phase protein synthesis in adult human hepatocytes. *FEBS Letter* 242: 237–257.

Castelli, M., Black, P., Schneider, M., *et al.* 1988. Protective, restorative, and therapeutic properties of recombinant human IL-1 in rodent model. *Journal of Immunology* 140: 3830–3837.

Cetus Corporation. 1992. Proleukin® (aldesleukin) package insert. Emeryville, CA: Chiron Corporation.

Chen, Y., Shiao, R., Labayog, J., *et al.* 1997. Modulation of interleukin-6/interleukin-6 receptor cytokine loop in the treatment of multiple myeloma. *Leukemia and Lymphoma* 27(1–2): 11–23.

Chiron Corporation. 1994. Proleukin® (Aldesleukin) package insert. Emeryville, CA: Chiron Corporation.

Chiron Corporation. 1998. Press release: Chiron's Proleukin® granted a marketing license by the FDA for new metastatic melanoma indication. Emeryville, CA: Chiron Corporation.

Chizzonite, R., Gubler, U., Magram, J., *et al.* 1998. Interleukin-12. In Mire-Sluis, A., and Thorpe, R. (eds). *Cytokines.* San Diego, CA: Academic Press, pp. 183–203.

Chomarat, P., Rybak, M., and Banchereau, J. 1998. Interleukin-4. In Thomson, A. (ed). *The Cytokine Handbook*, 3rd edn. San Diego, CA: Academic Press, pp. 133–174.

Choyke, P., Miller, D., Lotze, M., *et al.* 1992. Delayed reactions to contrast media after IL-2 therapy. *Radiology* 183(1): 111–114.

Cohen, M., and Cohen, S. 1996. Cytokine function: A study of biological diversity. *American Journal of Clinical Pathology* 105(5): 589–598.

Colatta, F., Ghezzi, P., and Mantovani, A. 1998. Interleukin 1. In Mire-Sluis, A., and Thorpe, R. (eds). *Cytokines.* San Diego, CA: Academic Press, pp. 1–18.

Crawford, R., Finbloom, D., Ohara, J., *et al.* 1987. BSF-1: A new macrophage activation factor: B cell stimulatory factor-1 (interleukin-4) activates macrophages for increased tumoricidal activity and expression in Ia antigens. *Journal of Immunology* 139(1): 135–141.

Crown, J., Jakubowski, A., Kemeny, N., *et al.* 1991. A phase I trial of recombinant human interleukin-1β alone and in combination with myelosuppressive doses of 5-fluorouracil in patients with gastrointestinal cancer. *Blood* 78(6): 1420–1427.

Curti, B., and Smith, J. 1995. Interleukin-1 in the treatment of cancer. *Pharmacology and Therapeutics* 65(3): 291–302.

D'Andrea, A., Rengaraju, M., and Valiante, N. 1992.

Production of natural killer cell stimulatory factor (interleukin-12) by peripheral blood mononuclear cells. *Journal of Experimental Medicine* 176: 1387–1398.

D'Angelica, M., and Fong, Y. 1998. Cytokine gene therapy for human tumors. *Surgical Oncology Clinics of North America* 7(3): 537–563.

Dawson, M. (ed). 1991. *Lymphokines and Interleukins*. Boca Raton, FL: CRC Press.

Dereuddre-Bosquet, N., Clayette, P., Martin, M., *et al.* 1997. Lack of interleukin-10 expression in monocyte-derived macrophages in response to in vitro infection by HIV type 1 isolates. *Journal of AIDS Research in Human Retroviruses* 13: 961–966.

de Waal Melefyt, R., Abrams, J., Bennett, B., *et al.* 1991. IL-10 inhibits cytokine synthesis by human monocytes: An autoregulatory role of IL-10 produced by monocytes. *Journal of Experimental Medicine* 174: 1209–1220.

de Waal Malefyt, R., and Moore, K. 1998. Interleukin-10. In Thomson, A. (ed). *The Cytokine Handbook*, 3rd edn. San Diego, CA: Academic Press, pp. 333–364.

DeVita, V., Hellman, S., and Rosenberg, S. (eds). 1995. *Biologic Therapy of Cancer*, 2nd edn. Philadelphia, PA: J.B. Lippincott, p. 88.

Dillman, R., Church, C., Oldham, R., *et al.* 1993. Inpatient continuous-infusion interleukin-2 in 788 patients with cancer. *Cancer* 71(7): 2358–2370.

Dillman, R., Oldham, R., Barth, N., *et al.* 1991. Continuous interleukin-2 and tumor-infiltrating lymphocytes as treatment of advanced melanoma. *Cancer* 68(1): 1–8.

Dinarello, C. 1991. Interleukin-1 and interleukin-1 antagonism. *Blood* 77(8): 1625–1652.

Dinarello, C. 1998a. Interleukin-1. In Thomson, A. (ed). *The Cytokine Handbook,* 3rd edn. San Diego, CA: Academic Press, pp. 35–72.

Dinarello, C. 1998b. Interleukin-1, interleukin-1 receptors and interleukin-1 receptor antagonist. *International Reviews in Immunology* 16: 457–499.

Dinarello, C., and Wolff, S. 1993. The role of interleukin-1 in disease. *The New England Journal of Medicine* 328(2): 106–113.

Dosik, D., Chachoua, A., Oratz, R., *et al.* 1996. Phase I study of IL-1α combined with high dose cisplatinum (CDDP) in patients (PTS) with metastatic melanoma. *Proceedings of American Society of Clinical Oncology* 15: A1369, p. 440.

Dudjak, L. 1993. Rationale and therapeutic basis for patients receiving recombinant interleukin-2. *Seminars in Oncology Nursing* 9(3 suppl 1): 3–7.

Dutcher, J.P., Atkins, M., Fisher, R., *et al.* 1997. Interleukin-2 based therapy for metastatic renal cell cancer: The cytokine working group experience, 1989–1997. *The Cancer Journal from Scientific American* 3(suppl 1): S73–S78.

Edwards, M., Heniford, B., Klar, E., *et al.* 1992. Pentoxifylline inhibits interleukin-2 induced toxicity in C57BL/6 mice but preserves antitumor efficacy. *Journal of Clinical Investigations* 90(2): 637–641.

Eisenberg, S., Evans, R., Arend, W., *et al.* 1990. Primary structure and functional expression from complementary DNA of a human interleukin-1 receptor antagonism. *Nature* 343: 341–346.

Emilie, D., Zou, W., Fior, R., *et al.* 1997. Production and roles of IL-6, IL-10, and IL-13 in B-lymphocyte hyperactivity of HIV infection and autoimmunity. *Methods* 11: 133–142.

Farrell, M. 1992. The challenge of adult respiratory distress syndrome during interleukin-2 immunotherapy. *Oncology Nursing Forum* 19(3): 475–480.

Fay, J.W., Collins, R., Bheiro, L., *et al.* 1994. Concomitant administration of interleukin-6 and Leucomax following autologous bone marrow transplantation—A phase I trial update. *American Society of Clinical Oncology Program/Proceedings* 13: A247, p. 111.

Fefer, A. 1997. Interleukin-2 in the treatment of hematologic malignancies. *The Cancer Journal from Scientific American* 3(suppl 1): S35–S36.

Fefer, A., Benyunes, M., Higuchi, C., *et al.* 1993. Interleukin-2 ± lymphocytes as consolidative immunotherapy after autologous bone marrow transplantation. *Acta of Haematology* 89 (suppl 1): 2–7.

Feldmann, M., Brennan, F.M., Elliott, M., *et al.* 1994. TNF alpha as a therapeutic target in rheumatoid arthritis. *Circulatory and Shock* 43: 179–184.

Feldmann, M., and Male, D. 1989. Cell cooperation in the antibody response. In Roitt, I., Brostoff, J., and Male, D. (eds). *Immunology*. Philadelphia, PA: J.B. Lippincott, pp. 8.1–8.12.

Figlin, R.A. 1997. Renal cell carcinoma and interleukin-2: What are the endpoints? *The Cancer Journal from Scientific American* 3(suppl 1): S68–S69.

Figlin, R., Pierce, W., Kaboo, R., *et al.* 1997. Treatment of metastatic renal cell carcinoma with nephrectomy, interleukin-2 and cytokine-primed or CD8(+) selected tumor infiltrating lymphocytes from primary tumor. *Journal of Urology* 158(3 Pt 1): 740–745.

Figlin, R., Thompson, J.B.R., Bukowski, R. M., *et al.* 1999. A multicenter, randomized phase III trial of CD8+ tumor-infiltrating lymphocytes in combination with recombinant interleukin-2 in metastatic renal carcinoma. *Journal of Clinical Oncology* 17: 2521–2529.

Fiorentino, D., Zlotnik, A., Vieira, P., *et al.* 1991. IL-10 acts on the antigen presenting cell to inhibit cytokine production by T_{h1} cells. *Journal of Immunology* 146: 3444–3451.

Fisher, B., Keenan, A., Garra, B., *et al.* 1989. Interleukin-2 induces profound reversible cholestasis: A detailed analysis in treated cancer patients. *Journal of Clinical Oncology* 7(12): 1852–1862.

Fisher, R.I., Rosenberg, S.A., and Fyfe, G. 2000. Long-term survival update for high-dose recombinant interleukin-2 in patients with renal cell carcinoma. *The Cancer Journal from Scientific American* 6(suppl 1): S55–S57.

Fisher, C., and Zheng, Y. 1996. Potential strategies for inflammatory mediator manipulation: Retrospect and prospect. *World Journal of Surgery* 20(4): 447–453.

Fishman, J., Aberle, D., Moldawer, N., *et al.* 1991. A typical contrast reaction associated with systemic interleukin-2 therapy. *American Journal of Roentgenology* 156(4): 833–834.

Flaherty, L.E. 2000. Rationale for intergroup trial E-3695 comparing concurrent biochemotherapy with cisplatin, vinblastine, and DTIC alone in patients with metastatic melanoma. *The Cancer Journal of Scientific American* 6(suppl 1): 515–520.

Forman, A. 1994. Neurologic complications of cytokine therapy. *Oncology* 8(4): 105–110.

Futami, H., Jansen, R., MacPhee, M., *et al.* 1990. Chemoprotective effects of recombinant human IL-1α in cyclophosphamide-treated normal and tumor-bearing mice. *Journal of Immunology* 145: 4121–4130.

Gaffen, S., Goldsmith, M., and Greene, W. 1998. Interleukin-2 and the interleukin-2 receptor. In Thomson, A. (ed). *The Cytokine Handbook*, 3rd edn. San Diego, CA: Academic Press, pp. 73–103.

Gale, D. 1997. Part II: Nursing management guidelines. *Biotherapy: Considerations for Oncology Nurses* 2(1): 3–5.

Gately, M., Desai, B., Wolitzky, A., *et al.* 1991. Regulation of human lymphocyte proliferation by a heterodimeric cytokine, IL-12 (cytotoxic lymphocyte maturation factor). *Journal of Immunology* 147: 874–882.

Gaynor, E., and Fisher, R. 1993. Hemodynamic and cardiovascular effects of interleukin-2. In Atkins, M., and Mier, J. (eds). *Therapeutic Applications of Interleukin-2*. New York, NY: Marcel Dekker, pp. 381–388.

Germann, T., Gately, M., Schoenhaut, D., *et al.* 1993. Interleukin-12/T cell stimulating factor, a cytokine with multiple effects on T helper type 1 but not T helper type 2 cells. *European Journal of Immunology* 23: 1762–1770.

Gery, I., Gershon, R., and Waksman, B. 1972. Potentiation of the T-lymphocyte response to mitogens. I. The responding cell. *Journal of Experimental Medicine* 136(1): 128–142.

Gilleece, M., Scarffe, J., Ghosh, A., *et al.* 1992.

Recombinant human interleukin-4 (IL-4) given as daily subcutaneous injections—A phase I dose toxicity trial. *British Journal of Cancer* 66(1): 204–210.

Golab, J., and Zagozdon, R. 1999. Antitumor effects of interleukin-12 in pre-clinical and early clinical studies. *International Journal of Molecular Medicine* 3(5): 537–544.

Gold, P., Thompson, J., Markowitz, D., *et al.* 1997. Metastatic renal cell carcinoma: Long term survival after therapy with high-dose continuous-infusion interleukin-2. *The Cancer Journal from Scientific American* 3(suppl 1): S85–S91.

Grimm, E. 1993. Properties of IL-2 activated lymphocytes. In Atkins, M., and Mier, J. (eds). *Therapeutic Applications of Interleukin-2*. New York, NY: Marcel Dekker, pp. 27–38.

Guleria, A., Yang, J., Topalian, S., *et al.* 1994. Renal dysfunction associated with high-dose interleukin-2 in 199 consecutive patients with metastatic melanoma and renal cancer. *Journal of Clinical Oncology* 12: 2714–2722.

Haegeman, G., Content, J., Volckaert, G., *et al.* 1986. Structural analysis of the sequence encoding for an inducible 26-kDa protein in human fibroblasts. *European Journal of Biochemistry* 159: 625–632.

Hamm, J., Dimitrov, N., and Vogel, C. 1997. A phase III study utilizing recombinant human IL-6 with G-CSF versus placebo with G-CSF following high-dose cytoxan and Adriamycin in patients with advanced breast cancer. *American Society of Clinical Oncology Program/Proceedings* 16: 107a.

Hartman, L., Urba, W., Steis, R., *et al.* 1989. Use of prophylactic antibiotics for prevention of intravascular catheter-related infections in interleukin-2 treated patients. *Journal of the National Cancer Institute* 81(15): 1190–1193.

Herodin, F., Mestries, J., Janodet, D., *et al.* 1992. Recombinant glycosylated human interleukin-6 accelerates peripheral blood platelet count recovery in radiation-induced bone marrow depression in baboons. *Blood* 80(3): 688–695.

Hibi, M., Nakajima, K., and Hirano, T. 1996. IL-6 cytokine family and signal transduction: A model of the cytokine system. *Journal of Molecular Medicine* 74 (1): 1–12.

Higuchi, C., Thompson, J., Lindgren, C., *et al.* 1989. Induction of lymphokine-activated killer activity by interleukin-4 in human lymphocytes pre-activated by interleukin-2 in vivo or in vitro. *Cancer Research* 49(23): 6487–6492.

Higuchi, C., Thompson, J., Peterson, F., *et al.* 1991. Toxicity and immunomodulatory effects of interleukin-2 after autologous bone marrow transplantation for hematologic malignancies. *Blood* 77: 2561–2568.

Hirano, T. 1998. Interleukin-6. In Thomson, A. (ed). *The Cytokine Handbook*, 3rd edn. San Diego, CA: Academic Press, pp. 197–228.

Hochster, H., Speyer, J., Mandeli, J., *et al.* 1999. A phase II double-blind randomized study of the simultaneous administration of recombinant human interleukin-6 and recombinant human granulocyte colony-stimulating factor following paclitaxel and carboplatin chemotherapy in patients with advanced epithelial ovarian cancer. *Gynecologic Oncology* 72(3): 292–297.

Holcombe, R. 1994. Clinical applications of interleukins: Present and future. *Journal of the Louisiana State Medical Society* 146(11): 479–483.

Hossan, E., and Rieger, P. 1997. Interleukin-2 therapy: Nursing management plus education equals success in the ambulatory setting. *Biotherapy: Considerations for Oncology Nurses* 2(2): 1–7.

Howard, M., Farrar, J., Hilfiker, M., *et al.* 1982. Identification of a T-cell derived B-cell growth factor distinct from interleukin-2. *Journal of Experimental Medicine* 155(3): 914–923.

Huhn, R., Pennline, K., Radwanski, E., *et al.* 1999. Effects of single intravenous doses of recombinant human interleukin-10 on subsets of circulating leukocytes in humans. *Immunopharmacology* 41(2): 109–117.

Huhn, R., Radwanski, E., O'Connell, S., *et al.* 1996. Pharmacokinetics and immunomodulatory properties of intravenously administered recombinant human interleukin-10 to healthy volunteers. *Blood* 87: 699–705.

Huland, E., Heinzer, H., and Huland, H. 1999. Treatment of pulmonary metastatic renal-cell carcinoma in 116 patients using inhaled interleukin-2 (IL-2). *Anticancer Research* 19(4A): 2679–2683.

Ihle, J., Witthuln, B., Quelle, F., *et al.* 1994. Signaling by the cytokine receptor superfamily, JAKs and STATs. *Trends in Biochemical Science* 19: 222–227.

Isomaki, P., Luukkainen, R., Saario, R., *et al.* 1996. Interleukin-10 functions as an anti-inflammatory cytokine in rheumatoid arthritis. *Arthritis Rheumatology* 39: 386–395.

Itoh, K., and Balch, C. 1993. Properties of human tumor-infiltrating lymphocytes. In Atkins, M., and Mier, J. (eds). *Therapeutic Applications of Interleukin-2*. New York, NY: Marcel Dekker, pp. 39–48.

Jansen, J., Fibbe, W., Willemze, R., *et al.* 1990. Interleukin-4: A regulatory protein. *Blut* 60: 269–274.

Johnson, C. 1993. Interleukin-1: Therapeutic potential for solid tumors. *Cancer Investigation* 11(5): 600–608.

Kammuller, M. 1995. Recombinant human interleukin-6: Safety issues of a pleiotropic growth factor. *Toxicology* 105: 91–107.

Katsikes, P., Chu, C., Brennan F., *et al.* 1994. Immunoregulatory role of interleukin-10 in rheumatoid arthritis. *Journal of Experimental Medicine* 179: 1517–1527.

Kawakami, A., Eguchi, K., Matsuoka, N., *et al.* 1997. Inhibitory effects of interleukin-10 on synovial cells of rheumatoid arthritis. *Immunology* 91: 252–259.

Kawakami, Y., Rosenberg, S., and Lotze, M. 1988. Interleukin-4 promotes the growth of tumor infiltrating lymphocytes cytotoxic for human autologous melanoma. *Journal of Experimental Medicine* 168(6): 2183–2191.

Khatri, V., Baiocchi, R., Bernstein, Z., *et al.* 1997.

Immunotherapy with low-dose interleukin-2: Rationale for prevention of immune-deficiency-associated cancer. *Cancer Journal from Scientific American* 3(suppl 1): S128–S136.

Khayat, D., Borel, C., Tourani, J., *et al.* 1993. Sequential chemoimmunotherapy with cisplatin, interleukin-2 and interferon alfa-2a for metastatic melanoma. *Journal of Clinical Oncology* 11: 2172–2180.

Klempner, M., and Snydman, D. 1993. Infectious complications associated with interleukin-2. In Atkins, M., and Mier, J. (eds). *Therapeutic Applications of Interleukin-2*. New York, NY: Marcel Dekker, pp. 409–424.

Kluth, D., and Rees, A. 1996. Inhibiting inflammatory cytokines. *Seminars in Nephrology* 16(6): 576–582.

Kobayashi, M., Fitz, L., Ryan, M., *et al.* 1989. Identification and purification of natural killer cell stimulatory factor, a cytokine with multiple biologic effects on human lymphocytes. *Journal of Experimental Medicine* 170: 827–845.

Koostra, N., Van'tWout, A., Huisman, H., *et al.* 1994. Interference of interleukin-10 with human immunodeficiency virus type 1 replication in primary monocyte-derived macrophages. *Journal of Virology* 68: 6967–6975.

Kuby, J. 1997. Cytokines. In Kuby, J. (ed). *Immunology*, 3rd edn. New York, NY: W.H. Freeman, pp. 313–334.

Kucharzik, T., Lugering, N., Adolf, M., *et al.* 1997. Synergistic effect of immunoregulatory cytokines on peripheral blood monocytes from patients with inflammatory bowel disease. *Digestive Disease Science* 42: 805–812.

Kucharzik, T., Lugering, N., Weigelt, H., *et al.* 1996. Immunoregulatory properties of IL-13 in patients with inflammatory bowel disease, comparison with IL-4 and IL-10. *Clinics in Experimental Immunology* 104: 483–490.

Kucharzik, T., Stoll, R., Lugering, N., *et al.* 1995. Circulating anti-inflammatory cytokine IL-10 in patients with inflammatory bowel disease (IBD).

Clinics in Experimental Immunology 100: 452–456.

Laughlin, M., Kirkpatrick, G., Sabiston, N., *et al.* 1993. Hematopoietic recovery following high-dose combined alkylating-agent chemotherapy and autologous bone marrow support in patients in phase I clinical trials of colony stimulating factors: G-CSF, GM-CSF, IL-1, IL-2 and MCSF. *Annals in Hematology* 67: 267–276.

Leach, M., Rybak, M., and Rosenblum, I. 1997. Safety evaluation of recombinant human interleukin-4. II. Clinical studies. *Immunology and Immunopathology* 83(1): 12–14.

Legha, S., and Buzaid, A. 1993. Role of recombinant interleukin-2 in combination with interferon-alpha and chemotherapy in the treatment of advanced melanoma. *Seminars in Oncology* 20(6 suppl 9): 27–32.

Legha, S., Ring, S., Bedikian, A., *et al.* 1993. Biochemotherapy using interleukin-2 + interferon alpha-2a (IFN) in combination with cisplatin (C), vinblastine (V), and DTIC (D) in patients with metastatic melanoma. *Third International Conference on Melanoma: Abstracts* 3: 32–33.

Legha, S., Ring, S., Eton, O., *et al.* 1998. Development of a biochemotherapy regimen with concurrent administration of cisplatin, vinblastine, dacarbazine, interferon alfa, and interleukin-2 for patients with metastatic melanoma. *Journal of Clinical Oncology* 16(5): 1752–1759.

Leonard, J., Sherman, M., Fisher, G., *et al.* 1997. Effects of single-dose Interleukin-12 exposure on Interleukin-12 associated toxicity and interferon-γ production. *Journal of Blood* 90: 2541–2548.

Lestingi, T.M., Richards, J., Schulman, K., *et al.* 1994. Pilot phase II study of recombinant human interleukin-6 (rhIL-6) and chemotherapy (CT) in metastatic melanoma. *American Society of Clinical Oncology Program/Proceedings* 13: A1346, p. 395.

Lewko, W., Smalley, R., and Oldham, R. 1998. Lymphokines and cytokines. In Oldham, R. (ed). *Principles of Cancer Biotherapy*, 3rd edn. New York, NY: Marcel Dekker, pp. 211–265.

Lissoni, P., Barni, S., Ardizzoia, A., *et al.* 1994. Second line therapy with low dose subcutaneous interleukin-2 alone in advanced renal cancer patients resistant to interferon-alpha. *European Journal of Cancer* 51: 59–62.

Lotem, J., Shabo, Y., and Sachs, L. 1989. Regulation of megakaryocyte development by interleukin-6. *Blood* 77: 461–471.

Lotze, M. 1995. Biologic therapy with interleukin-2: Preclinical studies. In DeVita, V., Hellman, S., and Rosenberg, S. (eds). *Biologic Therapy of Cancer*, 2nd edn. Philadelphia, PA: J. B. Lippincott, pp. 74(5):1545–1551.

Malek, T., and Gutgsell, N. 1993. IL-2 and its receptor: Structure, function, and regulation of expression. In Atkins, M., and Mier, J. (eds). *Therapeutic Applications of Interleukin-2*. New York, NY: Marcel Dekker, pp. 3–25.

Mandrup-Poulsen, T., Helqvist, S., Molvig, J., *et al.* 1989. Cytokines as immune effector molecules in autoimmune endocrine diseases with special reference to insulin-dependent diabetes mellitus. *Autoimmunity* 4(3): 191–218.

Margolin, K. 1993. The clinical toxicities of high-dose interleukin-2. In Atkins, M., and Mier, J. (eds). *Therapeutic Applications of Interleukin-2*. New York, NY: Marcel Dekker, pp. 331–362.

Margolin, K., Aronson, F., Sznol, M., *et al.* 1994. Phase II studies of recombinant human interleukin-4 in advanced renal cancer and malignant melanoma. *Journal of Immunotherapy with Emphasis on Tumor Immunology* 15(2): 147–153.

Margolin, K., and Forman, S.J. 2000. Immunotherapy with interleukin-2 after hematopoietic cell transplantation for hematologic malignancy. *The Cancer Journal from Scientific American.* 6(suppl 1): S33–S38.

Maslak, P., and Nimer, S. 1998. The efficacy of IL-3, SCF, IL-6 and IL-11 in treating thrombocytopenia. *Seminars in Hematology* 35(3): 253–260.

Masood, R., Lunardi-Iskandar, Y., Moudgil, T., *et al.* 1994. IL-10 inhibits HIV-1 replication and is induced by tat. *Biochemistry and Biophysics Research Communication* 202: 374–383.

Mazumder, A. 1997. Experimental evidence of interleukin-2 activity in bone marrow transplantation. *The Cancer Journal from Scientific American* 3(suppl 1): S37–S42.

Meehan, K., Verma, U., Rajagopal, C., *et al.* 1995. Stem cell transplantation with high dose chemoradiotherapy myeloablation and interleukin-2. *Journal of Infusional Chemotherapy* 6: 28–32.

Meloni, G., Vignetti, M., Pogliani, E., *et al.* 1997. Interleukin-2 therapy in relapsed acute myelogenous leukemia. *The Cancer Journal from Scientific American* 3(suppl 1): S43–S47.

Metzger, D., Raeder, R., Van Cleave, V., *et al.* 1995. Protection of mice from group A streptococcal skin infection by interleukin-12. *Journal of Infectious Disease* 171: 1643–1645.

Mier, J. 1993a. Abrogation of interleukin-2 toxicity. In Atkins, M., and Mier, J. (eds). *Therapeutic Applications of Interleukin-2*. New York, NY: Marcel Dekker, pp. 455–475.

Mier, J. 1993b. Pathogenesis of the interleukin-2 induced vascular leak syndrome. In Atkins, M., and Mier, J. (eds). *Therapeutic Applications of Interleukin-2*. New York, NY: Marcel Dekker, pp. 363–379.

Mier, J., Vachino, G., van der Meer, J., *et al.* 1988. Induction of circulating tumor necrosis factor (TNF) alpha as the mechanism for the febrile response to Interleukin-2 (IL-2) in cancer patients. *Journal of Clinical Immunology* 8: 426–436.

Mitra, M., Judge, T., Nestle, F., *et al.* 1995. Psoriatic skin-derived dendritic cell function is inhibited by exogenous IL-10. Differential modulation of B7-1 (CD80) and B7-2 (CD86) expression. *Journal of Immunology* 154: 2668–2677.

Modiano, M. 1997. Phase II trial of recombinant interleukin-4 SCH 39400 in advanced non-small cell lung cancer (NSCLC): A dose ranging study. *Proceedings of American Society of Clinical Oncology* 16: A1711, p. 475a.

Mongan, A., Ramdahin, S., and Warrington, R. 1997. Interleukin-10 response abnormalities in systemic lupus erythematosus. *Scandinavian Journal of Immunology* 46: 406–412.

Moore, M. 1991. Clinical implications of positive and negative hematopoietic stem cell regulators. *Blood* 78: 1–19.

Morgan, D., Ruscetti, F., and Gallo, R. 1976. Selective in vitro growth of T lymphocytes from normal human bone marrows. *Science* 193(4257): 1007–1008.

Mossman, T. R., Cherwinski, H., Bond, M. W., *et al.* 1986. Two types of murine helper T cell clones. I. Definition according to profiles of lymphokine activities and secreted proteins. *Journal Immunology* 136: 2348–2357.

Motzer, R., Rakhit, A., Schwartz, L., *et al.* 1998. Phase I trial of subcutaneous recombinant human interleukin-12 in patients with advanced renal cell carcinoma. *Clinical Cancer Research* 4(5): 1183–1191.

Muir-Sluis, A. 1998. Interleukin-4. In Muir-Sluis, A., and Thorpe, R. (eds). *Cytokines*. San Diego, CA: Academic Press, pp. 53–68.

Mulé, J., McIntosh, J., Jablons, D., *et al.* 1990. Antitumor activity of recombinant interleukin-6 in mice. *Journal of Experimental Medicine* 171: 629–632.

Mussi, A., Bonifati, C., Carducci, M., *et al.* 1994. IL-10 levels are decreased in psoriatic lesional skin as compared to the psoriatic lesion-free and normal skin suction blister fluids. *Journal of Biological Regulation and Homeostatic Agents* 8: 117–120.

Naif, H., Chang, J., Ho-Shon, M., *et al.* 1996. Inhibition of human immunodeficiency virus replication in differentiating monocytes by Interleukin-10 occurs in parallel with inhibition of cellular RNA expression. *AIDS Research Human Retroviruses* 12: 1237–1245.

Naume, B., Gately, M., and Espevik, T. 1992. A

comparative study of IL-12 (cytotoxic lymphocyte maturation factor), IL-12, and IL-7 induced effects on immunomagnetically purified CD56+ NK cells. *Journal of Immunology* 148: 2429–2436.

Nemunaitis, J., Appelbaum, F., Lilleby, K., *et al.* 1994. Phase I study of recombinant interleukin-1 beta in patients undergoing autologous bone marrow transplant for acute myelogenous leukemia. *Blood* 83(12): 3473–3479.

Niederau, C., Backmerhoff, F., Schumacher, B., *et al.* 1997. Inflammatory mediators and acute phase proteins in patients with Crohn's disease and ulcerative colitis. *Journal of Hepatogastroenterology* 44: 90–107.

Nielsen, O., Koppen, T., Rudiger, N., *et al.* 1996. Involvement of interleukin-4 and -10 in inflammatory bowel disease. *Digest of Disease Science* 4: 1786–1793.

Nikolic-Paterson, D., Lan, H., and Atkins, R. 1996. Interleukin-1 receptor antagonism. *Seminars in Nephrology* 16(6): 583–590.

Ohara, J. 1989. Interleukin-4: Molecular structure and biochemical characteristics, biological function and receptor expression. In Cruse, J., and Lewis, R. (eds). *The Year in Immunology: Immunoregulatory Cytokines and Cell Growth*, vol. 5. Switzerland: Basel Karger, pp. 126–159.

Oldham, R., and Brogley, J. 1990. Contrast medium "recalls" interleukin-2 toxicity. *Journal of Clinical Oncology* 8(5): 942.

Oldham, R., Dillman, R., Yannelli, J., *et al.* 1991. Continuous infusion interleukin-2 and tumor-derived activated cells as treatment of advanced solid tumors. *Molecular Biotherapy* 3(2):68–73.

Oleksowicz, L., Paciucci, P., Zuckerman, D., *et al.* 1991. Alterations of platelet function induced by interleukin-2. *Journal of Immunotherapy* 10(5): 363–370.

Olencki, T., Finke, J., Tubbs, R., *et al.* 1996. Immunomodulatory effects of interleukin-2 and interleukin-4 in patients with malignancy. *Journal of Immunotherapy with Emphasis on Tumor Immunology* 19(1): 69–80.

Opal, S., Fisher, C., Jr., Dhainaut, J., *et al.* 1997. Confirmatory interleukin-1 receptor antagonist trial in severe sepsis: A phase III, randomized, double-blind, placebo-controlled, multicenter trial. The Interleukin-1 Receptor Antagonist Sepsis Investigator Group. *Critical Care Medicine* 25(7): 1115–1124.

Opal, S., Wherry, J., and Grint, P. 1998. Interleukin-10: Potential benefits and possible risks in clinical infectious diseases. *Clinical Infectious Disease* 27(6): 1497–1507.

Oppenheim, J. 1998. Forward. In Thomson, A. (ed). *The Cytokine Handbook*, 3rd edn. San Diego, CA: Academic Press, pp. xviii–xxii.

Oppenheim, J., Ruscetti, F., and Faltynek, C. 1991. Cytokines. In Stites, D., and Terr, A. (eds). *Basic and Clinical Immunology*. Norwalk, CT: Appleton and Lange, pp. 78–100.

Paciucci, P., Mandeli, J., Oleksowicz, L., *et al.* 1990. Thrombocytopenia during immunotherapy with interleukin-2 by constant infusion. *American Journal of Medicine* 89(3): 308–312.

Parkinson, D. 1989. The role of interleukin-2 in the biotherapy of cancer. *Oncology Nursing Forum* 16(6 suppl): 16–20.

Patarca, R., and Fletcher, M. 1997. Interleukin-1: Basic science and clinical applications. *Critical Reviews in Oncology* 8(2–3): 143–188.

Paul, W. 1991. Interleukin-4: A prototypic immunoregulatory lymphokine. *Blood* 77(9): 1859–1870.

Perussia, B., Chan, S. H., D'Andrea, A., *et al.* 1992. Natural killer (NK) cell stimulatory factor or IL-12 has differential effects on the proliferation of TCR-alpha beta+, TCR-gamma delta+ T lymphocytes, and NK cells. *Journal of Immunology* 149: 3495–3502.

Piper, B., Rieger, P., Brophy, L., *et al.* 1989. Recent advances in the management of biotherapy-related side effects: Fatigue. *Oncology Nursing Forum* 16(6 suppl): 27–34.

Pockaj, B., Topalian, S., Steinberg, S., *et al.* 1993. Infectious complications associated with interleukin-2 administration: A retrospective review of

935 treatment courses. *Journal of Clinical Oncology* 11(1): 136–147.

Poli, G. 1999. Laureate ESCI award for excellence in clinical science 1999. Cytokines and the human immunodeficiency virus: From bench to bedside. *European Journal of Clinical Investigation* 29(8): 723–732.

Porrini, A., Gambi, D., and Reder, A. 1995. Interferon effects on Interleukin-10 secretion. Mononuclear cell response to Interleukin-10 is normal in multiple sclerosis patients. *Journal of Neuroimmunology* 61: 27–34.

Prendiville, J., Thatcher, N., Lind, M., *et al.* 1993. Recombinant human interleukin-4 (rhu IL-4) administered by the intravenous and subcutaneous routes in patients with advanced cancer: A phase I toxicity study and pharmacokinetic analysis. *European Journal of Cancer* 29A(12): 1700–1707.

Puri, R., and Siegel, J. 1993. Interleukin-4 and cancer therapy. *Cancer Investigation* 11(4): 473–486.

Rambaldi, A., Torcia, M., Bettoni, S., *et al.* 1991. Modulation of cell proliferation and cytokine production in acute myeloblastic leukemia by interleukin-1 receptor antagonist and lack of its expression by leukemic cells. *Blood* 78: 3243–3253.

Rayman, P., Finke, J., Olencki, T., *et al.* 1994. Adoptive immunotherapy utilizing IL-2 and IL-4 for expansion of tumor infiltrating by lymphocytes in renal cell carcinoma. In Chang A., and Suyu, S. (eds). *Immunotherapy of Cancer with Sensitized Lymphocytes.* Austin, TX: R.G. Landes Company, pp. 123–131.

Redman, B., Abubakr, Y., Chou, T., *et al.* 1994. Phase II trial of recombinant interleukin-1 beta in patients with metastatic renal cell carcinoma. *Journal of Immunotherapy with Emphasis on Tumor Immunology* 16(3): 211–215.

Richards, C. 1998. Interleukin-6. In Mire-Sluis, A., and Thorpe, R. (eds). *Cytokines.* San Diego, CA: Academic Press, pp. 87–108.

Richards, J., Gale, D., Mehta, N., *et al.* 1999. Combination of chemotherapy with interleukin-2 and interferon alfa for the treatment of metastatic melanoma. *Journal of Clinical Oncology* 17(2): 651–657.

Richards, J., Mehta, N., Ramming, K., *et al.* 1992. Sequential chemoimmunotherapy in the treatment of metastatic melanoma. *Journal of Clinical Oncology* 10(8): 1338–1343.

Rieger, P. 1992. The pathophysiology of selected symptoms associated with BRM therapy. *Biological Response Modifiers: Perspectives for Oncology Nurses.* Monograph. Emeryville, CA: Cetus Corporation, pp. 4–10.

Rieger, P. 1997. Biotherapy. In Otto, S. (ed). *Oncology Nursing,* 3rd edn. St. Louis, MO: Mosby YearBook, pp. 573–613.

Rosenberg, S. 1997. Keynote address: Perspectives on the use of interleukin-2 in cancer treatment. *The Cancer Journal from Scientific American* 3(suppl 1): S2–S6.

Rosenberg, S., Lotze, M., Yang, J., *et al.* 1989. Experience with the use of high-dose interleukin-2 in the treatment of 652 cancer patients. *Annals of Surgery* 210(4): 474–485.

Rosenberg, S., Lotze, M., Yang, J., *et al.* 1993. Prospective randomized trial of high-dose interleukin-2 alone or in conjunction with lymphokine-activated killer cells for the treatment of patients with advanced cancer. *Journal of the National Cancer Institute* 85: 622–632.

Rosenberg, S., Packard, B., Aebersold, P., *et al.* 1988. Use of tumor-infiltrating lymphocytes and interleukin-2 in the immunotherapy of patients with metastatic melanoma. *The New England Journal of Medicine* 319(25): 1676–1680.

Rosenberg, S., Yang, J., Schwartzentruber, D., *et al.* 1999. Prospective randomized trial of the treatment of patients with metastatic melanoma using chemotherapy with cisplatin, dacarbazine, and tamoxifen alone or in combination with interleukin-2 and interferon alfa-2b. *Journal of Clinical Oncology* 17(3): 968–975.

Rosenberg, S., Yang, J., Topalian, S., *et al.* 1994. Treatment of 283 consecutive patients with metastatic melanoma or renal cell cancer using high-dose bolus interleukin-2. *Journal of the American Medical Association* 271(12): 907–913.

Rubin, J. 1993. Interleukin-2: Its biology and clinical application in patients with cancer. *Cancer Investigation* 11(4): 460–472.

Rubin, J., and Lotze, M. 1992. Acute gastric mucosal injury associated with the systemic administration of interleukin-4. *Surgery* 111(3):274–280.

Rudick, R.A., Ransohoff, R.M., Peppler, R., *et al.* 1996. Interferon beta induces interleukin-10 expression: Relevance to multiple sclerosis. *Annals of Neurology* 40: 618–627.

Rust, D., and Rosenzweig, M. 1997. Fatigue assessment and management of patients receiving biotherapy. *Biotherapy: Considerations for Oncology Nurses* 2(1): 6–11.

Salmaggi, A., Dufour, A., Eoli, M., *et al.* 1996. Low serum interleukin-10 levels in multiple sclerosis: Further evidence for decreased systemic immunosuppression? *Journal of Neurology* 243:13–17.

Sandoz Pharmaceuticals, 1991. Data on file.

Sands, B. 1999. Novel therapies for inflammatory bowel disease. *Gastroenterology Clinics of North America* 28(2): 323–351.

Sandstrom, S. 1996. Nursing management of patients receiving biological therapy. *Seminars in Oncology Nursing* 12(2): 152–162.

Schlaak, J., Buslau, M., Jochum, D., *et al.* 1994. T cells involved in psoriasis vulgaris belong to the Th1 subset. *Journal of Investigational Dermatology* 102: 145–149.

Scholz, W. 1996. Interleukin 6 in disease: Cause or cure? *Immunopharmacology* 31: 131–150.

Schreiber, S., Heinig, T., Thiele, H., *et al.* 1995. Immunoregulatory role of interleukin-10 in patients with inflammatory bowel disease. *Journal of Gastroenterology* 108: 1434–1444.

Schwartz, D., and Merigan, T. 1990. Interleukin-2 in the treatment of HIV disease. *Biotherapy* 2(2): 119–136.

Schwartz, D., Skowron, G., and Merigan, T. 1991. Safety and effects of interleukin-2 plus zidovudine in asymptomatic individuals infected with human immunodeficiency virus. *Journal of Acquired Deficiency Syndromes* 4(1): 11–23.

Schwartzentruber, D. 1997. Capillary leak syndrome in patients receiving immunotherapy. *Biotherapy: Considerations for Oncology Nurses*, 2(2). Washington Crossing, PA: Scientific Frontiers Inc., pp. 8–10.

Scott, P. 1993. Initiation cytokine for cell-mediated immunity. *Science* 260: 496–497.

Seipp, C.A. 1997. Capillary leak syndrome: Nursing considerations. *Biotherapy: Considerations for Oncology Nurses*, 2(2). Washington Crossing, PA: Scientific Frontiers Inc., pp. 11–15.

Sergi, J. 1991. The physiology of the flu-like syndrome and the cardiopulmonary and renal symptoms associated with BRM therapy. *Biological Response Modifiers: Perspectives for Oncology Nurses*. Monograph. Emeryville, CA: Cetus Corporation, pp. 4–10.

Shen, V., Bergeron, S., Krailo, M., *et al.* 1997. Enhanced hematological recovery but a high incidence of grade (GD) III/IV toxicities attributed to interleukin-6 (IL-6) in children with recurrent/refractory solid tumor treated with rIL-6 and G-CSF following ifosfamide, carboplatin, and etoposide (ICE). *American Society of Clinical Oncology Program/Proceedings* 16: 110a.

Shulman, K., Thompson, J., Benyunes, M., *et al.* 1993. Adverse reactions to intravenous contrast media in patients treated with interleukin-2. *Journal of Immunotherapy* 13(3): 208–212.

Silberstein, D., Schoof, M., Rodrick, M., *et al.* 1989. Activation of eosinophils in cancer patients treated with IL-2 and IL-2 generated lymphokine-activated killer cells. *Journal of Immunology* 142(6): 2162–2167.

Sleijfer, D., Janssen, R., Buter, J., *et al.* 1992. Phase II study of subcutaneous interleukin-2 in unselected patients with advanced renal cell cancer on an outpatient basis. *Journal of Clinical Oncology* 10(7): 1119–1123.

Smith, J., Longo, D., Alvord, W., *et al.* 1993. The effects of treatment with interleukin-1 on platelet recovery after high-dose carboplatin. *The New England Journal of Medicine* 328(11): 756–761.

Smith, J., Urba, W., Curti, B., *et al.* 1992. The toxic and hematologic effects of interleukin-1 alpha administered in a phase I trial to patients with advanced malignancies. *Journal of Clinical Oncology* 10(7): 1141–1152.

Smith, K. 1993. Lowest dose interleukin-2 immunotherapy. *Blood* 81(6): 1414—1423.

Smith, K. 1997. Rational interleukin-2 therapy. *Cancer Journal from Scientific American* 3(suppl 1): S137–S140.

Snydman, D., Sullivan, B., Gill, M., *et al.* 1990. Nosocomial sepsis associated with interleukin-2. *Annals of Internal Medicine* 112(2): 102–107.

Soiffer, R., Murray, C., Cochran, K., *et al.* 1992. Clinical and immunologic effects of prolonged infusion of low-dose recombinant interleukin-2 after autologous and T-cell-depleted allogenic bone marrow transplant. *Blood* 79: 517–526.

Sosman, J., Fisher, S., Kefer, C., *et al.* 1994. A phase I trial of continuous infusion interleukin-4 (IL-4) alone and following interleukin-2 (IL-2) in cancer patients. *Annals of Oncology* 5(5): 447–452.

Sparber, A., and Biller-Sparber, K. 1993. Immunotherapy and neuropsychiatric toxicity. *Cancer Nursing* 16(3): 188–192.

Spriggs, D. 1991. Tumor necrosis factor: Basic principles and preclinical studies. In DeVita, V., Hellman, S., and Rosenberg, S. (eds). *Biological Therapy of Cancer*. Philadelphia, PA: J.B. Lippincott, pp. 354–392.

Stadler, W., Rybak, M., and Vogelzang, N. 1995. A phase II study of subcutaneous recombinant human interleukin-4 in metastatic renal cell carcinoma. *Cancer* 76(9): 1629–1633.

Starnes, H. 1991. Biological effects and possible clinical applications of interleukin-1. *Seminars in Hematology* 29(2 suppl 2): 34–41.

Storkus, W., Tahar, H., and Lotze, M. 1998. Interleukin-12. In Thomson, A. (ed). *The Cytokine Handbook*, 3rd edn. San Diego, CA: Academic Press, pp. 391–425.

Suminami, Y., Elder, E., Lotze, M., *et al.* 1995. In situ interleukin-4 gene expression in cancer patients treated with genetically modified tumor vaccine. *Journal of Immunotherapy: Emphasis on Tumor Immunology* 17(4): 238–248.

Sundin, D., and Wolin, M. 1998. Toxicity management in patients receiving low-dose aldesleukin therapy. *Annals of Pharmacotherapy* 32(12): 1344–1352.

Sykes, M., Abraham, V., Harty, M., *et al.* 1993. IL-2 reduces graft-versus-host disease and preserves a graft-versus-leukemia effect by selectively inhibiting CD4$^+$ T cell activity. *Journal of Immunology* 150(1): 197–205.

Sznol, M., and Longo, D. 1993. Chemotherapy drug interactions with biological agents. *Seminars in Oncology* 20(1): 80–93.

Teranishi, T., Hirano, T., Arima, N., *et al.* 1982. Human helper T cell factor(s) (ThF). II. Induction of IgG production in B lymphoblastoid cell lines and identification of T cell replacing factor (TRF)-like factors(s). *Journal of Immunology* 128: 1903–1908.

Thompson, J., Gold, P., and Fefer, A. 1997. Outpatient chemoimmunotherapy for the treatment of metastatic melanoma. *Seminars in Oncology* 24(1 suppl 4): S44–S48.

Thompson, J., Lee, D., Lindgren, C., *et al.* 1988. Influence of dose and duration of infusion of interleukin-2 on toxicity and immunomodulation. *Journal of Clinical Oncology* 6(4): 669–678.

Thompson, J., Lindgren, C., Benyunes, J., *et al.* 1993. The effects of pentoxifylline on the generation of human lymphokine-activated killer cell cytotoxicity. *Journal of Immunotherapy* 13(2): 82–90.

Thorpe, R. 1998. Interleukin-2. In Muir-Sluis, A., and Thorpe, R. (eds). *Cytokines*. San Diego, CA: Academic Press, pp. 19–33.

Trehu, E., Isner, J., Mier, J., *et al.* 1993. Possible myocardial toxicity associated with interleukin-4 therapy. *Journal of Immunotherapy* 14(4): 348–351.

Tso, C., Duckett, J., deKernion, J., *et al.* 1992. Modulation of tumor-infiltrating lymphocytes derived from human renal cell carcinoma by interleukin-4. *Journal of Immunotherapy* 12(2): 82–89.

Tsuji-Takayama, K., Matsumoto, S., Koide, K., *et al.* 1997. Interleukin-18 induces activation and association of p56(lck) and MAPK in a murine

TH1 clone. *Biochemical and Biophysical Research Communications* 237(1): 126–130.

Uyemura, K., and Nickoloff, B. J. 1993. The cytokine network in lesional and lesion-free psoriatic skin is characterized by a T helper type 1 cell mediated response. *Journal of Infectious Disease* 101: 701–705.

Vadhan-Raj, S., Kudelka, A., Garrison, L., *et al.* 1994. Effects of interleukin-1α on carboplatin-induced thrombocytopenia in patients with recurrent ovarian cancer. *Journal of Clinical Oncology* 12(4): 707–714.

Vassilopoulou-Sellin, R. 1994. Endocrine effects of cytokines. *Oncology* 8(10): 43–46.

Veldhuis, G. J., Willemse, P. H. B., Mulder, N. H. *et al.* 1996. Potential use of recombinant human interleukin-6 in clinical oncology. *Leukemia and Lymphoma* 20: 373–379.

Veltri, S., and Smith, J. 1996. Interleukin 1 trials in cancer patients: A review of the toxicity, antitumor and hematopoietic effects. *Oncologist* 1(4): 190–200.

Venkatraj, U., Lee, S., and Logie, K. 1997. ECOG phase II trial of interleukin-4 (IL-4) in chronic lymphocytic leukemia (CLL) and indolent non-Hodgkin's lymphoma (NHL) (E5Y92). *Proceedings of American Society of Clinical Oncology* 16: abstract No. 445, p.126a.

Verma, U.N., Bagg, A., Brown, E., *et al.* 1994. Interleukin-2 activation of human bone marrow in long-term cultures: An effective strategy for purging and generation of anti-tumor cytotoxic effectors. *Bone Marrow Transplantation* 13: 115–123.

Verschraegen, C., Kudelka, A., Termrungruanglert, W., *et al.* 1996. Effects of interleukin-1 alpha on ovarian carcinoma in patients with recurrent disease. *European Journal of Cancer* 32A(9): 1609–1611.

Vetto, J., Papa, M., Lotze, M. *et al.* 1987. Reduction of toxicity of interleukin-2 and lymphokine activated killer cells in humans by the administration of corticosteroids. *Journal of Clinical Oncology* 5: 496–503.

Viele, C., and Moran, T. 1993. Nursing management of the nonhospitalized patient receiving recombinant interleukin-2. *Seminars in Oncology Nursing* 9(3 suppl 1): 20–24.

Vilček, J. 1998. The cytokines: An overview. In Thomson, A. (ed). *The Cytokine Handbook*, 3rd edn. San Diego, CA: Academic Press, pp. 1–20.

Vogelzang, N., Lipton, A., and Figlin, R. 1993. Subcutaneous interleukin-2 plus interferon alfa-2a in metastatic renal cancer: An outpatient multicenter trial. *Journal of Clinical Oncology* 11(9): 1809–1816.

Vokes, E., Figlin, R., Hochester, H., *et al.* 1998. A phase II study of recombinant human interleukin-4 for advanced or recurrent non-small cell lung cancer. *Cancer Journal from Scientific American* 4(1): 46–51.

Weidmann, E., Bergmann, L., Stock, J., *et al.* 1992. Rapid cytokine release in cancer patients treated with interleukin-2. *Journal of Immunotherapy* 12(2): 123–131.

Weisdorf, D., Katsanis, E., Verfaillie, C., *et al.* 1994. Interleukin-1 alpha administered after autologous transplantation: A phase I/II clinical trial. *Blood* 84(6): 2044–2049.

Weissenbach, J., Zeevi, M., Landau, T., *et al.* 1979. Identification of the translation products of human fibroblast interferon mRNA in reticulocyte lysates. *European Journal of Biochemistry* 98: 1–8.

Wheeler, V. 1996. Interleukins: The search for an anticancer therapy. *Seminars in Oncology Nursing* 12(2): 106–114.

Wheeler, V. 1997. Biotherapy. In Groenwald, S., Frogge, M., Goodman, M., and Yarbro, C. (eds). *Cancer Nursing: Principles and Practice*, 4th edn. Boston: Jones and Bartlett, pp. 426–458.

White, R., Jr., Schwartzentruber, D., Guleria, A., *et al.* 1994. Cardiopulmonary toxicity of treatment with high-dose interleukin-2 in 1999 consecutive patients with metastatic melanoma or renal cell carcinoma. *Cancer* 74: 3212–3222.

Whitehead, R., Unger, J., Goodwin, J., *et al.* 1998. Phase II trial of recombinant human interleukin-

4 in patients with disseminated malignant melanoma: A Southwest Oncology Group study. *Journal of Immunotherapy* 21(6): 440–446.

Whitehead, R., Wolf, M., Solanki, D., *et al.* 1995. A phase II trial of continuous infusion recombinant interleukin-2 in patients with advanced RCC: A Southwest Oncology Group study. *Journal of Immunotherapy* 18: 104–114.

Wolkenstein, P., Chosidow, O., Wechsler, J., *et al.* 1993. Cutaneous side effects associated with interleukin-2 administration for metastatic melanoma. *Journal of the American Academy of Dermatology* 28(1): 66–70.

Woodlock, T., Sahasrabudhe, D., Marquis, D., *et al.* 1996. Active specific immunotherapy for metastatic colorectal carcinoma (CRC): Phase I–II study of an allogeneic cell vaccine plus low dose interleukin-1 alpha (IL-1α). *Proceedings of the American Society of Clinical Oncology* 15: abstract no. 1810, p. 556.

Yang, J., and Rosenberg, S. 1997. An ongoing prospective randomized comparison of interleukin-2 regimes for the treatment of metastatic renal cell cancer. *The Cancer Journal from Scientific American* 3(suppl 1): S79–S78.

Yang, J., Topalian, S., Parkinson, D., *et al.* 1994. Randomized comparison of high-dose and low-dose interleukin-2 for the therapy of metastatic renal cell carcinoma: An interim report. *Journal of Clinical Oncology* 12(8): 1572–1576.

Yin, T., Taga, T., and Tsaang, ML-S. 1993. Involvement of IL-6 signal transducer gp130 in IL-11-mediated signal transduction. *Journal of Immunology* 151: 2555–2561.

Zukiwski, A., David, C., Coan, J., *et al.* 1990. Increased incidence of hypersensitivity to iodine containing radiographic contrast media after interleukin-2 administration. *Cancer* 65(2): 1521–1524.

Zurawski, S., Vega, F., Jr., Huyghe, B., *et al.* 1993. Receptors for interleukin-13 and interleukin-14 are complex and share a novel component that functions in signal transduction. *EMBO Journal* 12: 2663–2670.

Clinical Pearls

1. Pretreatment assessment: Because of toxicities related to the administration of IL-2, especially capillary-leak syndrome, it is important to establish baseline status/functioning of the renal, hepatic, hematologic, cardiovascular, and pulmonary systems.

2. Performance status should be ECOG 0 or 1 or Karnofsky Performance Score 70% to 100%.

3. Concomitant use of corticosteroids may reduce the effectiveness of aldesleukin and should therefore be avoided.

4. In-house studies at Chiron have demonstrated safety when a 5-day supply of medication is drawn into syringes in a sterile environment and stored at refrigerated temperatures. Consult package insert or manufacturer for details.

5. For subcutaneous and continuous infusion regimens designed for the ambulatory setting, patients must have ready access to the health care team for response to questions or to manage adverse events.

6. Even in regimens designed for the ambulatory setting, adverse events stemming from capillary-leak syndrome may become problematic. Patients should be monitored on a regular basis for symptomatic hypotension, tachycardia, weight gain of 5 to 10 pounds over several days, shortness of breath, and significantly decreased urine

Reportable Signs and Symptoms

System	Sign or Symptom
General	Overwhelming fatigue (spends majority of day in bed or unable to perform routine activities of daily living)
	Fever uncontrolled with antipyretics
Neurologic	Confusion or disorientation
	Extreme drowsiness
	Hallucinations
	Sleep disturbance
Gastrointestinal	Inability to maintain adequate hydration or food intake because of nausea/vomiting or stomatitis, or diarrhea
	Emesis uncontrolled with antiemetics
	Diarrhea (more than 2–3 loose stools per day or uncontrolled with antidiarrheal medication)
Cardiovascular	Weight gain of >5 to 10 pounds within a week
	Palpitations, chest pain
	Dizziness when changing position
Pulmonary	Shortness of breath, respiratory distress
	Cough with production of sputum
Renal	Voiding only small quantities of urine
	No urine output
Integument	Large, painful inflammatory reactions at the injection site
	Signs of infection (erythema, swelling)
	Severe desquamation

Source: Adapted with permission from Hossan, E., and Rieger, P. T. (1997). Interleukin-2 therapy: Nursing management + patient education = success in the ambulatory setting. *Biotherapy: Considerations for Oncology Nurses* 2(2): 1–7.

output. For high-dose inpatient regimens, patients should be monitored every 4 hours for changes in neurologic, pulmonary, cardiovascular, and renal function.

7. Patients with indwelling central lines should be placed on antibiotic coverage prophylactically to prevent infection from gram-positive organisms.

8. For patients receiving IL-2 in the ambulatory setting, education of the patient and family is vital to successful management. Self-care skills (e.g., either medication self-administration through subcutaneous injection or management of an ambulatory infusion pump), reportable signs and symptoms (see table), contact numbers to call for questions or management of adverse events, and when to report for laboratory and diagnostic tests and follow-up clinic visits are crucial to include in the teaching plan.

9. Aggressive management of toxicities such as flu-like symptoms, nausea and vomiting, stomatitis, pruritus, and dry desquamated skin with concomitant medications and nonpharmacologic interventions must be considered and planned for at the onset of therapy.

10. Once a cycle of therapy is completed, fluid is rapidly mobilized from the periphery and weight generally returns to pretreatment baseline. On occasion, furosemide is used to assist in the mobilization of fluid.

11. Instruct patients to avoid direct sunlight and to use sunscreen when outdoors.

12. Have patients keep a diary of symptoms and timing and placement of injections to assist with monitoring the occurrence of toxic effects and the success of management strategies.

Key References

Akira, S. 2000. The role of IL-18 in innate immunity. *Current Opinions in Immunology* 12(1): 59–63.

Atkins, M., and Mier, J. (eds). 1993. *Therapeutic Application of Interleukin-2.* New York, NY: Marcel Dekker, pp. 3–476.

Atkins, M. B., Lotze, M. T., Dutcher, J. P., *et al.* 1999. High-dose recombinant interleukin-2 therapy for patients with metastatic melanoma: Analysis of 270 patients treated between 1985 and 1993. *Journal of Clinical Oncology* 17(7): 2105.

Car, B.D., Eng, V.M., Lipman, J.M., *et al.* 1999. The toxicology of interleukin-12: A review. *Toxicology and Pathology* 27(1): 58–63.

Castro, M., VanAuken, J., Spencer-Cisek, P., *et al.* 1999. Acute tumor lysis syndrome associated with concurrent biochemotherapy of metastatic melanoma: A case report and review of the literature. *Cancer* 85(5): 1055–1059.

De Vita, V.T., Hellman, S., and Rosenberg, S.A. 2000. Interleukin-2. *The Cancer Journal from Scientific American* 6(suppl 1): S1–S112.

Dillman, R.O. 1999. What to do with IL-2? *Cancer Biotherapy and Radiopharmacy* 14(6):423–434.

Dinarello, C.A. 1999. IL-18: A TH1-inducing, proinflammatory cytokine and new member of the IL-1 family. *Journal of Allergy and Clinical Immunology* 103(1 Pt 1): 11–24.

Green, R.J., and Schuchter, L.M. 1998. Systemic treatment of metastatic melanoma with chemotherapy. *Hematology Oncology Clinics of North America* 12(4): 863–875, viii.

Hellstrand, K., Hansson, M., and Hermodsson, S. 2000. Adjuvant histamine in cancer immunotherapy. *Seminars in Cancer Biology* 10(1):29–39.

Kammula, U.S., White, D.E., and Rosenberg, S. A. 1998. Trends in the safety of high dose bolus interleukin-2 administration in patients with metastatic cancer. *Cancer* 83(4): 797–805.

Mackiewicz, A., Koj, A. and Sehgal, P.B. (eds). 1995 Interleukin-6-type cytokines. *Annals of the New York Academy of Sciences* 762: 1–507.

Moldawer, N., and Carr, E. 2000. The promise of recombinant interleukin-2. *American Journal of Nursing* 100(5): 35–40.

Stordeur, P., and Goldman, M. 1998. Interleukin-10 as a regulatory cytokine induced by cellular stress: Molecular aspects. *International Reviews in Immunology* 16(5–6): 501–522.

Wheeler, V. 1996. Interleukins: The search for an anticancer therapy. *Seminars in Oncology Nursing* 12(2): 106–114.

CHAPTER 7 | Hematopoietic Growth Factors

Debra Wujcik, RN, MSN, AOCN®

Hematopoietic growth factors (HGFs) constitute a large family of glycosylated proteins that interact with specific receptors to regulate the reproduction, maturation, and functional activity of blood cells (Crosier and Clark, 1992; Williams and Quesenberry, 1992). These proteins attach to receptors on the surface membrane of the target cell, and in response, the cell proliferates, differentiates, and matures. Although some HGFs stimulate a single response, others stimulate a cascade effect. Because HGFs are produced only in minute amounts in humans, studying their effects was difficult until recombinant technology made it possible for HGFs to be cloned, reproduced in large quantities, and made available for clinical trials.

HGFs were first identified through **colony assays** in the laboratory (Golde and Gasson, 1988; Metcalf and Morstyn, 1991). Bone marrow cells, which included **pluripotent stem cells (PPSCs)**, were added to culture dishes containing **feeder layers** consisting of various types of leukocytes and semisolid medium. Colonies of leukocytes formed in response to incubation. When the feeder layers were varied, different types of colonies formed, suggesting that the cells grew in response to specific growth factors. A number of these growth factors have now been identified (Bociek and Armitage, 1996).

Originally discovered in the 1950s, HGFs are hormone-like proteins that mediate intracellular communication. They are similar to hormones, but they have some distinct differences. First, HGFs may be produced by several different types of cells, whereas hormones are produced only by specialized cells. Second, HGFs usually have only a local effect rather than affecting distant organs as hormones do (Metcalf and Morstyn, 1991). Originally, HGFs were named colony-stimulating factors (CSFs) because of their ability to induce growth and maturation of specific colonies of cells *in vitro*. The 4 classic CSFs are **granulocyte colony-stimulating factor (G-CSF)**, **granulocyte-macrophage colony-stimulating factor (GM-CSF)**, **macrophage colony-stimulating factor (M-CSF)**, and **interleukin (IL)-3**, which is called the **multipotential colony-stimulating factor**. These CSFs are the major regulatory molecules controlling the formation of neutrophils and monocyte/macrophages and are part of the larger HGF family of specific hematopoietic regulators.

Four HGFs have been approved for use by the Food and Drug Administration (FDA) (see Table 7.1). The efficacy of G-CSF and GM-CSF in minimizing the myelosuppression of chemotherapy is well established. **Erythropoietin (Epo)** was initially indicated for patients with anemia due to chronic renal failure who were dependent on transfusions. In 1994, another indication was added, the treatment of anemia resulting from cancer chemotherapy. IL-11 was approved for the prevention of severe thrombocytopenia following myelosuppressive chemotherapy. Other HGFs, including IL-3, M-CSF, stem cell factor (SCF), and thrombopoietin (Tpo), are being studied in clinical trials (Bockheim and Jassak, 1993; Kaushansky *et al.*, 1995).

There are several clinical applications for HGFs (see Table 7.2). They are used most frequently in patients who are receiving chemotherapy. HGFs are used to hasten engraftment after autologous bone marrow transplant (BMT) and for patients with delayed engraftment after allogeneic BMT. HGFs are effective in mobilizing the release of bone marrow stem cells into the peripheral circulation where they are easily collected. Additional indications, such as differentiation therapy or stimulation of dendritic cells, are under investigation. Combinations of HGFs are being studied to determine whether the combination approach maximizes the effect of the proteins. Some HGFs, such as G-CSF and M-CSF, may be useful in treating patients with infection.

Classification

HGFs are synthesized by a wide variety of cells and they are classified according to the type of mature cells that grow in the colonies produced in response to these proteins. Class I HGFs are **multilineage**, acting on the pluripotent and immature progenitors. Class II HGFs act on more mature progenitor cells and are **lineage restricted** (see Table 7.3).

Lineage-Restricted Hematopoietic Growth Factors

G-CSF, Epo, M-CSF, Tpo, and IL-11 are class II lineage-restricted HGF proteins. G-CSF stimulates neutrophil production and maturation (Crosier and Clark, 1992; Wujcik, 1992). The effect occurs further along in the differentiation cascade on maturing progenitor cells. (See the following section entitled "Hematopoiesis.") G-CSF enhances the function of mature neutrophils as well.

Epo is produced in response to decreased levels of oxygen in the blood circulating through the kidneys. The presence of Epo allows a proliferating pool of committed erythroid progenitors to be maintained, permits erythroblast differentiation, and recruits immature progenitors (Bociek and Armitage, 1996).

M-CSF activates monocytes, prompting macrophage production. It also stimulates enhanced cytotoxicity against fungi. Tpo has a direct effect on megakaryocytopoiesis and

Table 7.1 Side effects of FDA-approved and investigational hematopoietic growth factors

	HGF	Generic Name (Trade Name)	Manufacturer	Side Effects
FDA-Approved HGFs	Epo	epoetin-alfa (Epogen®)	Amgen	Flu-like symptoms with arthralgias and myalgias
		epoetin-alfa (Procrit®)	Ortho Biotech	Occasional headache and bloodshot eyes
	G-CSF	filgrastim (Neupogen®)	Amgen	Bone pain in areas of high bone marrow reserve
	GM-CSF	sargramostim (Leukine®)	Immunex	Rare allergic reactions with rash, urticaria, facial edema, dyspnea, hypotension, and tachycardia
	IL-11	interleukin-11 (Neumega®)	Genetics Institute	Fever, dose-related fluid retention, dyspnea, myalgias, joint pain, and bone pain
Investigational HGFs	GM-CSF	molgrastim (Leucomax®)	Sandoz/Schering	Fluid retention with edema, tachycardia, dyspnea, and conjunctival redness
	M-CSF	M-CSF (Macstim®) (Macrolim®)	Genetics Institute/ Sandoz/Schering Chiron Therapeutics	Fever, fluid retention, dyspnea, myalgias, joint pain, and bone pain
	IL-3	IL-3	Sandoz	Fever, headache, rash, facial flushing, myalgias, photophobia; may cause thrombocytopenia, chest tightness, wheezing with *E. coli* product
	SCF	SCF	Amgen and Systemix	Dose-related fever, chills, headache, bone pain, facial flushing, nausea, and vomiting
	PIXY321 (fusion protein)	GM-CSF and IL-3 (Pixikine)	Immunex	Local injection-site reaction, dermatologic reactions, occasional cough, sore throat, throat tightness, and hypotension; Local injection-site reaction, headache, chest pain, and asthenia
	Tpo	Tpo	Genentech	Headache
	MGDF	MGDF	Amgen	Rash, deep-vein thrombosis, and pulmonary emboli

Abbreviations: Epo, erythropoietin; G-CSF, granulocyte colony-stimulating factor; GM-CSF, granulocyte-macrophage colony-stimulating factor; IL, interleukin; M-CSF, macrophage colony-stimulating factor; MGDF, megakaryocyte growth and development factor; SCF, stem cell factor; Tpo, thrombopoietin

Table 7.2   Clinical applications for hematopoietic growth factors

- Decrease chemotherapy-induced myelosuppression
- Stimulate hematopoiesis in marrow failure
- Promote cellular differentiation
- Support peripheral stem cell harvesting
- Enhance antibiotic therapy

platelet formation. IL-11 acts on stem cells and early and late progenitors. In addition, IL-11 plays a role in immune modulation by downregulating inflammatory products such as tumor necrosis factor (TNF), IL-1 beta, and IL-12

(Kaushansky, 1997; Prow and Vadhan-Raj, 1998).

Multilineage Hematopoietic Growth Factors

GM-CSF, IL-3, and SCF are class I multilineage HGF proteins. GM-CSF preferentially supports neutrophil, eosinophil, and macrophage development and interacts with progenitors at an earlier stage than G-CSF. It has both direct and indirect cellular effects. Direct effects on mature cells include inhibition of neutrophil migration, degranulation, changes in receptor expression, and effects on cytoskeleton and cell shape (Gasson *et al.*, 1990). Indirect

Table 7.3   Source and function of hematopoietic growth factors

HGF	Classification	Source	Function
Epo	Lineage-restricted	Kidney and liver	Stimulates erythrocyte progenitors
G-CSF	Lineage-restricted	Macrophages, fibroblasts, and endothelial cells	Stimulates neutrophil progenitors
M-CSF	Lineage-restricted	Many cell types	Stimulates progenitors of monocytes/macrophages
Tpo	Lineage-restricted	Liver, bone marrow, and kidneys	Stimulates megakaryocytopoiesis and platelets
IL-11	Lineage-restricted	Fibroblasts, endothelial cells, adipocytes, and monocytes	Stimulates platelet progenitors
GM-CSF	Multilineage	T lymphocytes, macrophages, endothelial cells, and fibroblasts	Stimulates progenitors of neutrophils, eosinophils, monocytes, and basophils
IL-3	Multilineage	T lymphocytes	Stimulates early progenitors for neutrophils, monocytes, platelets, eosinophils, basophils, and stem cells
SCF	Multilineage	Bone marrow stroma, many cell types	Stimulates pluripotent stem cell and progenitors for all cell lines

Abbreviations: Epo, erythropoietin; G-CSF, granulocyte colony-stimulating factor; GM-CSF, granulocyte-macrophage colony-stimulating factor; IL, interleukin; M-CSF, macrophage colony-stimulating factor; Tpo, thrombopoietin; SCF, stem cell factor.

effects have been referred to as priming effects because they enhance the ability of neutrophils to respond to secondary triggering signals and allow amplification of the immune response (Crosier and Clark, 1992). This includes enhancing the phagocytic function of neutrophils, macrophages, and eosinophils and increasing antibody-dependent, cell-mediated cytotoxicity toward tumor cells.

IL-3 causes stem cells to differentiate into granulocytes, macrophages, megakaryocytes, erythrocytes, and lymphocytes (Prow and Vadhan-Raj, 1998). SCF works at the earliest level of commitment to promote cell survival, proliferation, differentiation, adhesion, and functional activation (Ashman, 1999).

Biological Actions

HGFs are usually given in supraphysiologic dosages. However, a basic understanding of the role of HGFs in normal **hematopoiesis** is required in order to understand the role of HGFs in patient care.

Hematopoiesis

The process of hematopoiesis or blood cell production begins with the PPSC and culminates with the production of fully functional circulating cells (Appelbaum, 1989; Metcalf and Morstyn, 1991) (Figure 7.1). The PPSC is an uncommitted cell with the potential to become any cell of the blood. Although PPSCs are small in number within the marrow (1 to 2 million or 0.1% of marrow cells), they possess a unique characteristic. Each PPSC produces 2 daughter cells: one that enters a differentiation pathway and another that returns to a resting pool of cells. This allows self-renewal of the stem cell pool and provides a supply of cells to replace dying mature cells of the periphery. Production

of PPSCs can be increased by stress, infection, hemorrhage, or bone marrow depletion.

Hematopoiesis occurs in the extravascular spaces. The PPSCs grow and develop in sinusoidal spaces surrounded by bone marrow stroma, which consists of endothelial cells, fibroblasts, adipocytes, and macrophages that produce collagen and adhesive proteins. The **progenitor** cells stick to the collagen and adhesive proteins, ensuring maturation and development in the presence of the appropriate growth factors. Many of the HGFs necessary for hematopoiesis are produced by these stromal cells (Spangrude, 1994).

COMMITTED PROGENITOR CELLS

Once a cell leaves the stem cell pool, it begins the commitment process. The first level of commitment is to the myeloid or lymphoid lineage. These cells are somewhat pluripotent as they can commit to one of several cell lineages. The cells become more differentiated, that is, more committed to a single cell line, as they change from pluripotent cells to unipotent cells.

Each of the cell lineages that produces a mature functioning cell follows the same maturation process: from progenitor cell to precursor cell to mature cell. Progenitors are the earliest committed cells in each lineage. **Precursors** are immature cells. As the cells mature, their proliferative capacity becomes progressively restricted (Metcalf and Morstyn, 1991).

The lymphoid stem cells mature first into pre-B and pre-T progenitor cells and eventually mature into B and T lymphocytes. Myeloid stem cells, under the influence of HGFs, become the multilineage colony-forming unit that can produce granulocytes, erythrocytes, macrophages, and megakaryocytes (CFU-GEMM).

GRANULOCYTES

Granulocytes, which include neutrophils, eosinophils, and basophils, constitute the body's main defense against bacterial infection.

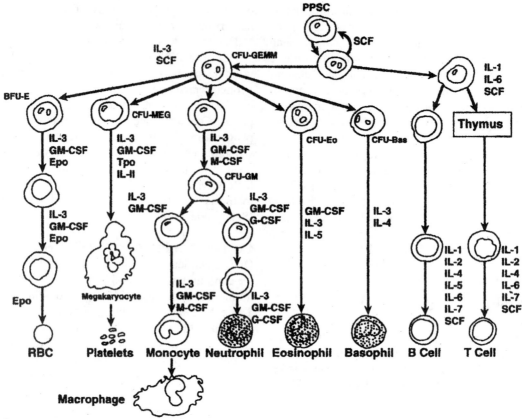

Figure 7.1 Hematopoietic cascade. BFU-E, burst-forming unit-erythrocyte; CFU-Bas, colony forming unit-basophil; CFU-Eo, colony forming unit-eosinophil; CFU-GEMM, colony forming unit-granulocyte, erythrocyte, macrophage, megakaryocyte; CFU-GM, colony forming unit-granulocyte/macrophage; CFU-Meg, colony forming unit-megakaryocyte; Epo, erythropoietin; G-CSF, granulocyte-colony stimulating factor; GM-CSF, granulocyte-macrophage colony-stimulating factor; IL, interleukin; M-CSF, macrophage-colony stimulating factor; PPSC, pluripotent stem cell; RBC, red blood cell; SCF, stem cell factor; Tpo, thrombopoietin.

Source: Reprinted with permission from: Wujick, D. 1993. Infection control in oncology patients. *Nursing Clinics of North America* 28(3): 639–650.

Neutrophils

Neutrophils are the most numerous type of granulocyte, accounting for 50% to 70% of the total white blood cell (WBC) count. Neutrophils are mature white blood cells containing neutrophil granules that attack and destroy bacteria. They are the first and most numerous cells to arrive at any area of disease or tissue injury. Because there are usually 3 times as many neu-

trophils stored in the bone marrow as there are circulating, a reserve pool is always ready.

Neutrophils go through 6 stages of maturation. The first 3 cell types, the myeloblasts, promyelocytes, and myelocytes, undergo cellular division over 4 to 5 days. At the metamyelocyte level, cells are no longer capable of mitosis, but maturation continues for approximately six more days. Mature cells are released into the peripheral blood where half circulate freely and the other half adhere to vessel walls. Neutrophils remain in the circulation 6 to 8 hours, then move into the tissues where they survive for 2 to 3 days. In times of serious injury, the total life span of a neutrophil decreases to several hours.

Eosinophils

Eosinophils comprise up to 4% of the total WBC count. The committed eosinophil progenitor, colony-forming unit-eosinophil (CFU-Eo), descends from the CFU-GEMM. There are 3 immature forms of eosinophils that precede the mature eosinophil: myeloblasts, promyelocytes, and myelocytes. Eosinophils circulate for about 8 hours, then migrate into the tissue. Eosinophils ingest bacteria and release factors that alter the inflammatory response. The eosinophil level is generally increased in patients who have parasitic infections and allergic reactions.

Basophils

Basophils differentiate in a manner parallel to that of eosinophils: colony-forming unit basophil (CFU-Bas); basophilic myeloblast, promyelocyte, and myelocyte; metamyelocyte; and basophil. Unlike neutrophils and eosinophils, basophils do not phagocytize bacteria. Rather, they release substances (including heparin and histamine) following stimulation, contributing to hypersensitivity reactions. Basophils account for up to 0.05% of the WBC count and may be elevated in patients with asthma, allergies, and some carcinomas.

ERYTHROCYTES

Erythrocyte development begins with the burst-forming unit-erythroid (BFU-E). The proliferating immature forms are proerythroblast and erythroblast. The normoblast, or next level of differentiation, loses the ability to divide. The **reticulocyte** is released into the bloodstream where it circulates for 1 to 2 days until it is a fully matured erythrocyte. The function of the erythrocyte is to transport oxygen to the tissues and carry carbon dioxide from the tissues to the lungs via the hemoglobin molecule.

MONOCYTES/MACROPHAGES

Monocytes and neutrophils share a common progenitor cell, colony-forming-unit granulocyte-macrophage (CFU-GM). Upon stimulation by certain HGFs, these cells produce monoblasts. Further maturation results in promonocytes and monocytes. The mature monocyte is released into the bloodstream, where it circulates for one to three days. After entering the tissue, the monocyte matures into a macrophage, which provides nonspecific immunity against parasitic, protozoan, and fungal infections. Normal monocyte levels are 6% to 8% of the WBC count.

MEGAKARYOCYTES

The committed megakaryocyte progenitor cell is the colony-forming unit-megakaryocyte (CFU-Meg). The earliest thrombocyte progenitor detected in the bone marrow is the megakaryoblast. The next level of differentiation is the megakaryocyte, which releases many platelets. Through a complex process, platelets form hemostatic plugs at the site of injured blood vessels. They also release factors that initiate clotting. Thrombocytes usually survive 7 to 8 days in the blood.

LYMPHOCYTES

Lymphocytes account for 30% to 35% of the total WBC count. The lymphoid stem cell arises from the PPSC and differentiates into one of two cell lineages, T or B lymphocytes. Pre-T lymphocytes mature in the thymus into prothymocytes, lymphoblasts, and T lymphocytes. T lymphocytes mediate cellular immunity, circulating freely between tissue and peripheral blood. When stimulated by specific antigens,

T lymphocytes produce many cytokines that regulate the specific immune response.

Pre-B lymphocytes migrate to lymph tissue, such as the spleen and lymph nodes, to mature. The B lymphoblast, responding to the antigen-antibody binding on its surface, matures into the B lymphocyte, and this cell eventually matures into a plasma cell capable of secreting specific antibodies (i.e., Igs). B lymphocytes comprise 20% to 25% of the lymphocyte count.

Hematopoietic Growth Factors in Hematopoiesis

The entire process of hematopoiesis is controlled by a complex feedback system. The HGFs regulate hematopoiesis by stimulating the cells to divide and mature in an orderly manner. Some HGFs have a specific influence on precursor and mature cells, whereas others affect cell differentiation and proliferation at the progenitor level (Crosier and Clark, 1992).

In a patient with an infection, HGF levels increase to stimulate neutrophil production and activity. When the T-cell receptor is activated by an antigen, one of the major responses is the production of multiple cytokines, including IL-2, IL-3, IL-4, IL-5, and IL-9; GM-CSF; TNF; and interferon (IFN-γ) (Crosier and Clark, 1992). Monocytes and macrophages respond to bacteria, bacterial cell-wall products, and other cytokines by releasing other cytokines such as IL-1 and IL-6, TNF, G-CSF, M-CSF, and GM-CSF (Wimperis et al., 1989). As the infection resolves, HGF levels return to normal.

In vivo studies have shown that endogenous levels of G-CSF are high in persons with chemotherapy-induced neutropenia and that these levels decline as the neutrophil count recovers (Layton et al., 1989; Watari et al., 1989). It has been shown that M-CSF and IL-6 are also elevated in patients who are febrile and neutropenic.

Cell Surface Receptors

HGFs work at the cellular level by binding to specific cell-surface-membrane receptors. Each receptor appears to receive only a single type of HGF, but receptors for more than 1 type of growth factor may be expressed on a given cell. The direct actions of HGFs are initiated by the binding of the particular HGF to cell-surface receptors. After binding to its specific receptor, the protein and its receptor are internalized into the cell and direct the cell to divide or mature. The remaining cell-surface receptors specific for the HGF are internalized or inactivated.

Moreover, the HGF can act indirectly on cells. The protein product released from the initial action can bind to a different cell and stimulate it, initiating a secondary cytokine cascade. For example, GM-CSF stimulates the release of macrophages, TNF, and IFN-γ. These cytokines are known to cause symptoms such as fever and chills (Traynor, 1992). Individual cells express more than 1 receptor. There are relatively few receptors on the cells (a few hundred per cell), and the biological effects are elicited with a low level of receptor occupancy, around 10% (Nicola, 1989; Metcalf and Morstyn, 1991). Receptors are present on both mature and immature cells.

Genetics

Genes that encode for GM-CSF, M-CSF, and IL-3 have been localized to a closely clustered region of the distal long arm of chromosome 5 (Yang, et al., 1988; van Leeuwen, et al., 1989). Of interest is the fact that this chromosome region is frequently deleted in patients with myelodysplastic syndromes (MDSs). Designated the 5q-syndromes, MDSs are also the chromosomal abnormalities seen most frequently in acute myeloid leukemia secondary to radiation exposure. The gene that encodes G-CSF has been mapped to chromosome 17

(Simmers *et al.*, 1987). The gene for Epo is on chromosome 7 in the region of q11–q22 (Spivak, 1989).

In 1994, several laboratories reported the discovery of the c-Mpl ligand that when bound to the Mpl receptors on the committed megakaryocyte progenitor promotes the proliferation and maturation of megakaryocytes (Schick, 1994). The Mpl ligand gene is mapped to chromosome 3q27, which consists of 7 exons linked to 6 introns. The human c-Mpl ligand has been identified and cloned into a full-length form (Tpo) and a truncated form (megakaryoctye growth and development factor or MGDF). The pegylated formulation is bound to polyethylene glycol to prolong its time in circulation (Fanucchi *et al.*, 1997). Recombinant IL-11 was isolated from a bone marrow stromal line and mapped to chromosome 19q13.3–13.4.

Once the genes for specific HGFs were identified, researchers were able to use recombinant techniques to produce them in large quantities. To do so, specific genes are isolated and combined with a DNA strand from another organism, which then serves as a factory, continuing to produce DNA identical to that in the original molecule (Jaramilla, 1992).

Animal Studies

Regulation of erythropoiesis was first demonstrated in 1950 (Reissman, 1950). Epo was purified in 1977, and by 1979, an assay for the protein was developed (Sherwood and Goldwasser, 1979; Miyake *et al.*, 1997). The physiology of Epo is not as well studied as the physiology of HGFs that were later identified (Spivak, 1989).

Preclinical studies of G-CSF began with intraperitoneal administration in mice (Fujisawa *et al.*, 1986; Kobayashi *et al.*, 1987). When given alone, G-CSF induced neutrophilia. When given after 5-fluorouracil and

total-body irradiation, neutrophil recovery was accelerated.

A study in which monkeys received subcutaneously administered G-CSF for 28 days resulted in neutrophilia with marrow hypercellularity and extramedullary hematopoiesis in lymph nodes (Welte *et al.*, 1987). When administered after cyclophosphamide and continued for 14 days, G-CSF restored the neutrophil count to pretreatment levels within 10 days. After the G-CSF was discontinued, the neutrophil count remained higher than that of the control group for another week. When G-CSF was also given before and concomitant to cyclophosphamide, neutropenia was more severe than in the control group, but neutrophil recovery was not affected. It was postulated that the G-CSF recruited responsive cells into the cell cycle, causing them to be more sensitive to the cytotoxic effects of the chemotherapy (Welte *et al.*, 1987).

Murine studies with GM-CSF demonstrated multilineage response that included neutrophils, macrophages, and eosinophils in addition to erythrocyte and megakaryocyte precursors (Metcalf, 1980; Metcalf *et al.*, 1980; Metcalf *et al.*, 1986). This factor has activity at both the progenitor level (CFU-GEMM) and in the differentiation of mature cells.

Further studies in monkeys have shown an acute and sustained rise in leukocytes in response to intravenous infusion of GM-CSF. Leukocytosis occurred within 24 to 72 hours following the initiation of the infusion, and bone marrow cellularity was increased by day 7 (Donahue *et al.*, 1986). Further studies demonstrated dose-dependent leukocytosis. Dosages have ranged from 4 to 300 mcg/kg/day (Demetri and Antman, 1992). Two early studies on primates demonstrated a nadir that occurred sooner than expected after chemotherapy, and combinations of HGFs were more effective than single HGFs in producing cellular response (Bonilla *et al.*, 1987; Donahue *et al.*, 1987).

Positive results in these studies led to clinical trials evaluating the effectiveness of HGFs in patients.

A number of HGFs, including IL-1, IL-3, GM-CSF, IL-6, GM-CSF + IL-3 (PIXY 321), and SCF, have been studied in the hope of ameliorating chemotherapy-induced thrombocytopenia. Each of these HGFs has minimal efficacy and moderate-to-excess toxicity (Ishibashi *et al.,* 1989; Asano *et al.,* 1990; Kaushansky, 1996). Preclinical trials with Tpo and MGDF have demonstrated a dose-response effect in platelets similar to that seen with neutrophils in response to G-CSF or GM-CSF. Miyazaki (1996) reported that recombinant human (rh) Tpo supported megakaryocyte colonies in rat marrow cultures. Daily administration of Tpo produced dose-dependent thrombocytosis and decreased the severity of thrombocytopenia in mice treated with mitomycin C.

Akahori *et al.* (1996) administered rhTpo intravenously to monkeys every day for 28 days beginning the day after nimustine. Doses of rhTpo were given at 0.04, 0.2, or 1.0 mcg/kg/day, with the highest dose completely preventing thrombocytopenia. There was also a reduction in neutropenia but no effect on anemia.

Farese *et al.* (1995) studied the effect of pegylated (PEG)-MGDF on platelet counts in normal rhesus monkeys. Daily administration for 10 days at doses of 2.5, 25, or 250 mcg/kg produced a significant increase in platelets. Ulich *et al.* (1991) evaluated PEG-MGDF on murine platelet recovery after carboplatin. The platelet count increased significantly by 6 days and peaked at 12 to 14 days after the completion of the cytokine.

Hokom *et al.* (1995) investigated a murine model of carboplatin and radiation therapy that produced a 94% mortality rate. Administration of PEG-MGDF decreased the mortality rate to less than 15% and also decreased the depth and duration of thrombocytopenia. Adding PEG-MGDF and G-CSF prevented any deaths and further reduced neutropenia and thrombocytopenia.

Clinical Trials

Clinical trials with HGFs began in 1986. Phase I studies sought to identify adverse effects and to define a dose-response relationship. Phase II studies endeavored to optimize the dose needed to achieve the desired biological effect (e.g., with G-CSF and GM-CSF, the dose needed to reduce neutropenia following chemotherapy). Phase III studies attempted to measure not only the biological effects of the HGFs but also to confirm clinical benefits.

Erythropoietin

Epo was first identified in 1906, was isolated in 1977, and is now produced by recombinant technology (Metcalf and Morstyn, 1991). Because the kidneys produce 90% of endogenous Epo, patients with chronic renal failure suffer from decreased Epo production and subsequent chronic anemia. Initial clinical trials demonstrated that administration of Epo stimulated erythropoiesis in these patients, usually increasing the reticulocyte count within 10 days and increasing the hematocrit level 2 to 6 weeks after initiation of therapy. Patients with renal failure typically became independent of transfusions on dosages of 50 to 300 mcg/kg 3 times weekly (Eschbach *et al.,* 1987).

Subsequent studies demonstrated that patients who are infected with the human immunodeficiency virus also responded to Epo according to their serum level of endogenous Epo prior to treatment (Eschbach *et al.,* 1987). Patients with Epo levels less than or equal to

500 mU/mL generally responded to Epo therapy, whereas those with Epo levels greater than or equal to 500 mU/mL did not seem to respond.

In patients with cancer, anemia may be related to the disease process itself or to the myelosuppressive effects of chemotherapy. A series of clinical trials evaluated 131 anemic patients who were receiving cyclic chemotherapy containing cisplatin or therapies that did not include cisplatin (Doweiko and Goldberg, 1991; Means and Krantz, 1991; Platanias *et al.*, 1991). Patients with lower endogenous Epo levels responded to the therapy as demonstrated by increased hematocrit levels and a decrease in the need for transfusions.

Epo has been studied in patients scheduled for surgery who would normally require blood transfusions and would not or could not participate in autologous blood donation programs. In a double-blind study of 318 patients scheduled for hip or knee surgery, the patients were stratified according to their preoperative hemoglobin (Hgb) level and then randomized to receive Epo or placebo (DeAndrade and Jove, 1996). There was a significant decrease in the need for an allogeneic transfusion in the group with Hgb greater than 10 and less than or equal to 13 g/dL. A later open-label study of 145 participants with Hgb levels greater than 10 and less than or equal to 13 g/dL who were also scheduled for hip or knee surgery resulted in fewer transfusions than were expected (Goldberg and McCutchen, 1996). The 2 groups received either: (1) 600 U/kg Epo weekly for 3 weeks prior to surgery and on the day of surgery or (2) 300 U/kg Epo once daily for 10 days prior to surgery, on the day of surgery, and 4 days after surgery. Postoperative mean Hgb levels were similar for the 2 treatment groups.

Recent studies have evaluated the effect of Epo on quality of life (QOL). In an open trial of 2,342 patients undergoing cytotoxic chemotherapy, patients reported an increase in mean self-rated scores for energy level, activity level, and overall QOL. These improvements correlated positively with increased Hgb levels (Glaspy *et al.*, 1997).

Bociek and Armitage (1996) reviewed a series of randomized, double-blind studies that demonstrated significant increases in hematocrit (defined as 6% or more) and in QOL measures in 50% of patients. They concluded that with only 50% of patients responding to Epo it is difficult to conclude that Epo therapy is cost-effective when compared with conventional transfusion therapy.

Cremieux *et al.* (1999) assessed whether quality-adjusted life-years (QALYs) of patients receiving Epo for chemotherapy-induced anemia provide a basis for measuring the value of supportive care interventions. Because Epo has been shown to improve QOL but not the length of life, the conclusion was the QALYs have limited value.

Ludwig *et al.* (1994) proposed an algorithm to identify patients who would benefit from Epo therapy. If after 2 weeks of Epo the serum Epo level is greater than 100 U/L and there is less than 0.5 g/dL improvement in Hgb levels, there is a 93% rate of nonresponse. If the serum Epo level is less than 100 U/L and the Hgb increase is greater than or equal to 0.5 g/dL, there is a 95% response rate. There is an 88% rate of nonresponse if the serum ferritin level is 400 mg/mL or greater after 2 weeks of therapy, although 75% of patients do respond if the ferritin level is less than 400 mg/mL.

Granulocyte-Macrophage Colony-Stimulating Factor

Early clinical trials of GM-CSF were conducted in patients with acquired immunodeficiency syndrome (AIDS) and MDS and in patients who were receiving myelosuppressive chemotherapy. Receiving HGFs allowed patients with

AIDS to continue receiving therapeutic but myelosuppressive drugs such as zidovudine, gancyclovir, or pentamidine. Groopman *et al.* (1987) administered GM-CSF as an intravenous bolus and as a continuous infusion to patients with AIDS. Increased WBC counts were documented along with edema, weight gain, and myalgias. Baldwin *et al.* (1987) demonstrated an increase in the number and the functionality of circulating neutrophils in these patients when GM-CSF was administered intravenously.

GM-CSF factor was used to induce differentiation of dysplastic cells in MDS. In 1987, Vadhan-Raj *et al.* (1987) administered GM-CSF to patients with MDS and noted an increase in neutrophil levels and a subsequent decrease in the incidence of infections and transfusions in these patients. A later study (Thompson *et al.*, 1989) verified the increased neutrophil levels but noted that the increase was temporary. Patients experienced fever and flu-like symptoms. Demetri and Antman (1992) reviewed 11 studies of GM-CSF in MDS. Overall, there was an increase in leukocyte levels in 50% to 75% of patients, but 10% to 25% of patients had concurrent increases in peripheral blood blast counts (Demetri and Antman, 1992). No significant risk of HGF-induced transformation to acute leukemia has been documented. The current recommendation is that HGFs should be used intermittently in a subset of patients with MDS who have neutropenia and recurrent infection (ASCO, 1994).

In early studies of HGFs administered following chemotherapy, patients with sarcoma who received mesna, doxorubicin, ifosfamide, and dacarbazine (MAID) received intravenous GM-CSF for 5 to 14 days after the first course of therapy (Antman *et al.*, 1987). The response of the WBC count to this regimen was compared with the response after the second cycle when no HGF was given. The WBC count was higher, and the nadir period was 4 days shorter

in the first than in the second cycle. This study has been criticized because a longer nadir period is expected after the second cycle of therapy. At doses of 4 to 32 mcg/kg/day, side effects were mild, but at 64 mcg/kg/day, fluid retention, and pericardial and pleural effusions were reported.

In studies with GM-CSF, dose-response-induced leukocytosis has been achieved reliably with continuous intravenous infusion, bolus intravenous infusion, and subcutaneous injection. In placebo-controlled randomized studies of patients who were receiving myelosuppressive chemotherapy, the number of days of neutropenic fever, the number of days of antibiotic treatment for infection, and the number of days of hospitalization were reduced with this factor (Antman *et al.*, 1988; Herrman *et al.*, 1990).

The use of GM-CSF has also been evaluated after high-dose chemotherapy followed by autologous BMT (Nemunaitis *et al.*, 1988a; Nemunaitis *et al.*, 1990b). The period of neutropenia was reduced in these patients from 18 to 12 days, but platelet recovery did not seem to occur earlier. The initial studies of GM-CSF in BMT were conducted in patients with lymphoid malignancies because of the hypothetical concern that GM-CSF would stimulate growth of neoplastic myeloid cells. Aurer *et al.* (1990) reviewed 8 autologous BMT studies and summarized the findings. Neutrophil recovery after BMT was accelerated by 7 days in those receiving GM-CSF, although the interval before neutrophils appeared in the peripheral blood after BMT was the same both for patients receiving GM-CSF and the control group. In addition, patients receiving GM-CSF had fewer days of fever, fewer platelet transfusions, and fewer days in the hospital after BMT. These benefits do not hold true for patients receiving marrow purged with 4 hydroperoxycyclophosphamide and anti-T- or anti-B-cell antibodies (Blazer *et al.*, 1989; Singer, 1992). There is no acceleration of neutrophil recovery by GM-CSF. This seems to demonstrate a need to preserve adequate numbers of CFUs in order to have a response to GM-CSF (Blazer *et al.*, 1989).

GM-CSF used in allogeneic BMT is also well tolerated (Mertelsmann *et al.*, 1990). Another theoretical concern was that GM-CSF would increase graft-versus-host disease (GVHD) due to the release of IL-1 and TNF, which stimulate T lymphocytes. This has not been demonstrated, and there has been no increase in acute GVHD. GM-CSF is more effective in patients who receive GVHD prophylaxis with cyclosporine and prednisone versus cyclosporine and methotrexate (Singer, 1992). Patients who have a matched unrelated donor (MUD) BMT have an increased risk of GVHD and graft failure. In a study using yeast-derived GM-CSF in 40 patients receiving a MUD BMT, there was no significant effect on neutrophil recovery, but there was decreased risk of infection (8% versus 24%). Although there was no difference in overall incidence of GVHD, there was a decreased risk of more severe grades III and IV GVHD (Singer *et al.*, 1990). Graft failure, defined as no engraftment of cells by day 28 after BMT, occurs in about 10% of BMT patients. GM-CSF stimulates marrow recovery in patients with graft failure with no increase in the incidence of GVHD (Nemunaitis *et al.*, 1988b).

Both G-CSF and GM-CSF have been effective in promoting neutrophil recovery after chemotherapy for acute myelogenous leukemia (AML) without evidence of CSF-induced blast-cell acceleration (Ohno *et al.*, 1990; Buchner *et al.*, 1991). GM-CSF has been administered to a high-risk population of elderly patients who were newly diagnosed with AML in an attempt to decrease the period of neutropenia. Although the period of absolute neutropenia was 6 to 9 days shorter in the group treated with GM-CSF, 2 patients experienced rapid regrowth of leukemic cells. This leukemia cell growth slowed in 1 patient after discontinuation of the HGF (Buchner *et al.*, 1991). Studies have been conducted in which growth factors were used to recruit AML blast cells into the S phase of the cell cycle, followed immediately by high-dose chemotherapy. This therapy significantly increased cell kill (Cannistra *et al.*, 1989; Estey, 1990).

Clinical trials have addressed the issue of whether the use of HGFs will allow for administration of dose-intensified therapy and thereby contribute to improved patient survival. Logothetis and colleagues (1990) studied the effect of GM-CSF in 32 patients with metastatic urothelial tumors who were refractory to methotrexate, vinblastine, doxorubicin, and cisplatin (MVAC). Unglycosylated rhGM-CSF allowed for escalation of chemotherapy doses even in heavily pretreated patients. Demetri and Antman (1992) studied patients with metastatic breast cancer who were receiving cyclophosphamide, doxorubicin, and 5-fluorouracil (CAF) and found that GM-CSF support allowed increases in the doses of cyclophosphamide and doxorubicin. In phase II trials, 40% of the treated patients responded with 23% achieving a complete remission (Demetri and Antman, 1992).

Although studies have suggested improvement in response rates and treatment results, few randomized studies have demonstrated the benefits of HGF-induced dose intensification. A study by Pujol *et al.* (1997) evaluated the dose intensity of a 4-drug regimen with and without GM-CSF in patients with extensive small-cell lung cancer. The 50% increase in dose could not be achieved because of excessive toxicity. However, the use of HGFs to mobilize stem cells from marrow to hasten myeloid recovery after high-dose chemotherapy and transplantation have been recommended (ASCO, 1994).

Granulocyte Colony-Stimulating Factor

Patients with MDS who were treated with intravenous G-CSF have also been found to have rapid increases in peripheral leukocyte and marrow granulocyte precursor levels with no increase in blast-cell level (Kobayashi et al., 1989). When subcutaneous G-CSF was used in patients with MDS (Negrin et al., 1989), 10 of 12 patients had 5- to 40-fold increases in neutrophil counts. No patient had converted to acute leukemia, and several had some differentiation of granulocyte precursors.

Gabrilove et al. (1988) administered G-CSF subcutaneously to patients with bladder cancer who were being treated with MVAC. The HGF was given on days 4 through 11 at a dose of 200 mcg/m². In addition to a shorter, less-severe nadir period, Gabrilove and colleagues noted decreased incidence of mucositis. Transient bone pain was also reported.

Crawford et al. (1991) described a study of 211 patients who received G-CSF or placebo after chemotherapy for small-cell lung cancer. The standard therapy for this disease is a chemotherapy regimen of cyclophosphamide, doxorubicin, and etoposide given in 6 cycles. The incidence of febrile neutropenia was 57% in the study group receiving placebo and 28% in the group receiving G-CSF. The G-CSF group had a 47% reduction in the number of days on antibiotics and spent 45% less time in the hospital.

In another classic study, patients with advanced cancer who received continuous subcutaneous infusion of G-CSF or GM-CSF experienced less myelosuppression than the control group (Morstyn et al., 1989a). The subcutaneous route was shown to be more effective than intravenous bolus infusion.

Dose-response leukocytosis may also result from continuous intravenous infusion (Bron-chud et al., 1987), bolus intravenous infusion (Gabrilove et al., 1988; Morstyn et al., 1988), and subcutaneous administration (Morstyn et al., 1989b) of G-CSF. In placebo-controlled randomized studies of patients who were receiving myelosuppressive chemotherapy, the number of days of neutropenic fever, of antibiotic treatment of infection, and of hospitalization were reduced with the use of G-CSF (Bronchud et al., 1987; Gabrilove et al., 1988; Morstyn et al., 1988; Neidhart et al., 1989; Crawford et al., 1991).

G-CSF has also been evaluated after high-dose chemotherapy followed by autologous BMT (Kodo et al., 1988; Taylor et al., 1989). A study by Sheridan et al. (1989) showed tendencies toward shorter hospital stays, fewer days of fever, shorter periods of total parenteral nutrition, and fewer days in a protected environment in patients who received G-CSF, but none of these differences achieved statistical significance.

G-CSF has been shown to increase levels of circulating peripheral blood stem cells (PBSCs). These cells are harvested by leukapheresis and used as an alternative to bone marrow for hematopoietic rescue after high-dose chemotherapy (To et al., 1987). HGFs can be used to predictably increase the number of progenitor cells available for harvest. One study demonstrated that the number of PBSCs collected increased a median 83 times (Sheridan, 1990). Patients who received PBSC and HGFs had periods of neutrophil recovery similar to those of the control group who received BMT and G-CSF or GM-CSF. Platelet recovery was significantly faster in the patients who received PBSCs than in the control group of BMT patients.

Several studies have demonstrated the impact of G-CSF on chemotherapy dose intensification (Bronchud et al., 1987; Neidhart et al., 1989). Bronchud et al. (1989) doubled or tripled the normal dosage of doxorubicin given to patients with advanced breast or ovarian cancer. Administration of G-CSF allowed the cytotoxic drugs to be administered at 14-day intervals. The dose-limiting toxic effects were mucositis and skin toxicity.

In another study, 65 patients with small-cell lung cancer who were receiving chemotherapy were randomized to receive G-CSF or no HGF. Dose reductions were not allowed in the study, but the interval between cycles was variable. The G-CSF group had a shorter interval between treatments, and there was an apparent increase in the 2-year survival rate that was not significant (Woll *et al.,* 1995).

Interleukin-11 and Thrombopoietin

Chang *et al.* (1996) studied endogenous IL-11, Tpo, and IL-6 levels in patients with bone marrow depression following chemoradiation. They found an inverse correlation of Tpo and IL-11 levels to platelet levels but not the same relationship of IL-6 to platelet levels. However, in patients with idiopathic thrombocytic purpura, where platelet production is normal but survival is not, IL-11 was increased but Tpo was not. The results suggest that IL-11 may be regulated by a negative feedback loop based on circulating platelet counts and that there are other regulatory factors involved in production of Tpo.

Phase I and II clinical trials have been conducted with Tpo and MGDF. Vadhan-Raj *et al.* (1996) reported on patients with sarcoma who received doxorubicin and ifosfamide every 21 days or thiotepa every 28 days for advanced cancer. Tpo was given in doses of 0.3, 0.6, 1.2, or 2.4 mcg/kg. Platelet counts increased from 60% to 200%, peaking on day 12. The platelet count was still significantly higher than baseline at day 21. There was no change in the WBC or red blood cell (RBC) counts. The most common

side effect in one third of patients was mild transient headache.

Basser *et al.* (1996) studied the use of MGDF before and after chemotherapy in patients with advanced cancer. Patients received placebo or MGDF daily for up to 10 days. MGDF was given subcutaneously in doses of 0.03, 0.1, or 1.0 mcg/kg. The median increases in dose-related response were 12% for the placebo and 39%, 51%, and 84%, respectively, for the different doses of MGDF. Patients receiving drug had a dose-responsive increase in platelets beginning on day 6; the platelet count continued to rise after the drug was stopped. Platelet recovery was complete at 18 days after chemotherapy for the MGDF group versus 26 days for the placebo group with no change in WBC or RBC counts. A low rate of toxic effects was reported.

Fanucchi *et al.* (1997) conducted a randomized, double-blind, placebo-controlled, dose-escalation study with MGDF. Fifty-three patients with lung cancer treated with carboplatin and paclitaxel received subcutaneous MGDF at 0.03, 0.1, 0.3, 1.0, 3.0, or 5.0 mcg/kg. Thirty-eight patients had a median platelet count of 189,000/mm^3 compared with 111,000/mm^3 in the placebo group. The platelet count recovered to baseline at 14 days for the MGDF group versus 21 days for the placebo group. Of the 40 patients receiving MGDF, 1 had pulmonary embolus and deep-vein thrombosis and another had superficial thrombophlebitis.

Interleukin-11

Schlerman *et al.* (1996) studied IL-11 in doses of 10, 30, and 100 mcg/kg in normal monkeys, and a dose-response effect was demonstrated. A dose of 125 mcg/kg/day was given after 3 days of carboplatin. Severe thrombocytopenia was prevented, and a more rapid recovery of platelet count was demonstrated.

Orazi *et al.* (1996) evaluated 12 women with breast cancer and no bone marrow involvement who were given 10, 25, 50, or 75 mcg/kg of IL-11 subcutaneously for 14 days. All doses of IL-11 stimulated precursor cells of different lineages.

A phase I trial of 16 women with stage IIIB or IV breast cancer utilized 5 dose levels of IL-11 (10, 25, 50, 75, and 100 mcg/kg/day) given subcutaneously for 14 days before chemotherapy (Gordon *et al.,* 1996). The women then received 1.5 gm/m^2 cyclophosphamide and doxorubicin. They then received the assigned dose of IL-11 on days 3 to 14. The prechemotherapy results showed an increased platelet count by day 4. The maximum tolerated dose was 75 mcg with grade 2 myalgias reported. There was a dose-dependent increase in platelets, no increase in WBC, and a 19% decrease in hematocrit. The study concluded that IL-11 is well tolerated at doses of 10, 25, and 50 mcg/kg/day and decreases thrombocytopenia at 25 mcg/kg/day and higher doses.

Tepler *et al.* (1996) conducted a multicenter, randomized, phase II trial in 93 patients who had received transfusions for low platelet counts. The patients were randomized to receive placebo or IL-11 at 50 or 25 mcg/kg/day for 14 to 21 days, beginning 1 day after chemotherapy. The end point of this study was the number of transfusions needed. In the study group, 8 of 27 patients did not need a transfusion, whereas 1 of 27 participants in the placebo group did not receive a transfusion. Fatigue and cardiovascular symptoms (e.g., tachycardia and atrial arrhythmia) were reported.

Isaacs *et al.* (1997) conducted a randomized trial of IL-11 after multicycle chemotherapy in 77 women with breast cancer. Primary efficacy was measured as preventing the need for a transfusion. The placebo group had a 41% success rate versus a 68% success rate in the IL-11 group. Patients received 2 blinded cycles after transfusions and recovered earlier. The

study conclusion was that IL-11 accelerated platelet recovery and was well tolerated.

Regulatory-Approved Agents

Granulocyte Colony-Stimulating Factor

G-CSF (filgrastim) was approved by the FDA for commercial use in 1991 to decrease the incidence of infections in patients with nonmyeloid malignancies receiving myelosuppressive chemotherapy. The recommended starting dose is 5 mcg/kg/day administered as a subcutaneous injection. If the desired response is not seen, the dosage may be doubled after the subsequent course of chemotherapy.

In 1994, G-CSF was approved for use after BMT in treatment of nonmyeloid malignancies and for patients with severe chronic neutropenia. The dose is 10 mcg/kg/day given intravenously over 4 to 24 hours and starting 24 hours after BMT. The most recent indication for G-CSF is for the mobilization of hematopoietic progenitor cells in PBSC transplantation. The dose is 10 mcg/kg/day given subcutaneously or by continuous infusion for at least 4 days. Apheresis begins on the fourth day. The optimal dose and duration of HGFs for PBSC transplantation remains under investigation (ASCO, 1996).

G-CSF may be given intravenously but is given over at least 30 minutes and must be diluted to less than 2 mcg/mL with 5% dextrose; G-CSF is not compatible with saline. Because levels of neutrophils decrease by about 50% in the first 24 hours after G-CSF is discontinued, it must be administered past the expected nadir (Figure 7.2). It is administered daily past the expected nadir for up to 2 weeks or until the absolute neutrophil count (ANC) exceeds 10,000 cells/mm^3. Comley *et al.* (1999) demonstrated no difference in ANC recovery, indura-

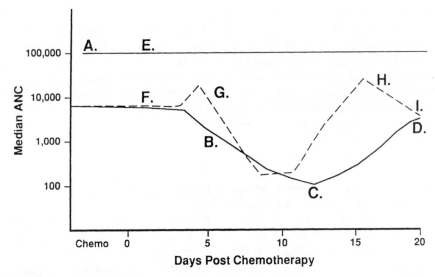

Figure 7.2 Infection risk and prophylaxis in a patient who was receiving myelosuppressive chemotherapy. (A) Chemotherapy is administered with varying numbers and combinations of drugs. (B) In response to interrupted blood cell production, the absolute neutrophil count (ANC) begins to decrease (solid line). (C) The nadir, or lowest ANC, usually occurs 10 to 14 days after chemotherapy begins. (D) Recovery of ANC is seen three to four weeks after chemotherapy begins. (E) Prophylactic antibiotics may be given to protect the patient throughout the period of neutropenia. (F) Colony-stimulating factors may be administered daily beginning 24 hours after therapy ends. (G) A rise in the ANC was due to the release of reserve cells from the marrow (broken line). (H) The nadir occurs earlier than expected, is of a shorter duration, and is less severe, and the ANC recovers rapidly. The colony-stimulating factor therapy is discontinued when the ANC exceeds 10,000/mm³. (I) The ANC decreases by half within 24 hours after discontinuation; the patient continues to produce neutrophils at normal levels.

Source: Reprinted with permission from Wujick, D. 1993. Infection control in oncology patients. *Nursing Clinics of North America* 28(3): 639–650.

tion, bruises, erythema, or patient discomfort when giving 1.6 mL in one or two subcutaneous injections. Monitoring recommendations include a baseline and then twice-weekly complete blood count and platelet count. Uric acid levels should be monitored in patients with malignancies associated with high uric acid levels.

Granulocyte-Macrophage Colony-Stimulating Factor

GM-CSF was approved by the FDA in 1991 under the generic name sargramostim and is indicated to accelerate myeloid recovery in selected patients who are undergoing autologous BMT. These are patients with non-Hodgkin's lymphoma, Hodgkin's disease, or acute lymphocytic leukemia. Additional approvals include its use after allogeneic BMT from human-leukocyte-antigen-matched donors, after BMT graft failure or engraftment delay, following induction chemotherapy in AML, and to mobilize hematopoietic progenitor cells for collection or further acceleration of myeloid reconstitution following PBSC transplantation.

GM-CSF is available in a powdered form along with diluent in a 250-mcg or 500-mcg size. The recommended dose is 250-mcg/kg/day, given as a daily infusion over 2 hours for 21 days or until myeloid recovery is achieved. Administration of GM-CSF is discontinued when the ANC exceeds 20,000 cells/mm³ or the platelet count exceeds 500,000 cells/mm³. This factor is compatible with saline or 5% dextrose in water if concentrations are greater than or equal to 10 mcg/mL (Immunex Corporation, 1997). Human serum albumin must be added to solutions with dilutions less than 10 mcg/mL.

The dose is the same for all indications but administration guidelines differ. For graft failure or delay, GM-CSF is given for 14 days, then stopped for 7 days. If needed, GM-CSF is repeated for 14 days and stopped for another 7 days. If indicated again, the dose is doubled and given for another 14 days. For PBSC pheresis, GM-CSF is given intravenously for 24 hours or subcutaneously each day for 4 days. It is administered daily beginning immediately after PBSC transplant until the ANC is greater than 1,500 for 3 days.

Monitoring includes complete blood count, differential, platelet count, and reticulocyte count at baseline, then twice weekly. Patients with preexisting renal dysfunction, hepatic dysfunction, or both require monitoring of liver enzymes and creatinine.

Recombinant GM-CSF is expressed in yeast, bacteria, and mammalian cells. Sargramostim, the GM-CSF expressed by yeast, is most like native GM-CSF as both are glycosylated (i.e., attached to a sugar molecule). Molgrastim is nonglycosylated. It is produced by *Escherichia coli* and remains investigational. Although the natural and recombinant products are similar, there are differences in the pharmacokinetics, biological activity, and immunogenicity. Dorr (1993) reviewed 32 clinical trials to compare frequency of adverse events experienced by pa-tients who received *E. coli*-derived GM-CSF and those who received yeast-derived GM-CSF and concluded that the *E. coli* product is associated with more side effects (Table 7.1). In addition, a "first-dose reaction" occurs with the *E. coli* product, characterized by flushing, hypotension, fever, dyspnea, musculoskeletal pain, transient hypoxia, diaphoresis, nausea, vomiting, and tachycardia (Morstyn *et al.*, 1989b).

Erythropoietin

Two recombinant Epo (epoetin alfa) products were approved by the FDA in 1989. Epogen® is indicated for use in patients with anemia associated with chronic renal failure. Procrit® is approved for use in patients with anemia due to chronic renal failure requiring dialysis, HIV infection requiring myelosuppressive therapy, and nonmyeloid malignancy and for the reduction of allogeneic transfusions in surgery patients. Administration of Epo enables these patients to become independent of transfusions and to continue therapy, respectively. The dose for renal failure is 50 to 100 U/kg administered subcutaneously 3 times per week.

The recommended dosage for treatment of anemia caused by cancer chemotherapy is 150 U/kg subcutaneously 3 times weekly. If a satisfactory response (defined as an increase of hematocrit by 5% to 6% points) is not obtained after 4 weeks of therapy, the dose is increased up to 300 U/kg. If the hematocrit increases by more than 4 points in a two-week period, the frequency is decreased to twice weekly (see Figure 7.3). It is important to rule out other causes of anemia such as iron, B_{12}, and folate deficiencies prior to starting Epo therapy (Worrall *et al.*, 1999).

Procrit also has an indication for surgery patients with an Hgb level greater than 10 and less than or equal to 13 g/dL. The recommended dosage is 300 U/kg/day subcutaneously for 10

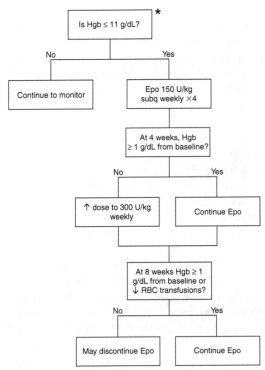

Figure 7.3   Algorithm for erythropoietin (Epo) administration

*Consider iron supplements if transferrin saturation is less than 20% or serum ferritin level is less than 100 ng/mL. Hgb, hemoglobin; RBC, red blood cell; ↑, increase; ↓, decrease.

days prior to surgery, on the day of surgery, and for 4 days after surgery.

Interleukin-11

IL-11 was approved by the FDA as oprelvekin in November 1998. The indication for IL-11 is the prevention of severe thrombocytopenia and a reduction in the need for platelet transfusions following myelosuppressive chemotherapy in patients with nonmyeloid malignancy who are at high risk for severe thrombocytopenia. IL-11 is administered once daily by subcutaneous injection 6 to 24 hours following chemotherapy

at a dose of 50 mcg/kg. IL-11, available in single-use vials of 5 mg, is reconstituted with 1 mL of sterile water. It is recommended that it be used within 3 hours.

Patient monitoring includes complete blood cell and platelet counts prior to starting chemotherapy and at regular intervals throughout the expected nadir. Daily injections are continued until platelet recovery is demonstrated.

Side Effects

For a complete review of side effects seen with HGF administration, see Table 7.1.

G-CSF is usually well tolerated. In phase II/III studies, bone pain was reported in 20% to 24% of patients and was described as mild to moderate, brief, and easily controlled with non-narcotic analgesia (Gabrilove *et al.*, 1988; Crawford *et al.*, 1991). The most common sites of bone pain were sternum, back, pelvis, and limbs, which are all bones with large marrow reserves. The pain typically occurs 2 to 3 days after administration of G-CSF begins and right before the WBC counts begin to rise, suggesting an association with rapid myelopoiesis.

Common side effects seen with GM-CSF administration include low-grade fever and bone pain. The dose-limiting toxic effects of this agent (pericarditis and atrial arrhythmias) were identified at doses greater than or equal to 20 mcg/kg/day. At doses ranging from 30 to 64 mcg/kg/day, pulmonary emboli, severe weight gain with pleural and pericardial effusions, and capillary leak syndrome were reported (Antman *et al.*, 1988; Brandt *et al.*, 1988; Hartmann and Edmonson, 1990). Doses of 2 to 20 mcg/kg/day were associated with milder side effects such as skin rashes, anorexia, fevers with chills, arthralgias, myalgias, and headaches. A "first-dose" reaction has been described with bolus intravenous administration that includes flushing, hypotension, transient hypoxia, and tachycardia. Subsequent administrations do not generally elicit this same response.

Epo is well tolerated, although blood pressure must be controlled prior to therapy and iron supplements may be needed to maintain iron stores in patients who receive this agent over long periods.

The side effects of IL-11 are symptoms associated with fluid retention. These symptoms disappear after the drug is discontinued. Patients may experience mild to moderate peripheral edema, dyspnea, and tachycardia. Conjunctival redness is also seen with IL-11 administration.

Clinical Issues

CLINICAL GUIDELINES
The American Society of Clinical Oncology (ASCO) convened an ad hoc Colony-Stimulating Factor Guideline Expert Panel that published guidelines for the use of HGFs in 1994 and 1996 (ASCO, 1994; ASCO, 1996). The format for development of the guidelines was consensus with high agreement on some issues and no agreement on others. Table 7.4 summarizes the main guidelines. Members of ASCO were surveyed in 1994 and 1997 to determine whether more appropriate patterns of CSF use occurred after the publication of the ASCO guidelines. Although decreased and more appropriate use occurred, many oncologists still use CSFs in scenarios and with scheduling criteria that the guidelines do not support (Bennett et al., 1999). Figure 7.4 is an algorithm for use in the administration of HGFs (Demetri, 1997).

TIMING
It is recommended that HGFs be administered 24 to 72 hours after chemotherapy. There is concern that increasing the number of divisions of the neutrophil progenitors and then destroying them with chemotherapy will result in severe myelosuppression. Timing of CSF administration was explored by Crawford et al. (1993). In patients with lung cancer who were receiving cyclophosphamide, doxorubicin, and etoposide, G-CSF was administered on day 4, 6, or 8. It is not yet clear whether it is better to start earlier or later. The results remain controversial.

Morstyn et al. (1989a) gave G-CSF before melphalan, and they were unable to prove that the HGF gave an advantage. One study showed that if G-CSF was delayed for up to 7 days after chemotherapy and administered for a short period (days 8 through 13 after chemotherapy), it would still shorten the nadir period. Meropol et al. (1992) administered G-CSF along with 5-fluorouracil and leucovorin and found that patients who received G-CSF experienced more severe neutropenia. Vadhan-Raj et al. (1992) evaluated the dose, schedule, and timing of GM-CSF administered with cyclophosphamide, doxorubicin, and dacarbazine (CyADIC) chemotherapy. The modified schedule, which allowed for earlier administration of GM-CSF (immediately following discontinuation of chemotherapy), improved the beneficial effects of GM-CSF by enhancing myeloprotection and permitting dose-intensification of chemotherapy.

A more recent study by Crawford et al. (1997) studied the effects of G-CSF given beginning on day 4, 6, or 8 after 3 days of chemotherapy. Initiating G-CSF on day 8 produced suboptimal hematologic recovery, whereas initiation on day 4 and day 6 produced a similar pattern of hematologic recovery.

The timing of HGFs after transplantation has also been evaluated. One retrospective analysis showed that delaying HGFs until 6 to 8 days after reinfusion of bone marrow instead of 24 hours after reinfusion did not significantly change the time to neutrophil recovery (Khwaja et al., 1993). In another study of 96 patients with stage II to IV breast cancer, the delay of

Table 7.4   Practice guidelines for granulocyte colony-stimulating factor and granulocyte-macrophage colony-stimulating factor

Indication	Recommendation
Primary administration (before neutropenia or fever)	Not recommended on a routine basis Use if risk of febrile neutropenia in 40% or greater Use if patient has preexisting or active fever
Secondary administration (protection against new episodes of febrile neutropenia or chemotherapy dose reductions)	
Afebrile patients	Not recommended
Febrile patients	Not recommended unless certain risk factors indicating poor outcome are present, such as pneumonia, hypotension, multiorgan dysfunction, or fungal infection
Dose intensification	Not recommended unless in clinical trial
PBSC transplantation	Recommended to enhance PBSC mobilization and hasten myeloid recovery after transplantation
Myeloid malignancies	Not recommended for priming effect before induction chemotherapy unless in clinical trial Recommended for decreasing duration of neutropenia when given right after induction therapy in older patients ($\geq$55 years)
Myelodysplastic syndromes	Intermittent use in neutropenic patients with infection
Patients receiving concomitant chemotherapy and radiation therapy	Not recommended

PBSC, peripheral blood stem cell.

Source: Data from ASCO. 1994. American Society of Clinical Oncology recommendations for the use of hematopoietic colony-stimulating factors: Evidence-based clinical practice guidelines. *Journal of Clinical Oncology* 12(11): 2471–2508; ASCO 1996. Update of recommendations for the use of hematopoietic colony-stimulating factors: Evidence-based clinical practice guidelines. *Journal of Clinical Oncology* 14(6): 1957–1960.

G-CSF for up to 7 days after autologous PBSC transplantation did not alter the time to neutrophil recovery after starting G-CSF but did add to the time to full recovery (Schwartzberg *et al.*, 1994). Further study of G-CSF administration at day 1 or day 7 after PBSC transplantation did not show a significant difference in the amount or length of supportive treatment during hospitalization (Piccirillo *et al.*, 1999).

LENGTH OF THERAPY

The optimal length of HGF therapy remains unclear. The optimal ANC (greater than 1,000, 5,000, or 10,000/mm^3) is not apparent. In dose-intensive regimens, stopping at 10,000 mm^3 does not always ensure that counts will not drop lower. A priming effect has been observed: neutropenia is less severe in some patients during the second and subsequent cycles of chemo-

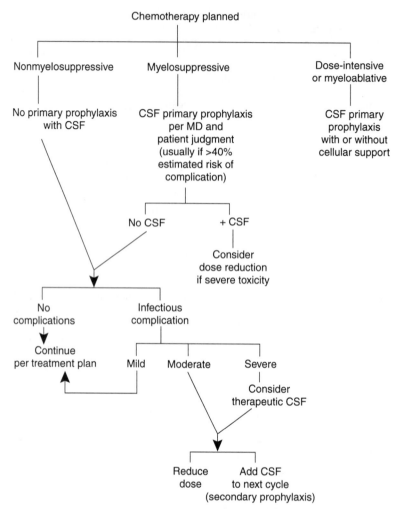

Figure 7.4 Algorithm for use in the administration of hematopoietic growth factors. CSF, colony-stimulating factor(s).

Source: Reprinted with permission from Demetri, G.O. 1997. Hematopoietic Growth Factors. In Holland, J., Bast, R., Morton, D., Frei, E., Kufe, D. and Weichselbaum, R. (eds.). *Cancer Medicine* 4th edn. Baltimore: Williams and Wilkins, pp 1227-1243.

therapy (Crawford *et al.*, 1991). The ASCO guidelines recommend continuing HGF therapy until the ANC is greater than or equal to 10,000/mm³ (ASCO, 1994).

DOSE INTENSIFICATION

HGFs have demonstrated the ability to reduce morbidity and make present chemotherapy regi-

mens more tolerable. However, an even greater question is whether the use of HGFs will allow for dose-intensification of therapy that could ultimately translate into improved patient survival. Studies exploring this question have been conducted with mixed results.

Phase I and II studies in patients with non-Hodgkin's lymphoma showed successful dose intensification using G-CSF. Doses of epirubicin and cyclophosphamide were doubled (Talbot *et al.*, 1999) and doses of cyclophosphamide, doxorubicin, vincristine, and prednisone (CHOP) were increased by 1.8 times (Santoro *et al.*, 1999).

A phase I and II trial of intensification of the MAID regimen enabled a 25% increase (Chevreau *et al.*, 1999). Patients with limited-stage small-cell lung cancer achieved a 5-year progression-free survival of 53% with high-dose cyclophosphamide, cisplatin, and carmustine followed by stem cell support (Elias *et al.*, 1999). A phase III study in patients with small-cell lung cancer demonstrated that the ACE protocol (doxorubicin, cyclophosphamide, etoposide) with G-CSF could be given every two weeks instead of three weeks, with improved survival (Thatcher *et al.*, 2000).

Other studies have negative results. Font *et al.* (1999) conducted a randomized trial in patients with advanced non-small-cell lung cancer. Although a 32% increase in dose intensification was achieved, comparable improvements in survival were not demonstrated. An intensification regimen for patients with advanced head and neck cancer with radiation therapy, chemotherapy with routine G-CSF support, and surgical resection produced unacceptable systemic toxicity (Grecula *et al.*, 1999). Another study of dose intensification using GM-CSF for adults with acute lymphoblastic leukemia found no major improvements in outcome (Ifrah *et al.*, 1999). At this time, ASCO guidelines do not recommend HGFs to augment dose intensification (ASCO, 1996).

Investigational Agents

Stem Cell Factor

SCF is an HGF that acts on the earliest progenitors and possibly the PPSCs. It is also known as the "Steel factor," so named because it is the HGF missing in Steel mutant mice, which have an aberrant hematopoietic process (Bernstein and Kufe, 1992). This HGF was simultaneously identified and named by other investigators as "kit ligand" (Williams *et al.*, 1990b), "mast cell growth factor" (Anderson *et al.*, 1990; Huang *et al.*, 1990), and SCF (Zsebo *et al.*, 1990).

SCF interacts with the most primitive cell forms and supports growth of various colonies when used in combination with other HGFs (Anderson *et al.*, 1990). When compared with GM-CSF and IL-3, SCF produces a greater number of cell colonies and greater colony sizes (Bernstein *et al.*, 1991). However, exposure of bone marrow cultures to SCF alone does not result in significant colony formation. When administered in combination with G-CSF, GM-CSF, or IL-3, both colony size and number increase (Bernstein *et al.*, 1991; McNiece *et al.*, 1991).

SCF continues to be studied in the mobilization of stem cells for PBSC transplantation, especially in combination with other cytokines (McNiece *et al.*, 1991; Andrews *et al.*, 1995). Glaspy *et al.* (1995) administered SCF and G-CSF daily for 7 days to women with metastatic or localized breast cancer. All had previously received multiple cycles of chemotherapy. The results showed enhanced mobilization compared with controls using G-CSF alone. Weaver *et al.* (1996) investigated the mobilization of long-term, culture-initiating cells (LTC-IC) in the blood of women with ovarian cancer receiving G-CSF plus escalating doses of SCF versus G-CSF alone after chemotherapy. Enhanced mobilization of both LTC-IC and committed progenitors was seen with the SCF/G-CSF group.

There are several potential clinical applications for SCF. Expansion of a progenitor population that is responsive to a later, more lineage-restricted hematopoietin is one possibility. Use of SCF may decrease the dosage of a second growth factor needed to stimulate an appropriate number of colonies. Another potential application is to accelerate marrow regeneration in BMT. It has been proposed that if SCF does stimulate the PPSC, a single stem cell could be selected, stimulated with SCF, and used for BMT.

The FDA Biological Response Modifiers Advisory Committee in July 1998 recommended the approval of stemgen (Ancestim, r-metHuSCF), an SCF recommended for use in the treatment of cancer patients receiving stem cell transplants. Full licensing is pending (Cancer Economics, 1998).

Macrophage Colony-Stimulating Factor

M-CSF is a lineage-specific HGF that supports proliferation and activation of monocytes and their committed progenitors. It has been shown in animal studies to stimulate the numbers and size of monocytes (Garnick and Stoudemire, 1990; Bajorin et al., 1991; Stoudemire and Garnick, 1991). In a phase I study, patients with metastatic melanoma received 7-day infusions of M-CSF ranging from 12 to 120 mcg/kg/day. Increased numbers of circulating monocytes were noted, and there was also a decrease in platelet counts that reversed upon drug cessation. One patient showed tumor regression. Overall, M-CSF was well tolerated.

M-CSF has been given with IFN-γ to induce proliferation of peripheral monocytes and differentiation into circulating macrophages. It was administered by continuous intravenous infusion for 14 days at doses of 10 to 140 mcg/kg/day and subcutaneously on days 8 through 14 (Weiner et al., 1993). Some tumor regression was noted in 3 of 28 patients, and all had increased levels of macrophages.

Monocytes stimulated by M-CSF have greater cytotoxicity in fungal infections than normal monocytes. M-CSF has been shown to be useful in treating fungal infections refractory to amphotericin B therapy (Nemunaitis et al., 1990a). A phase I/II trial of recombinant M-CSF explored the use of this HGF in patients with invasive fungal infections. Sixteen patients were treated, 13 who had had BMT and 3 who were too ill to undergo BMT. The 3 very ill patients had complete resolution of infection. Ten of the 13 BMT patients had improvement or resolution (Nemunaitis et al., 1993).

More recently, Ohno et al. (1997) reported a study of 198 patients with AML in remission who received 3 courses of consolidation chemotherapy and M-CSF or placebo. The M-CSF was given at 8 $\times$ 10^6 U/day daily beginning after the last chemotherapy dose and continuing for 14 days. The M-CSF group had 34% fewer days of febrile neutropenia and a shorter overall time to completion of consolidation therapy. However, no significant difference in survival was reported.

Maruhashi et al. (1997) evaluated the usefulness of M-CSF in decreasing chemotherapy-induced neutropenia in women with ovarian cancer. M-CSF at a dose of 1 $\times$ 10^6 U/day was infused intravenously for 7 days after chemotherapy in a randomized, double-blind, controlled study. The drug was well tolerated, and the period between cycles was shorter for the M-CSF group.

Interleukin-3

IL-3 is also known as "multi-CSF." This multi-lineage HGF acts on early progenitors (Lindemann and Mertelsmann, 1993). Alone, it is the most effective cytokine in supporting CFU-GEMM formation in humans and, specifically, is a more potent stimulator of megakaryocytopoiesis than other HGFs. IL-3 produces a multi-lineage response, with increases in leukocytes, platelets, and reticulocytes. The response is delayed in platelets and erythrocytes, probably indicating that IL-3 should be administered continuously for prolonged periods.

IL-3 has been studied in patients with advanced malignancy, patients with prolonged myelosuppression secondary to chemotherapy or radiation therapy, and patients with MDS or aplastic anemia (Ganser *et al.*, 1990a; Ganser *et al.*, 1990b; Hoelzer *et al.*, 1991). Treatment consisted of 30 to 500 mcg/m² IL-3 given as a subcutaneous bolus injection daily for 15 days. The first doses were given intravenously over 5 minutes. The intravenous injection produced an increase in neutrophil counts within 30 minutes that peaked at 4 to 6 hours.

The toxic effects of subcutaneously administered IL-3 were mild. Seventy percent of patients had fever that was more pronounced during the first few days of therapy and was associated with higher dosages. Headache, chills, and bone pain were also reported.

IL-3 continues to be evaluated in clinical trials. In a study by Lemoli *et al.* (1996), patients with Hodgkin's disease and non-Hodgkin's lymphoma were randomly assigned to receive G-CSF alone, G-CSF combined with IL-3, or sequential G-CSF and IL-3 after autologous BMT. Patients receiving both G-CSF and IL-3 recovered more quickly and had lower transfusion requirements and shorter durations of hospitalization. There was no significant difference in results based on sequential versus concomitant administration; however, data suggest a possible trend toward faster hematologic recovery when the drugs are given concomitantly.

Novel Erythropoiesis-Stimulating Protein

Novel erythropoiesis-stimulating protein (NESP) is being evaluated for its potential to stimulate the production of RBCs. NESP has demonstrated an increased circulating serum half-life compared with Epo. This may indicate that NESP has a clinical advantage over Epo, because NESP would require less-frequent dosing. However, less-frequent dosing with Epo, is also being evaluated (Gabrilove *et al.*, 1999).

As of July 2000, Amgen had submitted regulatory license applications for NESP in the United States.

Combinations of Hematopoietic Growth Factors

There is enhancement of early progenitors *in vitro* when early- and late-acting HGFs are combined (Brugger *et al.*, 1992a; Brugger *et al.*, 1992b). G-CSF plus Epo prevented anemia and neutropenia in AIDS patients who were receiving zidovudine (Miles *et al.*, 1991). Other combinations of HGFs, such as IL-3 plus GM-CSF, have also been studied. Preclinical studies indicate that sequential administration produces better results than simultaneous administration. Molecules administered simultaneously may compete for the same receptors, altering the number of functional receptors for each CSF (Hoelzer *et al.*, 1991; Brugger *et al.*, 1992a).

Another application for cytokine combinations is the *ex vivo* expansion and maintenance of bone marrow cells prior to BMT. Hassan (1996) found that a combination of Epo, SCF, and IL-3 or Epo, SCF, and IL-11 was sufficient for maintaining erythropoiesis in long-term human bone marrow cultures that previously could not sustain erythropoiesis.

Growth factors can be fused together using molecular techniques. IL-3 and GM-CSF have been combined into a molecule, PIXY321, that has greater bioactivity than either IL-3 or GM-CSF alone (Williams *et al.*, 1990a). PIXY321 is 10- to 20-fold more potent on a weight basis than GM-CSF or IL-3 given alone or sequentially. This molecule is administered subcutaneously once or twice daily or intravenously over 2 hours. It is unknown whether the fusion protein provides a better therapeutic response than sequential administration of the 2 CSFs (Bernstein *et al.*, 1991).

Three studies of PIXY321 in patients who

were receiving myelosuppressive chemotherapy have been reported. In 1 study, patients with sarcoma treated with cyclophosphamide, doxorubicin, and dacarbazine received PIXY321 subcutaneously twice daily before the first dosages of chemotherapy and after the second cycle 3 weeks later (Vadhan-Raj *et al.*, 1992). A dose of 750 mcg/m^2 was determined to be optimal for decreasing myelosuppression and reducing cumulative thrombocytopenia. Local skin reactions and mild constitutional symptoms were the only side effects reported. Other studies evaluated PIXY321 in patients with breast cancer who are receiving doxorubicin and thiotepa (Reptis *et al.*, 1993) and in patients with advanced cancer who are receiving high-dose carboplatin (Miller *et al.*, 1993).

Broxmeyer *et al.* (1995) reported the success of PIXY321 administration for stimulation of multipotential and lineage-restricted progenitors. In doses less than 1,000 mcg, the results were similar to those seen previously with GM-CSF. At higher doses of PIXY321, the cells remained in a cycling state even after cessation of the agent.

Jones *et al.* (1999) conducted a double-blind, placebo-controlled trial to evaluate PIXY321 in stage II and III breast cancer. Although there was decreased incidence and duration of chemotherapy-induced neutropenia in cycles 1 and 2, there was more systemic toxicity and thrombocytopenia in cycles 3 and 4.

The role of combination HGFs in clinical practice and the impact on patient survival are not yet known. The results of phase III and IV studies will provide the evidence to support or refute the use of combinations of HGFs.

Future Directions

Many clinical issues remain in determining the optimal use of HGFs. Several hematopoietic and nonhematopoietic cell lines have receptors for HGFs. Colonic adenocarcinoma (Berdel *et al.*, 1989), small-cell lung cancer (Avalos *et al.*, 1990), breast cancer, osteosarcoma (Baldwin *et al.*, 1989; Berdel *et al.*, 1989), and leukemia cells have been identified as having receptors for HGFs. A clinical implication is that these factors may stimulate rather than retard growth of malignant cells, but this has not yet been known to occur.

Dosing schedules continue to be evaluated. Dose increases are recommended if the time to response by WBC count or the magnitude of neutrophil response are unacceptable, for example, in patients with prior irradiation of bone marrow areas, patients who have had a BMT, and patients whose doses have been intensified. Thus far, the maximum tolerated dose has not been identified. Patients have received up to 115 mcg/kg/day of G-CSF.

A number of different trials are looking at HGFs in combination with other agents. A novel agent, PSK, a protein-bound polysaccharide, is being combined with various cytokines. In preclinical evaluation, the addition of PSK seems to improve myelosuppression (Kohgo *et al.*, 1994). An IL-3 receptor agonist, daniplestim (SC-55494), was combined with G-CSF for PBSC mobilization and was found to be superior to G-CSF alone (DiPersio *et al.*, 1997). Long-acting forms of G-CSF have been identified as well. A single dose of Ro25-8315, a pegylated derivative of nartograstim, a human G-CSF, has been shown to achieve pharmacodynamic effects equivalent to G-CSF at 5 mcg/kg/day or 10 mcg/kg/day over 5 to 7 days for PBSC mobilization (Xu *et al.*, 1997). One dose of sustained duration filgrastim appears equivalent to daily filgrastim before and after chemotherapy (Johnston *et al.*, 1998). A phase I trial combining M-CSF and anti-GD3 ganglioside monoclonal antibody in patients with metastatic melanoma demonstrated tumor regression (Minasian *et al.*, 1995). Further investigation of M-CSF continues. The use of fusion products leads researchers to wonder about the possibility of HGF cocktails that combine specific HGFs to elicit a specific response. Some speculate that neutralizing antibodies may develop secondary to an immune response to the synthetic genetic linkage (Bernstein and Kufe, 1992).

Clinicians continue to evaluate which patients undergoing specific protocols will benefit from the use of HGFs. To date, CSFs have not been evaluated with drugs that cause delayed myelosuppression, such as the nitrosoureas or mitomycin C. Cost and QOL remain important issues to consider when using HGFs in the therapy of the patient with cancer.

References

Akahori, H., Shibuya, K., Obuchi, M., *et al.* 1996. Effect of recombinant human thrombopoietin in nonhuman primates with chemotherapy-induced thrombocytopenia. *British Journal of Haematology* 94(4): 722–728.

Anderson, D., Lyman, S., Baird, A., *et al.* 1990. Molecular cloning of mast cell growth factor, a hematopoietin that is active in both membrane bound and soluble forms. *Cell* 63(1): 235–243.

Andrews, R., Briddell, R., Knitter, G., *et al.* 1995. Rapid engraftment by peripheral blood progenitor cells mobilized by recombinant human stem cell factor and recombinant human granulocyte colony-stimulating factor in nonhuman primates. *Blood* 85: 15–20.

Antman, K., Griffin, J., Elias, A., *et al.* 1987. Use of rhGM-CSF to ameliorate chemotherapy induced myelosuppression in sarcoma patients. *Blood* 70(5 suppl 1): 129a (abstract).

Antmann, K., Griffin, J., Levine, J., *et al.* 1988. Effect of recombinant human GM-CSF on chemotherapy induced myelosuppression. *The New England Journal of Medicine* 319(10): 593–598.

Applebaum, F. 1989. The clinical use of hematopoietic growth factors. *Seminars in Hematology* 26(3 suppl 3): 7–13.

Asano, S., Okano, A., Ozawa, K., *et al.* 1990. *In vivo* effects of recombinant human interleukin-6 in primates: Stimulated production of platelets. *Blood* 75(8): 1602–1605.

ASCO. 1994. American Society of Clinical Oncology recommendations for the use of hematopoietic colony-stimulating factors: Evidence-based on clinical practice guidelines. *Journal of Clinical Oncology* 12(11): 2471–2508.

ASCO. 1996. Update of recommendations for the use of hematopoietic colony-stimulating factors: Evidence-based on clinical practice guidelines. *Journal of Clinical Oncology* 14(6): 1957–1960.

Ashman, L. 1999. The biology of stem cell factor and its receptor C-kit. *International Journal of Biochemistry and Cell Biology* 31: 1037–1051.

Aurer, I., Ribas, A., Gale, R., *et al.* 1990. What is the role of recombinant colony stimulating factors in bone marrow transplantation? *Bone Marrow Transplantation* 6: 79–87.

Avalos, B., Gasson, J., Hedvat, C., *et al.* 1990. Human granulocyte colony-stimulating factor: Biologic activities and receptor characterization on hematopoietic cells and small cell lung cancer cell lines. *Blood* 75(4): 851–857.

Bajorin, D., Nai-Kong, V., and Houghton, A. 1991. Macrophage colony stimulating factor: Biological effects and potential applications for cancer therapy. *Seminars in Hematology* 28(2 suppl 2): 42–48.

Baldwin, G., Gasson, J., Kaufman, S., *et al.* 1989. Nonhematopoietic tumor cells express functional GM-CSF receptors. *Blood* 73(2): 1033–1037.

Baldwin, G., Gasson, J., Quan, S., *et al.* 1987. GM-CSF enhances neutrophil function in AIDS patients. *Blood* 70(5 suppl 1): 130a (abstract).

Basser, R., Rasko, J., Clarke, K., *et al.* 1996. Thrombopoietic effects of pegylated recombinant human megakaryocyte growth and development factor (PEG-rHuMGDF) in patients with advanced cancer. *The Lancet* 348(9037): 1279–1281.

Bennett, C., Weeks, J., Somerfield, M., *et al.* 1999. Use of hematopoietic colony-stimulating factors:

Comparison of the 1994 and 1997 American Society of Clinical Oncology surveys regarding ASCO clinical practice guidelines. *Journal of Clinical Oncology* 17: 3676–3681.

Berdel, W., Danhauser-Riedl, S., Steinhauser, G., *et al.* 1989. Various human hematopoietic growth factors (interleukin-3, GM-CSF, G-CSF) stimulate clonal growth of nonhematopoietic tumor cells. *Blood* 73(1): 80–83.

Bernstein, I., Andrews, R., and Zsebo, K. 1991. Recombinant human stem cell factor enhances the formation of colonies by CD34+ and CD34+ lin-cells, and the generation of colony-forming cell progeny from CD34+ lin-cells cultured with IL-3, G-CSF, or GM-CSF. *Blood* 77(7): 2316–2321.

Bernstein, S., and Kufe, D. 1992. Future of basic/clinical hematopoiesis research in the era of hematopoietic growth factor availability. *Seminars in Oncology* 19(4): 441–448.

Blazer, B., Kersy, J., McGlave, P., *et al.* 1989. *In vivo* administration of recombinant human granulocyte-macrophage colony-stimulating factor in acute lymphoblastic leukemia patients receiving purged autografts. *Blood* 73: 849–857.

Bociek, R., and Armitage, J. 1996. Hematopoietic growth factors. *CA: A Cancer Journal for Clinicians* 46: 165–184.

Bockheim, C., and Jassak, P. 1993. The expanding world of colony-stimulating factors. *Cancer Practice* 1(3): 205–216.

Bonilla, M., Gillio, A., Porter, G., *et al.* 1987. Effects of recombinant human granulocyte colony stimulating factor and granulocyte-macrophage colony stimulating factor on cytopenias associated with repeated cycles of chemotherapy in primates. *Blood* 70(5): 377a (abstract).

Brandt, S., Peters, W., Atwater, S., *et al.* 1988. Effect of recombinant human GM-CSF on hematopoietic reconstitution after high-dose chemotherapy and autologous bone marrow transplantation. *The New England Journal of Medicine* 318(14): 869–876.

Bronchud, M., Howell, A., Crowther, D., *et al.* 1989.

The use of granulocyte colony-stimulating factor to increase the intensity of treatment with doxorubicin in patients with advanced breast and ovarian cancer. *British Journal of Cancer* 60(1): 121–125.

Bronchud, M., Scargge, J., Thatcher, N., *et al.* 1987. Phase I/II study of recombinant human G-CSF in patients receiving intensive chemotherapy for small-cell lung cancer. *British Journal of Cancer* 56(6): 809–813.

Broxmeyer, H., Benninger, L., Cooper, S., *et al.* 1995. Effects of *in vivo* treatment with PIXY321 (GM-CSF/IL-3 fusion protein) on proliferation kinetics of bone marrow and blood myeloid progenitor cells in patients with sarcoma. *Experimental Hematology* 23(4): 335–340.

Brugger, W., Frisch, J., Schulz, G., *et al.* 1992a. Sequential administration of interleukin-3 and granulocyte-macrophage colony-stimulating factor following standard dose combination chemotherapy with etoposide, ifosfamide, and cisplatin. *Journal of Clinical Oncology* 18(9): 1452–1459.

Brugger, W., Klaus-J, B., Lindemann, A., *et al.* 1992b. Role of hematopoietic growth factor combinations in experimental and clinical oncology. *Seminars in Oncology* 19(2 suppl 4): 8–15.

Buchner, T., Hidemann, W., Koenigsmann, M., *et al.* 1991. Recombinant human granulocyte-macrophage colony-stimulating factor after chemotherapy in patients with acute myeloid leukemia at higher age or after relapse. *Blood* 78(5): 1190–1197.

Cancer Economics. 1998. FDA advisors recommend approval of Stemgen for SCT. "Cancer Economics" is a supplement to *The Cancer Letter, Inc.*: 4–5.

Cannistra, S., Groshek, P., and Griffin, J. 1989. Granulocyte-macrophage colony-stimulating factor enhances the cytotoxic effects of cytosine arabinoside in acute myeloblastic leukemia and in the myeloid blast crisis phase of chronic myeloid leukemia. *Leukemia* 3(5): 328–334.

Chang, M., Suen, Y., Meng, G., *et al.* 1996. Differential mechanisms in the regulation of endogenous levels of thrombopoietin and interleukin-11 during thrombocytopenia: Insight into the regulation of platelet production. *Blood* 88(9): 3354–3362.

Chevreau, C., Bui, B., Chevallier, B., *et al.* 1999. Phase I–II trial of intensification of the MAID regimen with support of lenograstim (rHuG-CSF) in patients with advanced soft-tissue sarcoma (STS). *American Journal of Clinical Oncology* 22: 267–272.

Comley, A., DeMeyer, E., Adams, N., *et al.* 1999. Effect of subcutaneous granulocyte colony-stimulating factor injectate volume on drug efficacy, site complications, and client comfort. *Oncology Nursing Forum* 26: 87–94.

Crawford, J., Kreisman, H., Garewal, H., *et al.* 1997. The impact of filgrastim schedule variation on hematopoeitic recovery post-chemotherapy. *Annals of Oncology* 8: 1117–1124.

Crawford, J., Ozer, H., Stoller, R., *et al.* 1991. Reduction by granulocyte colony-stimulating factor of fever and neutropenia induced by chemotherapy in patients with small-cell lung cancer. *The New England Journal of Medicine* 325(3): 164–170.

Crawford, J., Streisman, H., Garewal, H., *et al.* 1993. A pharmacodynamic investigation of the recombinant human granulocyte colony-stimulating factor (r-metHuG-CSF) schedule variation in patients with small cell lung cancer (SCLC) given CAE chemotherapy. *Proceedings of the American Society of Clinical Oncology* 11: 299 (abstract 1005).

Cremieux, P., Finkelstein, S., Berndt, E., *et al.* 1999. Cost effectiveness, quality-adjusted life-years and supportive care. Recombinant human erythropoietin as a treatment of cancer-associated anaemia. *Pharmacoeconomics* 16: 459–472.

Crosier, P., and Clark, S. 1992. Basic biology of the hematopoietic growth factors. *Seminars in Oncology* 19(4): 349–361.

DeAndrade, J., and Jove, M. 1996. Baseline hemoglobin as a predictor of risk of transfusion and response to epoetin alfa in orthopedic surgery patients. *American Journal of Orthopedics* 25(8): 524–532.

Demetri, G.D. 1997. Hematopoietic Growth Factors.

In Holland, J., Bast, R., Morton, D., Frei, E., Kufe, D., and Weichselbaum, R. (eds). *Cancer Medicine*, 4th edn. Baltimore: Williams and Wilkins, pp. 1227–1243.

Demetri, G., and Antman, K. 1992. Granulocyte-macrophage colony-stimulating factor (GM-CSF): Preclinical and clinical investigations. *Seminars in Oncology* 19(4): 362–385.

DiPersio, J., Abboud, C., Schuster, M., *et al.* 1997. Phase II study of mobilization of PBSC by administration of daniplestim (SC-55494) and G-CSF in patients with breast cancer or lymphoma. *Proceedings of the American Society of Clinical Oncology* 16: 87 (abstract 306).

Donahue, R., Seehra, J., Norton, C., *et al.* 1987. Stimulation of hematopoiesis in primates with human interleukin-3 and granulocyte-macrophage colony stimulating factor. *Blood* 70(5): 133a (abstract).

Donahue, R., Wang, E., Stone, D., *et al.* 1986. Stimulation of hematopoiesis in primates by continuous infusion of recombinant human GM-CSF. *Nature* 321(6037): 872–875.

Dorr, R. 1993. Clinical properties of yeast derived versus *Escherichia coli*-derived granulocyte-macrophage colony-stimulating factor. *Clinical Therapeutics* 15(1): 19–29.

Doweiko, J., and Goldberg, M. 1991. Erythropoietin therapy in cancer patients. *Oncology* 5(8): 31–37.

Elias, A., Ibrahim, J., Skarin, A., *et al.* 1999. Dose-intensive therapy for limited-stage small-cell lung cancer: Long-term outcome. *Journal of Clinical Oncology* 17: 1175–1178.

Eschbach, J., Egrie, J., Downing, M., *et al.* 1987. Correction of the anemia of end-stage renal disease with recombinant human erythropoietin. *The New England Journal of Medicine* 316(2): 73–78.

Estey, E., Dixon, D., Hagop, M., *et al.* 1990. Treatment of poor-prognosis, newly diagnosed acute myeloid leukemia with Ara-C and recombinant granulocyte-macrophage colony-stimulating factor. *Blood* 75(5): 1766–1769.

Fanucchi, M., Glaspy, J., Crawford, J., *et al.* 1997. Effects of polyethylene glycol-conjugated recombinant human megakaryocyte growth and development factor on platelet counts after chemotherapy for lung cancer. *The New England Journal of Medicine* 336(6): 404–409.

Farese, A., Hunt, P., Boone, T., *et al.* 1995. Recombinant human megakaryocyte growth and development factor stimulates thrombocytopoiesis in normal nonhuman primates. *Blood* 86(1): 54–59.

Font, A., Moyano, A., Puerto, J., *et al.* 1999. Increasing dose intensity of cisplatin-etoposide in advanced non-small-cell lung carcinoma: A phase III randomized trial of the Spanish Lung Cancer Group. *Cancer* 85: 855–863.

Fujisawa, M., Kobayashi, Y., Okabe, T., *et al.* 1986. Recombinant human granulocyte colony-stimulating factor induces granulocytosis *in vivo*. *Japanese Journal of Cancer Research* 77(9): 866–869.

Gabrilove, J., Einhorn, L., Livingston, R., *et al.* 1999. Once weekly dosing of epoetin alfa is similar to three-times-weekly dosing in increasing hemoglobin and quality of life. *Proceedings of the American Society of Clinical Oncology* 18: 574 (abstract).

Gabrilove, J., Jakubowski, A., Scher, H., *et al.* 1988. Effect of G-CSF on neutropenia and associated morbidity due to chemotherapy for transitional-cell carcinoma of the urothelium. *The New England Journal of Medicine* 318(22): 1414–1422.

Ganser, A., Lindemann, A., Seipelt, G., *et al.* 1990a. Effects of recombinant human interleukin-3 in patients with normal hematopoiesis and in patients with bone marrow failure. *Blood* 76(4): 666–676.

Ganser, A., Lindemann, A., Seipelt, G., *et al.* 1990b. Effects of recombinant human interleukin-3 in aplastic anemia. *Blood* 76 (7): 1287–1292.

Garnick, M., and Stoudemire, J. 1990. Preclinical and clinical evaluation of recombinant human macrophage colony-stimulating factor (rhM-CSF). *International Journal of Cell Cloning* 8(suppl 1): 356–371.

Gasson, J., Baldwin, G., Sakamoto, K., *et al.* 1990. The biology of human granulocyte-macrophage colony-stimulating factor (GM-CSF). *Progress in Clinical and Biological Research* 352: 375–384.

Glaspy, J., Bukowski, R., Steinberg, D., *et al.* 1997. Impact of therapy with epoetin alfa on clinical outcomes in patients with nonmyeloid malignancies during cancer chemotherapy in community oncology practice. *Journal of Clinical Oncology* 15(3): 1218–1234.

Glaspy, J., Chap, L., Menchaca, D., *et al.* 1995. Effect of prior chemotherapy on peripheral blood progenitor cell (PBPC) harvests in patients with breast cancer. *Proceedings of the American Society of Clinical Oncology* 14: 319 (abstract).

Goldberg, M., and McCutchen, J. 1996. A safety and efficacy comparison study of two dosing regimens of epoetin alfa in patients undergoing major orthopedic surgery. *American Journal of Orthopedics* 25(8): 544–552.

Golde, D., and Gasson, J. 1988. Hormones that stimulate the growth of blood cells. *Scientific American* 259(1): 62–70.

Gordon, M., McCaskill-Stevens, W., Battiato, L., *et al.* 1996. A phase I trial of recombinant human interleukin-11 (neumega rhIL-11 growth factor) in women with breast cancer receiving chemotherapy. *Blood* 87(9): 3615–3624.

Grecula, J., Schuller, D., Rhoades, C., *et al.* 1999. Intensification regimen 2 for advanced head and neck squamous cell carcinomas. *Archives of Otolaryngology Head and Neck Surgery* 125: 1313–1318.

Groopman, J., Mitsujasu, R., DeLeo, M., *et al.* 1987. Effects of recombinant human granulocyte-macrophage colony-stimulating factor in patients on myelopoiesis in the acquired deficiency syndrome. *The New England Journal of Medicine* 317(10): 1545–1552.

Hartmann, L., and Edmonson, J. 1990. Atrial fibrillation during treatment with granulocyte-macrophage colony stimulating factor (GM-CSF). *Proceedings of the American Society of Clinical Oncology* 9: 194 (abstract).

Hassan, H. 1996. Maintenance and expansion of erythropoiesis in human long-term bone marrow cultures in the presence of erythropoietin plus stem cell factor and interleukin-3 or interleukin-11. *European Cytokine Network* 7(2): 129–136.

Herrman, F., Schulz, G., Wieser, M., *et al.* 1990. Effect of GM-CSF in neutropenia and related morbidity induced by myelotoxic chemotherapy. *American Journal of Medicine* 88: 619–624.

Hoelzer, D., Seipelt, G., and Ganser, A. 1991. Interleukin 3 alone and in combination with GM-CSF in the treatment of patients with neoplastic disease. *Seminars in Hematology* 28(2 suppl 2): 17–24.

Hokom, M., Lacey, D., Kinstler, O., *et al.* 1995. Pegylated megakaryocyte growth and development factor abrogates the lethal thrombocytopenia associated with carboplatin and irradiation in mice. *Blood* 86(12): 4486–4492.

Huang, E., Nocka, K., Beier, D., *et al.* 1990. The hematopoietic growth factor KL is encoded at the S1 locus and is the ligand of the c-kit receptor, the gene product of the W locus. *Cell* 63(1): 225–233.

Ifrah, N., Witz, F., Jouet, J., *et al.* 1999. Intensive short term therapy with granulocyte-macrophage colony-stimulating factor support, similar to therapy for acute myeloblastic leukemia, does not improve overall results for adults with acute lymphoblastic leukemia. GOELAMS Group. *Cancer* 86: 1496–1505.

Immunex Corporation. 1997. Leukine package insert. Seattle, WA: Immunex Corporation.

Isaacs, C., Robert, N., Bailey, F., *et al.* 1997. Randomized placebo-controlled study of recombinant human interleukin-11 to prevent chemotherapy-induced thrombocytopenia in patients with breast cancer receiving dose-intensive cyclophosphamide and doxorubicin. *Journal of Clinical Oncology* 15: 3368–3377.

Ishibashi, T., Kiumra, H., Shikama, Y., *et al.* 1989. Interleukin-6 is a potent thrombopoietic factor *in vivo* in mice. *Blood* 74: 1241–1244.

Jaramilla, J. 1992. Biotechnology overview. *Pharmacy and Therapeutics* 17: 1372–1377.

Johnston, E., Crawford, J., Lockbaum, P., *et al.* 1998. Single-dose subcutaneous (SC), sustained-duration filgrastim (SD) versus daily filgrastim in non-small-cell lung cancer patients (NSCLC): A randomized, controlled, dose escalation study. *Proceedings of the American Society of Clinical Oncology* 17: 73 (abstract 284).

Jones, S., Khandelwal, P., McIntyre, K., *et al.* 1999. Randomized, double-blind, placebo-controlled trial to evaluate the hematopoietic growth factor PIXY321 after moderate-dose fluorouracil, doxorubicin, and cyclophosphamide in stage II and III breast cancer. *Journal of Clinical Oncology* 17: 3025–3032.

Kaushansky, K. 1996. The thrombocytopenia of cancer: Prospects for effective cytokine therapy. *Hematology-Oncology Clinics of North America.* 10(2): 341–355.

Kaushansky, K. 1997. Thrombopoietin: Platelets on demand? *Annals of Internal Medicine* 126(9): 731–733.

Kaushansky, K., Broudy, V., Grossmann, A., *et al.* 1995. Thrombopoietin expands erythroid progenitors, increases red cell production, and enhances erythroid recovery after myelosuppressive therapy. *Journal of Clinical Investigation* 96: 1683–1687.

Khwaja, A., Mills, W., Leveridge, K., *et al.* 1993. Efficacy of delayed granulocyte colony-stimulating factor after autologous BMT. *Bone Marrow Transplant* 11: 479–482.

Kobayashi, Y., Okabe, T., Urabe, A., *et al.* 1987. Human granulocyte colony-stimulating factor shortens the period of granulocytopenia induced by irradiation in mice. *Japanese Journal of Cancer Research* 78(8): 763–766.

Kobayashi, Y., Okabe, T., Urabe, A., *et al.* 1989. Treatment of myelodysplastic syndromes with recombinant human granulocyte colony-stimulating factor: A preliminary report. *American Journal of Medicine* 86(2): 178–181.

Kodo, H., Tajika, K., Takahashi S., *et al.* 1988. Acceleration of neutrophil granulocyte recovery after bone-marrow transplantation by administration of recombinant human granulocyte colony stimulating factor. *The Lancet* 2(8601): 38–39.

Kohgo, Y., Hirayama, Y., Sakami, S., *et al.* 1994. Improved recovery of myelosuppression following chemotherapy in mice by combined administration of PSK and various cytokines. *Acta Hematologica* 92(3): 130–135.

Layton, J., Hockman, J., Sheridan, W., *et al.* 1989. Evidence for a novel *in vivo* control mechanism of granulopoiesis: Mature cell related control of a regulatory growth factor. *Blood* 74(4): 1303–1307.

Lemoli, R., Rosti, G., Gherlinzoni, F., *et al.* 1996. Concomitant and sequential administration of recombinant human granulocyte colony-stimulating factor and recombinant human interleukin-3 to accelerate hematopoietic recovery after autologous bone marrow transplantation for malignant lymphoma. *Journal of Clinical Oncology* 14(11): 3018–3025.

Lindemann, A., and Mertelsmann, R. 1993. Interleukin-3: Structure and function. *Cancer Investigation* 11(5): 609–623.

Logothetis, C., Dexeus, F., Sella, A., *et al.* 1990. Escalated therapy for refractory urothelial tumors: Methotrexate-vinblastine-doxorubicin-cisplatin plus unglycosylated recombinant human granulocyte-macrophage colony-stimulating factor. *Journal of the National Cancer Institute* 82(8): 662–672.

Ludwig, H., Fritz, E., Leitgeb, C., *et al.* 1994. Prediction of response to erythropoietin treatment in chronic anemia of cancer. *Blood* 84: 1056–1063.

Maruhashi, T., Takahashi, T., Yakushiji, M., *et al.* 1997. Clinical usefulness of macrophage colony-stimulating factor (M-CSF) after chemotherapy for ovarian cancer: A well-controlled randomized study. *Proceedings of the American Society of Clinical Oncology* 16:123 (abstract 432).

McNiece, I., Briddell, R., Yan, X., *et al.* 1994. The role of stem cell factor in mobilization of peripheral blood progenitor cells. *Leukemia and Lymphoma* 15: 405–409.

McNiece, J., Langley, K., Zsebo, K., *et al.* 1991. Recombinant human stem cell factor synergized with GM-CSF, G-CSF, IL-3, and Epo to stimulate human progenitor cells of the myeloid and erythroid lineages. *Journal of Experimental Hematology* 19(3): 226–231.

Means, R., and Krantz, S. 1991. Erythropoietin in cancer therapy. *Biologic Therapy of Cancer Updates* 1(4): 1–7.

Meropol, N., Miller, L., Korn, E., *et al.* 1992. Severe myelosuppression resulting from concurrent administration of G-CSF and cytotoxic chemotherapy. *Journal of the National Cancer Institute* 84(15): 1201–1203.

Mertelsmann, R., Herrmann, F., Hecht, T., *et al.* 1990. Hematopoietic growth factors in bone marrow transplantation. *Bone Marrow Transplantation* 6: 73–77.

Metcalf, D. 1980. Clonal analysis of proliferation and differentiation of paired daughter cells: Action of granulocyte-macrophage colony-stimulating factor on granulocyte-macrophage precursors. *Proceedings of the National Academy of Sciences* 77: 5327–5330.

Metcalf, D., Burgess, A., Johnson, G., *et al.* 1986. In vitro actions on hemopoietic cells of recombinant murine GM-CSF purified after production in *Escherichia coli:* Comparison with purified native GM-CSF. *Journal of Cellular Physiology* 128(3): 421–431.

Metcalf, D., Johnson, G., and Burgess, A. 1980. Direct stimulation of purified GM-CSF on the proliferation of multipotential and erythroid precursor cells. *Blood* 55(2): 138–147.

Metcalf, D., and Morstyn, G. 1991. Colony-stimulating factors: General biology. In DeVita, V., Hellman, S., and Rosenberg, S. (eds). *Biologic Therapy of Cancer.* Philadelphia, PA: J.B. Lippincott, pp. 417–444.

Miles, S., Mitsuyasu, R., and Moreno, J. 1991. Combined therapy with recombinant granulocyte colony-stimulating factor and erythropoietin decreases hematologic toxicity from zidovudine. *Blood* 77(10): 2109–2117.

Miller, L., Smith, J., Urba, W., *et al.* 1993. A phase I study of an IL-3/GM-CSF fusion protein (PIXY321) and high dose carboplatin (CBCDA) in patients with advanced cancer. *Proceedings of the American Society of Clinical Oncology* 12: 353 (abstract).

Minasian, L., Yao, T., Steffens, T., *et al.* 1995. A phase I study of anti-GD3 ganglioside monoclonal antibody R24 and recombinant human macrophage-colony stimulating factor in patients with metastatic melanoma. *Cancer* 75(9): 2251–2257.

Miyake, T., Jung, C., and Goldwasser, E. 1977. Purification of human erythropoietin. *Journal of Biology and Chemistry* 252: 5538–5564.

Miyazaki, H. 1996. Cloning of thrombopoietin and its therapeutic potential. *Cancer Chemotherapy and Pharmacology* 38 (suppl): 74–77.

Morstyn G., Campbell, L., Lieschke, G., *et al.* 1989a. Treatment of chemotherapy induced neutropenia by subcutaneously administered granulocyte colony-stimulating factor (G-CSF) with optimization of dose and duration of therapy. *Journal of Clinical Oncology* 7(10): 1554–1562.

Morstyn, G., Campbell, L., Souza, L., *et al.* 1988. Effect of G-CSF on neutropenia induced by cytotoxic chemotherapy. *The Lancet* 1(8587): 667–672.

Morstyn, G., Lieschke, G.L., Sheridan, W., *et al.* 1989b. Clinical experience with recombinant human granulocyte colony stimulating factor and granulocyte-macrophage colony stimulating factor. *Seminars in Hematology* 26(2 suppl 2): 9–13.

Negrin, R., Hauber, D., Nagler, A., *et al.* 1989. Treatment of myelodysplastic syndrome with recombinant human granulocyte colony stimulating factor: A phase I–II trial. *Annals of Internal Medicine* 110(12): 967–984.

Neidhart, J., Mangalik, A., Kohler, W., *et al.* 1989. Granulocyte-colony stimulating factor stimulates recovery of granulocytes in patients receiving dose intensive chemotherapy without bone marrow transplantation. *Journal of Clinical Oncology* 7(11): 1685–1692.

Nemunaitis, J., Meyers, J., Buckner, C., *et al.* 1990a. Phase I/II trial of recombinant macrophage colony stimulating factor (M-CSF) in patients with invasive fungal infection. *Blood* 76(10 suppl 1): 159.

Nemunaitis, J., Meyers, J., Buckner, C., *et al.* 1993. Phase I/II trial of recombinant human macrophage-colony stimulating factor (M-CSF) in patients with invasive fungal infection. *Proceedings of the American Society of Clinical Oncology* 12: 159 (abstract).

Nemunaitis, J., Singer, J., Buckner, C., *et al.* 1988a. Use of recombinant human granulocyte-macrophage colony-stimulating factor in autologous marrow transplantation for lymphoid malignancies. *Blood* 72(2): 834–836.

Nemunaitis, J., Singer, J., Buckner, C., *et al.* 1988b. The use of rHuGM-CSF for graft failure in patients after autologous, allogeneic, or syngeneic bone marrow transplantation (BMT). *Blood* 72(suppl 1): 398a (abstract).

Nemunaitis, J., Singer, J., Buckner, C., *et al.* 1990b. Use of recombinant human granulocyte-macrophage colony-stimulating factor in graft failure after bone marrow transplantation. *Blood* 76(1): 245–253.

Nicola, N. 1989. Hemopoietic cell growth factors and their receptors. *Annual Review of Biochemistry* 58: 45–77.

Ohno, R., Miyawaki, S., Hatake, K., *et al.* 1997. Human urinary macrophage colony-stimulating factor reduces the incidence and duration of febrile neutropenia and shortens the period required to finish three courses of intensive consolidation therapy in acute myeloid leukemia: A double-blind controlled study. *Journal of Clinical Oncology* 15(8): 2954–2965.

Ohno, R., Tomonoaga, M., and Kogayashi, T. 1990. Effect of G-CSF after intensive induction therapy in relapsed or refractory acute leukemia. *The New England Journal of Medicine* 323(13): 871–877.

Orazi, A., Cooper, R., Tong, J., *et al.* 1996. Effects of recombinant human interleukin-11 (Neumega rhIL-11 growth factor) on megakaryocytopoiesis in human bone marrow. *Experimental Hematology* 24(11): 1289–1297.

Piccirillo, N., Sica, S., Laurenti, L., *et al.* 1999. Optimal timing of G-CSF administration after CD34$^+$ immunoselected peripheral blood progenitor cell transplantation. *Bone Marrow Transplantation* 23: 1245–1250.

Platanias, L., Miller, C., Mick, R., *et al.* 1991. Treatment of chemotherapy-induced anemia with recombinant human erythropoietin in cancer patients. *Journal of Clinical Oncology* 9(11): 2021–2026.

Prow, D., and Vadhan-Raj, S. 1998. Thrombopoietin: Biology and potential applications. *Oncology* 12: 1597–1607.

Pujol, J., Douillard, J., Riviere, A., *et al.* 1997. Dose-intensity of a four-drug chemotherapy regimen with or without recombinant human granulocyte-macrophage colony-stimulating factor in extensive-stage small-cell lung cancer: A multicenter randomized phase III study. *Journal of Clinical Oncology* 15(5): 2082–2089.

Reissman, K. 1950. Studies on the mechanism of erythropoietic stimulation in parabiotic rats during hypoxia. *Blood* 5: 372–380.

Reptis, G., Gilewski, T., Gabrilove, J., *et al.* 1993. Evaluation of PIXY321 (PIXY) as a myeloprotective agent in patients (pts) with metastatic breast cancer receiving doxorubicin and thiotepa. *Proceedings of the American Society of Clinical Oncology* 12: 235 (abstract).

Santoro, A., Balzarotti, M., Tondini, C., *et al.* 1999. Dose-escalation of CHOP in non-Hodgkin's lymphoma. *Annals of Oncology* 10: 519–525.

Schick, B. 1994. Clinical implications of basic research: Hope for treatment of thrombocytopenia. *The New England Journal of Medicine* 331: 13–14.

Schlerman, F., Bree, A., Kaviani, M., *et al.* 1996. Hematopoietic activity of recombinant human interleukin 11 (rHuIL-11) in normal and myelosuppressed nonhuman primates. *Stem Cells* 14(5): 517–532.

Schwartzberg, L., Birch, R., Weaver, C., *et al.* 1994. The effect of varying durations of granulocyte colony stimulating factor (G-CSF) on neutrophil engraftment and supportive care following peripheral blood progenitor cell (PBPC) infusion. *Blood* 84: 91 (abstract).

Sheridan, W., Juttner, C., Szer, J., *et al.* 1990. Granulocyte colony-stimulating factor (G-CSF) in peripheral blood stem cell (PBSC) and bone marrow (BM) transplantation. *Blood* 76(5): 2251a.

Sheridan, W., Morstyn, G., Wolf, M., *et al.* 1989. Granulocyte colony-stimulating factor and neu-

trophil recovery after high-dose chemotherapy and bone marrow transplantation. *The Lancet* 2(8668): 891–895.

Sherwood, J., and Goldwasser, E. 1979. A radioimmunoassay for erythropoietin. *Blood* 54: 885–893.

Simmers, R., Webber, L., Shannon, M., *et al.* 1987. Localization of the G-CSF gene on chromosome 17 proximal to the breakpoint in the t(15;17) in acute promyelocytic leukemia. *Blood* 70(1): 330–332.

Singer, J. 1992. Role of colony-stimulating factors in bone marrow transplantation. *Seminars in Oncology* 19(suppl 3): 27–31.

Singer, J., Nemunaitis, J., Bianco, J., *et al.* 1990. RhGM-CSF following allogeneic bone marrow transplantation from unrelated marrow donors: A phase II study. *Blood* 76(suppl): 566a (abstract).

Spangrude, G. 1994. Biological and clinical aspects of hematopoietic stem cells. *Annual Reviews in Medicine* 45: 93–104.

Spivak, J. 1989. Erythropoietin. *Blood Reviews* 3(20): 130–135.

Stoudemire, J., and Garnick, M. 1991. Effects of recombinant human macrophage colony-stimulating factor on plasma cholesterol levels. *Blood* 77(4): 750–755.

Talbot, S., Westerman, D., Grigg, A., *et al.* 1999. Phase I and subsequent phase II study of filgrastim (R-met-HuG-CSF) and dose intensified cyclophosphamide plus epirubicin in patients with non-Hodgkin's lymphoma and advanced solid tumors. *Annals of Oncology* 10: 907–914.

Taylor, K., Jagannath, S., Spitzer, G., *et al.* 1989. Recombinant human granulocyte colony-stimulating factor hastens granulocyte recovery after high-dose chemotherapy and autologous bone marrow transplantation in Hodgkin's disease. *Journal of Clinical Oncology* 7(12): 1791–1799.

Tepler, I., Elias, L., Smith, J., *et al.* 1996. A randomized placebo-controlled trial of recombinant human interleukin-11 in cancer patients with severe thrombocytopenia due to chemotherapy. *Blood* 87(9): 3607–3614.

Thatcher, N., Girling, D., Hopwook, P., *et al.* 2000.

Improving survival without reducing quality of life in small-cell lung cancer patients by increasing dose-intensity of chemotherapy with granulocyte colony-stimulating factor support: Results of a British Medical Research Council multicenter randomized trial. Medical Research Council Lung Cancer Working Party. *Journal of Clinical Oncology* 18: 395–404.

Thompson, J., Lee, D., Kidd, P., *et al*. 1989. Subcutaneous granulocyte-macrophage colony-stimulating factor in patients with myelodysplastic syndrome: Toxicity, pharmacokinetics and hematological effects. *Journal of Clinical Oncology* 7(5): 629–637.

To, L., Dyson, P., Branford, A., *et al*. 1987. Peripheral blood stem cells collected in very early remission produce rapid and sustained autologous hematopoietic reconstitution in acute non-lymphoblastic leukemia. *Bone Marrow Transplantation* 2(1): 103–108.

Traynor, B. 1992. The cytokine network. *Proceedings of the 7th International Conference on Cancer Nursing* 6–10.

Ulich, T., delCastillo, J., Yin, S., *et al*. 1991. Megakaryocyte growth and development factor ameliorates carboplatin-induced thrombocytopenia in mice. *Blood* 86(3): 971–976.

Vadhan-Raj, S., Broxmeyer, H., Hittelman, W., *et al*. 1992. Abrogating chemotherapy-induced myelosuppression by recombinant granulocyte-macrophage colony-stimulating factor on patients with sarcoma: Protection at the progenitor level. *Journal of Clinical Oncology* 10(8): 1266–1277.

Vadhan-Raj, S., Keating, M., LaMaistre, A., *et al*. 1987. Effects of recombinant human granulocyte-macrophage colony-stimulating factor in patients with myelodysplastic syndrome. *The New England Journal of Medicine* 17(25): 1545–1552.

Vadhan-Raj, S., Papadoupoulos, N., Burgess, M., *et al*. 1994. Effects of PIXY321, a granulocyte-macrophage colony-stimulating factor/interleukin-3 protein, on chemotherapy-induced multilineage myelosuppression in patients with sarcoma. *Journal of Clinical Oncology* 12(4): 715–724.

Vadhan-Raj, S., Patel, S., Broxmeyer, H., *et al*. 1996.

Phase I–II investigation of recombinant human thrombopoietin (rhTPO) in patients with sarcoma receiving high dose chemotherapy (CT) with adriamycin (A) and ifosfamide (I). *Proceedings of the American Society of Clinical Oncology* 15: 48a (abstract).

van Leeuwen, B., Martinson, M., Webb, G., *et al*. 1989. Molecular organization of the cytokine gene cluster, involving the human IL-3, IL-4, IL-5, and GM-CSF genes, on chromosome 5. *Blood* 73(5): 1142–1148.

Watari, K., Asano, S., Shirafuji, N., *et al*. 1989. Serum granulocyte colony-stimulating factor levels in healthy volunteers and various disorders estimated by enzyme immunoassay. *Blood* 73(1): 117–122.

Weaver, A., Ryder, D., Crowther, D., *et al*. 1996. Increased numbers of long-term culture-initiating cells in the apheresis product of patients randomized to receive increasing doses of stem cell factor administered in combination with chemotherapy and a standard dose of granulocyte colony-stimulating factor. *Blood* 88(9): 3323–3328.

Weiner, L., Li, W., Catalano, R., *et al*. 1993. Phase I trial of recombinant macrophage colony-stimulating factor (M-CSF) and recombinant gamma-interferon (γ-IFN): Peripheral blood mononuclear phagocyte proliferation and differentiation. *Proceedings of the American Society of Clinical Oncology* 12: 291 (abstract 947).

Welte, K., Bonilla, M., Gillio, A., *et al*. 1987. Recombinant human granulocyte colony-stimulating factor. Effects on hematopoiesis in normal and cyclophosphamide-treated primates. *Journal of Experimental Medicine* 165(4): 941–948.

Williams, D., Broxmeier, H., Curtis, B., *et al*. 1990a. Enhanced biological activity of a human GM-CSF/IL-3 fusion protein. *Experimental Hematology* 18(2): 256a (abstract).

Williams, D., Eisenman, J., Baird, A., *et al*. 1990b. Identification of a ligand for the c-kit proto-oncogene. *Cell* 63(1): 167–174.

Williams, M., and Quesenberry, P. 1992. Hematopoietic growth factors. *Hematologic Pathology* 6(3): 105–124.

Wimperis, J., Niemeyer, C., Sieff, C., *et al.* 1989. Granulocyte-macrophage colony-stimulating factor and interleukin-3 mRNAs are produced by a small fraction of blood mononuclear cells. *Blood* 74(5): 1525–1530.

Woll, P., Hodgetts, J., Lomax, L., *et al.* 1995. Can cytotoxic dose intensity be increased by using colony stimulating factor? A randomised controlled trial of lenograstim in small-cell lung cancer. *Journal of Clinical Oncology* 13: 652–659.

Worrall, L., Thompkins, C., and Rust, D. 1999. Recognizing and managing anemia. *Clinical Journal of Oncology Nursing* 3: 153–160.

Wujcik, D. 1992. Overview of colony-stimulating factors: Focus on the neutrophil. *A Case Management Approach to Patients Receiving G-CSF.* Pittsburgh, PA: Oncology Nursing Society, pp. 8–11.

Xu, Z.-X., Capdeville, R., Faugeas, R., *et al.* 1997. Safety/tolerability and pharmacokinetics/pharmacodynamics (PK/PD) following administration of ascending subcutaneous doses of a long-acting (5–7 days), chemically modified G-CSF mutein (Ro 25-8315) to healthy subjects. *Proceedings of the American Society of Clinical Oncology* 16: 87 (abstract 305).

Yang, Y.-C., Kovacic, S., Kriz, R., *et al.* 1988. The human genes for GM-CSF and IL-3 are closely linked in tandem on chromosome 5. *Blood* 71(4): 958–961.

Zsebo, K., Wypych, J., McNiece, I., *et al.* 1990. Identification, purification, and biological characterization of hematopoietic stem cell factor from Buffalo rat liver-conditioned medium. *Cell* 63(1): 195–201.

Clinical Pearls

1. Currently, the majority of HGFs are used as supportive therapy in the oncology setting to decrease sequelae of hematopoietic toxicity following chemotherapy or BMT or to enhance yield during pheresis for stem cells to be used in peripheral blood stem cell transplantation.

2. The majority of HGFs are well tolerated with minimal side effects. In general, multi-lineage growth factors such IL-11 or GM-CSF tend to have more toxicity, perhaps related to the induction of other cytokines in the body.

3. In the majority of cases, HGFs are given by the subcutaneous route in the ambulatory setting. Patients and family members must therefore learn medication self-administration and subcutaneous injection skills. Reimbursement for the drug may be problematic, especially for those patients on Medicare, in the ambulatory setting.

4. In general, with WBC growth factors, an increase in WBCs is seen very quickly following administration. It is important, therefore, to administer the HGF through the expected nadir. For example, an initial rise in WBCs will be seen, followed by a drop, then recovery.

5. With HGFs for cell lines other than WBCs, such as RBCs, it may take more time for the clinical effect to be seen. With epoetin alfa, it often requires 4 to 8 weeks before clinical results are seen. Therefore, when possible, it is wise to pro-actively plan for the need for epoetin alfa to avoid severe anemia in patients.

6. Determine whether the institution or clinical setting has guidelines in place for the use of HGFs in patients with cancer. Many institutions have adopted guidelines set forth by ASCO.

7. Patients should be educated concerning reportable signs and symptoms such as fever (e.g., the temperature threshold for reporting fever to the health care team) and signs and symptoms of infection.

Key References

American Society of Clinical Oncology. 1994. American Society of Clinical Oncology recommendations for the use of hematopoietic colony-stimulating factors: Evidence-based clinical practice guidelines. *Journal of Clinical Oncology* 12(11): 2471–2508.

Ashman, L. 1999. The biology of stem cell factor and its receptor C-kit. *International Journal of Biochemistry and Cell Biology* 31: 1037–1051.

Bennett, C., Weeks, J., Somerfield, M., *et al.* 1999. Use of hematopoietic colony-stimulating factors: Comparison of the 1994 and 1997 American Society of Clinical Oncology surveys regarding ASCO clinical practice guidelines. *Journal of Clinical Oncology* 17: 3676–3681.

Crawford, J., Foote, M., and Morstyn, G. 1999. Hematopoietic growth factors in cancer chemotherapy. *Cancer Chemotherapy and Biological Response Modifiers* 18: 250–267.

Fetscher, S., and Mertelsmann, R. 2000. Supportive care in hematologic malignancies: hematopoietic growth factors, infections, transfusion therapy. *Current Opinions in Hematology* 7(4):255–260.

Kaushansky, K. 2000. Use of thrombopoietic growth factors in acute leukemia. *Leukemia* 14(3): 505–508.

Kurzrock, R. 2000. Hematopoietic growth factors. In Bast, R., Kufe, D.W., Pollock, R.E., Weischelbaum, R.R., Holland, J.F., and Frei, E. (eds). *Cancer Medicine* 5th edn. Hamilton, Ontario: B.C. Decker, pp. 835–859.

Pecorelli, S. (ed). 2000. Suboptimal hemoglobin levels: Do they impact patients and their therapy? *Seminars in Oncology* 27(2 suppl 4): 1–19.

Rieger, P.T., and Haeuber, D. 1995. A new approach to managing chemotherapy-related anemia: Nursing implications of epoetin alfa. *Oncology Nursing Forum* 22(1): 71–81.

Rust, D.M., Wood, L.S., and Battiato, L.A. 1999. Oprelevekin: an alternative treatment for thrombocytopenia. *Clinical Journal of Oncology Nursing* 3(2): 57–62.

Seipelt, G., Ottmann, O.G., and Hoelzer, D. 2000. Cytokine therapy for myelodysplastic syndrome. *Current Opinions in Hematology* 7(3): 156–160.

Swanson, G., Bergstrom, K., Stump, E., *et al.* 2000. Growth factor usage patterns and outcomes in the community setting: Collection through a practice-based computerized clinical information system. *Journal of Clinical Oncology* 18(8): 1764–1770.

Vadhan-Raj S. 1998. Recombinant human thrombo-poietin: Clinical experience and *in vivo* biology. *Seminars in Hematology* 35(3): 261–268.

Worrall, L.M., Tompkins, C.A., and Rust, D.M. 1999. Recognizing and managing anemia. *Clinical Journal of Oncology Nursing* 3(4): 153–160.

CHAPTER 8

Monoclonal Antibodies: Overview and Use in Hematologic Malignancies

Janet E. DiJulio, RN, MSN

Antibodies are naturally occurring proteins that are elicited in response to foreign antigens to protect the host. The immune system is able to develop antibodies that are unique to any antigen encountered by the host. Speculation about the theory that **passive antibody therapy** could be used to control and eradicate tumors has been ongoing for decades; however, testing this theory has been fraught with problems. Early studies of passive antibody therapy used heterologous antisera that were either obtained from animals or humans immunized with whole tumor cells or cell extracts. Unfortunately, immunization in this fashion resulted in a mixture of antibodies (**polyclonal antibodies**), many of which were not specific for tumor antigens. Not surprisingly, early attempts at passive immunotherapy showed little promise (Rosenberg and Terry, 1977).

In the mid-1970s, Nobel Prize winners

Köhler and Milstein (1975) developed a technique to fuse antibody-producing cells with a myeloma cell line that resulted in an "immortal" hybrid cell that produced a single antibody recognizing a single antigen. This **hybridoma** technique made it possible to produce unlimited amounts of pure monoclonal antibody (MAB) that varied little from batch to batch and that was highly specific for a single **antigenic determinant** (Schlom, 1995). Because of this discovery, researchers can now develop MABs from a variety of sources for essentially all antigens. The primary source of antibody production has been the mouse (Lotze and Rosenberg, 1988). Since the early 1990s, these murine antibodies have been modified to increase their usefulness in humans while reducing the immunogenicity of the mouse protein (LoBuglio and Saleh, 1992; Rybak *et al.*, 1992).

However, the search for tumor-specific

antigens to use as targets for the antibodies has proved troublesome. Most of the MABs are targeted to antigens that are present on normal as well as malignant cells. These targets include **oncofetal** antigens, differentiation antigens, tissue-specific antigens, growth factor receptors, oncogene products, and **idiotypes**. As mentioned previously, these proteins are present on all normal cells but may be present in a higher concentration on malignant cells (Lotze and Rosenberg, 1988; Mendelsohn and Baselga, 1995; Schlom, 1995). The one exception to this is B-cell malignancy. When B cells undergo malignant transformation, they provide an excellent target for antibody therapy (DeVita and Canellos, 1999). Because the lymphoma arises from a single clone of cells, the immunoglobulin (Ig) expressed is unique to the tumor. Thus, the antibody secreted by the B cell can be used as a target for antibody production. This unique binding region is called the "idiotype." In essence, the idiotype is a true "tumor-specific" antigen because it is not present on normal B cells (Maloney *et al.*, 1992b).

Molecular biologists have also identified cell-surface receptors that are products of cellular oncogenes, and several of these receptors are for growth factors, including platelet-derived growth factor and epidermal growth factor. These receptor sites have been used primarily as targets for antibodies in solid tumors (LoBuglio and Saleh, 1992; Mendelsohn and Baselga, 1995) and are beyond the scope of discussion in this chapter. (See Chapter 9 for a discussion of antibodies targeted toward cell-surface receptors.)

The name of an antibody typically correlates with the antigen it targets, the specific clone from which it originates, or the corporation that developed it and it usually consists of only numbers and letters. Once the MAB receives Food and Drug Administration (FDA) approval, a generic name and a trade name are assigned.

MABs are now used in the diagnosis and treatment of many diseases. This chapter will cover the technology involved in manufacturing antibodies and the use of MABs in the diagnosis and treatment of the lymphomas and leukemias. Clinical trials of MABs conjugated to drugs, toxins, and isotopes will be reviewed and common toxicities involved in the use of these therapies will be discussed. How these biological agents differ from other drugs submitted for FDA approval will be identified. Finally, the factors affecting successful use of this unique biological agent will be presented.

Hybridoma Technology

Köhler and Milstein (1975) capitalized on the properties of two different murine cell populations: antibody-forming B lymphocytes and malignant plasma cells. If one attempts to develop a specific antibody by immunizing a mouse and harvesting the antibody-forming lymphocytes, the cells can be maintained in culture for only a very short time, and the antibody yield is low. If, on the other hand, that cell line is fused with a malignant plasma cell that, although it is a poor antibody producer, possesses the malignant properties of immortality, the cell culture can be maintained for years. Figure 8.1 is a schematic representation of Köhler and Milstein's hybridoma technology. The mouse is first immunized with the desired antigen and an antibody response is allowed to develop. The mouse's spleen is harvested, and the lymphocytes from the spleen are placed in solution with the myeloma cells selected from a culture that is deficient in the enzyme hypoxanthine phosphoribosyl transferase (HPRT). Fusion is chemically induced using polyethylene glycol. Because myeloma cells need the HPRT enzyme to survive, only those that fuse with the mouse lymphocytes that possess the necessary enzyme will survive in culture. Suc-

HYBRIDOMA TECHNOLOGY

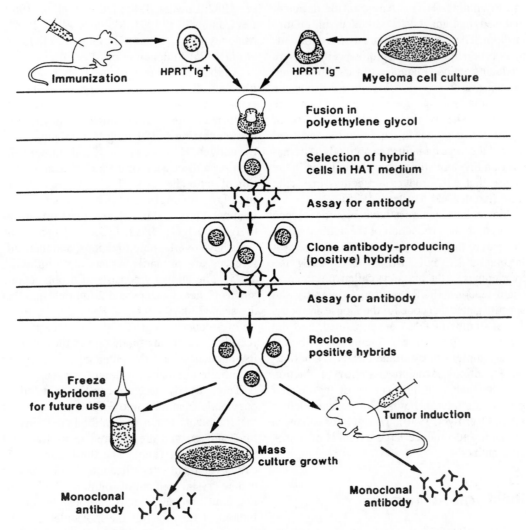

Figure 8.1 Schematic representation of hybridoma technique for the production of monoclonal antibodies. The mouse is immunized with the desired antigen, and an antibody response is allowed to develop. The mouse's spleen is harvested and the lymphocytes from the spleen are placed in solution with myeloma cells from a culture that is deficient in the enzyme hypoxanthine phosphoribosyl transferase (HPRT). Only the fused cells will survive in the hypoxanthine, aminopterin, and thymidine (HAT) media. Assay for antibody production is done, and those cells producing antibody are cloned. The hybridoma may be frozen for future use, it may be grown in mass culture, or it may be used to induce a tumor in the mouse that results in antibody production.

Source: Reprinted with permission from DiJulio, J. 1986. Treatment of B-cell and T-cell lymphomas with monoclonal antibodies. *Seminars in Oncology Nursing* 4: 103.

cessfully fused cells are selected and grown in a medium containing hypoxanthine, aminopterin, and thymidine (HAT). Any enzyme-deficient (unfused) malignant cells will die in this culture medium. The selected cells are assayed for antibody production, and only those cells that are producing antibody targeted toward the selected antigen are cloned. These cells constitute the hybridoma. At this point several options are available. The hybridoma may be frozen for future use or grown in mass cutures and used to produce large quantities of antibody. Alternatively, a myeloma tumor may be induced in the mouse that will produce antibodies in ascitic fluid (Köhler and Milstein, 1975).

Molecular techniques have been developed to speed up the production of the antibody. The first part of the process is identical to that shown in Figure 8.1, but instead of culturing the hybridomas, a technology called polymerase chain reaction (PCR) is used to amplify the specific genes that code for the mouse antibody. The 2 strands of DNA are separated, and the separated strands serve as a template for building a complementary strand of DNA. Continuous repetitions of the process allow production of more than 2 million copies of the desired gene in a matter of hours (Cooper and Flaum, 1988; Overmyer, 1990). This greatly enhances the ability to produce large amounts of a specific antibody.

Biological Actions

Native MABs, those that are not bound to drugs, toxins, or isotopes, have been used to treat human cancer since 1979. Although a variety of malignancies have been treated, only tumors that include the lymphomas and leukemias will be discussed in this chapter. Hematologic tumors treated with MABs include B-cell lymphoma, chronic lymphocytic leukemia (CLL), cutaneous T-cell lymphoma (CTCL),

Hodgkin's disease, and acute lymphocytic leukemia (ALL) (Nadler *et al.*, 1980; Dillman *et al.*, 1982; Lowder, 1985; Dillman *et al.*, 1989; Levy and Miller, 1991; Maloney *et al.*, 1992a; Maloney *et al.*, 1992b; Horning, 1994; Jurcic *et al.*, 1995; Maloney *et al.*, 1997a).

Antibodies are part of the body's humoral immune response. The function of antibodies is to rid the host organism of harmful substances identified as nonself, or antigens. They do this by recognizing and binding to a unique site on the antigen. How the antibody kills tumor cells requires a discussion of the structure and function of antibodies or Ig. The 5 classes of Ig are IgG, IgA, IgD, IgM, and IgE. IgG is the most common class, and in humans, the 4 subclasses of IgG are IgG1, IgG2, IgG3, and IgG4. The IgGs have overlapping functions, and their differences are primarily structural (Smith-Gill, 1995). The antibody consists of 4 polypeptide chains (2 heavy chains and 2 light chains) that are shaped like the letter *Y.* Each chain is made up of a constant region and a variable region. It is the variable region that gives the antibody its uniqueness and the potential to react with an infinite number of different antigens.

The antibody structure can be separated by enzymatic treatment into 3 fragments. Two of the fragments retain the antibody's ability to bind antigen and are referred to as fragment antigen binding (Fab). The third fragment is called fragment crystallization (Fc) because it can be crystallized out of solution. The Fc cannot bind antigens, but is responsible for the biological functions of the molecule once the antigen has been bound to the Fab of the intact molecule (Benjamini and Leskowitz, 1988). See Figure 8.2 for a schematic diagram of an Ig molecule (Abbas *et al.*, 1991).

Antibody-induced cytotoxicity is thought to happen in several ways. The first is through the recruitment of the host's immune function. This mechanism includes activation of the human complement-dependent cascade. Some classes

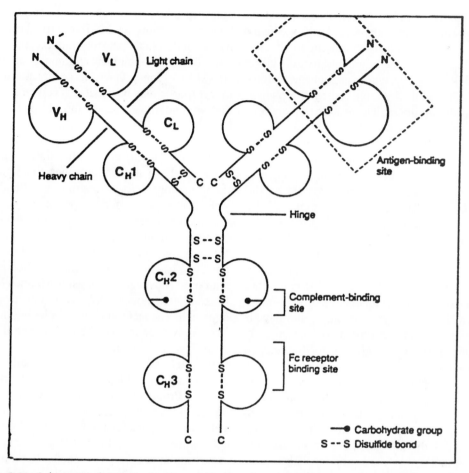

Figure 8.2   Schematic diagram of an Ig molecule. The antigen-binding sites are formed by the juxtaposition of the variable light (VL) and variable heavy (VH) domains. The locations of complement and Fc receptor-binding sites within the heavy chain constant regions are approximations. S—S refers to intrachain and interchain disulfide bonds; N and C refer to amino and carboxy termini of the polypeptide chains.

Source: Reprinted with permission from Abbas, A., Lichtman, M., and Prober, J. 1991. Antibodies and antigens. In Abbas, A., Lichtman, M., and Prober, J. (eds). *Cellular and Molecular Immunology.* Philadelphia, PA: W. B. Saunders, p. 51.

of antibody have the ability to firmly fix the complement subcomponent **C1q**. Antibodies may vary in their ability to mediate the complement cascade. For example, IgM appears to be a better activator of complement than IgG2a and IgG2b (Lotze and Rosenberg, 1988). Once this protein is bound, the antibody-C1q com-

plexes may trigger phagocytosis of the tumor cells via the host's reticuloendothelial system. A bond between the antibody and C1q also induces the remaining steps in the complement cascade, which causes cell lysis by disruption of the cell membrane. The second mechanism of host immune function is antibody-dependent cell-mediated cytotoxicity, which occurs when the Fc portion of antibody-coated cells mediates killing of malignant cells by binding to effector cells. The effector cells include natural killer cells, killer T cells, and macrophages. Antibody-coated cells are engulfed by the phagocytic cells in the reticuloendothelial system (Benjamini and Leskowitz, 1988; Lotze and Rosenberg, 1988; Scheinberg, 1991; Smith-Gill, 1995). Another mechanism of tumor destruction by antibodies is altering the function of physiologically important receptors on the cell surface. This can be accomplished by blocking the growth factor receptor sites or by directly inducing programmed cell death (**apoptosis**) (Maloney *et al.*, 1996).

For the antibody to locate and destroy the tumor, several critical factors must come into play. First, it is important that the surface-membrane antigens are present on all the tumor cells and are distributed in high density. The antibody should possess a high affinity for the antigen target, and the antigen should remain on the surface of the tumor, providing a specific target for the antibody. Optimally, there should be little circulating antigen to react with the antibody before it reaches the tumor. It is also ideal if the antibody does not have cross-reactivity with normal tissue. The tumor should be highly vascular so that the antibody can be delivered to the site, and there should be no mutations or variants in antigen expression. Tumor size and tumor burden also must be considered. If the tumor volume is too great it may not be possible to deliver enough antibody to effectively treat the tumor. The antigen should have a critical biological function and should be necessary for tumor survival. Finally, in order to provide optimum binding to the tumor, the antigen should not be internalized or shed (Maloney, 1998).

Native MABs derived from mice can be potent antigens when used in humans. This is particularly true after repeated treatments. The murine product may elicit a human antiglobulin response. Because the MAB is derived from the mouse, individuals who are immunocompetent may develop a human antimouse antibody (HAMA) response. Once this occurs, the antitumor response may be negated. There is concern that with continued use of the MAB, immune complexes could form, resulting in rapid clearance and possible tissue damage (Jurcic *et al.*, 1996). In order to negate this limitation, researchers have used approaches to minimize the immunogenicity of the mouse antibody.

Researchers are studying ways to overcome the HAMA response. One suggestion has been the use of immunosuppressive therapy prior to antibody treatment. The most prevalent method, however, has been through modification of the antibody. The potential for using a human MAB instead of a mouse antibody is one possible approach. The technique for developing human MABs involves immortalizing immune B cells with Epstein-Barr virus. The immune B cell is then fused with a human myeloma cell line or a human lymphoblastoid cell line (Dorfman, 1985). Problems encountered with human MABs include the paucity of human myeloma cell lines that are fusion efficient and the lack of readily available human B cells that have been immunized with tumor cells. To immunize human subjects with tumor cells or products is not a viable option (LoBuglio and Saleh, 1992). The few human antibodies available do not allow for wide-scale clinical trials.

A second method of antibody modification is to try reducing the amount of mouse protein in the antibody by inserting the human gene that codes for the constant region. Technology has made it possible to produce antibodies with a murine variable region combined with a human constant region through use of genetic engineering techniques. The gene for the human constant region is isolated and amplified by PCR in the same fashion as the mouse variable-region genes. Both genes are inserted into a virus that is allowed to infect *Escherichia coli* (*E. coli*). The viral DNA is inserted into the cellular DNA of the *E. coli*, and the cell produces the desired mouse-human antibody. Growing *E. coli* in cultures is much easier than growing the antibody in the mouse and yields large volumes of pure antibody. This type of antibody is called a chimeric antibody and is named after a mythical beast, the chimera, which has the head of a lion, the body of a goat, and the tail of a dragon (Overmyer, 1990). Potential advantages of this type of antibody include less immunogenicity, longer circulation of the antibody, and better cell killing. Cell killing is enhanced because the chimeric antibody maintains the antigenic specificity of the murine antibody and the effector properties of the human Fc receptor (LoBuglio and Saleh, 1992; Hozumi and Sandhu, 1993). It is believed that these antibodies mediate antibody-dependent cell-mediated cytotoxicity with human effector cells, causing lysis of the tumor cells.

Of course, there is still a possibility that the patient receiving a chimeric MAB would be at risk for developing a human antihuman antibody response (HAHA) or a human antichimeric antibody response (HACA). Studies using chimeric antibodies will be discussed later in the chapter.

A third technique for reducing the immunogenicity of the MAB is to include even more human portions in the engineered antibody. MABs thus adapted are termed "humanized" and are differentiated from chimeric antibodies in that they contain a human constant region and a variable region that contains both the murine complementarity-determining regions and the human V-region framework determinants (LoBuglio and Saleh, 1992). Therefore, only a very small portion of the humanized MAB contains genetic material from the mouse. There is insufficient information thus far to determine whether these MABs decrease the incidence of a HAMA response. Figure 8.3 is a schematic representation of the murine, human, chimeric, and humanized antibodies.

Clinical Studies

Clinical studies of MABs in the leukemias and lymphomas involve the use of (1) unconjugated MABs, (2) combination therapies with cytotoxic drugs or other biological agents, and (3) MABs conjugated with radionuclides, toxins, or drugs. This section will include an overview of some of the historical studies as well as the current approaches to MAB therapy. All 3 methods of treatment will be addressed. However, given the increasing recognition of target antigens for MABs and the ever-expanding number of studies, it is not possible to include all of the major advances.

In early studies of MABs in the treatment of malignancies, they were used in their native form (unconjugated). However, in an attempt to utilize the unique targeting properties of MABs and enhance their cytotoxicity, investigators have subsequently coupled antibodies with therapeutic agents such as α-, β-, and γ-emitting radionuclides; with protein toxins such as pokeweed antiviral protein (PAP), *Pseudomonas,* diphtheria, ricin, and saporin; and with antineoplastic drugs such as doxorubicin and methotrexate (Houston and Nowinski, 1981; Pimm *et al.*, 1982; Thorpe and Ross, 1982; Vitetta *et al.*, 1982; Redwood *et al.*, 1984; Lotze and Rosenberg, 1988; Kreitman and Pastan, 1995; Myers and Uckun, 1995). Newer drugs such as maytansinoids and calicheamicins are now being conjugated with MABs. These drugs have a much higher toxicity than conventional antineoplastics; therefore, they need to be linked to an MAB to minimize the toxicity to normal tissues (Hinman *et al.*, 1993; Hinman *et al.*, 1994; Vitetta *et al.*, 1998).

These agents, known as immunoconjugates are frequently termed "magic bullets" because

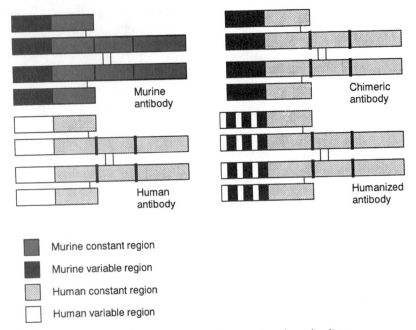

Murine constant region

Murine variable region

Human constant region

Human variable region

Figure 8.3   Schematic diagram of various types of monoclonal antibodies

Source: Reprinted with permission from LoBuglio, A., and Saleh, M. 1992. Monoclonal antibody therapy of cancer. *Critical Reviews in Oncology/Hematology* 13: 273.

of their ability to target the malignant cell and deliver a toxic insult. A primary disadvantage of immunoconjugates thus far has been in the stability of the binding to the antibody. This is particularly troublesome when using **immunotoxins** and radioisotope conjugates because damage to normal tissue can occur if the toxin or radioisotope is freed prior to reaching the tumor site. Both toxins and drugs must be internalized by the cell to cause cell death (Vitetta *et al.*, 1998).

Toxins make an excellent choice for conjugates in that they are extremely potent and have well-defined chemistry. Toxins are transported to the tumor-cell surface by the MAB, which is targeted to a specific antigen. After binding to the antigen, the complex is internalized. At this point the toxin escapes to the cytosol, crossing the cell membrane, and mediates the inhibi-

tion of protein synthesis, leading to cell kill (Gould *et al.*, 1989). Because they inhibit protein synthesis, toxins not only kill dividing cells but resting cells as well (Pai and Pastan, 1995). Figure 8.4 provides a schematic representation of the difference between native ricin and an altered form of the same toxin. In this diagram, the B-chain of the native ricin binds indiscriminately to the galactose residues on a non-B cell, to a B lymphocyte, and to a tumor cell. Once internalized, the toxic A-chain acts at the ribosome to inhibit protein synthesis. The altered toxin, also called blocked ricin, has affinity ligands that are attached to the B-chain and that block nonspecific binding of the toxin. Furthermore, the blocked ricin is conjugated to the anti-CD19 MAB. The MAB binds with CD19 on the surface of the B lymphocyte as well as the B lymphoma. The conjugated toxin is

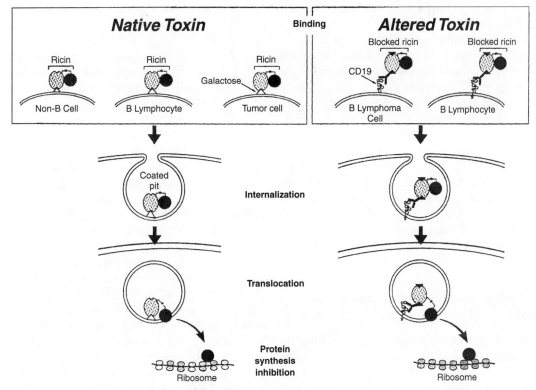

Figure 8.4   Pathway of immunotoxin entry. Cytotoxic mechanism of native ricin and anti-B4-bR. Native ricin consists of 2 chains. The B-chain binds to galactose residues on the cell membrane. In blocked ricin, affinity ligands (▼) are covalently attached to the B-chain and block nonspecific binding of the toxin. Binding is now conferred by the anti-CD19 antibody to which the altered toxin is conjugated. The toxic A-chain acts at the ribosome to inhibit protein synthesis.

Source: Reprinted with permission from Grossbard, M., Press, O., Appelbaum, F., *et al.* 1992c. Monoclonal antibody-based therapy of leukemia and lymphoma. *Blood* 80: 867.

internalized, and the A-chain is released to block protein synthesis. Toxins are chosen based on their ability to internalize to the cytosol and to initiate the catalysis of proteins (Grossbard *et al.*, 1992a; Grossbard *et al.*, 1992c). The trials using ricin A-chain and anti-B4 blocked ricin are also under investigation and will be discussed later in this chapter.

The historical basis for using radionuclides for treatment of malignancies has been well established. Tumor-specific antibodies when conjugated to a radioisotope (**radioimmunoconjugates**) have the advantage of providing both diagnostic and treatment capabilities. The most common radionuclides used for the treatment of non-Hodgkin's lymphoma include iodine (^{131}I), yttrium (^{90}Y), and copper ([67]Cu) (Davis and Knox, 1998). The advantages of using radioisotopes for immunoconjugates are that they radiate beyond a single cell and generally do not require internalization by the target cell.

Because the MABs are able to target tumors, linking chemotherapeutic drugs with the antibody (**chemoimmunoconjugates**) is a logical step in achieving the "magic bullet" approach to killing tumors. Antineoplastic drugs have a proven record in cancer therapy; their toxicity and maximum tolerated dose are well known. Although a number of agents such as doxorubicin, methotrexate, chlorambucil, vinca alkaloids, and mitomycin have been conjugated with MABs, no significant responses have been observed in clinical trials (LoBuglia and Saleh, 1992). This approach has been used more in solid tumors and will be reviewed in Chapter 9. A more common approach in the hematologic malignancies is to administer the chemotherapy as adjuvant rather than as conjugate therapy.

Clinical Studies of the Leukemias and Lymphomas

One of the first antibodies to be studied in humans was anti-CD5 (Leu-1, T101) (Miller *et al.*, 1981; Miller *et al.*, 1983; Dillman *et al.*, 1984). This antibody is directed against the surface antigen CD5, which is present on both normal and malignant mature T cells and a subset of B cells. Although clinical responses varied, there was transient clearing of cells in patients with chronic B-cell lymphocytic leukemia (Lowder *et al.*, 1985). The MAB anti-CD5 was also conjugated to ricin A-toxin and used to treat patients with chronic lymphocytic T-cell leukemia. Although these patients experienced a rapid fall in circulating leukemic cells, no clinical responses were observed (Laurent *et al.*, 1986; Blakey and Thorpe, 1988; Hertler *et al.*, 1988).

Observable tumor responses also occurred in the patients with T-cell lymphoma. Responses lasted from 1.4 to 4 months; however, many of the responses were interrupted by the development of HAMA (Dillman *et al.*, 1982; Foon *et al.*, 1982; Foon *et al.*, 1983; Miller *et al.*, 1983; Dillman *et al.*, 1984; Lowder *et al.*, 1985). Chimeric MABs that are part human and part mouse were developed to the CD4 antigen to minimize the HAMA response. Reports of 15 patients with T-cell lymphoma mycosis fungoides treated with this antibody showed only partial responses of short duration (Knox *et al.*, 1996b).

Leukemia cells express several potential targets for antibody therapy although none are leukemia-specific. Table 8.1 lists the potential targets for MAB-based treatment of leukemia that have been investigated in both preclinical or clinical studies (Multani and Flavell, 1998). Unfortunately, none of these targets are leukemia-specific. When antibody therapies are directed against normal tissue-differentiation antigens, the competition for binding of the antibody with the normal cell greatly reduces the effectiveness of the MAB. Multani and Flavell (1998) state that there are 3 absolute requirements that a MAB must meet if it is to be of practical value in treating leukemia: (1) the leukemia cells should have a homogeneous expression of the antigen on the surface, (2) the antigen should not be expressed on any life-sustaining normal tissue or stem cells, and finally, (3) if using unconjugated antibodies, the antigen should remain on the surface rather than modulating.

CD10 is the common acute lymphoblastic leukemia antigen (CALLA) expressed by over 65% of leukemic cells. In a study of an unconjugated J-5 antibody (anti-CALLA), 4 patients were treated with the MAB (Ritz *et al.*, 1980). Although 3 of the patients experienced a reduction in the number of circulating CALLA-positive blasts, those leukemic cells that were CALLA negative persisted. It was also reported that when the levels of MAB in the circulation were no longer detectable, the CALLA-positive blasts reappeared. In studies in which the antibody was conjugated to ricin A-chain, it was found that the antibody was more potent than the unconjugated MAB; however, because the

Table 8.1   Target molecules for antibody-based treatment of leukemia

Target Molecule	Normal Expression	Indicated Disease	Mean Reactivity %*		
			cALL	T-ALL	AML
CD2	T cells, NK cells, thymocytes	T-ALL	18	60	<10
CD5[+]	Mature T cells, thymocytes, subset B cells	cALL, T-ALL	21	<10	<10
CD7[+]	Early and late T cells	T-ALL	<5	50	<10
CD10[+]	Early B- and T-cell precursors, stromal cells, kidney, and gut	cALL	66	14	<10
CD19[+]	All B cells, follicular dendritic cells	cALL	78	<5	<10
CD22[+]	Subset of mature B cells: cytoplasmic in pro-B and pre-B cells	cALL	26	0	<10
CD24	Early and late B cells; absent from plasma cells	cALL	78	<5	<10
CD33[+]	Myeloid precursors in bone marrow; not on pluripotent stem cell	AML	<5	<5	40
CD38	Early B and T cells; activated B and T cells; myeloid precursors	Myeloma, cALL, T-ALL, AML	52	72	50
CD40	All mature B cells; absent from plasma cells	cALL	32	<5	16
CD72	All B cells; absent from plasma cells	cALL	30	<5	<10

*Data from Leukocyte Typing IV (Boston Workshop).
[+]Studied clinically.

AML, acute myelocytic leukemia; cALL, common acute lymphoblastic leukemia; NK, natural killer; T-ALL, T-cell lymphocytic leukemia.

Source: Reprinted with permission from Multani, P., and Flavel, D. 1998. Antibody-based therapies for treatment of acute leukemia. In Grossbard, M. (ed). *Monoclonal Antibody-Based Therapy of Cancer.* New York, NY: Marcel Dekker, p. 193.

CD10 antigen is expressed on normal tissues, including the kidney, the potential toxicity severely limits its application (Luo and Seon, 1990).

CD19 is a differentiation antigen present on all B cells. It is one of the most widely utilized markers for targeting B cells. Twenty-five patients with B-cell lymphoma were treated with the anti-CD19 immunotoxin MAB conjugated to ricin. The galactose binding sites of the ricin were blocked in an effort to reduce toxicity to normal cells (Grossbard *et al.*, 1992a). Nine patients had partial or mixed responses, and 1 patient had a complete response. In a second trial of B-cell lymphoma, 15 patients received the anti-CD19 blocked ricin immunotoxin (anti-B4-bR). One third of these heavily pretreated patients demonstrated a clinical response (Vitetta *et al.*, 1991). Although the response rates are modestly higher for patients with non-Hodgkin's lymphoma compared with solid tumors, durable remissions are infrequent.

A phase I study by Uckun and colleagues (1993) used the anti-CD19 immunotoxin (B43-PAP). Seventeen patients were treated with escalating doses. Although the primary end point was determination of the maximum tolerated dose, there were 4 complete responders. Phase II studies are currently in progress.

CD25, the interleukin-2 (IL-2) receptor "Tac," has also been identified as a target for MAB anti-Tac therapy. This receptor shows increased expression in the HTLV-1-induced T-cell ALL (Waldmann et al., 1992). In a study of 19 patients with adult T-cell ALL treated with the MAB anti-Tac, there were 6 responses, 2 of which were complete responses that lasted 2 months to 3 years (Waldmann et al., 1988; Waldmann, 1995). The advantage of targeting the IL-2 receptor is that resting T and B cells do not express the antigen. Furthermore, anti-Tac has been used to treat individuals who are rejecting allografts and to target abnormal T cells in selected patients with autoimmune diseases. Anti-Tac has also been coupled with the immunotoxins *Pseudomonas* and diphtheria as well as radionuclides such as ^{90}Y and has shown promising results in the phase II trials (Waldmann, 1995).

CD33 is an antigen expressed by myeloid precursors in the bone marrow but not on pluripotent stem cells. In some cases, it is also expressed on the surface of acute myelogenous leukemia (AML) cells. A study utilizing the anti-CD33 MAB (M195) in 10 patients with AML showed little response; however, when the antibody was labeled with trace-iodine, the bone marrow showed rapid uptake (Scheinberg et al., 1991). Based on the fact that the antibody did reach the bone marrow, studies were conducted to determine the effectiveness of a radioimmunoconjugate with ^{131}I. Twenty-five patients with relapsed or refractory AML were treated. Responses included a decrease in the number of blast cells in the bone marrow in 23 of the 25 patients. Three patients were complete

responders and 8 went on to bone marrow transplant. Unfortunately, 37% of the patients treated developed a HAMA response to the M195 antibody (Schwartz et al., 1993). To reduce the immunogenicity to the mouse protein, a humanized version of M195 has been developed (see earlier discussion of humanized antibodies). Thus far, the humanized M195 has been combined with ^{131}I and a potent toxin, calicheamicin (Hinman et al., 1993; Multani and Flavell, 1998). Phase I testing of these agents is ongoing, and investigors are hopeful that the CD33 antigen may prove to be a critical target for AML therapies. Phase I testing of the immunoconjugate (CMA-676) has recently been concluded. Forty patients with refractory or recurrent AML received the recombinant humanized anti-CD33 antibody conjugated with the potent antitumor antibiotic calicheamicin. In this phase I dose escalation study, 8 (20%) patients had clearing of AML cells from the bone marrow and peripheral blood. Three of these 8 patients had complete restoration of normal hematopoiesis. The most common toxicity of the immunoconjugate was myelosuppression. Nonhematologic toxicity included the infusion-related complex of chills and fever. Nausea and vomiting was reported in approximately one third of the study patients (Sievers et al., 1999; Sievers, 2000). In May 2000, gemtuzumab ozogamicin (Mylotarg™; American Home Products, Madison, NJ) received FDA approval for the use of this antibody for the treatment of patients with CD33-positive acute myeloid leukemia in first relapse who are 60 years or older and who are not considered candidates for cytotoxic chemotherapy (Wyeth Ayerst, 2000).

CD52 is another cell-surface antigen that has been used to target lymphoid malignancies and some cases of AML. The antibody CAMPATH-1 is from a family of rat antibodies that recognizes CD52. Early studies of this antibody showed promising results; however, repeated treatments were limited because of the development of human anti-rat antibody (Dyer *et al.*, 1989). A humanized version of the antibody (CAMPATH-1H) was developed and studied in phase I/II trials in over 113 patients with non-Hodgkin's lymphoma or CLL. Although there were major responses, the unconjugated antibody had a significant toxicity profile with 2 documented cases of pneumocystis pneumonia, 3 cases of cytomegalovirus-related disease, and multiple cases of recurrent herpes zoster and herpes simplex (Clendenin *et al.*, 1992). In a follow-up of 50 patients in a phase II trial, grade IV neutropenia occurred in 28% of the study group. Seven patients developed opportunistic infections, 9 had bacterial infections, and there were 3 deaths related to infectious complications (Lundin *et al.*, 1998). The immunosuppression-related toxicities are thought to be related to the rapid and profound decrease in the lymphocytes following antibody infusion.

ANTI-IDIOTYPE MABS

The B-cell malignances have served as a prototype for many of the ongoing studies of MABs. In B-cell malignancies, the Ig produced by the tumor provides an ideal tumor marker. The antibody binding site, also called the idiotype, serves as a tumor-specific marker on the surface of the B cell. Taking advantage of the unique nature of these malignancies, investigators have developed MABs to the variable region or idiotype. These antibodies are called **anti-idiotypes**. Miller *et al.* (1982) reported the first study with a "tailor-made" antibody for each patient with low-grade B-cell lymphoma. These "private" antibodies have been studied extensively *in vivo* (Maloney *et al.*, 1992b). The anti-idiotype studies have been updated by Davis *et al.* (1998). Between 1981 and 1993, 45 patients with low-grade B-cell lymphoma received 52 courses of anti-idiotype MAB in 4 different trials. Sixteen patients received antibody alone (2 patients received a second course of anti-

body). The remainder received antibody with an immunomodulating agent (interferon [IFN]-α or IL-2) (Brown *et al.*, 1989b) or chemotherapy (chlorambucil) (Maloney *et al.*, 1992a). Anti-idiotype MAB was infused on an average of 3 times a week. Cumulative doses ranged from 400 to 15,000 mg. Dose escalation was used to achieve sustained antibody levels in the serum of greater than 25 mcg/mL. An overall response rate of 66% has been documented; 18% achieved complete response. Of those 8 complete responders, 6 have had durable responses of greater than 4 years; 5 have had continued responses from 4 to 10 years. The results of these trials are summarized in Table 8.2 (Davis *et al.*, 1998).

The first patient treated on the anti-idiotype study in 1981 has provoked interest as to the role of infection or circulation in sustained remission. The initial response lasted for 7 years. Following surgery for coronary artery disease, the patient developed an infection at the saphenous vein harvest site. A localized recurrence of his lymphoma in the lower portion of the infected leg was also noted. This recurrence responded to local irradiation. He remained in continuous remission for an additional 9 years (Davis *et al.*, 1998). Davis and colleagues (1998) attempted to determine whether 5 of the patients with sustained remissions had residual disease. At the time of analysis, the patients had been in remission for 3 to 8 years. The tests used to determine residual disease included enzyme-linked immunoabsorbent assay for detection of idiotype protein or anti-idiotype antibodies in the serum; flow cytometry of blood and bone marrow samples for idiotype positive cells; and PCR for clonal gene rearrangement or translocation [t(14,8)]. Despite the fact that these patients showed no evidence of clinical disease, 4 of 5 patients had molecular evidence of residual disease. These 4 patients have had no symptomatic recurrence for 3 years since the analysis.

Table 8.2 Results of therapeutic trials using anti-idiotype antibodies

Therapy	Patients Treated	PR	CR	CR Duration (years)
Anti-id	18	8	4	1.4, 4+, 7,* 9.5+
Anti-id + IFN-α	12	7	2	9.5+, 10+
Anti-id + Chl	13	8	1	2.5
Anti-id + IL-2	9	2	1	4.5
Total	52	25	8	

Antibodies were given either alone or in combination with other agents.
* Patient 1 received local radiation therapy after a local relapse at 7 years and subsequently has been in continuous and ongoing remission for an additional 9 years. Chl, chlorambucil; CR, complete remission; id, idiotype; IFN, interferon; IL-2, interleukin-2; PR, partial remission.

Source: Reprinted with permission from Davis, T., Maloney, D., Czerwinski, D., *et al.* 1998. Anti-idiotype antibodies can induce long-term complete remissions in non-Hodgkin's lymphoma without eradicating the malignant clone. *Blood* 92(4): 1184–1190.

These studies established that anti-idiotype antibodies are active therapeutic agents in both heavily treated patients and patients who have progressed to higher-grade lymphomas. Unfortunately, the time to develop and customize the antibodies, coupled with the cost, led researchers to search for other options.

SHARED IDIOTYPE MABS

The aforementioned limitations of producing individual therapeutic MABs led researchers to the discovery that it was possible to identify shared idiotypes (SIDs). These SIDS were reactive to lymphoma cells from more than 1 patient (Miller *et al.*, 1989; Maloney *et al.*, 1992b). IDEC Pharmaceutical Corporation (San Diego, CA) produced 15 anti-idiotype antibodies that reacted with the tumors of 20% of the patients with low-grade B-cell lymphoma (Maloney *et al.*, 1992b). The early use of SIDs was one of the first steps in overcoming many of the problems of private anti-idiotypes. They were available for immediate use and could be used to treat many different patients (Maloney *et al.*, 1992b).

CHIMERIC MABS

In the ongoing attempt to find an antibody therapy with broader implications than the idiotypes and SIDs, a chimeric anti-CD20 (IDEC-C2B8) was investigated in patients with recurrent B-cell lymphoma. CD20 is expressed on both normal B cells and nearly all B-cell malignancies. In a phase I clinical trial, 15 patients received a single dose of MAB in escalating doses (10, 50, 100, 250, and 500 mg/m^2). Despite the fact that each patient received only 1 dose of antibody, tumor regression occurred in 6 of the 15 patients (2 partial and 4 minor responses). The responses were seen in patients receiving doses of 100 mg/m^2 or greater (Maloney *et al.*, 1994). Building on this early study, a phase I study of IDEC-C2B8 was conducted in 20 patients to evaluate the effects of weekly infusions in dosages of 125 mg/m^2 ($n = 3$), 250 mg/m^2 ($n = 7$), or 375 mg/m^2 ($n = 10$). Of the 18 assessable patients, 6 had a partial remission, with a range of disease progression from 3 to 21.7 months. Minor responses were seen in 5 patients, and 7 patients had disease progression (Maloney *et al.*, 1997a). This study led to a phase II trial in 37 patients with relapsed low-grade or follicular B-cell lymphoma. Antibody dosage was 375 mg/m^2 repeated weekly for 4 weeks. Seventeen (46%) of the 37 patients had a clinical response. Two patients were withdrawn from the study for adverse events following the first antibody infusion, and one patient had a high-grade B-cell malignancy. Thirty-four patients were evaluable. Three patients had a complete response (9%) and 14 had a partial response (41%). Eight additional patients had some evidence of tumor response (Maloney et al., 1997b).

A multicenter, open-label single-arm study was conducted with 166 patients with relapsed low-grade lymphoma or follicular B-cell non-Hodgkin's lymphoma. The overall response rate was 48% (80/166 patients). The median time to onset of response was 50 days, and the median duration of response was 12 months (McLaughlin et al., 1998). This study was the pivotal trial that led to FDA approval in 1997 of the C2B8 antibody rituximab (Rituxan®; IDEC Pharmaceuticals Corporation and Genentech, Inc., South San Franciso, CA). Rituximab became the first MAB approved for clinical treatment of malignancy (Maloney, 1998). Rituximab is now being evaluated in other B-cell malignancies as well as in combination therapy (chemotherapy plus IFN) (Maloney, 1998). In a trial with CHOP chemotherapy (cyclophosphamide, doxorubicin, vincristine, and prednisone) and 6 infusions of rituximab, the evaluable patients tested with PCR showed a negative t(14:18) translocation (Czuzman et al., 1996).

Unlike the responses to chemotherapy or radiation therapy, the onset of response with MAB therapy in the B-cell lymphoma trials is generally 1 to 2 months following therapy, although some patients can exhibit regression for many months following therapy (Maloney et al., 1992b; Maloney et al., 1997b; Davis et al., 1998; Kostis and Callaghan, 2000). This suggests that the treatment induced an immune response in the patient against the tumor.

Hodgkin's disease has presented a different challenge in the use of MABs for treatment. This tumor is characterized by the diagnostic presence of Reed-Sternberg cells and surrounded by a larger diverse population of cells such as macrophages, lymphocytes, and granulocytes. Because of the diversity of the cell population, it is difficult to identify antigens that could be used as targets. The Reed-Sternberg cell is frequently negative for B- and T-cell markers but positive for CD15, DR (class II major histocompatibility antigens), transferrin receptor, CD30, and CD25. Unmodifed MABs to these target antigens have shown little clinical efficacy (Morein and Junghans, 1998).

RADIOIMMUNODETECTION/ RADIOIMMUNOTHERAPY

Radioimmunoconjugates consisting of monoclonal antibodies conjugated with radioactive isotopes have been developed both as a treatment modality and as a method of imaging tumors. **Radioimmunodetection** or RAID uses low doses of beta-emitting radionuclides attached to an antibody to image disease sites. In studies of B-cell lymphoma, Kaminski and colleagues (1993; 1996) reported successful imaging of all disease sites greater than 2 cm with ^{131}I anti-CD20 MAB. Press and colleagues found a 73% rate of tumor visualization in a review of 173 patients with B-cell and T-cell lymphomas (Press et al., 1993). This technique allows investigators to determine the biodistribution of the antibody and to estimate tumor burden.

When using radioimmunotherapy or RIT, there are several critical issues in the application that must be addressed. The first issue is the biodistribution of the radiolabeled antibody. Because the antibody is usually cleared by the liver, it is imperative that the dosage not cause liver toxicity and damage. The second issue is the stability of radioimmunoconjugates in vivo, which has been a problem. Occasionally, the MAB and the radionuclide separate before reaching the intended target (Eary et al., 1990). This has been especially true for iodine, which is readily cleaved from the antibody. The ability of the MAB to reach the intended target is the third issue. Despite the specificity of MABs, only a small fraction of the radiolabeled antibody may reach the tumor. A technique of pre-administering unlabeled MABs prior to RIT has become a widespread practice because unlabeled antibodies appear to be taken up by the nonspecific cells, thus leaving the radioimmunoconjugate to target the primary tumor (Kaminski et al., 1996; Davis and Knox, 1998). Fourth, the antibody must be freshly labeled and exposure to radiation must be controlled (Larson et al., 1995).

In studies of non-Hodgkin's lymphomas and Hodgkin's disease, investigators have shown that these tumors respond to the RIT (DeNardo et al., 1987, 1998, 1999; Rosen et al., 1987; Press et al., 1989). Bone marrow toxicity is the most significant problem; however, an approach used to circumvent this toxicity is to harvest autologous bone marrow prior to treatment and reinfuse it if necessary (Press et al., 1989). Several studies now use RIT as myeloablative therapy for either autologous bone marrow or peripheral stem cell transplant for lymphoma. This therapy is then followed by reinfusion of bone marrow or peripheral stem cells (Press et al., 1995; Kaminski et al., 1997).

The radioisotope most frequently used in phase I trials has been [131]I. Antitumor activity has been demonstrated in lymphoma with the ^{131}I-labeled antibody Lym-1 (DeNardo et al., 1987, 1998) and with ^{131}I-labeled LL2 (EPB-2) (Goldenberg et al., 1991). Most trials use high doses of radioisotopes conjugated to MABs (232 to 608 mCi of ^{131}I). In contrast to the above-mentioned trials, Kaminski et al. (1996) showed promising results with low-dose therapy using doses of 34 to 161 mCi of ^{131}I in patients with B-cell lymphoma. Each patient received only a single dose of anti-B1 MAB, which targets the CD20 antigen. Documented responses were reported in 22 of 28 patients. Fourteen patients had complete remissions and 8 patients had partial remissions. The median duration of response was 16.5 months. Six of

the complete responders had ongoing responses of 16 to 31 months at the time of the report. The researchers theorize that the "low-dose" radiation induced apoptosis in lymphoid cell lines and that binding of the MAB was synergistic in the induction of this effect. They also noted that the anti-CD20 may be a superior targeting agent for B-cell lymphomas. As of July 2000, a phase II study of [131]I -labeled anti-B1 MAB (Coulter Pharmaceutical, South San Francisco, CA) with an accrual goal of 60 had shown positive results. In 1998, Kaminski et al. (1998) reported on 21 evaluable patients. The initial response was 100%, with 15 of the 21 patients achieving a complete response and 6 patients achieving a partial response. Two patients with a complete response have relapsed, and 5 of the 6 partial responders have progressed (Kaminski et al., 1998). These results are encouraging and offer new insight into the use of radiolabeled antibodies. These results were encouraging and offered new insight into the use of radiolabeled antibodies. In March 2000, Vose et al. (2000) reported an update on this multicenter phase II study evaluated the efficacy, dosimetry methodology, and safety of ^{131}I-labeled anti-B1 MAB (tositumomab) in patients with chemotherapy-relapsed/refractory low-grade or transformed low-grade non-Hodgkin's lymphoma. Tositumomab produced a high overall response rate, and approximately one third of patients had a CR despite having chemotherapy-relapsed or refractory low-grade or transformed low-grade NHL.

Another radionuclide, ^{90}Y has been used in treatment of patients with B-cell lymphoma (LoBuglio and Saleh, 1992). In a group of patients with refractory Hodgkin's disease, complete remissions were observed in 30% of evaluable patients treated with ^{90}Y-labeled polyclonal antiferritin Ig (Vriesendorp et al., 1991). A phase I/II study of 18 patients with relapsed low-grade or intermittent-grade non-Hodgkin's lymphoma with ^{90}Y-labeled anti-CD20 was conducted by Knox and colleagues (1996a). Patients received a single dose of the MAB. Overall response rates were 72%, with 6 complete responses and 7 partial responses. Freedom from progression ranged from 3 to more than 29 months. In 1999, Witzig and colleagues reported on the use of ^{90}Y (ibritumomab tiuxetan; IDEC-Y2B8). This MAB is a murine IgG1-κ MAB that covalently binds MX-DTPA (tiuxetan), which chelates the radioisotope ^{90}Y. The antibody targets CD20, a B-lymphocyte antigen. A multicenter phase I/II trial was conducted to compare 2 doses of unlabeled rituximab given before radiolabeled antibody to determine the maximum tolerated single dose of IDEC-Y2B8 that could be administered without stem cell support and to evaluate safety and efficacy. The maximum tolerated dose was 0.4 mCi/kg IDEC-Y2B8. A lower dose, 0.3 mCi/kg, was given for patients with baseline platelet counts of 100 to 149,000/μL. The overall response rate for the intent-to-treat population (n = 51) was 67% (26% complete response and 41% partial response). These phase I/II data demonstrate that IDEC-Y2B8 radioimmunotherapy is a safe and effective alternative for outpatient therapy of patients with relapsed or refractory NHL. A phase III study is ongoing (Witzig et al., 1999).

In a review of several studies with chimeric MABs labeled with ^{131}I, Davis and Knox (1998) reported complete remissions ranging from 33% to 85%. This form of therapy has shown great promise in the non-Hodgkin's lymphoma population, but there are areas that need further evaluation. For example, RIT may be useful as a replacement for the conditioning regimen of total-body irradiation for bone marrow or stem cell transplants. Clearly, this promising method of therapy needs further study. There are several clinical trials, both myeloablative and nonmyeloablative (^{131}I-Lym-1 and ^{131}I-B1) that are considered pivotal for FDA approval (Davis and Knox, 1998).

BONE MARROW PURGING

Monoclonal antibodies have been used *in vitro* to perform immunologic purging of malignant cells from the harvested bone marrow. The patient's marrow is harvested prior to receiving high-dose ablative therapy. Following therapy, the purged marrow is then used for autologous bone marrow transplantation. The use of this technique in the management of advanced cancers is increasing, but the technique has been studied most in leukemias and lymphomas (Ball et al., 1990; Freedman et al., 1990; Gribben et al., 1991). Gribben and colleagues (1991) attempted to determine whether the removal of residual tumor cells from the bone marrow prolongs disease-free survival. Because the lymphoma cells may lack the targeted antigen, it is frequently difficult to determine whether occult lymphoma cells remain in the marrow after purging. These investigators used PCR to detect the 14:18 chromosome translocation t(14:18) observed in 85% of follicular lymphomas and 30% of diffuse lymphomas. This method is sensitive enough to detect 1 lymphoma cell in 1 million normal cells. The bone marrow was purged *ex vivo* with a cocktail of three B-cell antibodies. Rabbit complement was added to enhance tumor-cell destruction. Residual lymphoma cells were detected by PCR in the bone marrow of all of the patients prior to immunologic purging. Following the purging, no lymphoma cells were detected in 57 of the 114 treated patients. Disease-free survival was significantly longer ($p < 0.00001$) in these patients than in the patients whose marrow still had detectable lymphoma cells after treatment (Gribben et al., 1991).

Negrin and colleagues (1991) confirmed the usefulness of PCR in detecting minimal residual disease before and after bone marrow purging. In an *ex vivo* study they used mixtures of either 4 B-cell antibodies or 8 T-cell antibodies combined with rabbit complement to purge the marrow. They also noted increased disease-free survival in those patients where no residual malignant cells could be detected in the purged marrow.

In 2 separate studies, Press and colleagues (1989, 1995) purged autologous bone marrow with either anti-CD37 MAB or anti-CD20 MAB and complement prior to treatment with ^{131}I radiolabeled antibody in a trial of refractory non-Hodgkin's lymphoma. Nineteen patients received therapeutic infusions ranging from 237 to 777 mCi of ^{131}I MAB followed by autologous marrow reinfusion. Complete remission was reported in 15 patients and partial remission in 2 patients; 9 patients remained in complete remission ranging from 3 to 53 months.

Combinations of MABs directed at T-cell and B-cell antigens along with immunomagnetic beads have also been used to increase the efficacy of the removal of the malignant cells. These beads utilize magnetic microspheres that have been coated either with a purified sheep or goat antimouse antibody directed against the Fc portion of the MAB or attached directly to the primary MAB (Gribben and Nadler, 1995). Figure 8.5 provides an overview of the purging process in B-cell non-Hodgkin's lymphoma. The bone marrow is harvested and the antigens that are expressed on the lymphoma cells but not on the surface of the hematopoietic progenitors are targeted. These harvested bone marrow cells, which express the antigens CD10, CD19, and CD20, are then incubated *ex vivo* with the MABs chosen to target these antigens. The antibody-coated lymphoma cells are removed in the presence of complement, immunotoxins, and magnetic beads. The marrow is then reinfused. Those lymphoma cells that weakly express the target antigen may escape removal and be reinfused (Gribben and Nadler, 1995).

An alternative approach to purging the bone marrow of malignant cells is to try to selectively administer normal stem cells and progenitor cells. This would eliminate the need to purge the negative cells. The antigen CD34 is expressed on early normal progenitor cells but not on the mature cells of non-Hodgkin's lymphoma. Unfortunately, it is expressed on the neoplastic cells of AML, chronic myelogenous leukemia, B-lineage ALL, and some T-lineage ALL (Beauger and Roy, 1998). Although successful engraftment has resulted through the selection of CD34-positive cells, the malignant cells persisted (Gorin *et al.*, 1995).

Adverse Effects

MAB therapy is a desirable approach to the treatment of leukemias and lymphomas because the antibody directly targets the tumor-associated antigen and, in most cases, preserves the integrity of normal cells. This targeting allows many of the acute and long-term toxic effects to be avoided; however, the MABs are not without adverse events. The type and severity of adverse reactions will depend on whether the antibody is administered unconjugated or conjugated to radioisotopes, chemotherapy drugs, or immunotoxins.

Early trials involving treatment of lymphoid malignancies with nonspecific antibodies, which recognized not only tumor-cell antigens but also the tissues from which they arise, revealed many more cases of allergic reaction and anaphylaxis than are currently seen. Dillman and colleagues (1982) were first to report significant toxic effects with monoclonal antibody infusions. In their studies of patients with B-cell CLL, they noted anaphylaxis, bronchospasm, and allergic reactions that required cessation of therapy. It should be noted that in these early trials the antibody was administered by bolus or rapid infusion. It has been shown that with slower infusion, many of these acute toxic effects can be alleviated (Miller *et al.*, 1982).

Adverse effects with unconjugated MABs show a similar pattern whether the antibody is

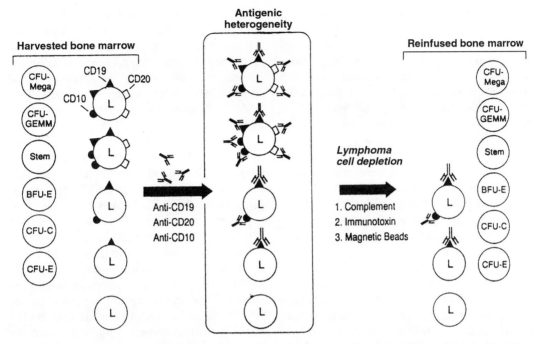

Figure 8.5   Principle of immunologic purging illustrated in B-cell non-Hodgkin's lymphoma. The targeted antigens are expressed on the surface of the lymphoma cell (L) but are not expressed on the hematopoietic progenitors. Monoclonal antibodies are incubated *ex vivo* with the harvested bone marrow mononuclear cell fraction. Antibody-coated cells are removed and marrow is reinfused. The remaining lymphoma cells are likely to lack or to weakly express the targeted antigens.

BFU-E, burst-forming unit–erythrocyte; CFU-C, colony-forming unit–cells; CFU-E, colony-forming unit–erythrocyte; CFU-GEMM, colony-forming unit–granulocytes, erythrocytes, macrophages, and megakaryocytes; CFU-Mega, colony-forming unit–megakaryocytes.

Source: Reprinted with permission from Gribben, J., and Nadler, L. 1995. Purging of bone marrow. In Devita, V., Hellman, S., and Rosenberg, S. (eds). *Biologic Therapy of Cancer: Principles and Practice*, 2nd edn. Philadelphia, PA: J. B. Lippincott, p. 598.

targeted to a normal cell-differentiation antigen or to an idiotype. Patients treated with rituximab for non-Hodgkin's B-cell lymphomas experienced a set of symptoms now commonly called infusion-related symptom complex. These symptoms included fever, chills, and rigor. They usually occur with the initial antibody infusion and are dramatically reduced or absent in subsequent treatments (Maloney *et al.*, 1997a, 1997b). The response is believed to be related to the antibody-antigen equilibration in the circulation. Maloney *et al.* (1997b) speculate that the rapid depletion of B cells from the circulation that has been observed during the first treatment may be the cause of this reaction. B-cell lysis or binding of immune complexes to Fc receptors may lead to the release of cytokines that produce these symptoms. The presence of infusion-related symptoms is not serious enough to discontinue treatment and is easily managed with temporary halting of the infusion and symptomatic treatment with diphenhydramine and acetominophen. Other symptoms have included hypotension, nausea, asthenia, headache, rash, urticaria, pruritis, and a sensation of tongue or throat swelling (Maloney et al., 1994, 1997b). Because there is a rapid and prolonged depletion of the B cells from the circulation, which may last up to 6 months posttreatment, followed by a slow recovery, there was a concern that infection could present a problem. In the pivotal trial, 50 patients ($n = 166$) developed infections. Of those patients, only 9% were grade 3 in severity, and none were grade 4 (McLaughlin et al., 1998). It appears that infections are no higher than what is normally seen in this patient population undergoing cytotoxic chemotherapy (Maloney et al., 1997b).

Tailoring antibodies to the specific antigenic-binding site of the tumor cell, which is different from the host's normal B cells, reduces the frequency of toxic effects. In a review of 45 non-Hodgkin's lymphoma patients receiving MAB directed against the tumor Ig idiotype, there were no reported cases of anaphylaxis or allergic reactions (Davis et al., 1998). Furthermore, the most significant toxic effects have been seen in patients with prolymphocytic leukemia, CLL, or in patients with a high level of circulating idiotype. Toxic reactions are typically associated with high levels of circulating tumor cells or antigen and are most often observed during the first treatment. It has been noted that a few patients in whom the desirable amount of antibody cannot be achieved experience toxic effects throughout the course of treatment. Once the free antigen or antigen-positive cells have been cleared from the serum and an excess of antibody can be achieved, side effects resolve (Brown et al., 1989b).

In addition to fever, chills, and rigor, myalgias and arthralgias have been observed in the anti-idiotype studies. More severe toxic effects, although rare, have included bronchospasm, increased respiratory secretions, and hypotension (Miller et al., 1982; Meeker et al., 1985; Maloney et al., 1992a, 1992b). It has been postulated that respiratory symptoms may occur as a result of pulmonary leukostasis, which is a consequence of sequestration of antibody-coated tumor cells in the pulmonary vasculature. This leads to wheezing, dyspnea, and in some cases hypotension (Press et al., 1987).

In the group of patients treated with rituximab, hematologic toxicities were rare. With anti-idiotype antibody, hematologic toxic effects were also less common. Thrombocytopenia (platelets $< 50,000/mm^3$) was observed in patients whose baseline counts were less than $100,000/mm^3$. In early trials, transient thrombocytopenia was associated with high levels of circulating idiotype protein (Meeker et al., 1985). The cause of thrombocytopenia remains unclear; however, according to Press et al. (1987), the reduction in platelets may be the result of small quantities of antibody being absorbed by the Fc receptors to these cells and removed from circulation by the reticuloendothelial system. Granulocytopenia has also been documented, again in patients whose baseline counts were less than $1,000$ cells/mm^3 (Maloney et al., 1992b). This, too, was a transient phenomenon.

An interesting observation, although probably not a toxic effect, is tumor flare, which has been observed in the anti-idiotype MAB studies. Tumor flare is characterized by swelling, tenderness, and warmth of lymph nodes. This typically occurred between 7 and 14 days after treatment and resolved within 2 to 7 days. Although the etiology of this effect is not certain, it is believed to have been a result of effector cells penetrating the lymph node. This effect was also noted in early trials that combined anti-idiotype antibody with IFN. Brown et al. (1989a) documented swelling in one or more lymph nodes in several patients within the first week of treatment. All tumor sites that exhibited this reaction had major regressions following treatment. Anecdotal reports of patients receiving rituximab have also indicated that they have experienced pain at the tumor sites.

Acute reactions to the murine MABs have been reported; however, immediate allergic reactions are rare. Because it takes time for the body to develop a HAMA reaction, symptoms may occur in subsequent treatments. The reaction is usually manifested by fever, rigors, rash, and neutropenia (Meeker et al., 1985). Meeker and colleagues noted the onset of symptoms within 1 to 2 hours of receiving treatment, with resolution within several days. Prolonged treatment with the MAB, however, usually leads to the development of HAMA in the immunocompetent patient. Other clinical symptoms associated with a HAMA reaction include serum sickness and hypersensitivity reactions (Tjandra et al., 1990). The more troublesome effect of HAMA is that once it develops, continuation of treatment is no longer an option.

Myelosuppression has been a dose-limiting factor when administering radiolabeled antibodies. Goldenberg et al. (1991) found grade 3 or 4 marrow toxicities even at low doses that were not considered therapeutic (59 mCi of ^{131}I). To overcome this adversity, Press et al. (1989) have harvested, purged, and reinfused bone marrow to patients in a dose-escalation trial. In this phase I trial, doses of ^{131}I ranged from 232 to 608 mCi, with myelosuppression occurring between 3 to 5 weeks following treatment. In a subsequent study, Press et al. (1995) treated 19 patients with doses of ^{131}I escalating to 777 mCi. Seventy-eight percent of the patients required bone marrow reinfusion between 13 and 31 days following therapy. Bone marrow toxicity was caused by prolonged circulating antibody-isotope conjugates or free ^{131}I that had been released from the conjugate (Davis and Knox, 1998). Kaminiski et al. (1996), however, have reported the opposite effects with low doses of ^{131}I (34 to 66 mCi) conjugated to the anti-B1 MAB. In their studies, hematologic toxicities were reported as only grade 1 or 2, and no patients required bone marrow reinfusion.

Nonhematologic toxic effects of radiolabeled antibodies have been mild and include fever, urticaria, pruritus, malaise, and asymptomatic hypothyroidism. The latter was observed 1 year after completion of therapy and reflects the inability to achieve complete blockage of ^{131}I uptake in the thyroid by the administration of the protective agent potassium iodide (Press et al., 1989). Gastrointestinal toxic effects in the form of nausea are thought to be caused by gastric irradiation from the excretion of free iodine from the stomach. Press et al. (1995), in a study of 19 patients, have also noted alopecia (21%), elevated liver function (42%), hyperbilirubinemia (37%), and severe cardiopulmonary toxicity (10%).

When antibody and chemotherapy drugs are conjugated, one can expect the usual toxic effects related to antibody alone, and if circulating free drug is present, all of the usual side effects and complications of the chemotherapy drug given alone may also occur. Unusual toxic effects resulting from nonspecific binding of the chemoimmunoconjugate to normal tissues may also occur. Myelosuppression is usually the dose-limiting toxic effect.

The most severe toxic effects have been attributed to immunotoxin-conjugated MABs. These effects, which were shown to be reversible, were noted even at doses too low to yield detectable binding of the immunoconjugate to the target antigen (Pai and Pastan, 1995). Weiner et al. (1989) described vascular-leak syndrome as an effect of treatment with a recombinant ricin A-chain linked to MAB. This syndrome is characterized by weight gain, edema, dyspnea, decreased albumin levels, and, in some cases, hypotension. They suggest the probability that the immunoconjugate was delivering recombinant ricin A-chain to unintended targets. They also showed that ricin

A-toxin contains immunotoxins that bind to the human monocyte Fc receptors. Others postulate that monocyte activation or cell death may lead to the release of mediators that bring about capillary leakage (Gould et al., 1989).

Grossbard et al. (1992b) reported clinically significant hepatotoxicity associated with treatment with B4-blocked ricin. This has also been documented with diphtheria toxin (Pai and Pastan, 1995). The onset of hepatic toxic effects was noted within 24 to 48 hours after infusion and resolved within 7 to 14 days. Elevated SGOT and SGPT levels rose as high as 10 times the upper limit of normal. They postulate these elevated serum levels were caused by the clearance of the immunotoxin by the reticuloendothelial system rather than to nonspecific antibody binding or free blocked ricin. Interestingly, they did not report capillary leak syndrome or neurotoxicity. Tolerable toxic effects such as fevers, malaise, fatigue, nausea, hypoalbuminemia, and thrombocytopenia were also noted.

Given the historical and current data, one can see that adverse reactions vary according to the type and specificity of the MAB used. Most toxic effects are transient and respond to standard interventions.

Obstacles to Treatment

Human Antimurine Antibodies

As mentioned previously, a major limitation associated with murine MABs has been the development of HAMA response. The development of host antibodies against the protein has a neutralizing effect and inhibits antibody binding (Schroff et al., 1985). Meeker et al. (1985) noted that once an immune response had begun, further infusions of antibody were incapable of reaching the tumor. Those patients who had an immune response did not demonstrate a clinical response. Serum assays of antibody levels also indicated that this neutralizing effect occurs. Meeker et al. (1985) reported decreased serum half-life as well as lower antibody levels with a HAMA response, which correlate with the clearance of administered antibody. The onset of a HAMA response in hematologic malignancies has been variable and can occur from 10 to 24 days after treatment (Levy, 1985). As previously discussed, toxic effects related to the HAMA response are characterized by allergic reactions or other immune reactions, such as the formation of immune complexes (Schroff et al., 1985).

Although more prevalent in patients with solid tumors, HAMA response has been observed in patients with hematologic malignancies. There were higher incidences of a HAMA response in early trials with anti-idiotype antibodies for B-cell lymphomas than in later trials. In 1982, Miller and colleagues reported that during treatment with anti-idiotype antibodies, 5 of 11 patients developed a HAMA response; whereas in the later trials reported by Brown et al. (1989b) only 2 of 11 patients had positive immune responses. Subsequent trials revealed no detectable HAMA responses in 13 patients (Maloney et al., 1992b). The lack of a HAMA response in these patients may be related to the purity of the antibodies, to prior immunosuppressive therapy, or to immunosuppression by their disease (Brown et al., 1989b).

The development of chimeric antibodies (discussed earlier) is an attempt to overcome the HAMA response. Of course, there is still a possibility that the patient receiving a chimeric MAB would be at risk for developing a HACA. There have been reports of HACA responses in patients treated with chimerized antibodies, and it has been noted that these responses were to the murine variable regions rather than the human constant region (Khazaeli et al., 1991). Because studies are ongoing in this area, it remains to be seen whether the risk of developing an immune response to the humanized portion will be a salient issue.

Clinical trials with the chimeric anti-CD20 (C2B8), rituximab, which were discussed earlier, showed no quantifiable levels of either HAMA or HACA in those patients treated for relapsed lymphoma. Patients were treated with weekly doses of 375 mg/m^2 for a total of 4 weeks (Maloney et al., 1997b).

The third technique for reducing the immunogenicity of the MAB is to include even more human portions in the engineered antibody. These MABs contain a human constant region and a variable region that includes both the murine complementarity-determining regions and the human V-region framework determinants (LoBuglio and Saleh, 1992). There is insufficient information thus far to determine whether these MABs decrease the incidence of a HAHA response.

Antigenic Modulation

Over the years, researchers have been concerned with how tumor cells escape antibody destruction. One of the defense mechanisms of the tumor cells is antigenic modulation. The antigen disappears from the cell surface either by shedding or internalization (Oldham, 1983). If therapeutic antibody is administered during this modulation, there may not be sufficient opportunity for the MAB to bind to the target cell to effect elimination (Dillman, 1984).

Antigenic modulation can occur within hours after antibody administration. Once the antibody stimulus is removed, the antigen is reexpressed, usually within 24 hours. In in vivo tests conducted by Miller et al. (1981) leukemic cells underwent antigenic modulation as a result of antibody binding to the cell surface. The researchers noted the onset of modulation at 1, 6, and 12 hours after treatment, but no change was observed during the first hour after treatment. In vitro experiments indicated that modu-

lation was time and dose dependent; that is, the longer the cells are exposed to the antibody, the more susceptible they become to modulation (Miller et al., 1981). Additional in vitro studies confirmed that modulation resulted in the loss of both antibody and antigen from the cell surface but was reversible once the antibody disappeared (Ritz et al., 1980).

Careful scheduling of the antibody doses is one method of circumventing the effects of modulation (Miller et al., 1981). Other attempts to control modulation have included the use of biological agents such as IFN-α to induce the expression of tumor-associated antigens on the cell surface, which leads to better binding (Schlom, 1995).

Interestingly, not all surface antigens modulate. For instance, CALLA and surface Ig have a high propensity to modulate, whereas histocompatibility antigens do not (Ritz and Schlossman, 1982). Modulation also occurs more often with hematopoietic cells than in solid tumor cells (Levy, 1985). Many of the targeted tumor antigens in the leukemias and lymphomas are capable of modulation (Maloney, 1998). In designing therapies with MABs, modulation can be used to advantage with immunotoxins, especially if the antigen is internalized (Maloney, 1998).

Antigen Blockade

High levels of circulating antigen can act as a blockade to prevent antibody from reaching the targeted tumor cells. Of course, this will depend on the normal secretion of the antigen as well as the type of antibody and its affinity (Dillman, 1984). When the circulating antigen is freely secreted, there is a blocking effect on the administered antibody that prevents the MAB from reaching the tumor cell and binding (Brown et al., 1989b). Because serum idiotype from the malignant B-cell clone can be used as a marker, it is easier to measure the amount of free antigen in the circulation. One approach to clearing excess antigen has been the infusion of large quantities of MAB. As already noted, however, this poses a risk of increased toxic effects. Alternatively, Meeker *et al.* (1985) employed the technique of plasmapheresis prior to and during therapy to clear free idiotype from the serum. In this trial, no tumor showed a significant response until excess serum idiotype was depleted and free antibody could persist. Unfortunately, clearing was only transient. Miller *et al.* (1981) reported an interesting phenomenon in which a patient with T-cell leukemia developed circulating antigen after the first dose of therapy. This suggested that the antigen was released as a result of antibody-induced tumor cell lysis. This has not been a problem in later trials.

Tumor Heterogeneity

Idiotype-negative variants, or tumor heterogeneity, has also been a difficult problem to overcome when studying and treating hematologic malignancies. In this process, tumor cells secrete mutant forms of surface Ig that eludes the effect of the antibody and allows continued tumor growth. Meeker *et al.* (1985) studied idiotype-negative variants in patients with B-cell lymphoma and found that the change seemed to be related to a somatic mutation in the variable region of the active Ig genes. This results in amino acid changes in the Ig molecule and subsequent alteration in the idiotype. Following treatment with anti-idiotype therapy, these variant cells become the prominent population. This is one possible explanation for some of the relapse or progression of disease that is observed (Maloney *et al.*, 1992b). Combined modality trials were undertaken to overcome this variance. Unfortunately, the addition of the synergistic agents did not prevent the emergence of idiotype-negative variance (Brown *et al.*, 1989a; Maloney *et al.*, 1992a). Another possible solution would be to treat with multiple

antibodies, each recognizing a different portion of the tumor population (Levy, 1985).

Cost

Finally, because of the extensive research and technology needed to develop MABs and MAB conjugates, cost is often identified as an obstacle to treatment. Because many of the antibody trials are still experimental, major funding has been provided by grants supported by the National Cancer Institute. At this time, patients receiving antibody therapy on these studies do not incur charges for the antibody. For those antibodies that have received FDA approval, cost for the patient may be a problem. Fortunately, the fact that the course of therapy is short and can be safely administered in an outpatient setting helps minimize the cost. Furthermore, the toxicity profile is low and patients usually do not require hospitalization to treat the side effects of therapy. For those patients with insurance, coverage of the therapy is usually not a problem. The pharmaceutical companies who manufacture these agents also provide toll-free numbers to patients who need assistance with reimbursement.

Other Uses of Monoclonal Antibodies

MABs have greatly enhanced the pathologist's ability to differentiate among the hematopoietic subsets of tumors. By utilizing antibodies to surface proteins, predominantly differentiation antigens, the pathologist is able to distinguish cell types and thus the origin of tumors. For example, lymphocytes look the same under the microscope, but when stained with antibodies that have affinity to the surface markers, it is easy to identify the subsets of T and B cells (Schlom, 1995).

As discussed previously, radiolabeled MABs

can be used to determine the amount and distribution of the tumor. This approach is more effective in solid tumors than in the hematopoietic malignancies because the target antigens are not found exclusively on the malignant cells.

Resistance of malignant tumors to chemotherapy drugs has been attributed to a multigene family designated *Mdr-1*. These genes encode the membrane proteins called P-glycoproteins 1 through 5 (Arceci *et al.*, 1993). The murine MAB 4E3, which is directed to the human *Mdr-1*-encoded P-glycoprotein, has been used to identify cells that produce this protein. The MAB is thus useful in studying the phenomenon of multidrug resistance in normal and malignant cells (Arceci *et al.*, 1993). Future applications of this antibody may include conjugation to biological toxins or cytotoxic drugs.

Regulatory Approval

As a form of biotherapy, MABs are subject to the same FDA approval process as other biological agents (Middleton, 1992). In the United States, the development of biological agents for therapeutic use is regulated in the FDA's Center for Biologics Evaluation and Research (CBER). Because of the nature of biological products, the control of the manufacturing involves multiple steps. The law regulating biological agents was actually enacted in July 1902 as the Virus-Toxin Law. The law specifies manufacturing, inspection, licensing, and labeling requirements. The National Institutes of Health maintained regulatory control of biological agents until 1972, when control was transferred to the FDA. On January 4, 1983, the Orphan Drug Act was signed into law and is designed to provide financial incentives for companies to develop new products that might be used in the treatment, diagnosis, or prevention of rare diseases. It was also designed to reduce regulatory barriers (Wandres and Lau,

1992). Most of the MABs currently in testing fall under the category of orphan drugs.

Procedures for MAB development are outlined in documents prepared by the CBER (1993, 1994) and include requirements that the cell banks be free of infectious agents. In addition, MABs used for purging of tumor cells *ex vivo* must meet the same standards for purity, potency, safety, and freedom from adventitious viruses (Siegel *et al.*, 1995).

The first approval of a MAB for treatment of cancer was granted for rituximab in November 1997. This antibody is jointly manufactured by IDEC Pharmaceuticals Corporation and Genentech, Inc. This approval process took approximately 7 years from the start of clinical trials until the pivotal trial was completed in 1997 (Maloney *et al.*, 1997a; 1997b). Rituximab is approved for the treatment of patients with relapsed or refractory, low-grade or follicular CD20-positive B-cell non-Hodgkin's lymphoma. Clinical trials evaluating rituximab in intermediate and high-grade lymphomas are ongoing as well as evaluations of the antibody with other therapy modalities. In May 2000, gemtuzumab ozogamicin (American Home Products, Madison, NJ) was approved to treat patients at least 60 years of age who are in first relapse with CD33-positive AML and who are not candidates for cytotoxic chemotherapy.

Future Directions

MABs have assumed an increasing role in the treatment of the hematologic malignancies. The growth of studies utilizing both conjugated and unconjugated MABs has been exponential. It is likely that this work will continue as researchers attempt to overcome many of the obstacles mentioned earlier. For example, further development and refinement of chimeric or humanized antibodies that have higher affinity for tumor cells and a reduced risk of causing an immune response represent two possibilities. Human antibodies could be developed using severe combined immunodeficient mice that have been reconstituted with human lymphocytes. These mice could then serve as the factories for the development of human antitumor antibodies. Recombinant DNA technology could be used to produce modified toxins that retain tumoricidal potential but have reduced nonspecific binding. Improvements in the cytotoxicity of the immunotoxins are underway as well. Laboratory studies that focus on new, more potent toxins with decreased side effects and immunogenicity are continuing (Gadina *et al.*, 1994). Antibody-drug conjugates, more stable than those now available, would allow drug release at the tumor site and spare the surrounding healthy tissue. A second type of antibody-drug conjugate could allow the antibody to carry multiple non-cross-reacting drugs (LoBuglio and Saleh, 1992; Russell *et al.*, 1992).

It is likely that studies evaluating the use of MABs as adjuvant treatment will continue as timing and dose schedules are refined. Much like adjuvant chemotherapy, MABs will be administered at a time when patients are in a complete remission following initial chemotherapy. The goal would be to "mop up" residual cancer cells.

It is clear that the hybridoma technology developed by Köhler and Milstein has a wide range of applications for the entire medical field. MABs have been derived that can react with proteins, carbohydrates, nucleic acids, or haptenated forms of these molecules (Kummer and Staerz, 1993). MABs have been used in cancer treatment and detection for almost 2 decades, but the potential of these agents has only begun to be understood. Ongoing studies are needed to evaluate combinations of antibodies as well as the multitude of immunoconjugates still in development. Many predict that immunotoxins and MAB-based drugs will eventually take their place alongside chemotherapy and radiation therapy as one of the primary modalities in the treatment of cancer.

References

Abbas, A., Lichtman, M., and Prober, J. 1991. Antibodies and antigens. In Abbas, A., Lichtman, M., and Prober, J. (eds). *Cellular and Molecular Immunology*, Philadelphia, PA: W.B. Saunders, p. 51.

Arceci, R., Stieglitz, K., Bras, J., *et al.* 1993. Monoclonal antibody to an external epitope of the human *mdr1* P-glycoprotein. *Cancer Research* 53: 310–317.

Ball, E., Mills, L., and Cornwell, C. 1990. Autologous bone marrow transplantation for acute myeloid leukemia using monoclonal antibody-purged bone marrow. *Blood* 75: 1199–1206.

Beauger, N., and Roy, D. 1998. Hematopoietic progenitor-cell graft processing and treatment. In Grossbard, M. (ed). *Monoclonal Antibody-based Therapy of Cancer*. New York, NY: Marcel Dekker, pp. 229–280.

Benjamini, E., and Leskowitz, S. 1988. *Immunology: A Short Course*. New York, NY: Alan R. Liss, Inc.

Blakey, D., and Thorpe, P. 1988. An overview of therapy with immunotoxins containing ricin or its A chain. *Antibody Immunoconjugate Radiopharmacology* 1: 1–16.

Brown S., Miller R., Horning, S., *et al.* 1989a. Treatment of B-cell lymphoma alone and in combination with alpha interferon. *Blood* 73(3): 651–661.

Brown, S., Miller, R., and Levy, R. 1989b. Antiidiotype antibody therapy of B-cell lymphoma. *Seminars in Oncology* 16(3): 199–210.

Center for Biologics Evaluation and Research. 1993. *Points To Consider in the Characterization of Cell Lines Used to Produce Biologicals*. Bethesda, MD, 7/12/93.

Center for Biologics Evaluation and Research, 1994. *Points To Consider in the Manufacture of Monoclonal Antibody Products For Human Use.* Bethesda, MD, 6/01/87; updated 1994.

Clendenin, N., Nethersell, A., Senti, J., *et al.* 1992. Phase I/II trials of CAMPATH-1H, a humanized anti-lymphocyte monoclonal antibody (MnAb) in non-Hodgkin's lymphoma (NHL) and chronic lymphocytic leukemia (CLL). *Blood* 80 (suppl 1): 158A.

Cooper, E., and Flaum, M. 1988. The use of monoclonal antibodies in blood testing and typing. *Modern Medicine* 56(5): 46–52.

Czuzman, M., Grillo-Lopez, A., and Saleh, M. 1996. IDEC-C2B8/CHOP chemoimmunotherapy in patients with low-grade lymphoma: Interim clinical and bcl-2 (PCR) results. *Annals of Oncology* 7(suppl 1): 56.

Davis, T., and Knox, S. 1998. Radioimmunoconjugate therapy of NHL. In Grossbard, M. (ed). *Monoclonal Antibody-based Therapy of Cancer.* New York, NY: Marcel Dekker, pp. 113–136.

Davis, T., Maloney, D., Czerwinski, D., *et al.* 1998. Anti-idiotype antibodies can induce long-term complete remissions in non-Hodgkin's lymphoma without eradicating the malignant clone. *Blood* 92(4): 1184–1190.

DeNardo, G., DeNardo, S., Goldstein, D., *et al.* 1998. Maximum-tolerated dose, toxicity, and efficacy of (131)I-Lym-1 antibody for fractionated radioimmunotherapy of non-Hodgkin's lymphoma. *Journal of Clinical Oncology* (10): 3246–3256.

DeNardo, S., DeNardo, G., O'Grady, *et al.* 1987. Treatment of a patient with B-cell lymphoma using I-131 Lym-1 monoclonal antibodies. *International Journal of Biological Markers* 2(1): 49–53.

DeNardo, S., Kroger, L., and DeNardo, G. 1999. A new era for radiolabeled antibodies in cancer. *Current Opinion in Immunology* 11(5): 563–569.

De Vita, V., and Canellos, G. 1999. The lymphomas. *Seminars in Hematology* 36 (4 suppl 7): 84–94.

DiJulio, J. 1988. Treatment of B-cell lymphomas with monoclonal antibodies. *Seminars in Oncology Nursing* 4: 102–106.

Dillman, R., 1984. Monoclonal antibody in the treatment of cancer. *Critical Review in Oncology/Hematology* 1(4): 357–385.

Dillman, R., Shawler, D., Dillman, J., *et al.* 1984. Therapy of chronic lymphocytic leukemia and cutaneous T-cell lymphoma with T 101 monoclonal antibody. *Journal of Clinical Oncology* 2: 881–891.

Dillman, R., Shawler, D., Dillman, J., *et al.* 1985. Monoclonal antibodies in patients with CLL and CTCL. *Journal of Cellular Biochemistry* 9A: 48 (abstract).

Dillman, R., Shawler, D., Sobol, R., *et al.* 1982. Murine monoclonal antibody therapy in two patients with chronic lymphocytic leukemia. *Blood* 59: 1036–1045.

Dorfman, N. 1985. The optimal technological approach to the development of human hybridomas. *Journal of Biologic Response Modifiers* 4: 213–239.

Dyer, M., Hale, G., Hayhoe, F., *et al.* 1989. Effects of CAMPATH-1 antibodies *in vivo* in patients with lymphoid malignancies: Influence of antibody isotype. *Blood* 73: 1431–1439.

Eary, J., Press, O., Badger, C., *et al.* 1990. Imaging and treatment of B-cell lymphoma. *Journal of Nuclear Medicine* 31: 1257–1268.

Foon, K., Schroff, R., and Gale, R. 1982. Surface markers on leukemia and lymphoma cells: Recent advances. *Blood* 60: 1–19.

Foon, K., Schroff, R., Mayer, D. *et al.* 1983. Monoclonal antibody therapy of chronic lymphocytic leukemia and cutaneous T-cell lymphoma: Preliminary observations. In Boss, B., Langman, R., Trowbridge, I., and Dulbecco, R. (eds). *Monoclonal Antibodies and Cancer.* Orlando, FL: Academic Press, pp. 32–39.

Freedman, A., Takvorian, T., Anderson, K., *et al.* 1990. Autologous bone marrow transplantation in B-cell non-Hodgkin's lymphoma: Very low treatment related mortality in 100 patients in sensitive relapse. *Journal of Clinical Oncology* 7: 1821–1829.

Gadina, M., Newton, D., Rybak, S., *et al.* 1994. Humanized immunotoxins. *Therapeutic Immunology* 1: 59–64.

Goldenberg, D., Horowitz, J., Sharkey, R., *et al.* 1991. Targeting dosimetry and radioimmunotherapy of B-cell lymphomas with iodine-131-labeled LL2 monoclonal antibody. *Journal of Clinical Oncology* 4: 548–564.

Gorin, N., Lopez, M., Laporte, J., *et al.* 1995. Preparation and successful engraftment of purified CD34$^+$ bone marrow progenitor cells in patients with non-Hodgkin's lymphoma. *Blood* 85: 1647–1654.

Gould, B., Borowitz, M., Groves, E., *et al.* 1989. Phase I study of an anti-breast cancer immunotoxin by continuous infusion: Report of a targeted toxic effect not predicted by animal studies. *Journal of Clinical Investigation* 81(10): 775–781.

Gribben, J., and Nadler, L. 1995. Purging of bone marrow. In DeVita, V., Hellman, S., and Rosenberg, S. (eds). *Biologic Therapy of Cancer: Principles and Practice*, 2nd edn. Philadelphia, PA: J. B. Lippincott, pp. 596–606.

Gribben, J., Freedman, A., Neuberg, D., *et al.* 1991. Immunologic purging of marrow assessed by PCR before autologous bone marrow transplant. *The New England Journal of Medicine* 22: 1525–1533.

Grossbard, M., Freedman, A., Ritz, J., *et al.* 1992a. Serotherapy of B-cell neoplasms with anti-B4 blocked ricin: A phase I trial of daily bolus infusion. *Blood* 79: 576–585.

Grossbard, M., Lambert, J., Goldmacher, V., *et al.* 1992b. Correlation between *in vivo* toxicity and preclinical *in vitro* parameters for the immunotoxin anti-B4-blocked ricin. *Cancer Research* 51: 5461.

Grossbard, M., Press, O., Appelbaum, F., *et al.* 1992c. Monoclonal antibody-based therapy of leukemia and lymphoma. *Blood* 80: 863–878.

Hertler, A., Schlossman, D., Borowitz, M., *et al.* 1988. A phase I study of T101-ricin A chain immunotoxin in refractory chronic lymphocytic leukemia. *Journal of Biologic Response Modifiers* 7: 97–113.

Hinman, L., Hamman, P., Beyer, C., *et al.* 1994. Calicheamicin conjugates of the anti-CD33 antibody, p67, shows potent selective antitumor effects in models of acute myeloid leukemia and against human leukemic bone marrow cells. *Proceedings of the American Society of Cancer Research* 35: 507.

Hinman, L., Hamman, P., Wallace, R., *et al.* 1993. Preparation and characterization of monoclonal antibody conjugates of the calicheamicins: A novel and potent family of antitumor antibiotics. *Cancer Research* 52: 3336–3342.

Horning, S. 1994. Treatment approaches to the low-grade lymphomas. *Blood* 83: 881–884.

Houston, L., and Nowinski, R. 1981. Cell-specific cytotoxicity expressed by a conjugate of ricin and murine monoclonal antibody directed against the 1.1 antigen. *Cancer Research* 41: 3913–3917.

Hozumi, N., and Sandhu, J. 1993. Recombinant antibody technology: Its advent and advances. *Cancer Investigation* 11(6): 714–723.

Jurcic, J., Caron, P., Miller, W., *et al.* 1995. Sequential targeted therapy for relapsed acute promyelocytic leukemia with all-transretinoic acid and anti-CD33 monoclonal antibody M195. *Leukemia* 9: 244–248.

Jurcic, J., Scheinberg, D., and Houghton, A. 1996. In Pindo, H., Longo, D., and Chabner, B. (eds). *Cancer Chemotherapy and Biological Response Modifiers Annual* 16. New York, NY: Elsevier Science B.V., pp. 168–188.

Kaminski, M., Estes, M., Regan, M., *et al.* 1997. Frontline treatment of advanced B cell low-grade lymphoma with radiolabeled anti-B1 antibody: Initial experience. *Proceedings of the American Society of Clinical Oncology*, 15: (abstract 51).

Kaminski, M., Gribben, T., and Estes, J. 1998. I-131 anti-B1 antibody for previously untreated follicular lymphoma (FL): Clinical and molecular remissions. *Proceedings of the American Society of Clinical Oncology*, 16: (abstract 6).

Kaminski, M., Zasadny, K., Francis, I., *et al.* 1993. Radioimmunotherapy of B-cell lymphoma with [131] anti-B1 (Anti-CD20) antibody. *The New England Journal of Medicine* 329(7): 459–465.

Kaminski, M., Zasadny, K., Francis, I., *et al.* 1996. Iodine-131 anti-B1 radioimmunotherapy for B-cell lymphoma. *Journal of Clinical Oncology* 14: 1974–1981.

Khazaeli, M., Saleh, M., Liu, T., *et al.* 1991. Pharmacokinetic immune response of 131I-chimeric mouse/human B 72.3 (human gamma 4) monoclonal antibody in humans. *Cancer Research* 51(20): 5461–5466.

Knox, S., Goris, M., Trisler, K., *et al.* 1996a. Yttrium 90-labeled anti-CD20 MAB therapy of recurrent B-cell lymphoma. *Clinical Cancer Research* 2(3): 457–470.

Knox, S., Hoppe, R., Maloney, D., *et al.* 1996b. Treatment of cutaneous T-cell lymphoma with chimeric anti-CD4 monoclonal antibody. *Blood* 87(3): 893–899.

Köhler G., and Milstein, C. 1975. Continuous cultures of fused cells secreting antibody of predefined specificity. *Nature* 256: 495–496.

Kostis, C., and Callaghan, M. 2000. Rituximab: A new monoclonal antibody therapy for non-Hodgkin's lymphoma. *Oncology Nursing Forum* 27(1): 51–59.

Kreitman, R., and Pastan, I. 1995. Targeting pseudomonas exotoxin to hematologic malignancies. *Seminars in Cancer Biology* 6: 297–306.

Kummer, U., and Staerz, U. 1993. Concepts of antibody-mediated cancer therapy. *Cancer Investigation* 11: 174–184.

Larson, S., Sgouras, G., and Cheung, N. 1995. Radioisotope conjugates. In DeVita, V., Hellman, S., and Rosenberg, S. (eds). *Biologic Therapy of Cancer*. Philadelphia, PA: J.B. Lippincott, pp. 534–552.

Laurent, G., Pris, J., and Farcet, J. 1986. Effects of therapy with T101 ricin A-chain immunotoxin in two leukemia patients. *Blood* 67: 1680–1687.

Levy, R. 1985. Biologicals for cancer treatment: Monoclonal antibodies. *Hospital Practice* 20(11): 67–74, 77, 80–84.

Levy, R., and Miller, R. 1991. Antibodies in cancer therapy. Section 22.1. B-cell lymphomas. In De Vita, V., Hellman, S., and Rosenberg, S. (eds). *Biological Therapy of Cancer*. Philadelphia, PA: J.B. Lippincott, pp. 512–522.

LoBuglio, A., and Saleh, M. 1992. Monoclonal antibody therapy of cancer. *Critical Reviews in Oncology/Hematology* 13: 271–282.

LoBuglio, A., Saleh, M., Lee, J., *et al.* 1988. Phase I trial of multiple large doses of murine monoclonal antibody CO17-1A. Clinical aspects. *Journal of the National Cancer Institute* 80: 932–936.

Lotze, M., and Rosenberg, S. 1988. The immunologic treatment of cancer. *CA-A Cancer Journal for Clinicians* 3(2): 68–95.

Lowder, J., Meeker, T., and Levy, R. 1985. Monoclonal antibody therapy of lymphoid malignancy. *Cancer Surveys* 4(2): 360–375.

Lundin, J., Osterborg, A., Brittinger, G., *et al.* 1998. CAMPATH-1H monoclonal antibody in therapy for previously treated low-grade non-Hodgkin's lymphomas: A phase II multicenter study. *Journal of Clinical Oncology* 16(10): 3247–3263.

Luo, Y., and Seon, B. 1990. Marked difference in the in vivo antitumor efficacy between two immunotoxins targeted to different epitopes of common acute lymphoblastic leukemia antigen (CD10). Mechanisms involved in the differential activities of immunotoxins. *Journal of Immunology* 145: 1974–1982.

Maloney, D. 1998. Unconjugated monoclonal antibody therapy of lymphoma. In Grossbard, L. (ed). *Monoclonal Antibody-based Therapy of Cancer*. New York, NY: Marcel Dekker, pp. 53–79.

Maloney, D., Brown, S., Czerwinski, D., *et al.* 1992a. Monoclonal anti-idiotype antibody therapy of B-cell lymphoma: The addition of a short course of chemotherapy does not interfere with the antitumor effect nor prevent the emergence of idiotype negative variant cells. *Blood* 80(6): 1502–1510.

Maloney, D., Grillo-Lopez, A., White, C., *et al.*

1997a. IDEC-C2B8: Results of a phase I multiple-dose trial in patients with relapsed non-Hodgkin's lymphoma. *Journal of Clinical Oncology* 15(10): 3266–3274.

Maloney, D., Grillo-Lopez, A., White, C., *et al.* 1997b. IDEC-C2B8 (Rituximab) anti-CD20 monoclonal antibody therapy in patients with relapsed low-grade non-Hodgkin's lymphoma. *Blood* 90(6): 2188–2195.

Maloney, D., Levy, R., and Miller, R. 1992b. Monoclonal anti-idiotype therapy of B-cell lymphoma. In DeVita, V., Hellman, S., and Rosenberg, S. (eds). *Biological Therapy of Cancer Updates* 2(6). Philadelphia, PA: J.B. Lippincott, pp. 1–10.

Maloney, D., Liles, T., Czerwinski, C., *et al.* 1994. Phase I clinical trial using escalating single-dose infusion of chimeric anti-CD20 monoclonal antibody (IDEC-C28) in patients with recurrent B-cell lymphoma. *Blood* 84(8): 2457–2466.

Maloney, D., Smith, B., and Appelbaum, F. 1996. The anti-tumor effect of monoclonal anti-CD20 antibody (mAb) therapy includes direct anti-proliferative activity and induction of apoptosis in CD20 positive non-Hodgkin's lymphoma (NHL) cell lines. *Blood* 88(10 suppl 1): 63 (abstract).

McLaughlin, P., Grillo-Lopez, A., Link, B., *et al.* 1998. Rituximab chimeric anti-CD20 monoclonal antibody therapy for relapsed indolent lymphoma: Half of patients respond to a 4-dose treatment program. *Journal of Clinical Oncology* 8: 2825–2833.

Meeker, T., Lowder, R., Maloney, D., *et al.* 1985. A clinical trial of anti-idiotype therapy for B cell malignancy. *Blood* 65: 1349–1353.

Mendelsohn, J., and Baselga, J. 1995. Antibodies to growth factors and receptors. In DeVita, V., Hellman, S., and Rosenberg, S. (eds). *Biologic Therapy of Cancer*, 2nd edn. Philadelphia, PA: J.B. Lippincott, pp. 607–623.

Middleton, R. 1992. The drug approval process: An introduction. *California Journal of Hospital Pharmacy* 4: 5–11.

Miller, R., Hart, S., Samoszuk, M., *et al.* 1989. Shared idiotypes expressed by the human B-cell lymphomas. *The New England Journal of Medicine* 321: 851–857.

Miller, R., Maloney, D., McKillop, J., *et al.* 1981. In vivo effects of murine hybridoma monoclonal antibody in patients with T-cell leukemia. *Blood* 58(1): 78–86.

Miller, R., Maloney, D., Warnke, R., *et al.* 1982. Treatment of B-cell lymphoma with monoclonal anti-idiotype antibody. *The New England Journal of Medicine* 306: 517–522.

Miller, R., Oseroff, A., Stratte, P., *et al.* 1983. Monoclonal antibody therapeutic trials in seven patients with T-cell lymphoma. *Blood* 62: 988–995.

Morein, H., and Junghans, R. 1998. Antibody-based therapies for Hodgkin's disease. In Grossbard, L. (ed). *Monoclonal Antibody-Based Therapy of Cancer*. New York, NY: Marcel Dekker, pp. 149–188.

Multani, P., and Flavell, D. 1998. Antibody-based therapies for the treatment of acute leukemia. In Grossbard, M. (ed). *Monoclonal Antibody-Based Therapy of Cancer*. New York, NY: Marcel Dekker, pp. 189–209.

Myers, D., and Uckun, F. 1995. An anti-CD72 immunotoxin against therapy-refractory B-lineage acute lymphoblastic leukemia. *Leukemia Lymphoma* 18: 119–122.

Nadler, L., Stashenko, P., Hardy, R. *et al.* 1980. Serotherapy of a patient with a monoclonal antibody directed against a human lymphoma-associated antigen. *Cancer Research* 40: 3147–3154.

Negrin, R., Kiem, H., Schmidt-Wolf, H., *et al.* 1991. Use of polymerase chain reaction to monitor the effectiveness of *ex vivo* tumor cell purging. *Blood* 77(3): 654–660.

Oldham, R. 1983. Monoclonal antibody in cancer therapy. *Journal of Clinical Oncology* 1(9): 582–590.

Overmyer, R. 1990. Genetically engineered antibodies improve the therapeutic efficacy of drugs. *Modern Medicine* 58: 38–45.

Pai, L., and Pastan, I. 1995. Immunotoxins and recombinant toxins. In DeVita, V., Hellman, S., and Rosenberg, S. (eds). *Biologic Therapy of Cancer*,

2nd edn. Philadelphia, PA: J.B. Lippincott, pp. 521–531.

Pimm, M., Jones, J., Price, M., *et al.* 1982. Tumor localization of monoclonal antibody against a rat mammary carcinoma and suppression of tumor growth with adriamycin-antibody conjugates. *Cancer Immunology Immunotherapy* 12: 125–134.

Press, O., Appelbaum, F., Ledbetter, J., *et al.* 1987. Monoclonal antibody 1F5 (anti-CD20) serotherapy of human B cell lymphomas. *Blood* 6(9): 584–591.

Press, O., Eary, J., Appelbaum, F., *et al.* 1995. Phase II trial of 131I-B1 (anti-CD20) antibody therapy with autologous stem cell transplantation for relapsed B cell lymphomas. *The Lancet* 346: 336–340.

Press, O., Eary, J., Badger, C., *et al.* 1989. Treatment of refractory non-Hodgkin's lymphoma with radiolabeled MB-1 (anti-CD37) antibody. *Journal of Clinical Oncology* 7: 1027–1038.

Redwood, W., Tom, T., and Strand, M. 1984. Specificity, efficacy, and toxicity of radioimmunotherapy in erythroleukemic mice. *Cancer Research* 44: 5681–5687.

Ritz, J., and Schlossman, S. 1982. Utilization of monoclonal antibodies in the treatment of leukemia and lymphoma. *Blood* 59(1): 1–11.

Ritz, J., Pesando, J., Notis-McConarty, J., *et al.* 1980. Modulation of human acute lymphoblastic leukemia antigen induced by monoclonal antibody in vitro. *Journal of Immunology* 125(4): 1506–1514.

Rosen, S., Zimmer, A., Goldman-Leiken, R., *et al.* 1987. Radioimmunodetection and radioimmunotherapy of cutaneous T-cell lymphomas using an 131 I-labeled monoclonal antibody: An Illinois Cancer Council Study. *Journal of Clinical Oncology* 5: 562–573.

Rosenberg, S., and Terry W. 1977. Passive immunotherapy of cancer in animals and man. *Advances in Cancer Research* 25: 323–388.

Russell, S., Llewelyn, M., and Hawkins, R. 1992. Principles of antibody therapy. *British Medical Journal* 305: 1424–1429.

Rybak, S., Hoogenboom, H., Meade, H., *et al.* 1992. Humanization of immunotoxins. *Proceedings of the National Academy of Sciences USA* 89: 3165–3169.

Scheinberg, D. 1991. Current application of monoclonal antibodies for the therapy of hematopoietic cancers. *Current Opinion in Immunology* 3: 679–684.

Scheinberg, D., Lovett, D., Divgi, C., *et al.* 1991. A phase I trial of monoclonal antibody M195 in acute myelogenous leukemia: Specific bone marrow targeting and internalization of radionuclide. *Journal of Clinical Oncology* 9: 478–490.

Schlom, J. 1995. Monoclonal antibodies in cancer therapy: Basic principles. In DeVita, V., Hellman, S., and Rosenberg, S. (eds). *Biologic Therapy of Cancer*. Philadelphia, PA: J.B. Lippincott, pp. 507–521.

Schroff, R., Foon, K., Beatty, S., *et al.* 1985. Human anti-murine immunoglobulin responses in patients receiving monoclonal antibody therapy. *Cancer Research Update* 45: 879–885.

Schwartz, M., Lovett, D., Redner, A., *et al.* 1993. Dose-escalation trial of M195 labeled with iodine 131 for cytoreduction and marrow ablation in relapsed or refractory myeloid leukemias. *Journal of Clinical Oncology* 11: 294–303.

Siegel, J., Gerrard, T., Cavagnaro, J., *et al.* 1995. Development of biological therapeutics for oncologic use. In DeVita, V., Hellman, S., and Rosenberg, S. (eds). *Biologic Therapy of Cancer* 2nd edn. Philadelphia, PA: J.B. Lippincott, pp. 566–575.

Sievers, E. 2000. Clinical studies of new "biologic" approaches to therapy of acute myeloid leukemia with monoclonal antibodies and immunoconjugates. *Current Opinion in Oncology* 12(1): 30–35.

Sievers, E., Appelbaum, R., Spielberger, S., *et al.* 1999. Selective ablation of acute myeloid leukemia using antibody-targeted chemotherapy: A phase I study of an anti-CD33 calicheamicin immunoconjugate. *Blood* 93(11): 3678–3684.

Smith-Gill, S. 1995. Biology of antibody-mediated responses. In DeVita, V., Hellman, S., and Rosenberg, S. (eds). *Biologic Therapy of Cancer* 2nd edn. Philadelphia, PA: J.B. Lippincott, pp. 39–51.

Thorpe, P., and Ross, W. 1982. The preparation and cytotoxic properties of antibody-toxin conjugates. *Immunology Review* 62: 119–158.

Tjandra, J., Ramidi, L., and McKenzie, I. 1990. Development of human anti-murine antibody (HAMA) response in patients. *Immunology Cell Biology* 68: 367–376.

Uckun, F. 1993. Immunotoxins for the treatment of leukaemia. *British Journal of Haematology* 85: 435–438.

Vitetta, E., Frolick, K., and Uhr, J. 1982. Neoplastic B- cells as targets for antibody-ricin A chain immunotoxins. *Immunology Review* 62: 9–183.

Vitteta, E., Ghetie, M., and Ghetie, V. 1998. Immunotoxin therapy: Past lessons and future directions. In Grossbard, M. (ed). *Monoclonal Antibody-Based Therapy of Cancer*. New York, NY: Marcel Dekker, pp. 417–432.

Vitetta, E., Stone, M., Amlot, P., *et al.* 1991. Phase I immunotoxin trial in patients with B-cell lymphoma. *Cancer Research* 51: 4052–4058.

Vriesendorp, H., Herpst, J., Germack, M., *et al.* 1991. Phase I/II studies of yttrium-labeled antiferritin treatment for end-stage Hodgkin's disease, including Radiation Therapy Oncology Group 87-01. *Journal of Clinical Oncology* 9: 918–928.

Vose, J.M., Wahl, R.L., Saleh, M., *et al.* 2000. Multicenter phase II study of iodine-131 tositumomab for chemotherapy-relapsed/refractory low-grade and transformed low-grade B-cell non-Hodgkin's lymphomas. *Journal of Clinical Oncology* 18(6): 1316–1323.

Waldmann, T. 1995. Antibodies in cancer therapy. Section 21.2. T-cell leukemia/lymphoma. In DeVita, V., Hellman, S., and Rosenberg, S. (eds). *Biologic Therapy of Cancer* 2nd edn. Philadelphia, PA: J. B. Lippincott, pp. 566–575.

Waldmann, T., Goldman, C., Bongiovanni, K., *et al.* 1988. Therapy of patients with human T-cell lymphotrophic virus I-induced adult T-cell leukemia with anti-Tac, a monoclonal antibody to the receptor for interleukin-1. *Blood* 72: 1805–1816.

Waldmann, T., Pastan, I., Gansow, O., et al. 1992. The multichain interleukin-2 receptor: A target for immunotherapy. *Annals of Internal Medicine* 116: 148–160.

Wandres, D., and Lau, J. 1992. An overview of orphan drugs. *California Journal of Hospital Pharmacy* 4: 12–13.

Weiner, L., O'Dwyer, J., Kitson, J., *et al.* 1989. Phase I evaluation of an anti-breast carcinoma monoclonal antibody 260F-6 recombinant ricin A chain immunoconjugate. *Cancer Research* 49: 4062–4067.

Witzig, T.E., White, C.A., Wiseman, G.A., *et al.* 1999. Phase I/II trial of IDEC-Y2B8 radioimmunotherapy for treatment of relapsed or refractory CD20(+) B-cell non-Hodgkin's lymphoma. *Journal of Clinical Oncology* 17(12):3793–3803.

Wyeth-Ayerst. 2000. Package Insert for Mylotarg™, Philadelphia, PA: Wyeth-Ayerst.

Clinical Pearls

1. It is important to determine the origin of the MAB being administered (i.e., murine [derived solely from mouse immunoglobulin] or chimeric [part human, part mouse]). Newer-generation chimeric antibodies will have less tendency to cause allergic reaction due to the decreased portion of the antibody that is of murine origin.

2. Emergency drugs should be kept at the bedside (e.g., epinephrine, corticosteroids, and diphenhydramine) for the treatment of potential allergic reactions. Although extremely rare, the potential for an anaphylactic reaction to occur is ever present.

3. If an anaphylactic reaction occurs, the infusion should be stopped immediately, fluids started, the physician paged, and emergency drugs administered as ordered.

4. Patients should be monitored closely at the onset of infusion for the potential of an allergic reaction or infusion-related symptom complex.

5. The occurrence of an infusion-related symptom complex is believed to be related to the interaction of the MAB with circulating white blood cells and the subsequent release of cytokines. It is more commonly seen with MABs targeted toward white blood cells. Concomitant administration of diphenhydramine or acetaminophen is useful in the management of these symptoms. Some clinicians may withhold antihypertensive medication for 12 hours prior to infusion with MABs known to cause infusion-related events (e.g., rituximab).

6. Resolution of infusion-related events usually occurs by slowing or interrupting the infusion and providing supportive care (e.g., intravenous saline, bronchodilators, diphenhydramine, or acetaminophen) as required.

7. In general, in the oncology setting, the MAB is administered as a controlled infusion not as a bolus infusion. The use of an infusion pump is recommended.

8. An infusion worksheet may be helpful in the clinical setting to infuse MABs that are administered by incrementally increasing the infusion rate. Depending on the concentration of the MAB supplied by the pharmacy (mg/mL), the infusion rate used to provide a set amount of mg/hour will vary. It is helpful to work with pharmacy personnel to ensure that the MAB is given in a concentration that facilitates this process (i.e., makes calculations less difficult).

9. Antibodies conjugated to other substances such as chemotherapy or radioisotopes will require additional precautions and handling procedures appropriate for the conjugate. For example, an MAB conjugated to ^{131}I requires appropriate precautions and handling for the radioactive isotope [131]I.

10. MABs given as anti-idiotypic vaccines may produce local reactions and a flu-like syndrome, especially when given in conjunction with adjuvants.

11. It is important to determine whether the antibody is being given for a diagnostic/detection purpose (e.g., OncoScint®) or for a therapeutic reason (e.g., rituximab). This will assist in educating the patient concerning the goals of therapy.

Key Resources

References

Bast, R.C., Zalutsky, M.R., Kreitman, R.J., *et al.* 2000. Monoclonal serotherapy. In Bast, R.C., Kufe, D.W., Pollock, R.E., Weischelbaum, R.R., Holland, J.F., and Frei, E. (eds). *Cancer Medicine* 5th edn. Hamilton, Ontario: B.C. Decker, Inc., pp. 860–875.

Bodey, B., Bodey B. Jr., and Siegel, S. 2000. Genetically engineered monoclonal antibodies for direct anti-neoplastic treatment and cancer cell specific delivery of chemotherapeutic agents. *Current Pharmaceutical Design* 6(3): 261–276.

Coiffier, B., Haioun, C., Ketterer, N., *et al.* 1998. Rituximab (anti-CD20 monoclonal antibody) for the treatment of patients with relapsing or refractory aggressive lymphoma: A multicenter phase II study. *Blood* 92(6): 1927–1932.

DeVita Jr., V., and Canellos, G. 1999. The lymphomas. *Seminars in Hematology* 36 (4 suppl 7): 84–94.

Karius, D., and Marriott, M. 1997. Immunologic advances in monoclonal antibody therapy: Implications for oncology nursing. *Oncology Nursing Forum* 24: 483–494.

Kosits, C., and Callaghan, M. 2000. Rituximab: A new monoclonal antibody therapy for non-Hodgkin's lymphoma. *Oncology Nursing Forum* 27(1): 51–59.

Press, O. 1999. Radiolabeled antibody therapy of B-cell lymphomas. *Seminars in Oncology* 26 (5 suppl 14): 58–65.

Rosen, S. (guest ed). 1999. Recent advances and future directions using monoclonal antibodies for B-cell malignancies. *Seminars in Oncology* 26 (5 suppl 14): 1–120.

Trail, P., and Bianchi, A. 1999. Monoclonal antibody drug conjugates in the treatment of cancer. *Current Opinions in Immunology* 11(5): 584–588.

Weiner, M. 1999. Monoclonal antibody therapy of cancer. *Seminars in Oncology* 26 (5 suppl 14): 43–51.

Monograph and Videotape

"Exploring the Promise of Monoclonal Antibody Therapy in Non-Hodgkin's Lymphoma"—Monograph and videotapes contain excerpts from a presentation given May 8, 1998 at the 23rd Annual Congress of the Oncology Nursing Society in San Francisco, CA. This continuing education activity is accredited for 1.2 contact hours by the Oncology Nursing Society. Copies may be obtained by calling GenQuest Biomedical Education Services, Inc. or faxing a request to 858-623-3557.

Videotape

Stepping Stones—"Person to Person"—Patients talk about their treatment with rituximab.

Slide Set

Monoclonal Antibody Nursing Slide Program—Slide kit with lecture notes for oncology nurses. GenQuest Biomedical Education Services, Inc. Phone: 858-597-6756

Web Sites

http://www.rituxan.com/
BioOncology OnLine Oncology Resource Center. Here you will find a growing source of information focusing on the many aspects of biologic oncology.

- Monoclonal antibody therapy information for professionals
  Color teaching slides
  Clinical reviews
- Calendar of upcoming events, i.e., oncology/immunology meetings.
- Resources for professionals to use in patient counseling:
  Contact information for cancer centers and associations, information pages about monoclonal antibodies, basic cancer treatments, and other topics and an oncology glossary.
- Hot links
- Bibliography

CHAPTER 9 | Monoclonal Antibodies: Applications in Solid Tumors and Other Diseases

Paula Trahan Rieger, RN, MSN, CS, AOCN®, FAAN

Marjorie Green, MD

James Lee Murray III, MD

The limitations of traditional cancer therapy (e.g., surgery, chemotherapy, and radiation therapy) have driven researchers to develop new strategies to help decrease treatment toxicity and improve overall survival rates for cancer patients. In particular, the quest to develop therapies that will selectively target cancer cells and spare normal cells is of prime importance. Therefore, the use of monoclonal antibody (MAB) therapy for solid tumors has many attractions.

The theory behind biological treatment of malignancy has been around for almost 100 years. With observations in the 1950s of tumor regression after administration of pooled sera, scientists were encouraged to explore methods of harnessing the power of the immune system to fight cancer (Wright *et al.*, 1976). The goal was development of a specific antibody directed against a unique target that would negatively affect tumor cells while sparing normal tissue. However, the use of pooled sera did not provide a consistent source of antibody to be used in clinical trials. Mass production of specific murine antibodies became possible in the 1970s with the development of hybridoma technology (Köhler and Milstein, 1975; also see Chapter 8). The first clinical trial of MAB therapy in solid tumors was published in the early 1980s (Sears *et al.*, 1982). Unfortunately, this trial did not establish MAB therapy as the "magic bullet" for cancer, as some had previously hoped. In addition to having minimal clinical efficacy, there were toxicities associated with these treatments.

Since then, many trials have been conducted to evaluate the efficacy of MABs in the treatment of solid tumors, in the diagnosis and detection of solid tumors, and in their use as cancer vaccines (Bast *et al.*, 2000). Clinical responses have been seen, however, that have encouraged the continued development of MAB therapy. As of July 2000, several MABs have received regulatory approval for use in solid tumors. In the 1990s, three MABs received regulatory approval for the detection of cancer when attached to a low-dose radioisotope. Indium-111 (^{111}In)-labeled satumomab pendetide (OncoScint®; Cytogen Corp., Princeton, NJ) is approved for the detection of disease in patients with colorectal or ovarian cancers; technetium 99m (^{99}mTc)-labeled arcitumomab (CEA-Scan®), the fraction antigen-binding (Fab) fragment of a murine MAB, is approved for the detection of colorectal cancer; and ^{111}In-labeled capromab pendetide (ProstaScint®, Cytogen) is approved for the detection of prostate cancer. In the fall of 1998, the first MAB for the treatment of a solid tumor received regulatory approval. Trastuzumab (Herceptin®; Genentech, Inc., San Francisco, CA) was approved for the treatment of patients with metastatic breast cancer whose tumors overexpress the human epidermal growth factor receptor 2 (HER-2) protein.

This chapter will briefly review the biology of MABs, their mechanism of action when used therapeutically in solid tumors, the barriers to successful therapy, the major clinical trials evaluating both unconjugated and conjugated MABs in solid tumors, clinical toxicities, and future directions for the use of MABs in solid tumors.

Biological Actions

To generalize, treatment with antibodies attempts to target antigens that are not immunogenic and to use the body's own defense mechanisms to eradicate tumors. As reviewed in Chapter 2, the generation of an immune response involves multiple factors. Antigens, broadly defined as components of cells or other substances that can be recognized by the immune system, interact with B lymphocytes, macrophages, and other cells (antigen-presenting cells). These cells present the molecules in conjunction with major histocompatibility antigens (e.g., MHC II) for recognition by the immune system. Once an antigen is recognized, a cascade of activity ensues with cytokine production, proliferation of B-cell clones, and eventually production of antibodies. Not all antigens are capable of producing an immune response. Tumor cells, in general, have a decreased ability to produce an immune response (not immunogenic) (Khazaeli *et al.*, 1994). Tumor cells often do not have antigens that differ from normal tissue, and they "escape" the normal mechanisms that fight many pathogens. In addition, for the tumor antigens that differ from normal tissue antigens, there may be impediments for tumor antigen presentation to effector cells, possibly decreasing usual immune responses (Schlom and Abrams, 2000).

There are many possible ways that antibody therapy works to fight cancer, and it is plausible that several mechanisms of action occur with the administration of a specific antibody. MABs may be used in either the unconjugated form (alone) or the conjugated form (attached to other substances, e.g., radioisotopes or toxins).

Unconjugated Antibody Therapy: Direct and Indirect Effects

Antibodies can interact with antigens/**epitopes** on cells and have direct cytotoxic effects. One proposed mechanism for how antibodies can directly kill cells is by the induction of programmed cell death (apoptosis) (Ishizuka *et al.*, 1998). Alternatively, when used alone, antibodies can have an indirect effect that leads to the death of tumor cells. One important mechanism is the induction of antibody-dependent cellular cytotoxicity (ADCC). When an antibody binds to a cell, the crystallizable fragment (Fc) portion of the immunoglobulin (Ig) can be bound by an effector cell (e.g., lymphocytes, monocytes, or macrophages), leading to destruction of the intended target cell (Steplewski *et al.*, 1983).

The ability of an antibody to produce ADCC depends on a number of factors, including the amount of antigen present on tumor cells, the type of effector cell that is activated by the antibody, and the subclass of the antibody (Ortaldo *et al.*, 1987). An emerging approach to heighten this response involves bifunctional antibodies. These antibodies have two antigenic receptors, that is, each arm of the antibody recognizes a different antigen. One of the receptors binds tumor antigen, and the other receptor binds to an effector cell, thereby helping to increase the likelihood of ADCC (Zeidler *et al.*, 1999). The interaction of antibody and antigen can also produce cell death through complement-mediated cytotoxicity. The Fc portion of the antibody, in this case, interacts with complement, thereby activating the complement

cascade and leading ultimately to complement-mediated lysis of the cell (Ballare *et al.*, 1995).

Another approach to the use of antibodies alone has been termed "regulatory" in contrast to "cytotoxic." Cells are dependent upon cellular receptors for proliferation and interactions with other cells. Thus, it is known that tumor cells have a variety of receptors that are important for growth or proliferative advantages. Examples of targets for regulatory therapy include the epidermal growth factor receptor (EGFR), the HER-2 receptor, idiotypic Igs (see Chapter 8), the interleukin-2 (IL-2) receptor, the transferrin receptor, and the platelet-derived growth factor receptor. Theoretically, antibodies directed against growth factor receptors may either directly block these receptors, which are vital for cell function and growth, leading ultimately to cell death (Baselga and Mendelsohn, 1994) or they may downregulate the number of receptors available on the cell surface. This would ultimately impair the cell's ability to differentiate, divide, or both. Many receptors may internalize their ligand, which presents the opportunity for use of receptor-targeted MABs with immunoconjugates. See Table 9.1

Table 9.1   Biological actions induced by unconjugated monoclonal antibodies

Biological Action	Example
Induction of the anti-idiotype network	Vaccines
Complement-mediated cytotoxicity	17-1A
Antibody-directed cellular cytotoxicity	Trastuzumab
Direct antitumor effects	
Apoptosis	Anti-EGF MABs
Interference with ligand-receptor interactions	Anti-EGF MABs
Enhancement of the cytotoxic effects of a second agent	Anti-EGF MABs
	Anti-HER-2 MABs
Induction of biological effects	Anti-CD3 receptor

EGF, epidermal growth factor; MAB, monoclonal antibody.

Source: Adapted with permission from Weiner, L. M. 1999. An overview of monoclonal antibody therapy. *Seminars in Oncology* 26(4 suppl 12): 44 (Table 3).

for a review of the biological actions of unconjugated MABs.

Conjugated Antibody Therapy: Isotopes, Immunotoxins, and More

Often the direct actions of antibodies are not enough to provide sufficient cytotoxicity. Tumors are heterogeneous in composition, that is, not all cells express the same antigen, and some express only small amounts of antigen, decreasing antibody effectiveness (Carlsson *et al.*, 1989). To increase the lethality of MAB therapy to tumor cells, scientists have engineered antibodies that will carry toxic substances to tumor cells. The MABs are used to provide target specificity in cytotoxic processes. In a sense, the MAB serves as a "magic bullet" that delivers a toxic payload to the surface of a cancerous cell. See Table 9.2 for a review of the advantages and benefits of conjugated MABs.

One such approach is to combine isotopes with antibodies to allow focused delivery of radiation doses to tumors. In addition to affecting the primary target cells, the radiation affects surrounding cells that may not have adequate expression of the target antigen. Radioisotopes are often chosen for their pattern and distribution of emissions. For example, iodine-131 (^{131}I) emits beta particles that travel millimeters to a few centimeters in radius. Other radioisotopes give off emissions with an even smaller radius of effect so that the radioisotope can be chosen based on clinical need (Wilder *et al.*, 1996). Toxicity can occur if the antibody-isotope stays in the circulation too long or has a volume of distribution that allows damage to hematopoietic cells in the marrow. Toxicity can also take place if the antigen is expressed on normal tissue.

Toxins such as plant-derived ricin and bacteria-derived *Pseudomonas* exotoxin A are also

Table 9.2   Benefits of conjugated monoclonal antibodies

Immunotoxins
- Use of toxins that are exceptionally potent
- Allows for one toxin molecule per MAB to kill tumor
- Toxins have well-defined biology and chemistry
- Toxins are internalized, thus will not affect nontargeted cells

Chemoimmunoconjugates
- Proven efficacy of antineoplastic drugs in cancer therapy
- Well-defined spectrum of toxicity with chemotherapy
- Non-cross-reactive toxicity with MAB
- Possibility of a bystander effect
- Internalization of conjugate not required for therapeutic effect

Radioimmunoconjugates
- Multiple available isotopes permit a customized approach
- Address the problem of heterogeneity as a result of isotopes having a multiple cell radius of action
- Internalization is generally not required for a toxic effect
- Dosimetry allows for predictable toxicity

MAB, monoclonal antibody.

Source: Adapted with permission from Weiner, L. M. 1999. An overview of monoclonal antibody therapy. *Seminars in Oncology* 26(4 suppl 12): 41–50.

combined with antibodies to enable increased cell kill (Reiter and Pastan, 1998). Most toxins require transport and intracellular processing to exert their effects. Toxins generally contain two chains: one chain facilitates cell binding and transport to the interior of the cell; the second is responsible for the catalytic activity of the toxin. With respect to MAB-toxin conjugates, the antibody-binding domain replaces the cell-binding chain of the toxin creating an immnotoxin with antibody-directed specificity. *Pseudomonas* exotoxin A is a bacterial toxin that kills cells by inhibiting protein synthesis. This toxin has been engineered so that it will kill cells only when directed to them by an antibody. Once the toxin has been directed to the target cell, the toxin is internalized by the cell, where it inhibits protein synthesis. Ricin is a toxin derived from the castor bean. The active chain of ricin (the A-chain) also acts through inhibition of protein synthesis; however, it has its primary effect via changes in ribosomal activity. This toxin also requires internalization by the target cell. Rather than removing the portion of the toxin that normally enables ricin to enter most cells, scientists have blocked the normal binding sites with the antibody that provides tumor specificity. Each of these toxins is extremely potent—one toxin molecule can kill a cell. Because of the effectiveness of these toxins, specificity of antibody for tumor antigen again is of utmost importance in helping limit damage to normal cells.

Antibodies can similarly be linked with individual chemotherapy molecules to help deliver toxic agents locally to tumors (Panchagnula and Dey, 1997). The BR96 antigen is expressed on many cancerous cells, including breast, lung, and colon cancers. Numerous clinical trials have evaluated the efficacy of BR96 conjugated to doxorubicin (BR96-doxorubicin), but to date, little clinical activity has been seen. Alternatively, delivery of enzymes to tumors could allow conversion of pro-drugs into active chemotherapeutic agents in individual tumor cells to again decrease systemic impairment (Blakey *et al.*, 1995).

Targeting Antibodies for Clinical Use

The therapeutic use of MABs has been evaluated in clinical trials since early 1980. (See Table 9.3 for a review of the advantages of

Table 9.3   Advantages of using MABs in cancer therapy

- Allows for therapy that is specifically targeted toward a chosen tumor antigen
- Low cross-reactivity with normal cells
- Highly purified proteins of known specificity
- Technology allows for alteration of design to suit clinical needs
- Customized effector functions based on class of antibody chosen
- Ability to specifically target toxic payloads

Source: Adapted with permission from Weiner, L. M. 1999. An overview of monoclonal antibody therapy. *Seminars in Oncology* 26(4 suppl 12): 41–50.

using MAB therapy.) Several advances have occurred in the use of MABs to treat hematologic malignancies, including the development and widespread use of rituximab (Rituxan®, Genentech) for relapsed or refractory CD20+ non-Hodgkin's lymphoma (see Chapter 8). With the exception of trastuzumab, MAB treatment of solid tumors has not gained widespread clinical use despite the many advances seen in oncology. There are many reasons why treatment of solid tumors with antibodies has not had significant success. Table 9.4 reviews the obstacles to successful therapy with MABs in solid tumors and possible solutions for overcoming these barriers.

One problem with MAB therapy of established solid tumors is the heterogeneous distribution of antibodies in tumors. Some of this is related to the variable expression of tumor antigen on the surface of cancer cells. There is also nonhomogenous blood flow to tumors and, in tumors themselves, high interstitial pressure that decreases the ability of antibodies to infiltrate tumors (Jain and Baxter, 1988). Once antibody has left the circulation, diffusion of the antibody to individual cells is also inconsistent. There is also evidence that unbound antigen can bind administered antibody, decreasing the

Table 9.4   Obstacles to effective treatment of solid tumors with monoclonal antibodies

Obstacle	Possible Solutions
Induction of human antimouse antibody (HAMA) response with murine monoclonal antibodies (MABs)	• Treat patients with depressed humoral immunity • Use humanized or chimeric antibodies • Administer immunosuppressive agents such as cyclosporin A • Complex circulating levels of HAMA with MABs • Plasmapheresis prior to treatment
Inadequate trafficking of potential cellular effector cells to the tumor	• Use humanized or chimeric antibodies • Use bifunctional antibodies
Inability of murine MABs to interact with human effector cells	• Use humanized or chimeric antibodies
Insufficient targeting specificity	• Use other biological agents such as interferon to upregulate antigen expression • Use conjugates that will have a bystander effect
Antigenic heterogeneity of the tumor	• Use a cocktail of MABs that will recognize different antigens • Use conjugates that will have a bystander effect
Modulation (e.g., shedding or internalization) of the antigen	• Target antigens that do not modulate • Use sequential infusions of antibody so that tumor cells may be targeted once antigen is reexpressed
Inadequate blood flow to deliver MAB to the tumor	• Use antibody fragments or other small molecules • Combine with radiation therapy, hyperthermia, or other cytokines to increase blood flow • Inject MAB directly into the tumor

total dose seen by tumor cells. The unbound antibody can be both in the tumor interstitium as well as in the circulation.

Moreover, some of the earlier clinical trials with MABs revealed unexpected side effects caused by cross-reactivity with antigen on normal tissue in addition to MAB targeting the desired tumor antigen. For example, a trial evaluating an anti-GD_2 antibody in metastatic melanoma found that patients developed neuropathic pain and motor neuropathy, revealing probable cross-reactivity with neurologic tissue (Saleh

et al., 1992). Although this is an extreme example of cross-reactivity, it helps illustrate difficulties in the development of MAB therapy for solid tumors.

Overcoming Barriers to Effective Treatment

To help reduce the possible cross-reactivity of antibody with normal tissue antigen, researchers have focused efforts on finding tumor-specific targets. Investigations have tended to focus on two broad areas for further antibody development (Schlom, 1990). Researchers have tried to focus on two types of potential antigen targets: oncofetal antigens and tumor-specific antigens. Oncofetal antigens are expressed on some fetal tissues, many tumors, and some normal tissue. These antigens can often be found on more than one tumor cell type, broadening their possible applications. Included in this category are carcinoembryonic antigen (CEA), CA 19-9, L6, and 17-1A. Identification of antigens that are found solely on tumors or expressed to a greater degree than the corresponding benign tissue are also being investigated. One well-described tumor-specific antigen is the human milk fat globule mucin found primarily in breast cancers.

Another approach to overcoming barriers to effective therapy has been to genetically engineer antibodies. As previously stated, hybridoma technology developed in the 1970s enabled the mass production of murine antibodies directed against human antigens. Murine antibodies have many disadvantages that keep them from having increased efficacy. Because they are "nonhuman," the antibodies themselves are capable of eliciting an immune response. Human antibodies can form against the therapeutic antibodies as human anti-mouse antibodies (HAMA), decreasing the ability to treat patients multiple times with the same therapy. The development of HAMA occurs usually after repeated exposure to the administered antibody (Khazaeli *et al.*, 1994). Once an immune response occurs, administered antibodies can be rapidly cleared from the circulation. To help decrease the immunogenicity of the murine antibodies, chimeric and humanized antibodies were developed. These antibodies are theoretically less immunogenic and interact more effectively with human immune cells (see Chapter 8).

Scientists have also tailored antibodies to improve performance. For example, an antibody

subclass can be chosen to optimize immune response. The IgG3 class of immunoglobulins mediate ADCC to a greater degree than IgG2a, IgG2b, or IgG1 in laboratory testing (Anasetti *et al.*, 1987). Making antibody fragments containing decreased amounts of the constant portion of the Ig can change the size of the antibody product. These smaller particles have the same binding affinity for an antigen but can have improved ability to reach tumors and are also capable of enhancing delivery of isotopes, toxins, and other agents to tumors (Rodwell, 1989). Manipulation of the antibodies can also change the pharmacokinetics of the therapy. For example, alterations in antibody half-life and volume of distribution can change toxicities.

Clinical Trials of Unconjugated Antibodies

Growth Factor Receptor Blockade: A Model for Antibody Development

Whereas decreasing toxicity to normal tissue is an ideal goal, other targets found universally on cells are also being explored. Significant interest has focused on the development of antibodies against growth factor receptors. Growth factor receptors are vital for cell function, cell growth, and interaction among cells. Examples of this type of receptor are the EGFR, the HER-2 receptor, the transferrin receptor, and the insulin-like growth factor receptor (IGFR). Activation of many of these receptors can initiate the cell cycle and, therefore, cell division in the right environment. These receptors are found on normal cells, and there is evidence that they are overexpressed on many tumor types (Slamon *et al.*, 1987; Rusch *et al.*, 1993). In addition, tumor cells can be stimulated to grow through these receptors by way of paracrine and autocrine pathways (Ruck and Paulie, 1998). The blockade of these receptors could consequently help stop cell division and tumor growth and possibly cause cell death via induction of immune response or through initiation of apoptosis.

The EGFR has been an active target for antibody development. EGFR is overexpressed on many different types of tumors, including breast, lung, and head and neck cancers. Overexpression of EGFR often portends a worse prognosis (Slamon *et al.*, 1987). This receptor, like many growth factor receptors, has intrinsic tyrosine kinase activity that is responsible for transmitting cellular signals (Aaronson, 1991). Preclinical studies with the anti-EGFR murine 225 and the chimeric C225 show significant antitumor effect in *in vitro* and *in vivo* laboratory experiments. C225 is being investigated clinically as a therapeutic agent, both as monotherapy and in combination with other modalities, primarily in head and neck, renal cell, lung, and breast cancers. Preliminary results of a trial that evaluated the use of C225 as monotherapy for patients with metastatic renal cell cancer show the ability of the antibody to have biological activity in a historically poorly responsive malignancy. Of 54 patients enrolled, 47 had received more than 1 dose of antibody. The time to progression varied between 98 and 332 days, with 1 partial response, 2 complete responses, and more than 25% of patients with stable disease (Gunnett *et al.*, 1999).

Several reports of *in vitro* synergistic cytotoxicity with chemotherapy have stimulated clinical trials evaluating combination therapy of C225 plus cisplatin (Baselga and Mendelsohn, 1994). A phase I trial of C225 in combination with cisplatin in patients with recurrent squamous cell carcinoma of the head and neck evaluated weekly doses of C225 given concurrently with 100 mg/m² of cisplatin administered every 3 weeks. Although this was primarily a study to evaluate safety and ideal dose of antibody, tumor responses were seen. Of the 7 patients that could be evaluated, there were 1 complete response, 3 partial responses, and 1 mixed response. Three of the patients with clinical benefit from the combination therapy had failed previous cisplatin-based chemotherapy (Mendelsohn *et al.*, 1999). The precise mechanism of increased efficacy with combination therapy is unknown; however, data from experiments of the tyrosine kinase inhibitor suggest that concomitant use of chemotherapy with blockade of EGFR activation (in this case via inhibition of the tyrosine kinase activity of the receptor) induces apoptosis (Lei *et al.*, 1999).

C225 has also been combined with radiation therapy as treatment for locally advanced head and neck tumors. Preclinical studies have shown that C225 increases radiosensitivity in squamous cell carcinoma cells. C225 increased the number of cells in G_1 and decreased the number of cells in S phase, heightening the ability of radiation to cause cellular damage. In addition, there was enhancement of the antibody's ability to induce apoptosis when combined with radiation (Huang *et al.*, 1999). A phase I trial evaluated the optimal safe dose of intravenous C225 given weekly for 7 weeks when combined with daily or twice-daily radiation therapy. Of 15 evaluable patients with stage IV (81%) and stage III disease, 14 (93%) had clinical complete remissions (Ezekiel *et al.*, 1999).

Additional antibodies are being developed against the EGFR. ICR62, a rat MAB, has shown activity against breast cancer and several squamous cell carcinoma cell lines *in vitro* and *in vivo*. This antibody effectively blocks the binding of EGF, transforming growth factor (TGF)-α, and heparin-binding-EGF to the EGFR; inhibits the *in vitro* growth of tumor cell lines that overexpress the EGFR; and eradicates such tumors when grown as xenografts in athymic mice. In one trial, 11 patients with squamous cell carcinoma of the head and neck and 9 patients with squamous cell carcinoma of the lung whose tumors expressed EGFR were recruited. Groups of 3 patients were treated with 2.5 mg, 10 mg, 20 mg, or 40 mg of ICR62, and an additional 8 patients received 100 mg of ICR62. All patients were evaluated for toxicity using World Health Organizaton (WHO) criteria. Patients' sera were tested for the clearance of MAB ICR62 and the development of human anti-rat antibodies (HARA). No serious (WHO grade 3–4) toxicity was observed in patients treated with up to 100 mg of ICR62. Only 4 of 20 patients showed HARA responses (1 at 20 mg, 1 at 40, and 2 at 100-mg doses), and of these, only the first 2 were anti-idiotypic responses. On the basis of these study results, the authors concluded that MAB ICR62 can be administered safely to patients with squamous cell carcinomas and that it can localize efficiently to metastases even at relatively low doses (Modjtahedi et al., 1996).

A fully humanized MAB E7.6.3 has also been produced and recently described. This antibody is generated from a strain of mice (Xeno-Mouse™) engineered to be deficient in murine antibody production. These mice were then injected with yeast artificial chromosomes containing a large portion of the human heavy and kappa light chain loci. In vivo lab experiments have shown the ability of E7.6.3 to eradicate large tumors without concurrent chemotherapy or radiation therapy, and it appears to be a good candidate for use in clinical trials assessing the full therapeutic potential of anti-EGFR antibody in the therapy of multiple patient populations with EGFR-expressing solid tumors (Yang et al., 1999).

In addition to EGFR, another growth factor receptor has been a major focus of current research. HER-2 is a proto-oncogene found on the short arm of chromosome 17 (17q21) that encodes a transmembrane glycoprotein receptor with tyrosine kinase activity. This receptor is homologous to EGFR; however, it has different stimuli (ligands) involved in its activation (Baselga and Mendelsohn, 1994). As with other growth factor receptors, the receptor encoded by HER-2 is involved with growth regulation of normal cells. Amplification of the proto-oncogene can result in increased levels or overexpression of the growth factor receptor on the surface of malignant cells. The proto-oncogene HER-2 is amplified or the encoded growth factor receptor (p185^{Her-2} or HER-2) is overexpressed on many cells, including breast, lung, ovarian, and prostate cancers (Cline and Battifora, 1987; Slamon et al., 1987; Berchuck et al., 1990; Gu et al., 1996). For breast cancer cells, amplification of HER-2 is usually correlated with overexpression of the gene product. With overexpression of the receptor, the normal balance of growth regulation is altered, leading to increased opportunity for uncontrolled growth.

HER-2 is overexpressed in approximately 20% to 30% of breast cancers (Slamon et al., 1987). Preclinical work in vitro and in vivo has shown that amplification of HER-2 endows tumor cells with the increased ability to grow, synthesize DNA, form tumors, and develop metastatic lesions. In humans, positive HER-2 status is also associated with increased aggressiveness of tumors. Kallioniemi et al. (1991) found that high expression of HER-2 was associated with pathological indications of increased aggressiveness, including high nuclear grade, DNA aneuploidy, high tumor S-phase fraction, and lack of estrogen and progesterone receptors. In addition, this group correlated high levels of HER-2 expression with a statistically significant increased relative risk of death when compared with controls with low levels of HER-2 expression.

Similar to EGFR, amplification of the HER-2 or overexpression of its product is often correlated with a poor prognosis. For patients with breast cancer, HER-2 status has been evaluated as a prognostic indicator of clinical outcome (Slamon et al., 1987). A review by Ross and Fletcher (1999) discussed the relative advantages and disadvantages of methods used for assessing HER-2 overexpression (e.g., immunohistochemistry, Southern blot analysis, polymerase chain reaction amplification, and fluorescence *in situ* hybridization assays) designed to detect HER-2 gene amplification as compared with HER-2 protein overexpression assays performed with immunohistochemical techniques applied to frozen and paraffin-embedded tissues and enzyme immunoassays performed on tumor cytosols. The potential value of HER-2 protein status for the prediction of response to therapy in breast cancer is presented for standard hormone therapy, cytotoxic chemotherapy, and radiation therapy. Also evaluated is the status of serum-based testing for circulating HER-2 receptor protein and its ability to predict disease outcome and response to therapy. Although it is clear that amplification of HER-2 can imply a worse prognosis for some patients, it is still uncertain whether all patients are equally at risk. Several studies have suggested that overexpression of HER-2 predicts decreased benefit to certain systemic therapy (e.g., cyclophosphamide, methotrexate, and 5-fluorouracil [CMF]), whereas other studies have suggested improved response in anthracycline-based therapy.

A trial presented to the American Society of Clinical Oncology (ASCO) in 1999 helped confirm the idea that patients who overexpress HER-2 might have improved response and survival if they are treated with anthracycline-based therapy. A study in Spain, which evaluated the efficacy of CMF versus 5-fluorouracil, doxorubicin, and cyclophosphamide (FAC) was retrospectively analyzed for information regarding HER-2 overexpression and response. These researchers found that survival for HER-2-positive patients was worse if they received CMF compared with similar HER-2-negative patients. This difference in response was not seen with the anthracycline-based FAC regimen, in which HER-2-positive and -nega-

tive patients had similar results. In addition, it was suggested that HER-2-positive patients who received FAC had improved overall survival compared with those who received CMF; however, the difference was not statistically significant ($p = .3$) (Vera *et al.*, 1999).

In the trials conducted to date, it is evident that the ability of HER-2 to predict response to systemic therapy is debatable. These trials were not originally designed to answer the questions currently being posed. In addition, these groups used a variety of methods to evaluate HER-2 amplification and HER-2 overexpression. These varied techniques combined with differing definitions of what constitutes elevation of HER-2 or its product make direct comparisons of the above outcomes difficult. Some of the currently ongoing trials designed to evaluate the role of HER-2 in response to chemotherapy may help answer some of these questions.

As with EGFR, antibodies against the protein product of HER-2 have been developed and researched. Around the time that HER-2 was associated with prognosis in breast cancer, evidence that murine MABs against HER-2 could suppress tumor growth *in vitro* was released. The antibody 4D5 was found to have partial or weak agonist properties, but overall, it was able to inhibit cell proliferation in cells that overexpressed HER-2 (Sarup *et al.*, 1991). Of interest was the fact that this inhibition occurred only in cells that overexpressed HER-2. The murine MAB 4D5 caused a human antimouse antibody response *in vivo* and also lacked activation of effector cell function. Therefore, this antibody was further engineered to a humanized MAB that had less immunogenicity and increased ability to mediate ADCC (Carter *et al.*, 1992). The resulting antibody, trastuzumab, began evaluation in clinical trials. Findings from one of the first phase II trials evaluating the use of trastuzumab as monotherapy for breast cancer were published in 1996

(Baselga *et al.*, 1996). In this trial, the subjects were women with metastatic breast cancer whose tumors overexpressed HER-2 (80% of tumors had >50% positive membrane staining for HER-2). The overall response rate (complete and partial responses combined) was 11.6%. Two patients had minor responses, and 14 had stable disease at day 77 of treatment. Of note is that this patient population had visceral metastases in 80% of the cases and a history of extensive prior therapy, possibly enhancing the significance of the results achieved. Overall, the median time to progression for patients with minor response or stable disease was 5.1 months.

A second trial evaluating the benefit of trastuzumab as monotherapy for patients with metastatic breast cancer was presented at ASCO in 1998. This trial was a larger, single-arm trial that enrolled 222 women. Over 60% of patients had more than 2 prior therapies for metastatic disease. Of the women enrolled, 213 received trastuzumab, and at 11 months, the overall response rate was found to be 15% by an independent response committee. The median duration of response was 8.4 months with an estimated median survival duration of 13 months. Treatment was well tolerated; only 2 patients discontinued therapy because of toxicity. Nine patients, however, had reduction (>10%) in ejection fraction. Of these, 6 patients were symptomatic due to compromised cardiac function (Cobleigh *et al.*, 1998). These results show that trastuzumab has impressive efficacy in heavily pretreated patients. In addition, side effects were minimal, with the prominent effects being fever and chills during the first infusion.

Attempts to take advantage of preclinical data showing synergy between chemotherapy and MAB to HER-2 were seen in a phase II trial investigating the combination of trastuzumab and cisplatin. In this study, 39 patients were treated with weekly doses of trastuzumab, with cisplatin administration every 4 weeks.

These patients were also heavily pretreated, with 90% of patients having received 2 or more cycles of chemotherapy for metastatic disease. Of 37 patients evaluable for tumor response, 9 (24.3%) had a partial remission, 3 (8%) had a minor response, and 16 (16%) had stable disease. The median duration of response was 5.3 months. Toxicity was increased in this trial compared with trastuzumab monotherapy; however, toxicities were similar to those expected from monotherapy with cisplatin. This trial showed that the combination of trastuzumab and chemotherapy was not only possible but of greater efficacy than MAB therapy or chemotherapy alone (Pegram *et al.*, 1998).

Additional preclinical work found that trastuzumab enhances the efficacy of paclitaxel and doxorubicin against HER-2-overexpressing breast cancer cells. The greatest effect *in vitro* and *in vivo* was seen with the combination of paclitaxel and trastuzumab (Baselga *et al.*, 1998). This and other preclinical work was used to assist in the design of a randomized trial comparing the addition of trastuzumab to standard chemotherapy as front-line treatment for metastatic breast cancer. Four hundred sixty-nine patients with overexpression of HER-2 were randomized to chemotherapy based on prior treatments. Patients without anthracycline exposure were given doxorubicin and cyclophosphamide (AC) with or without trastuzumab. Those patients previously treated with doxorubicin were given paclitaxel with or without trastuzumab. With a median follow-up of 10.5 months, results were presented in 1998. Investigators found an overall benefit with the combination of chemotherapy and trastuzumab versus chemotherapy alone without a significant increase in severe adverse events. For both groups receiving chemotherapy, time to progression was 8.6 months for the combination of chemotherapy and trastuzumab versus 5.5 months for treatment with chemotherapy alone. The response rate was also improved with the combination of chemotherapy and trastuzumab (62%) versus chemotherapy alone (36.2%) (Slamon *et al.*, 1998a). An update of this trial was provided in 1999, and at a median follow-up of 25 months the combination of chemotherapy with trastuzumab resulted in a statistically significant superior overall survival duration (25.4 months) versus chemotherapy alone (20.9 months) (Norton *et al.*, 1999).

As with the initial trials investigating trastuzumab, the combination of this drug with chemotherapy was associated with an increased risk of cardiotoxicity. Grade 3 or 4 cardiotoxicity occurred more often in patients receiving doxorubicin and trastuzumab (18%) than in patients receiving paclitaxel and trastuzumab (2%) (Slamon *et al.*, 1998b). The combination of anthracycline and trastuzumab caused greater toxicity than would be expected from either medication alone. In the phase III trial evaluating trastuzumab as monotherapy for breast cancer, 5% of patients had grade 3/4 cardiotoxicity. In general, this population had previous exposure to anthracyclines, again implicating the combination of trastuzumab and doxorubicin as the significant contributor to cardiac dysfunction.

The success with trastuzumab as treatment for metastatic breast cancer, both as monotherapy and in combination with other medications, led to its regulatory approval in late 1998. The success of the early clinical trials has inspired many more studies evaluating the role of trastuzumab in the adjuvant as well as metastatic setting. As more information is discovered about this antibody, it is anticipated that new applications can be implemented (Shak, 1999). In addition, a review of clinical trials listed in the National Cancer Institute's clinical trial database shows that clinical trials are currently evaluating the efficacy of trastuzumab as monotherapy or in combination with chemotherapy in lung, pancreatic, prostate, and ovarian cancers.

Prior to receiving therapy with trastuzumab, a patient's tumor must be assessed for overexpression of HER-2. Standardization of the methodologies for performing and evaluating a laboratory-based test has been needed to ensure wide adoption in clinical practice. Immunohistochemical methods are broadly used because they are simple and rapid and the equipment required is generally available in pathology laboratories. Ideally, this methodology would be used on fresh, frozen tissue. A multitude of HER-2 antibody and antisera preparations are available, which may account for the significant differences seen in sensitivity and specificity. Additionally, scoring criteria for overexpression may also vary according to factors such as cellular localization of the stain, the percentage of cells that stain, the intensity of staining, or a combination thereof. In the United States, DAKO Corp. (Carpenteria, CA) markets the only immunohistochemical kit approved by the Food and Drug Administration (FDA) for the determination of HER-2 protein overexpression in breast cancer tissues. HercepTest™ is indicated as an aid in assessing patients for whom trastuzumab treatment is being considered. Staining levels are scored on a range of 0 for "no staining" to 3+ for "strongly positive." It is hoped that further research and experience with these tests will address issues such as standardization of methods, quality control, agreement on common grading criteria and scoring systems, standardized reporting systems, and comparability of results obtained with different assays and among different laboratories (Albain *et al.*, 1999). Many centers are now beginning to use fluorescence *in situ* hybridization as a method of evaluating the overexpression of the HER-2-*neu* gene.

Breast Cancer: Other Options for Therapy

With the development of antibody therapy against HER-2, other antigens on breast cancer cells have been explored as the focus for MAB development. BR96 Ag is an antigen expressed on many cancerous cells, including those from breast, lung, and colon cancers, but it has limited expression on normal cells. This antigen is a variant of the Lewis Y antigen, which is also expressed on normal tissues to a lesser degree. Murine monoclonal and chimeric antibodies against the BR96 Ag have been developed that show ability to kill cells via ADCC.

L6 Ag is an antigen also found on many tumor types, including adenocarcinoma of the lung, breast, and colon. A murine MAB against this antigen has been developed and tested in patients with metastatic breast cancer. This antibody was found to mediate ADCC, complement-dependent cytotoxicity, or both in addition to direct growth inhibition of tumor cells (Hellstrom et al., 1986). A phase I trial evaluating L6 as monotherapy found localization of the antibody to tumors and clinical efficacy in 1 patient with breast cancer. This treatment was associated with minimal side effects; however, the majority of patients did develop HAMA, suggesting limited application for repeated use (Goodman et al., 1990). A chimeric form of L6 was developed that showed similar binding properties in tumors with decreased but still present development of HAMA (Goodman et al., 1993).

Additional antigens targeted for therapy in breast cancer include Ag-2.15 and the epithelial cell adhesion molecule, both seen on many different carcinomas as well as breast cancer (Mordoh et al., 1994; Braun et al., 1999). The human milk fat globule antigen and the M_r 400,000 breast epithelial mucin epitope are also under investigation, which may lead to increased selectivity for breast cancer tumor cells (Kramer et al., 1998; Tripathy et al., 1999).

Colon Cancer

Immunological therapy for gastrointestinal malignancies has been approached from several different directions. An excellent review of this broad topic, including the use of antibodies in radioimmunodiagnostics, was published by Foon et al. (1999). MAB therapy as monotherapy has had some success in the management of colon cancer. Much of the work in this field has pivoted around development of anti-idiotype vaccines against CEA and other tumor-associated antigens.

One of the antigenic targets currently under investigation, and the most extensively studied MAB in the treatment of colorectal cancer, is the CD17-1A antigen. This antigen is overexpressed by many epithelial tumors and is believed to play a role in epithelial cell adhesion. In preclinical work, the murine MAB to this antigen, 17-1A (edrecolomab/Panorex™), was able to induce ADCC. In addition, there is evidence that 17-1A directly inhibited growth of tumors *in vivo* when the antibody was administered close to the time of cell implantation. In initial phase I and II trials of this antibody in metastatic colon cancer, toxicities have been minimal, consisting primarily of mild allergic reactions and development of HAMA. Clinical responses were seen, with reports of objective response (including stable disease) in 10% to 27% of patients (Adkins and Spencer, 1998).

Given evidence of clinical responses in patients with widely metastatic disease, investigators moved this therapy into the adjuvant setting with the goal of targeting micrometastases before they could become clinically apparent and possibly more difficult to treat. Initially published in 1994 and updated in 1998, a randomized trial evaluated the benefit of 17-1A as adjuvant therapy in stage III Duke's C colon adenocarcinoma. Patients were randomized to receive either 17-1A or close observation after curative-intent surgery. Treatment with 17-1A reduced the overall mortality rate by 32% and the recurrence rate by 23% at 7 years median follow-up. The greatest effect of antibody therapy was seen in deterring distant metastases. Side effects were tolerable, with signs and symptoms such as malaise, low-grade fever and chills, diarrhea, and allergic reactions being most prominent. In all, only 45 adverse reactions were seen in 371 total doses administered (Riethmuller *et al.*, 1998).

Currently, 2 randomized studies are further evaluating the use of 17-1A in the adjuvant setting. Study 157-001, being conducted in North and South America, is evaluating adjuvant chemotherapy with a 5-fluorouracil (5-FU) regimen alone versus chemotherapy plus 17-1A antibody. Study 157-002, ongoing in Europe, is similarly designed; however, in this trial, a third arm of monotherapy with antibody will be included. The primary end point in both studies will be overall survival. Safety data presented in 1999 revealed that the addition of antibody therapy to a fluorouracil-based adjuvant chemotherapy does not significantly worsen side effects (Fields *et al.*, 1999).

An additional target for MAB therapy for colon cancer is the tumor-associated glycoprotein (TAG)-72. This antigen is found on many carcinomas of epithelial origin and to a minor extent on normal tissue. Given that almost 90% of colon adenocarcinomas express this antigen, it has been explored as a serum tumor marker, a marker of early neoplastic transformation or of malignancy in effusions, and as a target for immunodiagnostics and immunotherapy (Guadagni *et al.*, 1996). Murine and chimeric antibodies have been developed that are targeted toward this antigen and have been evaluated in clinical trials coupled to various radioisotopes (see section on "Radioimmunotherapy").

Lung Cancer

The diversity of cell types and tumor antigens in lung cancer create challenges for creating antibody monotherapy for this disease. As with breast cancer, our knowledge about the role of growth factors in non-small-cell lung cancer continues to grow. This area is an active subject for research and clinical trials. In addition to

EGFR and HER-2, other growth factor receptors are being investigated, including c-*erB*-3 and IGFR-1 (Zia *et al.*, 1996; Yi *et al.*, 1997).

One unique area of research in the development of MAB therapy for squamous cell carcinoma of the lung is the investigation of a particular antigen identified by the antibody Po66. After a patient's squamous cell carcinoma cell line was used to induce several murine antibodies, Po66 was found to target xenografts of human lung cancers in laboratory animals. Further investigation revealed that the target of the antibody is an intracellular antigen found in squamous cell carcinoma, esophageal carcinoma, and inconsistently in adenocarcinoma of the lung. This antigen is also seen in normal tissue, including the esophagus, and in distal and collecting tubules in the kidney (Martin *et al.*, 1989).

Given that the majority of targets for immunotherapy with antibodies are superficial antigens/epitopes, the identification of a purely intracellular antigen created interesting avenues for exploration. One of the difficulties that can be encountered in the administration of MAB is the phenomenon termed "modulation" (see Chapter 8). With modulation, antigen binding by antibody causes internalization of the complex, therefore decreasing the ability of the antibody to have cytotoxic effects through ADCC or complement-mediated cytotoxicity. Antigen modulation can be inconsistent; therefore, the discovery of a continuously internal antigen provides a unique opportunity for the use of MABs, especially in the delivery of immunoconjugates.

Neural-cell adhesion molecules (NCAMs) are a family of markers indicating neuroendocrine differentiation in lung cancer. These markers are implicated in intercellular interactions and can also be found on a variety of normal tissues. MABs have been developed against these antigens that have been found to be active *in vitro* against both non-small-cell lung cancers and small-cell lung cancer (SCLC) cell lines (Moolenaar *et al.*, 1990). These markers are expressed to a high degree on SCLCs, making them an attractive target for antibody therapy. Because of the heterogeneous nature of NCAMs, the multiple antibodies developed against this mixture of antigens are referred to as the cluster 1 antibodies (Gilks *et al.*, 1994). These antibodies have been evaluated for their efficacy in the immunodetection of tumor cells in bone marrow of SCLC patients (Pelosi *et al.*, 1999).

In addition to the studies with antibodies formed against multiple different antigens encompassed by over 11 different clusters, another interesting approach has developed. Observations that gastrin-releasing peptide was involved in an autocrine stimulatory loop in SCLC prompted researchers to develop antibodies that block this loop. One of the MABs developed, 2A11, binds to gastrin-releasing peptide and prohibits the molecule from further stimulating malignant cells. Of 12 evaluable patients in a phase II trial evaluating this antibody in previously treated SCLC, 1 had a complete response and 4 had stable disease. No patients developed HAMA while on therapy, and no grade 3 or 4 toxicities were seen (Johnson and Kelley, 1998). These results are encouraging and will hopefully stimulate further research into new ways to direct antibody therapy.

Malignant Melanoma

Significant studies in melanoma have been performed using MABs reactive with antigens called gangliosides. Gangliosides consist of a carbohydrate, a spingosome, and a fatty acid. Tumors that express gangliosides include those of neuroectodermal origin, such as SCLC, neuroblastoma, osteosarcoma, and melanoma. The 4 most frequently expressed gangliosides (GM3, GM2, GD3, and GD2) are sequentially expressed during melanoma differentiation and are characterized by varying numbers of sialic acid residues (Ravindranath and Irie, 1988).

Antibodies to each of the above gangliosides have been produced. MAB R24, a murine antibody reactive with GD3, was administered to melanoma patients by Houghton and colleagues with minimal toxicity and a response rate of 15% to 20% (Houghton *et al.*, 1985). Since this pioneering study, R24 has been used in combination with cytokines and growth factors without a significant improvement in tumor responses (Bajorin *et al.*, 1990; Caulfield *et al.*, 1990; Chachoua *et al.*, 1994). Anti-idiotype MABs against GD3 and GD2 are also being investigated in clinical trials (McCaffrey *et al.*, 1996; Foon *et al.*, 1999).

MABs to GD2, a ganglioside that differs from GD3 by an additional sialic acid residue, have also been tested clinically (Saleh *et al.*, 1992). To date, higher response rates have been observed in neuroblastoma than in melanoma because of the extremely high antigen expression in GD2 (Mujoo *et al.*, 1986). Unfortunately, murine anti-GD2 MABs bind to peripheral nerves, causing transient severe pain and occasionally other neurologic side effects (Murray *et al.*, 1994).

Vaccines

Another approach with unconjugated MABs has been the use of MABs as vaccines. The theory behind this approach capitalizes on the induction of the idiotypic network. The antigen-combining site of each antibody is known as the "idiotype," a unique clonally derived structure that is capable of stimulating the production of antibodies against it. In this response, the Ab1 antibody is formed against an antigen/epitope on a tumor cell. Ab1 is generally a murine or chimeric antibody. This idiotype-containing antibody can be used to cause the formation of an anti-idiotype antibody, Ab2, against Ab1.

Ab2 is targeted toward the idiotype of Ab1, and it mirrors the image of the original antigen. Ab2 is then used to immunize the patients, leading to the production of anti-anti-idiotype antibodies (Ab3). Ab3 in part binds the tumor antigen against which the original antibody, Ab1, was targeted. The benefit is that Ab3 is produced by the patient and will hopefully interact to a greater degree with other components of the patient's immune system to destroy tumor cells. These anti-idiotype antibodies mimic a number of tumor antigens and are under investigation as cancer vaccines in a number of clinical trials (see Table 9.5). The majority of these trials have demonstrated limited clinical responses or prolongation of survival. Increased titers of Ab3 and Ab1 antibodies, in some cases, have correlated with response or remission. In some studies, the induction of T-cell immunity characterized by increased lymphocyte proliferation to antibody or cytotoxic T cells has been observed.

Monoclonal Antibodies as Biological Response Modifiers

Another approach for the use of unconjugated MABs has been as biological response modifiers to, in a sense, modulate or induce an indirect antitumor action through activation of the immune system. The best example to date for this approach is the use of the muromonab (Orthoclone®, OKT3; Ortho Biotech, Raritan, NJ) MAB, which reacts with the T-cell receptor CD3. OKT3 is approved for the treatment of rejection episodes in kidney transplantation. Several trials have evaluated the use of OKT3 in activating T cells in the hope of promoting immune response against the tumor. Other investigators have evaluated this approach in combination with IL-2 administration in the hope of obtaining synergistic stimulation of the immune system. OKT3 also has T-cell activating properties that are thought to be caused by

cross-linking of T cells via CD3 to Fc receptor-bearing cells, leading to massive cytokine release. To date, no significant clinical benefit has been demonstrated with this approach. Of note, the dose-limiting toxicity associated with OKT3 appears to be neurotoxicity exhibited as headache and confusion (Dillman, 1998).

Conjugate Therapy

In many instances, the results of clinical trials using unconjugated MABs have been disappointing, especially in the treatment of solid tumors. An additional approach to using MABs in this group of patients has been to attach another substance with cytotoxic capabilities to the MAB. The MAB then serves as a delivery system to selectively target the tumor cells with these "lethal" substances. Examples of substances that have been attached to MABs include α-, β-, and γ-emitting radionuclides (radioimmunoconjugates); protein toxins such as ricin, diptheria, or *P. exotoxin* (immunotoxins); and chemotherapeutic drugs such as doxorubicin or methotrexate (chemoimmunoconjugates). To date, none of these MABs has received regulatory approval. The majority of success has been seen in the use of radioimmunoconjugates in the hematologic malignancies (see Chapter 8). This section will provide a brief overview of each of these approaches.

Radioimmunoconjugates

Radionuclides attached to MABs have several potential uses in the management of patients with cancer: for detection of disease as a nuclear scan (radioimmunodetection) or during surgery (radioimmunoguided surgery or RIGS) and in the treatment of cancer (radioimmunotherapy or RIT). See Table 9.6 for a review of isotopes commonly attached to MABs for both diagnostic and therapeutic purposes. Three MABs have

Table 9.5 Clinical trials of anti-idiotype antibodies

Study	Tumor AB	No. Patients	Results	Year	Immune Response
Herlyn et al.	Colorectal Carcinoma 171A	30	13 PRs	1987	Ab3 and Ab1'
Mittelman et al.	Melanoma 228	37	7 PRs	1990	Ab3 and Ab1' Induction
Mittelman et al.	Melanoma 228	25	3 PRs; survival relatively longer in 14	1992	Survival increase in patients with Ab1'
Miller et al. Meeker et al.	B-cell lymphoma Anti-idiotype	11	5 PRs	1982 1985	—
Kwak et al.	B-cell lymphoma Idiotype	9	PRs and tumor regression in 8	1992	Increase T cell function, Ab2
Foon et al.	Colon cancer CEA	12	None	1997	Ab3, Ab1' increase lymphocyte proliferation to Ab2
Saleh et al.	Melanoma (MELIMMUNE)	21	—	1998	Increase in Ab3 but not Ab1'
Pride et al.	Melanoma (MELIMMUNE)	32	Adjuvant	1998	Increase CTL + Ab3
Foon et al.	Melanoma Anti-GD2	47	PR	2000	Increase survival in Ab3+ patients
McCaffrey et al.	Melanoma BEC2 (Anti-GD3)	20	Possible survival advantage	1996	Increase Ab1' in 3/14

Ab, antibody; CTL, cytotoxic T lymphocyte; PR, partial response

Table 9.6   Isotopes used in radioimmunotherapy and radioimmunoscintigraphy

Radionuclide	Particles Emitted	Half-life	Common Usage	Disadvantages
^{67}Cu	Beta, gamma	6.2 hours	RIT, also images	Scarce
^{177}Lu	Beta, gamma	6.7 days	RIT, also images	Scarce, seeks bone
^{131}I	Beta, gamma	8.0 days	RIT	Radiation safety concerns
^{125}I	Electron capture	60 days	RIT	Does not image, very long half-life
^{90}Y	Beta	64 hours	RIT	Does not image well, seeks bone
^{111}In	Gamma		RIS	Liver seeking
^{99m}Tc	Gamma		RIS	Very short half-life

Cu, Copper; I, iodine; In, indium; Lu, Lutetium; RIS, radioscintigraphy; RIT, radioimmunotherapy; Tc, technetium; Y, yttrium.

Source: Adapted with permission from Wilder, R. B. 1996. Radioimmunotherapy: Recent results and future directions. *Journal of Clinical Oncology* 14(4): 1383–1400.

received regulatory approval for use in radioimmunodetection (RAID): satumomab pendetide for detection of colorectal and ovarian cancer, capromab pendetide for detection of prostate cancer, and anti-CEA Fab for the detection of colon cancer.

RADIOIMMUNOTHERAPY

Many antigens have heterogeneous distribution on tumor cells; therefore, one of the challenges in the treatment of solid tumors with MABs has been to devise immunotherapy that will treat antigen-positive and antigen-negative cells. The use of radiolabeled MABs may overcome this difficulty. This approach has been used in a variety of solid tumors. Dosimetry is an important component of RIT and is dependent on the kinetics of uptake and clearance of radiolabeled antibodies, the distribution of the radiolabeled antibodies, and the radioisotope attached to the antibody. To date, over 100 trials have evaluated this approach in both hematologic malignancies and solid tumors (Wilder *et al.*, 1996).

One example is CC49, a high-affinity anti-TAG-72 murine antibody that has been labeled with Lutetium-177 (^{177}Lu) and ^{131}I and that has

been tested in clinical trials. Phase I studies with ^{177}Lu-CC49 revealed the compound to have prolonged half-life *in vivo*, leading to unexpected bone marrow toxicity. No tumor responses were seen; however, this could possibly be related to the pharmacokinetic restrictions on the maximal dose of Lu given (Mulligan *et al.*, 1995). A phase II trial of ^{131}I-CC49 showed reversible grade 3 to 4 thrombocytopenia and granulocytopenia in over 40% of patients. Estimated tumor doses ranged from 19 to 667 rads; however, no tumor responses were observed with this trial. It was noted that over 60% of the patients treated with the radiolabeled antibody a second time had altered pharmacokinetics, with increased antibody clearance associated with the development of HAMA (Murray *et al.*, 1994). Investigators have attempted to increase efficacy of this antibody in several ways. Khazaeli *et al.* (1991) performed a phase I study with ^{131}I-chimeric B72.3 and demonstrated little if any HAMA response. CC49 has also been humanized to help decrease HAMA, and it is hoped that this will allow repeated administration of the antibody (Kashmiri *et al.*, 1995).

CC49 attached to ^{131}I has also been evaluated in patients with breast cancer. In a study reported by Macey *et al.* (1997), 15 women with breast cancer were randomized to receive daily injections of recombinant interferon (rIFN)-α 3 × 10⁶ U/m² for 14 days beginning on day 1 (group 1 = 7 patients) or on day 6 (group 2 = 8 patients). On day 3, all patients received a 10 to 20 mCi tracer dose of ¹³¹I-CC49, a high-affinity murine MAB reactive against TAG-72, followed by a therapeutic dose of 60 to 75 mCi/m² of ¹³¹I-CC49 on day 6. Preclinical studies have demonstrated that rIFN-α can enhance the TAG-72 on tumors. Whole-body and single-photon-emission computed tomography (CT) scans along with whole-blood pharmacokinetics were performed following the tracer and therapeutic phases. Hematological toxicity was considerable: reversible grade 3 to 4 neutropenia and thrombocytopenia were observed in 12 of 15 patients. Twelve of 14 patients tested developed HAMA 3 to 6 weeks after treatment. Treatment with rIFN-α was found to enhance TAG-72 expression in tumors from patients receiving rIFN-α (group 1) by 46 ± 19% ($p <$ .05) compared with only 1.3 ± 0.95% in patients not initially receiving IFN (group 2). The uptake of CC49 in tumors was also significantly increased in rIFN-α-treated patients. One partial and 2 minor tumor responses were seen. In summary, rIFN-α treatment altered the pharmacokinetics and tumor uptake of ¹³¹I-CC49 in patients at the expense of increased toxicity (Macey *et al.*, 1997).

The TAG-72 antigen is also expressed in ovarian cancer. A phase I study using the murine MAB B72.3 tagged with yttrium-90 (⁹⁰Y) as peritoneal therapy for ovarian cancer has been reported. The maximum tolerated dose was determined to be 10 mCi of yttrium because of hematological toxicity and platelet suppression, which typically occurred on day 29 following the initial infusion. EDTA administration was used as a pretreatment to suppress bone uptake and decrease myelosuppression. This approach allowed for escalation of the dose

to 40 mCi, with dose-limiting thrombocytopenia and neutropenia. Four responses were noted in patients who received between 15 and 30 mCi of ⁹⁰Y-labeled B72.3, with durations of 1 to 2 months. The authors concluded that further study, especially in patients with minimal residual disease after standard chemotherapy or for the palliation of refractory ascites, is warranted (Rosenblum *et al.*, 1999).

Taking advantage of the intracellular antigen location, a compound combining Po66 and ¹³¹I was engineered and tested in laboratory animals as monotherapy and in combination with chemotherapy. It was discovered that most of the antibody was bound in necrotic cells, making ¹³¹I therapy less effective for large tumors, where some cells could escape beta emissions. Researchers found, however, that administration of fractionated doses of radiolabeled antibody in combination with chemotherapy provided significant cytotoxicity against tumors and prolonged survival. They proposed that doxorubicin further enhanced the ability of ¹³¹I to be taken into cells, thereby enhancing kill in more viable tumor tissue (Desrues *et al.*, 1996). Their findings provide insight into newer possible avenues to explore in antibody therapy of solid tumors to enhance standard and novel treatment applications.

L6 was labeled with ¹³¹I and administered to heavily pretreated patients with metastatic breast cancer to evaluate the possible synergy of antibody-induced inflammatory response and radiation. Six of 10 patients did have objective tumor responses (minor response or better) with therapy, and 5 of 10 patients had responses lasting longer than 1 month. Toxicity was primarily hematologic, with temporary grade 3 to 4 neutropenia and thrombocytopenia seen in 90% of patients. HAMA occurred in 80% of the patients, despite the use of the chimeric form of L6 (DeNardo *et al.*, 1997). The ability of this modality to induce clinical response in patients failing standard therapy is encouraging.

Additional work to modify this antibody might provide greater benefits in the future.

In summary, the use of RIT for solid tumors has demonstrated only occasional responses, and these have not been persistent. One of the major obstacles remains hematopoietic toxicity, primarily thrombocytopenia. This limits the ability to provide sufficient doses of radiation for curative treatment of solid tumors. The number of clinical trials exploring this approach will continue to increase and will integrate the use of alternative isotopes and new generations of antibodies to improve tumor deposition and reduce nonspecific targeting of normal tissues.

RADIOIMMUNOGUIDED SURGERY

RIGS is an intraoperative procedure for the detection of carcinoma lesions that are targeted with a radiolabeled MAB to provide the surgeon with immediate intraoperative definition of tumor margins and identification of occult disease. This approach is based on the tissue characteristics, the radioactive tracer and its carrying molecule, or the affinity of both and represents the addition of an exciting new tool to the inspection and palpation traditionally used by the surgeon to determine the extent of disease. Current clinical applications for radioguided surgery are RIGS for detection of colon cancer; sentinel-node mapping for malignant melanoma (which has become state-of-the-art); sentinel-node mapping for breast, vulvar, and penile cancer; and detection of parathyroid adenoma and bone tumor (such as osteoid osteoma). Although the same gamma-detecting probe may be used for all these applications, the carrier substance and the radionuclide differ. As a carrier, MAB and peptides are used for RIGS, and sulphur colloid is used for sentinel-node mapping. The radionuclides used include iodine-125 for RIGS and technetium-99m (^{99m}Tc) for sentinel node, parathyroid, and bone. The mode of injection also differs, but

there are some common principles of gamma-guided surgery.

RIGS enables the surgeon to corroborate tumor existence, find occult metastases, and assess the margins of resection. This may result in a change in the surgical plan. The RIGS system works by injecting a low-level, radioactive, cancer-specific targeting agent into a cancer patient before surgery. The study generally uses a radiolabeled antibody fragment. During the operation, the surgeon uses a hand-held gamma-radiation-detecting probe to lactate diseased tissue that contains a significant amount of the radioisotope. Sentinel lymph-node scintigraphy for melanoma guides the surgeon to find the involved lymph nodes for lymph node dissection. Sentinel lymph node scintigraphy for breast cancer is being investigated, with promising results. This procedure has also changed the outlook of lymph node pathology by giving the pathologist designated tissue samples for more comprehensive examination. Gamma-guided surgery will result in more accurate and fewer unnecessary surgeries, better pathology, and, possibly, better patient survival (Bakalakos and Burak, 1999; Schneebaum et al., 1999).

A recent study evaluated the combination of radioimmunoscintigraphy and RIGS in patients with colorectal carcinoma. Twenty-nine patients (18 primary tumors, 10 with a suspicion of recurrence) received an injection of anti-TAG-72 MAB (CT-103) labeled with ^{111}In and were scanned at 48 and 72 hours after injection. RIGS was performed between 72 and 96 hours after injection by systematic screening with a hand-held gamma-detecting probe. A surgical index (tumor-to-normal tissue) was obtained. There were statistically significant differences between counts in normal tissue versus tumor, and RIGS was considered positive for the detection of tumor if the ratio between the counts in the area suspicious for tumor and the counts in the normal tissue was greater than 1.5. This study concluded that RIGS, as a complementary technique to radioimmunoscintigraphy, was particularly useful in detecting recurrences and was of benefit to surgeons in the resection of small tumor deposits, which are difficult to localize (Muxi *et al.*, 1999).

RADIOIMMUNODETECTION

RAID, also known as radioimmunoscintigraphy (RIS), involves the attachment of low-dose radioisotopes to MABs for the purpose of imaging tumor deposits. Once patients are dosed with the radiolabeled MABs, detection of tumors occurs by scanning with a gamma camera. In many instances, radiolabeled MABs are able to locate occult disease that is missed by more conventional scans such as magnetic resonance imaging (MRI) and CT. As of July 2000, 2 MABs and 1 MAB fragment had received regulatory approval for this indication.

The first antibody to receive regulatory approval for the detection of disease was MAB B72.3, which is used to diagnose colorectal and ovarian cancers. Satumomab pendetide is a conjugate produced from the murine MAB CYT-099 (MAB B72.3). MAB B72.3 is a murine MAB directed to TAG-72, a high-molecular-weight, tumor-associated glycoprotein expressed differentially by adenocarcinomas. *In vitro* diagnostic studies have demonstrated that MAB B72.3 is reactive with about 83% of colorectal adenocarcinomas; 97% of common epithelial ovarian carcinomas; and the majority of breast, non-small-cell lung, pancreatic, gastric, and esophageal cancers evaluated.

[111]In-labeled satumomab pendetide (Onco-Scint® CR/OV-In) is a diagnostic imaging agent that is indicated for determining the extent and location of extrahepatic malignant disease in patients with known colorectal or ovarian cancer. Clinical studies suggest that this imaging agent should be used after completion of standard diagnostic tests when additional information regarding disease extent could aid in patient management. The diagnostic images acquired with OncoScint CR/OV-In should be interpreted in conjunction with a review of information obtained from other appropriate tests. OncoScint CR/OV-In is also indicated for readministration to HAMA-negative patients who are at risk of recurrence. It is important to remember that the negative predictive value of an OncoScint CR/OV-In scan is 19% in colorectal cancer patients and 29% in recurrent ovarian cancer patients. Therefore, a negative antibody scan result is not informative about disease, and negative scan results should not be used to guide clinical practice.

The safety and imaging efficacy of OncoScint CR/OV-In were evaluated in patients with colorectal ($n = 192$) and ovarian ($n = 103$) cancer who received a single 1-mg intravenous dose. These clinical trials were performed in presurgical patients so that scan results could be scored positive or negative based on tissue confirmation of disease at the site of the lesion shown on the scan. Using this approach, OncoScint images detected disease in approximately 69% of patients with surgically confirmed colorectal or ovarian cancer; sensitivity was higher for extrahepatic lesions (71%) than for liver lesions (43%). Although a threshold for detection of disease based on lesion size has not been determined, clinical trial results suggest that there is a correlation between the size of tumor deposits and the probability of detection with OncoScint CR/OV-In.

Current trials continue to evaluate RIS in colorectal cancer by using [99mTc] antibody fragments and human MABs to achieve improvement in imaging efficacy and repeated or serial imaging and a significant further improvement in the accuracy of clinical decision making in oncology patients (Moffat *et al.*, 1999).

Arcitumomab labeled with [99mTc] pertechnetate (CEA-Scan®) was approved to assess the extent and location of disease in patients with colorectal cancer following a pivotal phase III trial conducted by the Immunomedics Study Group (Moffatt *et al.*, 1996). CEA-Scan, an anti-CEA Fab antibody fragment labeled with ^{99m}Tc was injected intravenously into 210 patients with advanced recurrent or metastatic colorectal carcinomas before they underwent surgery. External scintigraphy was performed 2 to 5 and 18 to 24 hours later. Imaging with conventional diagnostic modalities (CDM) was also performed, and findings were confirmed by surgery and histology. Potential clinical benefit from arcitumomab was demonstrated in 89 of 210 patients. Only 2 patients developed HAMA to CEA-Scan after a single injection. The sensitivity of CEA-Scan was superior to that of CDM in the extrahepatic abdomen (55% versus 32%; $p = .007$) and pelvis (69% versus 48%; $p = .005$), and CEA-Scan findings complemented those of CDM in the liver. This trial led to the regulatory approval of this agent for imaging disease in patients with colorectal cancer.

Prostate-specific membrane antigen (PSMA) is expressed in many primary and metastatic prostate cancer lesions. *In vitro* immunohistologic studies have shown the MAB 7E11-C5.3, targeted toward PSMA, to be reactive with over 95% of the prostate adenocarcinomas evaluated. In addition, the 7E11-C5.3 antibody is also immunoreactive with normal and hypertrophic adult prostate tissue. ^{111}In-labeled capromab pendetide (ProstaScint®) has been administered in single doses to over 600 patients in clinical studies and in repeat administrations (2 to 4 infusions) to 61 patients. A 0.5-mg dose was determined to be the lowest effective dose. The imaging performance of ProstaScint was evaluated in a phase II and a phase III trial in each of 2 clinical settings: (1) patients with clinically localized prostate cancer who were at high risk for metastases and (2) patients with a high clinical suspicion for occult recurrent or residual prostate cancer.

In clinical studies of patients with prostate cancer, ProstaScint localized to the prostate and some known primary and metastatic tumor sites. In 1 of 2 open-label, pivotal phase III trials, 160 patients with a tissue diagnosis of prostate cancer who were considered at high risk for lymph node metastasis underwent ^{111}In ProstaScint immunoscintigraphy prior to scheduled pelvic lymphadenectomy. High risk was defined as at least one of the following: (1) prostate specific antigen (PSA) 10 times the upper limit of normal and Gleason score 7, (2) prostatic acid phosphatase above the upper limit of normal, (3) equivocal evidence of lymph node metastases on CT or ultrasound and PSA 8 times the upper limit of normal, (4) Gleason score 8, or (5) clinical stage C and Gleason score 6. All patients had been evaluated for metastatic disease using standard noninvasive imaging techniques and were considered to have clinically localized prostate cancer. The ProstaScint images were interpreted onsite, and the reader had access to all clinical data. The interpretations were correlated with the results of surgical staging; however, a correlation of specific areas of ^{111}In ProstaScint uptake to specific sites of tumor involvement was not performed. ProstaScint proved effective in localizing to deposits of tumor in the lymph nodes (Manyak *et al.*, 1999).

In the second open-label, pivotal phase III trial, 183 patients with a high clinical suspicion of residual or recurrent prostate cancer following radical prostatectomy were evaluated. Patients with a rising PSA, a negative bone scan, and negative or equivocal standard diagnostic techniques (e.g., transrectal ultrasound, CT scan, or MRI) underwent ^{111}In ProstaScint immunoscintigraphy prior to biopsy of the prostatic fossa. ^{111}In ProstaScint images were interpreted onsite, and the reader had access to all clinical data. The interpretations were correlated with the results of histopathologic analysis of the prostatic fossa biopsy specimens. One hundred fifty-eight patients had an interpretable scan and prostatic fossa biopsy. Twenty-nine scans were classified as true positive, 29 as false positive, 70 as true negative, and 30 as false negative (Kahn *et al.*, 1998).

ProstaScint received regulatory approval in October 1996 for use as a diagnostic imaging agent in newly diagnosed patients with biopsy-proven prostate cancer thought to be clinically localized after standard diagnostic evaluation (e.g., chest x-ray, bone scan, CT scan, or MRI), who are at high risk for pelvic lymph node metastases. ProstaScint is also indicated as a diagnostic imaging agent in postprostatectomy patients with a rising PSA and a negative or equivocal standard metastatic evaluation in whom there is a high clinical suspicion of occult metastatic disease. A retrospective study published by Murphy *et al.* (2000) was done to evaluate the ability of ProstaScint scan to detect prostatic bed recurrence and metastases to regional and distant lymph nodes. One hundred sequential patients were evaluated with repeated ProstaScint scans because of evidence of recurrence during the course of their disease. These 100 patients were followed closely from November 1994 and April 1999 and had concurrent bone scans and serum PSA evaluations. The patients had received initial treatment ranging from hormone therapy to radical prostatectomy or radiation therapy. In each patient, the uptake of the follow-up scan or scans was compared with that of the initial scan. There were 257 scans representing 100 patients. All patients had at least 2 scans, 35 patients had 3 scans, and 11 patients had 4 scans. No individual exhibited detectable adverse clinical reactions during or after the scan. The authors concluded that the consistency on repeating the scan (79%) and the high percentage of patients showing persistent uptake at the prostate bed (43%) as well as the percentage of detection of regional nodes (20%) and distant nodes (32%) reflect the importance of using the ProstaScint scan in finding occult recurrences after primary treatment failure of prostate cancer.

Basic and clinical research currently in progress promises to yield agents and methods that provide rapid high-resolution imaging, high tumor-to-background ratios in all organs at risk for tumor recurrence or metastasis, negligible immunogenicity and toxicity, and a significant further improvement in the accuracy of clinical decision making in oncology patients.

Immunotoxins

Immunotoxins are a class of targeted therapeutic agents under development by many research groups. Immunotoxins are actually hybrid proteins in which the potent cytocidal action of a toxin is harnessed for the selective destruction of target cells by attachment to a specific MAB or growth factor such as IL-2 (see Chapter 22). Highly potent peptide toxins that catalytically inactivate protein synthesis have been linked both chemically and genetically to these ligands to produce this new class of cancer therapeutic agents. Examples of toxins under clinical investigation include diphtheria, *Pseudomonas exotoxin,* ricin, and gelonin. To date, this approach remains highly investigational, with trials having been performed in patients with breast cancer, ovarian cancer, colorectal cancer, melanoma, and lymphoproliferative disorders (Weiner, 1999). The following is a brief review of several MAB toxin studies.

N901 is an antibody directed against the NKH1 antigen (CD56). In addition to being found on several malignancies, this antigen is found on selected lymphocytes, peripheral nerve tissue, myocardium, and skeletal muscle. N901 has some modest activity in experiments with laboratory animals and was combined with the toxin ricin to help increase cytotoxicity.

Phase I studies evaluating N901-bR (antibody-ricin) immunotoxin revealed some biological evidence of activity in patients with SCLC, including one patient with a partial response and 6 patients with stable disease (Lynch *et al.*, 1997). Although the responses are encouraging, toxicities, including cardiac toxicity (atrial fibrillation in one patient and myocardial infarctions in 2 patients), capillary leak syndrome, and hypotension will require continued investigation for improved methods to target this antigen.

Immunotoxin LMB-1 is composed of MAB B3 chemically linked to PE38, a genetically engineered form of *Pseudomonas exotoxin.* B3 recognizes the carbohydrate antigen Lewis(y) or Le(y), which is present on many human solid tumors. Pai and colleagues (1996) conducted a phase I study of 38 patients with solid tumors who failed conventional therapy and whose tumors expressed the Le(y) antigen. Objective antitumor activity was observed in 5 patients, 18 had stable disease, and 15 progressed. A complete remission was observed in a patient with breast cancer that had metastasized to supraclavicular nodes. A greater than 75% tumor reduction and resolution of all clinical symptoms lasting for more than 6 months was observed in a patient with colon cancer with extensive retroperitoneal and cervical metastasis. Three patients (2 colon cancer, 1 breast cancer) had minor responses. The maximum tolerated dose of LMB-1 is 75 mcg/kg given intravenously 3 times every other day. The major toxicity is vascular leak syndrome manifested by hypoalbuminemia, fluid retention, hypotension, and, in one case, pulmonary edema. This was the first report of antitumor activity in epithelial tumors (Pai *et al.*, 1996).

BR96 sFv-PE40 is a recombinant DNA-derived fusion protein composed of the heavy- and light-chain variable-region domains of the MAB BR96 and the translocation and catalytic domains of *Pseudomonas exotoxin* A, which is being developed for the treatment of solid tumors expressing cell surface Le(y)-related antigens. It is hoped that the use of a smaller antibody fragment will decrease the problem of immunogenicity. Single- and repeat-dose intravenous toxicity studies in rats and dogs and a comparative *ex vivo* tissue-binding study with rat, dog, and human tissues were conducted to assess the toxicity of BR96 sFv-PE40 and to estimate a safe starting dose in humans. In rats, vascular leak syndrome was primarily confined to the lungs; in dogs, however, the primary toxicity was seen in the pancreas (Haggerty *et al.*, 1999).

Chemoimmunoconjugates

Antibodies can be internalized by target cells, making them ideal candidates for delivery of toxins. A key hurdle to overcome in the use of chemoimmunoconjugates has been the design of stable conjugates that will not release free drug (i.e., chemotherapy) into the circulation yet will release the drug inside the cell, where the MAB conjugate is internalized and degraded. *In vitro* and *in vivo* lab experiments with a BR96-doxorubicin conjugate were found to cure athymic mice and rats of xenografted lung, breast, and colon cancers. This conjugate was seen to bind to normal tissues of the gastrointestinal tract in rats; however, it was not associated with significant toxicities (Trail *et al.*, 1993). This immunoconjugate was tested in humans in a phase II trial published in 1999 (Tolcher *et al.*, 1999). BR96-doxorubicin immunoconjugate is a chimeric human/mouse MAB linked to approximately 8 doxorubicin molecules. The antibody is directed against the Le(y) antigen, which is expressed on 75% of all breast cancers but is limited in expression on normal tissues. Patients with metastatic breast cancer were randomly assigned to receive either monotherapy with doxorubicin or the immunoconjugate. There was unfortunately little clinical activity seen (1 partial response) with the BR96-doxorubicin conjugate, and this group developed significant gastrointestinal toxicities.

Future approaches will be the development of stronger cytotoxic agents that can be linked to the MAB. These agents, although too toxic for use as free drug, are perfect for use as chemoimmunoconjugates. Substances under development include the enediynes, maytansinoids, tricothecenes, and analogues of CC-1065. Calicheamicin, a member of the enediynes, has been conjugated to an anti-PEM antibody (CTM01, carcinoma-associated antigen, the *MUC1* gene product) and has shown curative effect against established breast and ovarian tumor xenografts in nude mice (King, 1998). Clinical trials are now under way with a conjugate of humanized CTM01-calicheamicin in patients with ovarian cancer (Kaye *et al.*, 1999).

Adverse Effects

For a review of the toxic effects seen with MABs, see Chapter 8. Toxicity with MABs in solid tumors may be broadly classified as allergic or nonallergic in nature and relate to several factors. The first is the derivation of the antibody. Allergic reactions are more likely to be seen in patients receiving murine antibodies. Because of the problem of HAMA production with repeated infusions, the risk for allergic reactions increases. Allergic reactions may be immediate or delayed. Immediate reactions may manifest from mild hives or rash with itching to allergic shock and anaphylaxis, where the patient experiences hypotension, bronchospasm, swelling of the throat or lips, shortness of breath, skin erythema, and circulatory and/or pulmonary collapse. With the introduction of chimeric or humanized MABs, allergic reactions and repeated infusions have been less problematic. Dermatologic symptoms alone may resolve without treatment or with diphen-

hydramine. For more severe reactions, the use of corticosteroids, epinephrine, or both may be required.

Delayed allergic reactions may also be seen. Immune complex complications (serum sickness) related to HAMA have, fortunately, been rare. This complication may manifest as fever, malaise, arthralgias/arthritis, myalgias, maculopapular erythematous skin rash, and fatigue and may occur 2 to 3 weeks following an infusion. Rarely, proteinuria may be observed. Serum sickness can be managed with nonsteroidal, anti-inflammatory agents and corticosteroids in more severe cases.

Patients may experience an infusion-associated symptom complex most commonly consisting of chills and fever and primarily observed with the first infusion. The symptoms may be managed by premedication with diphenhydramine, acetaminophen, or both and a decrease in the infusion rate. This is more commonly seen when MABs are used in patients with hematologic malignancies, as the MAB reacts with circulating cells and causes a release of cytokines when cells are destroyed. This may also be seen in patients with solid tumors who receive MABs that work by inciting ADCC or complement-dependent cytotoxicity. Other side effects may include gastrointestinal disturbance (e.g., nausea and vomiting), headache, and pain at the tumor site.

On occasion, unexpected toxicity may occur due to cross-reactivity with normal tissues. For example, in MABs targeted toward the GD_2 ganglioside, patients in clinical trials experienced severe pain during the infusion that resolved quickly when the infusion was completed. Rarely, patients developed postural hypotension. It has been hypothesized that this toxicity resulted from the MAB cross-reacting with the autonomic nervous system.

Toxicity may also result when different substances are attached to the MAB. As previously noted, radioisotopes cause hematopoietic toxicity, primarily thrombocytopenia. Immuno-toxins cause a vascular leak-type syndrome consisting of hypotension, weight gain, hypoal-buminemia, fevers, rigors, malaise, and rare but potentially devastating central nervous system effects. With the chemoimmunoconjugate BR96-doxorubicin, gastritis was the primary toxic effect and was felt to result from cross-reactivity to the gastrointestinal mucosa. If the conjugate were to become disassociated, the toxicity normally seen with the chemotherapuetic agent may be seen (Dillman, 1998).

In May 2000, a letter from Genentech Inc. (South San Francisco, CA) was sent to physicians reporting the adverse events associated with trastuzumab therapy, which included hypersensitivity reactions, infusion reactions, and pulmonary events. At that time, 15 deaths had been associated with trastuzumab therapy, and of those deaths, 9 occurred within 24 hours of the infusion. New product labels on trastuzumab packaging will include adverse reactions, warnings about hypersensitivity reactions, including fatal anaphylaxis; infusion reactions, including some with a fatal outcome; and pulmonary events, including adult respiratory distress syndrome and death. It is important to note that since the approval of trastuzumab in September of 1998, over 25,000 women have been treated. Most patients who died had significant preexisting pulmonary compromise secondary to intrinsic lung disease or malignant pulmonary involvement. Hence, it is important to include pulmonary assessment as part of the pretreatment workup for trastuzumab therapy.

The Use of MABs Outside of Cancer

As the field of biotherapy has progressed, its use as therapy in a variety of diseases has been investigated (see Chapter 22). Many MABs have now received regulatory approval for uses outside of cancer, primarily the treatment of

rejection episodes in solid organ transplantation and autoimmune diseases. The following is a brief review of approved agents or those that have received intensive investigation.

Infliximab (Remicade®; Centocor, Malvern, PA), a chimeric MAB to tumor necrosis factor-α (TNF-α), is approved for the treatment of Crohn's disease. Crohn's disease is a chronic inflammatory bowel disease of unknown cause that is characterized by segmental transmural inflammation and granulomatous lesions of the intestinal mucosa. The disease is complicated by the development of fistulas in approximately one third of patients. Fistulas are a complication and may be internal (e.g., bowel to bowel, bowel to bladder, or rectovaginal) or enterocutaneous (e.g., extending through the abdominal wall or into the perineum). The local production of TNF-α has been investigated as having a key role in the initiation and propagation of Crohn's disease. Strategies to neutralize TNF have therefore been actively investigated as treatment of Crohn's disease. In August 1998, infliximab received regulatory approval for use in relieving the symptoms in patients with moderately to severely active Crohn's disease who do not respond well to conventional therapies. The drug is indicated in patients with fistulizing Crohn's disease. The antibody is generally used as adjunctive therapy in patients who continue to receive corticosteroids, antibiotics, aminosalicylates, or other immunomodulators. In nonfistulizing patients, infliximab is used as a single infusion of 5 mg/kg. In clinical trials, about one half of nonfistulizing patients entered remission about 4 weeks after infliximab treatment. For fistulas, doses of 5 mg/kg are administered initially and at 2 and 6 weeks later. Therapy beyond these time periods has not been studied.

Infliximab is also being studied as treatment for rheumatoid arthritis (RA). In a 26-week, double-blind, placebo-controlled, multicenter trial, 101 patients with active RA exhibiting an incomplete response or flare of disease activity while receiving low-dose methotrexate were randomized to 1 of 7 groups of 14 to 15 patients each. The patients received either intravenous infliximab at 1, 3, or 10 mg/kg with or without methotrexate (7.5 mg/week) or intravenous placebo plus methotrexate 7.5 mg/week at weeks 0, 2, 6, 10, and 14; follow-up was done through week 26. Approximately 60% of patients receiving infliximab at 3 or 10 mg/kg with or without methotrexate achieved the 20% response based on Paulus criteria for median duration of 10.4 to more than 18.1 weeks ($p <$ .001 versus placebo). Multiple infusions of infliximab were effective and well tolerated, with the best results occurring at 3 and 10 mg/kg either alone or in combination with methotrexate in approximately 60% of patients with active RA despite therapy with low-dose methotrexate. When infliximab at 1 mg/kg was given with low-dose methotrexate, synergy was observed. The results of the trial provide a strategy for further evaluation of the efficacy and safety of long-term treatment with infliximab in RA (Maini *et al.*, 1998). On January 26, 1999, Centocor submitted a supplemental application to the FDA for infliximab to treat rheumatoid arthritis. This request was based on the results of a trial presented in San Diego in 1998 at the annual meeting of the American College of Rheumatology. A 30-week phase III RA trial with infliximab (the Anti-TNF Trial in Rheumatoid Arthritis with Concomitant Therapy [ATTRACT]) showed that infliximab reduced signs and symptoms of RA in 52% of patients receiving the drug compared with 20% of those on placebo *(http://www.centocor.com)*. In November 1999, Remicade, in conjunction with methotrexate, was approved for treatment of the signs and symptoms of RA in patients who have had an inadequate response to methotrexate.

Abciximab (ReoPro®, Centocor, Malvern, PA) is the Fab fragment of the chimeric human-murine MAB 7E3. Abciximab binds to the glycoprotein Iib/IIIa (a-IIbb-3) receptor of human platelets and inhibits platelet aggregation. Abciximab is effective in inhibiting blood clotting by inhibiting the aggregation of platelets. Anticoagulation agents such as abciximab are used in the treatment of cardiovascular disease to prevent blood clots. This antibody is currently used as adjunctive therapy to prevent cardiac ischemic complications in a broad range of patients undergoing percutaneous coronary intervention (PCI) as well as in patients with angina who are unstable and not responding to conventional medical therapy when PCI is planned within 24 hours. PCI includes balloon angioplasty, atherectomy, and stent placement. In the hallmark clinical trial, 2,009 patients treated at 56 centers received bolus and an infusion of placebo, a bolus of c7e3 Fab and an infusion of placebo, or a bolus and an infusion of c7E3 Fab. These patients were scheduled to undergo coronary angioplasty or atherectomy in high-risk clinical situations. The study end point was defined as any of the following: death, nonfatal myocardial infarction, unplanned surgical revascularization, unplanned repeat percutaneous procedure, unplanned implantation of a coronary stent, or insertion of an intra-aortic balloon pump for refractory ischemia. The use of the c7E3 Fab bolus and infusion resulted in a 35% reduction in the rate of the primary end point. The study concluded that ischemic complications of coronary angioplasty and atherectomy were reduced with the MAB. The primary toxic effect was an increased risk of bleeding (EPIC Study Group, 1994). Abciximab was cleared for marketing in the United States and Europe in December 1994.

A number of MABs have received regulatory approval for the treatment of rejection in organ transplantation. The first to receive such regulatory approval was OKT3, which has been used in the treatment of acute cell-mediated rejection in organ transplant. OKT3 is a murine MAB.

It has received regulatory approval for the treatment of acute organ rejection following renal transplant and in cardiac/hepatic allograft rejection for the treatment of steroid-resistant acute allograft rejection. The antibody reacts with a subunit of the surface antigen complex CD3 on human T cells and removes the antigen-bearing T cells from circulation, rendering them ineffective in mounting an immune response (Goldstein, 1987). The side effects seen in this setting are similar to those observed with patients being treated for malignancies. Fever, chills, nausea, vomiting, and diarrhea are not uncommon (Farrell, 1987; Moir, 1989). Adverse reactions are more typical during the first hour of infusion and less frequent with the second and third doses. As with the early antibody trials in malignancy, pulmonary edema has also been observed. Ensuring that the patient was not in fluid overload prior to treatment helped lessen this side effect (Moir, 1989). Generalized aches and malaise are also common symptoms. Because this MAB suppresses the immune system, patients receiving this form of treatment are at risk for bacterial, fungal, and viral infections. Fevers may not always be a reaction to the antibody but may herald an infection (Moir, 1989). The development of HAMA is problematic with this antibody; thus, current research has focused on the development of humanized forms.

Daclizumab (Zenapax®; Roche Laboratories, Nutley, NJ) received regulatory approval in December 1997 as a prophylaxis for organ rejection in patients receiving renal transplant. It is generally used as part of an immunosuppressive regimen that includes cyclosporin and corticosteroids. Daclizumab is a humanized MAB that reacts with the alpha subunit of the IL-2 receptor (CD25). This receptor is expressed in high concentration on the surface of activated T lymphocytes. The MAB thus inhibits IL-2-mediated activation of lympho-

cytes, a critical pathway in the cellular immune response involved in allograft rejection. Two well-controlled randomized trials led to the approval of daclizumab. In general, the MAB was well tolerated, with the most commonly reported adverse effects being gastrointestinal in nature. Patients complained of constipation, nausea, diarrhea, and abdominal pain. Also, the incidence of infections in patients who were receiving daclizumab generally was not higher than that in patients who were receiving placebo (Waldmann and O'Shea, 1998).

A third MAB also has regulatory approval for use in organ transplantation. Basiliximab (Simulect®; Novartis, East Hanover, NJ) has regulatory approval as a prophylaxis of acute organ rejection in patients receiving renal transplantation when used as part of an immunosuppressive regimen that includes cyclosporine and corticosteroids. A chimeric MAB, basiliximab specifically binds the alpha subunit of the IL-2 receptor on activated T lymphocytes. Hours after a single 2.5- to 25-mg intravenous dose of basiliximab, approximately 90% of available IL-2 receptors on T lymphocytes were complexed with the drug. This level of basiliximab binding was maintained for 4 to 6 weeks when patients receiving renal transplant received 20 mg of basiliximab 2 hours before and then 4 days after transplantation surgery. In 2 large, well-designed trials, the percentage of patients with biopsy-confirmed acute rejection episodes after renal transplantation was significantly lower with 20 mg of basiliximab administered 2 hours before and then 4 days after transplantation surgery (30% and 33%, respectively) than placebo (44% and 46%, respectively) at 6 months after surgery. Basiliximab was well tolerated during clinical trials. The incidence of infections (including active cytomegalovirus infection) and posttransplant lymphoproliferative disorders was similar with basiliximab and placebo. Cytokine-release syndrome was not observed in patients who received basiliximab (Onrust and Wiseman, 1999).

Palivizumab (Synagis™; MedImmune, Inc., Gaithersburg, MD) is a humanized MAB produced by recombinant DNA technology that is directed toward the respiratory syncytial virus (RSV). It is used as prophylaxis for serious lower-respiratory-tract disease caused by the RSV in pediatric patients at high risk for RSV. In a large multicenter trial, palivizumab given intramuscularly at 15 mg/kg more than halved the incidence of RSV-attributable hospitalization in 1,502 infants at high risk for RSV infection from 4.8% compared with 10.6% in placebo recipients. In the same group of high-risk infants, palivizumab significantly decreased total days in the hospital attributable to RSV infection, days with increased supplemental oxygen requirement, days with moderate to severe lower-respiratory-tract infections, and the incidence of admissions to the intensive care unit. However, the drug had no effect on the incidence or total number of days of ventilation. Palivizumab was well tolerated during clinical trials in infants at risk for RSV infection. The incidence of adverse events was similar in the placebo (10%) and palivizumab (11%) groups. Fever, irritability, and injection-site reaction were the most commonly reported adverse events (Scott and Lamb, 1999).

The use of MABs for the treatment of septic shock has been extensively studied. Bacterial sepsis is a clinical syndrome associated with severe bacterial infection from a wide variety of conditions. Once infected, bacterial products such as the cell-wall component lipopolysaccharide (endotoxin) elicit an inflammatory response that results in activation of an array of host defense systems and the release of a complex series of inflammatory mediators. These mediators include such cytokines as TNF and IL-1. In conjunction with the bacterial prod-

ucts, overactivation of these systems can lead to shock, organ failure, and death. Thus, significant research efforts have been targeted toward developing antibodies to endotoxin or to mediator cytokines such as TNF and IL-1. Several antibodies (e.g., murine IgM E5 and human IgM HA-1A) targeted toward lipid A have been developed. Both of these antibodies have demonstrated improved survival in animal models and progressed to large-scale clinical trials. In each case, although initial trials showed positive results, subsequent trials were unable to substantiate the initial successes in either E5 (Bone et al., 1995) or HA-1A (Natanson et al., 1994). HA-1A did appear effective in reducing the mortality rate in patients dying from endotoxemia but not in those with septic shock (McCloskey et al., 1994). A comprehensive review of these studies by Quezado et al. (1995) discussed the variability of the results. Quezado and colleagues contend that perhaps in the future a better understanding of sepsis will lead to the development of both laboratory and clinical predictors that will identify when and which patients may benefit from such therapy.

Regulatory Approvals

As of July 2000, one MAB has received regulatory approval for use in the treatment of solid tumors. Trastuzumab was approved in the fall of 1998 for the treatment of patients with metastatic breast cancer whose tumors overexpress the HER-2 protein. Three MABs have regulatory approval for the detection of cancer when attached to a low-dose radioisotope: OncoScint is approved for the detection of disease in patients with colorectal or ovarian cancers, CEA-Scan is approved for the detection of disease in patients with colorectal cancer, and ProstaScint is approved for the detection of prostate cancer.

Future Directions

In reviewing the studies above, it appears that MABs demonstrate considerable promise in specific diseases and under special circumstances. Antibody therapy has rapidly grown from the theoretical idea of cancer's "magic bullet" to active therapy that is making a difference in patients' lives. The examples of the changing vision of antibody therapy described here are only a small picture of the possibilities being explored in clinics and laboratories. Historically, antibody therapy of solid tumors has met with limited success. Studies were often restricted to patients with overwhelming, end-stage disease. It is possible that multiple—rather than single—dose antibody therapy will help improve results. Earlier trials also encountered limitations in repeated therapy because of unwanted immune responses such as HAMA. In addition, the goal of antibody therapy for solid tumors has been similar to that of conventional chemotherapy: effective cytoreduction of established tumors to obtain cure. Although this goal should continue to help shape our investigations, new paradigms of treatment should also be used.

These new paradigms include the idea that manipulation of cellular interactions or pathways, such as the work with growth factor receptors, can lead to tumor stabilization and eventually cytoreduction as cell turnover occurs. Use of antibodies as adjuvant therapy for solid tumors could also help increase their efficacy by limiting the volume of disease the antibody and immune system must fight. Combining traditional therapy (radiation therapy and chemotherapy) with antibody therapy can lead to increased efficacy, as seen in several of the examples cited above. Also, as our knowledge of tumor antigens (with their role in inter- and intracellular function), the immune system, and the mechanisms of tumorgenicity grows, new targets for therapy will arise. For example, anti-

bodies developed to directly block angiogenesis are already under investigation (Schlaeppi *et al.*, 1999).

The rapid growth of molecular techniques will permit the synthesis of novel single-chain antibodies (Bird *et al.*, 1998) as well as bifunctional constructs. For example, bivalent single-chain antibodies containing amino acid sequences for antibody-binding domains and cytokine domains can permit highly specific tumor targeting of the latter. The identification of MABs that bind to novel targets such as vascular endothelial growth factors (Ryan *et al.*, 1999) or antibodies that target necrotic tumors (Epstein *et al.*, 1988) are of interest. Finally, the route of administration (e.g., intratumoral or intraperitoneal) may be extremely important in allowing for a greater concentration of MABs in tumor. Trials of intraperitoneal ^{177}Lu- and ^{90}Y-labeled MABs in ovarian cancer patients with limited disease have shown promise (Meredith *et al.*, 1996; Rosenblum *et al.*, 1999), as have direct intratumoral injections of radiolabeled MABs in brain cancer (Brown *et al.*, 1996). Based on these novel approaches, the future of MAB therapy appears bright.

References

Aaronson, S. 1991. Growth factors and cancer. *Science* 254: 1146–1152.

Adkins, J., and Spencer, C. 1998. Edrecolomab (monoclonal antibody 17-1A). *Drugs* 56(4): 619–626.

Albain, K. S., Hortobagyi, G., Radvin, P., and Slamon, D. (eds). 1999. *HER2 Overexpression in Breast Cancer*. Monograph from Genentech Biooncology. Emeryville, CA: Genentech Biooncology, pp. 12, 14–16.

Albetini, M., Gan, J., Jaeger, P., *et al.* 1996. Systemic interleukin-2 modulates the anti-idiotypic response to chimeric anti-GD2 antibody in patients with melanoma. *Journal of Immunology* 19: 278–295.

Anasetti, C., Martin, P., Morishita, Y., *et al.* 1987. Human large granular lymphocytes express high affinity receptors for murine monoclonal antibodies of the IgG3 subclass. *Journal of Immunology* 138(9): 2979–2981.

Bajorin, D.F., Chapman, P. B., Wong, G., *et al.* 1990. Phase I evaluation of a combination of monoclonal antibody R24 and interleukin-2 in patients with metastatic melanoma. *Cancer Research* 50(23): 7490–7495.

Bakalakos, E., and Burak, W. 1999. The radioimmunoguided surgery (RIGS) system as a diagnostic tool. *Surgical Oncology Clinics of North America* 8(1): 129–144.

Ballare, C., Barrio, M., Portela, P., *et al.* 1995. Functional properties of FC-2.15, a monoclonal antibody that mediates human complement cytotoxicity against breast cancer cells. *Cancer Immunology Immunotherapy* 41: 15–22.

Baselga, J., and Mendelsohn, J. 1994. Receptor blockade with monoclonal antibodies as anticancer therapy. *Pharmacologic Therapy* 64(1): 127–154.

Baselga, J., Norton, L., Mendelsohn, J., *et al.* 1998. Recombinant humanized anti-HER2 antibody (Herceptin) enhances the antitumor activity of paclitaxel and doxorubicin against HER-2/*neu* overexpressing human breast cancer xenografts. *Cancer Research* 58: 2825–2831.

Baselga, J., Tripathy, T., Mendelsohn, J., *et al.* 1996. Phase II study of weekly intravenous recombinant humanized anti-p185HER2 monoclonal antibody in patients with HER2/neu overexpressing metastatic breast cancer. *Journal of Clinical Oncology* 14(3): 737–744.

Bast, R.C., Zalutsky, M., Kreitman, R., *et al.* 2000. Monoclonal serotherapy. In Bast, R.C., Kufe, D.W., Pollock, R.E., Weichselbaum, R.R., Holland, J.F., and Frei, E., III, (eds). *Cancer Medicine* 5th edn. Hamilton, Ontario: B.C. Decker, Inc., pp. 876-889.

Berchuck, A., Kamel, A., Whitaker, R., *et al.* 1990.

Overexpression of Her-2/neu is associated with poor survival in advanced epithelial ovarian cancer. *Cancer Research* 50(13): 4087–4091.

Bird, R., Hardman, K., Jacobson, J., *et al.* 1998. Single-chain antigen-binding proteins. *Science* 242: 423–426.

Blakey, D., Burke, P., Davies, D., *et al.* 1995. Antibody-directed enzyme prodrug therapy for treatment of major solid tumor disease. *Biochemical Society Transactions* 23: 1047–1050.

Bone, R., Balk, R., Fein, A., *et al.* 1995. A second large controlled clinical study of E5, a monoclonal antibody to endotoxin. *Critical Care Medicine* 23: 994–1006.

Braun, S., Janni, W., Hepp, F., *et al.* 1999. Monitoring of reduction of 17-1A expressing breast cancer micrometastases during antibody therapy with Edrecolomab—A pilot study. *Proceedings of the American Society of Clinical Oncology* 18: 448a (abstract 1728).

Brown, M., Coleman, R., Friedman, A., *et al.* 1996. Intrathecal 131I-labeled antitenascin monoclonal antibody 81C6 treatment of patients with leptomeningeal neoplasms or primary brain tumor resection cavities with subarachnoid communication: Phase I trial results. *Clinical Cancer Research* 2: 963–972.

Carlsson, J., Daniel-Szolgay, E., Frykholm, G., *et al.* 1989. Homogenous penetration but heterogeneous binding of antibodies to carcinoembryonic antigen in human colon carcinoma HT-29 spheroids. *Cancer Immunology Immunotherapy* 30(5): 269–276.

Carter, P., Presta, L., Gorman, C., *et al.* 1992. Humanization of an anti-p185HER2 antibody for human cancer therapy. *Proceedings of the National Academy of Sciences USA.* 89(10): 4285–4289.

Caulfield, M.J., Barna, B., Murthy, S., *et al.* 1990. Phase Ia-Ib trial of an anti-GD3 monoclonal antibody in combination with interferon-alpha in patients with malignant melanoma. *Journal of Biological Response Modifiers* 9(3): 319–328.

Chachoua, A., Oratz, R., Liebes, L., *et al.* 1994.

Phase Ib trial of granulocyte-macrophage colony-stimulating factor combined with massive monoclonal antibody R24 in patients with metastatic melanoma. *Journal of Immunotherapy and Emphasis on Tumor Immunology* 16(2): 132–141.

Cline, M., and Battifora, H. 1987. Abnormalities of proto-oncogenes in non-small-cell lung cancer. Correlations with tumor type and clinical characteristics. *Cancer* 61(5): 2669–2674.

Cobleigh, M., Vogel, C., Tripathy, D., *et al.* 1998. Efficacy and safety of Herceptin (humanized anti-HER2 antibody) as a single agent in 222 women with HER2 overexpression who had relapsed following chemotherapy for metastatic breast cancer. *Proceedings of the American Society of Clinical Oncology* 17: 97a (abstract 376).

Denardo, S., O'Grady, L., Richman, C., *et al.* 1997. Radioimmunotherapy for advanced breast cancer using I-131-ChL6 antibody. *Anticancer Research* 17(3B): 1745–1751.

Desrues, B., Brichory, F., Lena, H., *et al.* 1996. Treatment of human lung carcinoma xenografts with a combination of ^{131}I-labeled monoclonal antibody Po66 and doxorubicin. *Cancer Immunology and Immunotherapy* 43(5): 269–274.

Dillman, R. 1998. Antibody therapy. In Oldham, R. (ed). *Principles of Cancer Biotherapy*, 3rd edn. Boston: Kluwer Academic Press, pp. 284–317.

EPIC Study Group. 1994. Use of a monoclonal antibody directed against the platelet glycoprotein Iib/IIa receptor in high-risk coronary angioplasty. The EPIC Investigation. *The New England Journal of Medicine* 330: 956–961.

Epstein, A., Chen, F., and Taylor, C. 1988. A novel method for the detection of necrotic lesions in human cancers. *Cancer Research* 48: 5842–5848.

Ezekiel, M.P., Bonner, J.A., Robert, F., *et al.* 1999. Phase I trial of chimerized anti-epidermal growth factor receptor (anti-EGFR) antibody in combination with either once-daily or twice-daily irradiation for locally advanced head and neck malignancies. *Proceedings of the American Society of Clinical Oncology* 18: (abstract 1501).

Farrell, M. 1987. Orthoclone OKT 3: A treatment for acute renal allograft rejection. *ANNA Journal* 14: 373–376.

Fields, A., Nagy, A., Schwartzberg, L., *et al.* 1999. Edrecolomab (Panorex™, 17-1a antibody) alone or in combination with 5-FU based chemotherapy in adjuvant treatment of stage III colon cancer: A safety review. *Proceedings of the American Society of Clinical Oncology* 18: 435a (abstract 1676).

Foon, K., John, W., and Chakrabarty, M. 1997. Clinical and immune responses in advanced colorectal cancer patients treated with anti-idiotype monoclonal antibody vaccine that mimics the carcinoembryonic antigen. *Clinical Cancer Research* 3: 1267–1276.

Foon, K.A., Lutzky, J., Baral, R.N., *et al.* 2000. Clinical and immune responses in advanced melanoma patients immunized with an anti-idiotype antibody mimicking disialoganglioside GD2. *Journal of Clinical Oncology* 18(2): 376–384.

Foon, K., Yannelli, J., Bhattacharya-Chatterjee, M. 1999. Colorectal cancer as a model for immunotherapy. *Clinical Cancer Research* 5(2): 225–236.

Gilks, W., Stahel, R., Walker, N., *et al.* 1994. Statistical analysis of data from the third international IALSC workshop on lung tumor and differentiation antigens. *International Journal of Cancer* 8(suppl): 2–5.

Goldstein, G. 1987. Monoclonal antibody specificity: Orthoclone OKT3 T-cell blocker. *Nephron* 46(suppl) 1: 5–11.

Goodman, G., Hellstrom, I., Brodzinsky, L., *et al.* 1990. Phase I trial of murine monoclonal antibody L6 in breast, colon, ovarian, and lung cancer. *Journal of Clinical Oncology* 8(6): 1083–1092.

Goodman, G., Hellstrom, I., Yelton, D., *et al.* 1993. Phase I trial of chimeric (human-mouse) monoclonal antibody L6 in patients with non-small-cell lung, colon and breast cancer. *Cancer Immunology and Immunotherapy* 36(4): 267–273.

Gu, K., Mes-Masson, A., Gauthier, J., *et al.* 1996. Overexpression of her-2/neu in human prostate cancer and benign hyperplasia. *Cancer Letters* 99(2): 185–189.

Guadagni, F., Roselli, M., Cosimelli, M., *et al.* 1996. TAG-72 expression and its role in the biological evaluation of human colorectal cancer. *Anticancer Research* 16: 2141–2148.

Gunnett, K., Motzer, R., Amato, R., *et al.* 1999. Phase II study of anti-epidermal growth factor receptor antibody C225 alone in patients with metastatic renal cell carcinoma. *Proceedings of the American Society of Clinical Oncology* 18: 340a (abstract 1309).

Haggerty, H., Warner, W., Comereski, C., *et al.* 1999. BR96 sFv-PE40 immunotoxin: Nonclinical safety assessment. *Toxicology and Pathology* 27(1): 87–94.

Hellstrom, I., Beaumier, P., and Hellstrom, K. 1986. Antitumor effects of L6, an IgG2a antibody that reacts with most human carcinomas. *Proceedings of the National Academy of Sciences* 83: 7059–7063.

Herlyn, D., Wettendorff, M., Schmoll, E., *et al.* 1987. Anti-idiotype immunization of cancer patients modulation of the immune response. *Proceedings of the National Academy of Sciences USA* 84: 8055.

Houghton, A., Mintzer, D., Cordon-Cardo, C., *et al.* 1985. Mouse monoclonal IgG3 antibody detecting GD3 ganglioside: A phase I trial in patients with malignant melanoma. *Proceedings of the National Academy of Sciences USA* 82(4): 1242–1246.

Huang, S., Bock, J., and Harari, P. 1999. Epidermal growth factor receptor blockade with C225 modulates proliferation, apoptosis, and radiosensitivity in squamous cell carcinomas of the head and neck. *Cancer Research* 59(8): 1935–1940.

Ishizuka, H., Watananbe, M., Kubota, T., *et al.* 1998. Antitumor activity of murine monoclonal antibody NCC-ST-421 on human cancer cells by inducing apoptosis. *Anticancer Research* 18(4A): 2513–2518.

Jain, R., and Baxter, L. 1988. Mechanisms of heterogeneous distribution of monoclonal antibodies and other macromolecules in tumors: Significance of elevated interstitial pressure. *Cancer Research* 48: 7022–7031.

Johnson, B., and Kelley, M. 1998. Autocrine growth factors and neuroendocrine markers in the development of small-cell lung cancer. *Oncology* 12(1 suppl 2): 11–14.

Kahn, D., Williams, R.D., Manyak, M.J., *et al.* 1998. [111]Indium-capromab pendetide in the evaluation of patients with residual or recurrent prostate cancer after radical prostatectomy. The ProstaScint Study Group. *Urology* 159(6): 2041–2046.

Kallioniemi, O., Holli, K., Visakorpi, T., *et al.* 1991. Association of c-erbB-2 protein overexpression with high rate of cell proliferation, increased risk of visceral metastasis and poor long-term survival in breast cancer. *International Journal of Cancer* 49(5): 650–655.

Kashmiri, S., Shu, L., Padlan, E., *et al.* 1995. Generation, characterization, and in vivo studies of humanized anticarcinoma antibody CC49. *Hybridoma* 14(5): 461–473.

Kaye, S., Eisenhauer, E., and Hamilton, T. 1999. New non-cytotoxic approaches to ovarian cancer. *Annals of Oncology* 10(suppl 1): 65–68.

Khazaeli, M., Conry, R., and LoBuglio, A. 1994. Human immune response to monoclonal antibodies. *Journal of Immunology* 15(1): 42–52.

Khazaeli, M., Mansoor, N., Saleh, T., *et al.* 1991. Pharmacokinetics and immune response of ^{131}I-Chimeric mouse/human B72.3 (Human γ4) monoclonal antibody in humans. *Cancer Research* 51: 5461–5466.

King, D. 1998. Monoclonal antibodies in therapeutic applications. In King, D. (ed). *Applications and Engineering of Monoclonal Antibodies*. Philadelphia, PA: Taylor & Francis, pp. 119–159.

Köhler, G., and Milstein, C. 1975. Continuous culture of fused cells secreting antibody of predefined specificity. *Nature* 256: 495–497.

Kramer, E., Liebes, L., Wasserheit, C., *et al.* 1998. Initial clinical evaluation of radiolabeled MX-DTPA humanized BrE-3 antibody in patients with advanced breast cancer. *Clinical Cancer Research* 4(7): 1679–1688.

Kwak, L., Campbell, M., Czerwinsky, D., *et al.* 1992. Induction of immune responses in patients with

B-cell lymphoma against the surface-immuno-globulin idiotype expressed by their tumors. *The New England Journal of Medicine* 327: 1209–1215.

Lei, W., Mayotte, J., and Levitt, M. 1999. Enhancement of chemosensitivity and programmed cell death by tyrosine kinase inhibitors correlates with EGFR expression in non-small cell lung cancer cells. *Anticancer Research* 19(1A): 221–228.

Lynch, T., Lambert, J., Coral, F., *et al.* 1997. Immunotoxin therapy of small cell lung cancer: A phase I study of N901-blocked ricin. *Journal of Clinical Oncology* 15: 723–734.

Macey, D., Grant, E., Kasi, L., *et al.* 1997. Effect of recombinant alpha-interferon on pharmacokinetics, biodistribution, toxicity, and efficacy of ^{131}I-labeled monoclonal antibody CC49 in breast cancer: A phase II trial. *Clinical Cancer Research* 3(9): 1547–1555.

Maini, R., Breedveld, F., Kalden, J., *et al.* 1998. Therapeutic efficacy of multiple intravenous infusions of anti-tumor necrosis factor alpha monoclonal antibody combined with low-dose weekly methotrexate in rheumatoid arthritis. *Arthritis and Rheumatology* 41(9): 1552–1563.

Manyak, M. J., Hinkle, G. H., Olsen, J. O., *et al.* 1999. Immunoscintigraphy with Indium-111 capromab pendetide: Evaluation before definitive therapy in patients with prostate cancer. *Urology* 54(6): 1058–1063.

Martin, A., Pellen, P., Guitton, C., *et al.* 1989. Characterization of the antigen identified by Po66. A monoclonal antibody raised against a lung squamous cell carcinoma. *Cancer Immunology and Immunotherapy* 29(2): 118–124.

McCaffery, M., Yao, T., Williams, L., *et al.* 1996. Immunization of melanoma patients with BEC2 anti-idiotypic monoclonal antibody that mimics GD2 ganglioside: Enhanced immunogenicity when combined with adjuvant. *Clinical Cancer Research* 2: 679–686.

McCloskey, R., Straube, R., Sanders, C., *et al.* 1994. Treatment of septic shock with human monoclonal antibody HA-1A. A randomized, double-blind, placebo-controlled trial. CHESS Trail

Study Group. *Annals of Internal Medicine* 121(1): 1–5.

Meeker, T., Lowder, J., Maloney, D., *et al.* 1985. A clinical trial of anti-idiotype therapy for B cell malignancy. *Blood* 65: 1349–1363.

Mendelsohn, J., Shin, D., Donato, N., *et al.* 1999. A phase I study of the chimerized anti-epidermal growth factor receptor monoclonal antibody, C225, in combination with cisplatin in patients with recurrent head and neck squamous cell carcinoma. *Proceedings of the American Society of Clinical Oncology* 18: 389a (abstract 1502).

Meredith, R., Partridge, E., Alvarez, R., *et al.* 1996. Intraperitoneal radioimmunotherapy of ovarian cancer with lutetium-177Lu-CC49. *Journal of Nuclear Medicine* 37: 1491–1496.

Miller, R., Maloney, D., Warnke, R., *et al.* 1982. Treatment of B cell lymphoma with monoclonal anti-idiotype antibody. *The New England Journal of Medicine* 306: 517–522.

Mittelman, A., Chen, Z., Kageshita, T., *et al.* 1990. Active specific immunotherapy in patients with melanoma. A clinical trial with mouse antiidiotypic monoclonal antibodies elicited with syngeneic anti-high-molecular-weight melanoma-associated antigen monoclonal antibodies. *Journal of Clinical Investigation* 86: 2136–2144.

Mittelman, A., Chen, Z., Yang, H., *et al.* 1992. Human high molecular weight melanoma-associated antigen (HMW-MAA) mimicry by mouse anti-idiotypic monoclonal antibody MK2-23: Induction of humoral anti-HMW-MAA immunity and prolongation of survival in patients with stage IV melanoma. *Proceedings of the National Academy of Sciences USA* 89: 466–470.

Modjtahedi, H., Hickish, T., Nicolson, M., *et al.* 1996. Phase I trial and tumour localisation of the anti-EGFR monoclonal antibody ICR62 in head and neck or lung cancer. *British Journal of Cancer* 73(2): 228–235.

Moffat, F., Gulee, S., Serafini, A., *et al.* 1999. A thousand points of light or just dim bulbs? Radio-labeled antibodies and colorectal cancer imaging. *Cancer Investigations* 17(5): 322–334.

Moffat, F., Pinsky, C., Hammershaimb, L., *et al.* 1996. Clinical utility of external immunoscintigraphy with the IMMU-4 technetium-99m Fab' antibody fragment in patients undergoing surgery for carcinoma of the colon and rectum: Results of a pivotal, phase III trial. The Immunomedics Study Group. *Journal of Clinical Oncology* 14(8): 2295–2305.

Moir, E. 1989. Nursing care of patients receiving orthoclone OKT3. *ANNA Journal* 16(5): 327–328, 366.

Moolenaar, C., Muller, E., Schol, D., *et al.* 1990. Expression of neural cell adhesion molecule-related sialoglycoprotien in small cell lung cancer and in neuroblastoma cell lines H69 and CHP-212. *Cancer Research* 50(4): 1102–1106.

Mordoh, J., Leis, S., Bravo, A., *et al.* 1994. Description of a new monoclonal antibody FC-2.15, reactive with human breast cancer and other neoplasms. *International Journal of Biological Markers* 9(3): 125–134.

Mujoo, K., Spiro, R.C., and Reisfeld, R. A. 1986. Characterization of the unique glycoprotein antigen expressed on the surface of human neuroblastoma cells. *Journal of Biological Chemistry* 261(22): 10299–10305.

Mulligan, T., Carrasquillo, J., Curt, G., *et al.* 1995. Phase I study of intravenous Lu-labeled CC49 murine monoclonal antibody in patients with advanced adenocarcinoma. *Clinical Cancer Research* 1(12): 1447–1454.

Murray, J., Macey, D., Podoloff, D., *et al.* 1994. Phase II radioimmunotherapy trial with ^{131}I-CC49 in colorectal cancer. *Cancer* 73(suppl 3): 1057–1066.

Muxi, A., Pons, F., Vidal-Sicart, S., *et al.* 1999. *Nuclear Medicine Communications* 20: 123–130.

Natanson, C., Hoffman, W., Suffredoni, A., *et al.* 1994. Selected treatment strategies for septic shock based on proposed mechanisms of pathogenesis. *Annals of Internal Medicine* 120: 771–783.

Norton, L., Slamon, D., Leyland-Jones, B., *et al.* 1999. Overall survival (OS) advantage to simultaneous chemotherapy (CRx) plus the humanized anti-HER2 monoclonal antibody Herceptin (H) in HER2 overexpressing (HER2⁺) metastatic breast cancer (MBC). *Proceedings of the American Society of Clinical Oncology* 18: 127a (abstract 483).

Onrust, S., and Wiseman, L. (1999). Basiliximab. *Drugs* 57(2): 207–213.

Ortaldo, J., Woodhouse, C., Morgan, A., *et al.* 1987. Analysis of effector cells in human antibody dependent cellular cytotoxicity with murine monoclonal antibodies. *Journal of Immunology* 138: 3566–3572.

Pai, L., Wittes, R., Setser, A., *et al.* 1996. Treatment of advanced solid tumors with immunotoxin LMB-1: An antibody linked to Pseudomonas exotoxin. *Nature Medicine* 2(3): 350–353.

Panchagnula, R., and Dey, C. 1997. Monoclonal antibodies in drug targeting. *Journal of Clinical Pharmacology and Therapeutics* 22(1): 7–19.

Pegram, M., Lipton, A., Hayes, D., *et al.* 1998. Phase II study of receptor-enhanced chemosensitivity using recombinant humanized anti-p185HER2/*neu* monoclonal antibody plus cisplatin in patients with HER2/*neu* overexpressing metastatic breast cancer refractory to chemotherapy treatment. *Journal of Clinical Oncology* 16(8): 2659–2671.

Pelosi, G., Pasini, F., Pavanel, F., *et al.* 1999. Effects of different immunolabeling techniques on the detection of small-cell lung cancer cells in bone marrow. *Journal of Histochemistry and Cytochemistry* 47(8): 1075–1088.

Pride, M., Shuey, S., Grillo-Lopez, A., *et al.* 1998. Enhancement of cell-mediated immunity in melanoma patients immunized with murine anti-idiotypic Mabs (Melimmune®) that mimic the higher molecular weight proteoglycan antigen. *Clinical Cancer Research* 10: 2363–2370.

Quezado, Z., Banks, S., and Natanson, C. 1995. New strategies for combatting sepsis: The magic bullets missed the mark . . . but the search continues. *Trends in Biotechnology* 13(2): 56–63.

Ravindranath, M. H., and Irie, R. F. 1988. Gangliosides as antigens of human melanoma. *Cancer Treatment and Research* 43: 17–43.

Reissmann, P., Koga, H., Figlin, R., *et al.* 1999. Amplification and overexpression of the cyclin D1 and epidermal growth factor receptor genes in non-small-cell lung cancer. Lung Cancer Study Group. *Journal of Cancer Research in Clinical Oncology* 125(2): 61–70.

Reiter, Y., and Pastan, A. 1998. Recombinant Fv immunotoxins and Fv fragments as novel agents for cancer therapy and cancer diagnosis. *Trends in Biotechnology* 16(12): 513–520.

Riethmuller, G., Holz, E., Schlimok, G., *et al.* 1998. Monoclonal antibody therapy for resected Dukes' C colorectal cancer: Seven-year outcome of a multicenter randomized trial. *Journal of Clinical Oncology* 16(5): 1788–1794.

Riethmuller, G., Schneider-Gadicke, E., Schlimok, G., *et al.* 1994. Randomized trial of monoclonal antibody for adjuvant therapy of resected Dukes' C colorectal carcinoma. German Cancer Aid 17-1A Study Group. *Lancet* 343(8907): 1177–1183.

Rodwell, J. 1989. Engineering monoclonal antibodies. *Nature* 342: 99–100.

Rosenblum, M., Verschraegen, C., Murray, J., *et al.* 1999. Phase I study of 90Y-labeled B72.3 intraperitoneal administration in patients with ovarian cancer: Effect of dose and EDTA coadministration on pharmacokinetics and toxicity. *Clinical Cancer Research* 5(5): 953–961.

Ruck, A., and Paulie, S. 1998. EGF, TGF alpha, AR and HG-EGF are autocrine growth factors for human bladder carcinoma cell lines. *Anticancer Research* 18(3A): 1447–1452.

Rusch, V., Baselga, J., Cordon-Cardo, C., *et al.* 1993. Differential expression of the epidermal growth factor receptor and its ligands in primary non-small cell lung cancers and adjacent benign lung. *Cancer Research* 53(10 suppl): 2379–2385.

Ryan, A., Eppler, D., Haggler, K., *et al.* 1999. Preclinical safety evaluation of rhuMAbVEGF, an antiangiogenic humanized monoclonal antibody. *Toxicology and Pathology* 27: 78–86.

Sakahara, H., Saga, T., Onodera, H., Konishi, J., *et al.* 1997. Anti-murine antibody response to mouse monoclonal antibodies in cancer patients. *Japanese Journal of Cancer Research* 88: 895–899.

Saleh, M., Khazaeli, M., Wheeler, R., *et al.* 1992. Phase I trial of the murine monoclonal anti-GD2 antibody 14G2a in metastatic melanoma. *Cancer Research* 52(16): 35294–35300.

Saleh, M., Lilisan D., Jr., Pride, M., *et al.* 1998. Immunologic response to the dual murine anti-id vaccine melimmune-1 and melimmune-2 in patients with high-risk melanoma without evidence of systematic disease. *Journal of Immunology* 21: 379–388.

Sarup, J., Johnson, R., King, K., *et al.* 1991. Characterization of an anti-p185HER2 monoclonal antibody that stimulates receptor function and inhibits tumor cell growth. *Growth Regulation* 1(2): 72–82.

Schlaeppi, J., Siemeister, G., Wood, J., *et al.* 1999. Characterization of a new potent, in vivo neutralizing monoclonal antibody to human vascular endothelial growth factor. *Journal of Cancer Research and Clinical Oncology* 125(6): 336–342.

Schlom, J. 1990. Monoclonal antibodies: They are more and less than you think. In Broder S. (ed). *Molecular and Cellular Research for Future Diagnosis and Therapy.* Baltimore, MD: Williams and Wilkins, pp. 95–97.

Schlom, J., and Abrams, S.I. 2000. Tumor immunology. In Bast, R.C., Kufe, D.W., Pollock, R.E., Weichselbaum, R.R., Holland, J.F., and Frie, E., III, (eds). *Cancer Medicine* 5th edn. Hamilton, Ontario: B.C. Decker, Inc., pp. 153–167.

Schneebaum, S., Even-Sapir, E., Cohen, M., *et al.* 1999. Clinical applications of gamma-detection probes—Radioguided surgery. *European Journal of Nuclear Medicine* 26(4 suppl): S26–S35.

Scott, L., and Lamb, H. 1999. Palivizumab. *Drugs* 58(2): 305–311.

Sears, H., Atkinson, B., Mattis, J., *et al.* 1982. Phase I clinical trial of monoclonal antibody in treatment of gastrointestinal tumors. *Lancet* 1(8275): 762–765.

Shak, S. (1999). Overview of the trastuzumab (Herceptin) anti-HER2 monoclonal antibody clinical program in HER2-overexpressing metastatic breast cancer. Herceptin Multinational Investigator Study Group. *Seminars in Oncology* 26(4 suppl 12): 71–77.

Siegall, C., Chace, D., Mixan, B., *et al.* 1994. In vitro and in vivo characteristics of BR96 sFv-PE40. *Journal of Immunology* 152(5): 2377–2384.

Slamon, D., Clark, G., Wong, S., *et al.* 1987. Human breast cancer: Correlation of relapse and survival with amplification of the Her-2/neu oncogene. *Science* 235: 177–181.

Slamon, D., Leyland-Jones, B., Shak, S., *et al.* 1998b. Addition of Herceptin (humanized anti-HER2 antibody) to first line chemotherapy for HER2 overexpressing metastatic breast cancer (HER2$^+$/MBC) markedly increases anticancer activity: A randomized, multinational controlled phase III trial. *Proceedings of the American Society of Clinical Oncology* 17: 98a (abstract 377).

Steplewski, Z., Lubeck, M., and Koprowski, H. 1983. Human macrophages armed with murine immunoglobulin G2a antibodies to tumors destroy human cancer cells. *Science* 221: 865–868.

Tolcher, A., Sugarman, S., Gelmon, K., *et al.* 1999. Randomized phase II study of BR96-doxorubicin conjugate in patients with metastatic breast cancer. *Journal of Clinical Oncology* 17(2): 478–484.

Trail, P.A., Willner, D., Lasch, S.J., *et al.* 1993. Cure of xenografted human carcinomas by BR96-doxorubicin immunoconjugates. *Science* 261(5118): 212–215.

Tripathi, P., Qin, H., Chatterjee, S., *et al.* 1999. Construction and characterization of a chimeric fusion protein consisting of an anti-idiotype antibody mimicking a breast cancer-associated antigen and the cytokine GM-CSF. *Hybridoma* 18(2): 193–202.

Van Zaanen, H., Lokhorsti, H., Aarden, L., and van Oers, M. 1998. Chimaeric anti-interleukin 6 monoclonal antibodies in the treatment of an advanced multiple myeloma: A phase I dose-escalating study. *British Journal of Haematology* 102(3): 783–790.

Vera, R., Albanell, J., Lirola, J., *et al.* 1999. HER2 overexpression as a predictor of survival in a trial comparing adjuvant FAC and CMF in breast cancer. *Proceedings of the American Society of Clinical Oncology* 18: 71a (abstract 265).

Waldmann, T., and O'Shea, J. 1998. The use of antibodies against the IL-2 receptor in transplantation. *Current Opinion in Immunology* 10(5): 507–512.

Wilder, R., DeNardo, G., and DeNardo, S. 1996. Radioimmunotherapy: Recent results and future directions. *Journal of Clinical Oncology* 14: 1383–1400.

Wright, P., Hellstrom, K., Hellstrom, E., *et al.* 1976. Serotherapy of malignant disease. *Medical Clinics of North America* 60: 607–622.

Yang, X., Jia, X., Corvalan, J., *et al.* 1999. Eradication of established tumors by a fully human monoclonal antibody to the epidermal growth factor receptor without concomitant chemotherapy. *Cancer Research* 59(6): 1236–1243.

Yi, E., Harclerode, D., Gondo, M., *et al.* 1997. High c-erB-3 protein expression is associated with shorter survival in advanced non-small cell lung carcinomas. *Modern Pathology* 10(2): 142–148.

Zeidler, R., Reisbach, G., Lindhofer, H., *et al.* 1999. Simultaneous activation of T cells and accessory cells by a new class of intact bispecific antibody results in efficient tumor cell killing. *Journal of Immunology* 163(3): 1246–1252.

Zia, F., Jacobs, S., Kull, F., *et al.* 1996. Monoclonal antibody alpha IR-3 inhibits non-small cell lung cancer growth *in vitro* and *in vivo*. *Journal of Cellular Biochemistry Suppl.* 24: 269–275.

Clinical Pearls

1. It is important to determine the origin of the MAB being administered (i.e., murine, derived solely from mouse immunoglobulin, or chimeric, part human, part mouse. Newer-generation chimeric antibodies will have less tendency to cause allergic reaction because a decreased portion of the antibody is of murine origin.
2. Emergency drugs should be kept at the bedside (e.g., epinephrine, corticosteroids, and diphenhydramine) for the treatment of potential allergic reactions. Although extremely rare, the potential for an anaphylactic reaction is ever present.
3. If an anaphylactic reaction occurs, the infusion should be stopped immediately, fluids started, the physician paged, and emergency drugs administered as ordered.
4. Patients should be monitored closely at the onset of infusion for the potential for an allergic reaction or infusion-related symptom complex.
5. The occurrence of infusion-related symptom complex is believed to be related to the interaction of the MAB with circulating white blood cells and the subsequent release of cytokines. It is more commonly seen with MABs targeted toward white blood cells. Concomitant administration of diphenhydramine or acetaminophen is useful in the management of these symptoms.
6. In general, with most MABs used in the oncology setting, the MAB is administered as a controlled infusion not as a bolus infusion. The use of an infusion pump for administration is recommended.
7. Antibodies conjugated to other substances such as chemotherapy or radioisotopes will require additional precautions and handling procedures appropriate for the conjugate. For example, an MAB conjugated to iodine[131] (^{131}I) requires appropriate precautions and handling for the radioactive isotope [131]I.
8. MABs given as anti-idiotypic vaccines may produce local reactions and a flu-like syndrome, especially when given in conjunction with adjuvants.

9. It is important to determine whether the antibody is being given for a diagnostic purpose (e.g., OncoScint) or for a therapeutic reason (e.g., Rituxan®). This will assist in educating the patient about the goals of therapy.

Key References

Albain, K.S., Hortobagyi, G., Radvin, P., and Slamon, D. (eds). 1999. *HER2 Overexpression in Breast Cancer*. Monograph from Genentech Biooncology. Emeryville, CA: Genentech Biooncology.

Bacquiran, D., Dantis, L., and McKerrow, J. 1996. Monoclonal antibodies: Innovations in diagnosis and therapy. *Seminars in Oncology Nursing* 12: 130–141.

Breedveld, F.C. 2000. Therapeutic monoclonal antibodies. *The Lancet* 355(9205): 735–740.

Cao, Y., and Suresh, M. 1998. Bispecific antibodies as novel bioconjugates. *Bioconjugate Chemistry* 9(6): 635–644.

Davis, T., Streicher, H., Blatner, G., *et al.* 1998. Clinical trials referral resource. Clinical trials using monoclonal antibodies. *Oncology* 12(10): 1479, 1482, 1487.

Dillman, R. 1998. Antibody therapy. In Oldham, R. (ed). *Principles of Cancer Biotherapy*, 3rd edn. Boston: Kluwer Academic Press, pp. 284–317.

Fox, D.A. Cytokine blockade as a new strategy to treat rheumatoid arthritis: Inhibition of tumor necrosis factor. *Archives of Internal Medicine* 160(4): 437–444.

Genentech Biooncology. 1999. *Herceptin–anti-HER2 monoclonal antibody. Targeted Biological Therapy for the Treatment of HER2 Protein Overexpressing Metastatic Breast Cancer. Clinical Overview*. Monograph. Emeryville, CA: Genentech Biooncology.

Genentech Biooncology. 1999. A Mini Slide Kit for Healthcare Professionals.

Hall, S.S. 1995. Monoclonal antibodies at age 20: Promise at last? *Science* 270(5238): 915–916.

Hinkle, G., Burgers, J., Neal, C., *et al.* 1998.

Multicenter radioimmunoscintigraphic evaluation of patients with prostate carcinoma using indium-111 capromab pendetide. *Cancer* 83(4): 739–747.

Karius, D., and Marriott, M. 1997. Immunologic advances in monoclonal antibody therapy: Implications for oncology nursing. *Oncology Nursing Forum* 24: 483–496.

King, D. 1998. Monoclonal antibodies in therapeutic applications. In King, D. (ed). *Applications and Engineering of Monoclonal Antibodies*. Philadelphia, PA: Taylor & Francis, pp. 119–159.

Koelemij, R., Kuppen, P., van de Velde, C., *et al.* 1999. Bispecific antibodies in cancer therapy, from the laboratory to the clinic. *Journal of Immunotherapy* 22(6): 514–524.

Present, D. 1999. Review article: The efficacy of infliximab in Crohn's disease—healing of fistulae. *Alimentary Pharmacology and Therapy* 13(supp 14): 23–28.

Wiseman, L., and Faulds, D. 1999. Daclizumab: A review of its use in the prevention of acute rejection in renal transplant recipients. *Drugs* 58(6): 1029–1042.

Vitetta, E. (ed). 1999. Cancer. *Current Opinion in Immunology* 11(5): 539–588. Reviews the entire field of monoclonal antibodies in cancer care including immunotoxins, antibody drug conjugates, targeting enzymes, and bispecific antibodies.

CHAPTER 10 | Cancer Vaccines

Donna M. Kinzler, RN, MSN, CRNP, OCN®

Charles K. Brown, MD, PhD

Although the field of tumor immunology is a relatively young science, the concept of using cancer vaccines has been in practice for over 100 years. In the 1890s, Coley used an unfiltered bacteria mixture to treat inoperable malignancies. Although some patients did respond to the injection of Coley's toxin into their tumors, most patients ultimately succumbed to their disease. Since the advent of this crude form of vaccination, substantial new knowledge regarding tumor immunology has been delineated, and there has been significant progress in the field. These advances have allowed for the development of a multitude of cancer vaccines. The purpose of this chapter is to give an overview of various tumor vaccines and immunoadjuvants that are employed to augment the immune response against cancer. The basic mechanisms of how tumor vaccines work will be summarized along with data gathered through many years of trials.

Rationale for the Use of Cancer Vaccines

Tumor cells are different from normal cells. These differences are minute with regard to the whole repertoire of normal molecules that are still produced by the tumor cell in order to maintain itself as a metabolizing and living cell. Some of these differences result from variations in the expression of protein molecules—manifesting either as a higher level of production or as expression of "newly" mutated molecules. However minute, the differences in these molecules can be recognized by the immune system as tumor-specific factors; consequently, these antigens have been termed tumor-associated antigens (TAAs).

TAAs may be grouped into several categories. The first category is neoantigens. These are antigens not expressed by the normal cell from which the cancer cells are derived; they are, however, found on other normal cells. Examples of neoantigens are the human melanoma-associated ganglioside GD_2, which is normally expressed on neural tissue, and melanoma-associated protein antigens MAGE-1 and MAGE-3, which are expressed in testes tissues but not on normal melanocytes. The second category of TAAs is oncofetal antigens. These antigens, which include the carcinoembryonic antigen, are expressed by fetal tissues but are not generally seen in normal cells. Some tumors do express what are termed tumor-specific antigens. These antigens are not found on normal or fetal cells but are uniquely expressed in tumors. This last category is newly emerging and includes tumor antigens recognized by T cells that arise from specific mutations that result in altered proteins in neoplastic cells. The antigens are shared by normal tissues but may become overexpressed or contain alterations within the protein sequence, thus allowing for immune recognition. An example would be MUC-1, an antigen commonly expressed in pancreatic and breast cancers. There is evidence that the protein core of the mucin MUC-1, expressed by abnormal glycosylation in tumor cells, can be recognized by T cells (Barnd *et al.*, 1989; Jerome *et al.*, 1991).

Tumor vaccines differ from the classical vaccines, such as smallpox or polio vaccines, in that tumor vaccines act not to prevent the onset of disease, but rather as treatment of hosts with established disease. A cancer vaccine is a preparation containing TAA that when given to a host allows the host to mount an immune response against the tumor. This immune response can be humoral, cellular, or both. But ultimately, to achieve significant therapeutic response, specific antitumor T-cell immunity must be established. The generation of cells with the appropriate T-cell receptor (TCR), allowing for the interaction between the T cell and the tumor cell, is the goal in using tumor vaccines as a therapeutic modality. Increasingly, new approaches with cancer vaccines are also being used to treat patients with tumors with the hope of eradicating the tumors.

Antigen presentation initiates the pathway toward generating a tumor-specific T-cell clone. In this process, antigen is first encountered by antigen-presenting cells (APCs) such as macrophages or dendritic cells (DCs). The APCs then internalize the antigen, process it, and present it in the context of a major histocompatibility complex (MHC) molecule for immune recognition by the host. Without APCs, the process of antigen presentation is at least inefficient, if not ineffective. The manner in which the cancer vaccine is taken up by the APC for presentation of the TAA can be used to group all cancer vaccines into 1 of the following 3 categories (Figure 10.1). First, the cancer vaccine can be a preparation in which an exogenous source of TAA is internalized by the APC, processed, and then presented in the context of an MHC (Figure 10.1a). Tumor apoptotic bodies, tumor cells, tumor lysate, and purified tumor antigens belong in this category. Second, a cancer vaccine can be one that transduces the APC, leading to endogenous expression, processing, and subsequent presentation of the TAA in the context of an MHC (Figure 10.1b). Members of this group include recombinant viruses, bacteria, and naked nucleic acid molecules. Third, the vaccine can be peptides, which are pulsed onto empty MHC molecules on the surface of APCs for presentation (Figure 10.1c).

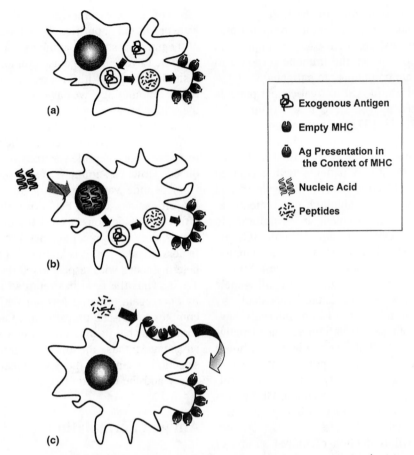

Figure 10.1   Three major classifications of cancer vaccines. A cancer vaccine can be (a) an exogenous source of supply of tumor-associated antigens (TAAs), or (b) a genetic material that is used to transduce cells for endogenous expression of the TAA, or (c) peptides pulsed onto empty MHC molecules of cells.

Source: Reprinted with permission of author.

Historical Overview of the Use and Development of Cancer Vaccines

The history of cancer vaccines dates back to over a century ago when Dr. William B. Coley, a surgeon, used bacterial extracts to induce immune responses in cancer patients (Coley, 1898). Patients with inoperable sarcomas were given heat-inactivated cultures of *Streptococcus erysipelas* and *Bacillus prodigious* (now called *Serratia marcescens*) after surgery to prevent recurrence (Coley, 1900). In the last century, multiple attempts to utilize cancer vaccination to generate immune responses have been made, based on an increasing understanding of immune reactivity. The purpose of **active specific immunity** (**ASI**) is to introduce into the tumor-bearing host TAAs in a way that will be more immunogenic. The goal of this therapy is to achieve rejection of tumor through augmentation or stimulation of the host's nascent immune response. Nonspecific immunostimulants (adjuvants) are often used in conjunction with ASI to enhance the immune response to otherwise nonimmunogenic antigens.

The first use of ASI to treat cancer patients was reported by von Leyden and Blumenthal in 1902 (Currie, 1972). An **autologous** tumor-cell preparation, a vaccine produced from the patient's own tumor, was used to stimulate an immune response in patients with advanced cancer. No objective improvement was found following treatment, although two patients reported some improvement in symptoms. In 1912, Coca, Dorrance, and Lebredo (Currie, 1972) used large quantities of macerated tumor, containing live tumor cells, to create a "tumor vaccine." Both autologous and **allogeneic** tumor cells were administered repeatedly by subcutaneous injection at 14-day intervals. Seventy-nine patients with various advanced malignancies were treated. One patient with breast cancer had a clinical response that lasted 4 months. Remarkably, only one patient developed a tumor at the site of injection. The authors reluctantly concluded that their approach was impractical and ineffective.

With the introduction of inbred strains of mice came the capability to immunize mice with small doses of **syngeneic** tumor cells. When later challenged with larger doses of tumor cells, the immunized mice were protected, whereas nonimmunized mice developed tumors that eventually led to their demise (Gross, 1943). These results suggested that the immunity of the inbred mice was specific for the tumor used for inoculation. This work, as well as the work of others in animal models (Foley, 1953; Prehn and Maine, 1957), established a firm basis for the existence of tumor-specific immunity.

In our endeavor to better understand the interplay between tumor cells and the immune system, we have seen the development of different types of cancer vaccines (Figure 10.2). Early forms of cancer vaccines, such as Coley's toxin, were crude and unpurified. With the delineation of the tumor-associated antigens, it has become possible to vaccinate against a tumor using just a single protein. With progress in the field of tumor immunology, we have come to learn that the entire protein molecule is not needed for the immune response; rather, a portion of the larger molecule is sufficient to elicit the same response. Thus, peptide vaccines are now introduced. However, immune responses resulting from peptide vaccination can be narrow and less efficacious. Often, better overall antitumor effect can be demonstrated if the immune system is allowed to react against multiple tumor factors. In addition, it is known that tumors are heterogeneous with respect to expression of the TAAs. Thus the field has returned to its roots by once again utilizing less purified and more complex tumor-cell preparations. Each vaccine formulation has its inherent advantages and disadvantages; thus, the optimal tumor vaccine selection depends on the desired method of delivery and the desired effects.

Antigen Formulations

Regulation of the immune system occurs at many levels: by antigens, cytokines, and the neuroendocrine system. The identification of antigens has opened up new therapies for treatment of cancer. Antigen can be presented in the form of a cancer vaccine when the TAA is known and can be delivered in the form of protein, peptide, and nucleic acid sequences. However, antigen can be susceptible to resistance mechanisms in which the tumor escapes immunologic recognition through downregulation of antigen. One mechanism for bypassing downregulation of a specific antigen is to vaccinate with multiple antigens, which can be achieved by using cellular preparations. Additionally, when the TAA is not known, cellular preparations from tumor cells contain all the

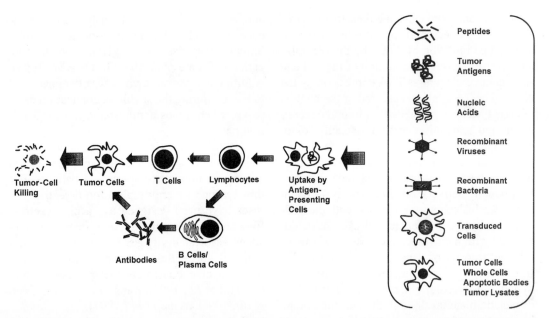

Figure 10.2 Types of cancer vaccines. TAA is supplied or expressed by the cancer vaccine. This is then presented by the antigen-presenting cell (APC) to the immune system. The subsequent interaction between the APC and lymphocytes allows for generation of both cellular and humoral immune responses. Although both immune responses can lead to tumor-cell killing, the cytotoxic T lymphocytes are considered to be the major effector cells.

Source: Reprinted with permission of author.

possible antigens that can be recognized by the immune system. Thus, without previously identifying the TAAs, effective vaccination preparation can still be delivered.

Antigen-Specific Preparations

In order to understand vaccines, it is important to understand the concept of MHC restriction. Briefly, there are 3 classes of MHC molecules in humans: class I, class II, and class III. Class III molecules are complement proteins and, as such, do not actively participate in antigen presentation. Class I and II molecules have molecular clefts that will bind an antigen epitope in the form of a peptide. There are absolute protein sequence requirements in order for a peptide to bind to an MHC molecule. Frequently, a peptide

that binds to one MHC molecule will not bind to a different MHC molecule with different sequence-binding requirements. If a peptide is not presented for immune recognition in the form of a peptide/MHC complex, an immune response may not be elicited. This is what is meant by MHC restriction. For example, a histocompatibility leukocyte antigen (HLA, the human version of MHC), type A_2 restricted peptide will not induce an immune response in an individual who is not HLA A_2.

VIRAL AGENTS

The identification of TAA has allowed for the development of recombinant anticancer viral vaccines. Deoxyribonucleic acid (DNA) sequences encoding the TAA are integrated into the viral genome using standard recombination and selection approaches adapted to the virus of interest. A recombinant virus is then produced. The infection of APCs by the recombinant viruses causes transduction of the cell and subsequent endogenous TAA expression by the APCs. The TAA, now expressed in the context of class I MHC, is presented for immune recognition and generation of tumor-specific cytotoxic lymphocytes (CTLs). In the context of delivery of tumor antigen to elicit an anticancer immune response, viral agents have become very popular delivery vehicles. This is the result of two intrinsic factors associated with the biology of viruses. In general, viruses have co-evolved with their respective hosts to allow for efficient transfer of genetic material into cells. In essence, the virus functions as a molecular hypodermic needle, allowing the introduction of genetic material through the cell-membrane barrier. Second, the proteins that make up the virus particle are foreign to the host and thus generate a significant associated inflammatory response. This associated inflammatory response is a "danger signal" that in turn stimulates the immune system and improves the immune response toward the tumor antigen. Thus, in this manner, viruses function not only as vaccine vectors but also as immuno-adjuvants.

Currently, members of the pox-, herpes-, adeno-, and adeno-associated viridae and retroviridae are the more popular vehicles for tumor vaccine construction. A unique quality of poxviruses is the large available capacity within their genomes for the insertion of exogenous coding sequences (Moss et al., 1984). In other words, multiple genes can be cloned into this vector as opposed to the other viral vectors, which are usually limited to carrying the coding sequences of one or two genes. The induction of potent cellular and humoral immune responses with recombinant poxviruses has been observed in several tumor models. Vaccinia virus, one of numerous poxviruses, encoding melanoma antigens such as MART-1, gp100, and tyrosinase, has induced both humoral and cellular immune responses when given to melanoma patients (Bronte et al., 1995; Irvine et al., 1995). Additionally, vaccinia virus was demonstrated to be safe during the smallpox eradication campaign, when it was administered to over 1 billion people.

Vaccinia virus is a replication-competent virus and as such can induce disseminated viremia in immunocompromised patients. For this reason, several replication-defective viruses have been designed as vaccine vectors: fowl pox, replication-defective adenovirus, and adeno-associated viruses. Efficient and lasting humoral and cellular responses are observed from vaccine constructs using these vectors (Juillard et al., 1995; Wang et al., 1995; Chen et al., 1996; Irvine et al., 1997).

Recombinant pox-, adeno-, and adeno-associated viruses only lead to transient expression of the cloned antigen. The reason is that these viral strains do not integrate their DNA into the host genome and so are eventually cleared from the host. Retroviruses, however, integrate their DNA molecule into the genome of the host and can therefore allow for continued expression of the cloned gene even when the virus is cleared from the host. But this unique quality of the retrovirus is also its weakness. Fear of inappropriate integration of the recombinant retroviral DNA and possible transformation of normal cells has curtailed some of its uses.

NUCLEIC ACIDS

Recombinant DNA vectors have been developed to allow for the expression of large amounts of tumor antigens. In this type of tumor vaccine, a recombinant plasmid DNA molecule encoding for the TAA is used to transduce cells. Plasmids are small, circularized, double-stranded DNA, originally derived from bacteria, that are used to carry genes specifying one or more antigenic proteins. Genes encoding for

TAAs can be spliced into plasmids and then delivered into small groups of cells. The antigen-encoding genes are ultimately transcribed, and the RNA transcripts are then translated into antigenic proteins. The proteins may leave the cell and circulate as free antigen or may be digested into smaller fragments within the cell and expressed on the surface in conjunction with MHC molecules. The cells that are transduced may be normal mesenchymal cells that are in the periphery of nucleic-acid injection or APCs such as macrophages or dendritic cells. The result is that the cells transduced by the DNA vector containing the tumor antigen-coding sequences express large amounts of the antigen. The expressed antigen is then detected by the immune system and results in an immune response evidenced by both detectable humoral and cellular immunity. Intramuscular injection of plasmid-DNA-encoding TAA has been demonstrated to induce MHC class I-restricted cytotoxic T lymphocytes and antibody responses. In 1993, Ulmer *et al.* achieved heterologous protection against influenza by injecting DNA encoding an influenza viral protein in a murine model. Later, the same group was able to show that this protection is the result of generating MHC class I-restricted CTL against the viral protein (Ulmer *et al.*, 1996). DNA vaccinations with protective response against subsequent challenges have also been demonstrated in tumor models (Donnelly *et al.*, 1994; Donnelly *et al.*, 1997). Irvine *et al.* (1997) showed that vaccinating with DNA encoding the β-galactosidase gene in mice protected against subsequent challenges from β-galactosidase-expressing tumors.

The major advantage of DNA vaccination is that it is easy to use and can induce long-lasting immune responses (Fu *et al.*, 1997). Advances in recombinant DNA technology have made construction of TAA genes a relatively uncomplicated and straightforward task. Consequently, large amounts of DNA constructs defining the anticancer vaccine can be obtained in a relatively short period of time and at a very reasonable cost. Another advantage is that DNA vaccination is not associated with an **anamnestic** immune response, which in the case of viral vaccines causes rapid clearance of the recombinant viruses following subsequent challenges. The major caveat with this system, however, is the relative inefficiency at which cells are transduced. Overall, cells—even APCs—take up exogenous DNA at a very low rate. Much of the delivered DNA is usually degraded once it enters the body. Consequently, naked DNA constructs like tumor vaccines have remained limited, and immunologists have favored viral vectors as a more efficient means of delivering the recombinant TAA genes.

BACTERIAL AGENTS

Recombinant bacterial vaccines fall into a unique category of cancer vaccines. As a group, they are not as frequently utilized as the other vaccine vectors. There are two organisms that have been modified and used as tumor vaccine constructs. These are *Listeria monocytogenes* and *Salmonella*. *L. monocytogenes* and *Salmonella* will infect macrophages and monocytes and, therefore, can be used to target antigen to these **professional APCs** (Poirier *et al.*, 1988; Sadoff *et al.*, 1988; Pan *et al.*, 1995). Additionally, these two bacteria can infect the host enterically, which has the advantage of a simple and efficient administration route. While both organisms can replicate intracellularly, *L. monocytogenes* has the added utility of a two-phase intracellular life cycle (Kaufmann, 1993). This dual intracellular life cycle is instrumental in the efficacy of *L. monocytogenes* as a vaccine vector.

The entry of *L. monocytogenes* into monocytes occurs via phagocytosis, and a phagolysosome is formed. While in this phagolysosomal phase, antigen(s) produced by the organism are processed via the MHC class II pathway. *L.*

monocytogenes then enzymatically destabilizes the phagolysosome, thus allowing for escape and initiation of the second intracellular phase—the cytosolic phase. While in this second phase, antigens expressed by *L. monocytogenes* are processed via the MHC class I pathway. It is believed that this dual antigenic processing can maximize antigen presentation for immune recognition. Indeed, Pan *et al.* (1995) have demonstrated the efficacy of utilizing *L. monocytogenes* by inducing regression of established macroscopic tumors in mice mediated by the oral administration of a recombinant *L. monocytogenes* vaccine.

PEPTIDES/PROTEINS

Nominal tumor-associated antigens expressed in cancer cells can stimulate potent tumor-protective immune responses in humans (Bystryn *et al.*, 1995). The immune response at the T-cell level relies on costimulatory signals present on antigen-presenting cells such as dendritic cells. In 1963, Anderer demonstrated that a T-cell immune response using the minimal synthetic peptide fragments of an ovalbumin carrier joined with the hexapeptide (string of six amino acid sequences) of the tobacco-mosaic virus could be obtained. This seminal paper helped demonstrate for the first time that peptides represent the minimal target required for T-cell recognition. Subsequent peptide-based vaccines revealed that naturally processed and presented cytotoxic T-lymphocyte epitopes can be duplicated by 9- to 12-amino acid (AA) synthetic peptides (Townsend *et al.*, 1986). Vaccines using such peptides can be used to elicit T-cell–mediated immunity. These peptide-specific T-cell responses are induced from synthetic peptides that bind to the restricting MHC molecules of antigen-presenting cells (DeBruijn *et al.*, 1991; DeBruijn *et al.*, 1992).

During the last several years, a number of studies have been conducted on the autologous CD8[+] T-cell–mediated response to human melanoma (Parmiani *et al.*, 1990). The emerging picture indicates that melanomas express multiple T-cell–defined epitopes, some of which are unique to a given tumor, whereas others are shared by allogeneic, HLA-matched melanomas (Anichini *et al.*, 1989; Van den Eynde *et al.*, 1989; Wolfel *et al.*, 1989). These epitopes represent short, 9- to 10-AA peptides derived from TAAs that are presented by MHC class I antigens to CD8[+] T cells (Hom *et al.*, 1991; Traversari *et al.*, 1992; Cox *et al.*, 1994; Gaugler *et al.*, 1994; Kawakami *et al.*, 1994; Mandelboim *et al.*, 1994; Wolfel *et al.*, 1994). Whereas many class I alleles have been reported to represent restriction elements for tumor-reactive CD8[+] T cells, the HLA-A2.1 allele (expressed by 45% of melanoma patients) appears to play an immunodominant role in presenting melanoma epitopes (Crowley *et al.*, 1991). At least six different CD8[+] T-cell–defined epitopes appear to be expressed by multiple HLA-A2[+] melanomas (Slingluff *et al.*, 1993; Storkus *et al.*, 1993; Wolfel *et al.*, 1994). Many of these peptide epitopes have recently been identified using both cDNA expression cloning and protein biochemical approaches (Maeurer *et al.*, 1995). Thus, peptides delivered from Melan A-associated, gp100, and tyrosinase sequences appear to represent the *immunodominant* melanoma epitopes (see Table 10.1).

Cellular Preparations

WHOLE CELLS

Whole-cell, autologous, irradiated tumor cells used in a vaccine may be obtained from fresh tumor. Many investigators have used this method to treat patients with advanced melanoma, renal cell carcinoma, or microscopic residual colon cancer. With autologous vaccination, treatment is limited to patients with advanced disease in whom sufficient numbers of cells are available to enable preparation of a series of vaccine injections. This process re-

Table 10.1   Peptide epitopes defined by human CD8$^+$ cytolytic T cells

Melanoma Antigen	Class I Restriction	Amino Acid Sequence
Melan-A	**HLA-A2**	**ILTVILGVL***
gp100	**HLA-A2**	**YLEPGPVTA**
Tyrosinase	**HLA-A2**	**YMDGTMSQV**
Melan-A	HLA-A2	AAGIGILTV
Melan-A	HLA-A2	GIGILTVIL
gp100	HLA-A2	LLDGTATLRL
Tyrosinase	HLA-A2	MLLAVLYCL
MAGE-I	HLA-A1	EADPTGHSY

* Three Melan-A/MART-1 epitopes recognized by T cells appear to be contained in the p27-40, 14-mer peptide AAGIGILT-VILGVL. The boldface sequences represent the only defined naturally processed melanoma epitopes recognized by T cells.

quires surgical excision to obtain the cells and substantial laboratory support to process and store the material for future use. Since the cells are used as the vaccine, the cells are irradiated so that the tumor cells are not able to regrow when given back to the patient. An advantage of whole-cell vaccines is that all of the antigens present on the tumor cells are presented to the immune system, thus maximizing presentation of all TAA for tumor recognition. Prehn and Main (1957) initially demonstrated that normal mice developed immunity in reaction to the existence of an antigenic tumor. Although inadequate to stop the growth of an established tumor, this immunity prevented the progression of challenge inoculations of the same tumor cells.

TUMOR LYSATES

Tumor lysates are produced by mechanically disrupting whole cells. The cells may also be irradiated prior to lysis. Lysates have multiple tumor antigens and may enhance a polyvalent immune response. Polyvalent vaccines are derived from more than one cell line but do not seem to be as immunogenic as whole-cell vaccines (Haigh *et al.,* 1999). With tumor lysates, there is the potential to create a standard (generic) product that can be used as treatment for

many patients and to prevent recurrence in those with microscopic residual disease.

Immune response to tumor lysates can be enhanced by oncolytic preparations. Oncolysates are tumor cells that have been infected and lysed by viruses. The process of viral infection causes release of costimulatory molecules by tumor cells. Additionally, immune response by the host to the foreign viral antigens causes more cytokine release by leukocytes, that is, more costimulation. The costimulatory molecules serve as "danger signals," which enhance the immune response, a concept that will be defined more clearly in the immunoadjuvant section of this chapter. Vaccinia has been used in the groundwork of viral oncolysates because this virus can infect and lyse tumor cells easily. Wallack and Michaelides, (1984) augmented a vaccinia melanoma oncolysate vaccine by infecting four allogeneic melanoma cell lines with live vaccinia virus. Hersey (1993) employed a vaccinia melanoma cell lysate comprised of a single melanoma cell line infected with vaccinia. Allogeneic tumor cells are utilized in oncolysates for consistency in the preparation of the vaccine. In order to encompass as many of the antigens as possible, more than one allogeneic tumor cell line may be used in the preparation of the oncolysate vaccine.

APOPTOTIC BODIES

A third cellular preparation that has gained much interest as a potential anticancer vaccine is the apoptotic tumor cell—apoptotic bodies. Apoptosis is programmed cell death mediated by internal cellular elements (Hockenbery, 1995). As a tumor cell undergoes apoptosis, it also releases costimulatory molecules, which enhance the immune response. Onier *et al.* (1999) hypothesized that a lipid, OM 174, induced tumor cell apoptosis, stimulated phagocytosis of apoptotic bodies, and activated the immune system by antigen presentation. Peritoneal carcinomatosis was induced in BDIX rats by intraperitoneal injection of syngeneic PROb cancer cells. The rats developed macroscopic peritoneal nodules 2 weeks after injection of the cancer cells. The rats were then injected intraperitoneally with OM 174; an intravenous treatment was later developed. The treated rats experienced complete regression of tumors, whereas the untreated rats died from their tumors.

Vaccination with apoptotic bodies can be done using different methods of preparation. One approach is to vaccinate directly with apoptotic bodies. Another is to vaccinate with a mix of apoptotic bodies and autologous dendritic cells. Both techniques have been shown to yield detectable humoral and cellular responses specific for tumor *in vivo* in rats (Henry *et al.*, 1999).

Cancer Vaccine Clinical Trials

Cancer vaccines have greater specificity for tumor cells with diminished adverse effects to normal cells, and several vaccine strategies will be discussed here. The understanding of molecular biology with regard to cancer vaccines has increased over the years. The information obtained from prior clinical trials informs the next generation of clinical researchers. The earliest

trials, initiated by Rosenberg and colleagues, investigated the treatment of patients with metastatic melanoma using melanoma tumor antigen peptide vaccines (Seipp, 1998). Immunodominant peptides from the gp100 melanoma-associated antigen were identified, and a synthetic peptide, designed to increase binding to HLA-A2 molecules, was used as a cancer vaccine. The researchers reported tumor responses in 13 patients (42%) of 31 receiving peptide administered in combination with interleukin-2 (IL-2) (Rosenberg *et al.*, 1998). This 42% response rate appeared to be an increase from the 17% response rate seen in the previous 134 patients treated in the surgery branch with the same dose of IL-2 alone and is attributed to the addition of peptide vaccination.

Scoggin and colleagues (1992) treated patients with high-risk stage I and II melanoma with a vaccinia melanoma oncolysate, a cell-membrane preparation of allogeneic melanoma cells infected with vaccinia virus. Each dose was administered intradermally near major lymph node drainage areas. Forty-eight patients were treated, and 24 remained disease-free at the conclusion of that study. The mean disease-free interval was 22 months (range, 17 to 28 months).

CancerVax is a polyvalent melanoma cell vaccine developed at the John Wayne Cancer Institute (Chan and Morton, 1998). The vaccine's active ingredients are three irradiated melanoma cell lines that express antigens that are commonly shared among other melanomas and can induce a cross-reactive immune response against the patient's tumor. The vaccination schedule used in a phase II study of CancerVax consisted of an induction phase, with injections every 2 weeks for 5 doses over a 2-month period. This was followed by a maintenance phase, with vaccine administration every 4 weeks for the remainder of the first year, every 2 months for 1 year, and then every 3 months for a total of 5 years (Chan and Morton,

1998). Side effects included fever, fatigue, and musculoskeletal discomfort. The results of this phase II trial for patients with stage IV melanoma revealed a 5-year survival rate of 25% for 157 patients treated with the vaccine. Phase III trials are underway to determine whether adjuvant BCG plus CancerVax will prolong survival compared to BCG plus placebo in stage III and stage IV melanoma patients who are without evidence of disease after surgical resection.

A cancer vaccine trial involving patients with metastatic renal cell carcinoma was reported by Fenton *et al.* in 1996. Seventeen patients with metastatic renal cell carcinoma went through surgical resection of tumor for preparation of an autologous tumor cell vaccine. Patients received intradermal injections twice at weekly intervals with 10^7 irradiated tumor cells plus BCG and once with 10^7 tumor cells alone. Simultaneously, patients were randomized to receive no adjuvant IL-2, low-dose IL-2, or high-dose IL-2. The IL-2 was given by the subcutaneous route on the first day of vaccination and for 4 consecutive days. Sixteen of 17 patients received the vaccine. Four patients developed cellular immunity specific for autologous tumor cells according to delayed-type hypersensitivity (DTH) responses. Two of these patients had not received IL-2, and 2 patients had received high-dose IL-2. The 2 patients who received high-dose IL-2 experienced partial responses. One of these patients was DTH$^+$ and the other patient was DTH$^-$. Another patient who did not receive IL-2 and had a partial response was DTH$^+$ after vaccination and after receiving IL-2 subcutaneously in another protocol. Fenton *et al.* noted that subcutaneously administered adjuvant IL-2 does not significantly enhance the immunologic response to autologous renal cell vaccines as determined by the development of tumor-specific DTH response.

A phase II vaccine study of autologous tumor cells and adoptive transfer of OKT3-activated autologous T lymphocytes following surgery and chemotherapy in patients with stage III or IV colon cancer is being conducted by the National Cancer Institute. This protocol evaluates in terms of response rate the efficacy of immunotherapy with irradiated autologous tumor cell vaccine and granulocyte-macrophage colony-stimulating factor (GM-CSF) followed by OKT3-activated T lymphocytes and IL-2 in combination with standard therapy. A phase III study using Theratope is underway for women with breast cancer. The vaccine consists of synthetic antigens that imitate natural cancer antigens. An objective of the study is to compare the time-to-disease progression and survival in patients receiving the vaccine to that in patients receiving a control vaccine (*http://www.biomira.com*).

Cancer vaccines have been shown to have immunologic and clinical responses. Melanoma peptide and lysate vaccines have been associated with good responses. As we increase our knowledge in this area, we have found that peptides are not sufficient by themselves and that the addition of other immunoadjuvants may provide benefit.

Immunoadjuvants

The goal of tumor vaccination is to generate reactive T-cell population(s) against the tumor. But in a host harboring an established tumor, often there is already ongoing interaction between native T cells and tumor cells; however, the desired effect of tumor killing is not observed. The question is, Why? Interactions between T cells and the tumor cells are mediated by the TCR. Molecularly, this interaction is defined by the binding of the TCR with the tumor antigen on the surface of the tumor cell as a peptide/MHC complex. This interaction can have two consequences. The desired effect is that a signal is transduced to the tumor cells, and death mediated by apoptosis of the tumor ensues. However, this is not always the outcome. Interaction of the T cell and the tumor cell mediated by the binding of the TCR with the tumor antigen can also lead to tolerance. That is, rather than tumor cells being killed, either the T cell dies or the tumor cell is not harmed. Biologically, this is the scenario when a patient presents clinically with cancer. Thus, the function of tumor vaccines may be more accurately depicted as trying to break tolerance rather than generating a new reactive T-cell clone—for all too often tumor-specific T-cell clones are already present, but they are just ineffective at eradicating the tumor.

It is believed that the environment surrounding T cells during their association with tumor cells is important in deciding the outcome: killing of tumor cells or tolerance. Costimulatory molecules, cytokines, chemokines, or other stimulants of inflammation may mediate this environment. The presence of these molecules represents a "danger signal" to the T cells, and interaction of T cells with tumor cells in such an environment results in the killing of the tumor cells. Even though the mechanisms of immunoadjuvants were not known in the early era of their usage, it is now postulated that they help to elicit this "danger signal" and lead to a more efficacious immune response to the vaccine.

The use of immunoadjuvants promotes recruitment of antigen-presenting cells as well as other inflammatory cells, thereby enhancing initiation of the immune response. Immunoadjuvants also activate nonspecific immune effectors, which results in activation of the reticuloendothelial system, and are used to stimulate recruitment of innate immune effectors. Responses are broad because they do not unequivocally involve tumor-specific T cells that distinguish either specific tumor-asso-ciated antigens or B cells that produce antibodies directly at tumor-antigen epitopes. Rather, the immunoadjuvants activate nonspecific responses to cytokines and lymphokines (Akporiaye and Hersh, 1995). These secondary stimuli amplify the immune response generally by stimulating macrophages, T cells, and natural killer (NK) cells. These substances can furnish the host with a formerly nonexistent immune response or intensify an existing one. Bacillus Calmett Guérin (BCG), *Corynebacterium parvum*, DETOX™ (Ribi Immunochem Research, Inc., Hamilton, MT), Freund's complete adjuvant, and IL-12 are several immunoadjuvants that have been used or are currently being tested in clinical trials. Figure 10.3 depicts the purported pathways where some of these adjuvants mediate their effects.

Adjuvant Formulations

IMMUNOADJUVANTS OF BACTERIAL ORIGIN

BCG is a microbial material made in 1922 from an attenuated strain of *Mycobacterium bovis*. It has been used for decades as immunization against tuberculosis and as a nonspecific immunopotentiating agent in cancer treatment. As with other biological agents, it is important to have an immunocompetent host, and a small tumor burden is believed to be necessary for this type of treatment to be effective (Zbar *et al.*, 1972).

In the treatment of cancer, BCG acts as a nonspecific immunostimulatory agent. This effect is believed to be initiated by a cascade of immunologic events involving both humoral and cellular immunity. T cells, B cells, macrophages, and NK cells are all activated by a variety of lymphokines, cytokines, and chemokines induced as a result of BCG administration (Murahata and Mitchell, 1976; Mitchell and Murntz, 1979). The exact mechanism by which

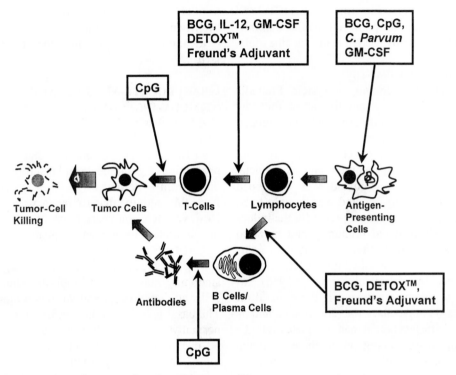

Figure 10.3   Site(s) of action of various immunoadjuvants.

Abbreviations: BCG, bacillus Calmette-Guérin; CpG, sequences of the nucleotides cytosine and guanine; IL, interleukin; GM-CSF, granulocyte-macrophage colony-stimulating factor.

Source: Reprinted with permission of author.

BCG causes tumor regression remains poorly understood, but the local presence of BCG and the development of a granuloma are believed to be important components (Hanna *et al.*, 1972; Snodgrass and Hanna, 1973).

Mathé *et al.* (1969) used BCG as an adjuvant in the treatment of acute lymphoblastic leukemia. Intensive weekly multisite scarifications with BCG were administered during both the induction and maintenance phases of chemotherapy. Improved survival over historical controls stimulated much interest in this treatment. Similar improvement in survival was demonstrated when BCG was used as therapy for acute myeloid leukemia (Freeman *et al.*, 1973). How-

ever, it had little effect on the duration of remission, and subsequent controlled clinical trials (other than in the setting of bladder cancer, where it is now approved) failed to show benefit.

C. parvum is a gram-positive formalin-killed bacterium that was first used in humans in the mid-1970s (Scott, 1975). A strong stimulator of the reticuloendothelial system, *C. parvum* also activates macrophages (Howard *et al.*, 1973); it is, however, no longer available for use in the clinical setting. DETOX™ (detoxified endotoxin) is a pyrogen-free preparation formulated from *Salmonella minnesota* and cell-wall skeletons of *Mycobacterium phlei* (Ribi *et al.*,

1984). A nonspecific stimulator, DETOX™ triggers both antibody and cell-mediated immunity and is currently used in many vaccine trials.

FREUND'S ADJUVANTS

Used to enhance the immune system, Freund's adjuvants are preparations that allow for slow antigen release from the adjuvant and extended exposure of the antigen to the immunoresponsive cells (Couch, 1996). There are two types of Freund's adjuvants: complete and incomplete. Freund's complete adjuvant was developed more than 30 years ago and was thought to be the most potent immunoadjuvant for the induction of cell-mediated immunity and humoral antibody formation. Freund's complete adjuvant consists of heat-killed mycobacterial cells suspended in mineral oil (Freund, 1956). Incomplete Freund's adjuvant is the mineral oil without the mycobacterial constituent and is thought to be less potent than complete Freund's adjuvant for enhancing cell-mediated immune responses. Montanide, an oil-based adjuvant similar to incomplete Freund's adjuvant, is currently used in several peptide vaccine strategies (Rosenberg, 1998).

INTERLEUKIN-12

IL-12, a heterodimeric cytokine originally termed cytotoxic lymphocyte maturation factor, T-cell stimulating factor, and NK-cell–stimulating factor (Lotze, 1996), was initially identified by its capacity to synergize effectively with IL-2 in activating NK cells and to facilitate the generation of allospecific cytolytic T lymphocytes (CTL). More recently, IL-12 has been shown to preferentially induce and enhance $CD8^+$ cellular immune responses against viral, bacterial, and protozoan infections as well as soluble peptide/protein antigens (Afonso et al., 1994; Ghalib et al., 1995; Pearlman et al., 1995; Wynn et al., 1995). IL-12 also serves as a potent adjuvant for the generation of T_{h1}-associated cellular immune responses (Wynn et al., 1995).

Similar T_{h1} immune responses are believed to be critical to the successful generation of long-term antitumor cellular immune response in vivo.

GRANULOCYTE-MACROPHAGE COLONY-STIMULATING FACTOR (GM-CSF)

GM-CSF was initially discovered in 1977 by Metcalf and colleagues (Burgess et al., 1977). It is an 18 to 30-kDa glycoprotein that stimulates production of granulocyte and macrophage colonies from bone marrow cells. It is primarily from this activity that its name was derived. However, in recent years, many other functions of this protein have been delineated.

GM-CSF is produced by many cell types: $CD4^+$ T_h cells, monocytes, macrophages, eosinophils, mast cells, fibroblasts, endothelial cells, epithelial cells, and various tumor cells. The basal level of production by these cells is normally quite low. However, production can be increased by ultraviolet irradiation, tissue injury, and secondary stimulation by cytokines released during an inflammatory process: IL-1, IL-2, IFN-α, and IFN-γ (Tarr, 1996). GM-CSF can also up-regulate MHC class II molecules and stimulate antigen presentation by DCs (Fischer et al., 1988). It is this latter function that has resulted in newer applications of this molecule in cancer therapeutics.

Currently, the most common clinical application of GM-CSF is in increasing granulocyte counts after chemotherapy. However, because of the more recently identified function of augmenting MHC class II expression and stimulating DC functions, GM-CSF has seen novel applications in immunotherapy. GM-CSF can function as an immunoadjuvant because it potentiates antigen presentation by DCs. In 1993, Dranoff et al. showed that the secretion of GM-CSF by tumor cells leads to increased specific-tumor immunity. In 1998, the same team also demonstrated that irradiated autologous melanoma cells genetically modified to secrete

GM-CSF showed specific-tumor regression in 11 of 16 patients (Soiffer *et al.*, 1998). Additionally, DCs transfected with the GM-CSF gene showed enhanced *in vivo* antigen-presenting capacity. Thus, it appears that GM-CSF may have several novel applications in the clinical arena in the future.

CpG Oligonucleotides

Although DNA is not generally considered to be an immunostimulatory agent, several structural differences exist between bacterial and vertebrate DNA that may render the bacterial DNA stimulatory in a vertebrate host. One of these differences is the frequency of CpG motifs, which are at least 20 times more common in bacteria than in vertebrates. Another difference is that in vetebrates CpG sequences are frequently methylated, whereas those of bacteria are not. It has been shown that oligodeoxynucleotides (ODNs) as short as 15 bases and containing nonmethylated CpG will have immunostimulatory activities (Krieg, 2000).

CpG ODNs stimulate various aspects of the immune system. Ballas and colleagues first described the effect of CpG motifs in ODNs in murine and human NK cells from induction of IL-12, TNF-α, and IFN-α production by macrophages and dendritic cells (Ballas *et al.*, 1996). Additionally, CpG ODNs are capable of promoting B-cell responses to protein antigens. They can induce class switching from immunoglobulin Ig-M toward IgG 2a and 2b (Lipford *et al.*, 1997). When combined with specific antigens *in vivo*, CpG ODNs can serve as a strong stimulus for T-cell activation as well as proliferation of antigen-specific CTLs (Jakob *et al.*, 1998). Also CpG ODNs can promote survival and maturation of human DCs by increasing expression of MHC class II and costimulatory molecules CD40, CD54, and CD86 (Hartmann *et al.*, 1999). Thus, by virtue of their stimulatory effect on many arms of the immune system, CpG ODNs have a tremendous potential for use in immunotherapy trials against cancer. Specifically, their effects on DCs make them a potentially useful adjuvant in DC-based immunotherapy for weakly immunogenic tumors.

Clinical Studies Using Immunoadjuvants

Earlier vaccine studies were limited to the use of BCG. Developments in biotechnology have led to an expanded arsenal of immunoadjuvants for use in cancer vaccines. Much of the work has just begun and will need to be investigated over the next several years.

McCune *et al.* (1981) treated 14 patients with metastatic renal cell carcinoma with a combination of autologous, irradiated tumor cells admixed with *C. parvum*. The vaccine preparation was injected intracutaneously in the shoulder on a weekly basis for 4 to 14 weeks, depending on the amount of available tumor tissue. Tenderness at the injection site, slight chills, and fatigue were the reported side effects. Four patients had complete or partial responses of some of their metastatic lesions, but the lesions in other patients remained stable or progressed. The authors concluded that the most likely cause for the mixed response was the presence of antigen-distinct subpopulations in metastatic cells that may not have been represented in the vaccine (McCune *et al.*, 1981).

In an effort to improve the rate of long-term, disease-free survival in postsurgical patients with colorectal cancer, Hoover *et al.* (1985) conducted a randomized two-armed clinical trial of ASI with a total of 40 patients, 20 in each arm. In the treatment group, autologous, irradiated tumor cells plus BCG were administered intradermally once a week for 3 weeks (4 to 5 weeks after surgery). Patients in the control group received surgery only. All ASI-treated patients developed ulcerations where BCG had been administered. Ulcerations began 3 weeks after the injection and were resolved within 3 months. In 60% of the ASI-treated patients, palpable ipsilateral inguinal lymphadenopathy also developed; it resolved within 3 months. At a mean follow-up period of 28 months, 9 recurrences and 4 deaths were noted in the control arm, whereas in the ASI arm there were 3 recurrences and no deaths. In this small trial, ASI significantly improved survival rates and reduced recurrence rates. In a subsequent adjuvant trial conducted in the Netherlands by Vermorken and colleagues (1999), patients with colon cancer were randomized prospectively to receive either ASI with an autologous tumor-cell vaccine plus BCG following surgical resection or no adjuvant treatment. A benefit was seen, but only in patients with Duke's B, not C (nodal metastatic), disease. The authors concluded that ASI has minimal adverse reaction and should be considered in the management of stage II colon cancer.

Berd *et al.* (1990) reported their experience using ASI in treating melanoma. An autologous, irradiated tumor vaccine mixed with BCG was administered intradermally in the upper arms or legs 3 days after intravenous administration of cyclophosphamide (300 mg/m²), a drug which augments the acquisition of immunity to new antigens and breaks immunological tolerance. This treatment schedule was repeated every 28 days. Fifty percent of the patients experienced nausea and vomiting after receiving the drug. All patients had local inflammatory reactions that developed into ulcers and drained clear fluid for 3 to 4 weeks after treatment. The number of treatments administered ranged from 2 to 16 (median, 5). Among 40 evaluable patients, there were 4 complete responses and 1 partial response. The median duration of response was 10 months. The investigators also reported that 6 of the nonresponders had delayed tumor regressions several months after ASI began. This phenomenon is similar to that reported by McCune *et al.* (1981) with their mixed responders (i.e., some lesions

regressed whereas others were stable or progressed). The authors postulated a delayed immune reaction or the presence of shared antigens between the metastatic lesions and the vaccine.

An allogeneic melanoma lysate administered with the adjuvant DETOX™ was used in 25 patients with measurable malignant melanoma (Mitchell *et al.*, 1990). Patients were treated with a low intravenous dose of cyclophosphamide (300 mg/m²) given 5 to 7 days before the first vaccine. Five injections of the vaccine were administered once a week for 6 weeks. Each vaccine was administered subcutaneously in two sites, deep in the deltoid or upper buttocks. Fatigue was reported in about one third of the patients. One patient reported flu-like symptoms lasting 4 to 5 days. Granulomas developed at the injection site in 5 patients, 1 of whom had developed a local abscess at the site. There was 1 complete response, 3 partial responses, and 1 case of long-term (17 months) disease stability. The median duration of response in this study was 16 months.

Dendritic Cells

Dendritic Cell Biology

According to Grabbe *et al.* (1995), DCs, named for their star-like morphology, are uncommon leukocytes. They stem from the bone marrow, flow through the bloodstream, and travel into tissues. DCs are the most potent antigen-presenting cells and are critical to the regulation, maturation, and maintenance of a cellular immune response to tumor (Lotze, 1997). They capture and take up antigens in the tissues and carry these antigens from peripheral sites to primary and secondary lymphoid sites. In the lymphoid organs, DCs express high levels of MHC class I and class II molecules and present the processed antigen epitopes to naive and memory T cells for the priming of antigen-specific responses. DCs also express high levels of costimulatory molecules (CD80 and CD86) that are required to activate antigen-specific T cells. Additionally, DCs may be induced to synthesize IL-12 and IFN-α, which are important immunostimulatory cytokines.

Dendritic cells are derived from many lineages, including myeloid, monocyte, granulocyte, T-cell, and B-cell lineages. The phenotype of DCs differs in relation to the cytokines added to the media in culture. DCs cultured in IL-4 and GM-CSF seem to stimulate immature DCs, which take up antigen and process it in tissues (Baar, 1999). DCs cultured in TNF-α stimulate mature DCs responsible for priming T cells in lymphoid tissues. Clinical trials involving infusion of DCs have become possible by the expansion of methods for acquiring large numbers of DCs. According to Timmerman and Levy (1999), the purification of immature DC precursors from peripheral blood and the *in vitro* differentiation of DCs from peripheral blood monocytes or CD34$^+$-hematopoietic progenitor cells are two approaches that have been used. The young DC precursors can be separated from T-cell and monocyte-depleted peripheral blood cells after 1 to 2 days of *in vitro* culture (Timmerman and Levy, 1999). Large numbers of DCs can also be generated by *in vitro* culture of monocytes or CD34$^+$ progenitor cells expanded in cytokines such as IL-4 and GM-CSF.

Of significant clinical interest, the histologic infiltration of DCs into primary tumor lesions has been associated with significantly prolonged patient survival and a reduced incidence of metastatic disease in patients with bladder, lung, esophageal, and nasopharyngeal carcinoma (Tsujitani *et al.*, 1990; Giannini *et al.*, 1991; Furihata *et al.*, 1992; Becker, 1993; Zeid *et al.*, 1993). In contrast, a comparatively poorer clinical prognosis has been observed for patients with lesions that exhibit a sparse infiltration of DCs and whose metastatic lesions are frequently deficient in DC infiltration (Tsujitani *et al.*, 1990; Giannini *et al.*, 1991; Furihata *et al.*, 1992; Becker, 1993; Murphy *et al.*, 1993; Zeid *et al.*, 1993). Patients treated with IL-2 show differentiation of CTL and DC from the peripheral blood. Thus, it has been hypothesized that co-localization of DCs and tumor cells may provide APCs capable of efficient rejection of tumor.

Dendritic Cell Clinical Studies

Many clinical studies performed with dendritic cells have yielded good clinical responses. Hsu *et al.* (1996) treated 4 patients with follicular B-cell lymphoma using DCs isolated from peripheral blood by leukapheresis and pulsed with antigen, followed 2 weeks later with subcutaneous injections of soluble antigens. One patient experienced a complete response, and a second patient had a partial response.

Reichardt *et al.* (1999) also reported on 12 multiple-myeloma patients treated with high-dose therapy and peripheral-blood stem cell transplantation followed by idiotype (Id) immunizations. Three to 7 months after high-dose therapy, the patients received monthly immunizations of 2 intravenous infusions of Id-pulsed autologous DCs, and then 5 subcutaneous injections of Id/keyhole limpet hemocyanin (KLH) given with adjuvant. The administration of Id-pulsed DC and Id/KLH vaccines were tolerated well, with minor transient side effects experienced. Two of 12 patients developed an Id-specific, cellular proliferative immune response, and 1 of 3 patients developed a transient Id-specific CTL response. Of the 12 patients, 11 revealed strong KLH-specific cellular proliferative immune responses, which demonstrates the patients' immunocompetence at vaccination.

Salgaller *et al.* (1998) treated 51 men with hormone-refractory prostate cancer with autologous DCs pulsed with prostate-specific membrane antigen. The patients received either 4 or 5 infusions of autologous DCs, peptide alone, or peptide-pulsed DCs. The toxic effect of this therapy was mild to moderate hypotension. Seven patients exhibited partial response from 150 to 225 days, based on positive prostate-specific antigen scores.

Sixteen patients with advanced melanoma received DCs generated from peripheral blood with GM-CSF and IL-4 (Nestle *et al.*, 1998). Depending on the patient's HLA haplotype, DCs were stimulated either with peptide or tumor lysate. KLH was added as a CD4 helper antigen and immunological tracer molecule. Five of 16 patients had objective responses to the DC vaccination.

Investigators at the University of Pittsburgh Cancer Institute are treating patients with HLA-A2$^+$ melanoma with peptide-pulsed DCs. Peripheral-blood–derived DCs were cultured with IL-4 and GM-CSF for 1 week and then pulsed with synthetic melanoma peptides, Melan A/MART-1, gp100, and tyrosinase. The patients were infused weekly for 4 weeks. The major side effect was fever. Two complete responses and 1 partial response were observed in 28 patients was in this trial, which has now been completed (M. Lotze, Personal Communication).

Regulatory Approval

Excluding BCG, as of July 2000, no vaccine to date has been approved by the Food and Drug Administration as a nonspecific treatment strategy for cancer. Vaccine trials are regulated by the Center for Biologics Evaluation and Research, the Food and Drug Administration (FDA), and the institutional review boards of individual centers. The clinical trials are regulated for safety by toxicity monitoring. In addi-

tion, all vaccine trials that involve gene transfer using one of the transduction vectors (viruses, DNA, or bacteria) also require approval from the Recombinant DNA Advisory Committee and local institutional biosafety committees.

Administration and Side Effects

Vaccines are administered subcutaneously, intradermally, intravenously, and intramuscularly. As many vaccines are given by local injection, regional site reactions as well as systemic side effects are monitored. Pain, tenderness, erythema, itching, granuloma, and ulceration may occur. Vaccines containing adjuvants have a greater likelihood of causing effects such as nausea, fatigue, myalgias, arthralgias, and fever. No evidence of organ dysfunction secondary to autoimmune effects has been noted. In general, vaccine therapy is considered outpatient therapy and is associated with low-grade toxicity and no reported mortality.

Nursing Management

Many vaccine strategies may require multiple injections. Prophylactic analgesia may be indicated for multiple intradermal injections prior to vaccination (Weber, 1998). Patient evaluation and documentation after vaccine injection should include the timing of the assessment (i.e., the number of hours postinjection); measurement of induration, erythema, or edema at the vaccination site; assessment for site-specific symptoms or systemic symptoms such as fever; determination of the effectiveness of symptom-control measures; and assessment for lymphadenopathy in the draining lymph node at the injection site. An acute reaction within the first 15 minutes, either local or systemic, may suggest an allergic reaction as opposed to the expected cellular inflammatory response.

Obstacles to Therapy

Active specific immunotherapy has tremendous potential as a cancer treatment modality. However, it is difficult for immunotherapy alone to have great impact in the setting of advanced disease. The ideal patients for vaccine therapy seemingly are patients with disease in the early phases, when immune competence is greatest, or those who have minimal residual tumor following therapeutic debulking. Whole-cell autologous vaccination is limited in patients with advanced disease to those possessing enough cells to support vaccine preparations. Frequently, patients who have advanced disease lack adequate viable tumor tissue, which precludes production of large quantities of autologous vaccine for large clinical trials. This factor has remained a significant challenge. Another problem with whole-cell therapy is that the tumor-processing procedure is time-consuming and difficult and can result in cells that fail to grow or that become contaminated. Patients must be made aware of this potential for treatment failure before cells are harvested.

Peptide vaccination depends on the specificity of CTL reactivity against the relevant tumor epitope. Peptide-based immunization requires that the majority of identified tumor peptides are presented in an HLA-restricted manner. Thus, these vaccines are accessible only to patients with specific HLA haplotypes.

Proximity to the study institution performing the clinical trial also needs to be considered. Many of these specialized therapies are offered at specific locations and oftentimes surgery for tumor harvesting has to be done at the designated institution. Patients need to be informed about their upcoming schedule and the time and cost associated with their travels during study enrollment.

Conclusion

Significant progress has been made over the last century in the use of vaccines as therapy for cancer; however, much work remains to be done. Although vaccines have been studied in a variety of solid tumors and hematologic malignancies, perhaps the best-studied tumor is melanoma. Investigation into the therapeutic use of vaccines in patients with metastatic melanoma has been critically important because of the lack of effective conventional therapeutic modalities. The most extensively studied melanoma vaccines in clinical trials to date have been whole-cell preparations or cell lysates that contain multiple antigens capable of stimulating an immune response. Unfortunately, in the majority of studies, immune responses to these vaccines have not translated into a survival advantage. Advances in tumor-cell immunology have led to the identification of candidate tumor-cell antigens that can stimulate an immune response. This discovery has allowed for refinements in vaccine design, but it is difficult to determine the precise tumor antigens that should be targeted with a specific vaccine. The univalent antigen vaccines, which have greater purity,are easier to manufacture and have greater reproducibility compared with polyvalent vaccines, may suffer from poorer results due to immunoselection and the appearance of antigen-negative clones within the tumor. Novel approaches discussed in this chapter, such as transfection of cells with cytokine genes and costimulatory molecules, may be promising, but the induction of immune responses does not necessarily confer a therapeutic benefit. Therefore, these elegant newer strategies need to be studied in carefully designed clinical trials so that outcomes can be compared objectively with standard therapy (Haigh *et al.*, 1999). If survival is improved with these vaccine approaches, their ease of administration and lack of toxicity will firmly entrench active specific vaccine immunotherapy as a standard modality in the treatment of the melanoma patient.

We are at the threshold of developing novel immunotherapeutic cancer treatment strategies. As cost containment continues to be emphasized by the managed health care industry, cancer vaccines hold out the promise of a safe and effective outpatient approach to cancer therapy. Vaccines are being investigated as a modality that can be combined with chemotherapy, immunotherapy, or surgery. Advances in our knowledge of adjuvants and vaccine dosing and administration may enable us to design more effective vaccine therapeutic approaches. Learning how to induce an effective T-cell response to antigens as our predecessors did is one of the great challenges to be addressed.

References

Afonso, L.C., Scharton, T.M., Vieira, M., *et al.* 1994. The adjuvant effect of interleukin-12 in a vaccine against Leishmania major. *Science* 263(5144): 235–237.

Akporiaye, E.T., and Hersh, E.M. 1995. Cancer Vaccines: Clinical applications. In DeVita, V.T., Hellman, S., and Rosenberg, S.A. (eds). *Biologic Therapy of Cancer,* 2nd edn. Philadelphia, PA: J.B. Lippincott Company, pp. 635–647.

Anderer, F.A. 1963. Preparation and properties of an artificial antigen immunologically related to tobacco mosaic virus. *Biochemica Biophysica Acta* 71: 246–249.

Anichini, A., Mazzocchi, A., Fossati, G., *et al.* 1989. Cytotoxic T lymphocyte clones from peripheral blood and from tumor site detect intratumoral heterogeneity of melanoma cells. Analysis of

specificity and mechanisms of interaction. *Journal of Immunology* 142(10): 3692–3701.

Baar, J. 1999. Clinical applications of dendritic cell cancer vaccines. *The Oncologist* 4(2): 140–144.

Ballas, Z.K., Rassmussen, W.L., and Krieg, A.M. 1996. Induction of NK activity in murine and human cells by CpG motifs in oligodeoxynucleotides and bacterial DNA. *Journal of Immunology* 157(5): 1840–1845.

Barnd, D.L., Lan, M.S., Metzgar, R.S., *et al.* 1989. Specific, major histocompatibility complex-unrestricted recognition of tumor-associated mucins by human cytotoxic T cells. *Proceedings of the National Academy of Sciences of the USA* 86(18): 7159–7163.

Becker, Y. 1993. Dendritic cell activity against primary tumors: An overview. *In Vivo* 7(3): 187–191.

Berd, D., Maguire, H., McCue, P., *et al.* 1990. Treatment of metastatic melanoma with an autologous tumor-cell vaccine: Clinical and immunologic results in 64 patients. *Journal of Clinical Oncology* 8(11): 1858–1867.

Bronte, V., Tsung, K., Rao, J.B., *et al.* 1995. IL-2 enhances the function of recombinant poxvirus-based vaccines in the treatment of established pulmonary metastases. *Journal of Immunology* 154(10): 5282–5292.

Burgess, A.W., Camakaris, J., and Metcalf, D. 1977. Purification and properties of colony-stimulating factor from mouse lung conditioned medium. *Journal of Biological Chemistry* 252(6): 1998–2003.

Bystryn, J.C., Shapiro, R.L., and Oratz, R. 1995. Partially purified tumor antigen vaccines. In De Vita, V.T., Hellman, S., and Rosenberg, S.A. (eds). *Biologic Therapy of Cancer,* 2nd edn. Philadelphia, PA: J.B. Lippincott Company, pp. 668–679.

Chan, A.D., and Morton, D.L. 1998. Active immunotherapy with allogeneic tumor cell vaccines: Present status. *Seminars in Oncology* 25(6): 611–622.

Chen, P.W., Wang, M., Bronte, V., *et al.* 1996. Therapeutic antitumor response after immunization with a recombinant adenovirus encoding a model tumor-associated antigen. *Journal of Immunology* 156(1): 224–231.

Coley, W.B. 1898. The treatment of inoperable sarcoma with the mixed toxins of erysipelas and bacillus prodigiosus. *Journal of the American Medical Association* 31: 389–395.

Coley, W.B. 1900. The mixed toxins of erysipelas and bacillus prodigiosus in the treatment of sarcoma. *Journal of the American Medical Association* 34: 906–908.

Couch, R.B. 1996. Vaccines. In Fleisher, T.A., Schwartz, B.D., Shearer, W.T., and Strober, W. (eds). *Clinical Immunology*. St. Louis, MO: Mosby-Year Book pp. 594–608.

Cox, A.L., Skipper, J., Chen, Y., *et al.* 1994. Identification of a peptide recognized by five melanoma-specific human cytotoxic T cell lines. *Science* 264(5159): 716–719.

Crowley, N.J., Darrow, T.L., Quinn-Allen, M.A., *et al.* 1991. MHC-restricted recognition of autologous melanoma by tumor-specific cytotoxic T cells. Evidence for restriction by a dominant HLA-A allele. *Journal of Immunology* 146(5): 1692–1699.

Currie, G. 1972. Eighty years of immunotherapy: A review of immunological methods used for the treatment of human cancer. *British Journal of Cancer* 26: 141–153.

DeBruijn, M., Nieland, J.D., Schumacher, T., *et al.* 1992. Mechanisms of induction of primary virus-specific cytotoxic T lymphocyte responses. *European Journal of Immunology* 22(11): 3013–3020.

DeBruijn, M., Schumacher, T., Nieland, J.D., *et al.* 1991. Peptide loading of empty major histocompatibility complex molecules on RMA-S cells allows the induction of primary cytotoxic T-lymphocyte responses. *European Journal of Immunology* 21(12): 2963–2970.

Donnelly, J.J., Ulmer, J.B., and Liu, M.A. 1994. Immunization with DNA. *Journal of Immunological Methods* 176(2): 145–152.

Donnelly, J.J., Ulmer, J.B., Shiver, J.W., *et al.* 1997.

DNA vaccines. *Annual Review of Immunology* 15: 617–648.

Dranoff, G., Jaffee, E., Lazenby, A., *et al.* 1993. Vaccination with irradiated tumor cells engineered to secrete murine granulocyte-macrophage colony-stimulating factor stimulates potent, specific, and long-lasting anti-tumor immunity. *Proceedings of the National Academy of Sciences of the USA* 90(8): 3539–3543.

Fenton, R.G., Steis, R.G., Madara, K., *et al.* 1996. A phase I randomized study of subcutaneous adjuvant IL-2 in combination with an autologous tumor vaccine in patients with advanced renal cell carcinoma. *Journal of Immunotherapy with Emphasis on Tumor Immunology* 19(5): 364–374.

Fischer, H.G., Frosch, S., Reske, K., *et al.* 1988. Granulocyte-macrophage colony-stimulating factor activates macrophages derived from bone marrow cultures to synthesis of MHC class II molecules and to augmented antigen presentation function. *Journal of Immunology* 141(11): 3882–3888.

Foley, E. 1953. Antigenic properties of methylcholanthrene induced tumors in mice of the same strain of origin. *Cancer Research* 13: 835–837.

Freeman, C., Harris, R., Geary, C., *et al.* 1973. Active immunotherapy used alone for maintenance of patients with acute myeloid leukaemia. *British Medical Journal* 4(892): 571–573.

Freund, J. 1956. The mode of action of immunological adjuvants. *Advanced Tubercle Research* 1: 130–148.

Fu, T., Ulmer, J.B., Caulfield, M.J., *et al.* 1997. Priming of cytotoxic T lymphocytes by DNA vaccines: Requirement for professional antigen presenting cells and evidence for antigen transfer from myocytes. *Molecular Medicine* 3(6): 362–371.

Furihata, M., Ohtsuki, Y., Ido, E., *et al.* 1992. HLA-DR antigen- and S-100 protein-positive dendritic cells in esophageal squamous cell carcinoma—their distribution in relation to prognosis. *Virchows Archives B, Cell Pathology Including Molecular Pathology* 61(6): 409–414.

Gaugler, B., Van den Eynde, B., van der Bruggen,

P., *et al.* 1994. Human gene MAGE-3 codes for an antigen recognized on a melanoma by autologous cytolytic T lymphocytes. *Journal of Experimental Medicine* 179(3): 921–930.

Ghalib, H.W., Whittle, J.A., Kubin, M., *et al.* 1995. IL-12 enhances Th 1-type responses in human Leishmania donovani infections. *Journal of Immunology* 154(9): 4623–4629.

Giannini, A., Bianchi, S., Messerini, L., *et al.* 1991. Prognostic significance of accessory cells and lymphocytes in nasopharyngeal carcinoma. *Pathology Research and Practice* 187(4): 496–502.

Grabbe, S., Beissert, S., Schwarz, T., *et al.* 1995. Dendritic cells as initiators of tumor immune responses: A possible strategy for tumor immunotherapy? *Immunology Today* 16(3): 117–121.

Gross, L. 1943. Intradermal immunization of C3H mice against a sarcoma that originated in an animal of the same line. *Cancer Research* 3: 326–333.

Haigh, P., Difronzo, L.A., Gammon, G., *et al.* 1999. Vaccine therapy for patients with melanoma. *Oncology* 13(11): 1561–1574.

Hanna, M., Jr., Snodgrass, M., Zbar, B., *et al.* 1972. Histopathology of tumor regression after intralesional injection of *Mycobacterium bovis*. IV. Development of immunity to tumor cells and to BCG. *Journal of the National Cancer Institute* 48: 245–257.

Hartmann, G., Weiner, G., and Krieg, A.M. 1999. CpG DNA: A potent signal for growth, activation, and maturation of human dendritic cells. *Proceedings of the National Academy of Sciences of the USA* 96: 9305–9310.

Henry F., Boisteau, O., Bretaudeau, L., *et al.* 1999. Antigen-presenting cells that phagocytose apoptotic tumor-derived cells are potent tumor vaccines. *Cancer Research* 59(14): 3329–3332.

Hersey, P. 1993. Evaluation of vaccinia viral lysates as therapeutic vaccines in the treatment of melanoma. *Annals of the New York Academy of Sciences* 690: 167–177.

Hockenbery, D.M., 1995. Principles of cell killing by biologic agents. In DeVita, V.T., Hellman, S., and Rosenberg, S.A. (eds). *Biologic Therapy of Cancer,* 2nd edn. Philadelphia, PA: J.B. Lippincott Company, pp. 95–102.

Hom, S.S., Topalian, S.L., Simonis, T., *et al.* 1991. Common expression of melanoma tumor-associated antigens recognized by human tumor infiltrating lymphocytes: Analysis by human lymphocyte antigen restriction. *Journal of Immunotherapy* 10(3): 153–164.

Hoover, H., Surdyke, M., Dangel, R., *et al.* 1985. Prospectively randomized trial of adjuvant active-specific immunotherapy for human colorectal cancer. *Cancer* 55(6): 1236–1243.

Howard, J., Christie, G., and Scott, M. 1973. Biological effects of *Corynebacterium parvum*. IV. Adjuvant and inhibitory activities on B-lymphocytes. *Cellular Immunology* 7(2): 290–301.

Hsu, F.J., Benike, C., Fagnoni, F., *et al.* 1996. Vaccination of patients with B-cell lymphoma using autologous antigen-pulsed dendritic cells. *Nature Medicine* 2(1): 52–58.

Irvine, K.R., Chamberlain, R.S., Shulman, E.P., *et al.* 1997. Enhancing efficacy of recombinant anticancer vaccines with prime/boost regimens that use two different vectors. *Journal of the National Cancer Institute* 89(21): 1595–1601.

Irvine, K.R., McCabe, B.J., Rosenberg, S.A., *et al.* 1995. Synthetic oligonucleotide expressed by a recombinant vaccinia virus elicits therapeutic CTL. *Journal of Immunology* 154(9): 4651–4657.

Jakob, T., Walker, P.S., Krieg, A.M., *et al.* 1998. Activation of cutaneous dendritic cells by CpG-containing oligodeoxynucleotides: A role for dendritic cells in the augmentation of T_{h1} responses of immunostimulatory DNA. *Journal of Immunology* 161(6): 3042–3049.

Jerome, K.R., Barnd, D.L., Bendt, K.M., *et al.* 1991. Cytotoxic T-lymphocytes derived from patients with breast adenocarcinoma recognize an epitope present on the protein core of a mucin molecule preferentially expressed by malignant cells. *Cancer Research* 51(11): 2908–2916.

Juillard, V., Villefroy, P., Godfrin, D., *et al.* 1995. Long-term humoral and cellular immunity induced by a single immunization with replication-defective adenovirus recombinant vector. *European Journal of Immunology* 25(12): 3467–3473.

Kaufmann, S. 1993. Immunity to intracellular bacteria. *Annual Review of Immunology* 11: 129–163.

Kawakami, Y., Eliyahu, S.R., Delgado, C.H., *et al.* 1994. Cloning of the gene coding for a shared human melanoma antigen recognized by autologous T cells infiltrating into tumor. *Proceedings of the National Academy of Sciences of the USA* 91(14): 6458–6462.

Krieg, A. M. 2000. The role of CpG motifs in innate immunity. *Current Opinion in Immunology* 12(1): 35–43.

Lipford, G. B., Bauer, M., Blank, C., *et al.* 1997. CpG containing synthetic oligonucleotides promote B and cytotoxic T cell responses to protein antigen: A new class of vaccine adjuvants. *European Journal of Immunology* 27(9): 2340–2344.

Lotze, M.T. 1997. Getting to the source: Dendritic cells as therapeutic reagents for the treatment of patients with cancer. *Annals of Surgery* 226(1): 1–5 (editorial).

Lotze, M.T., Interlenkintz: Cellular and molecular immunology of an important regulatory cytokine. Introduction. 1996. *Annals of the New York Academy of Sciences* 795: xiii–xix.

Maeurer, M., Hurd, S., and Martin, D. 1995. Cytolytic T-cell clones define HLA-A2 restricted human cutaneous melanoma peptide epitopes—correlation with T-cell receptor usage. *The Cancer Journal* 2: 162–170.

Mandelboim, O., Berke, G., Fridkin, M., *et al.* 1994. CTL induction by a tumor-associated antigen octapeptide derived from a murine lung carcinoma. *Nature* 369(6475): 67–71.

Mathé, G., Amiel, J., Schwarzenberg, L., *et al.* 1969. Active immunotherapy for acute lymphocytic leukemia. *Lancet* 1(7597): 697–699.

McCune, C., Schapira, D., and Henshaw, E. 1981. Specific immunotherapy of advanced renal carcinoma: Evidence for the polyclonality of metastases. *Cancer* 47(8): 1984–1987.

Mitchell, M., Harel, W., Kempf, R., *et al.* 1990. Active-specific immunotherapy for melanoma. *Journal of Clinical Oncology* 8(5): 856–869.

Mitchell, M., and Murahata, R. 1979. Modulation of immunity by bacillus Calmette-Guérin (BCG). *Pharmacology & Therapeutics* 4(2): 329–353.

Moss, B., Smith, G.L., Gerin, J.L., *et al.* 1984. Live recombinant vaccinia virus protects chimpanzees against hepatitis B. *Nature* 311(5981): 67–69.

Murahata, R., and Mitchell, M. 1976. Modulation of the immune response by BCG: A review. *The Yale Journal of Biology and Medicine* 49(3): 283–291.

Murphy, G., Radu, A., and Kaminer, M. 1993. Autologous melanoma vaccine induces inflammatory responses in melanoma metastases: Relevance to immunologic regression and immunotherapy. *Journal of Investigative Dermatology* 100(3): 335S–341S.

Nestle, F.O., Alijagic, S., Gilliet, M., *et al.* 1998. Vaccination of melanoma patients with peptide- or tumor lysate-pulsed dendritic cells. *Nature Medicine* 4(3): 328–332.

Onier, N., Hilpert, S., Arnould, L., *et al.* 1999. Cure of colon cancer metastasis in rats with the new lipid A OM 174. Apoptosis of tumor cells and immunization of rats. *Clinical and Experimental Metastases* 17(4): 299–306.

Pan, Z.K., Ikonomidis, G., Lazenby, A., *et al.* 1995. A recombinant *Listeria monocytogenes* vaccine expressing a model tumour antigen protects mice against lethal tumour challenge and causes regression of established tumours. *Nature Medicine* 1(5): 471–477.

Pan, Z.K., Ikonomidis, G., Pardoll, D., *et al.* 1995. Regression of established tumors in mice mediated by the oral administration of a recombinant *Listeria monocytogenes* vaccine. *Cancer Research* 55(21): 4776–4779.

Parmiani, G., Anichini, A., and Fossati, G. 1990. Cellular immune response against autologous human malignant melanoma: Are in vitro studies providing a framework for a more effective immunotherapy? *Journal of the National Cancer Institute* 82(5): 361–370.

Pearlman, E., Heinzel, F. P., Hazlett, F. E., *et al.* 1995. IL-12 modulation of T helper responses to the filarial helminth *Brugia malayi. Journal of Immunology* 154(9): 4658–4664.

Poirier, T.P., Kehoe, M.A., and Beachey, E.H. 1988. Protective immunity evoked by oral administration of attenuated *aroA Salmonella typhimurium* expressing cloned streptococcal M protein. *Journal of Experimental Medicine* 168(1): 25–32.

Prehn, R., and Maine, J. 1957. Immunity to methylcholanthrene-induced sarcomas. *Journal of the National Cancer Institute* 18: 769–778.

Reichardt, V.L., Okada, C.Y., Liso, A., *et al.* 1999. Idiotype vaccination using dendritic cells after autologous peripheral blood stem cell transplantation for multiple myeloma—a feasibility study. *Blood* 93(7): 2411–2419.

Ribi, E., Cantrell, J., Takayaman, K., *et al.* 1984. Lipid A and immunotherapy. *Review of Infectious Diseases* 6(4): 567–572.

Rosenberg, S., Yang, J., Schwartzentruber, D. J., *et al.* 1998. Immunologic and therapeutic evaluation of a synthetic peptide vaccine for the treatment of patients with metastatic melanoma. *Nature Medicine* 4(3): 321–327.

Sadoff, J.C., Ballou, W.R., Baron, L.S., *et al.* 1988. Oral *Salmonella typhimurium* vaccine expressing circumsporozoite protein protects against malaria. *Science* 240(4850): 336–338.

Salgaller, M.L., Tjoa, B.A., Lodge, P.A., *et al.* 1998. Dendritic cell-based immunotherapy of prostate cancer. *Critical Reviews™ in Immunology* 18(1–2): 109–117.

Scoggin, S., Sivanandham, M., Sperry, R., *et al.* 1992. Active specific adjuvant immunotherapy with vaccinia melanoma oncolysate. *Annals of Plastic Surgery* 28(1): 108–109.

Scott, M. 1975. Potentiation of the tumor-specific immune response by *Corynebacterium parvum. Journal of the National Cancer Institute* 55(1): 65–72.

Seipp, C.A. 1998. National Cancer Institute conducts vaccine trials. *ONS Biotherapy SIG Newsletter* 9: 1–6.

Slingluff, C.L., Jr., Cox, A.L., Henderson, R.A., *et al.* 1993. Recognition of human melanoma cells by HLA-2.1–restricted cytotoxic T lymphocytes is mediated by at least six shared peptide epitopes. *Journal of Immunology* 150(7): 2955–2963.

Snodgrass, M., and Hanna, M., Jr. 1973. Ultrastructural studies of histiocyte-tumor cell interactions during tumor regression after intralesional injection of *Mycobacterium bovis. Cancer Research* 33(4): 701–716.

Soiffer, R., Lynch, T., Mihm, M., *et al.* 1998. Vaccination with irradiated autologous melanoma cells engineered to secrete human granulocyte-macrophage colony-stimulating factor generates potent antitumor immunity in patients with metastatic melanoma. *Proceedings of the National Academy of Sciences of the USA* 95(22): 13141–13146.

Storkus, W.J., Zeh, H.J., III, Maeurer, M.J., *et al.* 1993. Identification of human melanoma peptides recognized by class I-restricted tumor infiltrating T-lymphocytes. *Journal of Immunology* 151(7): 3719–3727.

Tarr, P.E. 1996. Granulocyte-macrophage colony-stimulating factor and the immune system. *Medical Oncology* 13(3): 133–140.

Timmerman, J.M., and Levy, R. 1999. Dendritic cell vaccines for cancer immunotherapy. *Annual Review of Medicine* 50: 507–529.

Townsend, A., Rothbard, J., Gotch, F.M., *et al.* 1986. The epitopes of influenza nucleoprotein recognized by cytotoxic T-lymphocytes can be defined with short synthetic peptides. *Cell* 44(6): 959–968.

Traversari, C., van der Bruggen, P., Luescher, I.F., *et al.* 1992. A nonapeptide encoded by human gene MAGE-1 is recognized on HLA-A1 by cytolytic T lymphocytes directed against tumor antigen MZ2-E. *Journal of Experimental Medicine* 176(5): 1453–1457.

Tsujitani, S., Kakeji, Y., Watanabe, A., *et al.* 1990. Infiltration of dendritic cells in relation to tumor invasion and lymph node metastasis in human gastric cancer. *Cancer* 66(9): 2012–2016.

Ulmer, J.B., Deck, R.R., DeWitt, C.M., *et al.* 1996.

Generation of MHC class I-restricted cytotoxic T lymphocytes by expression of a viral protein in muscle cells: Antigen presentation by non-muscle cells. *Immunology* 89(1): 59–67.

Ulmer, J.B., Donnelly, J.J., Parker, S.E., *et al.* 1993. Heterologous protection against influenza by injection of DNA encoding a viral protein. *Science* 259(5102): 1745–1749.

Van den Eynde, B., Hainat, P., Herin, M., *et al.* 1989. Presence on a human melanoma of multiple antigens recognized by autologous CTL. *International Journal of Cancer* 44(4): 634–640.

Vermorken, J.B., Claessen, A.M., Van Tinteren., *et al.* 1999. Active specific immunotherapy for Stage II and Stage III colon cancer: a randomised trial. *Lancet* 353(9150): 345–350.

Wallack, M.K. and Michaelides, M. 1987. Serologic response to human melanoma line from patients with melanoma undergoing treatment with vaccinia melanoma oncolysates *Surgery* 96(4): 791–800.

Wang, M., Bronte, V., Chen, P.W., *et al.* 1995. Active immunotherapy of cancer with a nonreplicating recombinant fowlpox virus encoding a model tumor-associated antigen. *Journal of Immunology* 154(9): 4685–4692.

Weber, C.E. 1998. Cytokine-modified tumor vaccines: An antitumor strategy revisited in the age of molecular medicine. *Cancer Nursing* 21(3): 167–177.

Wolfel, T., Klehmann, E., Muller, C., *et al.* 1989. Lysis of human melanoma cells by autologous cytolytic T cell clones. Identification of human histocompatibility leukocyte antigen A2 as a restriction element for three different antigens. *Journal of Experimental Medicine* 170(3): 797–810.

Wolfel, T., Schneider, J., Meyer Zum Buschenfelde, K.H., *et al.* 1994. Isolation of naturally processed peptides recognized by cytolytic T lymphocytes (CTL) on human melanoma cells in association with HLA-A2.1. *International Journal of Cancer* 57(3): 413–418.

Wynn, T.A., Jankovic, D., Hieny, S., *et al.* 1995. IL-12 enhances vaccine-induced immunity to *Schistosoma mansoni* in mice and decreases T-helper 2 cytokine expression, IgE production and tissue eosinophilia. *Journal of Immunology* 154(9): 4701–4709.

Zbar, B., Bernstein, I., Bartlett, G., *et al.* 1972. Immunotherapy of cancer: Regression of intradermal tumors and prevention of growth of lymph node metastases after intralesional injection of living *Mycobacterium bovis. Journal of the National Cancer Institute* 49(1): 119–130.

Zeid, N., and Muller, H. 1993. S100 positive dendritic cells in human lung tumors associated with cell differentiation and enhanced survival. *Pathology* 25(4): 338–343.

Clinical Pearls: Vaccines

1. Patient evaluation and documentation after vaccine injection should include:
   - timing of the assessment (i.e., the number of hours postinjection);
   - measurement of induration, erythema, or edema at the vaccination site;
   - assessment for site-specific symptoms or systemic symptoms such as fever;
   - determination of the effectiveness of symptom control measures;
   - assessment for lymphadenopathy in draining lymph node regions in the limb where the injection was made.
2. An acute reaction within the first 15 minutes (local or systemic) may suggest an allergic reaction as opposed to the expected cellular inflammatory response.
3. The patient's cellular immunity is often assessed before the use of vaccines by delayed-type hypersensitivity (DTH) skin testing.

Key References

Berd, D. (ed.). 1998. Cancer Tumor Vaccines. *Seminars in Oncology* 25(6): 605–706.

Herlyn, D., and Birebent, B. 1999. Advances in cancer vaccine development. *Annals of Medicine* 31(1): 66–78.

Minev, B.R., Chavez, F.L., and Mitchell, M.S. 1999. Cancer vaccines: Novel approaches and new promise. *Pharmacology Therapeutics* 81(2): 121–139.

Mitchell, M.S. 1997. A personal (biased) perspective on cancer "vaccines." *Oncology Research* 9(9): 459–465.

Oncology Education Services. 2000. *Dendritic Cells: The Sentry Cell of the Immune System.* Pittsburgh, PA: Oncology Education Services. Supported by an unrestricted educational grant from Immunex Corporation. Monograph and on-line CE available fall of 2000.

Pardoll, D.M. 1998. Cancer vaccines. *Nature Medicine* 4(5): 525–531.

Ravindranath, M.H., and Morton, D.L. 2000. Active specific immunotherapy with vaccines. In Bast, R.C., Kufe, D.W., Pollock, R.E., Weichselbaum, R.R., Holland, J.F., and Frei E. (eds). *Cancer Medicine,* 5th edn. Hamilton, Ontario: B.C. Decker, Inc., pp. 800–814.

Restifo, N.P., Ying, H., Hwang, L., *et al.* 2000. The promise of nucleic acid vaccines. *Gene Therapy* 7(2): 89–92.

Rosenberg, S.A. (ed.). 2000. *Principles and Practice of the Biologic Therapy of Cancer,* 3rd edn. Philadelphia, PA: Lippincott Williams & Wilkins, pp. 491–732 (Section IV: Principles and Practice of Cancer Vaccines).

Shu, S., Plautz, G.E., Krauss, J.C., *et al.* 1997. Tumor immunology. *Journal of the American Medical Association* 278(22): 1972–1981.

Shurin, M.R. 1996. Dendritic cells presenting tumor antigen. *Cancer Immunology and Immunotherapy* 43(3): 158–164.

Sinkovics, J.G., and Horvath, J.C. 2000. Vaccination against human cancers (review). *International Journal of Oncology* 16(1): 81–96.

Sorokin, P. 2000. Vaccine guide 1999. *Biotherapy-ONCBIO* (ONS Special Interest Group Newsletter) 11(1): 3, 4, 6.

Stockwell, L.H., McGonagle, D., Martin, I.G., *et al.* 2000. Dendritic cells: Immunological sentinels with a central role in health and disease. *Immunology and Cell Biology* 78(2): 91–102.

Weiner, D.B., and Kennedy, R.C. 1999. Genetic vaccines. *Scientific American* 281(1): 50–57.

CHAPTER 11 | Tumor Necrosis Factor

Lynne Brophy, RN, MSN

For centuries, spontaneous regression and even complete eradication of some tumors have been noticed in patients who have had fever or inflammation (Nauts *et al.*, 1953; Westphal, 1975; Westphal, 1987). These findings encouraged physicians in the 19th century to inject cancer patients with pus from patients with erysipelas to see whether their tumors would regress. In the late 19th century, Dr. William Coley, a surgeon practicing in New York City, recognized that people often died of sepsis after such treatment. He administered a mixture of gram-positive and gram-negative bacteria to patients with cutaneous, easily measurable, primary or metastatic tumors. Administration of "Coley's toxins" often elicited a tumor response, including some complete clinical responses (Coley, 1893).

A half century later, Hartwell and colleagues discovered that the active ingredient in Coley's toxins was endotoxin or lipopolysaccharide, a component of the bacterial cell wall (Hartwell *et al.*, 1943; Westphal *et al.*, 1975). Later, Old and others (Carswell *et al.*, 1975) isolated a substance that was produced by activated macrophages, monocytes, and lymphocytes after exposure to endotoxin and called it tumor necrosis factor (TNF) (Carswell *et al.*, 1975). TNF appeared to be responsible for the biological effects seen after a patient was exposed to endotoxin. The gene for TNF was cloned in 1984, making it possible to produce recombinant TNF in large quantities (Old, 1988). With an available supply of TNF, further delineation of its biological activities and evaluation of its efficacy in cancer patients began.

Two types of TNF exist and are nearly identical in molecular structure. The first, TNF-α, or cachectin is the cytokine produced by activated macrophages, monocytes, and lymphocytes (Tracey and Cerami, 1992). It plays a role in tumor necrosis and cell-mediated killing of bacteria, parasites, and neoplastic cells (Fraker *et al.*, 1992). The second, TNF-β, or lymphotoxin, is a cytokine produced only by lymphocytes and also has the ability to lyse tumor cells (Dinarello, 1999). Lymphotoxin has some of the same antiproliferative properties as TNF-α, and both have multiple effects on normal and tumor cells. Both are induced by other cytokines such as interferon (IFN)-γ and interleukin (IL)-1, and both play roles in hemostasis, tissue necrosis, tumor cell destruction, differentiation of leukocytes, septic shock, and cachexia. This chapter will focus on the biological and therapeutic effects of TNF-α, which will be referred to simply as TNF.

Biological Actions

Vascular Changes

TNF is named for its ability to cause necrosis in tumors and healthy tissue by reducing or stopping the flow of blood to these tissues. TNF functions by damaging the endothelial or inner lining of blood vessels, causing a narrowing or blockage of the lumen of the vessel, or by triggering intravascular coagulation. When normal endothelial cells lining blood vessel walls are exposed to TNF, procoagulant activity is increased. TNF augments secretion of inhibitors of the tissue-plasminogen activator (a substance capable of initiating fibrinolysis) and stimulates release of the platelet-activating factor, resulting in an increased risk for disseminated intravascular coagulation (DIC) (Medcalf *et al.*, 1988; Schleef and Loskutoff, 1988; Van den Berg *et al.*, 1988; Fiers, 1995). The platelet-activating factor increases platelet aggregation, causes bronchoconstriction, activates leuko-

cytes, increases capillary permeability, and decreases cardiac output, resulting in hypotension (Smith, 1998).

When blood begins to clot, inflammatory mediators are released, antigen expression increases, and the functioning of the blood vessel wall changes. After changes in antigen expression, neutrophils and platelets are able to adhere to the endothelial lining. After adherence takes place, cells such as neutrophils are able to migrate across the endothelium into the extravascular space (Fiers, 1995). These changes result in swelling (inflammation) in the extravascular space. When TNF levels are very high, as in the case of septic shock, the fluid leakage increases incrementally. This phenomenon is known as "capillary leak syndrome" and results in hypotension due to decreased intravascular volume.

Effects on Hematopoietic Cells

The activities of TNF in the body increase the number of white blood cells and augment the functioning of the immune system. TNF affects leukocytes, or white blood cells, in various ways. It induces monocyte differentiation such that a portion of the monocytes produced become macrophages, it activates monocytes, and it mediates monocyte cytotoxicity (Spriggs, 1991). When monocytes are exposed to TNF, their maturation and metabolism rates increase. After this exposure, monocytes secrete cytokines that increase antibody expression and cytokine secretion by other white blood cells. When the production of more lymphocytes is needed, TNF inhibits the proliferation of myeloid cells by decreasing production of white blood cell precursors (Piacibello *et al.*, 1990).

Activation of Immune Mechanisms

TNF has an indirect role in the production of the antibodies and cells needed for cell-mediated immunity by inducing IL-6. The changes in antibody expression begin when TNF stimulates production of IL-6 by lymphocytes. IL-6 then stimulates proliferation of B cells and has been shown to inhibit the growth of breast cancer and leukemia-lymphoma cells in animal studies (Chen et al., 1998). T cells exposed to TNF express more receptors for IL-2, resulting in greater proliferation of T cells (Scheurich et al., 1987), and they also produce more granulocyte colony-stimulating factor (G-CSF) and granulocyte-macrophage colony-stimulating factor (GM-CSF) (Lu et al., 1988). However, TNF-β can inhibit these activities of TNF. Logan and others (1996) measured GM-CSF, macrophage colony-stimulating factor (M-CSF), and G-CSF levels in patients receiving intravenous TNF and mitomycin C therapy. The investigators found M-CSF and G-CSF levels to be increased after TNF therapy, but GM-CSF could not be detected. These findings support the possibility of a positive feedback loop in which exposure to increased amounts of TNF results in M-CSF and G-CSF production. Production of these growth factors results in increased production of blood cells and early release of progenitors from the bone marrow. One specific example of an immune system function enhanced by TNF is the destruction of foreign or abnormal cells: natural killer cells and lymphokine-activated T cells triggered by TNF play leading roles in the destruction of tumor cells and pathogens.

Inflammation

As a cytokine, TNF assists in the process of destroying abnormal cells other than tumor cells, such as pathogens. It indirectly destroys pathogens by serving as a mediator in the process of inflammation. Inflammation begins when bacteria invade the tissues of the body. If local immune responses, including phagocytosis, do not stop infection at the site of invasion, the pathogen may invade the circulation and cause the release of endotoxin, enterotoxin, and gram-positive cell-wall products. Antigens may also be shed (Smith, 1998). Endotoxin, a lipopolysaccharide in the walls of gram-negative bacteria, activates monocytes and macrophages by binding to them. Activation of these cells then leads to the release of TNF (Glauser, 1996). TNF and TNF-β levels are also increased by other cytokines that are activated (e.g., increased IFN-γ and IL-2 levels) after bacterial invasion. As TNF levels rise, cytokines active in the inflammatory process, such as platelet-activating factor, colony-stimulating factors, neutrophil chemotactic factor, and IL-6, are also produced in increased quantities (Broudy et al., 1987; Hajjar et al., 1987; Seelentag et al., 1987; Bussolino et al., 1988; Lapierre et al., 1988). IL-1 and TNF work together to increase blood flow and initiate a series of reactions that lead to vascular congestion, increased cellular infiltration, and the formation of clots (Dinarello, 1999). These reactions increase the ability of leukocytes to migrate to the site of inflammation and adhere to the endothelial lining (Smith, 1998). After this process, which is called margination, has begun, the white blood cells flood the intravascular and extravascular sites of invasion by a pathogen, swelling increases, and the site becomes inflamed.

TNF has the ability to directly and indirectly increase the effectiveness of white blood cells involved in humoral and cell-mediated immunity. TNF activates endothelial cells to synthesize IL-8, a potent chemotactic protein. IL-8 encourages migration and adhesion to the site of inflammation by polymorphonuclear neutrophils (PMNs) (Leirisalo-Repo, 1994). This factor aids PMNs in attracting other PMNs to sites where activated monocytes are found, thereby increasing phagocytosis in the area. Exposure to TNF also increases the ability of PMNs to kill pathogens and tumor cells (Djeu et al., 1986; Djeu and Blanchard, 1987; Shau, 1988; Djeu et al., 1990). IL-1 and TNF activate natural killer cells, T cells, PMNs, and monocytes during the inflammatory process, and TNF amplifies and mediates antibody-dependent cell-mediated cytotoxicity by natural killer and lymphokine-activated killer T cells (Ortaldo, 1986; Lattime *et al.*, 1988). Newly produced antibodies then travel to the site of infection and inflammation and detect and destroy antigens. The increased production of these various cytokines is thought to contribute to the progression from localized inflammation to a systemic inflammatory response.

Systemic inflammatory responses occur in a progressive series of stages called the systemic inflammatory response syndrome (SIRS). Septic shock is a late stage of this syndrome. When infection occurs, early inflammatory changes are characterized by increased temperature, tachycardia, tachypnea, hypoxia, and leukopenia or leukocytosis (Ackerman, 1994). IL-1, or endogenous pyrogen, is one of the cytokines stimulated by TNF during SIRS. Table 11.1 compares the biological actions of TNF and IL-1, highlighting their many similarities. After an infectious agent such as a gram-negative bacteria enters the bloodstream, macrophages are stimulated by toxins produced by this agent. These macrophages produce TNF (Glauser, 1996). TNF induces fever by stimulating IL-1 production (fever is discussed in detail in Chapter 16) but this stimulation can be inhibited by the administration of dexamethasone. The activation of cytokine, complement, coagulation, and kinin cascades is manifested by the symptoms of late SIRS: fever, hypotension, intravascular coagulation, inflammation, and multisystem organ failure possibly accompanied by DIC (Toney and Parker, 1996). Efforts to blunt the negative effects of TNF during SIRS are described later in this chapter.

Immunologic Surveillance

TNF clearly plays an important role in the body's defense against tumor development and infection, but it also has a role in destroying

Table 11.1 Similarities between TNF and IL-1

	TNF	IL-1
Pyrogen	x	x
Bone resorption	x	x
Lipoprotein lipase inhibition	x	x
Procoagulant release	x	x
Endothelial-cell adhesion molecules expression	x	x
Induction of colony-stimulating factors	x	x
Induction of IL-1, IL-6, and TNF	x	x
Radioprotective effects	x	x
Induction of myeloid differentiation	x	x
Leukocyte chemotaxis	x/0	x
Neutrophil activation	x	x
Monocyte activation	x	x
T-cell activation	x	x
Direct tumor-cell cytotoxicity	x	0
Fibroblast proliferation	x	x
Thymocyte proliferation	0	x

x, effect present; 0, effect absent.

Source: Reprinted with permission from Spriggs, D. 1991. Tumor necrosis factor: Basic principles and preclinical studies. In DeVita, V., Hellman, S., and Rosenberg, S. (eds). *Biologic Therapy of Cancer.* Philadelphia, PA: J.B. Lippincott, p. 365 (Table 16-11).

tumors that already are in place. TNF can kill selected tumor cells directly and indirectly in 3 ways. First, it is known that TNF and IFN-γ act synergistically to destroy tumor cells (Old, 1988). When cells are exposed to TNF, they swell, demonstrate damaged cell organelles, and later die. This process leads to tumor necrosis (Mueller, 1998). Second, TNF, along with IL-2 and IL-1, plays an indirect role in tumor-cell killing by activating natural killer cells (Spriggs, 1991). Third, TNF can induce apoptotic cell death.

Lipid Metabolism

Another effect of TNF on the body is cachexia, or wasting of body fat and protein, which is caused by accelerated lipid metabolism and decreased appetite (Michie *et al.*, 1989). Cachexia results in weight loss and is accompanied by decreased dietary intake and wasting of the body tissues. TNF has the ability to mobilize fat stores. After bolus administration of TNF to rats, triglyceride levels rise within two hours (Darling *et al.*, 1990). As fat stores are mobilized, triglyceride levels rise (Darling *et al.*, 1990). TNF also influences the activity of lipase, the enzyme that assists with fat processing and storage in the body, in two ways. It increases lipase activity, thereby increasing the rate at which fats are used, and inhibits the activity of enzymes that lyse lipids (Pekala *et al.*, 1983; Min and Spiegelman, 1986; Zechner *et al.*, 1988). It also changes the basal metabolic rate by stimulating hepatic cells to synthesize more lipids, DNA, albumin, transferrin, and acute-phase proteins, including some forms of complement (Feinberg *et al.*, 1988; Memon *et al.*, 1992). It has been hypothesized that TNF acts as an endogenous antineoplastic agent by preventing the provision of energy (fat) to tumor cells in the body while they grow (Urban *et al.*, 1986).

Clinical Studies in Patients with Cancer

Tumor Necrosis Factor as a Single Agent

Because of its biological activities, recombinant TNF has been given as an antineoplastic agent in many clinical studies during the past decade. Researchers hoped that the effects seen in preclinical studies, such as its ability to survey and destroy tumor cells, block the blood supply to tumors, and indirectly induce fever, and its indirect role in antibody production would lead to tumor destruction in humans.

Recombinant TNF has been given as therapy for melanoma; colorectal carcinoma; acquired immunodeficiency syndrome (AIDS)–related Kaposi's sarcoma; B-cell lymphoma; non–small-cell lung cancer; gastric, endometrial, and bladder cancer; multiple myeloma; various sarcomas; ovarian cancer; breast cancer; pancreatic cancer; and glioma (Chapman *et al.*, 1987; Kahn *et al.*, 1989; Heim *et al.*, 1990; Kauffmann *et al.*, 1990; Kemeny *et al.*, 1990; Schaadt *et al.*, 1990; Whitehead *et al.*, 1990; Yang *et al.*, 1990; Brown *et al.*, 1991; Budd *et al.*, 1991; del Giglio *et al.*, 1991; Hersh *et al.*, 1991; Feldman *et al.*, 1992; Lienard *et al.*, 1992a; Lienard *et al.*, 1992b; Yoshida *et al.*, 1992; Hohenberger and Kettelhack, 1998). To date, systemic TNF given alone has not provided significant effective palliative or curative therapy for any type of cancer. Important clinical trials with recombinant human TNF are summarized in Tables 11.2 and 11.3. In a trial of TNF given intravesically, Glazier and others (1995) found TNF was well tolerated, with a side effect profile that included mild urologic symptoms, flu-like symptoms, and mild hematologic and gastrointestinal toxicity. Eight of 9 patients enrolled in this trial had a complete but temporary response to therapy. A maximum tolerated dose (MTD) level was not reached in this study; the final dose level was 1,000 mcg given via gravity flow into a urethral catheter and retained for 2 hours. Zamkoff and others (1989), in a study of 19 patients with a variety of malignancies, administered TNF subcutaneously for a 5-day period every other week for a total of 3 cycles. These patients experienced chills, fever, hypotension, and nausea, with skin ulceration and necrosis at the site. Because of significant thrombocytopenia, the MTD was set at 150 mcg/m^2/day. Regardless of route of administration, most phase I trials of TNF given as a single agent revealed no significant antitumor activity (Fraker *et al.*, 1995). It is known that some types of tumor cells are resistant to TNF; however, it is not clear why. Mueller (1998) noted that cellular proteins with major functions in the apoptotic process may be mutated and able to survive despite a lack of oxygen. Toxi-

Table 11.2 Trials of intravenous TNF defining maximal dose and dose-limiting toxicity

Investigator Name	Year of Publication	Number of Patients in Study	Trial Design	Dose Range (mcg/m²)	MTD (mcg/m²)
Creaven	1987	29	IV bolus dose q 3 weeks	4.5–218.0	218
Kimura	1987	31	Single bolus IV dose	45.0–727.0	227
Selby	1987	18	IV bolus dose q 2 weeks	4.1–545.0	410
Lenk	1988	15	Single IV bolus dose	23.0–1,454.0	818
Taguchi	1988	41	Single IV bolus dose	33.0–1,667.0	333
Schiller	1991	53	IV bolus dose 3 × week	5.0–275.0	225
Furman	1993	27	Daily IV bolus dose for 5 days	100.0–350.0	300
Creagan	1988	27	Daily IV bolus dose for 5 days	5.0–200.0	150
Feinberg	1988	39	Daily IV bolus dose for 5 days	5.0–250.0	200
Moritz	1989	19	Daily IV bolus dose for 5 days	40.0–280.0	200
Creaven	1989	33	Daily IV bolus dose for 5 days	23.0–364.0	273
Gamm	1991	62	Twice daily IV bolus doses	2.5–400.0	200
Kemeny	1990	16	Twice daily IV bolus doses	100–150.0*	N/A— phase II trial
Whitehead	1990	22	Once daily IV bolus dose	150.0	N/A— phase II trial
Hersh	1991	127	Once daily IV bolus dose	150.0	N/A— phase II trial
Feldman	1992	21	Once daily IV bolus dose	150.0	N/A— phase II trial
Brown	1991	22	Once daily IV bolus dose	150.0	N/A— phase II trial
Feinberg	1988	39	Once daily for 30 minute or once daily for 4 hour	5.0–250.0	200
Budd	1991	22	Daily IV bolus dose	150.0	N/A— phase II trial
Furman	1993	27	Daily IV bolus dose	100.0–350.0	300
Wiedenmann	1989	15	Single 24-hour continuous infusion	40.0–400.0	200
Spriggs	1988	50	Single 24-hour continuous infusion	4.5–645.0	545

Table 11.2 *Continued*

Investigator Name	Year of Publication	Number of Patients in Study	Trial Design	Dose Range (mcg/m²)	MTD (mcg/m²)
Steinmetz	1988	18	5-day continuous infusion	30.0–290.0	40
Mittelman	1992	19	5-day continuous infusion	40.0–200.0	160
Sherman	1988	19	5-day continuous infusion	22.7–136.0	109
Schwartz	1988	18	5-day continuous infusion		30–40[†]

* Patients in this study received 100 mcg/m² twice daily on day 1 of cycle 1 with escalation to 150 mcg/m² twice daily thereafter.

† Study included intrapatient dose escalation.
IV, intravenous; N/A, not applicable.

Source: Reprinted and adapted with permission from Alexander, R., and Rosenberg, S. 1991. Tumor necrosis factor: Clinical applications. In DeVita, V., Hellman, S., and Rosenberg, S. (eds). *Biologic Therapy of Cancer*. Philadelphia, PA: J.B. Lippincott, p. 380 (Table 17-1), p. 384 (Table 17-3).

city, MTD, and responses in these clinical trials may vary because of differences in the preparation of TNF, patient populations, treatment schedules, and side effect interventions (Alexander and Rosenberg, 1991).

Recombinant TNF has most commonly been administered intravenously, intra-arterially, intratumorally, intramuscularly, or subcutaneously. TNF has also been given into the peritoneal cavity and via isolated limb perfusion (ILP). Intravenous therapy can be given as a bolus or by continuous infusion. When given intravenously in lower doses, recombinant TNF has a half-life of 16 minutes; when given in higher doses (i.e., more than 150 mcg/m²), its half-life increases to 40 to 80 minutes. The short half-life of TNF accounts for the typical transience of its side effects (Fraker *et al.*, 1995). No one route or schedule for administering TNF has proven to be most successful. Long, continuous intravenous infusions may provide the highest blood levels and longest exposure to TNF. The MTDs of TNF in various clinical trials are highlighted in Tables 11.2 and 11.3. The dose-limiting toxicities in phase I

trials to date have been hypotension, nausea, and fatigue (Mueller, 1998). Posner and colleagues (1995) published the first and perhaps only study of ILP using TNF alone. Six patients were treated, each at a different TNF dose level: 1 patient each at total doses of 1 mg, 2 mg, and 3 mg, and 3 patients at a total dose of 4 mg of TNF. In this trial, 1 complete response (CR) (duration 7 months) was seen, and 4 mg was supported as the MTD of TNF. Lejeune (1995) contends that in order to isolate TNF within the area of perfusion, the MTD must be 4 mg. The results of trials in which TNF is given alone via isolated perfusion have not been as promising as results of trials in which TNF was used in combination with other agents. Therefore, research has focused on what agents or methods should be combined with TNF to effect the greatest response.

Tumor Necrosis Factor in Combination Therapy

With the goal of increasing its efficacy as an antineoplastic agent, TNF has been given in

Table 11.3 Phase I studies of recombinant TNF in patients with advanced malignancy—Intramuscular and mixed administration

Author	Manufacturer	N	Histologic Type*	Administration	MTD[†]	Dose-limiting Toxicity
Bartsch et al.	Genentech	30	Colorectal Renal Lung	IM thrice weekly for 8 weeks	150 mcg/m²	Hypotension, constitutional symptoms, local reaction at injection site
Jakubowski et al.	Genentech	19	Gastrointestinal Melanoma Breast	IM daily for 5 days every other week	150 mcg/m²	Local reaction at injection site, hepatotoxicity, leukopenia, thrombocytopenia
Blick et al.	Genentech	20	Colon Renal Multiple myeloma	Alternating IM and IV bolus twice weekly for 4 weeks	ND	NA
Chapman et al.	Genentech	26	Melanoma Renal Sarcoma Breast Colon	Alternating SQ and IV bolus twice weekly for 4 weeks	ND	NA

* Histologic type and site shown are the most frequent for each series.

[†] Maximum tolerated dose calculated from manufacturer's specific activity.

IM, intramuscularly; IV, intravenous; SQ, subcutaneous; NA, not applicable; ND, not determined.

Source: Reprinted with permission from Alexander, R., and Rosenberg, S. 1991. Tumor necrosis factor: Clinical applications. In DeVita, V., Hellman, S., and Rosenberg, S. (eds). *Biologic Therapy of Cancer.* Philadelphia, PA: J.B. Lippincott, p. 387 (Table 17-4).

clinical trials in combination with other agents with which it is known to be synergistic. The cytotoxic abilities of TNF were enhanced *in vitro* when TNF was combined with either the IFNs, mitotic inhibiting agents, dactinomycin, 5-fluorouracil, cyclophosphamide, cisplatin, doxorubicin, or etoposide or with ionizing radiation or induced hyperthermia (Williamson *et al.*, 1983; Spriggs, 1991; Sella *et al.*, 1995; Pass *et al.*, 1996). One of the difficulties in administering TNF in combination with other antineoplastic agents is the additive toxicities and, in some cases, a side effect pattern very different from that seen when TNF is given as a single-agent TNF therapy.

Human studies of TNF in combination with other cytokines have revealed some differences in side effect patterns (Kurzrock *et al.*, 1989; Yang *et al.*, 1990; Negrier *et al.*, 1992). Some of this activity may be caused by the ability of IFN-γ to increase the expression of TNF receptors on cell surfaces, thereby enhancing the effect of TNF on human cells (Aggarwal *et al.*, 1985). IFN-γ has the ability to make TNF-resistant cells sensitive to TNF's antiproliferative effects (Sugarman *et al.*, 1985; Fransen *et al.*, 1986). Abbruzzese and others (1989) administered intramuscular IFN-γ every day and recombinant TNF by intravenous bolus every 8 hours for 5 days to patients with advanced gastrointestinal cancer. Because of hyperbilirubinemia, the MTD was established at 150 mcg/m²/day for both agents.

The rationale for administering TNF and IL-2 together stems from preclinical studies. The need for participation of activated lymphocytes in the destruction of murine tumors (Asher *et al.*, 1989) during treatment with TNF suggested that strategies to augment antitumor effects of lymphocytes might increase the therapeutic response to TNF. IL-2 is known to play a pivotal role in stimulation of cytotoxic lymphocytes. Negrier and others (1992) conducted a clinical trial of continuous intravenous infusion of IL-2 (18 MIU/m²/day) for 6 days followed by single bolus infusions of TNF daily for 3 days. Patients on this trial had a variety of refractory malignancies. The side effect profile of TNF plus IL-2 is different from that of single-agent TNF therapy. The dose-limiting side effect on this trial was hypotension, and the MTD was judged to be 120 mcg/m². Despite the fact that all patients received an intravenous infusion of indomethacin during the entire duration of therapy, they experienced all the side effects seen with TNF and IL-2 when given as single agents. However, patients who received the combination regimen developed hypotension requiring dopamine therapy earlier in the treatment cycles and at lower doses of TNF (60 to 80 mcg/m²/day). One third of the patients treated on this study also experienced life-threatening pulmonary toxicity in the form of adult respiratory distress syndrome, anaphylaxis, or bronchospasm. Pulmonary toxicity was more common and severe in the group that received the combination treatment than in patients who received TNF or IL-2 alone. Only 2 partial remissions were seen in this study, one in a person with breast cancer and the other in a person with renal cell carcinoma. The authors reported they had started a phase II trial of TNF plus IL-2 for women with advanced breast cancer (Negrier *et al.*, 1992).

Schiller and others (1995) reported the results of 2 parallel pilot studies involving administration of TNF plus IL-2 to patients with advanced non–small-cell lung cancer. In one of these studies, 7 patients received IL-2 (6 × 10⁶ IU/m²/day) by continuous infusion for 5 days every 14 days. These patients also were given 50 mcg/m²/day of intramuscular TNF on days 1 through 5. Grade 3 or 4 pulmonary and/or cardiac toxicity was seen in 11 of 15 patients in these pilot studies. Like the study by Negrier and colleagues (1992), the most common grade 4 toxicity seen by Schiller was pulmonary, with 2 patients experiencing grade 4 renal and neurologic side effects. No responses were observed. The authors felt that further studies of IL-2 plus TNF should be conducted using a different treatment schedule, in the hope that this will decrease toxicity.

Some researchers have also attempted to combine TNF with chemotherapeutic agents in attempts to achieve synergistic toxicity. It has been given with etoposide and melphalan and as an accompaniment to induced hyperthermia. In one study of TNF plus etoposide, patients experienced not only the side effects seen with single-agent TNF and etoposide therapy but also a profound myelosuppression (Orr *et al.*, 1989; Sherman, 1992). The systemic administration of TNF in effective tumoricidal doses seems to be impossible because of significant systemic toxicities. For this reason, research about the regional perfusion of TNF with other therapies is ongoing.

Isolated Perfusion

Research investigating combination therapy administered via perfusion into isolated regions of the body has produced some very exciting results. TNF has been administered in combination with chemotherapy or biotherapy and hyperthermia into the limbs, lungs, and peritoneal cavity. TNF was initially combined with chemotherapy for limb perfusion in order to exploit TNF's ability to necrose sarcomas. TNF has been combined with chemotherapy and/or biotherapy and administered via ILP in a few studies (Lienard *et al.*, 1992a; Fraker *et al.*, 1996; Thom *et al.*, 1995; Eggermont *et al.*, 1996).

Lienard's work has been helpful in establishing the MTD of TNF and effective therapeutic combinations for regional perfusion. Lienard chose to add IFN-γ to TNF in order to exploit the synergy between these agents. In his study of TNF, IFN-γ, and melphalan via ILP with or without hyperthermia for patients with sarcoma and melanoma, the CR rate was 89%, and the

duration of the response was improved from that of melphalan alone (Lienard *et al.*, 1992a). The time until CR was shortened in the study, and duration of all responses in the trial was longer than previously seen. The MTD in this trial was 4 mg of TNF in the perfusate in order to avoid systemic toxicity; the dose-limiting toxicity was myelosuppression. This dose was still considered to be the MTD of TNF for regional perfusion in a review by Alexander *et al.*, (1996).

In their study of TNF and melphalan with or without IFN for patients with sarcomas, Eggermont and others (1996) noted flu-like symptoms, neurotoxicity, hypotension, transient myelosuppression, and transient rise in hepatic transaminases. There were a 29% CR rate and a 53% partial response (PR) rate in this trial. Fraker *et al.* (1996) found painful myopathy and neuropathy to be the dose-limiting toxic effects in their trial of ILP with melphalan, TNF, and IFN-γ plus hyperthermia for patients with melanoma. The CR rate was 76%. Thom *et al.* (1995) also treated patients with refractory melanoma and sarcoma using ILP with melphalan alone or ILP with melphalan, TNF, and IFN-γ. The most common toxic effects in the TNF combination treatment arm of this study were fever and hypotension. Response rates were lower in this trial: 50% of patients treated in the TNF arm had a CR and the other 50% had a PR. Patients in the melphalan-only arm had a CR rate of 57% and a PR rate of 43%. Patients in this trial who experienced hypotension had a greater evidence of leak from the perfusion circuit.

In 1999, Lev-Chelouche and others (1999) reported the encouraging results of a small trial of hyperthermia and ILP with melphalan (1 to 1.5 mg/kg) and TNF (3 to 4 mg) for patients with soft tissue sarcoma. Two patients experienced toxic effects in the form of redness and blistering of the treated extremities. The response rate was 92%, with 38% of these responses being CRs. This study offered more support for the hypothesis that ILP with TNF and melphalan plus hyperthermia may offer palliation for patients with soft tissue sarcomas.

Once interest was piqued in regional perfusion of TNF as part of a combination regimen, Pass and others (1996) administered moderate hyperthermia plus TNF plus IFN-γ in an attempt to determine whether isolated lung perfusion could be done safely with TNF. Twenty patients with lung metastases arising from several types of cancer were perfused with TNF (0.3 to 0.6 mg) and IFN-γ (0.2 mg) via an oxygenation pump circuit for 90 minutes during hyperthermia treatment. When TNF did not leak from the pump circuit, none of the cardiovascular side effects expected with TNF were seen. Short-term PRs were seen in 3 of 15 (20%) patients who ultimately received perfusions. Their trial was successful in demonstrating that it is possible to locally infuse into the lung high levels of cytokines, which if given systemically would result in multisystem organ failure. Zwaveling *et al.* (1996) noted SIRS in patients who received limb perfusion with TNF, IFN-γ, and hyperthermia. Patients in this study who developed SIRS had to be moved to intensive care. It was theorized that SIRS developed when TNF leaked from the limb via collateral blood flow. Once methods to control leakage or SIRS in the setting of lung perfusion are developed, localized perfusion of TNF will become a safer treatment option.

Bartlett and others (1998) chose to use continuous hyperthermic peritoneal infusion with cisplatin and with or without TNF for patients with a variety of cancers. The majority of patients on this trial (41%) had colon cancer. The dose-limiting toxicity in this trial was renal toxicity, which the investigators felt was caused by cisplatin, despite the use of sodium thiosulfate. No significant toxicities were attributed to TNF. The MTD in the perfusate was 0.1 mg/m² of TNF with 250 mg/m² of cisplatin. All patients' tumors in this trial were reduced to such a level that they were not visible on a computed tomography scan. Because of the location of the tumors, clinical observations were not possible and response rates could not be judged. Duration of survival was not reported because of the variety of tumor types treated in the trial and the differences in expected survival associated with each tumor.

Alexander and others (1998) administered TNF and melphalan via isolated hepatic perfusion in combination with hyperthermia in an attempt to provide a more effective therapy with less systemic toxicity to patients with primary or metastatic disease to the liver. The investigators administered TNF at 1.0 mg and melphalan at 1.5 mg/kg. The treatment proved to be quite toxic, with 75% of patients experiencing grade 3 or 4 hepatic toxicity such as veno-occlusive disease, elevated bilirubin levels, and elevated transaminase levels. TNF is strongly suspected of having major responsibility for these toxicities. Despite the high incidence of toxicity, 75% of patients treated experienced a response (1 CR and 26 PRs). These results moved the investigators to recommend further investigation into isolated hepatic perfusion with melphalan with and without TNF.

Isolated perfusion with anticancer agents is still not standard practice, and ILP is the most successful perfusion method thus far. At this time, ILP is not an accepted treatment for locally advanced sarcoma and melanoma, as stated by Mueller (1998), but rather a therapy still being investigated, which can be administered safely if MTDs are used and the proper perfusion technique is employed (Alexander *et al.*, 1996). Future research needs to include well-designed trials with standardized doses of drugs and TNF and controlled methods of limb perfusion and hyperthermia. The duration of limb perfusion in these studies must be set, and the Esmarch tourniquet must be applied carefully to avoid higher rates of neuropathies

(Alexander *et al.*, 1996). ILP and chemotherapy need to be compared with surgical techniques such as integumentectomy or excision with or without grafting of skin. Investigation of perfusion into the lung, liver, and peritoneum has just begun. In the future, we will see studies looking at the efficacy of combination therapies that include TNF infused into other areas of the body, such as the liver, kidneys, and peritoneum. It is hoped these strategies will bring promising results.

Regulatory Status

As of July 2000, TNF has not yet been approved by the Food and Drug Administration for open-label use as an antineoplastic agent in the United States. TNF is currently produced by Boehringer Ingelheim, Ingelheim, Germany (Boehringer Ingelheim, 2000). Boehringer Ingelheim became licensed as a producer of TNF-α (Beromune®) in 1999. TNF-α is currently under registration as a treatment for soft tissue sarcoma in Germany.

Adverse Effects

The multiple side effects associated with therapeutic administration of TNF reflect the protein's many physiological effects. The side effect profile associated with TNF therapy is very much dependent on the dose and route of administration. For example, patients receiving high-dose intravenous therapy are more likely to have hypotension, fever, severe rigors, and focal neurological deficits such as aphasia. Individuals receiving low-dose subcutaneous therapy may experience local skin reaction at the injection site and mild flu-like symptoms. It is very important for the clinician to be aware of the self-limiting transitory nature of the side effects associated with TNF therapy.

A transient but significant side effect of TNF therapy is chills, which can progress to severe rigors and are usually followed by fever. Flu-like symptoms accompany the development of fever during and after TNF therapy and may include fatigue, anorexia, nausea, vomiting, diarrhea, malaise, and headaches (Alexander and Rosenberg, 1991). Chills related to TNF are a part of the physiological stage of fever. Fever begins with TNF stimulating the production of IL-1; IL-1 then stimulates the hypothalamus to produce fever. While fever is developing, the patient may experience headache, fatigue, malaise, and transitory aching. Moldawer and Figlin (1988) reported TNF-associated headaches as being dull, aching, frontal in location, and decreasing in severity and frequency as therapy progressed. Vasoconstriction and piloerection of the skin are followed by shivering or chills. This chilling phase can be, but is not always, followed by rigors, the generalized and involuntary shaking of the body. The rigors or chills increase the body temperature, after which these sensations stop and a sensation of warmth returns.

Fever and chills may appear at all dose levels of TNF therapy. Severe chills or rigors are one of the hallmarks of high-dose TNF therapy and can be quite frightening to the patient and significant others. Chills can begin as soon as an hour after beginning TNF therapy and are followed by fever. The pattern of fever onset, duration, and curve associated with TNF therapy varies according to the dose and schedule of therapy (Blick *et al.*, 1987; Feinberg *et al.*, 1987; Creaven *et al.*, 1989). Mild chills associated with low-dose TNF therapy will last for only a short time and usually cause only minor discomfort. Severe rigors lasting longer than a few minutes and causing the patient and the bed to shake are quite uncomfortable and frightening. (Refer to Chapter 16 for information about handling chills and rigors.)

Flu-like symptoms can be accompanied by

hypotension and capillary leak syndrome. Hypotension occurs at different time points during therapy, depending on the route of administration and the dose of TNF, and has been the dose-limiting side effect in many clinical trials (Feinberg et al., 1987; Taguchi, 1988; Alexander and Rosenberg, 1991). Any patient who receives TNF may experience hypotension, but those with a history of cardiac disease are more susceptible. Hypotension is most common in persons receiving intravenous therapy in doses equal to or greater than 100 mcg/m^2, and it almost always occurs in patients who receive 200 mcg/m^2 or more of intravenous TNF. Because of this, 200 mcg/m^2 has often been considered the MTD in clinical trials. Persons receiving TNF and experiencing hypotension often appear to have capillary leak syndrome (Tracey and Cerami, 1992). When doses higher than 100 mcg/m^2 are given, patients are often prehydrated.

In an effort to control TNF-induced hypotension, Lissoni et al. (1996) administered the pineal hormone melatonin concomitantly during a trial of IL-2 or TNF. In this trial of 116 cancer patients with advanced disease, patients received either IL-2 (3×10^6 IU/day subcutaneously 6 days a week for 4 weeks) or TNF (0.75 mg/day intravenously for 5 days). Patients were randomized to receive either no additional therapy or melatonin (40 mg/day orally in the evening) starting 7 days before cytokine therapy. Patients receiving melatonin experienced statistically significantly lower rates of hypotension. The investigators felt this effect might be caused by melatonin blocking the synthesis of nitric oxide, an endogenous vasodilator. Further study is needed to learn more about the effects of melatonin.

Although TNF is not a vesicant, it can cause irritation of the skin, characterized by erythema with or without induration and tenderness (Moldawer and Figlin, 1988). Injection-site reactions are most common with intramuscular and sub-

cutaneous TNF therapy. Reactions to TNF doses less than 150 mcg/m^2 usually occur 24 to 48 hours after the injection, resolve within 2 to 3 days, and are self-limiting (Moldawer and Figlin, 1988; Jakubowski et al., 1989). No therapy is needed for these minor reactions. Patients who receive TNF doses equal to or more than 150 mcg/m^2 intramuscularly or 100 mcg/m^2 subcutaneously are at risk for more severe skin reactions, which may include bulla formation at the injection site followed by ulceration and ensuing necrosis. This side effect can be prevented by dividing the dose and administering it at two sites, preferably the deltoid areas (Zamkoff et al., 1989). The cause of this skin reaction is not known.

Like skin reactions, other transitory acute reactions to TNF, such as changes in laboratory values, usually prove to be harmless. Multiple transitory changes in laboratory parameters may be seen at some dose levels. Changes in the complete blood count may include leukopenia, thrombocytopenia, and transient leukocytosis, especially elevations in monocyte counts. Increases in white blood cell counts during and after administration of TNF have stimulated the production of colony-stimulating factors, which increase production of white blood cells. Leukocytosis is transient: the leukocyte count usually does not exceed 20,000/mm^3 for more than a day, and the elevated leukocyte count resolves completely within a few days after therapy has ended. Thrombocytopenia is most common in patients who receive continuous intravenous or lengthy intramuscular therapy and is a result of platelets being used during the process of capillary thrombosis and hemorrhagic necrosis (Moldawer and Figlin, 1988). Thrombocytopenia can be accompanied by elevated levels of fibrin degradation products and reduced levels of fibrinogen, both of which resolve within a few days (Creaven et al., 1987; Kimura et al., 1987). TNF stimulates acute-phase protein biosynthesis by the liver, resulting in increased hepatic transaminase levels, particularly SGOT, SGPT, and BUN, and severe hypophosphatemia, which may be accompanied by cardiac arrhythmias (Taguchi, 1988; del Giglio *et al.*, 1991; Tracey and Cerami, 1992). Administration of TNF may also affect other tests, such as lung diffusion capacity (DLCO).

Patients who receive TNF therapy, both those with and without previous lung disease, have experienced dyspnea during and after administration of TNF and, when tested during or after therapy, have been found to have decreased DLCO (Creaven *et al.*, 1987; Kimura *et al.*, 1987; Figlin *et al.*, 1988; Moldawer and Figlin, 1988; Taguchi, 1988). Morice and others (1987) noted dyspnea in patients who received TNF on a phase I clinical trial. Pulmonary function testing on these patients revealed that those who received moderate to high doses of TNF (>50 mcg/m^2) or greater cumulative doses had acute, reversible changes in respiratory function as evidenced by decreased DLCO values. The DLCO levels returned to near baseline levels in all patients within 2 weeks of discontinuing therapy. Morice and colleagues suggested that changes in respiratory function were caused by endothelial changes within the lung and by pulmonary edema. The potential for these changes makes it advisable to do pulmonary function testing before TNF therapy and to monitor the respiratory status of patients carefully for dyspnea while they are receiving TNF. Further research is needed to determine what level of baseline respiratory dysfunction indicates that a patient is not able to receive TNF therapy.

Patients with baseline neurological deficits also may not be good candidates for TNF therapy because of the risk of central nervous system toxicity. Toxic effects of the central nervous system can include focal neurological deficits, such as aphasia, confusion, seizures, and cerebral vascular accidents (Moldawer and Figlin, 1988). Patients who experience these side effects should have therapy discontinued imme-

diately and should be carefully evaluated to determine the cause of the symptoms.

Clinicians caring for persons who are receiving TNF must be vigilant in assessing for the toxic side effects of TNF therapy. When the treatment dose, route, and schedule have been chosen, patients should be educated to look for fever and flu-like symptoms (if known). In general, persons with a history of coagulation problems or cardiac, pulmonary, hepatic, renal, or neurological disorders may not be good candidates for TNF therapy. Clinicians administering TNF in combination with other antineoplastic agents must be aware that side effect profiles may change or side effects may worsen when combination therapy is given. For example, side effects in patients who received TNF and IFN-γ included fever and flu-like symptoms that differed from those in patients who received TNF alone. Although hepatic transaminase levels did not increase significantly in patients who received TNF alone, alkaline phosphatase and lactic acid dehydrogenase did increase in the patients who received the combination (Kurzrock *et al.*, 1989).

Future Directions

TNF has not proven to be the "magic bullet" many people hoped it would be. Of course, TNF, like other biological agents, is very different from chemotherapeutic agents in that it has a wide range of effects on both normal and cancer cells. For this reason, routes and schedules of administration traditionally used with chemotherapy to treat cancer have not been very effective with TNF. The route that currently shows some promise is ILP with TNF in combination with other agents, such as melphalan. As clinical trials with ILP continue, they will need to focus on standardization of methods, as discussed earlier in the chapter. Possibly TNF may have to be delivered directly to tumors (i.e., locoregional administration) in order to achieve the desired therapeutic effect. Monoclonal antibodies attached to TNF have been shown to target tumor cells rather than endothelial cells (Corti and Marcucci, 1998). These results encourage the further investigation of TNF fused with monoclonal antibodies with the hope that systemic toxicity will be avoided.

Several methods for increasing the tumor-cell–killing ability of TNF are under investigation and may lead to more clinical trials with systemic TNF in the future. One combination therapy that seems to hold promise is IFN-γ and TNF. When TNF is given with IFN-γ, cytotoxic activity is greatly increased (Fransen *et al.*, 1986). In the laboratory, cytotoxicity also appears to increase when TNF is given with inhibitors of intracellular signaling pathways, such as staurosporine, a prototypic protein kinase C inhibitor (Corti and Marcucci, 1998). Perhaps the systemic toxicity of TNF can be reduced by encasing it in a liposome (Corti and Marcucci, 1998). Liposomal TNF has been found to be just as effective as non–lipid-bound TNF (Corti and Marcucci, 1998). Others have suggested that prolongation of the half-life of TNF may enhance its antitumor effects. Sidhu and Bollon (1993) have suggested derivatization of TNF, with polyethylene glycol as a route to this end. All of these are exciting possibilities, and one of them may hold the key to successful systemic TNF therapy in sufficient cytostatic doses.

Efforts to block TNF's actions will most definitely continue in the future. After TNF was found to be one of the cytokines involved in the mucosal immune response, researchers began to administer anti-TNF antibodies to patients with inflammatory bowel disease in an attempt to block the proinflammatory effects of TNF (Rogler and Andus, 1998). Administration of the anti-TNF antibody resulted in improvement for patients with inflammatory bowel disease except when they were in an early stage of peritonitis (Van Dullemen *et al.*, 1995). Patients in early peritonitis tended to survive a shorter amount of time compared with patients who received the anti-TNF antibody in a later stage of peritonitis, which indicates that TNF must play an important role in the immune response in peritonitis (Echtenacher *et al.*, 1990). Blockage of the effects of TNF may also be the future of rheumatoid arthritis therapy. Monoclonal antibodies targeted to TNF used in clinical trials have resulted in marked improvement in symptoms and articulation (Sander and Rau, 1998). Agents such as the pyridinyl-imidazole compounds, which stop IL-1 and TNF release from human monocytes, and pentoxifylline, which indirectly stops TNF synthesis, may have the potential to block the development of pulmonary fibrosis (Coker and Laurent, 1998). Because of TNF's many helpful and harmful effects, future TNF-related research will focus on augmenting and blocking TNF's activities in patients with cancer and other diseases.

References

Abbruzzese, J., Levin, B., Ajani, J., *et al.* 1989. Phase I trial of recombinant human gamma interferon and recombinant human tumor necrosis factor in patients with advanced gastrointestinal cancer. *Cancer Research* 49(14): 4057–4061.

Ackerman, M.H. 1994. The systemic inflammatory response, sepsis, and multiple organ dysfunction. *Critical Care Nursing Clinics of North America* 6(2): 243–250.

Aggarwal, B., Eessalu, E., and Hass, P. 1985. Characterization of receptors for human tumor necrosis factor and their regulation by gamma-interferon. *Nature* 318(6047): 665–667.

Alexander, H.R., Bartlett, D.L., Libutti, S.K., *et al.* 1998. Isolated hepatic perfusion with tumor necrosis factor and melphalan for unresectable cancers confined to the liver. *Journal of Clinical Oncology* 4: 1479–1489.

Alexander, H.R., Fraker, D.L., and Bartlett, D.L.

1996. Isolated limb perfusion for malignant melanoma. *Seminars in Surgical Oncology* 12: 416–428.

Alexander, R., and Rosenberg, S. 1991. Tumor necrosis factor: Clinical applications. In DeVita, V., Hellman, S., and Rosenberg, S. (eds). *Biologic Therapy of Cancer.* Philadelphia, PA: J.B. Lippincott Co., pp. 378–392.

Asher, A., Mulé, J., and Rosenberg, S. 1989. Recombinant human tumor necrosis factor mediates regression of a murine sarcoma *in vivo* via Lyt-2⁺ cells. *Cancer Immunology and Immunotherapy* 28(2): 153–156.

Bartlett, D.L., Buell, J.F., Libutti, S.K., *et al.* 1998. A phase I trial of continuous hyperthermic peritoneal perfusion with tumor necrosis factor and cisplatin in the treatment of peritoneal carcinomatosis. *Cancer* 83(6): 1251–1261.

Bartsch, H., Nagel, G., Mull, R., *et al.* 1988. Phase I study of recombinant human tumor necrosis factor-alpha in patients with advanced malignancies. *Molecular Biotherapy* 1: 21–29.

Blick, M., Sherwin, S., and Rosenblum, M. 1987. Phase I study of recombinant tumor necrosis factor in cancer patients. *Cancer Research* 47: 2986–2989.

Boehringer Ingelheim. Web site *http://www.boehringer-ingelheim.com/.* Accessed July 1, 2000.

Broudy, V., Harlan, J., and Adamson, J. 1987. Disparate effects of tumor necrosis factor-alpha/ cachectin and tumor necrosis factor-beta/lymphotoxin on hematopoietic growth factor production and neutrophil adhesion molecule expression by cultured human endothelial cells. *Journal of Immunology* 138(12): 4298–4302.

Brown, T.D., Goodman, P., Fleming, T., *et al.* 1991. A phase II trial of recombinant tumor necrosis factor in patients with adenocarcinoma of the pancreas: A Southwest Oncology Group study. *Journal of Immunotherapy* 10(5): 376–378.

Budd, G.T., Green, S., Baker, L.H., *et al.* 1991. A Southwest Oncology Group phase II trial of recombinant tumor necrosis factor in metastatic breast cancer. *Cancer* 68(8): 1694–1695.

Bussolino, F., Cammussi, G., and Baglioni, C. 1988. Synthesis and release of platelet-activating factor by human vascular endothelial cells treated with tumor necrosis factor or interleukin-1 alpha. *Journal of Biological Chemistry* 263(24): 11856–11861.

Carswell, E., Old, L., Kassel, R., *et al.* 1975. An endotoxin-induced serum factor which causes necrosis of tumors. *Proceedings of the National Academy of Sciences of the USA* 72: 3666–3670.

Chapman, P., Lester, T., Casper, E., *et al.* 1987. Clinical pharmacology of recombinant human tumor necrosis factor in patients with advanced cancer. *Journal of Clinical Oncology* 2(12): 1942–1951.

Chen, L., Mory, Y., Zilbertein, A., *et al.* 1998. Growth inhibition of human breast carcinoma and leukemia/lymphoma cell lines by recombinant interferon-beta 2. *Proceedings of the National Academy of Sciences of the USA* 85: 8037–8041.

Coker, R.K., and Laurent, G.J. 1998. Pulmonary fibrosis: Cytokines in the balance. *European Respiratory Journal* 11: 1218–1221.

Coley, W. 1893. The treatment of malignant tumors by repeated inoculations of erysipelas, with a report of ten original cases. *American Journal of Medical Science* 105: 487–511.

Corti, A., and Marcucci, F. 1998. Tumor necrosis factor: Strategies for improving the therapeutic index. *Journal of Drug Targeting* 5(6): 403–413.

Creagan, E., Kovach, J., Moertel, C., *et al.* 1988. A phase I clinical trial of recombinant human tumor necrosis factor. *Cancer* 62: 2467–2471.

Creaven, P., Brenner, D., and Cowens, W. 1989. Phase I clinical trial of recombinant human tumor necrosis factor (rH-TNF) given on a daily × 5 schedule. *Cancer Chemotherapy and Pharmacology* 23(3): 186–191.

Creaven, P., Plager, J., Dupere, S., *et al.* 1987. Phase I clinical trial of recombinant human tumor necrosis factor. *Cancer Chemotherapy and Pharmacology* 20: 137–144.

Darling, G., Fraker, D.L., Jensen, C., *et al.* 1990. Cachectic effects of recombinant human tumor necrosis factor in rats. *Cancer Research* 50: 4008.

del Giglio, A., Zukiwski, A., Ali, K., *et al.* 1991. Severe, symptomatic, dose-limiting hypophosphatemia induced by hepatic arterial infusion of recombinant tumor necrosis factor in patients with liver metastases. *Cancer* 67(10): 2459–2461.

Dinarello, C.A. 1999. Cytokines as endogenous pyrogens. *The Journal of Infectious Diseases* 179(suppl 2): S294–S304.

Djeu, J., and Blanchard, D. 1987. Regulation of human polymorphonuclear neutrophil (PMN) activity against *Candida albicans* by large granular lymphocytes via release of a PMN-activating factor. *Journal of Immunology* 139(8): 2761–2767.

Djeu, J., Blanchard, D., Halkias, D., *et al.* 1986. Growth inhibition of *Candida albicans* by human polymorphonuclear neutrophils: Activation by interferon-gamma and tumor necrosis factor. *Journal of Immunology* 137(9): 2980–2984.

Djeu, J.Y., Servoubek, D., and Blanchard, D.K. 1990. Release of tumor necrosis factor by human polymorphonuclear leukocytes. *Blood* 76(7): 1405–1409.

Echtenacher, B., Falk, W., and Mannel, D.N., *et al.*, 1990. Requirement of endogenous tumor necrosis factor/cachectin for recovery from experimental peritonitis. *Journal of Immunology* 145: 3762.

Eggermont, A.M.M., Koops, H.S., Liernard, D., *et al.* 1996. Isolated limb perfusion with high-dose tumor necrosis factor-alpha in combination with interferon-gamma and melphalan for irresectable extremity soft tissue sarcomas: A multicenter trial. *Journal of Clinical Oncology* 14: 2653–2665.

Feinberg, B., Kurzrock, R., Blick, M., *et al.* 1987. Phase I study of recombinant tumor necrosis factor in patients with disseminated cancer. *Proceedings of the American Society of Clinical Oncology* 6: 238 (abstract).

Feinberg, B., Kurzrock, R., Talpaz, M., *et al.* 1988. A phase I trial of intravenously administered recombinant tumor necrosis factor-alpha in cancer patients. *Journal of Clinical Oncology* 6: 1328–1334.

Feldman, E.R., Creagan, E.T., Schaid, D.J., *et al.* 1992. Phase II trial of recombinant tumor necrosis factor in disseminated malignant melanoma. *American Journal of Clinical Oncology* 15(3): 256–259.

Fiers, W. 1995. Biologic therapy with TNF: Preclinical studies. In DeVita, V., Hellman, S., and Rosenberg, S. (eds). *Biologic Therapy of Cancer,* 2nd edn. Philadelphia, PA: J.B. Lippincott Co., pp. 295–327.

Figlin, R., de Kerion, J., and Sarna, G. 1988. Phase II study of recombinant tumor necrosis factor (rTNF) in patients with metastatic renal cell carcinoma (rCCa) and malignant melanoma (MM). *Proceedings of the American Society of Clinical Oncology* 7: 169 (abstract).

Fraker, D., Alexander, H., and Norton, J. 1992. Biologic therapy of sepsis: The role of antibodies to endotoxin and tumor necrosis factor and the interleukin-1 receptor antagonist. In DeVita, V., Hellman, S., and Rosenberg, S. (eds). *Biologic Therapy of Cancer Updates* 2(3). Philadelphia, PA: J.B. Lippincott Co., pp. 1–12.

Fraker, D., Alexander, H., and Pass, H. 1995. Biologic therapy with TNF: Systemic administration and isolation-perfusion. In DeVita, V., Hellman, S., and Rosenberg, S. (eds). *Biologic Therapy of Cancer,* 2nd edn . Philadelphia, PA: J.P. Lippincott Co., pp. 329–345.

Fraker, D., Alexander, H., Andrich, M., *et al.* 1996. Treatment of patients with melanoma of the extremity using hyperthermic isolated limb perfusion with melphalan, tumor necrosis factor, and interferon gamma: results of a tumor necrosis factor dose escalation study. *Journal of Clinical Oncology* 14(2): 479–489.

Fransen, L., Van, D., Ruysschaert, R., *et al.* 1986. Recombinant tumor necrosis factor: Its effect and its synergism with interferon-gamma on a variety of normal and transformed human cell lines. *European Journal of Cancer and Clinical Oncology* 22(4): 419–426.

Furman, W. L., Strother, D., McClain, K., *et al.* 1993. Phase I clinical trial of recombinant human tumor necrosis factor in children with refractory solid tumors: A Pediatric Oncology Group study.

Journal of Clinical Oncology 11(11): 2205–2210.

Gamm, H., Lindemann, A., Mertelsmann, R., *et al.* 1991. Phase I trial of recombinant human tumour necrosis factor alpha in patients with advanced malignancy. *European Journal of Cancer* 27(7): 856–863.

Glauser, M.P. 1996. The inflammatory cytokines. New developments in the pathophysiology and treatment of septic shock. *Drugs* 52(suppl 2): 9–17.

Glazier, D.B., Bahnson, R.R., McLeod, D.G., *et al.* 1995. Intravesical recombinant tumor necrosis factor in the treatment of superficial bladder cancer: An Eastern Cooperative Oncology Group study. *Journal of Urology* 154(1): 66–68.

Hajjar, K., Hajjar, D., Silverstein, R., *et al.* 1987. Tumor necrosis factor–mediated release of platelet-derived growth factor from cultured endothelial cells. *Journal of Experimental Medicine* 166(1): 1235–1245.

Hartwell, J., Shear, M., and Adams, J. 1943. Chemical treatment of tumors: Nature of the hemorrhage-producing fraction from *Serratia marcescens* (*B. prodiziosus*) culture filtrates. *Journal of the National Cancer Institute* 4: 107–122.

Heim, M., Siegund, R., Illiger, H., *et al.* 1990. Tumor necrosis factor in advanced colorectal cancer: A phase II study. A trial of the phase I/II study group of the Association for Medical Oncology of the German Cancer Society. *Onkologie* 13(6): 444–447.

Hersh, E.M., Metch, B.S., Muggia, F.M., *et al.* 1991. Phase II studies of recombinant human tumor necrosis factor alpha in patients with malignant disease: A summary of the Southwest Oncology Group experience. *Journal of Immunotherapy* 10(6): 426–431.

Hohenberger, P., and Kettelhack, C. 1998. Clinical management and current research in isolated limb perfusion for sarcoma and melanoma. *Oncology* 55: 89–102.

Jakubowski, A., Casper, E., Gabrilove, J., *et al.* 1989. Phase I trial of intramuscularly administered tumor necrosis factor in patients with advanced

cancer. *Journal of Clinical Oncology* 7(3): 298–303.

Kahn, J., Kaplan, L., Volderding, P., *et al.* 1989. Intralesional recombinant tumor necrosis factor-alpha for AIDS-associated Kaposi's sarcoma: A randomized, double-blind trial. *Journal of Acquired Immune Deficiency Syndrome* 2(3): 217–223.

Kauffmann, M., Schid, H., Raeth, U., *et al.* 1990. Therapy of ascites with tumor necrosis factor in ovarian cancer. *Geburtshilfe und Frauenheilkunde* 50(9): 678–682.

Kemeny, N., Childs, B., Larchian, W., *et al.* 1990. A phase II trial of recombinant tumor necrosis factor in patients with advanced colorectal carcinoma. *Cancer* 66(4): 659–663.

Kimura, K., Taguchi, T., Urushizaki, I., *et al.* 1987. Phase I study of recombinant human tumor necrosis factor. *Cancer Chemotherapy and Pharmacology* 20: 223–229.

Kurzrock, R., Feinberg, B., Talpaz, M., *et al.* 1989. Phase I study of a combination of recombinant tumor necrosis factor-alpha and recombinant interferon-gamma in cancer patients. *Journal of Interferon Research* 9(4): 435–444.

Lapierre, L., Fiers, W., and Pober, J. 1988. Three distinct classes of regulatory cytokines control endothelial cell MHC antigen expression. Interactions with immune gamma interferon differentiate the effects of tumor necrosis factor and lymphotoxin from those of leukocyte alpha and fibroblast beta interferons. *Journal of Experimental Medicine* 167(3): 794–804.

Lattime, E., Stoppacciaro, A., Khan, A., *et al.* 1988. Human natural cytotoxic activity mediated by tumor necrosis factor: Regulation by interleukin-2. *Journal of the National Cancer Institute* 80(13): 1035–1038.

Leirisalo-Repo, M. 1994. The present knowledge of the inflammatory process and the inflammatory mediators. *Pharmacology and Toxicology* 75(suppl 2): 1–3.

Lejeune, F.J. 1995. High dose recombinant tumor necrosis factor (rTHFa) administered by isolation perfusion for advanced tumours of the limbs: A model for biochemotherapy of cancer. *European Journal of Cancer* 31A: 1009–1016.

Lenk, H., Tanneberger, S., Müller, U., *et al.* 1988. Human pharmacological investigation of a human recombinant tumor necrosis factor preparation (PAC-4D), a phase-I trial. *Archives Geschwulstforsch* 58: 89–97.

Lev-Chelouche, D., Abu-Abeid, S., Kollander, Y., *et al.* 1999. Mulitfocal soft tissue sarcoma: Limb salvage following hyperthermic isolated limb perfusion with high-dose tumor necrosis factor and melphalan. *Journal of Surgical Oncology* 70: 185–189.

Lienard, D., Ewalenko, P., Delotte, J., *et al.* 1992a. High-dose recombinant tumor necrosis factor alpha in combination with interferon gamma and melphalan in isolation perfusion of the limbs for melanoma and sarcoma. *Journal of Clinical Oncology* 10: 52–60.

Lienard, D., Lejeune, F., and Ewalenko, P. 1992b. In transit metastases of malignant melanoma treated by high dose rTNF alpha in combination with interferon-gamma and melphalan in isolation perfusion. *World Journal of Surgery* 16(2): 234–240.

Lissoni, P., Pittalis, S., Ardizzoia, A., *et al.* 1996. Prevention of cytokine-induced hypotension in cancer patients by the pineal hormone melatonin. *Supportive Care in Cancer* 4(4): 313–316.

Logan, T.F., Gooding, W., Kirkwood, J., *et al.* 1996. Tumor necrosis factor administration is associated with increased endogenous production of M-CSF and G-CSF but not GM-CSF in human cancer patients. *Experimental Hematology* 24: 49–53.

Lu, L., Srour, E., Warren, D., *et al.* 1988. Enhancement of release of granulocyte- and granulocyte-macrophage colony-stimulating factors from phytohemagglutinin-stimulated sorted subsets of human T lymphocytes by recombinant human tumor necrosis factor-alpha. Synergism with recombinant human IFN-gamma. *Journal of Immunology* 141(1): 201–207.

Medcalf, R., Kruithof, E., and Schleuning, W. 1988. Plasminogen activator inhibitor 1 and 2 are tumor necrosis factor/cachectin-responsive genes. *Journal of Experimental Medicine* 168(2): 751–759.

Memon, R.A., Feingold, K.R., Moser, A.H., *et al.* 1992. Differential effects of interleukin-1 and tumor necrosis factor on ketogenesis. *American Journal of Physiology* 263: E301.

Michie, H.R., Sherman, M.L., Spriggs, D.R., *et al.* 1989. Chronic TNF infusion causes anorexia but not accelerated nitrogen loss. *Annals of Surgery* 209: 19.

Min, H., and Spiegelman, B. 1986. Adipsin, the adipocyte serine protease: Gene structure and control of expression by tumor necrosis factor. *Nucleic Acids Research* 14(22): 8879–8892.

Mittelman, A., Puccio, C., Gafney, E., *et al.* 1992. A phase I pharmacokinetic study of recombinant human tumor necrosis factor administered by a 5-day continuous infusion. *Investigational New Drugs* 10(3): 183–190.

Moldawer, N., and Figlin, R. 1988. Tumor necrosis factor: Current clinical status and implications for nursing management. *Seminars in Oncology Nursing* 4(2): 120–125.

Morice, R., Blick, M., Ali, M., *et al.* 1987. Pulmonary toxicity of recombinant tumor necrosis factor (rTNF). *Proceedings of the American Society of Clinical Oncology* 6: 29 (abstract).

Moritz, T., Niederle, N., Baumann, J., *et al.* 1989. Phase I study of recombinant human tumor necrosis factor alpha in advanced malignant disease. *Cancer Immunology and Immunotherapy* 29: 144–150.

Mueller, H. 1998. Tumor necrosis factor as an antineoplastic agent: Pitfalls and promises. *Cellular and Molecular Life Sciences* 54: 1291–1298.

Nauts, H., Fowler, G., and Bogatko, F. 1953. A review of the influence of bacterial infection and of bacterial products (Coley's toxins) on malignant tumors in man. *Acta Medica Scandinavica Supplementum* 276: 1–103.

Negrier, M., Pourreau, C., Paler, P., *et al.* 1992. Phase I trial of recombinant interleukin-2 followed by recombinant tumor necrosis factor in patients with metastatic cancer. *Journal of Immunotherapy* 11: 93–102.

Old, L. 1988. Tumor necrosis factor. *Scientific American* 141: 59–60, 69–75.

Orr, D., Oldham, R., Lewis, M., *et al.* 1989. Phase I study of the sequenced administration of etoposide (VP-16) and recombinant tumor necrosis factor (rTNF; Cetus) in patients with advanced malignancy. *Proceedings of the American Society of Clinical Oncology* 8: A741 (abstract).

Ortaldo, J. 1986. Comparison of natural killer and natural cytotoxic cells: Characteristics, regulation and mechanism of action. *Pathology and Immunopathology Research* 5(3–5): 203–218.

Pass, H.I., Mew, D.J., Kranda, K.C., *et al.* 1996. Isolated lung perfusion with tumor necrosis factor for pulmonary metastases. *Annals of Thoracic Surgery* 61(6): 1609–1617.

Pekala, P., Kawakai, M., Angus, C., *et al.* 1983. Selective inhibition of synthesis enzymes for de novo fatty acid biosynthesis by an endotoxin induced mediator from exudate cells. *Proceedings of the National Academy of Sciences of the USA* 80: 2743–2747.

Piacibello, W., Sanavio, F., Severino, A., *et al.* 1990. Opposite effect of tumor necrosis factor alpha on granulocyte colony-stimulating factor and granulocyte-macrophage colony-stimulating factor–dependent growth of normal and leukemic hemopoietic progenitors. *Cancer Research* 50(16): 5065–5071.

Posner, M.C., Lienard, D., Lejeune, F.J., *et al.* 1995. Hyperthermic isolated limb perfusion with tumor necrosis factor alone for melanoma. *Cancer Journal Scientific American* 1: 274–280.

Rogler, G., and Andus, T. 1998. Cytokines in inflammatory bowel disease. *World Journal of Surgery* 22: 382–389.

Sander, O., and Rau, R. 1998. Clinical trials on biologics in rheumatoid arthritis. *International Journal of Clinical Pharmacology and Therapeutics* 36(11): 621–624.

Schaadt, M., Pfreundschuh, M., Lorscheidt, G., *et al.* 1990. Phase II study of recombinant human tumor necrosis factor in colorectal carcinoma. *Journal of Biological Response Modifiers* 9: 247–250.

Scheurich, P., Thoa, B., Ucer, U., *et al.* 1987. Immunoregulatory activity of recombinant human tumor necrosis factor (TNF)-alpha: Induction of TNF receptors on human T cells and TNF-alpha–mediated enhancement of T cell responses. *Journal of Immunology* 138(6): 1786–1790.

Schiller, J.H., Morgan-Ihrig, C., and Levitt, M.L. 1995. Concomitant administration of interleukin-2 plus tumor necrosis factor in advanced non–small cell lung cancer. *American Journal of Clinical Oncology* 18(1): 47–51.

Schiller, J.H., Storer, B.E., Witt, P.L., *et al.* 1991. Biological and clinical effects of intravenous tumor necrosis factor-alpha administered three times weekly. *Cancer Research* 51(6): 1651–1658.

Schleef, R., and Loskutoff, D. 1988. Fibrinolytic system of vascular endothelial cells. Role of plasminogen activator inhibitors. *Haemostasis* 18(4–6): 328–341.

Schwartz, J., Hersh, E., Wiggins, C., *et al.* 1988. Phase I study of recombinant tumor necrosis factor administered by continuous infusion to cancer patients. *Proceedings of the American Society of Clinical Oncology* 7: 58 (abstract).

Seelentag, W., Mermod, J., Montesano, R., *et al.* 1987. Additive effects of interleukin-1 and tumour necrosis factor-alpha on the accumulation of the three granulocyte and macrophage colony-stimulating factor mRNAs in human endothelial cells. *EMBO Journal* 6(8): 2261–2265.

Selby, P., Hobbs, S., Viner, C., *et al.* 1987. Tumor necrosis factor in man: Clinical and biological observations. *British Journal of Cancer* 56: 803–808.

Sella, A., Aggarwal, B.B., Kilbourn, R.G., *et al.* 1995. Phase I study of tumor necrosis factor plus actinomycin D in patients with androgen-independent prostate cancer. *Cancer Biotherapy* 10(3): 225–235.

Shau, H. 1988. Characteristics and mechanisms of neutrophil-mediated cytostasis induced by tumor necrosis factor. *Journal of Immunology* 141(1): 234–240.

Sherman, M., Spriggs, D., Arthur, K., *et al.* 1988. Recombinant human tumor necrosis factor administered as a five day continuous infusion in cancer patients: Phase I toxicity and effects on lipid metabolism. *Journal of Clinical Oncology* 6(2): 344–350.

Sherman, M., Spriggs, D., Arthur, K., *et al.* 1992. Enhanced myelosuppression in a phase I trial of recombinant human tumor necrosis factor in combination with etoposide. *Proceedings of the American Association for Cancer Research* 33: A1468 (abstract).

Sidhu, R.S., and Bollon, A.P. 1993. Tumor necrosis factor activities and cancer therapy—a perspective. *Pharmacology and Therapeutics* 57(1): 79–128.

Smith, A.L. 1998. Treatment of septic shock with immunotherapy. *Pharmacotherapy* 18(3): 565–580.

Spriggs, D. 1991. Tumor necrosis factor: Basic principles and preclinical studies. In DeVita, V., Hellman, S., and Rosenberg, S. (eds). *Biologic Therapy of Cancer.* Philadelphia, PA: J.B. Lippincott Co., pp. 354–377.

Spriggs, D., Sherman, M., Michie, H., *et al.* 1988. Recombinant human tumor necrosis factor administered as a 24-hour intravenous infusion. A phase I and pharmacologic study. *Journal of the National Cancer Institute* 80: 1039–1044.

Steinmetz, T., Schaadt, M., Gähl, R., *et al.* 1988. Phase I study of 24-hour continuous intravenous infusion of recombinant human tumor necrosis factor. *Journal of Biological Response Modifiers* 7: 417–423.

Sugarman, B., Aggarwal, B., Hass, P., *et al.* 1985. Recombinant human tumor necrosis factor-alpha: Effects on proliferation of normal and transformed cells in vitro. *Science* 230(4728): 943–945.

Taguchi, T. 1988. Phase I study of recombinant human tumor necrosis factor (rHu-TNF:PT-050). *Cancer Detection and Prevention* 12: 561–572.

Thom, A.K., Alexander, R., Andrich, M.P., *et al.* 1995. Cytokine levels and systemic toxicity in patients undergoing isolated limb perfusion with high-dose tumor necrosis factor, interferon gamma, and melphalan. *Journal of Clinical Oncology* 13(1): 264–273.

Toney, J.F., and Parker, M.P. 1996. New perspectives on the management of septic shock in the cancer patient. *Infectious Disease Clinics of North America* 10(2): 239–250.

Tracey, K., and Cerami, A. 1992. Tumor necrosis factor in the malnutrition (cachexia) of infection and cancer. *American Journal of Tropical Medicine and Hygiene* 47(suppl 1): 2–7.

Urban, J., Shepard, H., Rothstein, J., *et al.* 1986. Tumor necrosis factor: A potent effector molecule for tumor cell killing by activated macrophages. *Proceedings of the National Academy of Sciences of the USA* 83: 8318.

van den Berg, E.A., Sprengers, E., Jaye, M., *et al.* 1988. Regulation of plasminogen activator inhibitor-1 mRNA in human endothelial cells. *Thrombosis and Haemostasis* 60(1): 63–67.

Van Dullemen, H.M., van Deventer, S.J., Hommes, D.W., *et al.* 1995. Treatment of Crohn's disease with anti-tumor necrosis factor chimeric monoclonal antibody (cA2). *Gastroenterology* 109: 129.

Westphal, O. 1975. Bacterial endotoxins. The second Carl Prausnitz Memorial Lecture. *International Archives of Allergy and Applied Immunology* 49(1–2): 1–43.

Westphal, O. 1987. Hommage à Valy Menkin. In Bonavida, B., Gifford, G., Kirchner, H., *et al.* (eds). *International Conference on Tumor Necrosis Factor and Related Cytokines.* Basel, Switzerland: Karger, pp. 1–6.

Whitehead, R.P., Fleming, T., Macdonald, J.S., *et al.* 1990. A phase II trial of recombinant tumor necrosis factor in patients with metastatic colorectal adenocarcinoma: A Southwest Oncology Group study. *Journal of Biological Response Modifiers* 9(6): 588–591.

Wiedenmann, B., Reichardt, P., Räth, U., *et al.* 1989. Phase-I trial of intravenous continuous infusion of tumor necrosis factor in advanced metastatic carcinomas. *Journal of Cancer Research and Clinical Oncology* 115: 189–192.

Williamson, B., Carswell, E., Rubin, B., *et al.* 1983. Human tumor necrosis factor produced by human B-cell lines: Synergistic cytotoxic interaction with human interferon. *Proceedings of the National Academy of Sciences of the USA* 80: 5397–5401.

Yang, S., Owen-Schaub, L., Mendiguren-Rodriguez, A., *et al.* 1990. Combination immunotherapy for non–small-cell lung cancer. Results with interleukin-2 and tumor necrosis factor-alpha. *Journal of Cardiothoracic Surgery* 99(1): 8–12.

Yoshida, J., Wakabayashi, T., Mizuno, M., *et al.* 1992. Clinical effect of intra-arterial tumor necrosis factor-alpha for malignant glioma. *Journal of Neurosurgery* 77(1): 78–83.

Zamkoff, K., Newman, N., Rudolph, A., *et al.* 1989. A phase I trial of subcutaneously administered recombinant tumor necrosis factor to patients with advanced malignancy. *Journal of Biological Response Modifiers* 8: 539–552.

Zechner, R., Newman, T., Sherry, B., *et al.* 1988. Recombinant human cachectin/tumor necrosis factor but not interleukin-1 alpha down-regulates lipoprotein lipase gene expression at the transcriptional level in mouse 3T3-L1 adipocytes. *Molecular and Cellular Biology* 8(6): 2394–2401.

Zwaveling, J.H., Maring, J.K., Clarke, F.L., *et al.* 1996. High plasma tumor necrosis factor (TNF)-alpha concentrations and a sepsis-like syndrome in patients undergoing hyperthermic isolated limb perfusion with recombinant TNF-alpha, interferon-gamma, and melphalan. *Critical Care Medicine* 24(5): 765–770.

Key References

Alexander, H.R., and Feldman, A.L. 2000. Tumor necrosis factor: Basic principles and clinical applications in systemic and regional cancer treatment. In Rosenberg, S.A. (ed). *Principles and Practice of the Biologic Therapy of Cancer*, 3rd edn. Philadelphia, PA: Lippincott Williams & Wilkins, pp. 174–193.

Corti, A., and Marcucci, F. 1998. Tumour necrosis factor: Strategies for improving the therapeutic index. *Journal of Drug Targeting* 5(6): 403–413.

Exley, A., Cohen J., Buurman, W., *et al.* 1990. Monoclonal antibody to TNF in severe septic shock. *The Lancet* 335: 1275–1277.

Fraser, M., Marentay, P., and Bertha, R. 1999. A collaborative approach to isolated limb perfusion. *Association of Operating Room Nurses Journal* 70(4): 642–647, 649, 651–653.

Frei, E., and Spriggs, D. 1989. Tumor necrosis factor: Still a promising agent. *Journal of Clinical Oncology* 7(3): 291–294.

Mueller, H. 1998. Tumor necrosis factor as an antineoplastic agent: Pitfalls and promises. *Cell and Molecular Life Sciences* 54(12): 1291–1298.

CHAPTER 12 | The Retinoids

Paula Trahan Rieger, RN, MSN, CS, AOCN®, FAAN

Fadlo R. Khuri, MD

The **retinoids** have been recognized for more than 50 years for their profound impact on biological functions (Smith *et al.*, 1992). The relationship between vitamin A and cancer was noted as early as the 1920s, when experimentally induced vitamin A deficiency was shown to lead to precancerous lesions and, ultimately, cancer. In the 1960s, studies in animal models and other experiments began to demonstrate the potential therapeutic effects of vitamin A in cancer (Sporn *et al.*, 1976a, 1976b). Dramatic results following treatment of acute promyelocytic leukemia (APL), metastatic squamous-cell cancer of the skin, and squamous-cell carcinoma of the cervix led cancer specialists in early 1990 to obtain **investigational new drug application (INDA)** status for the therapeutic use of retinoids (Smith *et al.*, 1992).

Retinoid research has increased significantly over the past 20 years as a result of an improved understanding of their basic biology, the powerful role they play in influencing **gene expression** and their potential impact on the malignant process. These factors have led to investigations of the retinoids as therapeutic and chemopreventive agents (Evans and Kaye, 1999; Lippman and Lotan, 2000; Sporn and Suh, 2000). To date, the retinoids have been investigated both alone and in combination for the treatment of various human cancers, including skin cancers, cervical cancer, APL, lung cancer, bladder cancer, and squamous-cell cancer of the head and neck as a chemopreventive agent in the management of oral leukoplakia, squamous metaplasia of the lung, and second primary cancers in the upper aerodigestive system, and skin cancer.

As of July 2000, 2 retinoids have received

approval for use in cancer therapy. Tretinoin (Vesanoid®) received regulatory approval in November 1995 for the treatment of APL, and bexarotene (Targretin®) received regulatory approval in December 1999 for the treatment of cutaneous T-cell lymphoma (CTCL). This chapter reviews the biology of the retinoids, the major clinical trial investigations of the clinical efficacy of the major types of retinoids, known toxicities associated with retinoids, and future directions for the use of the retinoids in the management of cancer.

Biological Activity

The retinoids are a family of naturally occurring compounds that include vitamin A (retinol) and related derivatives. Vitamin A is a nonspecific term that encompasses two families of dietary factors: preformed vitamin A (inclusive of retinol and its esters) and provitamin A carotenoids. The latter category includes β-carotene and other carotenoids that can serve as metabolic precursors of retinol. Preformed vitamin A is found primarily in foods of animal origin, such as liver, meat, eggs, and milk products, whereas the primary sources of vitamin A carotenoids are fruits and vegetables, especially cruciferous vegetables such as cabbage (Mayne and Lippman, 1997).

After dietary retinol is absorbed into the small intestine, it is transported to the liver, where it is stored. Bound to a retinol-binding protein, retinol is released from the liver at a constant rate and transported to the tissues via the bloodstream. There are 2 types of carrier proteins in the plasma: retinol-binding protein (RBP) and *trans*-thyretin. Cells transfer retinol from RBP to the apo (or unbound) form of cytoplasmic RBP (CRBP). This is the specific *intracellular*-binding protein for retinol. Once bound to CRBP, retinol can be **esterified** by lecithin-retinol acyltransferase or **oxidized** to

retinoic acid (RA). The RAs include all-*trans*-retinoic acid (ATRA) and its 2 isomers, 13-*cis*-retinoic acid (13cRA) and 9 *cis*-retinoic acid (9cRA) (Blaner and Olson, 1994; Soprano and Blaner, 1994; Lippman and Davies, 1997).

The best-studied agents in human chemoprevention and cancer therapy include these natural derivatives (i.e., esters and isomers of RA) and synthetic analogues of vitamin A. ATRA (i.e., vitamin A acid or tretinoin) is a natural retinol metabolite and the **photoisomer** of 13cRA (i.e., isotretinoin or Accutane®), a well-investigated agent used widely in dermatology (Parkinson *et al.*, 1992). Another natural retinoid isomer is 9cRA. These natural derivatives are produced synthetically for use in the treatment of disease (Table 12.1).

Long known for their effects on a variety of biological functions, retinoids normally perform significant roles in vision, growth, reproduction, epithelial-cell **differentiation**, immune function, and **apoptosis** (i.e., programmed cell death) (Smith *et al.*, 1992). It is now known that the retinoids exert most of their biological effects by modulating gene expression. Once transported into the cell, retinol acts on the nucleus by binding to nuclear RA receptors and then mediating gene expression (Figure 12.1). The potentially beneficial effects of RA include direct induction of differentiation, direct growth inhibition without differentiation, a paracrine-mediated growth inhibition or differentiation, and induction of apoptosis (Smith *et al.*, 1992). The primary physiological function of the retinoids is to control the growth and differentiation of normal cells during embryonic development. The retinoids are capable of inducing differentiation of some cells and arresting development and differentiation of others. The pharmacological effects of the retinoids in cancerous cells replicate the basic biological effects of the retinoids in embryonic cells. The complexity of retinoid action *in vivo* is now known to result from the complicated

Table 12.1 Types of retinoids

Name	Natural or Synthetic	Receptor Activated	Primary Clinical Use
Vitamin A (retinol)	Natural	Binds to extracellular retinol-binding proteins and is then rebound intracellularly to cellular retinol-binding proteins and is metabolized to retinoic acid	Evaluation in chemoprevention
Retinal (retinyl palmitate)	Natural; esterified compound of retinol	Same as above	None
ATRA (tretinoin)	Natural analogue*	Panagonist for the RAR	Regulatory approval for the treatment of APL
13-*cis*-retinoic acid (isotretinoin); isomer of ATRA	Natural analogue*	Does not bind to RAR or RXR; rapidly isomerized to ATRA within the cell	Chemoprevention
9-*cis*-retinoic acid (panretinide); isomer of ATRA	Natural analogue*	Panagonist for RAR and RXR	Chemoprevention and under study in APL Panretim® gel is approved for the topical treatment of lesions in patients with acquired immune deficiency syndrome-related Kaposi's sarcoma.
4-hydroxyphenyl retinamide (fenretinide)	Synthetic	May function independently of a receptor; induction of apoptosis	Chemoprevention
Bexarotene	Synthetic	RXR selective	Approved for the treatment of CTCL; under clinical investigation in treatment of cancer, diabetes, and hyperlipidemia and in chemoprevention
Etretinate	Synthetic	RAR selective	Chemoprevention

APL, acute promyelocytic leukemia; ATRA, all-*trans*-retinoic acid; CTCL, cutaneous T-cell lymphoma; RAR, retinoic acid receptors; RXR, retinoid X receptors.
* Produced synthetically for use in chemoprevention and treatment.

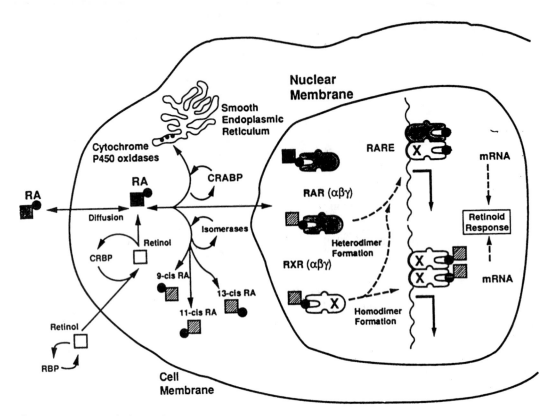

Figure 12.1   Metabolism of ATRA. Retinoic acid (RA) enters the cell by simple diffusion or by conversion from retinol (vitamin A) that has been absorbed from the gastrointestinal tract, bound in circulating form to retinol-binding proteins (RBP), and rebound intracellularly to cellular retinol-binding proteins (CRBP). RA can be immediately metabolized upon binding to cellular retinoic acid-binding proteins (CRABP) and oxidized by cytochrome P450 enzymes located in smooth endoplasmic reticulum. Alternatively, RA (or its isomer) enters the cell nucleus and binds to retinoic acid receptors (RARs) or retinoid X receptors (RXRs). Upon dimerization of these receptors (i.e., formation of a RAR-RXR heterodimer or RXR/RXR homodimer), RA-activated receptors bind with high affinity to specific DNA segments (the retinoic acid response element [RARE]) and effect mRNA transcription. Ultimately, the retinoid response is mediated by primary target genes, by interferences with other transcription factors, or by control of certain post-transcriptional actions.

Reprinted with permission from Warrell, R., de Thé, H., Wang, Z., *et al.* 1993. Acute promyelocytic leukemia. *New England Journal of Medicine* 329: 177–189.

biology of the nuclear receptors that mediate the biological effects of the retinoids (Chambon, 1996).

The nuclear retinoid receptors are members of a receptor superfamily that mediates the effects of numerous compounds such as steroid and thyroid hormones and vitamin D. There are two classes of retinoid receptors that act as transcription factors: RA receptors (RARs) and retinoid X receptors (RXRs). Each class includes 3 subclasses: alpha (α), beta (β), and gamma (γ). These subclasses are encoded by different genes and may be further divided into a large number of isoforms. Different RARs and RXRs appear to have distinct tissue-specific expression patterns and different biological functions (Mangelsdorf *et al.*, 1994 and 1995).

To exert their biological effect, the retinoid receptors must bind to one another to form either homodimers (the same) or heterodimers (different) that ultimately control gene expression. The retinoid responsiveness of a cell depends on both the quality and quantity of retinoid receptors active within that cell. Each retinoid receptor appears to be associated with a preferred pattern of target genes. There is evidence of considerable **redundancy** in the function of the individual receptors, which implies that there may be significant uses for retinoid therapy. The inactivation of retinoid-signalling pathways caused by mutations or functional inactivation may be potentially restored through activation of residual receptors and alternative signalling pathways. It also appears that the retinoids can suppress the activity of other transcription factors that are mediators of cellular proliferation. In sum, a growing list of genes have been shown to contain RA response elements, giving rise to both immediate and delayed effects (Clifford *et al.*, 1999).

Retinoids also have very definite effects on the immune system. They enhance humoral- and cell-mediated immune responses and **phagocytosis** by macrophages, and, according to extensive *in vivo* and *in vitro* studies, they induce prostaglandin synthesis. Interleukin-2 production by helper T cells, which leads to killer T-cell proliferation, is also augmented by RA (Dennert, 1985). These **immunomodulation** effects may be relevant to some oncologic uses of the retinoids (Smith *et al.*, 1992).

Clinical Studies

Chemoprevention

The term *chemoprevention*, first introduced in 1976 by Sporn *et al.*, may be defined as "the use of specific natural or synthetic chemical agents to reverse, suppress, or prevent carcinogenic progression to invasive cancer." A review by Lippman, Lee *et al.* (1998) states that there have been more than 60 randomized chemoprevention trials reported in the English language literature, with the results of 9 of those trials qualifying as definitive. The criteria used in the article to select definitive trials included factors such as the primary end point of cancer incidence, 2-sided hypothesis testing, randomization with placebo control versus interventions, large-scale trials, and a duration of more than 3 years. Of these nine trials, 4 evaluated the use of retinol.

Two trials were classified as positive (i.e., protective) definitive trials. The first positive trial evaluated the effect of tamoxifen in decreasing the incidence of breast cancer in women at increased risk for the disease. This trial evaluated the use of tamoxifen or placebo. More than 13,000 women were treated with tamoxifen or placebo for 5 years. A highly statistically significant reduction in breast cancer incidence was seen in the women on the tamoxifen arm of the trial, which led to the approval of tamoxifen in 1998 for use as a chemopreventive agent in women at increased risk for developing breast cancer. The second positive trial was the Skin Cancer Prevention-Actinic Keratosis trial. This trial evaluated the efficacy of retinol (25,000 IU/day) in preventing a first new squamous-cell carcinoma or a first new basal-cell carcinoma of the skin. The trial involved more than 2,200 subjects at moderate risk for skin cancer. Retinol treatment prevented squamous-cell carcinoma (at moderate statistical significance) but not basal-cell carcinoma. Although only 2 trials were classified as positive, much was learned that will guide the future use of the retinoids and other chemopreventive agents in cancer management.

Two basic concepts provide the rationale for the use of chemoprevention as part of cancer control: the multistep nature of cancer development and field **carcinogenesis**. It is now believed that cancer occurs as a result of the accumulation of successive mutations in the genes that control how cells grow, differentiate, repair genetic damage, and ultimately die (see Chapter 3). These multiple genetic alterations also results in the **phenotypic** alteration of cells. The use of chemoprevention is based on the premise that intervention is possible during the many steps of this process (Sporn *et al.*, 1976a).

In review, carcinogenesis has been broadly divided into 3 phases: initiation, promotion, and progression. With initiation, a carcinogen interacts with DNA, producing a fixed mutation. During promotion, the initiated cells proliferate.

This stage occurs over a long period and may be altered by agents that affect growth rates. Progression is the phase between a premalignant lesion and the development of invasive cancer. The rate of progression is based on the rate of genetic mutation and cell proliferation.

Field carcinogenesis describes the concept of a person being at risk for extensive, multifocal, genetically distinct premalignant and malignant lesions because of exposure of a region to carcinogens. An example would be exposure of the aerodigestive tract to the carcinogens in cigarette smoke. Table 12.2 reviews factors relevant to the design of chemoprevention trials.

As with biotherapy in general, the mechanisms of action of current chemopreventive agents are not well understood (Meyskens, 1999). For this reason, there is no widely accepted scheme for the classification of agents. One proposed classification scheme broadly places chemopreventive agents in 2 major groups: blocking agents and suppressing agents. Blocking agents prevent cancer-producing

Table 12.2   Issues relevant to the design of chemoprevention trials

Issue	Discussion
Level of risk	Strategies may be applied to the general population or to high-risk groups
Level of toxicity	The general assumption is that the toxicity level must be lower for acceptance by general population; high-risk groups may be more accepting of some toxicity
Sample size	The use of high-risk groups will allow for smaller sample sizes due to increased incidence rates
Study end points	Cancer incidence is the obvious end point for a chemoprevention trial; however, the low incidence of cancer often necessitates lengthy studies with thousands of patients enrolled. Biological indices of neoplasia, based on clinical, histologic, genetic, biochemical, proliferative, or differentiation-related properties, may be used to estimate the potential for progression to cancer and thus to determine the effect of the agent being tested. These biological indices are referred to as surrogate (intermediate) end point biomarkers.

Data from Singh, D.K., and Lippman, S. 1998. Cancer chemoprevention. Part 1 Retinoids and carotenoids and other classic antioxidants. *Oncology* 12 (11): 1643–1658.

compounds from reaching or reacting with critical target sites in the tissues. Suppressing agents prevent the progression of the neoplastic process in cells already altered by stimuli from carcinogens.

CHEMOPREVENTION TRIALS USING ATRA

Despite extensive studies revealing a significant degree of activity of ATRA in patients with myelodysplastic syndromes, the efficacy of this compound in the chemoprevention of human solid malignancies is quite limited. However, there remain compelling data to support a chemopreventive effect of ATRA against both cervical and skin malignancies. Topical ATRA was found to have a significant effect in the treatment of cervical dysplasia. In a study evaluating 301 patients with moderate (i.e., cervical intraepithelial neoplasia 2) and severe (i.e., cervical intraepithelial neoplasia 3) dysplasia who were randomized to receive either topical ATRA or placebo, a higher complete response rate was obtained in the ATRA group (43%) than in the placebo group (27%; $p = .041$) among the 141 patients with *moderate* dyspla-

sia (Meyskens *et al.*, 1994). Data also suggest that topical ATRA has significant dose-related activity in reversing premalignant skin lesions (e.g., actinic keratosis, which undergoes a malignant transformation rate of 5%). Systemic RA therapy has produced significant activity in the 2 reported randomized trials (Table 12.3). These randomized trials utilizing doses of either 0.05% or 0.1% of topical ATRA versus a vehicle control and encompassing more than 500 patients each revealed that at the higher dose, there was a significantly higher regression rate of actinic keratosis in the ATRA arm (55%) than in the vehicle-control arm (41%; $p < .001$). No prospective study has sought to evaluate intermediate end point **markers** in clinical trials of ATRA; therefore, no data exist to date on intermediate biomarkers other than cervical intraepithelial neoplasia and actinic keratosis in the treatment of cervical and skin premalignancies, respectively.

CHEMOPREVENTION TRIALS USING 9cRA

9cRA, a naturally occurring isomer of ATRA, was studied in several phase I trials. Limited

Table 12.3   Randomized intervention trials of ATRA in human cancer chemoprevention

Reference	Population	Intervention	Patients	End Point	Result	*p* Value
Kligman and Thorne, 1991	United States: actinic keratosis	Topical ATRA (0.05%)	266	Regression	42%	NS
		Vehicle control	261		34%	
Kligman and Thorne, 1991	United States: actinic keratosis	Topical ATRA (0.10%)	226	Regression	55%	<0.001
		Vehicle control	229		41%	
Meyskens *et al.*, 1994	United States: CIN 2,3	Topical ATRA (0.372%)	150	Complete response	43% (CIN 2); 25% (CIN 3)	.041 (CIN 2) NS (CIN 3)
		Placebo	151		27% (CIN 2); 31% (CIN 3)	

ATRA, all-*trans*-retinoic acid; CIN, cervical intrathelial neoplasia; NS, not significant.

studies established the maximum tolerated dose of 9cRA to be between 100 and 150 mg/m² in phase I studies; however, few clinical studies have evaluated the efficacy of 9cRA as a chemopreventive compound. An occasional complete response was achieved when 9cRA was used in the treatment of refractory promyelocytic leukemia that was no longer sensitive to ATRA (Miller *et al.*, 1995).

CHEMOPREVENTION TRIALS USING 13cRA

13cRA is, by far, the most-studied retinoid in clinical chemoprevention trials. The major areas of investigation have included single-arm trials in recurrent respiratory papillomatosis, dysplastic nevi of the skin, oral leukoplakia, and other areas, as well as randomized phase III studies in head and neck premalignancy and malignancy and lung premalignancy and malignancy. Other experience includes 2 randomized trials in nonmelanoma skin cancer: 1 in the prevention of second basal-cell carcinomas in individuals with prior basal-cell carcinoma and another in the prevention of basal- or squamous-cell carcinomas in patients with prior skin cancers. In this chapter, the focus is on the randomized trials completed to date while touching on some of the activity in uncontrolled trials.

Epithelial malignancies of the aerodigestive tract (i.e., head and neck, esophagus, and lungs) are the best-studied systems for chemoprevention. Premalignancy, second primary tumor (SPT) prevention, and primary prevention trials have all been conducted in this setting, and 13cRA has been studied in head and neck and esophageal cancers. Many of these investigations included the study of surrogate end point biomarkers.

Head and Neck Premalignancy

The oral premalignant lesion leukoplakia is a white patch that cannot be classified as any other disorder. The lesion is generally associated with tobacco use and is a precursor of squamous-cell carcinoma. Surgical removal or laser excision is the standard treatment for oral leukoplakia. Local therapy is rarely curative when multiple lesions exist or when dysplasia is found in the field. Small, hyperplastic leukoplakia lesions historically have a 30% to 40% spontaneous regression rate and are associated with a less than 5% risk of malignant transformation, as long as they are small, well demarcated, and have no evidence of dysplasia. On the other hand, erythroplakia (i.e., erythematous lesions) and dysplastic leukoplakia lesions have a less than 5% rate of spontaneous regression and are associated with a 30% to 40% lifetime risk of developing into oral cancers. This high-risk, diffuse, and multifocal disease accounts for approximately 10% to 15% of all oral premalignant lesions and is rarely controlled adequately with local therapy involving surgery or radiation therapy. Oral premalignant lesions often develop into squamous cancers at distant sites in the upper aerodigestive tract, as well as in the oral cavity. Thus, oral premalignant lesions represent an excellent model for testing chemoprevention.

Whereas there had been multiple prior studies evaluating the efficacy of 13cRA as a single agent in the reversal of leukoplakia, the first pivotal randomized trial of 13cRA in the reversal of oral premalignancy was conducted by Hong *et al.* (1986). Their report demonstrated that 3 months of high-dose 13cRA had significant activity in a prospective, randomized, double-blind, placebo-controlled clinical trial of oral leukoplakia. Oral premalignant lesions in this trial included both leukoplakia and erythroplakia. Patients with oral leukoplakia were treated with 1 to 2 mg/kg/day of 13cRA for 3 months and monitored for an additional 6 months. Clinical responses occurred in 16 (67%) of the 24 patients in the 13cRA group and in 2 (10%) of the 20 patients in the placebo group ($p = .002$). The histopathologic improvement (i.e., reversal of dysplasia) rate was also higher in the retinoid arm (54% versus 10%; $p = .01$). Major problems with the trial included substantial toxicity and a high rate of relapse with more than 50% of the patients experiencing a relapse within 2 to 3 months after discontinuing therapy.

In a subsequent study, Lippman et al. (1993) investigated the use of low-dose 13cRA to address the toxicity and relapse problems that occurred in the Hong study. Patients received a 3-month induction course of high-dose 13cRA (1.5 mg/kg/day), followed by a 9-month maintenance treatment with either low-dose 13cRA (0.5 mg/kg/day) or β-carotene (30 mg/day). Induction therapy produced a high rate of response (55%; 95% confidence interval, 42%–67%). During the maintenance phase, only 2 (8%) of the 24 patients who received low-dose 13cRA maintenance had progression of leukoplakia, compared with 16 (55%) of the 29 patients who had progression after receiving β-carotene maintenance ($p < .001$). Low-dose 13cRA was well tolerated, with no patients dropping out of the trial during the maintenance phase because of 13cRA toxicity. Follow-up was conducted for a median of 66 months to assess the long-term protective effect of 13cRA (Benner et al., 1994; Papadimitrakopoulou et al., 1997). The annual rates of cancer development in the two arms were not different after the chemopreventive effect of 13cRA had worn off approximately 18 to 24 months after treatment cessation. In addition, the clinical course of patients demonstrated a strong association between the short-term progression of oral premalignant lesions and the development of cancer. The strong correlation between long-term cancer development and short-term progression of premalignant lesions supports the validity of using oral premalignant lesion progression as

a surrogate end point in head and neck chemoprevention trials.

Lung Premalignancy

There have been two trials reported on the use of 13cRA in lung premalignancy. Adding to the difficulty in this area is the fact that there is less consensus about the definition of lung premalignancy than there is about oral leukoplakia as a reasonable model for head and neck premalignancy. Saccomanno et al. (1982) were among the first to use cytologic changes as a marker of premalignancy. Twenty-six patients with documented abnormalities and sputum samples ranging from moderate atypical metaplasia to overt carcinoma were treated with 1 to 2.5 mg/kg/day of 13cRA. Although Saccomanno et al. found no improvement in the degree of atypia after this treatment, they did note significant alterations in cellular morphology. In the only randomized study of 13cRA in lung premalignancy, Lee et al. (1994) evaluated a series of individuals who had a metaplasia index of 15% or greater, with the metaplasia index calculated by dividing the number of tissue samples with metaplasia by the number of tissue samples counted and then multiplying the sum by 100. They conducted a randomized, double-blind, placebo-controlled trial of 13cRA in chronic smokers. The volunteers in this study underwent bronchoscopy and had endobronchial biopsies taken from six specific anatomic sites within the proximate lung field. Of the 152 chronic smokers who were screened with bronchoscopic biopsies, 93 patients had squamous metaplasia or dysplasia. Eligible smokers with metaplasia or dysplasia were randomized to 6 months of treatment with 13cRA or placebo. Of the 86 patients randomized, 69 were assessable following completion of 6 months of therapy. The extent of metaplasia decreased similarly (in approximately 50% of the subjects) in both study arms. Only smoking cessation (confirmed biologically using cotinine levels), which occurred in 16 patients (10 in the 13cRA group, 6 in the placebo group) was associated significantly with a reduction in the metaplasia index during the 6-month intervention. Therefore, in this one trial, there did not appear to be any evidence that 13cRA can have a substantial effect on lung premalignancy, given the models used.

Head and Neck Second Primary Tumor Prevention Trials

The high likelihood of SPTs following treatment of early head and neck squamous-cell cancer makes this disease an excellent model for the chemoprevention of SPTs. Hong et al. (1990) conducted a randomized, double-blind, placebo-controlled trial of high-dose 13cRA as adjuvant therapy following definitive surgery, radiation therapy, or a combination of these treatments for patients with advanced primary head and neck squamous-cell cancer. One hundred and three patients were randomly assigned to receive either high-dose 13cRA (50 to 100 mg/m²/day) or placebo for 12 months. After a median follow-up of 32 months, SPTs developed in 2 (4%) of 49 patients treated with 13cRA compared with 12 (24%) of 51 patients receiving placebo ($p = .005$). A total of 14 SPTs occurred, with 13 (93%) located in the tobacco-smoke-exposed field of the upper aerodigestive tract, lungs, and esophagus. The limitations of the study were the substantial toxicity caused by high-dose 13cRA (i.e., one third of the retinoid-treated patients required dose reductions or discontinuation of therapy) and a lack of impact on recurrence or overall survival.

These data were reanalyzed after a median follow-up of 4.5 years (Benner et al., 1994). Retinoid-treated patients continued to have significantly fewer total SPTs: 7 (14%) in the 13cRA arm and 16 (31%) in the placebo arm ($p = .042$). When only the SPTs that developed in the tobacco-smoke-exposed field of the upper

aerodigestive tract or lungs were considered, the results were even more impressive—SPTs occurred in 3 of 49 13cRA-treated patients and in 13 of 51 assessable patients receiving placebo ($p = .008$). These provocative results suggest that the chemopreventive effect of 13cRA persisted for approximately 3 years after the completion of therapy. However, this effect appears to subsequently disappear, as demonstrated by the fact that the SPT rates in both arms were equivalent from that point onward.

As a follow-up to this trial, an intergroup, randomized, double-blind, placebo-controlled study of 13cRA in the prevention of SPTs using low-dose (30 mg/day) 13cRA was initiated in 1991. This trial, which closed to new-patient accrual in June 1999, has already accrued 1,384 patients, with 1,190 patients randomized, eligible, and evaluable as of November 1999. All patients are being followed for survival, SPT development, and recurrence. In addition, smoking status is assessed at time of entry into and during the study. Patients are randomized to receive either placebo or 13cRA for three years and then have an additional four years of follow-up. To date, this study has shown a significantly higher rate of SPTs in patients who were smokers as opposed to those who had never smoked. This is particularly striking when one evaluates smoking-related SPTs (1.6% versus 4.1% annual rate) in nonsmokers versus current smokers ($p < .01$) (Khuri et al., 1999; Kim et al., 2000).

Lung-Cancer Prevention of Second Primary Tumors

In a placebo-controlled clinical trial, Pastorino et al. (1993) tested retinyl palmitate (300,000 IU/day for 12 months) in 307 patients at risk for SPTs following definitive therapy for primary stage I non-small-cell lung cancer. After a median follow-up of 46 months, 56 (37%) patients in the retinoid arm and 75 (48%) in the control arm had either a recurrence or new primary tumors. Eighteen patients in the retinoid group developed an SPT, and 29 patients in the control group developed 1 or more SPTs. A statistically significant difference in favor of treatment was observed concerning time to new primary tumors in the involved field of prevention ($p = .045$, log-rank test). The treatment difference in terms of disease-free interval was close to statistical significance ($p = .054$, log-rank test) and significant only when adjusted for primary tumor classification ($p = .038$, Cox regression model).

On the basis of the promise of 13cRA in oral premalignancy, as well as the activity demonstrated by Pastorino et al. (1993), a large randomized trial was launched through the intergroup mechanism (a National Cancer Institute–supported, National Cooperative Oncology Group) to confirm the earlier promising results of retinoids in the prevention of head and neck and lung SPTs. Having completed accrual in mid-1997, the lung intergroup trial involved low-dose 13cRA in nearly 1,500 patients. Final results of this trial are expected by mid-2000 after treatment and follow-up of the final patients. The preliminary results revealed a striking difference in recurrence rates between T2 N0 M0 and T1 N0 M0 non-small-cell lung cancers, as well as a higher than expected overall recurrence rate (Lippman et al., 1998). After further follow-up, there were no differences seen in the rate of developing an SPT between the placebo and treatment arms (Lippman, personal communication, 2000).

Skin Cancer

The efficacies of various chemopreventive agents, including 13cRA, β-carotene, and selenium, were assessed in patients at risk for non-melanoma skin cancer. A study by Kraemer et al. (1988) found that high-dose 13cRA prevented new skin cancers in individuals with xeroderma pigmentosum. After 2 years of treatment, subjects had an average 63% reduction in skin cancers. After drug discontinuation, the frequency of tumor formation increased a mean of 8.5-fold compared with the frequency of tumor development during treatment (Kraemer et al., 1988).

In contrast, phase III trials using lower net doses in individuals at lower risk reported mixed results. In a randomized clinical trial of patients previously treated for basal-cell carcinoma, 36 months of treatment with low-dose 13cRA failed to produce a statistically significant difference in the occurrence of new basal-cell carcinomas. In addition, the treated group developed significant side effects associated with 13cRA (Tangrea et al., 1992).

Two additional chemoprevention trials were conducted to evaluate the effects of retinoids on 2 primary end points: squamous-cell carcinoma and basal-cell carcinoma. One of these studies, the skin-cancer prevention/squamous-cell skin cancer and basal-cell skin cancer (SKICAP-S/B) trial randomly assigned high-risk individuals with a history of 4 or more skin cancers to 1 of 3 treatment arms—25,000 IU/day of retinol, 5 or 10 mg/day of 13cRA, or placebo—all for a duration of 3 years. No significant benefits of retinoid treatment on the prevention of squamous-cell carcinoma or basal-cell skin cancer were observed in this high-risk group (Levine et al., 1997).

CHEMOPREVENTION TRIALS USING FENRETINIDE (FENRETINAMIDE 4-HPR)

An improved understanding of retinoid biology has allowed for the development of synthetic retinoids that are more selective, less toxic than the naturally occurring retinoids, or both. Perhaps no retinoid has provoked as much excitement as N-(4-hydroxyphenyl)retinamide (4-HPR), a synthetic retinoid unlike other retinoids in that it seems to exert its influence without significant binding to the nuclear retinoid receptors. 4-HPR has been studied in various settings, including oral premalignancy, second primary breast-cancer prevention, and in patients at risk for prostate adenocarcinoma and bladder cancer.

Oral Premalignant Lesions

A randomized study of 4-HPR in oral premalignancy was begun in 1988 at the Milan Cancer Institute in Milan, Italy, to evaluate the efficacy of 52 weeks of systemic 4-HPR maintenance therapy (compared with no intervention) after complete laser resection of oral premalignant lesions. The most recent report on this ongoing study included data from 153 randomized patients. A 3-day drug holiday was instituted at the end of each month to avoid the adverse effects (e.g., night blindness) of lowering serum retinol by 4-HPR treatment. The rate of treatment failure (i.e., recurrence rate plus new lesion rate) among those patients who completed the 12-month intervention was 6% in the 4-HPR group and 30% in the control group (Chiesa *et al.*, 1993). Ongoing investigations of 4-HPR currently include a study of 4-HPR in patients with oral leukoplakia who demonstrate disease progression after treatment with 13cRA or retinol palmitate. No reports from this study have been published.

4-HPR also was studied for its efficacy in reversing bronchial metaplasia in smokers (Kurie *et al.*, 1999) and in dose-escalation studies for the treatment of solid tumors. Whereas Kurie *et al.* saw no activity of 4-HPR in the reversal of lung premalignancy, preliminary data from Lippman *et al.* suggest that the agent does have a degree of activity in oral leukoplakia, with approximately 20% of patients to date who previously failed other retinoid therapy demonstrating evidence of response to 4-HPR (Lippman, personal communication, 2000).

Breast-Cancer Chemoprevention

Promising breast-cancer chemoprevention studies have been conducted with 4-HPR. Perhaps most striking are the preliminary reports from the large-scale randomized trial of 4-HPR (compared with no treatment) for 5 years in more than 3,000 women after definitive local therapy for a T1 or T2 N0 M0 breast cancer. The 4-HPR dose being used in this trial is 200 mg/day, with monthly 3-day drug holidays to avoid ocular toxicity. Between 1987 and 1993, 2,972 women between the ages of 30 and 70 were enrolled. A report of results from this study, with a median observation time of 97 months, found no statistically significant difference in the occurrence of contralateral or ipsilateral breast cancer between the two arms. When results were analyzed by menopausal status, a difference was detected in the occurrence of contralateral breast cancers among premenopausal women receiving 4-HPR compared with those receiving placebo (Veronesi *et al.*, 1999). Based on these preliminary findings, randomized trials have been launched or are in preparation for premenopausal women with prior histories of breast cancer or for women at high risk for developing breast cancer (Conley *et al.*, 2000).

Scientific rationale for the current and future studies that will be supported by the National Cancer Institute (NCI) in the prevention of contralateral breast cancer includes the fact that the combination of fenretinide and tamoxifen is well tolerated, as indicated in a recent phase I study in patients with advanced breast cancers. Furthermore, the combination appears to produce a substantial reduction in insulin-like growth factor I. Tamoxifen suppression of insulin-like growth factor I is thought to be a mechanism of this agent's anticarcinogenic effects in breast carcinogenesis.

Lung Cancer

No primary trials exist in the prevention of second primary lung cancer using 4-HPR. However, a recently reported study by Kurie *et al.* (1999) in 70 evaluable active smokers randomized patients to treatment with either 4-HPR at

200 mg/day or placebo. All patients on this trial had evidence of bronchial metaplasia and dysplasia and were active smokers. Individuals with a 15% or greater metaplasia index or any evidence of dysplasia were eligible. The study, which was reported at the American Society of Clinical Oncology in 1999, found no difference in the modulation of primary bronchial metaplasia or squamous dysplasia after evaluation with bronchoscopy scheduled at 6 and 12 months. At the present time, no plans exist through the NCI to proceed with randomized large phase III trials of 4-HPR in patients with previous lung cancers.

Prostate Cancer

To date, several small trials have used 4-HPR in patients at risk for adenocarcinoma of the prostate. In one such trial, 22 patients were entered into a clinical trial that involved taking 12 cycles of 4-HPR for 28 days each. Eight patients with negative results for pre-study biopsies had biopsies positive for prostate cancer prior to or at the time of their 12th-cycle evaluation. This, and difficulty with accruing patients, led to early closure of the study (Pienta *et al.*, 1997).

Bladder Cancer

4-HPR also has been investigated in the management of superficial bladder cancer using DNA-flow cytometry as an intermediate end point. In this randomized study, 12 patients were treated with oral 4-HPR at a dose of 200 mg/day and compared with 17 nonrandomized, untreated controls. The median interval between transurethral resection and 4-HPR administration was 5.5 months (range, 0 to 36 months). The proportion of patients with DNA aneuploid stem lines in bladder-washed cells decreased from 7 of 12 (58%) to 5 of 11 (45%) in the 4-HPR group, but increased from 7 of 17 (41%) to 10 of 17 (59%) in the control group. Perhaps more significantly, positive or

suspicious results for cytologic examinations in 3 of 12 treated cases prior to 4-HPR administration, and all subsequently returned to normal. In the control group, positive or suspicious results increased from 4 of 17 (24%) to 6 of 17 (35%) (Decensi *et al.*, 1994).

In summary, 4-HPR has demonstrated provocative activity in the prevention of progression of recurrence in oral leukoplakia, some possible activity in the prevention of contralateral breast cancers in premenopausal women, and possibly prevention of ovarian cancer in women with prior breast cancer. Whereas impressive activity exists to date in modulation of flow-cytometry biomarkers in the small bladder-cancer trial, the numbers are such that this trial bears repeating with a larger sample size.

Treatment of Cancer

The retinoids have been investigated both alone and in combination for the treatment of both hematologic malignancies and solid tumors (Warrell, 1994; Kurie and Hong, 1999). The most success thus far has been seen in the treatment of APL, an uncommon type of acute myeloid leukemia characterized by the presence of disseminated intravascular coagulation at diagnosis, which responds to oral ATRA therapy.

APL is also characterized by a reciprocal translocation between chromosomes 15 and 17 t(15;17). This translocation results in the union of portions of the promyelocytic leukemia (PML) gene on chromosome 15 and the gene for the RARα on chromosome 17 and severely disrupts the normal RARα receptor. This fusion protein is believed to interfere with normal differentiation of myeloid cells by preventing PML and RARα from binding with their natural partners. The use of ATRA in patients with APL who harbor this translocation can induce granulocytic differentiation (Fenaux and Chomienne, 1996).

In initial clinical studies using oral ATRA in patients with APL, differentiation-induced complete remissions were achieved (Miller, 1998). These initial studies led to the regulatory approval of ATRA for the treatment of APL in 1995. Although the initial response to exogenous ATRA in patients with APL was high, the duration of complete remission was short (i.e., median < 6 months). In addition, few patients were able to be maintained in complete remission on monotherapy with ATRA. The current standard for treatment of APL has become combination therapy with ATRA and chemotherapy, because this combination achieves complete remission rates of approximately 90% and, in randomized trials, has been shown to improve long-term survival (Tallman et al., 1997).

The retinoids have shown activity in certain other hematologic malignancies as well. Mycosis fungoides (i.e., T-cell lymphoma), a malignancy of the helper/inducer T-cell phenotype, typically involves the skin, with the potential for dissemination to the lymph nodes, spleen, liver, and other organs (Kuzel et al., 1991). Patients treated with starting doses of 1 to 2 mg/kg/day of 13cRA showed clinical improvement within 2 to 4 weeks of treatment initiation. Responses were documented in up to 44% of patients (including three clinical complete responses), most of whom had been treated previously (Kessler et al., 1987). In a pilot clinical trial by Cheng et al. (1994), 18 lymphoma patients were treated, 16 of whom did not respond previously to at least one regimen of intensive chemotherapy, with oral 13 cis RA being given at 1 mg/kg/day. In this pilot clinical trial, 5 complete remissions and 1 partial remission were observed in 12 patients with peripheral T-cell lymphoma, whereas no response was noted in the 6 patients with B-cell lymphoma.

Bexarotene (Targretin®), a member of a subclass of retinoids that selectively activate RXRs, also was studied in the treatment of CTCL. Miller et al. (1997) initially published the results of a study evaluating the safety, clinical tolerance, and pharmacokinetics of bexarotene in patients with advanced cancer. Fifty-two patients received bexarotene administered orally once daily at doses ranging from 5 to 500 mg/m^2 for 1 to 41 weeks. Two patients with CTCL experienced major antitumor responses. Based on results of this study, a dose of 300 mg/m^2 was recommended for single-agent trials. In December 1999, bexarotene received regulatory approval for the treatment of CTCL based on results of 2 multicenter, open-label, historically controlled clinical studies conducted in the United States, Canada, Europe, and Australia. These studies enrolled a total of 152 patients, 102 of whom had disease refractory to at least 1 prior systemic therapy. Although few patients had a complete response to therapy with bexarotene, 30% in 1 of the 2 studies experienced partial remissions. The recommended starting dose is 300 mg/m^2 by mouth per day (Ligand Pharmaceuticals, 1999).

Castleberry et al. (1994) evaluated the use of 13cRA in the treatment of juvenile chronic myelogenous leukemia (CML). Ten children (median age, 10 months) were enrolled in the study and were treated with 100 mg/m^2 of oral 13cRA. Four children had disease progression. Two children had complete responses to 13cRA (i.e., normalization of the white-cell count and disappearance of organomegaly), three had partial responses (more than a 50% reduction in the white-cell count and the degree of organomegaly), and one had a minimal response (more than a 50% reduction in the white-cell count, but a 26% to 50% reduction in the degree of organomegaly). The median duration of response was 37 months (range, 6 to 83 months). Three of the four children who had a complete or partial response and who did not undergo bone-marrow transplantation were alive 36 to 83 months after the diagnosis of juvenile CML.

In general, the retinoids have shown disappointing single-agent activity in established cancers (Miller, 1998; Clifford *et al.*, 1999). Presented here is a concise review of some of the initial clinical studies investigating the efficacy of the retinoids in solid tumors. The antiproliferative and differentiation effects of retinoids on squamous-cell carcinoma cell lines led investigators to evaluate their use in patients with this tumor. In surgically incurable head and neck squamous-cell carcinomas, administration of high-dose 13cRA (3 mg/kg/day) resulted in partial responses in 3 of 19 patients (Lippman *et al.*, 1987). Another study involving patients with locally advanced or metastatic squamous-cell carcinoma of the head and neck had similar results at the same dose (3 mg/kg/day for at least 6 weeks). Lippman *et al.* (1988) again reported three partial responses and one complete response among 19 total patients. Both tRA and cRA have been used to treat a variety of skin malignancies, including basal-cell carcinoma, squamous-cell carcinoma, and melanoma. In cutaneous basal-cell carcinoma, topical administration of both cRA and tRA resulted in complete or partial responses in most patients (Epstein, 1986; Sankowski *et al.*, 1987). Lippman and Meyskens (1987) used systemic administration of cRA for locally advanced squamous-cell carcinoma of the skin and achieved a 40 to 50% response rate. Topical administration of tRA was used on subcutaneous metastatic melanoma lesions and resulted in transient local regression of some tumors (Levine and Meyskens, 1987). Bonhomme *et al.* (1991) reported on the use of topically applied tRA (1% gel) to treat cutaneous lesions of patients with Kaposi's sarcoma; a 50% reduction in the size of cutaneous lesions was noted in 7 of 8 patients.

Combination trials also were conducted for treatment of advanced squamous-cell carcinoma of the skin and locally advanced squamous-cell carcinoma of the cervix. Interferon alpha (IFN-α) and 13cRA were used in 28 patients with either locally advanced or metastatic squamous-cell carcinoma of the skin (Lippman *et al.*, 1992a). Sixty-eight percent of the patients achieved response, with 7 of 19 responders achieving a complete response. In another study, previously untreated patients with locally advanced squamous-cell carcinoma of the cervix received cRA (1 mg/kg/day) and IFN-α (6 MIU/day subcutaneously) (Lippman *et al.*, 1992b). Half of the patients had at least a partial response, and the outpatient regimen was well tolerated. A phase II trial conducted at Memorial Sloan-Kettering Cancer Center evaluated the combination of 13cRA (1 mg/kg/day) and IFN-α (3 to 9 MIU/day) in patients with renal-cell cancer. A major response rate of 30% (13 patients) was obtained, including three complete responses (Motzer *et al.*, 1995). *In vitro* studies have shown that the retinoids and the IFNs cooperate supra-additively or synergistically to inhibit proliferation, induce apoptosis, or both in a large number of tumor cell lines. This work, along with the successes seen in early clinical trials, serves as the foundation for the continuing evaluation of this combination in solid tumors, especially in patients with advanced head and neck premalignant lesions, renal-cell carcinoma, and squamous-cell carcinomas of the skin and cervix (Lippman *et al.*, 1997; Clifford *et al.*, 1999; Papadimitrakopoulou *et al.*, 1999).

Regulatory Approval

Vitamin A capsules (15 mg retinol) have been approved as treatment for vitamin-A deficiency. Retin A® cream (tretinoin) has been approved for the treatment of acne vulgaris. Accutane® (isotretinoin), an orally administered retinoid, has been approved for treatment of cystic acne. In November 1995, tretinoin (Vesanoid®) was approved for the induction of remission in patients with APL, French-American-British classification M3 characterized by the presence of t(15;17) translocation, the presence of PML/RAR-α gene, or both, who are refractory to or have relapsed from anthracycline chemotherapy or for whom anthracycline-based chemotherapy is contraindicated. In December 1999, bexarotene (Targretin®) was approved for the treatment of CTCL in patients who are refractory to at least one prior systemic therapy. In June 2000, bexarotene gel (Targretin® gel) (1%) was approved for topical treatment of cutaneous lesions of early stage CTCL.

Toxicity

Acute hypervitaminosis A toxicity exhibits a well-known clinical presentation (Windhorst and Nigra, 1982). Drowsiness, irritability, headache, and vomiting are all symptoms of the toxic effects on the central nervous system (CNS). Dermatologic changes include desquamation, pruritus, alopecia, increased pigmentation, and drying and cracking of the lips, mucous membranes, and skin. Fatigue, anorexia, **arthralgias**, hepatosplenomegaly, and irritation of the eyes are also common. The chronic, low-grade toxic effects seen in the clinical trials of the natural retinoids (e.g., 9cRA, 13cRA, and ATRA) are similar to the acute effects just described, but serious CNS effects are rare. Signs and symptoms usually disappear within 1 to 4 weeks following discontinuation of treatment; however, bone toxicities and some visual disturbances may persist (Miller, 1998).

The major classes of retinoid toxicity are mucocutaneous, visual, skeletal, lipid, liver, and teratogenic. Although no randomized comparisons have been reported, toxicities appear to vary in incidence and intensity with respect to the specific retinoid prescribed, the dose, and the duration of administration. The major and most frequent toxicities observed in clinical trials include significant mucocutaneous drying (e.g., chelitis, skin dryness, and conjunctivitis),

headache, xerosis, lethargy, and fatigue. The mucocutaneous drying is the most troublesome toxicity with respect to long-term use of the retinoids, especially when used in the setting of chemoprevention, and often significantly affects patients' quality of life. CNS changes such as headache and dizziness generally are seen at higher doses and at a slightly increased frequency in patients receiving ATRA (Smith *et al.*, 1992) or 9cRA (Kurie *et al.*, 1996). Lipid abnormalities, such as hypertriglyceridemia, hypercholesterolemia, and elevation of liver enzymes, also are observed. In some patients, musculoskeletal toxicity, such as **myalgias** and arthralgias, may be significant.

The most significant toxic effect associated with both tRA and cRA is teratogenesis. Both retinoids have the potential to produce a 25-fold increase in the incidence of severe embryopathic changes, including spontaneous abortions and malformations that involve the craniofacial, cardiac, thymic, and CNS structures (Lammer *et al.*, 1985). Women of childbearing potential must be thoroughly counseled concerning the serious risks to the fetus if they should become pregnant while undergoing treatment. The length of time during which pregnancy must be avoided after treatment has ended has not been determined.

A hyperleukocytosis syndrome unique to ATRA therapy has been seen in approximately 25% to 30% of patients receiving systemic ATRA for the treatment of APL, and has been termed *retinoic-acid syndrome*. It is manifested as leukocytosis, thrombosis, fever, respiratory distress, pulmonary infiltrates, pleural effusions, and weight gain (Frankel *et al.*, 1992). It occurs within the first 2 to 3 weeks of treatment. The symptoms of this syndrome may be difficult to distinguish from the symptoms of a bacterial or fungal infection. This syndrome has been successfully treated with leukapheresis and high-dose corticosteroids, alone and in combination. At the first sign or symptom, patients generally are treated immediately with high-dose steroids (i.e., 10 mg of dexamethasone intravenously every 12 hours for 3 days or until resolution of the symptoms), irrespective of the white blood cell count. Most patients do not require discontinuation.

With some of the synthetic retinoids, such as fenretinide, more significant visual toxic effects have been observed. Fenretinide can produce reversible night blindness, although asymptomatic electroretinogram abnormalities are more common. The side effect is believed to result from the synthetic retinoid-lowering serum retinol levels and competition with the **endogenous** (physiologic) vitamin A metabolite retinal for the retinal receptor. This creates deficiency of necessary retinol in the ocular tissue, which can be avoided by the use of a drug holiday in fenretinide dosing schedules.

Future Directions

To date, the retinoids have demonstrated efficacy in the treatment and prevention of certain human cancers. However, with the exception of the use of ATRA in APL, no significant clinical successes have been seen. Future research must focus on overcoming the barriers to treatment success and optimizing the use of the retinoids in the clinical setting.

Although, in general, the retinoids do not cause life-threatening toxicities, the toxicities seen can significantly affect quality of life. This is a major concern when drugs are used in the chemoprevention setting. In a high-risk population being treated with chemoprevention agents, one of the goals is to keep toxicity to a minimum. Patients will be less likely to continue on chemopreventive agents for significant periods if the toxicities are too distressing and uncomfortable. This is especially true with retinoid-related toxicities such as mucocutaneous dryness, chelitis, headache, fatigue, and

arthralgias. Therefore, a goal of future studies and research is to maximize dosing schedules to diminish toxicity, or to design synthetic retinoids that selectively stimulate receptors to maximize clinical effectiveness and diminish toxicity. Fenretinide represents an example of such a "designer retinoid."

As noted previously, such selecting will be a key goal in trials of the future. As the underlying pathophysiology of certain cancers is better elucidated, specific retinoid receptors ultimately may be targeted for therapy and will likely differ between different diseases. Currently, the majority of retinoids are not receptor specific and bind to many receptors, either within a class (i.e., RARs) or across classes (i.e., both RARs and RXRs). Synthetic retinoids will continue to be developed and evaluated that have very specific binding capabilities, such as binding only to RAR-β or RAR-α receptors. This may further enhance clinical efficacy while diminishing unwanted toxicities.

Within chemoprevention trials, the selection of intermediate end point biomarkers will become increasingly important. The current challenge is to determine *which* markers should be measured and followed to determine clinical effectiveness of the drug. Within the old paradigm, the end point in cancer-prevention trials was the development of cancer. Within the emerging paradigm—the understanding that cancer is a result of a stepwise process of successive mutations—the end point may be the selection of biomarkers that are reflective of specific genetic changes. Table 12.4 is an overview of characteristics important in the selection of suitable biomarkers. Studies are beginning to incorporate measurement of biomarkers within the framework. For example, Xu *et al.* (1994) found RAR-β to be significantly **downregulated** in oral premalignant lesions. On the basis of suggestive findings of studies of nuclear retinoid receptors in squamous tumors in surrounding tissue, Lotan *et*

Table 12.4   Factors important in the selection of biomarkers

- Should be detectable in small tissue specimens that also will permit serial biopsies of the same site.
- Expression in high-risk (premalignant) sites should differ from expression in normal tissues in accordance with carcinogenic changes.
- Pattern and degree of expression should correlate with histopathologic state (e.g., hyperplasia, degree of dysplasia, cancer).
- The marker should be subject to modulation by chemoprevention agents.
- The marker should have a low rate of spontaneous change.
- Quality assurance and control measures should be well established.
- Evaluation of the marker should be cost-effective.

Source: Mayne, S., and Lippman, S. 1997. Cancer prevention: Chemoprevention agents. In DeVita, V., Dellman, S., and Rosenberg, S. (eds). *Cancer: Principles and Practice of Oncology,* 5th edn. Philadelphia, PA: Lippincott-Raven Publishers, pp. 585–597.

al. (1995) evaluated biopsy specimens of 52 patients with oral premalignant lesions for the expression of RARs and RXRs, both before and after 13cRA treatment. These receptor findings then were compared with receptor findings in normal control subjects. All normal specimens contained RAR-β messenger RNA (mRNA), but only 21 (40%) of the 52 pretreated oral premalignant lesions had detectable RAR-β mRNA levels at baseline. After the patients on the clinical trial completed 3 months of treatment with 13cRA, 35 (90%) of the 39 oral premalignant lesions available for evaluation expressed RAR-β. This statistically significant improvement of RAR-β expression after 13-CRA treatment ($p < .001$ by McNemar test) demonstrates both that

RAR-β is selectively downregulated in oral premalignant lesions and that treatment with 13cRA can **upregulate** RAR-β in these lesions. This illustrates not only how biomarkers may be used as intermediate biomarkers but also that they may well predict which patients are most likely to respond to a specific therapy.

Subsequently, Lippman *et al.* (1995) used the oral premalignant lesion's retinoid system to study p53 protein accumulation in relation to RAR-β expression and resistance to retinoid. p53 protein accumulation was statistically significantly associated with resistance to retinoid and with a lack of RAR-β upregulation. 13cRA did not attenuate p53 accumulation in oral premalignant lesions that overexpressed p53 protein in this study. Other studies of intermediate end point markers explored the roles of the epidermal growth factor, proliferating cell nuclear **antigen**, and micronuclei as biomarkers for chemoprevention trials. In summary, despite studies of multiple intermediate biological markers, premalignant lesions (e.g., oral leukoplakia), with the possible exception of RAR-β, remain the most carefully studied intermediate end points defined to date. Final validation with the ultimate markers of cancer development and prognosis await further study and will represent a major area of focus in future studies.

Finally, the investigation of the retinoids in combination with other chemopreventive agents such as tamoxifen or oltipraz, biological agents, and chemotherapy serves an important area of focus. The success seen in the treatment of APL, where ATRA is used in conjunction with chemotherapy, will serve as an important example of how effective combination regimens can be designed. Great promise in the future lies in testing combinations of agents with different mechanisms (e.g., agents that can modulate differentiation with agents that can induce apoptosis). This may facilitate approaches that are more effective in overcoming single-agent resistance and may require lower doses with resultant decreased toxicity (Lippman *et al.*, 1998).

References

Benner, S., Pajak, T., Lippman, S., *et al.* 1994. Prevention of second primary tumors with 13cRA in squamous-cell carcinoma of the head and neck: Long-term follow-up. *Journal of the National Cancer Institute* 86: 140–141.

Blaner, W., and Olson, J. 1994. Retinol and retinoic-acid metabolism. In Sporn, M., Roberts, A., and Goodman, D. (eds). *The Retinoids: Biology, Chemistry and Medicine,* 2nd edn. New York, NY: Raven Press, pp. 229–257.

Bonhomme, L., Fredj, G., and Averous, S. 1991. Topical treatment of epidermic Kaposi's sarcoma with all-*trans*-retinoic acid. *Annals of Oncology* 2: 234–235.

Castleberry, R., Emanuel, P., Zuckerman, K., *et al.* 1994. A pilot study of isotretinoin in the treatment of juvenile chronic myelogenous leukemia. *New England Journal of Medicine* 331(25): 1680–1684.

Chambon, P. 1996. A decade of molecular biology of retinoic acid receptors. *Federation of American Societies for Experimental Biology (FASEB) Journal* 10(9): 940–954.

Cheng, A., Su, I., Chen, C., *et al.* 1994. Use of retinoic acids in the treatment of peripheral T-cell lymphoma: A pilot study. *Journal of Clinical Oncology* 12(6): 1185–1192.

Chiesa, F., Tradati, N., Marazza, M., *et al.* 1993. 4HPR in chemoprevention of oral leukoplakia. *Journal of Cell Biochemistry* 17(F): 255–261.

Clifford, J., Miano, J., and Lippman, S. 1999. Retinoids and interferons as antiangiogenic cancer drugs. In Teicher, B. (ed). *Antiangiogenic Agents in Cancer Therapy.* Totowa, NJ: Humana Press, Inc., pp. 355–370.

Conley, B., O'Shaughnessy, J., Prindiville, S., *et al.* 2000. Pilot trial of the safety, tolerability, and retinoid levels of N-(4-hydroxyphenyl) retinamide in combination with tamoxifen in patients at high risk for developing invasive breast cancer. *Journal of Clinical Oncology* 18(2): 275–283.

Decensi, A., Bruno, S., Costantini, M., *et al.* 1994. Phase IIa study of fenretinide in superficial bladder cancer, using DNA-flow cytometry as an intermediate end point. *Journal of the National Cancer Institute* 86(2): 138–140.

Dennert, G. 1985. Immunostimulation by retinoic acid. *Ciba Foundation Symposia* 113: 117–131.

Epstein, J. 1986. All-*trans*-retinoic acid and cutaneous cancers. *American Academy of Dermatology* 15(4 Pt 2): 772–778.

Evans, T., and Kaye, S. 1999. Retinoids: Present role and future potential. *British Journal of Cancer* 80(1–2): 1–8.

Fenaux, P., and Chomienne, C. 1996. Biology and treatment of acute promyelocytic leukemia. *Current Opinion in Oncology* 8: 3–12.

Frankel, S., Eardley, A., Lauwers, G., *et al.* 1992. The "retinoic acid syndrome" in acute promyelocytic leukemia. *Annals of Internal Medicine* 117(4): 292–296.

Hong, W., Endicott, J., Itri, L., *et al.* 1986. 13-*cis*-retinoic acid in the treatment of oral leukoplakia. *New England Journal of Medicine* 315: 1501–1505.

Hong, W., Lippman, S., Itri, L., *et al.* 1990. Prevention of second primary tumors with isotretinoin in squamous-cell carcinoma of the head and neck. *New England Journal of Medicine* 323: 795–801.

Kessler, J., Jones, S., and Levine, N. 1987. Isotretinoin and cutaneous helper T-cell lymphoma (mycosis fungoides). *Archives of Dermatology* 123: 201–204.

Khuri, F., Lee, J., Winn, R., *et al.* 1999. Interim analysis of randomized chemoprevention trial of HNSCC. *Proceedings of the American Society of Clinical Oncology* 18: abstract 1503.

Kim, E. S., Khuri, F. R., Lee, J. J., *et al.* 2000. Second

primary tumor incidence related to primary index tumor and smoking status in a randomized chemoprevention study of head and neck squamous cell cancer. *Proceedings of the American Society of Clinical Oncology* 19: abstract 1642.

Kligman, A., and Thorne, E. 1991. Topical therapy of actinic keratosis with tretinoin. In Marks, R. (ed). *Retinoids in Cutaneous Malignancy.* Cambridge, MA: Blackwell Scientific, p. 66.

Kraemer, K., DiGiovanna, J., Moshell, A., *et al.* 1988. Prevention of skin cancer in xeroderma pigmentosum with oral isotretinoin. *New England Journal of Medicine* 318: 1633–1637.

Kurie, J., and Hong, W. 1999. Commentary: Retinoids as antitumor agents: A new age of biological therapy. *The Cancer Journal from Scientific American* 5(3): 150–151.

Kurie, J., Lee, J., Griffin, T., *et al.* 1996. Phase I trial of 9-*cis*-retinoic acid in adults with solid tumors. *Clinical Cancer Research* 2(2): 287–293.

Kurie, J., Lee, J., Khuri, F., *et al.* 1999. 4-Hydroxy-phenylretinamide (4-HPR) in the reversal of bronchial metaplasia and dysplasia in smokers. *Proceedings of the American Society of Clinical Oncology* 18: abstract 1825.

Kuzel, T., Roenigk, H., and Rosen, S. 1991. Mycosis fungoides and the Sezary syndrome: A review of pathogenesis, diagnosis, and therapy. *Journal of Clinical Oncology* 9: 1298–1313.

Lammer, E., Chen, D., and Hoar, R. 1985. Retinoic acid embryopathy. *New England Journal of Medicine* 313: 837–841.

Lee, J., Lippman, S., Benner, S., *et al.* 1994. Randomized placebo-controlled trial of isotretinoin in chemoprevention of bronchial squamous metaplasia. *Journal of Clinical Oncology* 12(5): 937–945.

Levine, N., and Meyskens, F. 1987. Topical vitamin-A-acid therapy for cutaneous metastatic melanoma. *Lancet* 2(8188): 224–226.

Levine, N., Moon, T., Cartmel, B., *et al.* 1997. Trial of retinol and isotretinoin in skin cancer prevention: A randomized, double-blind, controlled trial. *Cancer Epidemiology Biomarkers and Prevention* 6: 957–961.

Ligand Pharmaceuticals. 1999. Packet insert. San Diego, CA: Ligand Pharmaceuticals Inc.

Lippman, S. 2000. Personal communication.

Lippman, S., Batsakis, J., Toth, B., *et al.* 1993. Comparison of low-dose isotretinoin with beta carotene to prevent oral carcinogenesis. *New England Journal of Medicine* 328: 15–20.

Lippman, S., and Davies, P. 1997. Retinoids, neoplasia, and differentiation therapy. In Pindeo, H., Longo, D., and Chabner, B. (eds). *Cancer Chemotherapy and Biological Response Modifiers Annual 17.* Elsevier Science B.V.: Amsterdam, The Netherlands, pp. 349–362.

Lippman, S., Kavanagh, J., Paredes-Espinoza, M., *et al.* 1992b. 13-*cis*-retinoic acid plus interferon-alpha-2a: Highly active systemic therapy for squamous-cell carcinoma of the cervix. *Journal of the National Cancer Institute* 84: 241–245.

Lippman, S., Kessler, J., Al-Sarraf, M., *et al.* 1988. Treatment of advanced squamous-cell carcinoma of the head and neck with isotretinion: A phase II randomized trial. *Investigational New Drugs* 6: 51–56.

Lippman, S., Kessler, J., and Meyskens, J. 1987. Retinoids as preventive and therapeutic anticancer agents. *Cancer Treatment Reports* 71: 391–405.

Lippman, S., Lee, J., Karp, D., *et al.* 1998. Phase-III intergroup trial of 13-*cis*-retinoic acid to prevent second primary tumors in stage I non-small-cell lung cancer (nsclc): Interim report of NCI #I91-0001. *Proceedings of the American Society of Clinical Oncology* 17(456a) abstract 1753.

Lippman, S., Lee, J., and Sabichi, A. 1998. Commentary: Cancer chemoprevention: Progress and promise. *Journal of the National Cancer Institute* 90(20): 1514–1528.

Lippman, S., and Lotan, R. 2000. Advances in the development of retinoids as chemopreventive agents. *Journal of Nutrition* 130(2S suppl): 479S–482S.

Lippman, S., Lotan, R., and Schleunicer, U. 1997. Retinoid-interferon therapy of solid tumors. *International Journal of Cancer* 70: 481–483.

Lippman, S., and Meyskens, F. 1987. Treatment of advanced squamous-cell carcinoma of the skin with isotretinoin. *Annals of Internal Medicine* 107: 499–502.

Lippman, S., Parkinson, D., Itri, L., *et al.* 1992a. 13-*cis*-retinoic acid and interferon alpha-2a: Effective combination therapy for advanced squamous-cell carcinoma of the skin. *Journal of the National Cancer Institute* 84: 235–241.

Lippman, S., Shin, D., Lee, J., *et al.* 1995. p53 and retinoid chemoprevention of oral carcinogenesis. *Cancer Research* 55(1): 16–19.

Lotan, R., Xu, X., Lippman, S., *et al.* 1995. Suppression of retinoic acid receptor-beta in premalignant oral lesions and its upregulation by isotretinoin. *New England Journal of Medicine* 332(21): 1405–1410.

Mangelsdorf, D., Thummel, C., Beato, M., *et al.* 1995. The nuclear receptor superfamily: The second decade. *Cell* 83: 835–839.

Mangelsdorf, D., Umesono, K., and Evans, R. 1994. The retinoid receptors. In Sporn, M., Roberts, A., and Goodman, D. (eds). *The Retinoids: Biology, Chemistry, and Medicine.* 2nd edn. New York, NY: Raven Press, pp. 319–350.

Mayne, S., and Lippman, S. 1997. Cancer prevention: Chemopreventive agents. In DeVita, V., Hellman, S., and Rosenberg, S. (eds). *Cancer: Principles & Practice of Oncology.* 5th edn. Philadelphia, PA: Lippincott-Raven Publishers, pp. 585–599.

Meyskens, F., Jr. 1999. Chemoprevention of human cancer: A reasonable strategy? *Recent Results in Cancer Research* 151: 113–121.

Meyskens, F., Jr., Surwit, E., Moon, T., *et al.* 1994. Enhancement of regression of cervical intraepithelial neoplasia II (moderate dysplasia) with topically applied all-*trans*-retinoic acid: A randomized trial. *Journal of the National Cancer Institute* 86: 539–543.

Miller, V., Benedetti, F., Rigas, J., *et al.* 1997. Initial clinical trial of a selective retinoid X receptor ligand, LGD1069. *Journal of Clinical Oncology* 15(2): 790–795.

Miller, W., Jr. 1998. The emerging role of retinoids and retinoic acid metabolism blocking agents in the treatment of cancer. *Cancer* 83(8): 1471–1482

Miller, W., Jr., Jakubowski, A., Tong, W., *et al.* 1995. 9-*cis*-retinoic acid induces complete remission but does not reverse clinically acquired retinoid resistance in acute promyelocytic leukemia. *Blood* 85(11): 3021–3027.

Motzer, R., Schwartz, L., Law, T., *et al.* 1995. Interferon alpha-2a and 13-*cis*-retinoic acid in renal-cell carcinoma: Antitumor activity in a phase II trial and interactions *in vitro. Journal of Clinical Oncology* 13: 1950–1957.

Papadimitrakopoulou, V., Clayman, G., Shin, D., *et al.* 1999. Biochemoprevention for dysplastic lesions of the upper aerodigestive tract. *Archives of Otolaryngology and Head Neck Surgery* 125(10): 1083–1089.

Papadimitrakopoulou, V., Lippman, S.M., and Lee, J.S. *et al.* 1997. Low-dose istretinoin versus beta-carotene to prevent oral carcinogenesis: Long-term follow-up. *Journal of the National Cancer Institute* 89: 257–258.

Parkinson, D., Smith, M., Cheson, B., *et al.* 1992. Trans-retinoic acid and related differentiation agents. *Seminars in Oncology* 19(6): 734–741.

Pastorino, U., Infante, M., Maioli, M., *et al.* 1993. Adjuvant treatment of stage I lung cancer with high-dose vitamin A. *Journal of Clinical Oncology* 11(7): 1216–1222.

Pienta, K., Esper, P., Zwas, F., *et al.* 1997. Phase II chemoprevention trial of oral fenretinide in patients at risk for adenocarcinoma of the prostate. *American Journal of Clinical Oncology* 20(1): 36–39.

Saccomanno, G., Moran, P., Schmidt, R., *et al.* 1982. Effects of 13-*cis* retinoids on premalignant and malignant cells of lung origin. *Acta Cytologica* 26: 78–85.

Sankowski, A., Janik, P., Jeziorska, M,. *et al.* 1987. The results of topical application of 13-*cis*-retinoic acid on basal-cell carcinoma. A correlation of the clinical effect with histopathological examination and serum retinol level. *Neoplasma* 34(4): 485–489.

Smith, M., Parkinson, D., Cheson, B., *et al.* 1992. Retinoids in cancer therapy. *Journal of Clinical Oncology* 10(5): 839–864.

Soprano, D., and Blaner, W. 1994. Plasma retinol binding protein. In Sporn, M., Roberts, A., and Goodman, D. (eds). *The Retinoids: Biology, Chemistry, and Medicine,* 2nd edn. New York, NY: Raven Press, pp. 257–282.

Sporn, M., Dunlop, N., Newton, D., *et al.* 1976a. Prevention of chemical carcinogenesis by vitamin A and its synthetic analogs (retinoids). *Federal Proceedings* 35: 1332–1338.

Sporn, M., Dunlop, N., Newton, D., *et al.* 1976b. Relationships between structure and activity of retinoids. *Nature* 263(5573): 110–113.

Sporn, M.B., and Suh, N. 2000. Chemoprevention of cancer. *Carcinogenesis* 21(3): 525–530.

Tallman, M., Anderson, J., Schiffer, C., *et al.* 1997. All-*trans*-retinoic acid in acute promyelocytic leukemia. *New England Journal of Medicine* 337: 1021–1028.

Tangrea, J., Edwards, B., Taylor, P., *et al.* 1992. Long-term therapy with low-dose isotretinoin for prevention of basal-cell carcinoma: A multicenter clinical trial. Isotretinoin-Basal Cell Carcinoma Study Group. *Journal of the National Cancer Institute* 84: 328–332.

Veronesi, U., DePalo, G., Marubini, E., *et al.* 1999. Randomized trial of fenretinide to prevent second breast malignancy in women with early breast cancer. *Journal of the National Cancer Institute* 91(21): 1847–1856.

Warrell, R. 1994. Introduction: Application for retinoids in cancer therapy. *Seminars in Hematology* 31(4 suppl 5): 1–13.

Warrell, R., de Thé, H., Wang, Z., *et al.* 1993. Acute promyelocytic leukemia. *New England Journal of Medicine* 329: 177–189.

Windhorst, D., and Nigra, T. 1982. General clinical toxicology of oral retinoids. *Journal of the American Academy of Dermatology* 6: 675–677.

Xu, X., Ro, J., Lee, J., *et al.* 1994. Differential expression of nuclear retinoid receptors in normal, premalignant, and malignant head and neck tissues. *Cancer Research* 54(13): 3580–3587.

Clinical Pearls

1. The retinoids are strongly teratogenic and should never be given in the first trimester of pregnancy. In addition, patients should be counseled to use effective methods of contraception (i.e., 2 reliable methods simultaneously) while on retinoid therapy to avoid pregnancy and for 1 month following cessation of therapy. (page 422)

2. Contraception must be used even when there is a history of infertility or menopause, unless a hysterectomy has been performed.

3. With use of ATRA in APL, confirmation of the t(15;17) genetic marker by cytogenetic studies or other molecular diagnostic techniques should occur prior to initiation of therapy.

4. With initiation of therapy for APL, monitor for signs of retinoic-acid syndrome (e.g., weight gain, radiographic pulmonary infiltrates, shortness of breath, and pleural or pericardial effusions).

5. For management of skin toxicity, instruct patient in use of nonperfumed soaps and lotions. Use lotions and emollients liberally on lips and skin to rehydrate.

6. Caution patients to avoid sun exposure. If out in the sun, use protective clothing such as a hat and sunglasses, and use sunscreen with a minimum SPF of 15.

7. For treatment of headaches, arthralgias, and myalgias, use acetaminophen or nonsteroidal anti-inflammatory agents. If these toxicities are grade II or higher, dose reduction may be considered.

8. Instruct patients to report visual disturbances, CNS symptoms such as severe headache or dizziness, shortness of breath, chest pain, and severe rashes.

9. In general, the following laboratory variables should be evaluated on a regular basis: liver-function, complete blood count with differential and platelets, and cholesterol and triglyceride levels.

Key References

Applications for Retinoids in Cancer Therapy. 1994. *Seminars in Hematology* 31(4 suppl 5): 1–40.

Armstrong, W.B., and Meyskens, F.L. Jr., 2000. Chemoprevention of head and neck cancer. *Otolaryngology Head and Neck Surgery* 122(5); 728–735.

Degos, L., and Parkinson, D. (eds). 1995. *Retinoids in Oncology.* New York: Springer Verlag, pp. 1–115.

Evans, T., and Kaye, S. 1999. Retinoids: Present role and future potential. *British Journal of Cancer* 80(1–2): 1–8.

Fenaux, P., and Chomienne, C. 1996. Biology and treatment of acute promyelocytic leukemia. *Current Opinion in Oncology* 8: 3–12.

Hong, W. 1999. Chemoprevention of lung cancer. *Oncology* (Huntington) 13(10 suppl 5): 135–141.

Khuri, F., and Lippman, S. 2000. Lung cancer chemoprevention. *Seminars in Surgical Oncology* 18(2): 100–105.

Kurie, J. 1999. The biologic basis for the use of retinoids in cancer prevention and treatment. *Current Opinions in Oncology* 11(6): 497–502.

Lippman, S., and Davies, P. 1997. Retinoids, neoplasia, and differentiation therapy. In Pindeo, H., Longo, D., and Chabner, B. (eds). *Cancer Chemotherapy and Biological Response Modifiers Annual 17.* Amsterdam, The Netherlands: Elsevier Science B.V., pp. 349–362.

Lippman, S., Lee, J., and Sabichi, A. 1998. Commentary: Cancer chemoprevention: Progress and promise. *Journal of the National Cancer Institute* 90(20): 1514–1528.

Miller, W., Jr. 1998. The emerging role of retinoids and retinoic acid metabolism blocking agents in the treatment of cancer. *Cancer* 83(8): 1471–1482.

Nau, H., and Blaner, W. (eds). 1999. *Retinoids: The biochemical and molecular basis of vitamin A and retinoid action.* New York, NY: Springer Verlag, pp. 1–619.

Nagpal, S., and Chandraratna, R.A. 2000. Recent

developments in receptor-selective retinoids. *Current Pharmaceutical Design* 6(9): 919–931.

Sabichi, A., Lerner, S.P., Grossman, H.B., *et al.* 1998. Retinoids in the chemoprevention of bladder cancer. *Current Opinions in Oncology* 10(5): 479–484.

Singh, D.K., and Lippman, S. 1998. Cancer chemo-prevention. Part 1 Retinoids and carotenoids and other classic antioxidants. *Oncology* 12(11): 1643–1658.

Swan, D., and Ford, B. 1997. Chemoprevention of cancer: Review of the literature. *Oncology Nursing Forum* 24(4): 719–727.

CHAPTER 13 | Gene Therapy

Yvette Payne, RN, MSN, MBA

Patricia Brusso, RN, MSN

Introduction

The role of genetic changes in the development of cancer has been studied for more than 100 years. The first systematic study was performed by David von Hansemann in 1890. He studied cell division in malignancy and found aberrant mitosis in cancer cells. In 1914, Theodore Boveri wrote a book suggesting that malignancy might result from the disturbance of normal **chromosomes**. This theory, known today as the **somatic mutation** theory of cancer, still exists as the principal paradigm of cancer pathogenesis (Culver, Blaese, and Anderson, 1992a). Technological changes over the past several decades, particularly the introduction of chromosome-banding techniques and the advent of molecular-genetic techniques, have led to a dra-

matic increase in knowledge about the **genetics** of cancer. The first human **gene** was cloned in 1977, and by late 1994, disease-producing mutations had been identified in almost 350 cloned genes (Conner and Ferguson-Smith, 1997).

Researchers with the Human Genome Project, a $3 billion international research effort begun in 1988, expect to identify the entire sequence of human genes by the year 2003 (Collins *et al.*, 1998). In late June 2000, it was announced that the rough draft of the **genome**, a scaffold of known DNA sequences across an estimated 90% of the genome, had been completed. Scientific and technologic advances made since the inception of the project have resulted in significant improvement in the speed and accuracy of the sequencing and mapping techniques. However, even after 15 years of intense research and the billions of dollars spent, a significant amount of work will remain once the entire human genome has been sequenced. Determining the function of each gene should make it possible to identify which genes malfunction and thereby cause various diseases. This will provide the rationale for the development of ever-expanding gene therapy trials that will seek to correct mutations in genes that result in disease. Preclinical research to learn more about genes and, ultimately, clinical trials evaluating optimal methods to deliver new genes into target cells and gene therapy strategies in human beings, will be necessary to move new information about genes from the laboratory to the clinical setting.

What Is Gene Therapy?

Despite the gaps in knowledge that will remain even after completion of the Human Genome Project, the advances in the fields of molecular biology and genetics that will result from the project will enable researchers to develop strategies to destroy cancers by correcting genetic defects, manipulating genes, or both. This approach, referred to as **gene therapy**, is a procedure in which a functioning gene is introduced into or transferred to a tumor host cell or effector cell to correct a genetic error, to sensitize tumor cells for destruction, to provide a cell with a new function, or to support other drug therapies (Culver *et al.*, 1992b; Blaese, 1997). Simply put, gene therapy is the deliberate transfer of **deoxyribonucleic acid (DNA)** for therapeutic purposes (Sikora, 1999).

The concept of gene therapy comes from the observation that certain diseases are caused by the inheritance of a single defect of a functional gene. In theory, a disease caused by a single genetic defect could be treated and even cured by the insertion and expression of a copy of the

normal counterpart of the dysfunctional gene. Today, however, most of the approved gene therapy protocols are designed to treat cancer, a disease involving multiple genetic defects, rather than diseases caused by a single genetic defect (Roth, 1996). Cancer arises as the culmination of a multistep process involving initiation, promotion, and a progression of genetic changes in key regulatory genes of a single normal cell (see Chapter 3). Initially, it might appear that successful gene therapy for cancer requires correction of all the genetic abnormalities in the cancer cell, many of which are still unknown. Tantalizing evidence exists, however, to suggest that this is not true.

Gene Therapy Strategies

Several gene therapy strategies are being investigated for their efficiency in the treatment of human cancers. These include the **transduction** (i.e., the transfer of genetic material from one cell to another or into a cell by a **vector**) of drug-resistance genes to protect bone marrow during chemotherapy, sensitization of tumor cells for destruction by other therapeutic agents, use of recombinant vaccines as a form of active specific immunotherapy, insertion of cytokine genes into immune cells to facilitate cytokine delivery to the tumor site or into tumor cells that serve as vaccines, and replacement of **tumor-suppressor genes** and inactivation of **oncogenes** (Table 13.1). Over the last decade, more than 300 phase I and phase II gene-based clinical trials have been conducted worldwide for the treatment of cancer and monogenic disorders (Romano *et al.*, 2000). As of July 2000, more than 180 gene therapy protocols had been reviewed by the U.S. Recombinant DNA Advisory Committee Office of Recombinant DNA and Gene Transfer Activities (*http://www.nih.gov/od/oba*).

Table 13.1 Selected oncology gene therapy strategies for treatment of cancer

Cancer Type	Protocol Title	Delivery Vehicle	Therapeutic Gene	Principle Investigator/ Institution/ Contact No.
Tumor-Suppressor Gene Replacement and/or Oncogene Inactivation				
NSCLC	Phase I pilot study of adenoviral *p53* administered by bronchoalveolar lavage in patients with bronchoalveolar cell lung carcinoma	Adenovirus	*p53*	David P. Carbone Eastern Cooperative Oncology Group 615-936-3524
TCC bladder	Phase I study of adenoviral *p53* in patients with locally advanced and metastatic bladder cancer	Adenovirus	*p53*	Lance C. Pagliaro the University of Texas M.D. Anderson Cancer Center 713-792-2830
Liver/colon with liver mets	Phase I study of gene therapy with SCH-58500 (adenoviral *p53*) via hepatic artery infusion in patients with primary and metastatic malignant tumors of the liver	Adenovirus	*p53*	Jo Ann Horowitz Schering-Plough Research Institute 888-223-4272
Breast	Phase I study of intralesional gene therapy plus chemotherapy for breast cancer	Adenovirus	*p53*	Margaret von Mehren Fox Chase Cancer Center 215-728-2626
Ovarian	Phase I study of intraperitoneal adenoviral *p53* gene therapy in patients with advanced recurrent or persistent ovarian cancer	Adenovirus	*p53*	Carolyn Y. Muller Simmons Cancer Center 214-648-3026

(continued)

Table 13.1 *Continued*

Cancer Type	Protocol Title	Delivery Vehicle	Therapeutic Gene	Principle Investigator/ Institution/ Contact No.
Glioblastoma	Phase I study of SCH-58500 in patients with recurrent or progressive resectable glioblastoma multiforme, anaplastic astrocytoma, or anaplastic mixed glioma	Adenovirus	*p53*	Jeffrey J. Olson Johns Hopkins Oncology Center 404-778-3091
Peritoneal carcinomatosis	Phase I study of SCH-58500 administered by intraperitoneal instillation in patients with peritoneal carcinomatosis	Adenovirus	*p53*	Jo Ann Horowitz Schering-Plough Research Institute 888-223-4272
Head and neck	Phase II study of Ad5CMV-53 for recurrent squamous-cell carcinoma of the head and neck	Adenovirus	*p53*	Lyndah Dreiling Rhone-Poulenc Rorer Pharmaceuticals, Inc. 610-454-5997
Drug Sensitivity				
Malignant glioma	Phase I study of adenovirus and herpes simplex virus thymidine kinase (*HSV-tk*) gene therapy for primary brain tumors	Adenovirus	*HSV-tk*	Jane B. Alavi University of Pennsylvania Cancer Center 215-662-6319
Ovarian	Phase I study of *in vivo* gene therapy with the herpes simplex thymidine kinase/ ganciclovir system for patients with refractory or relapsed ovarian adenocarcinoma	Herpes simplex virus	*HSV-tk*	Charles Joseph Link, Jr. Human Gene Therapy Research Institute 515-241-8787

Table 13.1 *Continued*

Cancer Type	Protocol Title	Delivery Vehicle	Therapeutic Gene	Principle Investigator/ Institution/ Contact No.
Drug Resistance				
Solid tumors and NHL	Phase I study of mutant *MGMT* gene transfer into human hematopoietic progenitors to protect hematopoiesis during 06-benzyguanine and carmustine therapy of advanced solid tumors and non-Hodgkin's lymphoma	Retrovirus	*MGMT-*G156A	Stanton L. Gerson Ireland Cancer Center 216-368-1176
Immunomodulatory				
Melanoma	Phase I study of adenovirus interferon (IFN)-γ in patients with locally recurrent or metastatic melanoma	Adenovirus	IFN	Joseph D. Rosenblatt University of Rochester Cancer Center 716-275-9484
Glioma	Phase I study of adenoviral *p53* gene therapy in patients with recurrent malignant gliomas	Adenovirus	*p53*	Frederick F. Lang, Jr. North American Brain Tumor Consortium 713-792-2400 Stuart A. Grossman Johns Hopkins Oncology Center 410-955-8837
Ovarian	Phase I study of anti-CD3-stimulated peripheral blood lymphocytes transduced with a gene encoding chimeric T-cell receptor reactive with folate-binding protein in patients with advanced ovarian epithelial cancer	Retrovirus	MOV-gamma chimeric (*MOV-PBL*)	Patrick Hwu Division of Clinical Sciences 301-402-1156

(continued)

Table 13.1   *Continued*

Cancer Type	Protocol Title	Delivery Vehicle	Therapeutic Gene	Principle Investigator/ Institution/ Contact No.
Neuroblastoma	Phase I study of interleukin (IL)-2 gene-modified autologous neuroblastoma cells for relapsed/refractory neuroblastoma	Adenovirus	*IL-2*	Laura C. Bowman St. Jude Children's Research Hospital 901-495-3519
Melanoma	Phase I/II study of intralesional immunotherapy with a recombinant vaccinia virus encoding the gene for granulocyte-macrophage colony-stimulating factor (GM-CSF) in metastatic melanoma	Vaccinia virus	*GM-CSF*	Michael Joseph Mastrangelo Kimmel Cancer Center of Thomas Jefferson University 215-955-8875
Melanoma	Phase II study of allovectin-7 as an immunotherapeutic agent in patients with stage III or IV melanoma	Direct gene transfer	Allovectin-7	Christine Siaton Covance Clinical and Periapproval Services, Inc. 609-716-6360
Melanoma	Phase III randomized study of dacarbazine with or without allovectin-7 in patients with metastatic melanoma	Direct gene transfer	Allovectin-7	Christine Siaton Covance Clinical and Periapproval Services, Inc. 609-716-6360

Data from *http://www.nih.gov/od/oba*.
NSCLC, non–small-cell lung cancer; TCC, transitional cell carcinoma.

Drug-Resistance Genes

The sensitivity of bone marrow to increasing doses of systemic chemotherapy agents is a limitation in the treatment of metastatic cancers. Protection of normal **hematopoietic** progenitor cells from the effects of chemotherapy would allow further dose escalation and possibly in-creased efficiency resulting in higher response rates. In ongoing research protocols, attempts are being made to enhance marrow protection by transducing the multiple-drug-resistance gene *(MDR-1)* into normal bone marrow or blood-derived stem cells (Clinical Protocols, 1995; ORDA Reports, 1995; Aran *et al.*, 1999). The protein product of the *MDR-1* gene is known as P-glycoprotein, which serves as an efflux pump for certain drugs. Insertion of the *MDR-1* gene into normal marrow stem cells produces a population of cells that can be selected for resistance to the effects of systemic chemotherapeutic agents, including the vinca alkaloids, dactinomycin, doxorubicin, and paclitaxel (Mastrangelo *et al.*, 1996; Roth and Cristiano, 1997). It is hoped that insertion of this gene into hematopoietic stem cells, would enable patients to tolerate higher doses of chemotherapy. The stem cells transduced with *MDR-1* would "pump out" chemotherapy and not be affected.

Some of the first research protocols for *MDR-1* were designed to treat patients with breast and ovarian cancers (Deisseroth *et al.*, 1994; 1996; Hesdorffer *et al.*, 1994). Although initial studies have shown this approach to be feasible, problems do remain. Potential problems with this study design are that higher doses of chemotherapy may not produce higher response rates; nonhematologic side effects (e.g., peripheral neuropathy or renal damage) may become the dose-limiting toxicity; and hematopoietic cancer cells in the marrow may be transduced and, therefore, protected (Roth and Cristiano, 1997). The overall transduction efficiency and stable engraftment of gene-modified hematopoietic stem cells must be improved before *MDR-1* gene therapy and *in vivo* selection with anticancer drugs can be used reliably to protect cancer patients from drug-related myelosuppression (Cowan *et al.*, 1999). Ultimately, if this approach proves efficacious, investigations comparing *MDR-1* therapy plus chemotherapy plus bone marrow transplantation with chemotherapy plus bone marrow transplantation would need to be initiated.

Drug-Sensitivity Genes

Another category of gene therapy is designed to sensitize tumor cells for destruction by other therapeutic agents. In this therapeutic strategy, drug sensitivity is conferred by transducing tumor cells with a gene whose product can metabolize a nontoxic **prodrug** to its toxic metabolite (i.e., suicide gene) (Mastrangelo *et al.*, 1996; Roth and Cristiano, 1997). The first protocol approved for this gene-therapy approach enabled brain tumors to be transduced with a retroviral vector expressing the herpes simplex **virus** thymidine kinase (HSV-*tk*) gene. The HSV-*tk* gene is able to phosphorylate a number of nucleotide analogues, such as acyclovir and ganciclovir. Once phosphorylated, the **nucleotide** analogue is incorporated into replicating DNA and causes termination of the DNA strand, resulting in cell death. When a patient is given systemic ganciclovir, an antiviral drug that works against the HSV that enters the tumor cells, the tumors are destroyed. Multiple studies have demonstrated that complete tumor regression can be accomplished even with only a minority of cells being transduced (Singhal and Kauser, 1998). This **cytotoxic** effect of transduced cells on nontransduced cells is called the "**bystander effect**" (Roth and Cristiano, 1997).

Several hypotheses have been put forward to explain the bystander effect; however, the true mechanism is still unknown. The bystander effect may be related to the observation that endothelial cells are susceptible to retrovirally mediated gene transfer, causing the endothelial cells to become sensitive to other drugs. Hemorrhagic areas within HSV–tk transduced tumors are noted after ganciclovir administration, suggesting that tumor regression may be caused by ischemia (Singhal and Kaiser, 1998). Secondary to this finding, new strategies are being investigated that will use **antiangiogenesis** gene therapy.

A review by Wildner (1999) discussed the clinical studies in patients with brain tumors. These studies revealed that the HSV-*tk*–ganciclovir approach is safe, but also that responses are observed only in very small brain tumors, indicating insufficient vector distribution and very low transduction efficiency with replication-deficient vector systems. To improve treatment efficacy, the use of replication-competent oncolytic vectors in combination with new or improved prodrug-suicide gene systems as a part of a multimodal approach is warranted. Techniques are being developed that will provide for the study of combination suicide-gene-therapy strategies in patients and allow for the introduction of a second therapeutic gene (Kuiper *et al.*, 2000).

Immunomodulatory Genes

Since the early 1980s, investigators have attempted to **modulate** the immune system to generate an effective anti-tumor response. Lack of success in clinical trials with human models led to a decline in interest in immunotherapy. However, recent identification of molecular models and the development of gene-transduction techniques have led to a renewed interest in immunotherapy for human cancers. Gene-transduction-based immunotherapy is based on 2 major assumptions: (1) that tumor-specific antigens exist and (2) that the host immune system is capable of recognizing these antigens and eradicating tumor cells (Kufe *et al.*, 2000). Failure of the natural host immune response is thought to result from the inability of the host to recognize tumors or to generate sufficient effector cells.

Following the cloning of various cytokine genes, it became apparent to a number of investigators that local tumor growth could be controlled and systemic antitumor immunity could be enhanced by these factors. In animal models, tumor cells were transduced *ex vivo* with a specific cytokine gene, and the cells were irradiated and then transplanted back into the host animal. In this manner, a number of cytokine genes were shown to reduce tumorigenicity or enhance systemic immunity. These genes include the interleukins (ILs) *IL-2, IL-4, IL-6, IL-7,* and *IL-12*; tumor necrosis factor *(TNF)*-α; **granulocyte colony-stimulating factor *(GCSF)*; granulocyte-macrophage colony-stimulating factor *(GM-CSF)***; and interferon-γ. Tumor cells obtained at resection of the primary tumor are grown in tissue culture and genetically modified with cytokine genes such that the vaccine cells, after injection, may stimulate immune recognition of tumor cells and generate immunologic memory to prevent future tumor recurrence. It is hoped that the local secretion of cytokines would increase the killing of tumor cells by inducing local infiltration of effector cells and other immune responses. Numerous clinical trials investigating this approach are under way, with an area of focus on patients with melanoma (Palmer *et al.*, 1999). Although this approach appears both safe and feasible, the clinical efficacy remains to be determined. This approach requires a significant investment in terms of effort, money, and resources to produce autologous-cell gene-modified vaccines. It is uncertain at this time whether this approach will offer a useful return on the investment or be feasible in the community setting (Vile *et al.*, 2000).

In many instances, tumor cells do not express cytokines after transduction, or tumor antigens are not appropriately presented to T cells, or the tumor antigens do not exist (Kufe *et al.*, 2000). Tumor cells may be defective in their expression of histocompatibility molecules, leading to defects in antigen presentation (Roth and Cristiano, 1997). In addition, co-stimulatory molecules may need to be present on the antigen-presenting cell to activate cytotoxic T cells.

Animals have shown that when the co-stimulatory **ligand** B7 is transduced into malignant melanoma cell lines and then into a mouse, tumors initially grow but then regress over 3 to 4 weeks (Townsend and Allison, 1993). Also, on challenge, these animals show protection against the tumor. A difficulty with this approach is the unpredictable effect of the loss of co-stimulatory molecules in human cancer. Hence, strategies are also now targeted toward transduction of tumor cells with co-stimulatory molecules and membrane proteins to more efficiently present antigens to T cells (Cavallo *et al.*, 1999).

Effective immunization against viruses was achieved through the expression of viral proteins in infected cells and the breakdown of these proteins in the cytoplasm. Peptide fragments from the breakdown of viral proteins are transported to the cell surface, where they are displayed in association with major histocompatibility complex antigens. Cytotoxic T cells are then activated to destroy the cell. It was shown that the inoculation of DNA-expression **plasmids** into animals can lead to a T-cell response to the expressed protein by the same mechanism that produced the antiviral response. This observation led to the investigation of DNA vaccination for the treatment of tumors. Direct injection of DNA into the livers and skeletal muscles of cats was shown to result in the expression of encoded genes in these specific areas (Benvensity and Reshef, 1986; Wolff *et al.*, 1990). Choosing the appropriate antigen is the principal challenge involved in producing an effective DNA vaccination. The optimal antigen to target will be one expressed exclusively on tumor cells or on tumor cells and nonessential normal tissue. Examples of these antigens include the carcinoembryonic antigen and the prostate-specific antigen (Conry *et al.*, 1994).

A similar strategy would be the induction of an **anti-idiotype** response against specific T-cell receptors in T-cell lymphomas and leukemias. It also may be possible to target new epitopes of mutations of normal cellular molecules such as *p53* (Kufe *et al.*, 2000). A concern with this strategy is the possibility of generating an immune response against normal tissue,

which could theoretically lead to an autoimmune disease, such as systemic lupus erythematosis—although this has not been seen in early clinical trials. For further discussion of genetic vaccine approaches, see Chapter 10.

Several assumptions exist regarding gene-transfer-mediated anti-tumor immunotherapy. It is not known whether tumor antigens exist for all tumors. It is an assumption that an effective immune response can be generated and that cancer patients do not develop immunologic tolerance to their tumor antigens. Few studies to date have demonstrated eradication of large, established tumors. Although the effectiveness of gene therapy in this setting remains to be proved, studies have been proposed that will use this approach to prevent tumor recurrence.

Tumor-Suppressor Gene Replacement and Oncogene Inactivation

Therapeutic gene transfer was originally envisioned as a method of replacing mutated or missing genes to treat disorders caused by defects in single genes. The identification of specific genes that contribute to the development of cancer presents an opportunity to use these genes as targets for prevention and treatment strategies. Two classes of genes implicated in carcinogenesis include oncogenes and tumor-suppressor genes. It is possible that modification of the expression of these genes, when mutated, may influence some characteristics that contribute to malignancy. For example, the *p53* tumor-suppressor gene is mutated in about 50% of human cancers (Fearon, 1997). The inactivation of this gene may contribute to tumor growth. Transduction of a **wild-type** *p53* gene can partially revert the malignant *p53* tumor cells, *in vivo,* and slow their growth substantially (Clayman *et al.*, 1995). The presence of a wild-type *p53* gene may be necessary for induction of **apoptosis** by some chemotherapeutic agents (Howe *et al.*, 1993). One *in vivo* study showed that in tumors treated directly with *p53*-expressing **adenovirus** (Ad-*p53*) and cisplatin, extensive areas of apoptosis were visualized, whereas tumors treated with either cisplatin or Ad-*p53* alone showed no apoptosis (Fujiwara *et al.*, 1994).

An alternative strategy, based on inactivating target molecules such as oncogenes that induce cellular proliferation and human cancer, also was suggested. There are several ways to inactivate these genes using gene-transfer techniques. One strategy involves transducing a dominant negative mutant of the oncogene. A dominant negative mutation would be one that is dominant in function. With respect to an oncogene, which is "on," the dominant negative usually binds to it, its regulators or, more frequently, its targets and shuts the system "off." The off signal is dominant over the on signal. Another strategy is to inhibit translation of the oncogene by transduction of the DNA molecule that encodes a specific ribozyme molecule. Ribozymes are **ribonucleic acid** (**RNA**) molecules that possess an RNA recognition site and enzymatic activity such that specific ribozyme-target RNA is cleaved and destroyed. Another method is to destroy specific intracellular proteins by transduction of a gene that encodes the single-chain variable region of an antibody specific to the target molecule. Following intracellular binding, the molecule is most often inactivated and then destroyed by intracellular proteases (Kufe *et al.*, 2000).

The most well-developed strategy to date for downregulation of intracellular targets is the use of antisense nucleic acids (Stein and Cheng, 1993). The gene to be downregulated is targeted. The antisense nucleic acids or antisense **oligodeoxy nucleotides** (**ODNs**) that are generated are complementary to specific sequences of messenger RNA derived from the target gene. The ODNs then bind to messenger RNA preventing its translation. The mechanism responsible for this effect is not clear. One advantage of this approach is its specificity. Expression of a specific gene can be targeted by choosing the appropriate ODN. The disadvantage is that most antisense strategies require prolonged duration of gene downregulation, leading to delivery problems and rapid degradation of the ODN (Kufe *et al.*, 2000). Gene therapy offers possible solutions to these problems by creating vectors that can stably express antisense or RNA transcripts over long periods (i.e., retroviral vectors).

The *ras* proto-oncogene is an example of a potential target for antisense ODNs. Activated *ras* is found in 20% to 30% of all cancers in more than 50% of colon cancers, and in more than 90% of pancreatic cancers (Kufe *et al.*, 2000). Inhibition of *ras* results in diminished tumor growth. Unfortunately, chronic suppression of *ras* is necessary or the tumor will begin to grow again. Antisense therapy is an active area of clinical research, with phase I trials in early stages. There are many points to be considered in the design of antisense therapy trials. Mani *et al.* (1999) proposed that trials should be designed to answer the questions specifically related to proof-of-concept for this new therapeutic modality. As of July 2000, more than a dozen compounds were in clinical trials in cancer and other diseases, such as **acquired immune deficiency syndrome** (**AIDS**). It is too early to determine the clinical effectiveness of this approach in the treatment of cancer (Marcusson *et al.*, 1999).

Delivery Methods

Regardless of why gene therapy is being delivered, special preparation is required to ensure that the gene is delivered to targeted cells accurately and efficiently. The steps involved in gene transfer are: (1) accessing the target cells, (2) binding of the gene to the target cells, (3) cytoplasmic transport to the nucleus, (4) DNA delivery and persistence in the nucleus, and (5) gene expression. The overall efficiency of a gene-transfer technique depends on the degree to which each step is completed (Vile and Russell, 1994). Because we are technically unable to insert genes into the genome, researchers have developed several methods for transporting genetic material using both viral and nonviral vectors. Vectors are often organisms, specifically viruses but sometimes liposomes or plasmids, into which foreign DNA can be inserted. The vector carries the gene product into the cell. Because they are more efficient, viral vectors are used more often than nonviral vectors in clinical trials. There are 2 basic approaches to deliver the vector to the cell: (1) *in vivo*, where the vector is introduced directly into the tissue to be treated; and (2) *ex vivo*, where the cells from a selected tissue are removed, exposed to the vectors in the laboratory, and then returned to the patient (Friedman, 1997).

Viral Vectors

Gene therapy based on viral vectors takes advantage of the fact that viruses can carry foreign genetic material directly into **eukaryotic** cells (Kufe *et al.*, 2000). The most commonly used technique is an *ex vivo* approach in which the defective target host cells are removed from the body, given normal copies of the affected DNA using a virus as the carrier, and then returned to the body. For example, early gene-therapy trials attempted to remove normal **tumor-infiltrating lymphocytes (TILs)** from the body and modified them by inserting the gene for TNF. The modified TILs then would be returned to the body intravenously, with the goal of providing higher concentrations of TNF in the area of the tumor, thereby achieving an increased tumor kill without dose-limiting TNF toxicity. Viral vectors are deliberately modified so they can carry genes into cells but cannot reproduce themselves. There are 3 main types of viral vectors: retroviral vectors, adenoviral vectors, and herpes simplex viral vectors. Clinical experience has been gained over the past decade with the use of different viral vectors, elucidating the advantages and disadvantages of each. Future research will be directed toward exploring new types of viruses such as adeno-associated viruses and herpes simplex viruses. In addition, the development of replicating-competent viruses (i.e., viruses that can replicate in tumor cells to enhance gene spread), the combination of components of different vectors into hybrid vectors with the beneficial properties of different systems, and the continued investigation of novel viral and nonviral delivery systems will be areas of focus (Vile *et al.*, 2000; Wu and Ataai, 2000).

Retroviral Vectors

Retroviral vectors are the most common vectors used in gene-therapy today (Robbins, 1999). Retroviruses contain RNA as their genetic material and convert RNA to DNA in the cells they infect. These very small single-stranded viruses were first discovered because of their propensity to cause tumors in animals. These simple viruses replicate after penetrating a cell. Their reverse-transcription process produces a double-stranded DNA intermediate called a "provirus." It is the provirus that enters the **nucleus** of the cell, integrating randomly into the host genome; this integration is essential to the retrovirus replication process (Miller, 1993). For use as vectors, retroviruses are altered so that they are not infectious. This occurs through the removal of structural genes vital for viral replication. Foreign genes can be placed into the altered virus for expression in the target cell. Following infection (i.e., transduction) of the target cell, the retrovirus is unable to produce infection because the deleted structural gene is not expressed in the target cell.

The advantages of retroviral vectors include their ability to infect a wide range of cell types and to carry large amounts of foreign nucleotides (i.e., large genes). Retroviruses have relatively simple structures, making it easy to construct various vectors (Kufe *et al.*, 2000). Vectors may be created that express no viral genes, which minimizes the chance of significant antiviral immune responses. Retroviruses integrate into the target DNA, achieving stable transduction.

There are several potential limitations of retroviral vectors. First, they insert genes only into actively dividing cells, such as T cells. This is important because in most solid tumors, fewer than 20% of the cells are actively dividing at any given time. Thus, retroviral vectors are then unlikely to be useful for transduction in solid tumors ((Kufe *et al.*, 2000). Second, the current **titers** able to be achieved in treatment (10^7) are lower than the titers needed to transduce all of the cells in large tumors (Roth and Cristiano, 1997). Third, cell-free infection is very inefficient. Direct cell-to-cell contact is required for optimal transduction efficiency. Finally, there are biosafety concerns about retroviruses. Retroviruses insert themselves at random into the host DNA, thus posing a small but certain risk of insertional mutagenesis, which could lead to malignancy (Marshall, 1995). If the vector positions itself upstream from a proto-oncogene, the promoter incorporated into the retrovirus then may turn on the proto-oncogene, moving the host cell closer to malignant transformation (Blaese, 1995). No retrovirus has ever been shown to be pathogenic in humans. However, lymphomas and leukemias have developed in nonhuman primates following treatment with high doses of retroviral vectors contaminated by helper viruses (Ahmad *et al.*, 1989). Viruses may not be selective about the cells they invade; therefore, it is difficult to direct the virus specifically to target cells. Despite these limitations, retroviral vectors remain noted for their stable transduction. Retroviral vectors may be best suited for *in vitro* transduction in which target cells can be isolated. *In vivo* use of these vectors appears to be less certain.

Adenoviral Vectors

In contrast to retroviruses, adenoviruses contain linear, double-stranded DNA complexed with core proteins surrounded by **capsid** proteins. There are almost 50 serotypes of adenovirus. The prototype vector is based on adenovirus types (Ad5), Class C (Kufe *et al.*, 2000). The adenovirus structure is described on the basis of the timing of the gene expression following infection. There is an early (E) phase that precedes viral DNA replication and a late (L) phase that starts about 6 hours later. E1A and E1B products are the first adenovirus proteins generated after infection and are critical for viral replication. Adenoviral-vector construction is based on the observation that deletion of the E1A and E1B genes renders the virus replication deficient (Kufe *et al.*, 2000).

Adenoviral vectors have several advantages over retroviral vectors. They can be produced at higher viral titers ($>10^{11}$) with little manipulation (Mittal *et al.*, 1995). Higher titers mean that a higher number of viruses are present for insertion into the host cell. Adenoviruses penetrate nondividing cells as well as dividing cells and may be frozen for later use. Some studies have shown that minimal amounts of adenovirus can generate high-level transduction of cells with efficient levels of gene expression in most tissues except hematopoietic cells (Li *et al.*, 1993; Kremer and Perricaudet, 1995). Because adenoviral vectors exist within the target-cell as **episomal** DNA, insertional mutagenesis is less of a concern than it is for retroviral vectors. In cancer therapy, adenoviral vectors are used in clinical trials to deliver drug-sensitivity genes, such as HSV-*tk*, to kill cancer cells in the brain or liver or to deliver the wild-type *p53* gene into the lung, head and neck, or liver cells through injection.

The major disadvantage of adenoviral vectors is that they express proteins that trigger immune responses, provoking inflammation and an immune attack. This may result in damage to the target tissue. For this reason, adenoviral-vector gene therapy is of short duration (Marshall, 1995). It may not be possible to administer the vector in a repeat dosing schedule or to previously treated recipients because of an immune response to viral antigens (Kufe *et al.*, 2000). Some investigators have suggested administering the different stereotypes sequentially to circumvent the neutralizing antibody response (Roth, 1996) or to create vectors that express few or no viral proteins.

Herpes Simplex Virus Vectors

HSV is a large double-stranded DNA virus that is naturally **neurotropic** but also highly infectious to a number of types of epithelial cells. Because it is able to establish infection in the brain, HSV has been used to deliver therapeutic genes to the central nervous system (CNS). HSV can follow a replicative or latency life cycle after infection. Infected cells release high titers of virus, which eventually result in cell **lysis** (Antman *et al.*, 1990). The latency period of the life cycle is associated with little viral-gene transcription and normal host-cell function. The 2 major types of HSV vectors are plasmid-derived vectors and **recombinant** vectors. Plasmid-derived vectors require a wild-type helper virus and, therefore, are not useful for most *in vivo* studies. Recombinant vectors are constructed by recombination of wild-type HSV and cloning vectors. By using cloning vectors, it is theoretically possible to control the degree of toxicity, replication, and virulence

(Kufe *et al.*, 2000) to "design" an HSV vector with the desired properties.

HSV vectors, in theory, offer a number of advantages for gene transfer. They are big and can carry a large amount of foreign DNA. In addition, as stated previously, they can infect the CNS. They are very efficient in cell transduction in a wide range of host cells, and they have demonstrated a remarkable latency period with possible long-term **transgene** expression (Kufe *et al.*, 2000).

HSV vectors also have a number of disadvantages. The herpes genome is not completely understood, and difficulties have arisen in generating stocks of replication-incompetent virus. Expression of *HSV* genes *in vivo* contributes to the potential for a significant antiviral immune response. There is concern that neuropathic effects may develop because of the high predilection of herpes infection in neuronal cells (Kufe *et al.*, 2000). Despite the many potential advantages of HSV vectors, much *in vitro* work must be completed to ensure that the vector is safe and reliable for clinical use.

Adeno-Associated and Vaccinia Virus

Adeno-associated virus (AAV) is a small, linear, single-stranded DNA virus dependent on helper viruses such as adenovirus, HSV, and vaccinia virus for its replication (Boulikas, 1997). Because AAV is small, it is easy to manipulate genetically. AAV stably integrates into the host genome with a special predilection for a region on chromosome 19 (Kotin *et al.*, 1992). It is unknown if site-specific integration offers an advantage over random integration, such as that found with retroviruses. A preliminary study showed that AAV is capable of infecting both dividing and nondividing cells, as well as hematopoietic cells (Flotte *et al.*, 1993). This property would distinguish AAV from other available viral vectors. The current generation of AAV recombination results in low viral titers (Roth and Cristiano, 1997). Recent advances in the production of high-titer purified AAV vector stocks have made the transition to human clinical trials a future reality (Monahan and Samulski, 2000).

Another large virus, vaccinia, also has received attention for its usefulness in gene delivery, particularly for delivery to the skin and subcutaneous tissues, for delivery of the IL genes. Although able to transduce both replicating and nonreplicating cells, vaccinia virus appears to have an affinity to localize to skin (Elkins *et al.*, 1994). Similar to the case with the adenovirus, the vaccinia genome does not stably integrate into the host-cell DNA, which may result in immune sensitization. Repeated exposure of humans to this vector may reduce its effectiveness due to immune elimination (Geraghty and Chang, 1995).

As the understanding of virology increases, a number of additional viruses likely will be used as gene vectors. Vectors based on pox viruses and bacillovirus already have been developed for use in cancer, and the use of other viruses (e.g., lentiviral vectors) are on the horizon (Trono, 2000). Vector selection also must be tailored to the disease being treated because there are specific requirements unique to the type of target tissue and the amount of gene-product required (Smith, 1999).

Nonviral Vectors

A number of strategies exist for delivering foreign genes to cells without the use of viral vectors. A promising area being developed is that of nonviral vectors. These vectors generally consist of **liposomes**, molecular conjugates, and naked DNA, which are delivered by mechanical methods. Substantial progress has occurred in the last 10 years in the development and application of nonviral vectors in gene therapy. How-

ever, many problems remain to be resolved before nonviral gene therapy can become a standard clinical practice (Felgner, 1997; Li and Huang, 2000).

Liposomes

Liposomes are bilipid membranes surrounding an aqueous center. **Hydrophilic** substances can be stably maintained within this aqueous environment. When combined with DNA, liposomes form a lipid-DNA complex to mediate both *in vitro* and *in vivo* gene transfer. Several **cationic** liposomal formulations have been used successfully for delivery of genes into tumors. Liposome vectors have the ability to pass DNA into the cell's nucleus and cause genes to be expressed. This system lacks the ability to target specific cell types and mediates gene transduction mainly at the site of administration (Roth and Cristiano, 1997). Some forms of lipids, such as glycolipids, may be used to target specific organs. In general, liposomes are much less efficient than most viral vectors for overall gene transduction.

Molecular Conjugates

The need for targeted gene delivery to a specific cell type has resulted in the investigation and development of molecular conjugates. Molecular conjugates consist of protein or polypeptide ligands to which a nucleic acid or DNA-binding agent has been attached to target specific cells, resulting in a protein-DNA complex. Wu and Wu developed this gene delivery system in 1991, and since then, multiple ligands have been successfully used for gene delivery to many cell types (Cristiano *et al.*, 1993). Initially, the level of transgene expression was low and the duration of expression was quite short (Kufe *et al.*, 2000). After binding of the polypeptide ligand to its cell-surface receptor, the complex is internalized by **endocytosis**. Much of the DNA within the endosome is degraded or damaged by the acidic environment of the nucleases. Current efforts to improve the transgene expression focus on mechanisms to disrupt the endocytic pathway; this has been achieved by binding inactivated adenoviruses to the DNA-ligand complex (Curiel *et al.*, 1991). Binding is achieved either chemically or with antibodies. This system introduced a mechanism of efficient gene delivery without the detrimental effects of intact viruses.

Naked DNA

The simplest method of gene transfer is the injection of naked DNA, that is, DNA without the use of a virus or synthetic vector. This is a tedious *in vitro* process. A microinjection technique is used to introduce DNA into individual cells, allowing for the transduction of only those cells near the injection site. Injection of naked DNA has been used to generate cancer vaccines in colon cancer and melanoma (Sobol and Scanlon, 1995). This technology has been improved by techniques that allow for more forceful injection of the DNA, like the "gene gun" strategy, by which naked DNA is coated into microprojectiles, most often gold pellets, and injected into the targeted tissue with a burst of air. This delivery method has been shown to generate gene expression in the liver, but requires a surgical procedure to allow access to the tissue (Nicolet *et al.*, 1995). A surprising finding is that naked plasmid DNA injected intravenously into animals results in a diffuse, multiorgan, transient expression of a transgene (Kufe *et al.*, 2000). Whereas this sounds advantageous, the technique may prove far too nonspecific and inefficient to be useful in most gene-therapy applications.

Comparison

Many gene delivery methods are being investigated, and each has its own advantages and disadvantages (Table 13.2). The functioning of each gene delivery system requires improvement. Nonviral vectors are a potentially safer method of human gene transfer than are viral vectors; however, nonviral approaches are not likely to generate a significant immune response compared with viral vectors. Currently, nonviral-vector gene transfer is less efficient than viral-vector gene transfer. Considering these factors, nonviral vectors must undergo significant development before they can replace virus-based vectors as the principal method of *in vivo* gene transduction.

Side-Effect Profile

To date, the side effects of virus or viral-vector gene therapy in phase I and II studies have been mild and self-limiting. The most common side effects observed are transient fevers, self-limiting flu-like symptoms, mild fatigue, and some pain with injection. The most common early side effect is minor pain at the injection site, which has been linked to the cold temperature of the injection. Improved stability of the gene solution has decreased the need to keep the solution very cold, and much of the pain has been minimized by injecting virus that is warmed to room temperature prior to administration. Pain from the injection is well managed with oral or intravenous pain medications, such as hydrocodone and acetaminophen combinations and intravenous meperidine hydrochloride (Demerol), promethazine (Phenergan), and chlorpromazine (Thorazine) in a 2-1-1 ratio. Anxiety related to the gene-therapy procedure is resolved with small doses of anxiolytics, such as lorazepam (Ativan) 1 mg orally.

Pain also may be caused by injection of too much fluid into too small a space. Injected local anesthesia (e.g., 1% lidocaine, plain or with epinephrine) should be used judiciously to treat tumors where the volume of injected virus may

Table 13.2 Delivery methods

Method	Advantages	Limitations
Retroviral vectors	Infect wide range of cell types Carry large amounts of foreign nucleotides; simple	Insert only into actively dividing cells; insert randomly into host DNA
Adenoviral vectors	Produce high viral titers ($>10^{11}$) Penetrate both nondividing and dividing cells	Express proteins that trigger immune responses
Herpes Simplex Virus vectors	Carry large amounts of foreign nucleotides; able to infect central nervous system; high-efficiency transduction in wide range of host cells; remarkable latency period	Difficult to generate stocks of replication–incompetent virus; concern over safety
Adeno-associated virus	Easy to manipulate because of small size; infects nondividing, dividing, and hematopoietic cells	Low viral titers
Vaccinia	Affinity to localize to the skin	Possible immune responses
Liposomes	Ability to pass DNA into the nucleus, leading to expression	Unable to target specific cell types
Molecular conjugates	Ability to deliver to a specific cell type	Low transgene expression
Naked DNA	Requires little preparation	Transduction of cells only near injection

overwhelm the space being injected. Too much local anesthesia (or any at all) may seriously limit the amount of gene solution that can be injected intratumorally. Vigilant follow-up is necessary to identify, diagnose, and prevent side effects.

The safety of the patient and the health care worker is well managed in the hospital setting, but becomes slightly more ambiguous in the ambulatory setting, which is where most patients are treated today. Patients with target tumors that are open, that are ulcerating, or that communicate with the oropharynx or nasopharynx or with tumors of the lung or aerodigestive tract are asked to wear masks or tracheostomy curtains during treatment and for 72 hours after the last treatment. These same patients are also asked to avoid people who are immunologically compromised (e.g., the very young, the elderly,

and organ-transplant patients) or who are pregnant for the entire duration of treatment (up to 6 months). It is difficult to ensure compliance with this requirement once the patient leaves the treatment area.

At present, scientists cannot predict the long-term risks of gene therapy to patients and their offspring. Some adverse effects may not be evident for years. Long-term follow-up of these patients is essential and was recommended early (Lea, 1997). Many practitioners recommend that patients or their partners not become pregnant for at least 1 year after treatment. During treatment, patients are urged to practice birth control with barrier contraception and spermicidal creams or jellies because it is unknown what type of effects the virus or viral vector could have on an unborn fetus; at present, no adverse effects due to gene therapy have been reported. Although not necessarily required by gene-therapy protocols, nurses must be aware that a patient has past exposure to a gene and monitor the patient carefully for long-term side effects that may have developed (Lea, 1997). The true human risk cannot be known until there is more experience.

Ethical Considerations

As early as 1967, the scientific community considered the possibility of altering the human genome. Now, more than 30 years later, genetic manipulation has reached the clinical setting. Researchers with the Human Genome Project are well on their way to mapping the entire human genome. As technology enables science to make the impossible possible, ethical issues are pushed to the forefront. The ethics of human genetic manipulation including cloning, and manipulation for diagnosis and treatment of disease, are important issues that warrant the immediate attention of researchers, clinical practitioners, medical ethicists, lawmakers, and the general public.

Examination of the types of genetic manipulation that are possible reveals that both somatic and germline interventions have been considered by researchers. Whereas somatic alterations (by which the genetic trait is not passed on to offspring) seem much less controversial than those of germline cells (by which the altered genetic trait is passed to future generations), both approaches have stimulated a great deal of debate in the scientific and medical communities of the United States and the rest of the world.

Interventions centered around somatic cells are the addition of cells (adding a gene or genetic material that may be missing from a cell) and the modification of cells (changing the current genetic material to produce more desired characteristics). Germline alterations include enhancement (placement of a gene into a cell to enhance a desirable characteristic), replacement (completely replacing a defective gene with a normal copy), and modification (Payne, 1996). In germline cells, genetic addition does not yield satisfactory results because it is not possible to predict the effects of a mix of normal genes and mutated genes on the regulatory signals necessary for normal cell growth and development (Wivel and Walters, 1993).

Ethical decision making in medicine is based on four basic principles: (1) nonmalfeasance, which involves issues of safety and doing no harm; (2) beneficence, which alludes to risk versus benefit or efficacy of the treatment; (3) autonomy, which refers to informed consent and patients' rights to make their own decisions; and (4) justice, which encompasses the availability, cost, and allocation of resources (Dyer, 1997). Although there are numerous definitions of clinical ethics, the common element among the definitions is that clinical ethics has to do with ethical problems associated with the care of particular patients (Ahronheim *et al.*, 2000). Ethical dilemmas in clinical practice may occur at any level, that is, with the patient, family, health care provider, and/or society. As both health educators and patient advocates, nurses have certain ethical responsibilities, and they must be prepared to justify decisions on more than just an intuitive basis (Meares, 1997). Nurses must ensure that the information provided to patients is unbiased and research based. They also must ensure that the meaning and significance of the information provided to the patient is well understood. Self-righteous and paternalistic behaviors by the nurse must be resisted (Aquilino, 1999). Nurses are responsible for protecting the rights of their patients, treating people equally, ensuring confidentiality, and obtaining informed consent.

Nurses must be cognizant of their ethical responsibility when caring for a patient undergoing gene therapy and must remember that different cultures may not conform to Western bioethics. The nurse must promote individual rights, self-determination, and privacy (Trippreimer *et al.*, 1999).

Prior to the mid-1960s, the principle of beneficence was the guiding force behind the actions of medical practitioners. Drawn from a statement in the Hippocratic Oath, "I will apply [treatment] for the sick according to my ability and judgment . . .," this principle suggested that the ethical dilemma was the purview of the physician and was to be resolved utilizing his or her own judgment. With the advent of new technologies, organ transplantation, artificial organs, genetic engineering, artificial life support, surgical techniques, and medical/research centers, it could no longer be assumed that the patient would always want what the physician felt was best for him or her. In the area of gene therapy, informed patients often desire the newest experimental therapies; they often want to try "cutting edge," unproven treatment over standard therapy. It is the responsibility of the multidisciplinary team to make recommendations to the patient that include the best choice of therapy, as well as other available options. Safety data from phase I trials indicate that gene therapy is associated with little risk, but the efficacy of this treatment strategy has yet to be determined. With risk small and benefits unknown, beneficence is currently not a big issue in the area of gene therapy in and of itself; it is a more important issue in the area of standard versus experimental therapies.

Explicit informed consent came into being as movements for social autonomy, including the civil and consumer rights movements, swept the nation. Issues surrounding informed consent for gene therapy trials include reproductive issues such as contraception, how long after treatment a patient or partner must wait to become pregnant, and late and long-term effects on reproduction. Another issue addresses a public health concern: Is the patient being treated ca-

pable of spreading viral disease and, if so, does the patient pose a public health hazard? This issue raises yet another concern: Who should be "protected" from exposure to these patients?

The principle of nonmalfeasance is also drawn directly from a principle of the Hippocratic Oath: *premium non nocere* ("First, do no harm"). Establishment of gene therapy trials for advanced end-stage cancer has not been difficult because there is a relatively small number of other therapies available for this group of patients. It will be more difficult to determine nonmalfeasance in areas such as chemoprevention of precancerous states. If chemopreventive treatment is withheld because of its cost and a nonmalignant site becomes cancerous as a result, does this constitute "causing harm"? This is a difficult question with no easy answer.

Issues of social justice have arisen along with the advent of new technologies, new ways of managing costs, and the increasing specialization of regional medical centers. When these gene therapies become available on the open market, costs may become prohibitive; great numbers of patients may not be able to afford these innovative therapies. With treatments now being concentrated in regional or specialty centers, more patients may automatically be excluded from receiving the benefits of gene therapy because they live far from these centers. Will managed care allow patients to receive treatment outside their local community? All these issues need to be examined and resolved before this new therapy leaves the clinical trial setting.

The four stages of medical and scientific decision-making are threshold, open conflict, extended debate, and adaptation. In terms of genetic intervention, the disclosure seems to be caught in the stages of open conflict and extended debate (Wivel and Walters, 1993). What might change the red light to green? What might change the unthinkable to thinkable and then to expected? Johnathan Glover, a medical ethicist, identifies a number of anxieties regarding genetic interventions (Glover, 1984), including possible fascist applications, discrimination, loss of confidentiality, unequal access, and the decline of social solidarity. He feels that to submit to these anxieties will impede progress (Glover, 1984).

We live in an age of astounding achievement in basic science, medicine, and biotechnology. Life is extended, improved, and changed forever by daily discoveries. The possibility of gene therapy and genetic engineering forces us to examine how we as individuals and as a society value technology and human life. The prospect of genetic engineering helps us put that relationship in perspective to understand what it means to be human. It means we are mortal, imperfect, and flawed. It also means we are wise enough to take the steps necessary to better ourselves (Dyer, 1997).

The gene therapy debate is carried out at medical ethics meetings, scientific symposia, and breakfast tables across the nation. The gene revolution has become integrated into our daily lives. In February 1997, researchers created Dolly, a lamb cloned from the DNA of an adult sheep. This was supposed to be impossible (or at least generations away), but suddenly it was here—a clone of a higher mammal. Whatever Dolly's ultimate significance, she conclusively demonstrated the growing power of biotechnology. By now, most people have heard of, or read about Dolly, but the ethical debate surrounding this accomplishment will continue well beyond our lifetimes (Zajtchuk, 1999).

Initially, every gene therapy protocol had to be reviewed by the governmental Recombinant DNA Advisory Committee. However, many protocols were being initiated with concepts only slightly different from those of protocols that were already approved. There is now an expedited review process for these protocols. On May 9, 1996, the Recombinant DNA Advisory Committee ceased to be involved in protocol-by-protocol reviews. The **Food and Drug Administration (FDA)** continues to regulate gene therapy in its traditional role of development of biologic products. The FDA is primarily concerned with protecting patients who will undergo gene therapy (Kessler *et al.*, 1993). As with any human research, institutional review boards must approve gene therapy protocols before their implementation.

In late 1999, Jesse Gelsinger, an 18-year-old Arizona man, died in an experiment at the University of Pennsylvania (Philadelphia, PA) after receiving a dose of corrective genes encased in a weakened cold virus. His death, the first attributed to gene therapy, led the FDA on January 21, 2000, to temporarily suspend human gene therapy experiments at the university when "serious deficiencies" in ensuring patient safety were found. This led to an intense national debate over gene therapy, government oversight, and the assurance of public safety. The National Institutes of Health (NIH) held an advisory committee hearing in December 1999 to consider tougher controls for gene-therapy experiments. In March 2000, as a result of those hearings, the FDA and NIH announced two initiatives that will strengthen the safeguards for individuals enrolled in gene therapy trials. The FDA will implement a "Gene Therapy Clinical Trial Monitoring Plan," which requires sponsors of gene-therapy trials to routinely submit their monitoring plans to the FDA. This initiative was developed to address evidence that monitoring by study sponsors of several recent gene-therapy trials had been less than adequate. The NIH and the FDA also plan to convene a conference of investigators to review appropriate monitoring practices. The second initiative, a series of Gene Transfer Safety Symposia, expected to be held four times per year, will bring together leading experts in gene transfer research and provide an opportunity to publicly discuss medical and scientific data germane to their specialties. The FDA and NIH also will provide support for professional organizations and academic centers interested in holding safety conferences focused on gene-therapy. It is hoped that these initiatives will contribute to the assurance of patient safety and help restore confidence in the integrity of gene-therapy trials (Cannon, 1999; Anonymous, 2000; Smaglik, 2000; Stein, 2000).

Nursing Considerations

The Role of the Nurse in Gene Therapy

Nurses have a multifaceted role in gene therapy investigation; that of direct caregivers, educators, and advocates. Nurses must actively participate in clinical trials and must read the literature and attend relevant seminars to become knowledgeable about the advances being made in gene therapy.

As direct caregivers, nurses may help plan the investigational study. They are often seen as consultants to the principal investigator in planning treatment. Nurses can provide information about the administration of the altered cells, compatibility questions, intravenous pumps and tubing, and safe handling. Nurses may be called upon to administer the gene or gene-altered cells to the patient and are the most likely observers of expected and unexpected side effects of the treatment, including acute and/or chronic side effects. Nurses are responsible for reporting all side effects accurately and promptly and for documenting all observations in detail. The nurse's assessment of the patient provides critical data that may influence current and future gene therapy investigations. Nurses are also instrumental in the development of symptom management guidelines.

As educators, nurses are in an ideal position to reinforce information about the protocol and to answer questions that arise as treatment progresses. In this role, the nurse must help the patient and family to fully understand the treatment so they can give truly informed consent for treatment. Nurses must understand the basic concepts of genetics to be able to address the patients' concerns: the who, what, when, where, how, and why of treatment. The responsibility to develop educational materials for patients, the community, and other health care professionals also lies with the nurse.

Patients undergoing cancer therapy are often anxious and fatigued, as are their family members, and they look to nurses for support. As advocates, nurses can provide support by listening, answering questions, and giving encouragement. In some instances, patients need to be protected from the media. Nurses must help ensure patient confidentiality.

The nurse's role is essential to the further development of the field of gene therapy in the oncology setting and they must remain knowledgeable about the advances being made in this field.

Safety Issues

As advances in technology lead to new methods of prevention, detection, diagnosis, and treatment, it is the responsibility of professional nurses to expand their knowledge base to keep up with all the changes going on in this environment. They need an understanding of the basic sciences such as molecular biology and issues regarding genetic counseling. For those providing direct care to patients undergoing genetic intervention, they need an understanding of side effects; risks to patients, families, and staff; and safety issues regarding patient management.

There appears to be little risk to staff caring for patients undergoing gene therapy with viral vectors, although this safety needs to be proven. Unlike the case with chemotherapeutic agents, there are no clear safety guidelines for persons who may be exposed to genetically altered products. It is unclear whether standard safety precautions, such as wearing masks, gloves, and gowns, should be taken when no known risks have been identified (Lea, 1997). Many of these issues were apparent when retroviruses were the most popular viral vector in use. Now, with the possibility of replication-competent adenovirus at 10^9, 10^{10}, 10^{11}, and 10^{12} plaque-forming units (i.e., a measure of viral numbers) being given routinely, the issue has been muddied. At The University of Texas M. D. Anderson Cancer Center (Houston, TX), the following precautions are taken. Procedures developed by the institute's biosafety group or input from biosafety are based on recommendations of the FDA's Office of Recombinant DNA, the Occupational Safety and Health Administration, and the Centers for Disease Control and Prevention.

1. Patients who are hospitalized for daily gene therapy—typically patients with head and neck, gynecologic, and genito-urinary cancers—are placed in negative-pressure rooms with isolation precautions. All injections are given in a negative-pressure environment.
2. When intraoperative gene therapy is administered, only the administering surgeon and anesthesiologist are in the surgical suite.
3. Pregnant staff should not care for inpatients undergoing gene therapy. Safe exposure times and hazards to the fetus are unknown.
4. Staff administering gene therapy observe respiratory spatter, contact, and spill precautions. Staff use N-100 respirators that have been fit-tested, protective-cover gowns and eyewear, and gloves. The room where the dose is prepared and administered is cleaned with Virucide, and biosafety personnel are available to clean up spills greater than 100 mL or with greater than 10^9 plaque-forming units of virus in the dose.
5. Ambulatory patients are treated in a negative-pressure environment. Patients with ulcerated open lesions and tumors of the aerodigestive tract wear a mask for 72 hours; patients with solid tumors of skin, prostate, breast, or bladder do not.

These policies were developed using Centers for Disease Control and Prevention guidelines by the Biological and Chemical Department of Environmental Health and Safety section of The University of Texas M. D. Anderson Cancer Center.

Education

The education of the nursing staff regarding gene therapy traditionally has been undertaken on an area-by-area basis as novel treatment has been introduced to various specialty areas. Uniform policies and procedures need to be developed to cover the common issues related to all treatment protocols, no matter what the specialty area, as well as general information for all nurses regardless of where they happen to practice. Specialized procedures will remain specific to the patient population being treated (e.g., peritoneal lavage versus bladder irrigation and direct intratumoral injections versus bronchoscopy with washings). Pharmacy personnel also need specialized education to prepare, handle, and dispense virus or viral vectors. M. D. Anderson pharmacy staff developed a course to train pharmacists and technologists to handle orders for gene therapy. The course is constantly being revised and updated to meet the growing clinical need to educate personnel in this area (see the course outline in Table 13.3).

Nurses can better perform as direct caregivers, patient advocates, and educators if they learn as much as they can while gene therapy is in its infancy, and then stay interested and connected as this area of research moves from the experimental stages into the standard therapeutic armamentarium.

Patients and families also need to be educated about all aspects of gene therapy and

Table 13.3   Course outline for gene therapy pharmacy procedures

---

   I.   Orientation to viral products
      A. Types
         • Adenoviral
         • Retroviral
         • Other gene therapy (*E1A*, *Her-2/neu*, etc.)
      B. Rationale for use
         • Gene replacement
         • Inactivation of harmful gene
         • Gene augmentation
      C. Definition of a viral vector
  II. Summary of current protocols
 III. Safety
      • Biosafety levels for infectious agents
      • Minimum biosafety requirements for adenoviral products
      • Personnel safety
      • Product safety
  IV. Receipt of orders
   V. Order entry
  VI. Viral products log
 VII. Drug sign out
VIII. Dose calculations
  IX. Disposal of contaminated items
      • Product preparation
      • Contaminated patient syringes
      • Spill procedures
   X. Written test
  XI. Process validation and competency checklist

Source: Reported with permission from The University of Texas M. D. Anderson Cancer Center Pharmacy.

experimental protocols. Many patients gather information from the Internet, where pharmaceutical companies and clinical research centers maintain web sites that describe their products and the research protocols offering treatment with gene products (Table 13.4).

Future Directions

Gene therapy is just one more type of treatment that soon may be offered as standard therapy for cancer. Gene therapy trials currently under way range from treatment in the adjuvant setting with a focus on microscopic disease to treatment in the metastatic setting with a focus on bulky disease. Many technical difficulties have to be overcome before effective gene therapy can be achieved. As with other novel cancer treatments, gene therapy likely will be best utilized along with surgery, chemotherapy, radiation therapy, or a combination of these. However, gene therapy will have a major impact on the health of our population only when vectors are developed that can be injected safely and efficiently directly into patients as drugs. A universal gene delivery system would be ideal. There is a need for scientists to identify ways to reduce toxicity and immunogenicity of viral vectors, increase the transduction efficiency of

Table 13.4   Gene-therapy Internet sites

http://www.mc.vanderbilt.edu/   Introduction to Gene Therapy
This page gives an introduction to the basic methods of gene therapy. It also discusses the application
of the techniques and gives information on other sites dealing with this developing area of research.
Vanderbilt University course "Pharmacology 32."
http://www.asgt.org/   The American Society of Gene Therapy
Official site for the American Society of Gene Therapy, is a nonprofit, voluntary, professional
organization founded in 1996.
http://www.humangenetherapy.com/   USC Human Gene Therapy
USC Human Gene Therapy is the premier online source for the latest information concerning
human gene therapy. Seven volumes of editorials by Dr. French Anderson along with summaries
of recent and past articles are available.
http://www.nhgri.nih.gov/   The National Human Genome Research Institute
Details the National Human Genome Research Institute's programs, resources, and investigators.
Offers news and laboratory information.
http://www.newsrx.com/   Gene Therapy Weekly
Weekly newspaper provides a fact sheet, an events calendar, and an archive of articles. Compiles
medical, biotechnology, pharmaceutical, and health information weekly.
http://www.nih.gov/od/oba
Office of Recombinant DNA and Gene Transfer Activities—Office of Biotechnology

accessed September 1, 2000

nonviral vectors, enhance tumor/vector specificity and targeting, regulate gene expression, and evaluate combination gene therapy. Completing this research will provide 1 more weapon to use in the war against cancer.

References

Ahmad, T., Ciavarella, D., Feldman, E., *et al.* 1989. High dose, potentially myeloablative chemotherapy and ABMT for patients with advanced Hodgkin's disease. *Leukemia* 3: 19.

Ahronheim, J., Moreno, J., and Zuckerman, C. 2000. *Ethics in Clinical Practice*, 2nd edn. Gaithersburg, MD. Aspen Publishers Inc., pp. 1–3.

Anonymous. 2000. Science Policy: Agencies announce plan to monitor gene therapy trials. *The Cancer Letter* 26(10): 6–7.

Antman, K., Bearman, S., and Davidson, N. 1990. Dose-intensive therapy in breast cancer: Current status. In Gale, R.P., and Champlin R.E. (eds).

New Strategies in Bone Marrow Transplantation. New York, NY: Alan R. Liss, pp. 423–436.

Aquilino, M. 1999. In Bulecheck, G., and McCloskey, J. (eds). *Nursing Interventions: Effective Nursing Treatments,* 3rd edn. Philadelphia, PA: W.B. Saunders Company, pp. 469–481.

Aran, J.M., Pastan, I., and Gottesman, M.M. 1999. Therapeutic strategies involving the multidrug resistance phenotype: The MDR1 gene as target, chemoprotectant, and selectable marker in gene therapy. *Advances in Pharmacology* 46: 1–42.

Benvensity, N., and Reshef, L. 1986. Direct introduction of genes into rats and expression of the genes. *Proceedings of the National Academy of Sciences of the USA* 83: 9951–9555.

Blaese, M. 1995 (Nov. 15). Steps toward gene therapy: The initial trials. *Hospital Practice* 33–40.

Blaese, R. 1997. Gene therapy for cancer. *Scientific American* 276(6): 111–115.

Boulikas, T. 1997. Gene therapy for prostate cancer: p53, suicidal genes, and other targets. *Anticancer Research* 17: 1471–1506.

Cannon, A. 1999. Humility at the frontier. A come-uppance for genetic therapy. *US News and World Reports* 127(24): 60.

Cavallo, F., Nanni, P., Dellabona, P., *et al.* 1999. Strategies for enhancing tumor immunogenicity (or how to transform a tumor cell in a Franken-stenian APC). In Blankenstein, T. (ed). *Gene Therapy: Principles and Applications*. Basel, Switzerland: Birkhäuser Verlag, pp. 267–282.

Clayman, G., El-Nagger, A., Roth J., *et al.* 1995. *In vivo* molecular therapy with p53 adenovirus for microscopic residual head and neck squamous carcinoma. *Cancer Research* 55: 1–6.

Clinical Protocols. 1995. *Cancer Gene Therapy* 2: 67–74.

Collins, F., Patrinos, A., Jordon, E., *et al.* 1998. New goals for the U.S. Human Genome Project: 1998–2003. *Science* 23: 282(5389): 682–689.

Conner, M., and Ferguson-Smith, M. 1997. *Medical Genetics*, 5th edn. Avon, Great Britain: Bath Press.

Conry, R., LoBuglio, A., Kantor, J., *et al.* 1994. Immune response to a carcinoembryonic antigen polynucleotide vaccine. *Cancer Research* 54: 1164–1168.

Cowan, K.H., Moscow, J.A., Huang, H., *et al.* 1999. Paclitaxel chemotherapy after autologous stem-cell transplantation and engraftment of hemato-poietic cells transduced with a retrovirus con-taining the multidrug resistance complementary DNA (MDR1) in metastatic breast-cancer pa-tients. *Clinical Cancer Research* 5(7): 1619–1628.

Cristiano, R., Smith, L., Kay, M., *et al.* 1993. Hepatic gene therapy: Effective gene delivery and expres-sion in primary hepatocytes utilizing a conjugated adeno virus—DNA complex. *Proceedings of the National Academy of Sciences of the USA* 90: 6094–6098.

Culver, K., Blaese, R., and Anderson, W. 1992a. Gene therapy: A new frontier in medicine. In *1993 Yearbook of Science and the Future*. Chi-cago, IL: Encyclopedia Brittanica, Inc. pp. 126–127.

Culver, K., Ram, Z., Wallbridge, S., *et al.* 1992b. *In vivo* gene transfer with retroviral vector-producer cells for treatment of experimental brain tumors. *Science* 256: 1550–1552.

Curiel, D., Agarwal, S., Wagner, E., and Cotton, M. 1991. Adenovirus enhancement of transferrin-polylysine-mediated gene delivery. *Proceedings of the National Academy of Sciences of the USA* 88: 8850–8854.

Deisseroth, A.B., Holmes, F., Hortobagyi, G., *et al.* 1996. Use of safety-modified retroviruses to in-troduce chemotherapy resistance sequences into normal hematopoietic cells for chemoprotection during the therapy of breast cancer: A pilot trial. *Human Gene Therapy* 7(3): 401–416.

Deisseroth, A.B., Kavanagh, J., and Champlin, R. 1994. Use of safety-modified retroviruses to in-troduce chemotherapy resistance sequences into normal hematopoietic cells for chemoprotection during therapy of ovarian cancer: A pilot trial. *Human Gene Therapy* 5(12): 1507–1522.

Dyer, A. 1997. The ethics of human genetic interven-tion: A postmodern perspective. *Experimental Neurology* 144: 168–172.

Elkins, K., Ennist, D., Winegar, R., *et al.* 1994. *In vivo* delivery of interleukin-4 by a recombinant vaccinia virus prevents tumor development in mice. *Human Gene Therapy* 5: 809–820.

Fearon, E. 1997. Human cancer syndromes: Clues to the origin and nature of cancer. *Science* 278(5340): 1043–1050.

Felgner, P.L. 1997. Nonviral strategies for gene ther-apy. *Scientific American* 276(6): 102–106.

Flotte, T., Afione, S., Conrad, C., *et al.* 1993. Stable *in vivo* expression of the cystic fibrosis transmem-brane conductance regulator with an adeno-asso-ciated virus vector. *National Academy of Sciences of the USA* 90: 10613–10617.

Friedman, T. 1997. Overcoming the obstacles: Gene therapy. *Scientific American* 276(6): 96–101.

Fujiwara, T., Grimm, E., Mukhopadhyay, T., *et al.* 1994. Induction of chemosensitivity in human lung cancer cells *in vivo* by adenoviral-mediated transfer of the wild-type p53 gene. *Cancer Re-search* 54: 2287–2291.

Geraghty, P., and Chang, A. 1995. Basic principles

associated with gene therapy of cancer. *Surgical Oncology* 4: 125–137.

Glover, L. 1984. What sort of people should there be? Genetic engineering, brain control, and their impact on our future world. *Penquin* (quoted in Dyer, A. 1997).

Hesdorffer, C., Antman, K., Bank, A., *et al.* 1994. Human MDR1 gene transfer in patients with advanced cancer. *Human Gene Therapy* 5: 1151–1160.

Howe, J., Lairmore T., Veile R., *et al.* 1993. Development of a sequence-tagged site for the centromere of chromosome 10: Its use in cytogenetic and physical mapping. *Human Genetics* 91(3): 199–204.

Kessler, D., Siegel, J., Noguchi P., *et al.* 1993. Regulating somatic-cell therapy and gene therapy by the Food and Drug Administration. *New England Journal of Medicine* 329: 1169.

Kotin, R., Linden, R., and Berns, K. 1992. Characterization of a preferred site on human chromosome 19q for integration of adeno-associated virus by non-homologous recombination. *EMBO Journal* 11: 5071–5078.

Kremer, E., and Perricaudet, M. 1995. Adenovirus and adeno-associated virus mediated gene transfer. *British Medical Bulletin* 512: 31–44.

Kufe, D.W., Advanti, S., and Weichselbaum, R. 2000. Cancer gene therapy. In Bast, R.C., Kufe, D.W., Pollock, Weichselbaum, R.R., Holland, J.F., Frei, E. (eds). *Cancer Medicine,* 5th edn. Hamilton, Ontario: B.C. Decker Inc. pp. 876–889.

Kuiper, M., Sanches, R., Gaken, J.A., *et al.* 2000. Cloning and characterization of a retroviral plasmid, pCC1, for combination suicide gene therapy. *Biotechniques* 28 (3):572–576.

Lea, D. 1997. Gene therapy: Current and future implications for oncology nursing practice. *Seminars in Oncology Nursing* 13(2): 115–122.

Li, Q., Kay, M., Finegold, M., *et al.* 1993. Assessment of recombinant adeno-viral vectors for hepatic gene therapy. *Human Gene Therapeutics* 3: 403–409.

Li, S., and Huang, L. 2000. Nonviral gene therapy: Promises and challenges. *Gene Therapy* 7(1): 31–34.

Mani, S., Gu, Y., Wadler, S., *et al.* 1999. Antisense therapeutics in oncology: Points to consider in their clinical evaluation. *Antisense Nucleic Acid Drug Development* 9(6): 543–547.

Marcusson, E.G., Yacyshyn, B.R., Shanahan, W.R., Jr., *et al.* 1999. Preclinical and clinical pharmacology of antisense oligonucleotides. *Molecular Biotechnology* 12(1): 1–11.

Marshall, E. 1995. Gene therapy's growing pains. *Science* 269: 1050–1055.

Mastrangelo, M., Berd, D., Nathan, F., *et al.* 1996. Gene therapy for human cancer: An essay for clinicians. *Seminars in Oncology* 23(1):4–21.

Meares, C. 1997. A case study of application of the integrated ethical/clinical judgment model. *Oncology Nursing Forum* 24(3): 513–518.

Miller, A. 1993. Retroviral vectors. *Current Topics in Microbiology and Immunology* 158: 1–24.

Mittal, S., Bett, A., Prevec, L., *et al.* 1995. Foreign gene expression by human adenovirus type 5-based vectors studied using firefly luciferase and bacterial beta galactosidase genes as reporters. *Virology* 210: 226–230.

Monahan, P.E., and Samulski, R.J. 2000. AAV vectors: Is clinical success on the horizon? *Gene Therapy* 7(1): 24–30.

Nicolet, C., Burkholder, J., Gan, J., *et al.* 1995. Expression of a tumor-reactive antibody-interleukin 2 fusion protein after *in vivo* particle-mediated gene delivery. *Cancer Gene Therapeutics* 2: 161–170.

ORDA Reports. 1995. Recombinant DNA Advisory Committee (RAC) data management report—December 1994. *Human Gene Therapy* 6: 535–548.

Palmer, K., Moore, J., Everard, M., *et al.* 1999. Gene therapy with autologous, interleukin 2-secreting tumor cells in patients with malignant melanoma. *Human Gene Therapy* 10(8): 1261–1268.

Payne, J. 1996. Will gene therapy revolutionize medicine? *Nursing Interventions in Oncology,* 9–12.

Robbins, P.D. 1999. Retroviral vectors. In Blankenstein, T. (ed). *Gene Therapy: Principles and*

Applications. Basel, Switzerland: Birkhäuser Verlag, pp. 13–28.

Romano, G., Michell, P., Pacilio, C., *et al.* 2000. Latest developments in gene transfer technology: achievements, perspectives, and controversies over therapeutic applications. *Stem Cells* 18(1): 19–39.

Roth, J. 1996. Modification of tumor-suppressor gene expression in non-small-cell lung cancer (NSCLC) with a retroviral vector expressing wild-type (normal) p53. *Human Gene Therapy* 7: 861–874.

Roth, J., and Cristiano, F. 1997. Gene therapy for cancer: What have we done and where are we going? *Journal of the National Cancer Institute* 89(1): 21–39.

Sikora, K. 1999. Introduction. In Blankenstein, T. (ed). *Gene Therapy: Principles and Applications.* Basel, Switzerland: Birkhäuser Verlag, pp. 1–10.

Singhal, S., and Kaiser, L. 1998. Cancer chemotherapy using suicide genes. *Surgical Oncology Clinics of North America* 7(3): 505–536.

Smaglik, P. 2000. Gene therapy institute denies that errors led to trial death. *Nature* 403(6772): 820.

Smith, A.E. 1999. Gene therapy—where are we? *Lancet* 354(suppl 1): 1–4.

Sobol, R., and Scanlon, K. 1995. Clinical protocols list. *Cancer Gene Therapeutics* 2: 225–234.

Stein, C., and Cheng, Y. 1993. Antisense oligonucleotides as therapeutic agents: Is the bullet really magical? *Science* 261: 1004–1012.

Stein, T. 2000. Quandry in a test tube: Death and other problems cloud the great expectations of gene therapy. *HealthWeek* 5(3): 13.

Townsend, S., and Allison, J. 1993. Tumor rejection after direct costimulation CD8 T-cells by B7 transfected melanoma cells. *Science* 259: 368–370.

Trippreimer, T., Burk, P., and Pinkham C. 1999. In Bulechnek, G., and McCloskey, J. (eds). *Nursing Interventions Effective Nursing Treatments,* 3rd edn. Philadelphia, PA: W.B. Saunders Company, pp. 637–649.

Trono, D. 2000. Lentiviral vectors: turning a deadly foe into a therapeutic agent. *Gene Therapy* 7(1): 20–23.

Vile, R., and Russell, S. 1994. Gene transfer technologies for the gene therapy of cancer. *Human Gene Therapy* 1: 88–98.

Vile, R.G., Russell, S.J., and Lemoine, N.R. 2000. Millennium review cancer gene therapy: Hard lessons and new courses. *Gene Therapy* 7: 2–8.

Wildner, O. 1999. *In situ* use of suicide genes for therapy of brain tumors. *Annals of Medicine* 31(6): 421–429.

Wivel, N., and Walters, L. 1993. Germ-line gene modification and disease prevention: Some medical and ethical perspectives. *Science* 262: 533–538.

Wolff, J., Malone, R., Williams, P., *et al.* 1990. Direct gene transfer into mouse muscle *in vivo. Science* 247: 1465–1468.

Wu, G.Y., and Wu, C.H. 1991. Delivery systems for gene therapy. *Biotherapy* 3(1): 87–95.

Wu, N., and Ataai, M.M. 2000. Production of viral vectors for gene therapy applications. *Current Opinion in Biotechnology* 11(2): 205–208.

Zajtchuk, R. 1999. New technologies in medicine: Biotechnology and nanotechnology. *Disease-A-Month* 45(11): 449–495.

Clinical Pearls

The following are key questions to ask before administering gene therapy to a patient.

- Has the informed consent been signed?
- Is the patient able to verbalize an understanding of the procedure, risks, and benefits?
- What area/tumor is to be injected?
- What is the name of the gene to be delivered and the delivery method?
- Does this gene-delivery method require a solution?
- Is a premedication required for the gene treatment?
- What are the expected side effects of treatment?
- Does the patient know what side effects need to be reported immediately?
- Does the patient have an after-hours or emergency contact name and number?

Key References

Gene Therapy

Baselga, J. 1999. New horizons: Gene therapy for cancer. *Anticancer Drugs* 10(suppl 1): 239–242.

Blaese, M. 1995. Steps toward gene therapy: The initial trials. *Hospital Practice* (Nov 15): 33–40.

Blaese, R. 1997. Gene therapy for cancer. *Scientific American* 276(6): 111–115.

Blankenstein, T. (ed). 1999. *Gene Therapy: Principles and Applications*. Basel, Switzerland: Birkhäuser Verlag.

Breau, R.L., and Clayman, G.L. 1996. Gene therapy for head and neck cancer. *Current Opinion in Oncology* 8: 227–231.

Caskey, C.T. 1997. Medical genetics. *JAMA* 277(23): 1869–1870.

Cusack, J.C., Jr., and Tanabe, K.K. 1998. Cancer gene therapy. *Surgical Oncology Clinics of North America* 7(3): 421–469.

Friedman, T. 1997. Overcoming the obstacles: Gene therapy. *Scientific American* 276(6): 96–101.

Gibson, I. 1996. Antisense approaches to the gene therapy of cancer—'recnac.' *Cancer and Metastasis Reviews* 15: 287–289.

Lea, D.H. 1997. Gene therapy: Current and future implications for oncology nursing practice. *Seminars in Oncology Nursing* 13(2): 115–122.

Peters, J. 1997. Applications of genetic technologies to cancer screening, prevention, diagnosis, prognosis, and treatment. *Seminars in Oncology Nursing* 13(2): 74–81.

Rosenberg, S.A., Blaese, R.M., Brenner, M.K., et al. 1999. Human gene marker/therapy clinical protocols. *Human Gene Therapy* 10(18): 3067–3123.

Shreeve, J. 1999. Secrets of the gene. *National Geographic* 196(4): 42–75.

Sikora, K. 1999. Introduction. In Blankenstein, T. (ed). *Gene Therapy: Principles and Applications*. Basel, Switzerland: Birkhäuser Verlag, pp. 1–10.

Smith, A.E. 1999. Gene therapy—Where are we? *Lancet* 354(suppl 1): 1–4.

Vile, R.G., Russell, S.J., and Lemoine, N.R. 2000. Millennium review—Cancer gene therapy: Hard lessons and new courses. *Gene Therapy* 7: 2–8.

PART III

Nursing Management and Future Perspectives

CHAPTER 14 | Patient Management

Paula Trahan Rieger, RN, MSN, CS, AOCN®, FAAN

The value of biotherapy as a treatment for cancer is gaining widespread acceptance. The integration of biotherapy into all aspects of cancer care and the continual introduction of new biological agents presents an ongoing challenge for both experienced and novice oncology nurses. To maintain competency, nurses need to continually increase their knowledge of the biology of cancer and the immune system, the mechanisms of action of biological agents (especially new categories of agents such as fusion proteins), and diseases and conditions for which biological agents have received Food and Drug Administration (FDA) approval. Nurses also need to develop the skills required to help ensure successful outcomes in the current health-care system, including how to manage toxic effects specific to biotherapy, administer biological agents appropriately, teach patients and

family caregivers how to administer therapy in the home setting, and resolve reimbursement problems.

This chapter covers issues relevant to the management of patients receiving biological agents and includes information about (1) assessing and planning therapy, (2) administering treatment, and (3) managing side effects. The most common toxic effects associated with biotherapy—flu-like syndrome (FLS), mental-status changes, anorexia, and fatigue—are covered in detail in other chapters. Additional chapters focus on patient and family education and issues that impact provision of care in the current health-care environment, including reimbursement concerns. Where applicable data were available, oncology nursing research related to the care of patients receiving biotherapy is highlighted.

Nursing Standards: A Foundation for Practice

The American Nurses Association (ANA) *Standards of Clinical Nursing Practice* outlines the scope of nursing practice and defines the minimum expectations for patient care (ANA, 1999b). These standards describe a competent level of nursing care as exhibited through assessment, diagnosis, outcome identification, planning, implementation, and evaluation (ANA, 1999b). *Standards of Oncology Nursing Practice,* jointly published by the ANA and the Oncology Nursing Society (Brandt, 1996), explains how to implement the generic standards described in *Standards of Clinical Nursing Practice* in the cancer setting. These two standards form the cornerstone for the management of patients who receive biotherapy. Standards of care also exist for advanced practice nurses (ANA, 1996; Lester, 1997), who are now an integral component of the health-care team that manages the care of patients in both the ambulatory and inpatient setting. Because a significant portion of health care has moved to the home setting, many home health-care nurses care for patients who are receiving biotherapy in the home. The ANA recently published standards that guide the provision of nursing care in the home-health setting (ANA, 1999a).

Nursing Assessment

Nurses have a major responsibility in the multidisciplinary management of patients who are receiving biotherapy. For the purposes of this chapter, the word *patient* will be used to refer to those receiving care and, where applicable, to family members and others who provide care. Before the initiation of therapy, explanation of the purpose of therapy and its appropriateness for the patient, the treatment schedule, associated side effects, the cost of care and reimbursement concerns, and the potential influence of care maps or inclusion in clinical pathways should occur.

Pretherapy Assessment

BASELINE ASSESSMENT

Prior to initiation of therapy, the nurse should use a body-systems approach to perform a baseline assessment (Table 14.1). This assessment should include a history of prior treatment; current symptoms related to the underlying disease process or prior treatment; prior medical history, including any chronic, intercurrent illnesses; functional status; psychosocial concerns; and hopes, fears, and expectations related to therapy (Rieger, 1998). Examples of factors that place the patient at a higher risk of developing side effects associated with biotherapy include preexisting cardiac or pulmonary problems, a history of autoimmune disease or thyroid problems, a history of psychiatric problems, poor functional status, poor nutritional status, or advanced age. A medication and allergy profile also should be obtained. Medications such as aspirin, steroids, nonsteroidal anti-inflammatory drugs, or sedatives may be contraindicated with certain biological agents.

Recommended baseline physiological measurements include height, weight, temperature, pulse, blood pressure (including orthostatic measures for patients receiving agents known to cause hypotension), and respiratory rate. Results of baseline chest x-rays and electrocardiograms should be reviewed, as should an initial laboratory profile to measure hematologic, renal, metabolic, and hepatic functions. This profile should include the following (Schwartzentruber, 1995):

- Complete blood count, differential count, platelet and reticulocyte count, prothrombin time, and partial thromboplastin time

Table 14.1   Body-system approach to physical assessment of patients on biotherapy

Body System	Assessment Factors
Cardiovascular System	• Heart rate and rhythm • Abnormal heart sounds • Blood pressure • Orthostatic blood pressure with agents known to cause hypotension (e.g., IL-2, monoclonal antibodies)
Pulmonary System	• Respiratory rate • Breath sounds • Shortness of breath • Cyanosis • Clubbing
Gastrointestinal/Nutritional Status	• Weight • Eating patterns • Abdominal girth • Cleanliness, moisture, and integrity of oral cavity • Presence of bowel sounds • Normal bowel patterns
Renal System	• Normal voiding patterns • Amount and color of urinary output
Musculoskeletal System	• Range of motion • Functional status • Presence and patterns of arthralgias
Neurological System	• Affect • Orientation • Memory • Attention span • Social engagement • Sensory perception • Presence of depressive symptoms
Integumentary System	• Erythema • Rash or lesions • Injection site reactions • Dryness • Turgor • Alopecia
General	• Presence of fever or flu-like symptoms • Fatigue

IL, interleukin

- Blood urea nitrogen, creatinine, and urine analyses
- Electrolytes (i.e., sodium, potassium, and carbon dioxide), calcium, magnesium, and Phosphorus
- Serum albumin, liver function tests (i.e., bilirubin, alkaline phosphatase, lactate dehydrogenase, serum aspartate aminotransferase, and serum alanine aminotransferase)
- Thyroid-stimulating hormone, T3 (i.e., total serum tri-iodothyronine), and T4 (total serum) with interleukin (IL-2) therapy

SPECIAL CONSIDERATIONS IN ASSESSING THE ELDERLY

Geriatric patients require special attention (Roach, 1998). In addition to the baseline factors, other factors that may affect dosage and tolerance of biotherapy for these patients include alterations in hepatic and renal function; decreased cardiovascular function; alterations in neurosensory-perception protective mechanisms (e.g., vision); and decreased integrity of tissue, skin, and mucous membranes (Boyle *et al.*, 1992; Rieger, 1997a). Examination of the medication profile is of particular importance for the elderly because they are often taking numerous medications for treatment of chronic illnesses and related symptoms.

ASSESSING THE TREATMENT PLAN

The therapeutic plan also should be fully assessed before treatment begins so that the oncology nurse can develop a care plan and intervene appropriately. Areas to consider in developing the care plan are as follows:

- Setting: Will therapy be given in the hospital, the ambulatory setting, or both? Will the patient be primarily responsible for administering the drug at home? Determination of the patient's compliance with and understanding of the treatment schedule is of prime importance in the ambulatory and home setting.

- Diagnostic Tests: What types of laboratory tests (e.g., routine lab work, special lab work, or pharmacology studies) and diagnostic procedures are required?
- Toxicity: What agent or agents will the patient receive? What are the associated side effects?
- Nature of Therapy: Is the therapy FDA-approved or investigational? If investigational, has consent been secured? Are there any special requirements for handling and storage?
- Therapeutic Regimen: At what dose and schedule will the agent or agents be administered? Will the patient receive the biological agent in combination with other biological agents, with chemotherapy, or following surgery?
- Monitoring: Will special monitoring be required (e.g., orthostatic blood pressure, special vital signs, central venous pressure, or intake and output measurements)?
- Education: What type of patient education will be required (e.g., medication self-administration or management of an ambulatory infusion pump)? What is the best time to deliver the teaching?

It is imperative to determine whether patients understand the therapeutic plan and their responsibility to adhere to that plan. Any misconceptions should be relayed to other members of the health-care team as appropriate. Nurses often find themselves answering many of the questions that the patient is either too embarrassed or too afraid to ask the physician, and serving as an advocate for the patient in the health-care system.

The use of biotherapy in many patients remains within the context of a clinical trial. The physician must obtain informed consent for patients before entering a clinical trial. It is important that nurses understand the ethical and legal foundations of informed consent so they can serve as both educator and advocate for the patient (McCabe and Padberg, 1999). Within the scope of nursing practice, the nurse can do much to address patient questions or concerns about the clinical trial. Many nurses also function as research nurses, playing key roles in the management of clinical trials (Klimaszewski *et al.*, 2000).

In many instances, biotherapy may be administered in the outpatient clinic or at the patient's home, and both settings should be fully assessed. Outpatient treatment may require the patient to travel across town or out of town. For patients who travel across town, there may be a concern about being able to procure transportation to the clinic. It is important to determine whether the patient has the necessary resources in the home, such as a refrigerator to store medication. Common concerns of patients who must travel away from home are finances, housing, separation from family and friends, and job security. Patients also may feel lonely and fearful of the outcome of their therapy. Allowing them to voice their concerns and assisting them with resolution of problems through appropriate referrals are important nursing interventions.

Patients should be able to verbalize the rationale for and nature of the therapy they are to receive. Because of the unique nature of biotherapy, several goals of treatment are possible: investigational, therapeutic, diagnostic, or supportive. In most cases, biotherapy is used to treat disease and will be either conventional (i.e., FDA-approved) or investigational. However, patients also may receive biotherapy for diagnostic purposes, as is the case with certain monoclonal antibodies (MABs) (e.g., OncoScint®, an antibody used to detect metastatic disease in patients with ovarian or colorectal cancer). Patients may receive biotherapy for supportive reasons, as is evidenced by the post-chemotherapy use of hematopoietic growth factors to abrogate myelosuppression, or during bone marrow transplantation to speed recovery of the bone marrow or to stimulate release of progenitor cells into the peripheral circulation prior to pheresis.

Assessment During Therapy

FREQUENCY OF ASSESSMENT

During therapy, the nurse performs a significant role in assessing the patient's adherence to and tolerance for the therapeutic plan. Especially with respect to investigational biological agents, any information the nurse obtains from the patient can be significant in delineating side effects associated with that agent. A basic understanding of the mode of action and side effects (acute and chronic) associated with the agent or agents forms the foundation for an ongoing assessment of biotherapy. This knowledge should be applied in a regular, systematic manner that includes monitoring of vital signs and review of body systems and pertinent laboratory values. At a minimum, these assessments should be done during every shift for hospitalized patients and at every clinic visit for outpatients. With some biological agents (e.g., IL-2 or MABs), the assessment interval may need to be more frequent. For example, during the first hour of the initial infusion of a MAB, vital signs may be taken as frequently as every 15 to 30 minutes. This ongoing assessment assists in formulating and updating the patient's plan of care.

EVALUATION OF SYMPTOMS AND SIDE EFFECTS

Symptoms should be evaluated in the context of timing (i.e., onset, duration, and frequency), location, setting, quality, quantity, aggravating and alleviating factors, and associated symptoms (Bickley *et al.*, 1999). However, few scales exist that reliably quantify common symptoms associated with biotherapy (e.g., fatigue, anorexia, and mental-status changes). In the past 5 years, advances have occurred in the development of tools for measuring fatigue in the clinical setting (see Chapter 17). Nevertheless, a form for self-reporting symptoms or a nursing-care flow sheet can be helpful in quantifying and recording the side effects experienced by patients. Strategies used to quantify the severity of symptoms can be as simple as using numerical codes to denote a mild, moderate, or severe symptom experience, or as sophisticated as using grading scales associated with clinical trials (Miller *et al.*, 1981; Oken *et al.*, 1982; White, 1992). The Cancer Therapeutic Evaluation Program (CTEP) of the National Cancer Institute also has common toxicity criteria that may be downloaded from its web site (CTEP, 1999). Over the years, the CTEP criteria have been updated to be more reflective of toxicities seen with newer treatment modalities such as biotherapy. The most current criteria include many of the common toxicities seen with biological agents, such as allergic reactions, injection-site reactions, and constitutional symptoms, including fever and fatigue. Whereas these criteria may be cumbersome for use in the clinical setting, they are frequently used in clinical trials.

Post-Therapy Assessment

Once patients have completed or have been removed from therapy, routine follow-up examinations should occur. Toxic effects that were experienced during therapy should be reassessed for resolution. Whereas most toxicities related to treatment with biological agents generally reverse within a few weeks of cessation of therapy, some toxic effects such as fatigue and mental-status changes may linger for longer periods. In addition, patients may continue to need assistance with managing symptoms associated with their disease and psychological support. In sum, patient assessment is crucial throughout the course of therapy and forms the basis for the plan of care. Table 14.2 is a list

Table 14.2   Potential nursing diagnoses for patients receiving biotherapy

Prevention and Detection
  Health-seeking behaviors
Information and Education
  Knowledge deficit
  Management of therapeutic regimen
    (individual), ineffective
Coping
  Anxiety
  Coping, ineffective individual
  Spiritual distress
  Body-image disturbance
  Social interaction (impaired)
  Role performance (altered)
Discomfort
  Pain
Nutrition
  Nutrition (altered; lower than body
    requirements)
Protective Mechanisms
  Infection (high risk for)
  Oral mucous membrane, altered
  Sensory/perceptual alterations
  Skin integrity (impaired)
  Skin integrity (impaired; risk for)
  Body temperature (altered; risk for)
  Thought process (altered)
  Protection (altered)
  Sleep-pattern disturbance
Mobility and Activity
  Fatigue
  Activity intolerance
Elimination
  Diarrhea
  Urinary elimination (altered)
Sexuality
  Sexuality patterns (altered)
Ventilation
  Gas exchange (impaired)
Circulation
  Fluid-volume deficit (risk for)
  Tissue perfusion (altered; specify)

of potential nursing diagnoses for patients who are receiving biotherapy.

Cultural Assessment

With the continued influx of immigrants from all parts of the world, the sociocultural diversity of the United States will continue to change in the coming years. It is estimated that in the next 20 to 30 years, whites will no longer represent the majority population in many states. To provide the best possible care for all patients, nurses will need to achieve competence in transcultural nursing care. Race, religion, and beliefs should be considered in the initial assessment to ensure that the care plan developed is tailored to the patient's culture and social system.

Culture represents the beliefs, knowledge, morals, laws, customs, and habits learned and acquired by individuals (Andrews and Boyle, 1995). In pursuit of cultural competence, it is helpful to know about different cultural beliefs; however, these beliefs and values must be validated with the patient and family so that stereotyping does not occur (Ersek *et al.*, 1998). One approach for developing cultural competence is to first gain an understanding of one's own culture, and then develop intercultural communication skills using a framework for assessing cultural beliefs and behavioral flexibility that will ultimately foster optimal working relationships with different groups (Lester, 1998; Zoucha, 2000). A cultural assessment is defined as a systematic appraisal or examination of the cultural beliefs, values, and practices of individuals, groups, and communities to determine nursing needs and intervention practices within the cultural context of the people being evaluated (Andrews and Boyle, 1997). There are six key areas in which cultural uniqueness should be assessed, as follows (Itano, 1998):

- communication patterns
- views on personal space
- social organization
- perception of time
- thoughts about one's ability to control the environment (including types of health beliefs)
- biologic variations among different racial groups

The nurse can use knowledge of transcultural nursing to guide the assessment and, ultimately, provision of care to those with beliefs that may differ from his or her own, and subsequently develop a successful relationship with patients and families from a variety of cultures. The Oncology Nursing Society (2000) has published *Oncology Nursing Society Multicultural Outcomes: Guidelines for Cultural Competence*. A copy may be obtained online at *http://www.ons.org* or by calling the national office at (412) 921-7373.

Psychosocial Assessment

The evaluation of psychosocial concerns should include the patient's usual coping patterns (Hogan, 1991; Barhamand, 1998; Sivesind and Rohaly-Davis, 1998), support systems, financial status, and related concerns. Increasingly, quality-of-life tools are being used to measure the value and outcomes of conventional treatments. The domains generally measured include health and functioning status, socioeconomic status, psychological/spiritual status, and family status (King *et al.*, 1997).

While psychosocial concerns are important to consider throughout therapy, they are especially important at the time therapy is discontinued. Therapy may be stopped for a variety of reasons, ranging from successful completion of a course of therapy with a good outcome to stopping therapy because of disease progression. Patients will have unique psychosocial needs depending on the situation. For example, patients frequently experience anxiety following completion of therapy. They may feel that "nothing is being done now" and that "the cancer may recur." They may miss seeing their health-care providers on a frequent basis and the support they provide. By being aware of the potential fears and anxieties related to what is generally considered a happy occasion (i.e., cessation of therapy), the nurse can help patients verbalize their concerns and develop strategies to cope with their feelings (Bush, 1998).

The decision to stop therapy because of progression of disease often represents a time of crisis for patients. Previous responses to original diagnosis, prognosis, or possible failure of prior treatment may recur. Emotions may be intense, especially with the addition of disappointment and dashed hopes. It is critical that the patient not feel abandoned by the health-care team. The simplest measures, such as touch and active listening, often will reassure the patient that they will not be abandoned (Soeken and Carson, 1987; Highfield, 1997; Radziewicz, 1997; Schlesselman, 1998). Even if cure is not possible, hope can be fostered by reassuring the patient that he or she will be cared for; that is, that symptoms will be managed and support provided during the terminal phase of disease. Radziewicz (1997) noted that:

> Nurses symbolically light candles for patients experiencing cancer to help them see through the darkness associated with disease and treatment. Nurses can spark the light of inner strength and courage that guides the human spirit. By their presence and guidance, nurses promote hope through the uncertain journey of cancer, reflect understanding to help promote growth, provide warmth to heal and melt frozen emotions, and celebrate moments of joy.

It might be necessary to refer the patient to the team psychologist, psychiatric clinical nurse specialist, clergy, or social worker. Referrals to support groups, lay volunteers, or cancer survivors trained to provide support also may be helpful.

A study by Hunt Raleigh (1992) identified and explored sources of hope in 90 patients with cancer or another chronic illness. In the study, no significant differences were found between patients with cancer and patients with other chronic illnesses. The most commonly reported sources for supporting hopefulness were family, friends, and religious beliefs. Patients also were able to describe specific cognitive or behavioral strategies used to maintain hope. Strategies such as keeping busy, talking to other people, praying or focusing on religious activities, and thinking of other things were employed to combat periods of decreased hope.

A conceptual model for assessing and developing hope (Penrod and Morse, 1997) is *The Hope Assessment Guide,* which provides strategies for assessment and stage-specific nursing to foster hope. The authors contend that hope is a dynamic process, not a static state that can be evaluated easily at one point in time; therefore, assessment must be brief and repeated as often as needed. Secondly, prescriptive clinical strategies must address the course of hope, including the fluctuations commonly encountered among people developing or sustaining hope. Table 14.3 outlines *The Hope Assessment Guide* and strategies for fostering hope.

A study by Koopmeiners *et al.* (1997) explored whether health-care professionals influence patients with cancer and, if so, how they influence their hope. Thirty-two men and women receiving active or supportive treatment or palliative care for cancer were interviewed by investigators in a semistructured format. Health-care professionals positively and negatively influenced hope in this sample. Hope was facilitated through the health-care providers' presence, sharing of information, and demonstration of caring behaviors. The most common response to how health-care professionals

Table 14.3 The HOPE Assessment Guide

Stages of Hope (Universal Components)	Nursing Assessment	Behavioral Signs	Strategies

1. Recognizing the threat (Realistic initial assessment of threat)	Did the impact of the event sink in?	• Reiteration—in speech and thoughts
		• Connecting—with others to reiterate or release
		• Stressed—at times overwhelmed by situation
		• One-way information flow—either reiterates or takes in information with no or few questions
			Provide information and monitor level of acknowledgment by
			1. Educating
			  • Content: condition/prognosis/usual outcomes of treatment
			  • Method: repeat the information at different times (repetition)/provide information in small increments/encourage audio recording, as appropriate/encourage questions
			  • Evaluate: ask patient to explain situation to you, assess degree of internalization and comprehension
			2. Responding to feelings
			  • Offer sympathy, consolation, or commiseration
			  • Listen attentively for changes in the story
			  • Provide time for rest or healthy releases

2. Making a plan (Envision alternatives and set goals/brace for negative outcomes)	Is there a plan? Is the patient prepared for the worst?	• Questioning statistical odds
		• Seeking direction on "next steps"
		• May acknowledge reality verbally, weighing options
		• Seeking others who have had experience
		• Entering two-way discussions
		• Physical envisioning
		• Articulating goals—global or focused
			Assist with formulation of a plan by
			1. Exploring options
			  • Encourage consideration of full array of available options.
			  • Discuss options not considered, including possible negative outcomes.
			  • Answer questions realistically, do not "protect" the patient from harsh realities.

(continued)

Table 14.3 *Continued*

Stages of Hope (Universal Components)	Nursing Assessment	Behavioral Signs	Strategies

		• Recognizing the possibility of negative outcomes, then compartmentalizing the possibility that it may eventuate
		• Conducting personal review of related past experiences/internal resources/external resources (human and material)
		• Checking the reputation of doctors and others involved in care
		• Eventuating the ability of friends to "be there"
			Provide both statistical and experiential information.
			2. Making connections
			  • Introduce patient to others who have managed successfully (successful role models).
			3. Supporting
			  • Provide emotional support and adequate time for contemplation, rest, and healthy releases.
			4. Sharing the plan
			  • Encourage the articulation of goals to facilitate mutual objectives in care.

3. Taking stock (Realistic assessment of personal/external resources and conditions)	What resources have been identified?	• Seeking out others who are sympathetic to the mission (new and existing relationships)
		• May change support persons as goals change
			Facilitate full assessment of resources by
			1. Supporting realistic self-assessment
			  • Point out personal resources or attributes that may be taken for granted.
			  • Engage patient in discussion regarding healthy releases.
			2. Orienting to external resources
			  • Explain services that may support the devised plan (including how to access them, eligibility requirements, and expected benefits).
			3. Monitoring support network
			  • Continue to monitor both the internal and external support network throughout course of treatment.
			  • Reinforce availability of community (external) resources as treatment progresses.

4. Reaching out (Solicitation of mutually supportive relationships)	Are there adequate supports?		Bolster supportive relationships by
			1. Setting the scene
			  • Allow liberal visiting time to permit supportive relationships to flourish.
			  • Orient to available support groups or networks.
			  • Recommend supportive counseling, as appropriate.
			2. Being there if needed
			  • Know the plan and reinforce it as needed.
			  • Listen attentively.
			  • Do not stereotypically assume supportive relationships.

5. Looking for signs (Continuous evaluation of signs of reinforcement)	What signs are being received?	• Seeking clarification of information—especially the odds of meeting hoped-for goals • May review previous history to determine "what ifs" • Conducting self-examination for signs of recurrence • Comparing self to other survivors	Point out the signs by opening channels of communication by 1. Discussing interpretation of "signs" and perspectives on progress. 2. Providing honest appraisal of progress toward goal. 3. Assisting with reformulation of goal or plans as indicated.

6. Holding on (A determination to persevere)	Does this person have stamina and will?	• Using techniques that help them get by (e.g., how to handle seeing deformed body in mirror)
		• Focusing energy
		• Expressing new perspective on life
			Provide encouragement by
			1. Monitoring energy levels
			  • Provide quiet time as desired by the person.
			  • Observe patterns with visitors—who energizes and who drains?
			  • Discuss the energy demands of hope work.
			2. Supporting endurance
			  • Provide honest praise and encouragement.
			  • Give "permission" to attend to personal needs.
			  • Teach healthy releases.

Note. Releases may occur at any stage of the process of developing or sustaining hope; therefore, they are not listed in each stage.

Source: Reprinted with permission from Penrod, J., and Morse, J. 1997. Strategies for assessing and fostering hope: *The Hope Assessment Guide. Oncology Nursing Forum* 24(6): 1055–1063.

increased patients' hope was by being present. The responses indicated that the most important way of "being present" was by "taking time to talk." Negative influences on hope primarily concerned the way in which health-care professionals gave information. Although most nursing actions are hope-enhancing, nurses can reduce a patient's sense of hope if the information they provide or their attitude toward patients is insensitive or disrespectful. Although the study is limited by its small sample size, it does provide useful implications for clinical practice, and the findings are consistent with other studies that evaluated hope in patients with cancer (Christman, 1990; Herth, 1990; Hunt Raleigh, 1992).

Administration of Biotherapy

Administration Routes, Modalities, and Techniques

Biotherapy may be administered via several routes and schedules (see Chapters 5 through 13). The most common routes are subcutaneous, intramuscular, or intravenous (i.e., single bolus, intermittent, or continuous infusions). Table 14.4 is a review of routes of administration, advantages, disadvantages, and nursing implications. The nurse should be aware that patients receiving IL-2 are often at high risk for catheter-related infections (Bock et al., 1990). Potential reasons for this risk include decreased neutrophil chemotaxis, transient impairment of T-cell immunity, and IL-2 skin toxicity. A strict aseptic technique should be used when caring for central-venous catheters in patients receiving IL-2. In addition, many institutions use prophylactic antibiotics to prevent infection (Bock et al., 1990; Snydman et al., 1990). Other routes such as intraperitoneal, intra-arterial, intrathecal, intravesical, intralesional, or scarification also may be used. Patients may be given a predetermined standard dose or a dose calcu-lated by body surface area (per m^2) or per kilogram of body weight. Increasingly, clinical guidelines are adhering to dosages that more closely match vial sizes in order to minimize drug waste. For example, a dosage calculated on a per-m^2 basis would be rounded up or down to match the closest vial size of the drug being used. Guidelines for adjusting the dosage based on hepatic or renal impairment or excessive toxicity generally can be found on the package insert.

The following safety measures should be used when administering biological agents:

- Use the proper aseptic technique during preparation and administration.
- Implement institutional procedures as appropriate for investigational agents.
- Identify the location of emergency equipment and supplies; this is especially important for the administration of MABs.
- Administer premedication (e.g., acetaminophen, diphenhydramine, or meperidine) as ordered.
- Educate patients about expected side effects and signs and symptoms that should be reported.
- Determine any special handling precautions or the need for special equipment or supplies.
- Verify the frequency at which certain vital signs are monitored (e.g., every 15 minutes for 1 hour), orthostatic blood pressures are taken, and injection sites are assessed.
- Use appropriate storage requirements. Many biological agents should be refrigerated—not frozen—at 36 to 46°F (2 to 8°C).

Some biological agents, such as interferon (IFN)-α, are manufactured by several different companies. Characteristics of the particular drug to be used, such as available vial size, solubility, stability, compatibility, filterability, and storage requirements, must be determined prior to administration because these factors differ based on the commercial brand. Any

Table 14.4 Routes of administration of biological agents

Route	Advantages	Disadvantages	Complications	Nursing Implications
Oral	Ease of administration	Inconsistency of absorption	Drug-specific complications	Evaluate compliance with medication schedule
Subcutaneous/ intramuscular	Ease of administration Decreased side effects	Adequate muscle mass and tissue required for absorption	Infection Bleeding	Evaluate platelet count (>50,000) Use smallest gauge needle possible Prepare injection site with an antiseptic solution Assess injection site for signs and symptoms of infection, inflammation
Intravenous	Consistent absorption	May require hospitalization Increased cost	Infection Phlebitis	Check for IV patency before and after administration of drugs
Intraarterial	Increased doses to tumor with decreased systemic toxic effects	Requires surgical procedure or special radiography for equipment placement	Bleeding Embolism	Monitor for signs/symptoms of bleeding Monitor prothrombin time (PT), partial thromboplastin time (PTT)
Intrathecal/ intraventricular	More consistent drug levels in cerebrospinal fluid	Requires lumbar puncture or surgical placement of reservoir or implanted pump for drug delivery	Headaches Confusion Lethargy Nausea and vomiting Seizures	Observe site for signs of infection Monitor reservoir or pump functioning

(continued)

Table 14.4 *Continued*

Route	Advantages	Disadvantages	Complications	Nursing Implications
Intraperitoneal	Direct exposure of intra-abdominal metastases to drug	Requires placement of Tenckhoff catheter or intraperitoneal port	Abdominal pain Abdominal distention Bleeding Ileus Intestinal perforation Infection	Warm chemotherapy solution to body temperature Check patency of catheter or port Instill solution according to protocol—infuse, dwell, and drain or continuous infusion
Intravesicular	Direct exposure of bladder surfaces to drug	Requires insertion of indwelling catheter	Urinary tract infection Cystitis Bladder contracture Urinary urgency Allergic drug reactions	Maintain sterile technique when inserting indwelling catheter Instill solution, clamp catheter for 1 hr., and unclamp to drain

Source: Adapted and reprinted with permission from Bender, C. 1998. Nursing implications of antineoplastic therapy. In Itano, J., and Taoko, K., (eds.). *Core Curriculum for Oncology Nursing*, 3rd edn. Philadelphia, PA: W.B. Saunders Co., p. 648.

special considerations, such as mixing with albumin or the need for special pumps or tubing also must be assessed. For example, with continuous infusions of IL-2, it is often difficult to simultaneously infuse vasopressor agents, concurrent fluids, and medications to control symptoms; therefore, a special intravenous tubing setup may be required. The vasopressor should be attached as close to the intravenous insertion site as possible or to a separate line to avoid the simultaneous bolus infusion of the biological agent and other drugs or fluids. See Appendix B, "Quick Summary Pages," for a review of special considerations for commonly used biological agents. Pharmacy personnel, package inserts, and drug-comapny websites are helpful resources for specific information on biological agents.

Increasingly, as biotherapy is given in conjunction with chemotherapy, therapeutic regimens are becoming more complex. Verification of dose and schedule is a critical step in the administration of both biotherapy and chemotherapy. Less than optimal dosing can result in reduced efficacy; however, an overdose can cause profound toxicity and, in the case of chemotherapy, even death. Reports in the media have highlighted cases of death due to incorrect administration of chemotherapy agents. In 2000, the Institute of Medicine (IOM) (an associated organization of the National Academy of Sciences) published a report, *To Err Is Human: Building a Safer Health System* (Kohn *et al.*, 2000). The report found that as many as 98,000 people die each year from medical errors that occur in hospitals. The IOM now spearheads an initiative to improve the quality of care in America by focusing on the facts and making wide-ranging recommendations. Central to the ideas proposed by the IOM is the premise that skilled and caring professionals can—and do—make mistakes. The IOM has proposed that this issue be placed at the top of our national agenda and that the nation seek ways to reduce these errors through the design of a safer health system. In early 2000, several bills were introduced in Congress proposing legislation that would address the concerns voiced in the IOM report.

The use of a systematic format for reviewing orders will reduce the potential for medication errors. This approach should include using current weights for dosage calculations, verifying all calculations, obtaining physician clarification when needed, and limiting administration of chemotherapy and biotherapy to those nurses certified in the procedure. Examining the system, policy, and procedures that govern administration of biotherapy and chemotherapy will enable staff to determine whether there are areas that need improvement to avoid potential errors. An example is the evaluation of the factors that have influenced the occurrence of a medication error or a potential medication error. Were the orders written illegibly? Was understaffing a factor? Was the chemotherapy/biotherapy vial label difficult to read? Does the dose seem exceptionally high compared with standard dosing? Examining these factors may prompt necessary changes in the system that could reduce the likelihood of a similar situation. Careful consideration of policies and procedures and verification of chemotherapy and biotherapy dosages and schedules will enhance patient safety (Schulmeister, 1997).

Handling and Disposal of Biological Agents

Policies and procedures governing the safe handling of cytotoxic agents during preparation, administration, and disposal are well established nationwide (Dana and Anderson, 1990; Fishman and Mrozek-Orlowski, 1999). However, there still has been no formal research to date regarding the safest way to handle biological agents. Although the majority of biological agents do not directly affect DNA and, therefore are not considered genotoxic substances (Dana,

1988), and although no published recommendations exist, the general rule has been to avoid direct contact with skin and generating aerosols (Conrad and Horrell, 1995). For simplicity, many institutions traditionally placed biological agents in the category of cytotoxic products requiring special handling. Nurses are advised to check institutional policy regarding handling of biological agents at their place of employment.

In response to numerous inquiries, the office of Occupational Health and Safety Administration (OSHA) first published guidelines for the management of cytotoxic (i.e., antineoplastic) drugs in the workplace in 1986. At that time, surveys indicated little standardization in the use of engineering controls and personal-protection equipment. Although practices have improved in subsequent years, problems still exist. In addition, the occupational management of these chemicals has been further clarified. These trends, in conjunction with many information requests, prompted OSHA to revise its recommendations for hazardous-drug handling (OSHA, 1999). To provide recommendations consistent with current scientific knowledge and practice, new guidelines were developed that expanded the original document to cover hazardous drugs. The recommendations apply to all settings where employees are occupationally exposed to hazardous drugs, such as hospitals, physicians' offices, and through home health-care services. It is recognized that sections dealing with work areas and prevention of employee exposure refer to workplaces where pharmaceuticals are used in concentrations appropriate for patient therapy. In those settings where employees work with drugs in a more potentially hazardous form (i.e., a more concentrated form than that encountered in certain components of pharmaceutical manufacturing), measures that afford employees a greater degree of protection from exposure are commonly employed and should be used.

A number of pharmaceuticals in the health-care setting may pose occupational risk to employees through acute and chronic workplace exposure. As noted in the 1986 guidelines, past attention mainly focused on drugs used to treat cancer. However, it is clear that many other agents also have toxicity profiles of concern. This recognition prompted the American Society of Health-System Pharmacists (ASHP) to define a class of agents as hazardous drugs. Its report specified concerns about antineoplastic and nonantineoplastic hazardous drugs in use in most institutions throughout the country. The *ASHP Technical Assistance Bulletin* (1990) described four drug characteristics, each of which could be considered hazardous: genotoxicity, carcinogenicity, teratogenicity or fertility impairment, and serious organ damage or other toxic manifestation at low doses in experimental animals or treated patients.

The OSHA guidelines list the drugs considered hazardous according to these criteria. There is no standardized reference for this information, nor is there complete consensus on all the agents listed (OSHA, 1999). In 1995, IFN-α was added to the list of hazardous drugs. Although not all institutions and health-care professionals are in agreement with this change, the addition of IFN-α to the hazardous drug list indicates that the same precautions applied in the use of cytotoxic drugs (e.g., gloves and gowns and special handling procedures) should be applied to the use of IFN-α (Gale, 1996). Again, it is recommended that nurses adhere to the policies in place at their workplace.

The combination of chemotherapeutic agents or toxins and biological agents necessitates special handling, and the addition of radioisotopes requires radiation safety precautions specific to the isotope used. Appropriate precautions regarding handling of blood and body fluids also should be adhered to per institutional policy, and patients should be taught these precautions.

Proper disposal of used vials and equipment used in biotherapy, especially in the home-care setting, is a topic of increasing importance. In some states, there are no laws requiring home health-care workers to take special precautions with waste such as sharps, whereas accrediting agencies require a well-defined medical-waste disposal policy. There are three ways that home health-care workers typically dispose of medical waste: by centralized waste-container disposal, by home pick-up by a licensed medical-waste hauler, or by individual contract with a hauler. Some companies provide waste-disposal services through the mail; for example, sharps may be disposed of this way. The mail-back containers have passed strict safety criteria imposed by the FDA and the U.S. Postal Service. The mail-back system provides a means for patients and clinicians to discard waste items generated during brief-stay home care, from treatment of a chronic condition such as diabetes, or from patients who practice self-injection of medication in the home (Carr, 1998). Thus, nurses should consult institutional and community policies regarding medical-waste disposal.

Many institutions and home health-care agencies allow patients to return sharps in a sealed container for appropriate disposal within the institution. The U.S. Environmental Protection Agency (USEPA) (1993) provides a card with instructions for disposal of medical equipment used at home. In general, used vials, needles, and syringes should be disposed of in a sealed, puncture-resistant container. Patients should be instructed not to recap needles. Occasionally, patients who are participating in a clinical trial may be required to return both empty and unused vials to the dispensing institution for purposes of accountability (Hahn and Jassak, 1988).

Management of Side Effects

The management of patients on therapy can represent a significant challenge. Not only may patients experience toxicities related to therapy, but they also may experience symptoms related to their disease and prior treatments. For every

one symptom reported, an average of two additional suboptimally controlled symptoms also may be identified. For example, an attempt to provide help in managing nausea may result in a recommendation for the management of concomitant problems such as anorexia, taste changes, or constipation. Therefore, symptoms cannot be managed in isolation or the resulting outcomes may be poor and evidenced by impaired quality of life, compromised survivorship, despair, caregiver burden, and decreased energy. By being aware of potential barriers to effective symptom management (e.g., cost, professional rivalries, lack of expertise, inadequate administrative support, inability to try new strategies and incorporate research-based interventions, and poor communication) and drawing on the expertise of their own knowledge, their colleagues, and their patients, oncology nurses play a powerful role in managing the majority of side effects associated with cancer and cancer treatment (Hogan, 1997). Figure 14.1 is a representation of sources that drive effective symptom management.

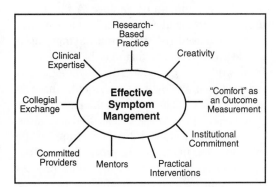

Figure 14.1   Effective Symptom Management
Effective symptom management practice is derived from many sources, including clinical expertise. This figure illustrates factors that contribute to the practice of effective symptom management.

Source: Reprinted with permission from Hogan, C. 1997. Cancer nursing: The art of symptom management. *Oncology Nursing Forum* 24(8): 1335–1341.

Managing side effects associated with biotherapy is one of the primary challenges facing the oncology nurse. Side effects commonly associated with biotherapy include constitutional or flu-like symptoms, fatigue, anorexia, weight changes (increase or decrease), mental-status changes, skin changes (erythema or rash), hypotension, and hematologic changes. The side effects unique to individual agents or approaches are reviewed in Chapters 5 through 13. Table 14.5 lists the toxicities associated with major biological agents used in clinical practice.

Symptom Management Model

The use of a framework for the assessment and management of symptoms is important for several reasons. First, it provides a systematic way to evaluate a variety of symptoms and should lead to a more thorough and complete assessment. Second, it provides a way of explaining the relationship between variables that may impact the symptom experience or the effect of one symptom on another. A framework may assist in the identification of patients who are at increased risk for certain symptoms or the degree of toxicity that may be expected. A framework also can guide the development of interventions. Following assessment, where the symptoms are evaluated from the patient's perspective, interventions are identified and implemented, and followed by evaluation of the outcomes the management process. Therefore, symptom management is a dynamic process, often requiring a change in strategy over time, depending on the efficacy of strategies chosen and patient acceptance. Two frameworks used to varying degrees by nurses are the University of California San Francisco (UCSF) Symptom Assessment and Management Model (UCSF Symptom Management Faculty Group, 1994) and the Middle-Range Theory of Unpleasant

Symptoms (Lenz *et al.*, 1997). A brief description of each follows.

The UCSF model was developed by the institution's nursing faculty and is based on the following three assumptions:

- The symptom experience is dynamic and involves the interaction of the patient's perception of a symptom, evaluation of a symptom, and response to a symptom.
- Management is a key and vital component of symptom control and should influence the symptom experience as well as symptom outcomes.
- Outcomes associated with the symptom experience are conceptualized as 10 multidimensional indicators: symptom status, self-care ability, financial status, morbidity, co-morbidity, mortality, quality of life, health-service utilization, emotional status, and functional status.

The Middle-Range Theory of Unpleasant Symptoms, developed by Lenz *et al.* (1997), is proposed as a means to integrate existing information about a variety of symptoms. This theory assumes that all symptoms have certain commonalities and that by recognizing those commonalities, research and practice may be appropriately guided. This theory also is based on three concepts, as follows:

- Each symptom is a multidimensional experience that can be conceptualized and measured separately or in combination with other symptoms.
- Certain physiological, psychological, and situational factors influence the occurrence, intensity, timing, distress level, and quality of symptoms.
- The consequences of the symptom experience are conceptualized in terms of their effect on functional and cognitive performance.

Table 14.5 Biotherapy-related side effects

Agent	Alteration in Hematologic Lab Value	Alteration in Mental Status	Anaphylaxis	Anorexia	Bone Pain	Bronchospasm	Capillary-Leak Syndrome	Chills	Desquamation	Diarrhea	Edema, Peripheral	Edema, Pulmonary	Fatigue	Fever	Fluid Retention	Flushing	Headache	Hives	Hypotension	Liver Enzymes	Mucositis	Myalgias	Nausea	Pruritus	Rash	Tachycardia	Weight Loss	Weight Gain	Other Side Effects
Interferon alpha and beta	+	O	R	+	O	R	R	+	R	O	R	R	+	+	R	O	+	R	O	+	R	+	O	O	O	O	+	R	Fever dissipates after first week
Interferon gamma	+	O	R	+	O	R	R	+	R	O	R	R	+	+	R	O	+	R	+	+	R	+	O	O	O	O	+	R	Fever higher and more persistent
Granulocyte-macrophage colony-stimulating factor (GM-CSF; sargramostim)	+	R	R	O	O	R	R	O*	R	O	R	R	O	+	O	O	O	R	+	O	R	O	O	O	O	O	O	O	Erythema at injection site; fever generally low grade; first pass effect
Granulocyte colony-stimulating factor (G-CSF; filgrastim)	+	R	R	R	R	R	R	R	R	R	R	R	R	R	R	R	R	R	R	O	R	R	R	R	R	R	R	R	Erythema at injection site
Erythropoietin; epoetin alfa	+	R	R	R	R	R	R	R	R	R	R	R	R	R	R	R	O	R	R	R	R	R	R	R	R	R	R	R	Occasional increase in blood pressure; hematocrit rises rapidly
Interleukin-11; oprelvekin	+	R	R	R	R	R	R	R	R	R	O	R	R	R	O	R	R	R	R	R	R	R	R	R	R	O	R	O	Dyspnea, conjunctival redness
Monoclonal antibodies (Rituximab)	O	R	R	O	R	O	R	+	R	O	R	R	O	+	R	+	O	O	O	O	R	O	R	O	O	O	R	R	Side effects also depend on what is attached; origin of antibody
Monoclonal antibodies (Trastuzumab)	O	R	R	O	R	O	R	+	R	O	R	R	O	+	R	+	O	O	O	O	R	O	R	O	O	O	R	R	Side effects also depend on what is attached; origin of antibody

(continued)

Table 14.5 Continued

Agent	Alteration in Hematologic Lab Value	Alteration in Mental Status	Anaphylaxis	Anorexia	Bone Pain	Bronchospasm	Capillary-Leak Syndrome	Chills	Desquamation	Diarrhea	Edema, Peripheral	Edema, Pulmonary	Fatigue	Fever	Fluid Retention	Flushing	Headache	Hives	Hypotension	Liver Enzymes	Mucositis	Myalgias	Nausea	Pruritus	Rash	Tachycardia	Weight Loss	Weight Gain	Other Side Effects
Tumor necrosis factor	+	O	R	+	R	R	R	+	R	O	R	R	+	+	R	R	+	R	O	O	R	+	O	R	R	O	+	R	Severe rigors
Interleukin-2	+	O	R	+	R	R	+	+	O	+	+	O	+	+	+	+	+	R	+	+	O	+	+	+	+	+	+	+	Weight gain during treatment and weight loss (occurs over time due to decrease in appetite)
Retinoids	O	R	R	O	O	R	R	R	+	O	R	R	+	O	R	R	+	R	R	+	O	+	O	O	O	R	R	R	Teratogenic, skin dryness, conjunctival irritation, vision changes, sensitivity to the sun
Vaccines	O	R	R	O	O	R	R	+	R	R	R	R	O	+	R	O	O	R	R	O	R	O	R	O	O	R	R	R	Inflammatory reactions at the injection site

+ = Common   O = Occasional   R = Rare

*Dose-dependent; as dose increases, chills are more regularly seen preceding fever.

•Patients may exhibit 10–20 mm/Hg decrease in systolic blood pressure; however, symptomatic hypotension is generally seen at higher doses given intravenously.

Source: Adapted and reprinted with permission from Rumsey, K., and Rieger, P. 1992. *Biological Response Modifiers: A Self-Instructed Manual for Health Professionals.* Chicago, IL: Precept Press, p. 6.

The Middle-Range Theory of Unpleasant Symptoms is designed to allow interventions that not only alleviate a given unpleasant symptom but also can alter factors that, when combined, influence the symptom experience.

Pathophysiology of Biotherapy-Related Side Effects

The pathophysiology underlying toxic effects associated with biological agents remains an active area of research that, it is hoped, will guide future interventions (Sergi, 1991; Rieger, 1992). Although management of biotherapy-related side effects may require the acquisition of new knowledge and skills, utilization of existing expertise in the care of oncology patients forms a foundation on which to build. Nurses are in a pivotal position to advance the management of side effects by creatively manipulating and building on the expertise they have in other areas of cancer care. In addition, the expertise of nurses in other specialty areas, such as nephrology and dialysis (i.e., use of erythropoietin for end-stage renal disease), can serve as a foundation to build on when agents previously used for one disease receive regulatory approval for another.

Select characteristics of biotherapy-related side effects differ from those associated with chemotherapy. As with chemotherapy, most biotherapy-related toxic effects are dose-related; that is, the intensity of the toxic effects increase as the dose is elevated. However, different from some chemotherapeutic agents such as doxorubicin, biotherapy-related toxic effects are typically noncumulative, in that there is not a ceiling dose beyond which a patient can receive no further therapy. Furthermore, most biotherapy-related side effects, myelosuppression included, are readily reversed on cessation of therapy. The timing of side effects also may differ from that of chemotherapy. For example, certain side effects may occur early in therapy and are often termed "acute." Others are manifested late in therapy and are classified as "chronic." Although most side effects are not life-threatening, they often have a tremendous impact on the patient's quality of life. Physical side effects such as FLS, gastrointestinal problems, fatigue, and mental-status changes may influence quality of life due to their alteration of social, physiological, and psychological functions (Brophy and Sharp, 1991). Lastly, signs and symptoms deemed reportable by the health-care team also differ for biological agents. Table 14.6 lists the critical indicators (i.e., signs and symptoms of side effects related to biotherapy) that should be reported.

Nursing Interventions

The nursing interventions described in this section represent the author's experience as well

Table 14.6   Critical indicators (symptoms) in biotherapy

Symptom/Signs
Excessive fatigue
Severe mental-status changes
Excessive somnolence
Confusion
Psychosis
Cardiac symptoms
Chest pain
Arrhythmias
Symptomatic hypotension
Weight changes
Losses greater than 10 pounds
Gains greater than 10 pounds
Allergic reactions
Anaphylaxis
Hives and itching
Dyspnea
Oliguria
Severe local inflammatory reactions
Fever
Uncontrolled with antipyretics
Unrelated to normal patterns of response

as the expertise of nurses across the country who have worked with patients receiving biotherapy. The reader is referred to the following references, both new and classic, for further information on care of the patient receiving biotherapy: Irwin, 1987; Dillman, 1988; Hahn and Jassak, 1988; Padavic-Shaller, 1988; Mayer, 1990; Brophy and Sharp, 1991; Rumsey and Rieger, 1992; White, 1992; Yarbro, 1993; Conrad and Horrell, 1995; Tomazewski, 1995; Rieger, 1996, 1977a, 1998, 1999; Wheeler, 1997; Coleman, 1998; Ignoffo et al., 1998; Kiley and Gale, 1998; and Battiato and Wheeler, 2000. In addition, many pharmaceutical companies provide educational resources to guide nurses in the care of patients who are receiving biotherapy. The local pharmaceutical sales representative for each company that markets oncology products is a valuable source of information on nursing and patient support materials available from his or her company. See the agent-specific Quick Summary Pages in Appendix B for a list of available resources. The Oncology Nursing Society has developed guidelines for the care of patients with cancer (McNally et al., 1991); textbooks focused on symptom management (Yarbro et al., 1999) are also available. The use of clinical expertise and creativity in practice also can be a powerful combination in devising new strategies to manage patients' symptoms (Cunningham, 1989).

GASTROINTESTINAL SIDE EFFECTS

Maintenance of nutritional status during therapy is of prime importance because anorexia and associated weight loss are common side effects of many biological agents (see Chapter 18). Patients often complain of a decreased desire for food or lack of motivation to eat. Taste changes that negatively affect food intake are also commonly reported. Recognizing the potential for problems associated with gastrointestinal side effects early on and providing early and regular nutritional assessments is key to implementing proactive interventions that may avert problems later in therapy. Therefore, baseline weight, nutritional status, and dietary intake should be assessed and documented.

Measures used with other types of oncology therapies (e.g., small, frequent meals and caloric supplements) are also appropriate in the biotherapy setting. Exploring which foods remain appealing and emphasizing those foods that the patient tolerates well rather than foods the patient no longer finds appealing can be helpful. Informing the family that the patient may not want to eat three meals a day will lessen the pressure they may place on the patient to eat. Encourage patients to consume more calories at breakfast, as their appetites tend to be better in the morning than later in the day. Encourage socialization during meals, which may increase oral intake (Rust et al., 1990). A dietary expert should be consulted if needed, and if weight loss becomes significant (i.e., 5% to 10% of body weight or greater), tube feedings or total parenteral nutrition may need to be considered, although it is generally not required.

Wickham et al., (1999) conducted a study to increase knowledge concerning the nature, frequency, and quality-of-life effects associated with taste changes following chemotherapy. They surveyed 284 adults who had received at least two chemotherapy cycles by having patients complete a taste-change questionnaire and the Functional Assessment of Cancer Therapy-General (a quality-of-life measure). They found taste changes to be frequent and at least moderately severe for many patients, who often reported dry mouth, decreased appetite, nausea, and vomiting. They found that oncology nurses and physicians rarely discussed the occurrence of taste changes with patients. Several questions were related to interventions that subjects chose themselves to manage taste changes (e.g., changing the way food was seasoned and avoiding certain foods) or that health-care providers had suggested. More subjects than not found that increasing seasonings (e.g., spices, herbs, pepper, condiments, peppers, hot sauce, and salt) was helpful.

Although the sample size was small and the study focused on patients who had received chemotherapy, the knowledge gained from patients regarding strategies that were helpful may be useful for patients who experience taste changes related to biotherapy. Because nurses play a key role in symptom management and should recognize that distressing taste changes are common after biotherapy, they should discuss this possibility with patients before biotherapy is initiated. In this way, nurses can help patients explore methods of coping with taste changes, which may increase comfort and self-control. Although nurses may not be able to change patients' risks for taste changes during therapy, continued assessment may lead to interventions that minimize the negative effects.

Nausea and vomiting are uncommon with most biological agents, except for IL-2. With IFN therapy, nausea and vomiting usually occur as a consequence associated with FLS and are seen more consistently at higher doses (Quesada et al., 1986). For example, nausea is a common side effect during the induction phase of IFN when the drug is used as adjuvant treatment for melanoma. The nausea and vomiting associated with IL-2 therapy more closely parallels that associated with chemotherapy and is seen in patients treated with both low and high doses of IL-2 (Foelber, 1998). Patients tend to be sensitive to food odors and unable to eat due to nausea. Scheduled prophylactic administration of antiemetics around the clock is often necessary to control this side effect. Table 14.7 lists the medications that can be used to treat toxic effects of IL-2, including antiemetics. Several classes of drugs may prove useful in controlling nausea and vomiting, including serotonin antagonists, dopamine antagonists, and benzodiazepines. Corticosteroids should not be

Table 14.7 Medications commonly used in the management of IL-2 toxicity

Toxic Effect	Medication
Fever and Inflammation	acetaminophen indomethacin sulindac naproxen
Hallucinations, Anxiety, and Sleeplessness	diphenhydramine diazepam fentanyl flurazepam haloperidol
Fluid Overload	furosemide metolazone
Gastritis	cimetidine ranitidine
Chills	meperidine HCL indomethacin dilaudid SL
Prevention of Line Sepsis	oxacillin clindamycin
Nausea	lorazepam prochlorperazine maleate promethazine HCL droperidol ondansetron ABH (lorazepam, diphenhydramine, haloperidol) scopolamine patches
Hypotension, Decreased Renal Perfusion, and Arrhythmia	dopamine HCL verapamil HCL atropine SO_4 phenylephrine
Diarrhea	codeine phosphate kaolin and pectin opium tincture diphenoxylate HCL with atropine SO_4 loperamide
Hypotension	0.9% sodium chloride boluses 5% N serum albumin
Itching	hydroxyzine HCl diphenhydramine colloidal oatmeal

HCl, hydrogen chemide; SL, sublingual; SO_4, sulfate

used to control nausea in patients receiving biological agents. Serotonin subtype 3 ($5HT_3$) is the newest class of antiemetics and includes ondansetron, dolasetron, and granisetron. These drugs have shown high efficacy in controlling nausea and vomiting associated with highly emetogenic chemotherapy regimens; however, they may not reliably control nausea and vomiting in all patients receiving IL-2. Serotonin antagonists will not be effective for nausea and vomiting induced by mechanisms other than $5HT_3$. The precise mechanism of IL-2–related nausea and vomiting remains unknown. The nausea associated with high-dose, adjuvant IFN-α is generally well controlled with premedication. Nonpharmacological interventions might include relaxation therapy, guided imagery, attentional distraction, acupressure and, as noted previously, dietary modification. Other practice measures include maintaining an odor-free environment and serving the patient cold foods (Grant, 1997; Hunt Johnson et al., 1997; Wickham, 1999). It is also important to assess patients for signs and symptoms indicative of complications associated with nausea and vomiting such as dehydration and electrolyte imbalance.

Mucositis also may occur with biotherapy, most commonly with IL-2 therapy. Symptoms typically include a dry, inflamed oral mucosa without ulceration. The oral cavity should be assessed and its condition should be documented at regular intervals using a valid and reliable scale. A pretreatment oral assessment by the dental oncologist to identify and treat preexisting oral disease may be recommended, especially when biotherapy will be given in conjunction with chemotherapy. Patients should practice meticulous oral hygiene with saline and baking-soda rinses and soft toothbrushes. Additional interventions include modifying the diet for comfort, avoiding food that could cause injury to the oral mucosa (e.g., spicy foods and hard foods such as tortilla chips), and avoiding the use of commercial mouthwash solutions that can exacerbate oral dryness. Frozen foods such as popsicles can reduce pain and soothe inflamed oral mucosa. Artificial saliva and foods with sauces may be helpful if oral dryness is extreme.

Diarrhea does not commonly occur with most biological agents, except for the severe diarrhea that may occur with IL-2 administration or diarrhea associated with high-dose IFN therapy during the occurrence of FLS. The description of diarrhea may be quite subjective and tends to vary even among experts. It is defined generally as an abnormal increase in stool liquid and frequency. Antidiarrheal medications generally control this side effect. The careful assessment of hydration status and electrolyte balance of patients with diarrhea is an important nursing responsibility. Fluid replacement and dietary modifications, such as avoidance of foods high in roughage or rich and highly seasoned foods, are helpful suggestions for symptom management. Patients should try to include foods high in pectin (e.g., apples and bananas) and bland foods such as white rice until symptoms resolve. It is also important that skin integrity in the perianal area be assessed in patients experiencing diarrhea. Hygienic measures and the use of prophylactic barrier creams to protect both damaged and intact skin is indicated (Hogan, 1998).

CARDIOVASCULAR/PULMONARY SYSTEMS

A thorough assessment of cardiopulmonary parameters is important with administration of all biological agents and is of extreme importance with IL-2 because of capillary-leak syndrome (see Chapter 6), which impacts the cardiopulmonary system. Capillary-leak syndrome, an escape of fluid from the vascular system into the tissues, also may be seen with immunotoxins such as ricin, saporin, or *Pseudomonas exotoxin*. Fluid retention may occur with oprelvekin and is related more to a secondary shift in plasma volume than capillary-leak syndrome. Symptoms observed may include tachycardia, dyspnea, and arrhythmias (Rust *et al.*, 1999). The majority of patients experiencing capillary-leak syndrome do not require therapy with diuretics; however, when used, the patient's fluid and electrolytes and blood pressure should be monitored carefully. Hypotension, which is also a component of capillary-leak syndrome, also may occur with MAB infusions such as rituximab. MAB-associated hypotension is more generally related to first-infusion-dose reaction or more rarely an allergic reaction.

For most biotherapy-related side effects that impact the cardiovascular system, nurses should monitor weight, heart rate and rhythm, and blood pressure. Nursing measures critical for management of IL-2-related capillary-leak syndrome will vary according to the dose of IL-2 used in the treatment regimen and the treatment setting (i.e., inpatient versus outpatient), but should include monitoring heart rate, blood pressure (including orthostatic checks), central venous pressure, and other cardiac indices. Accurate daily weights and strict fluid intake and output measures are of prime importance in evaluating fluid shifts, most specifically in higher-dose regimens in the inpatient setting (Sargent and Shelton, 1990; Schwartzentruber, 1995; Seipp, 1997), along with evaluation for edema and ascites. Daily measurement of abdominal girth also may be helpful in determining the quantity of fluid being retained. Capillary-leak syndrome manifests as peripheral edema of the soft tissues, ascites, or interstitial infiltrates of the lung. Patients may accumulate as much as 5 to 10 kg of extravascular fluid in just a few days.

Many patients with capillary-leak syndrome will be hypotensive. Safety measures include teaching patients to rise slowly from a lying position to a sitting or standing position to avoid dizziness. Bed rest may be needed if systolic blood pressure consistently runs less than 80 mm Hg and the patient is symptomatic. Medical management includes the use of vasopressors to maintain blood pressure, judicious use of fluid boluses and, if cardiovascular parameters are unstable, transfer to the intensive-care unit. The aggressive use of diuretics during treatment is generally not recommended because it may result in the depletion of intravascular volume and could lead to a hypotensive crisis. At the end of a treatment cycle, diuretics may be used to facilitate diuresis. Antihypertensive medications are often discontinued prior to initiation of IL-2 therapy.

Pulmonary complications with biotherapy are most commonly associated with fluid shifts related to IL-2 therapy or allergic reactions to a MAB. In some patients with existing pleural effusions, oprelvekin may cause an increase in the size of the effusion. Assessment for such complications includes auscultation of breath sounds, monitoring oxygenation, and evaluating complaints of shortness of breath or altered breathing patterns (Farrell, 1992). Nursing measures include positioning patients for minimal respiratory effort, adjusting the patient's physical activities, and reporting significant changes to the physician. Medical management includes administration of oxygen or diuretics or interruption of therapy. In extreme cases, with patients on high-dose IL-2 therapy, intubation and mechanical ventilation may be required. Within 24 hours of stopping IL-2, rapid diuresis will begin to clear many of the pulmonary-associated symptoms.

RENAL-SYSTEM SIDE EFFECTS

Of biological agents used in clinical practice, IL-2 most frequently causes renal toxicity, although renal changes also may be seen in patients receiving IFN therapy. Assessment for elevations in blood urea nitrogen (BUN), creatinine, decreased urine output, and significant weight gains should be made and changes should be reported to the physician. With IL-2, fluid shifts will cause urine output to decrease over time as a result of decreased perfusion of the kidneys. Intake and output will not balance; therefore, it is helpful if the physician defines a minimum fluid output (e.g., 10 to 30 mL/hour) that can be used as a guideline for reporting changes. Medical management includes judicious administration of fluids, diuretics, and low doses of vasopressors to maintain blood flow to the kidneys (Schwartzentruber, 1995).

HEMATOLOGIC-SYSTEM SIDE EFFECTS

Hematologic changes are not typically problematic in patients receiving biotherapy; however, blood-cell count (i.e., differential and platelets), coagulation profile, and reticulocyte count should be monitored to detect significant decreases in these levels. If myelosuppression, anemia, or thrombocytopenia develops, cessation of therapy generally will lead to rapid recovery of blood-cell counts. The patient should be taught how to recognize the signs and symptoms of thrombocytopenia, neutropenia, and anemia, and the appropriate precautions to take. Replacement of blood and platelets should be administered as ordered (Rieger, 1997b; Camp-Sorrell, 1998; Pruett, 1999; Wujcik, 1999). There are no specific therapeutic interventions for the rise in eosinophils that occurs with IL-2 administration. When hematopoietic growth factors are administered, hematologic parameters will increase according to the cell line being stimulated (e.g., filgrastim causes a dose-dependent increase primarily in neutrophils and erythropoietin in red bloods cells). With agents that cause fluid retention, patients may appear to have anemia that is actually dilutional in nature and that will resolve quickly upon cessation of therapy.

HEPATOLOGIC-SYSTEM SIDE EFFECTS

Changes in measures of hepatic function are common in patients who receive biotherapy, although the precise pathophysiology is unknown. Nursing measures include assessing patients for changes in liver function tests, hyperbilirubinemia, jaundice, or hepatomegaly and reporting significant changes to the physician. The total 24-hour dose of acetaminophen should be monitored carefully in patients receiving biotherapy because potential hepatotoxicity is related to its use, especially when higher doses are used.

Changes in liver function are commonly seen in patients receiving high-dose IFN therapy as adjuvant treatment for melanoma. These changes generally cause an alteration in the level of aspartate aminotransferase and are generally transient and not associated with permanent liver dysfunction. However, in the original clinical trials, two deaths related to hepatotoxicity were seen (Kirkwood *et al.*, 1996). These deaths occurred early in the trial in patients suspected to have a previous history of liver disease and whose liver function was not monitored. Therefore, it is important that liver function be monitored during therapy and that the dosage be adjusted if elevations are severe enough to warrant a decrease in dose. Patients with a history of prior liver disease should be monitored carefully (Kirkwood *et al.*, 1996; Donnelly, 1998).

METABOLIC SIDE EFFECTS

Metabolic changes such as hypothyroidism, hypomagnesemia, hypophosphatemia, and hypocalcemia also may be seen during treatment with biological agents, especially in patients receiving IL-2. Laboratory values should be monitored and significant changes should be reported to the physician. Medical interventions such as replacement therapy should be instituted as ordered.

INTEGUMENTARY-SYSTEM SIDE EFFECTS

The skin changes most frequently experienced with biotherapy are erythema, rashes, dryness with resultant desquamation, and an inflammatory reaction at injection sites. Rashes are commonly seen with IL-2 and also may occur with IFN and granulocyte-macrophage colony-stimulating factor (GM-CSF). The baseline assessment of skin condition should include evaluation of a history of underlying skin conditions such as psoriasis and any preexisting rashes or lesions. Skin should be carefully inspected for signs of breakdown or infection. Therapeutic measures for dry, pruritic skin include application of water-based lotions or creams several times daily, especially after bathing. Bath oils and mild soaps should be used. Cleansing should be gentle (avoid scrubbing the skin), and bath water should be tepid rather than hot. Clothing should be made of soft cotton. Perfumed lotions are to be avoided because they can further irritate already sensitive skin. Additional measures for treating pruritus include aggressive use of antipruritic medications, such as diphenhydramine or hydroxyzine hydrochloride (often on a scheduled basis), and colloidal oatmeal baths (Seiz and Yarbro, 1999). For some patients, room humidifiers help relieve pruritic skin conditions.

Patients who receive IL-2 should be cautioned against the use of topical steroids, which are contraindicated in most cases because of interference with the biological effects of IL-2. Patients also should be instructed to avoid exposure to the sun. In some patients, a reaction similar to radiation recall has been observed. Radiation recall occurs in response to the systemic administration of certain chemotherapeutic agents several months or a year or more after radiation was received. Typically, the patient will develop intraoral mucositis or a skin reaction in the exact pattern corresponding to the previously treated radiation portal (Hilderly, 1993). During administration of IL-2, areas where the patient received a prior severe sunburn may once again become erythemic. Patients experiencing severe skin changes in

addition to other side effects related to IL-2, such as edema and weight gain, often experience profound alterations in general appearance. The resulting changes in body image can cause significant distress for patients. Nursing interventions include encouraging patients to express their feelings and providing reassurance that changes will resolve when therapy is completed (Becker and Koutlas, 1990).

Inflammation with resultant erythema and swelling may occur at subcutaneous injection sites. These reactions generally resolve within 24 to 48 hours, but may be upsetting to patients. Further injections at inflamed sites must be avoided until healing is complete. Treatment is usually not necessary, but if applications of cold or heat are considered, their use should be verified with the physician because they may alter medication-absorption patterns. If pruritus occurs at the injection site, premedication with diphenhydramine may be helpful. Occasionally, patients complain of pain associated with subcutaneous injections. Topical application of a cream containing 50% lidocaine and 50% prilocaine (Emla®; Astra Pharmaceutical Products, Inc., Westborough, Massachusetts) may be useful. The syringe also may be held in the hand and warmed to room temperature. Many patients who receive IL-2 by subcutaneous injection develop subcutaneous nodules or indurations at the injection site. These nodules are transient, usually disappear within a few months after therapy, and generally do not present a reason to discontinue therapy.

With some biological agents that come as a liquid preparation, the volume of the injectate has been a concern. A study by Comley et al. (1999) evaluated the administration of filgrastim as either one injection (a volume of 1.6 mL = 480 mcg) or two injections of 0.8 mL each in a group of 76 women who received high-dose chemotherapy for breast cancer followed by hemopoietic rescue. The administration of 1.6-mL doses of filgrastim in one injection instead of two did not result in slower recovery of absolute neutrophils, induration, more frequent or larger bruises or areas of erythema, or greater discomfort. Although the sample size was small, this study represents one of the first of its kind to evaluate this issue in a systematic way. The nurse should use sound clinical judgment when weighing the volume of solution to be injected, the patient's body type, and the amount of subcutaneous tissue present in making a final determination of whether to give one or two injections.

Although rare, alopecia ocassionally may be experienced by patients who are receiving biotherapy. Patients will report a thinning of hair rather than actual hair loss. Use of wigs, scarves, and headwraps are appropriate with this population if thinning causes noticeable changes. Patients may be reassured that hair will regrow when therapy is complete.

ALLERGIC REACTIONS

Allergic reactions are most commonly associated with MAB infusions (Dillman, 1988). Symptoms may include fever, chills, hives, pruritus, shortness of breath, or hypotension. These reactions are seen more commonly when the MAB is of murine (mouse) origin rather than when chimeric or humanized antibodies are administered. Patients should be monitored regularly for vital signs, often as frequently as every 15 minutes for the first hour, and observed closely when therapy is initiated. Emergency drugs such as epinephrine, hydrocortisone, and diphenhydramine should be kept at the bedside, and a crash cart should be close at hand. Ideally, MAB should be administered via a side port so that if a severe allergic reaction occurs, the MAB infusion can be stopped and intravenous fluids can be initiated immediately. To avoid rapid bolus infusions, which tend to cause more side effects, an infusion pump should be used. An injection port also should be available on the intravenous tubing so that emergency drugs

can be injected if an allergic reaction occurs. To prevent or alleviate chills, fever, or urticaria, medication (e.g., meperidine or premedication with diphenhydramine, acetaminophen, or both) may need to be administered before or during therapy. With certain MABs, especially those used in treating the hematologic malignancies, fever is common, and its relationship to the course of therapy (i.e., early versus late) should be evaluated (Dillman, 1988). An infusion-related symptom complex is seen with the administration of some MABs, especially during the first dose. This symptom complex consists of fever, chills, hypotension, pain at the disease site, and shortness of breath. It is frequently seen with the administration of MABs targeted toward white blood cells (e.g., rituximab) and is thought to relate to the release of cytokines as white blood cells are destroyed. Symptoms are managed by careful assessment, premedication, and controlled administration of the MAB with step-wise increase in infusion rate according to patient tolerance (Karius and Marriott, 1997; Jonas, 1998b; Kosits and Callaghan, 2000).

Radiation Precautions

With radiolabeled MABs, appropriate radiation safety precautions, including the principles of time, distance, and shielding to minimize radiation exposure to the health-care team (Sitton, 1998; DeNardo *et al.*, 1999), should be observed. The particular precautions taken will be based on the isotope utilized and the dose the patient is to receive. Patients should be educated about the need for isolation with higher doses of radionuclides until radiation levels fall to state-regulated minima. Any special precautions to be utilized while in isolation, such as using disposable food trays, flushing the toilet three times after voiding, sitting while urinating (men) to avoid urine splashing, and avoiding bathing for 24 hours after administration of the isotope, should all be reviewed. Patients are often fearful of radiation therapy and may voice reluctance to be near family members once they are discharged from the hospital. To allay patient concerns, appropriate discharge precautions and issues related to sexuality should all be discussed prior to discharge (Jonas, 1998a; Penault, 1998).

Sexuality Concerns

Although nurses are often aware of the need to address sexual concerns, many are uncomfortable doing so, as are some patients. Patients who are receiving biotherapy may experience changes in sexuality due to factors such as fatigue, dryness of the mucous membranes, FLS, and change in body image. The following PLIS-SIT model (Annon, 1975) is frequently used in sexuality counseling or nursing intervention:

- P = *permission.* Discussion of patient concerns is promoted, and the couple is encouraged to continue in their present pattern of sexual activity.
- LI = *limited information.* New information is included to address sexual concerns.
- SS = *specific suggestions.* New sexual activities or techniques for the couple may be suggested.
- IT = *intensive therapy.* If necessary, the couple is referred to a therapist or counselor for intensive treatment.

Success at each step of this model depends on the nurse's knowledge and comfort level. Examples of interventions include encouraging the use of the supine position or a side-lying position during intercourse when patients are experiencing fatigue; using other expressions of intimacy such as cuddling or caressing; using water-based lubricants to relieve vaginal dryness; and using strategies such as long periods of foreplay, showering or bathing together, or making love in different rooms to help stimulate desire (Shell, 1997; Nishimoto, 1998). The American Cancer Society publishes books on sexuality for both men and women with cancer that are excellent resources (Schover, 1988a; 1988b).

Part of the concern regarding sexuality relates to prevention of pregnancy. The effect of biological agents on a fetus is unknown in many cases, yet absolutely contraindicated with others (e.g., the retinoids). The patient should be either informed of the potential for birth defects and appropriate methods of birth control, or referred to the proper specialist. Many research trials stipulate that the patient use an effective means of birth control.

Special Issues for Nursing Consideration

Novel Therapies

Novel treatments or approaches are frequently heralded by the media before efficacy has been determined. Scientific research is frequently reported in the newspaper and over the Internet as soon as it is published. Reports of preliminary research findings may be interpreted to be readily available in the clinical setting. Oncology nurses must be aware of information presented by the media so that they can answer patient questions, because it is often difficult for patients to put the information into perspective. Patients are often quite knowledgeable about ongoing clinical investigations across the country and frequently ask questions about the efficacy of those therapies. By actively listening to patient concerns and consulting with other members of the multidisciplinary care team, the nurse can help to clarify misconceptions. Oncology nurses are challenged to acquire the necessary skills to access information published on the Internet to be prepared to answer patients' questions and to help guide them to sites that provide appropriately monitored information (Carroll-Johnson, 1998). Many facilities also have patient libraries where patients can get answers to their questions. Nurses are in a key position to empower patients to become active partners in decision-making regarding their care (Mayer, 1999).

Alternative and Complementary Therapies

More and more patients are beginning to seek "complementary" and "alternative" therapies as treatment for symptoms associated with cancer and cancer treatments or for the cancer itself. A common misunderstanding is that complementary and alternative therapies are one and the same; in reality, they are not. The intent with which a therapy is used helps determine the proper terminology. If a therapy is used *instead* of conventional therapy, it is considered alternative. If it is used *in conjunction* with conventional therapy, it is considered complementary. As a result of the public's interest in and use of alternative and complementary therapies, the National Institutes of Health established the Office of Alternative Medicine by Congressional mandate in 1992. In 1998, a congressional mandate established the National Center for Complementary and Alternative Medicine (NCCAM), which now has 11 centers throughout the country to evaluate alternative therapies. The purpose of the NCCAM, according to Congressional mandate, was to "facilitate the evaluation of alternative medical-treatment modalities" to determine their effectiveness. The mandate also provides for a public information clearinghouse and a research training program. A working knowledge of herbal therapies can be very helpful in clinical practice or, at a minimum, in the ability to refer patients

to a colleague who is an expert in this area (Montbriand, 1999). Given the extensive use of herbal remedies by patients as complementary therapy, especially for symptom management, it indeed remains a challenge to be knowledgeable of all herbs currently in use by the public. The NCCAM web site (http://nccam.nih.gov/) serves as a valuable source of information about this rapidly expanding field. A recent survey by Richardson *et al.* (2000) found the use of complementary and alternative methods is common in outpatients. Over 80% of patients had used at least one approach.

Natural Therapies

Psychoneuroimmunology is the scientific field that investigates linkages between the brain, behavior, and the immune system, and the implications of these linkages for physical health and disease. Recent evidence suggests that both natural and laboratory-induced stressors can alter enumerative and functional aspects of the human immune system. Many believe that chronic stress may increase vulnerability to infectious disease; however, the role of stress in the course of other diseases such as inflammatory conditions or cancer remains unclear. There are large individual differences in psychological responses to stress; therefore, it is important to consider the role of cognitive and affective responses to stress. Cognitive states such as perceived control, views of self, and views of the future have been associated with immune parameters and health in some studies. Although the studies are few in number, research has begun to explore the benefit of such interventions as relaxation training, meditation, cognitive-behavioral stress management, and support groups on immune functions and ultimately on disease development. Very few controlled clinical trials have been conducted to assess whether psychosocial interventions can impact the immune system and the progression of medical conditions. Evidence-based discussion of this research literature with interested patients may help them make informed decisions regarding the use of such interventions and the state of the knowledge regarding the relationship between stress, the immune system, and cancer (Post-White, 1996; Kemeny and Greunewald, 1999).

Unconventional or Questionable Therapies

Patients often come to nurses with questions regarding unconventional or "questionable" therapies for cancer treatment. These may be defined as methods of cancer management (both diagnostic and therapeutic methods) that have not shown activity in animal-tumor models or in scientific clinical trials but are promoted for general use in cancer prevention, diagnosis, or treatment. Categories of unconventional therapy include dietary metabolic therapies, pharmacologic and biological approaches (e.g., antineoplaston therapy and oxymedicine), immunologic approaches, and behavioral and psychological approaches. The lines between what may be considered questionable, alternative, or complementary often are blurred. Patients are often hesitant to ask about treatments they have heard of or to admit to having used such strategies. The nurse is in an excellent position to establish rapport and trust with a patient so that he or she will feel comfortable asking about questionable methodologies. The nurse's role as a patient educator is one of the most powerful strategies for controlling questionable cancer remedies (Fletcher, 1992; Yarbro, 1997; Fitch *et al.*, 1999).

Nurse Stress

McCaffrey (1992) reviewed the issue of nurse stress associated with care of patients receiving investigational biological agents. Patients who enter clinical trials are faced with a host of coping challenges: resolution about feelings of prior aggressive, unsuccessful therapies; reactions of hope and fear surrounding the proposed therapy; learning new information and self-care skills; experiencing often difficult side effects; and concern about financial issues. The nurse is responsible for administering the agents that cause distressing side effects that may greatly affect the patient's quality of life. The nurse may feel powerless to lessen the severity of these side effects. Furthermore, the nurse's personal values regarding decisions to continue therapy may be in conflict with the patient's. In addition, the nurse may experience feelings of failure when therapy is unsuccessful. These elements all create stress for the nurse. Strategies for managing stress include assessing and understanding the problem (e.g., separating patient-related stress from nurse-related stress) and identifying measures to reduce both forms of stress (Table 14.8).

Ambulatory Care

Current trends in health care have mandated changes in the way care traditionally has been provided. The issues driving these changes include a shorter hospital stay, a move toward more ambulatory care, and scrutiny by third-party payors of services provided. These issues influence the manner in which care is provided (see Chapter 21). In addition, consumers are increasingly aware of and have a desire to control health-care costs. As a result of these trends, biotherapy is increasingly administered in the outpatient setting. Work continues to revise current inpatient therapies and design future strategies to ensure safe administration of biotherapy in the outpatient setting. All of these changes will continue to affect the role of the oncology nurse (Buchsel and Yarbro, 1993).

Table 14.8   Strategies for reducing nurse stress

Patient-Centered Strategies	Nurse-Centered Strategies
Set priorities with patients: • What bothers you the most right now? • What can I do to help you get through this difficult time? Use symptom distress scales to quantify the effect of nursing interventions. Implement a formal review process with peers of current caseload: • What went well? • What could we have done differently? • Extend mutual support and acknowledge the professional friend's contribution.	Critically examine the personal issues you bring to work and their coexistence in the health setting. Determine the extent of possible codependency: • Self-esteem derived heavily from patient interaction • "Only I can do it well" phenomenon • Puts others' needs before own • Represses feelings, then acts passively/aggressively • Seldom asks for help Delineate problems within the cancer-care team and the patient and use strategy to resolve difficult relationships. Personally identify mechanisms to "recharge your batteries": • List 30 stress reducers • Use one daily Reflect daily on successes in practice versus focus on the "I should have."

Source: Reprinted with permission from McCaffrey, D. 1992. Cancer nurse stress: A paradigm with relevance to investigational biotherapy. In Carroll-Johnson, R. (ed). *The Biotherapy of Cancer—V.* Pittsburgh, PA: Oncology Nursing Press, pp. 22–27.

In some instances, payor guidelines mandate that medications be given in the physician's office in order for physicians to be reimbursed for the drug. This is a common problem with patients on Medicare. Therefore, the administration of hematopoietic growth factors over a weekend becomes problematic because clinics are traditionally closed at this time. Some practices send patients to the hospital, which is expensive and often involves a significant wait time. Other practices rotate nurses so that the service can be available on weekends. Patients are generally asked to arrive early in the morning, and injections can be given quickly if no complications arise. In many facilities, the medications are drawn up on Friday afternoon to decrease work time on the weekend or a holi-day. Practices vary as to whether an oncologist must be present on-site or available by telephone during weekend or holiday hours of operation.

Considerations important to safe care of patients in the ambulatory setting also apply to preparing patients for discharge so that therapy may be continued in the outpatient setting. A primary goal for the patient with cancer is to develop or regain independence so that therapy may be managed successfully at home. In the ambulatory setting, planning begins immediately following the decision to start therapy so that the goal of self-sufficiency may be achieved. Major areas that need to be addressed include monitoring of patient reaction to initial administration of treatment, consistent assessment of tolerance to and compliance with therapy, patient education, use of support systems and referrals as appropriate, and financial concerns.

When therapy is initiated in the outpatient or home setting, patients should be monitored for tolerance to the first dose. The agent or agents being administered and the dose used will determine the length of time patients need to be monitored and the frequency at which vital signs should be checked. It is helpful if medical orders specify any necessary premedications, any parameters that should be reported to the physician (e.g., blood pressure less than 90 mm Hg), and discharge criteria.

Patients generally will require regular clinic follow-up visits or in-home nursing visits to assess tolerance to therapy. Scheduled follow-up visits allow nurses to determine patient adherence to and compliance with the therapeutic regimen (e.g., the medication schedule and laboratory and diagnostic tests). Any misunderstandings or problems can be addressed at the follow-up visit.

The use of symptom flow sheets, either as a self-reporting tool or nursing documentation form, can facilitate assessment and management of outpatients (White, 1992). Patient diaries or logbooks can be useful in reporting symptoms (Brophy and Sharp, 1991). In this manner, toxic effects can be reliably quantified and documented, and patient response to interventions can be assessed. A telephone triage system developed for use in the chemotherapy setting (Anastasia and Blevins, 1997) may be adapted for use in managing biotherapy-related symptoms.

Evaluation of patient or caregiver support systems is of utmost importance in planning outpatient therapy. Problems such as lack of financial resources or social support will need to be addressed by the multidisciplinary team to ensure successful implementation of therapy.

Some of the resources that may be considered are at-home care, provision of medical services as a partnership between the patient's local physician and the comprehensive cancer center, participation in support groups, financial assistance through community-based programs, and provision of food agencies such as the American Cancer Society or Meals-on-Wheels. Many health-care companies now provide affordable, cost-effective, patient-centered services to patients outside the acute-care setting, including parenteral nutrition, antibiotic therapy, hydration therapy, chemotherapy, and biotherapy. In some instances, the drugs can be dispensed in ready-to-inject form. These companies also provide pharmacist consultation and drug-interaction information.

As more care has shifted to the home, more attention has focused on the role of the caregiver. This role is complex and multifaceted and includes such functions as ensuring that the patient adheres to medication schedules; coordinating patient treatment and diagnostic appointments; performing medical/nursing procedures, including symptom management and physical-care duties; and providing emotional support. The oncology nurse faces many challenges in attempting to effectively prepare and educate caregivers in the day-to-day management of the patient with cancer. During the course of interactions with the patient and family members, the nurse should initiate assessment, develop a long-term plan for monitoring and evaluating the care being provided in the home, and formulate an educational plan to teach caregivers the skills they need to support the patient. The nurse serves as an educator by providing information, teaching psychomotor skills (e.g., injection techniques and management of ambulatory infusion pumps), and problem-solving. The nurse also may assist the family in brokering the caregiver task, counseling the patient and family, helping the family maintain open lines of communication, serving as the family's advocate in interactions with the health-care system, and coaching the family through the course of treatment (McNally, 1996; Kozachik et al., 1999).

Moore (1998) completed a study that determined the magnitude of out-of-pocket expenditures for patients undergoing chemotherapy in an outpatient setting. The setting was an urban outpatient chemotherapy clinic, and Moore used a sample of 20 adult patients. Although the sample size was small and the study focused on chemotherapy, the information gained can be used by nurses administering biotherapy in the ambulatory setting to heighten their awareness of the types of expenditures patients incur. Moore found that out-of-pocket expenses can be more costly than previously had been recognized. Examples of expenses incurred in this setting are the costs associated with clinic visits (e.g., transportation, meals/snacks, and child care); treatment of symptoms and side effects (e.g., medications, supplies, and special foods); support/assistance (e.g., maintenance and delivered-in or dine-out meals); administration (e.g., telephone and insurance costs); and quality of life (e.g., vacations and gifts). Moore also tried to capture patient estimates for lost income, which ranged from $20 to $2,600 for 1 month of chemotherapy. Although studies estimating costs have inherent limitations, this study does provide a glimpse of categorical expenses that patients incur during outpatient therapy.

Health-care policies that are formulated to shift the burden of cost to patients are unlikely to consider all of the costs that patients sustain. These costs may not be readily evident to providers, and patients may be embarrassed to discuss them with professionals. By being more knowledgeable of these costs, oncology nurses will be better prepared to assist patients and serve as patient advocates with policymakers and payors.

Nursing Research

Administration of biotherapy differs from that of chemotherapy. Biotherapy may be given daily and often lasts for months to years. The associated toxic effects are complex, frequently chronic, tend to be subjective in nature, and often have a major effect on the patient's quality of life. These factors are of major importance in the field of biotherapy nursing. Quality of life and symptom management are consistently ranked high among the research priorities of the Oncology Nursing Society surveys (Stetz et al., 1995).

The field of biotherapy, including clinical biotherapy, is ripe with possibilities for nursing research. Research studies of symptom management are beginning to be conducted, but further nursing studies are needed. One of the major problems in doing so has been the difficulty in accurately measuring symptoms experienced by patients. Although observer-rated toxicity scales used in clinical trials have been adapted to accommodate symptoms associated with biological agents, they are often not sensitive enough for research purposes. The subjective nature of most symptoms associated with biological agents also makes their measurement a challenge. To avoid these challenges, tools specific to biotherapy can be designed or existing tools can be adapted (Strauman, 1988). Although it is the most desirable approach, formulating tools specific to biotherapy requires a major investment of researcher time to validate scales. However, numerous questionnaires and tools are already available to assess symptoms, quality of life, functional status, fatigue, and depression in the general oncology setting (Frank-Stromberg and Olsen, 1997). It may be possible to adapt many of these instruments, such as the Symptom Distress Scale (McCorkle and Young, 1978) or the Sickness Impact Profile (SIP) (Bergner et al., 1981) for use with patients receiving biotherapy. A clearer understanding of the etiology of biotherapy-related side effects also will assist in the development of measurement strategies.

Nurses often feel unprepared to evaluate research findings and to integrate the findings into practice. Clinical nurse specialists and nurse researchers who can mentor and guide staff nurses in the research process may not be available in many settings. Nursing leaders can create environments that are conducive to research utilization by altering existing mechanisms, facilitating access to nursing research experts, creating an environment that supports time for research utilization efforts, authorizing for practice changes, and offering continuing education related to the research utilization process. It is a challenge to all nurses to become more familiar with research utilization practices as the profession aspires to research-based practice. Researchers must meet the challenge of communicating research findings in a manner that is "nurse friendly" and that clearly delineates applications to existing practice (Rutledge et al., 1998).

Research studies related to biotherapy, especially quality-of-life issues, have begun to appear in the literature. An exploratory, descriptive study of 30 patients by Longman et al. (1992) reported the care needs of home-based cancer patients receiving external-beam radiation therapy, biotherapy, or both, and the needs of their caregivers. For the purposes of the study, the home-based care needs of ambulatory cancer patients were defined as the physical, psychological, and health-service requirements necessary to maintain normal functioning at home. The caregivers' needs were reported in relation to the patients' situations. Data were presented for the group as a whole and were not separated according to individual therapeutic modalities. Scales were developed to assess patients' and caregivers' needs. All 30 patients reported needs in the areas of personal care, actual health care, activity management, and personal interaction. Areas reported by patients as requiring nursing attention, which was rated as very important (9 or 10) on a scale of 1 to 10 by more than 50% of patients, included use of a safe technique; competent and timely implementation of orders; being listened to by nurses; being kept informed about their condition, symptoms, and treatment in a way that was understandable; and being treated in a pleasant, cheerful, and respectful manner. Caregivers valued help in getting physician orders, being assured the patient was comfortable, being assured of the availability of emergency help, and being assured of the option of admitting the patient to the hospital. Although these results cannot be generalized to the cancer population at large, they do provide direction and guidance for oncology nurses whose patients are receiving biotherapy. It would be interesting to repeat the study with a larger population of patients who were receiving only biotherapy. Laizner et al. (1993) provide a review of research efforts regarding the needs of family caregivers of persons with cancer.

The long-term biological, psychological, and social effects of IL-2 therapy were reported by Jackson et al. (1991). Data were collected at baseline; during the treatment period; and at 1, 6, and 12 months after completion of therapy. Measures for the various aspects of quality of life were the SIP, the Inventory of Current Concerns (ICC), the Symptom Distress Scale, the Acute Physiology and Chronic Health Evaluation Scale (APACHE), and the Therapeutic Intervention Scoring System (TISS). Severity of illness, as measured by APACHE and TISS scores, showed a considerable increase during therapy, with a decline in severity beginning at cessation of therapy. This pattern reflected an increased need for nursing care during therapy. Emotional concerns, as measured by the ICC, and symptom distress also increased significantly during therapy, but returned to baseline within 1 month after the completion of therapy. Because of poor survival rates, analysis of quality of life (as measured by the SIP) was only possible at 1 month after completion of therapy. Mean SIP scores at 1 month did not differ significantly from pretherapy scores. This study presents important data regarding the biological, psychological, and social effects of IL-2 therapy. Increasingly, questions about the economic cost, changes in quality of life, and discomfort related to therapy are being viewed as equal in importance to the effects of therapy.

A retrospective, descriptive study by Rieker *et al.* (1992) reported perceptions of quality of life and quality of care for patients with cancer who were receiving biotherapy. The sample was drawn from patients with advanced cancer who had completed biotherapy from January 1986 through June 1988 at two biotherapy treatment centers in the southern United States or from close relatives of patients who had died. For the purposes of the study, quality of care and quality of life were evaluated subjectively and were considered to be multidimensional constructs. Quality of life was evaluated only for the patients alive at the end of data collection and was measured using the Profile of Mood States (POMS) and the Linear Analogue Self-Assessment scales. Quality of care was measured using a self-report questionnaire previously used in studies of survivors of cancer; the questionnaire was tailored to each of the sample subsets. The final sample consisted of 33 patients (response rate 60%) and 71 relatives (response rate 70%).

Despite the uncertainty concerning treatment outcomes, patients who had received biotherapy reported a relatively good quality of life. Available data indicated that the psychological status of the patient sample, as measured by the POMS, was similar to that of other groups of patients with advanced cancer and was within the range reported for healthy (e.g., noncancer) participants. The majority of patients and relatives gave positive reports about the quality of care that they had received; relatives of the deceased patients gave less positive reports about quality of care than did surviving patients and their relatives. The findings indicated that four components—symptom control, availability of support services, communication with the medical team, and adequate information about how medical care was proceeding—were significant to both patients' and family members' assessments of quality of care. These concerns should help provide direction for future research areas to help target interventions by the health-care team. Findings from the study are limited because of recall bias and a small, single-setting sample; however, the need to initiate prospective studies on quality of life and quality of care with patients receiving biotherapy should be an area of focus for future studies.

Fazio and Glaspy (1991) assessed quality of life in 10 patients with chronic neutropenia who were receiving therapy with filgrastim. The Ferrans & Powers Quality of Life Index was used to assess quality of life. Measurements were taken at three time points: pretherapy, after 4 months of therapy, and after 10 months of therapy. The mean overall quality of life had improved significantly by the second time point and was maintained through the third time point. Subjects reported feeling "more healthy" after treatment with filgrastim. The major limitations of this study were the small sample size, the lack of a control group, and the use of the quality-of-life index in the pediatric population. However, the study illustrates the importance of measuring both the efficacy and the impact on quality of life of a particular therapy.

There are many patient management issues to be addressed through nursing research of biotherapy. Efforts should focus on the development of tools to measure side effects and symptom distress, determination of the most effective time of drug administration to alleviate side effects, development of interventions to control or prevent toxicity, and the evaluation of and the development of current and new patient-education methodologies. Studies measuring quality of life have gained increasing importance in the field of oncology and should be incorporated into biotherapy research and clinical trials. It is exciting that nursing research is also beginning to explore issues of concern to those caring for patients who are receiving biotherapy; however, a great deal of work remains to be completed.

Summary

Biotherapy nursing represents an exciting area of specialization within the field of oncology nursing. Because of the rapid introduction of novel agents, treatment approaches, and combination therapies, nurses are needed who have a desire to learn about new therapeutic modalities and who have the creativity to develop new standards of care for patients who are receiving these therapies. By building on prior oncology experience, integrating new knowledge specific to biotherapy, and conducting research to generate innovative approaches to new problems, nurses who care for patients with cancer receiving biotherapy will be able to meet the challenge.

References

American Nurses Association (ANA). 1996. *Scope and Standards of Advanced Practice Registered Nursing*. Washington, DC: American Nurses' Publishing.

American Nurses Association (ANA). 1999a. *Scope and Standards of Home Health Nursing Practice*. Washington, DC: American Nurses' Publishing.

American Nurses Association (ANA). 1999b. *Standards of Clinical Nursing Practice*, 2nd edn. Washington, DC: American Nurses' Publishing.

American Society of Hospital Pharmacists (ASHP). 1990. ASHP technical assistance bulletin on handling cytotoxic and hazardous drugs. *American Journal of Hospital Pharmacy* 47: 1033–1049. (Also available from web site at *http://www.ashp.org*) (Accessed May 1, 2000).

Anastasia, P., and Blevins, M. 1997. Outpatient chemotherapy: Telephone triage for symptom management. *Oncology Nursing Forum* 24(1 suppl): 13–22.

Andrews, M., and Boyle, J. 1995. *Transcultural Concepts in Nursing Care*, 2nd edn. Philadelphia, PA: Lippincott, Williams and Wilkins.

Andrews, M., and Boyle, J. 1997. Competence in transcultural nursing care. *American Journal of Nursing* 97(8): 16AAA–16DDD.

Annon, J. 1975. *Behavioral Treatment of Sexual Problems: Brief Therapy*. Hagerstown, MD: Medical Department, Harper and Row.

Barhamand, B. 1998. Coping with cancer: Family issues. In Burke, C. (ed). *Psychosocial Dimensions of Oncology Nursing Care*. Pittsburgh, PA: Oncology Nursing Press, pp. 28–52.

Battiato, L., and Wheeler, V. 2000. Biotherapy. In Yarbro, C.H., Frogge, M.H., Goodman, M., and Groenwald, S.L. (eds). *Cancer Nursing: Principles and Practice*, 5th edn. Sudbury, MA: Jones and Bartlett Publishers, pp. 543–579.

Becker, K., and Koutlas, J. 1990. Alteration in body image for the patient undergoing RIL-2/LAK cell therapy. *Oncology Nursing Forum* 17(6): 965.

Bergner, M., Bobbitt, R., Carter, W., *et al.* 1981. The sickness impact profile: Development and final revision of a health status measure. *Medical Care* 19(8): 787–805.

Bickley, L., Hoekelman, R., and Bates, B. (eds). 1999. *Bates' Guide to Physical Examination and History Taking*, 7th edn. Philadelphia, PA: Lippincott.

Bock, S., Lee, R., Fisher, B., *et al.* 1990. A prospective randomized trial evaluating prophylactic antibiotics to prevent triple-lumen catheter-related sepsis in patients treated with immunotherapy. *Journal of Clinical Oncology* 8(1): 161–169.

Boyle, D., Engelking, C., Blesch, K., *et al.* 1992. ONS position paper on cancer and aging. *Oncology Nursing Forum* 19(6): 913–933.

Brandt, J. (ed). 1996. *Oncology Nursing Society and American Nurses' Association: Standards of Oncology Nursing Practice.* Pittsburgh, PA: Oncology Nursing Press.

Brophy, L., and Sharp, E. 1991. Physical symptoms of combination biotherapy: A quality-of-life issue. *Oncology Nursing Forum* 18(1 suppl): 25–30.

Buchsel, P., and Yarbro, C. (eds). 1993. *Oncology Nursing in the Ambulatory Setting.* Boston, MA: Jones & Bartlett Publishers, Inc.

Bush, N. 1998. Anxiety and the cancer experience. In Carroll-Johnson, R., Gorman, L., and Bush, N. (eds). *Psychosocial Nursing Care Along the Cancer Continuum.* Pittsburgh, PA: Oncology Nursing Press, pp. 125–138.

Camp-Sorrell, D. 1998. Myelosuppression. In Itano, J., and Taoka, K. (eds). *Core Curriculum for Oncology Nursing*, 3rd edn. Philadelphia, PA: W.B. Saunders, pp. 207–219.

Cancer Therapeutic Evaluation Program (CTEP). 1999. *Common Toxicity Criteria Manual.* Available at *http://ctep.info.nih.gov/CTC3/CTC-Manual.htm*

Carr, E. 1998. Waste not, want not. Home-care workers grapple with hazardous trash. *HealthWeek (Houston/San Antonio).* October 26, 1998: 17.

Carroll-Johnson, R. (ed). 1998. A toll for creating our future: The Internet. *Oncology Nursing Forum* 25(10 suppl): 3–32.

Christman, N. 1990. Uncertainty and adjustment during radiotherapy. *Nursing Research* 39: 17–20.

Coleman, C. 1998. Overview of biotherapy and nursing considerations. *Journal of Intravenous Nursing* 21(6): 367–373.

Comley, A., DeMeyer, E., Adams, N., *et al.* 1999. Effect of subcutaneous granulocyte colony-stim-

ulating factor injectate volume on drug efficacy, site complications, and client comfort. *Oncology Nursing Forum* 26: 87–94.

Conrad, K., and Horrell, C. 1995. *Recommendations for Nursing Practice Related to Biotherapy*, 2nd edn. Pittsburgh, PA: The Oncology Nursing Society.

Cunningham, M. 1989. Putting creativity into practice. *Oncology Nursing Forum* 16(4): 499–505.

Dana, W. 1988. Procedure for handling biological response modifiers. The University of Texas M.D. Anderson Cancer Center. *Pharmacy Bulletin* 6: 2.

Dana, W., and Anderson, R. 1990. Handling of cytotoxic agents. *Cancer Bulletin* 42(6): 399–404.

DeNardo, G., O'Donnell, R., Rose, L., *et al.* 1999. Milestones in the development of Lym-1 therapy. *Hybridoma* 18(1): 1–11.

Dillman, J. 1988. Toxicity of monoclonal antibodies in the treatment of cancer. *Seminars in Oncology Nursing* 4(2): 107–111.

Donnelly, S. 1998. Patient management strategies for interferon alfa-2b as adjuvant therapy in high-risk melanoma. *Oncology Nursing Forum* 25: 921–927.

Ersek, M., Kagawa-Singer, M., Barnes, D., *et al.* 1998. Multicultural considerations in the use of advance directives. *Oncology Nursing Forum* 25: 1683–1690.

Farrell, M. 1992. The challenge of adult respiratory distress syndrome during interleukin-2 therapy. *Oncology Nursing Forum* 19(3): 475–480.

Fazio, M., and Glaspy, J. 1991. The impact of granulocyte colony-stimulating factor on quality of life in patients with severe chronic neutropenia. *Oncology Nursing Forum* 18(8): 1411–1414.

Fishman, M., and Mrozek-Orlowski, M. (eds). 1999. *Oncology Nursing Society Cancer Chemotherapy Guidelines and Recommendations for Practice*, 2nd edn. Pittsburgh, PA: Oncology Nursing Press.

Fitch, M., Gray, R., Greenberg, M., *et al.* 1999. Nurses' perspectives on unconventional therapies. *Cancer Nursing* 22(3): 238–245.

Fletcher, D. 1992. Unconventional cancer treatments: Professional, legal, and ethical issues. *Oncology Nursing Forum* 19(9): 1351–1354.

Foelber, R. 1998. Autologous stem-cell transplant plus interleukin-2 for breast cancer: Review and nursing management. *Oncology Nursing Forum* 25: 563–568.

Frank-Stromberg, M., and Olsen, S. (eds). 1997. *Instruments for Clinical Nursing Research,* 2nd edn. Sudbury, MA: Jones & Bartlett Publishers, Inc.

Gale, D. 1996. Clinical practice update: Occupational Safety and Health Administration now includes alpha interferon on hazardous drug list. *Biotherapy Special Interest Group Newsletter.* September 1996: 3. Pittsburgh, PA: Oncology Nursing Press.

Grant, M. 1997. Therapeutic approaches to chemotherapy-induced nausea and vomiting. *Oncology Nursing Forum* 24(7 suppl): 1–45.

Hahn, M., and Jassak, P. 1988. Nursing management of patients receiving interferon. *Seminars in Oncology Nursing* 4(2): 95–101.

Herth, K. 1990. Fostering hope in terminally ill people. *Journal of Advanced Nursing* 15: 1250–1259.

Highfield, M. 1997. Spiritual assessment across the cancer trajectory: Methods and reflections. *Seminars in Oncology Nursing* 13(4): 237–241.

Hilderly, L. 1993. Radiotherapy. In Groenwald, S., Goodman, M., Hansen Frogge, M., and Yarbro, C.H. (eds). *Cancer Nursing: Principles and Practice,* 3rd edn. Boston: Jones & Bartlett Publishers, pp. 235–269.

Hogan, C. 1991. Coping with biotherapy: Physiological and psychosocial concerns. *Oncology Nursing Forum* 18(1 suppl): 19–23.

Hogan, C. 1997. Cancer nursing: The art of symptom management. *Oncology Nursing Forum* 24(8): 1335–1341.

Hogan, C. 1998. The nurse's role in diarrhea management. *Oncology Nursing Forum* 25: 879–886.

Hunt Johnson, M., Moroney, C., and Gay, C. 1997. Relieving nausea and vomiting in patients with cancer: A treatment algorithm. *Oncology Nursing Forum* 24(1): 51–57.

Hunt Raleigh, E. 1992. Sources of hope in chronic illness. *Oncology Nursing Forum* 19(3): 443–448.

Ignoffo, R., Viele, C., Damon, L., *et al.* (eds). 1998. *Cancer Chemotherapy Pocket Guide.* Philadelphia, PA: Lippincott-Raven.

Irwin, M. 1987. Patients receiving biological response modifiers: Overview of nursing care. *Oncology Nursing Forum* 14(6 suppl): 32–37.

Itano, J. 1998. Cultural issues. In Itano, J., and Taoka, K. (eds). *Core Curriculum for Oncology Nursing,* 3rd edn. Philadelphia, PA: W.B. Saunders Company, pp. 60–76.

Jackson, B., Strauman, J., Frederickson, K., *et al.* 1991. Long-term biopsychosocial effects of interleukin-2 therapy. *Oncology Nursing Forum* 18(4): 683–690.

Jonas, C. 1998a. Radioimmunotherapy: Special delivery. *Oncology Nursing Forum Practice Corner* 25: 668–669.

Jonas, C. 1998b. Rituxan™: The new kid on the block. *Oncology Nursing Forum Practice Corner* 25: 669.

Karius, D., and Marriott, M. 1997. Immunologic advances in monoclonal antibody therapy: Implications for oncology nursing. *Oncology Nursing Forum* 24: 483–494.

Kemeny, M., and Greunewald, T. 1999. Psychoneuroimmunology update. *Seminars in Gastrointestinal Diseases* 10(1): 20–29.

Kiley, K., and Gale, D. 1998. Nursing management of patients with malignant melanoma receiving adjuvant alpha interferon-2b. *Clinical Journal of Oncology Nursing* 2(1): 11–16.

King, C., Haberman, M., Berry, D., *et al.* 1997. Quality of life and the cancer experience: The state-of-the-knowledge. *Oncology Nursing Forum* 24(1): 27–41.

Kirkwood, J., Strawderman, M., Ernstoff, M., *et al.* 1996. Interferon alfa-2b adjuvant therapy of high-risk resected cutaneous melanoma: The Eastern

Cooperative Oncology Group Trial EST 1684. *Journal of Clinical Oncology* 14: 7–17.

Klimaszewski, A., Aikin, J., DiStasio, S., Ehrenberger, H., and Ford, B. (eds). 2000. *A Guide to Clinical Trials Nursing*. Pittsburgh, PA: Oncology Nursing Press.

Kohn, L.T., Corrigan, J.M., and Donaldson, M.S. (eds). Committee on Quality of Health Care in America, Institute of Medicine. 2000. *To Err Is Human: Building a Safer Health System*. Washington, DC: National Academy Press.

Koopmeiners, L., Post-White, J., Gutknecht, S., *et al.* 1997. How health-care professionals contribute to hope in patients with cancer. *Oncology Nursing Forum* 24(9): 1507–1513.

Kosits, C., and Callaghan, M. 2000. Rituximab: a new monoclonal antibody therapy for non-Hodgkin's lymphoma. *Oncology Nursing Forum* 27(1): 51–59.

Kozachik, S., Given, B., and Given, C. 1999. Cancer patients at home: Activating nurses to assist patients and to involve families in care at home. *Oncology Nursing Updates* 6(2): 1–11.

Laizner, A., Shegda Yost, L., Barg, F., *et al.* 1993. Needs of family caregivers of persons with cancer: A review. *Seminars in Oncology Nursing* 9(2): 114–120.

Lenz, E., Pugh, L., Milligan, R., *et al.* 1997. The Middle-Range Theory of Unpleasant Symptoms: An update. *Advances in Nursing Science* 14: 17–23.

Lester, J. (ed). 1997. *Oncology Nursing Society Statement on the Scope and Standards of Advanced Practice in Oncology Nursing*. Pittsburgh, PA: Oncology Nursing Press.

Lester, N. 1998. Cultural competence: A nursing dialogue. *American Journal of Nursing* 98(8): 26–33.

Longman, A., Atwood, J., Sherman, J., *et al.* 1992. Care needs of home-based cancer patients and their caregivers. *Cancer Nursing* 15(3): 182–190.

Mayer, D. 1990. Biotherapy: Recent advances and nursing implications. *Nursing Clinics of North America* 25(2): 291–308.

Mayer, D. 1999. Cancer Patient Empowerment. In Hubbard, S.M., Goodman, M., and Knobf, M.T. (eds). *Oncology Nursing Update: Patient Treatment and Support* 6(4) Cedar Knolls, NJ: Lippincott Williams & Wilkins Healthcare, pp. 1–9.

McCabe, M., and Padberg, R. (eds). 1999. Informed consent in clinical trials. *Seminars in Oncology Nursing* 15(2): 75–144.

McCaffrey, D. 1992. Cancer nurse stress: A paradigm with relevance to investigational biotherapy. In Carroll-Johnson, R. (ed). *The Biotherapy of Cancer–V*. Pittsburgh, PA: Oncology Nursing Press, pp. 22–27.

McCorkle, R., and Young, K. 1978. Development of a symptom distress scale. *Cancer Nursing* 1(3): 373–378.

McNally, J. (ed). 1996. Home care for oncology patients. *Seminars in Oncology Nursing* 12(3): 177–243.

McNally, J., Somerville, E., Miaskowski, C., *et al.* (eds). 1991. *Guidelines for Cancer Nursing Practice*. Philadelphia, PA: W.B. Saunders.

Miller, A., Hoogstraten, B., Staquet, M., *et al.* 1981. Reporting results of cancer treatment. *Cancer* 47: 207–214.

Montbriand, M. 1999. Past and present herbs used to treat cancer: Medicine, magic, or poison? *Oncology Nursing Forum* 26: 49–60.

Moore, K. 1998. Out-of-pocket expenditures of outpatients receiving chemotherapy. *Oncology Nursing Forum* 25: 1615–1622.

Nishimoto, P. 1998. Sexuality. In Itano, J., and Taoka, K. (eds). *Core Curriculum for Oncology Nursing*, 3rd edn. Philadelphia, PA: W.B. Saunders, pp. 85–95.

Occupational Safety and Health Administration (OSHA). 1999. *Controlling Occupational Exposure to Hazardous Drugs*. Washington, DC: OSHA Technical Manual (TED 1-0.15A), Section 6, Chapter 2. Also available at: *http://www.osha-slc.gov/dts/osta/otm/otm_vi/otm_vi_2.html* (July 2000)

Oken, M., Creech, R., Tormey, D., *et al.* 1982. Toxicity and response criteria of the Eastern Cooperative Oncology Group. *American Journal of Clinical Oncology* 5(6): 649–655.

Padavic-Shaller, K. 1988. Nursing applications in a developing science. *Seminars in Oncology Nursing* 4(2): 142–151.

Penault, R. 1998. Nursing care of the patient receiving radioactive 131I. *Oncology Nursing Forum Practice Corner* 25: 669.

Penrod, J., and Morse, J. 1997. Strategies for assessing and fostering hope: *The Hope Assessment Guide. Oncology Nursing Forum* 24: 1055–1063.

Post-White, J. 1996. The immune system. *Seminars in Oncology Nursing* 12(2): 89–96.

Pruett, J. 1999. Bleeding. In Yarbro, C., Hansen Frogge, M., and Goodman, M. (eds). *Cancer Symptom Management*, 2nd edn. Sudbury, MA: Jones & Bartlett Publishers, pp. 285–306.

Quesada, J., Talpaz, M., Rios, A., *et al.* 1986. Clinical toxicity of interferons in cancer patients: A review. *Journal of Clinical Oncology* 4(2): 234–243.

Radziewicz, R. 1997. Go light your world. *Oncology Nursing Forum* 24: 1689–1694.

Richardson, M.A., Sanders, T., Palmer, J.L., *et al.* 2000. Complementary/alternative medicine use in a comprehensive cancer center and the implications for oncology. *Journal of Clinical Oncology* 18(13): 2505–2514.

Rieger, P. 1992. The pathophysiology of selected symptoms associated with BRM therapy–monograph. Emeryville, CA: Cetus Corporation.

Rieger, P. (ed). 1996. Biotherapy: Present accomplishments and future projections. *Seminars in Oncology Nursing* 12(2): 81–171.

Rieger, P. 1997a. Biotherapy. In Otto, S. (ed). *Oncology Nursing*, 3rd edn. St. Louis, MO: Mosby Year Book, pp. 573–613.

Rieger, P. 1997b. Myelosuppression. In Varricchio, C., Pierce, M., Walker, C., and Ades, T. (eds). *A Cancer Source Book for Nurses*, 7th edn. Atlanta, GA: American Cancer Society, pp. 161–173.

Rieger, P. 1998. Nursing implications of biotherapy.

In Itano, J., and Taoka, K. (eds). *Core Curriculum for Oncology Nursing*, 3rd edn. Philadelphia, PA: W.B. Saunders Company, pp. 630–640.

Rieger, P. (ed). 1999. *Clinical Handbook for Biotherapy*. Sudbury, MA: Jones & Bartlett Publishers, Inc.

Rieker, P., Clark, E., and Fogelberg, P. 1992. Perceptions of quality of life and quality of care for patients with cancer receiving biological therapy. *Oncology Nursing Forum* 19(3): 433–440.

Roach, M. 1998. Nurses manage recombinant interleukin-2 side effects in elderly patients with leukemia. *Oncology Nursing Forum Practice Corner* 25: 29–30.

Rumsey, K., and Rieger, P. (eds). 1992. *Biological Response Modifiers: A Self-Instructional Module for Health-Care Professionals*. Chicago, IL: Precept Press.

Rust, D., Bell, D., Colao, D., *et al.* 1990. Symptom management for patients receiving biotherapy. *Oncology Nursing Forum* 17(6): 964.

Rust, D., Wood, L., and Battiato, L. 1999. Oprelvekin: An alternative treatment for thrombocytopenia. *Clinical Journal of Oncology Nursing* 3(2): 57–62.

Rutledge, D., Ropka, M., Greene, P., *et al.* 1998. Barriers to research utilization for oncology staff nurses and nurse managers/clinical nurse specialists. *Oncology Nursing Forum* 25: 497–506.

Sargent, C., and Shelton, B. 1990. Cardiotoxicities of interleukin-2 (IL-2): The nursing challenge. *Oncology Nursing Forum* 17(6): 964.

Schlesselman, S. 1998. The influence of hope on the psychosocial experience. In Carroll-Johnson, R., Gorman, L., and Bush, N. (eds). *Psychosocial Nursing Care Along the Cancer Continuum*. Pittsburgh, PA: Oncology Nursing Press.

Schover, L. 1988a. *Sexuality and Cancer: For the Man Who Has Cancer, and His Partner*. New York, NY: American Cancer Society.

Schover, L. 1988b. *Sexuality and Cancer: For the Woman Who Has Cancer, and Her Partner*. New York, NY: American Cancer Society.

Schulmeister, L. 1997. Preventing chemotherapy dose and schedule errors. *Clinical Journal of Oncology Nursing* 1(3): 79–85.

Schwartzentruber, D. 1995. Biologic therapy with interleukin-2: Clinical applications—principles of administration and management of side effects. In: DeVita, V.T., Hellman, S., and Rosenberg, S.A. (eds). *Biologic Therapy of Cancer,* 2nd edn. Philadelphia, PA: J.B. Lippincott, pp. 235–249.

Seipp, C. 1997. Capillary-leak syndrome: Nursing considerations. *Biotherapy: Considerations for Oncology Nurses* (CE accredited newsletter). 2(2): 11, 12, 15.

Seiz, A., and Yarbro, C. 1999. Pruritus. In Yarbro, C.H., Hansen Frogge, M., and Goodman, M. (eds). *Cancer Symptom Management*, 2nd edn. Sudbury, MA: Jones & Bartlett Publishers, Inc., pp. 148–160.

Sergi, J. 1991. The physiology of the flu-like syndrome and the cardiopulmonary and renal symptoms associated with BRM therapy—monograph. Emeryville, CA: Cetus Corporation.

Shell, J. 1997. Impact of cancer on sexuality. In Otto, S. (ed). *Oncology Nursing,* 3rd edn. St. Louis, MO: Mosby Year Book, pp. 835–858.

Sitton, E. 1998. Nursing implications of radiation therapy. In Itano, J., and Taoka, K. (eds). *Core Curriculum for Oncology Nursing*, 3rd edn. Philadelphia, PA: W.B. Saunders Company, pp. 616–629.

Sivesind, D., and Rohaly-Davis, J. 1998. Coping with cancer: Patient issues. In Burke, C. (ed). *Psychosocial Dimensions of Oncology Nursing Care*. Pittsburgh, PA: Oncology Nursing Press, pp. 3–26.

Snydman, D., Sullivan, B., Gill, M., *et al.* 1990. Nosocomial sepsis associated with IL-2. *Annals of Internal Medicine* 112(2): 102–107.

Soeken, K., and Carson, V. 1987. Responding to the spiritual needs of the chronically ill. *Nursing Clinics of North America* 22(3): 603–611.

Stetz, K., Haberman, M., Holcombe, J., *et al.* 1995. 1994 Oncology Nursing Society Research Priorities Survey. *Oncology Nursing Forum* 22(5): 785–789.

Strauman, J. 1988. The nurse's role in the biotherapy of cancer: Nursing research of side effects. *Oncology Nursing Forum* 15(6 suppl): 35–39.

Tomaszewski, J. 1995. Biotherapy module II. Overview of biotherapy. *Cancer Nursing* 18(5): 397–412.

U.S. Environmental Protection Agency (USEPA). 1993. *Disposal Tips for Home Health Care*. Washington, DC: USEPA. Publication #EPA530-F-93-027a.

University of California San Francisco (UCSF) School of Nursing Symptom Management Faculty Group. 1994. A model for symptom management. *Image* 26: 272–276.

Wheeler, V. 1997. Biotherapy. In Groenwald, S., Hansen Frogge, M., Goodman, M., and Yarbro, C. (eds). *Cancer Nursing: Principles and Practice*, 4th edn. Boston, MA: Jones & Bartlett Publishers, Inc., pp. 426–458.

White, C. 1992. Symptom assessment and management of outpatients receiving biotherapy: The application of a symptom report form. *Seminars in Oncology Nursing* 8(4 suppl 1): 23–28.

Wickham, R. 1999. Nausea and vomiting. In Yarbro, C., Hansen Frogge, M., and Goodman, M. (eds). *Cancer Symptom Management*, 2nd edn. Sudbury, MA: Jones & Bartlett Publishers, Inc., pp. 228–263.

Wickham, R., Rehwaldt, M., Kefer, C., *et al.* 1999. Taste changes experienced by patients receiving chemotherapy. *Oncology Nursing Forum* 26: 697–706.

Wujcik, D. 1999. Infection. In Yarbro, C., Hansen Frogge, M., and Goodman, M. (eds). *Cancer Symptom Management*, 2nd edn. Sudbury, MA: Jones & Bartlett Publishers, Inc., pp. 307–321.

Yarbro, C. (ed). 1993. Management of patients receiving interleukin-2 therapy. *Seminars in Oncology Nursing* 9(3 suppl 1): 1–35.

Yarbro, C. 1997. Questionable methods of cancer therapy. In Groenwald, S., Hansen Frogge, M.,

Goodman, M., and Yarbro, C.H. (eds). *Cancer Nursing: Principles and Practice*, 4th edn. Boston, MA: Jones & Bartlett Publishers, Inc., pp. 1625–1641.

Yarbro, C., Hansen Frogge, M., and Goodman, M. (eds). 1999. *Cancer Symptom Management*, 2nd edn. Sudbury, MA: Jones & Bartlett Publishers, Inc.

Zoucha, R. 2000. The keys to culturally sensitive care. *American Journal of Nursing* 100(2): 24GG, 24HH, 24KK.

Key Resources

Newsletters

Biotherapy: Considerations for Oncology Nurses. A CE-accredited newsletter published quarterly by Scientific Frontiers, Inc. (Washington Crossing, PA) and funded as a professional service by Chiron Therapeutics (Emeryville, CA).

Biotherapy (ONCBIO Newsletter). A newsletter published by the Oncology Nursing Society (ONS) Biotherapy Special Interest Group. To join special interest group, call 1-412-921-7373. You must be an ONS member.

Fatigue Forum Newsletter. A newsletter that focuses on fatigue-management strategies funded by Ortho Biotech (Raritan, NJ). Available on the Oncology Education Services web site: *http://www.oesweb.com/*

Supportive Solutions to Pain, Fatigue, and Nutrition. A quarterly newsletter made available by the Ambassador 2000 program, funded by the Supportive Care Division of Bristol-Myers Squibb Oncology/Immunology (Princeton, NJ). Available on the Oncology Education Services web site: *http://www.oesweb.com/*

Books

Carpenito, L.J. (ed). 2000. *Nursing Diagnosis: Application to Clinical Practice,* 8th edn. Philadelphia, PA: Lippincott.

Cohen, M.R. (ed). 2000. *Medication Errors: Causes, Prevention, Risk Management.* Sudbury, MA: Jones & Bartlett Publishers, Inc., American Pharmaceutical Association.

Decker, G. (ed). 1999. *An Introduction to Complementary and Alternative Therapies.* Pittsburgh, PA: Oncology Nursing Press.

King, C., and Hinds, P. (eds). 1998. *Quality of Life from Nursing and Patient Perspectives.* Sudbury, MA: Jones & Bartlett Publishers, Inc.

Klimaszewski, A., Aikin, J., Bacon, M., *et al.* (eds).

2000. *Manual for Clinical Trials Nursing.* Pittsburgh, PA: Oncology Nursing Press.

North American Nursing Diagnosis Association. 2000. *Nursing Diagnosis: Definitions and Classifications, 1999-2000,* 3rd edn. Philadelphia, PA: North American Nursing Diagnosis Association.

Yarbor, C., Hansen Frogge, M., and Goodman, M. (eds). 1999. *Cancer Symptom Management,* 2nd edn. Sudbury, MA: Jones & Bartlett Publishers, Inc.

Slide Sets

Biotherapy nursing curriculum. The basics: Agents and management. A slide kit with lecture notes for use in training oncology nurses in the field of biotherapy. This project is supported by an unrestricted educational grant from Chiron Therapeutics Corporation. (Emeryville, CA.) Available on the Oncology Nursing Society web site under education (nursing) (*www.ons.org/*) and by request in writing to the following address:

> Genquest Biomedical Education Services
> 4350 La Jolla Village Drive, Suite 205
> San Diego, CA 92122

Monographs

Yasko, J., Kearney, B., and Conrad, K. 1996. Biotherapy in cancer: Continuing education for oncology nurses. Heberman, R., and Ignoffo, R. (eds). Richmond, CA: Berlex Laboratories.

Web Sites

Oncology Nursing Society: *http://www.ons.org.* A discussion forum for biotherapy.

Cancer Education.com: *http://www.cancereducation.com.*

Cancer Source RN: *http://www.cancersourcern.com.*

Patient Materials

The Cancer Survival Toolbox™. A set of self-help audio tapes that teaches survivors skills they need to advocate for themselves when it comes to treatments, insurance, and employment issues. Call 1-877-TOOLS-4_US (1-877-866-5448). The web site address is: *www.cansearch.org/programs/toolboxs.htm*. Also available at the ONS web site.

Caregiver Materials

Strength for Caring: Education and support for family cancer caregivers. 1998. Ortho-Biotech (Raritan, NJ).

Pharmaceutical Company Support Programs

Clinical Support Specialists—Amgen (Thousand Oaks, CA).

Ambassador 2000 Program—Oncology nurses with special training who are available to disseminate state-of-the-art information about the management of pain, fatigue, and nausea to both professionals and the public. Bristol/Myers Squibb Oncology/Immunology (Princeton, NJ). For a list of current Ambassadors, contact Oncology Education Services at 1-412-921-1929.

Oncology Nurse Educators—Ortho-Biotech (Raritan, NJ)

Patient Care Coordinators—Schering Plough (New Brunswick, NJ)

CHAPTER 15 | Upside Down: Life with Lymphoma

Brian Stabler, PhD

This chapter is an anecdotal chronology of my experience with non-Hodgkin's lymphoma (NHL). But before I begin my story, let me explain that this type of writing is not something I do regularly; in fact, I am more than a little nervous in such personal territory because it is unfamiliar to me as a scientist. However, I wanted to give health professionals a glimpse at the peculiar psychology of a patient attempting to come to terms with an essentially incurable cancer. This is my account of how I dealt with my diagnosis, endured novel treatments, and, essentially, learned to live with lymphoma.

Life Before Lymphoma

It has been said that nobody can be lucky all the time; however, I have a sneaking suspicion that I might be the exception. When I arrived in the United States as a Rotary International graduate student in 1967, I was amazed and delighted to find the University of North Carolina at Chapel Hill to be, as the local guidebook claimed, "the southern part of heaven." This was my first bit of good luck.

Originally, my visit was to have been for 1 academic year, which is about 9 months. As it turned out, after receiving a master's degree, I was invited to enter the university's doctorate program, then to take a fellowship in clinical psychology, and then to join the faculty of the Department of Psychiatry, where I am now a professor. How many people are asked to join the faculty at the best state university in America after having been a student there? I could not believe my luck!

My professional interests have always been in the area of clinical psychology that deals with health, illness, and the stress of coping with chronic medical conditions. I originally focused on childhood health, but after about 10 years, my good luck popped up again when I was offered a sabbatical at Duke Medical Center in Durham, North Carolina, where I was introduced to the world of adult behavioral medicine. Since then, I have specialized in pediatric and adult clinical-health psychology. In my research, I have studied the psychological effects of diabetes, cystic fibrosis, cancer, stress, and growth hormone deficiency, a childhood condition that leads to short stature. In the past few years, I have been involved in delivering care to patients who have diseases and disorders that can be influenced by psychological stress. I have learned a lot about the psychophysiology of stress, the effect of thoughts on emotions, and the connections between thinking, feeling, and behaving. The knowledge I have gained through my professional endeavors prepared me for my own experience with cancer.

Hitting the Wall

I was on my way home from a medical meeting in Florence, Italy, in June 1990 when I realized that what I thought was just a bug that had endured for 2 weeks was coming on even stronger. Midway through the return flight, I began to feel lightheaded; I was also having trouble breathing. This was my first experience with panic.

When I got home, I called my internist to ask for a prescription. He was understandably hesitant to prescribe an antibiotic without seeing me, but because of my persistence, he relented and phoned in the order. Ten days later nothing had changed, and the doctor insisted I have a chest x-ray that day. I did, and an hour later, I received an ominous note from his office that sent a bolt through me: "Call me immediately." Perhaps, I thought, my luck is finally running out.

On the phone, the doctor's voice was calm and balanced, but what he told me was not. "You have a pretty big pleural effusion on the left side," he said. "We need to tap your lung to make a diagnosis."

Inwardly, I screamed, "Oh my God, I've got lung cancer!" Outwardly, I was almost as calm, intellectual, and cool as he had been. "What do you think it might be?"

He was noncommittal but reassuring. "It might be a chronic infection, perhaps even tuberculosis, since you do work in a large hospital. In any event, let's get it tapped and see what the sample tells us." I was getting dizzy just hearing this news, but I recall that he was a steady, unflappable presence on the other end of the line. "Don't worry," he said. "Whatever it is, you're in the right place with the best medical experts in the country. We'll figure this out."

A day later, I was in his office to hear the "verdict." My stomach was in a knot, my mouth was bone dry, and my skin was cold and clammy. I felt like I was going to throw up, but I maintained a focused, concerned expression. In later days, I would find myself continually showing this discrepancy between how I really felt and how I appeared to others. This facade failed me when I needed help, however, because others could not tell what I was thinking or feeling. I wonder whether other patients likewise keep their emotions bottled up, and whether their unspoken thoughts and unexpressed feelings hamper their ability to communicate well with doctors and other health care providers.

The tests indicated that I had advanced, stage IV, low-grade, follicular B-cell lymphoma with involvement of bone marrow and lymph nodes evident above and below the diaphragm. I did not want to hear this. I remember asking the same questions over and over in a vain attempt to change the answers. "Is this like Hodgkin's disease? They can cure that, can't they?" "Do I have to do something right now or can I wait?" "I must have had this thing for a long time. Do some people not treat it at all?" Finally, I looked at my favorite doctor and wailed, "My God, am I going to die soon?" I had been avoiding the inevitable but eventually I had to acknowledge the awful fear I felt.

Coping with cancer, especially during the early months when you are adjusting to the diagnosis, can be like continually running into a brick wall. It seems as though nothing you do can stop what is happening to you. Everything is changing. You have no idea what to do. Nothing goes your way. It is like driving a car that will not go in the direction you are steering—sooner or later, you are bound to hit a wall.

Facing Fears

Bad news can literally be a shock to your system. It is like being physically assaulted: you get the nervous jitters; your blood pressure and pulse rates increase; your muscles tighten; you begin to sweat; and you are ready to fight, flee, or both. This is definitely not your finest hour, and anything someone else can do to help you is usually very much appreciated.

One thing that I did not find helpful was being told not to worry; it is a request that simply cannot be honored. In fact, you actually **need** to worry. I also did not like having information about my diagnosis or treatment delayed, watered down, or in some way distorted in an attempt to make it easier for me to accept. I firmly believe that we should learn to deal with the unpleasant aspects of life as they occur; it is the best way to begin the coping process. By considering each situation we encounter a potential learning opportunity, we can focus our attention on the immediate struggle, which enables us to garner coping competence. If we put off dealing with our feelings or deny them,

> "I firmly believe that we should learn to deal with the unpleasant aspects of life as they occur; it is the best way to begin the coping process."

we miss opportunities to grow and change—and these opportunities may not be available at a later time or in another place. Throughout this experience, I found that when I dealt with issues *in vivo momenti*, the outcome was favorable as far as my personal feelings were concerned.

Overcoming the Dread

Unfortunately, our social perception and understanding of a cancer diagnosis is that it essentially constitutes an eviction order from life or a death sentence. Cancer, it is often said, is a terminal event—but so is life. Using a thinking-feeling-behaving philosophy, I chose to look at my cancer as a condition rather than a conclusion. Therefore, it should be managed like any of life's other calamities: figure out what needs to be done, look for help anywhere you can find it, and then set about trying to make change happen. I know it sounds trite and simplistic, but for me—and many of the patients I have counseled over the years—this approach seems to work better than more passive, dependent approaches to coping with cancer.

How can the proactive approach be initiated? For me, it was always a combination of things, including reading related articles, talking with someone who had traveled the same path, watching a videotape presentation on the topic,

> "Cancer [is] a condition rather than a conclusion; therefore, it should be managed like any other of life's calamities . . ."

and having ample time to ask questions and express my thoughts.

And while we are on the subject, why do we refer to the cancer experience with such aggressive metaphors: "war against cancer," "battle with cancer," "bout with cancer"? It seems to me that the more we make these kinds of pronouncements—that is, the more energy we spend getting ourselves psyched up for a "fight,"—the less likely we are to be prepared to do what actually needs to be done. Bad thoughts beget fearful emotions.

From one perspective, I guess it makes sense to react vigorously and aggressively against cancer because our society tells us that cancer is to be feared and dreaded. In a movie I saw some years ago, one of the main characters was diagnosed with leukemia. When telling others of the sick man's plight, his friend whispered, "He has the big C." This was followed by an extreme closeup of the speaker's pained and knowing expression to the accompaniment of funereal music. The "big C" was clearly the enemy and was surely going to win the battle. If we view cancer only as an "enemy," we make ourselves vulnerable to a do-or-die, win-or-lose scenario.

I am always surprised at how patients answer when I ask them what cancer is. They often equate it with a dark, evil presence. It is understandable, then, that patients develop an enormous fear and loathing for cancer, and are willing to go to "war" to rid themselves of this unwelcome intruder. I believe that cancer cells are simply our own biochemistry gone astray. The cancer cell is by definition an immature cell out of control—a juvenile delinquent who needs to be taken by the hand and given guidance. The sooner cancer patients begin to view their illness in these terms, the sooner the coping process and, indeed, self-healing can begin. This is where education and preparation become essential.

Accepting the Role of "Patient"

I had always believed that a patient was expected to display the virtue "patience." When I became ill, I looked up the definition of the word "patient" in the *Oxford English Dictionary* and found that it stems from the Latin word "patiens," which means a victim or a sufferer. In ancient times, this no doubt was a realistic viewpoint because it was likely that even people suffering from a case of influenza would have a painful, protracted experience—possibly even die.

Today, however, a patient does not have to be a passive, compliant sufferer who readily accepts illness and a possible doomed fate. Cancer patients who have more enduring remission rates and a functional lifestyle are said to have a "fighting spirit." These patients refuse to retreat to the role of victim; rather, they energize and empower themselves to manage their predicament. Health care workers may find it difficult to work with these patients. They ask many questions, challenge diagnoses, do not always follow protocol regimens, and constantly seek alternative solutions. In the long run, however, their nonacceptance of orthodox "patienthood" stands them in good stead, and they tend to live longer and better.

From the beginning, I was actively involved in my own care plans. It was empowering for me to be told that the decisions about my care

---

"Today . . . a patient does not have to be a passive, compliant sufferer who readily accepts illness and a possible doomed fate. . . . They ask many questions . . . and constantly seek alternative solutions. In the long run, however, their nonacceptance of orthodox 'patienthood' stands them in good stead, and they tend to live longer and better."

"It was empowering for me to be told that the decisions about my care were mine to make. At the same time, however, I did not want to be the final arbiter of my own fate. I needed to feel that I had strong input, but I welcomed direction from the medical experts; also this way, I felt included but not ultimately responsible."

were mine to make. At the same time, however, I did not want to be the final arbiter of my own fate. I needed to feel that I had strong input, but I also welcomed direction from the medical experts; this way, I felt included but not ultimately responsible.

As outlined in Dr. Abraham Maslow's theory of human needs, being able to participate in decisions about my health care gave me a sense of being affiliated with the health care team in working toward a common goal—my survival. My anxious fears and despair subsided, and my hope blossomed.

Discussions with my doctors regarding treatment options taught me a lot about the medical-care decision process that became critical to my survival. I learned that there is always another alternative, that sometimes "stay put" is better advice than "just do it," and that conversations with a doctor need not always be one-sided.

Round One

It was July 1990. I had been diagnosed with NHL a month earlier. My oncologist, Dr. John C. Parker, was explaining a treatment option involving alpha-interferon and a small daily dose of cyclophosphamide.

"It really is a pretty good option if you can handle the side effects of interferon," he said after examining my node sites.

"Side effects?" I wanted to know more.

"Nothing really serious, but some people say they get flu-like symptoms after an injection," he explained. "It usually gets better with time."

Nobody likes to hear they will have the flu, least of all that they have brought it on themselves. There had to be other options, I thought; preferably some with milder side effects. I had just read a book by the late Senator Paul Tsongas entitled *Heading Home*, in which he described his experience with lymphoma, including treatment with autologous bone marrow transplantation (BMT). So I asked, "What about trying something like a transplant where I can try to get rid of this thing?"

I could see that the doctor was not impressed with that idea, and he was very straightforward in his reply. "You don't need a transplant. We can treat what you have with standard methods, like chemotherapy. Bone marrow transplantation is still experimental. You may not even qualify for a protocol, and, if you do, you'd be crazy to take the risks."

I was insistent. "But if there is a chance it would clean out the lymphoma cells, I want to at least try."

He looked at me across the table with a warm grin. Shaking his head, he put his hand on my shoulder and said, "Let's keep our powder dry until we need the big guns, okay?"

I was somewhat comforted by what he said, especially because he had said "we." But I was still anxious about my situation for several reasons. First, with the treatment he was describing, my physical condition was going to become much worse. This seemed irrational to me, even absurd, because I was feeling relatively well at that time. Second, there seemed to be a ready acquiescence to the incurability of low-grade, follicular NHL, meaning that no matter what standard treatment I chose, the disease would always return. The standard therapies were, in essence, palliative treatments. I remember thinking, "Why is everyone so accepting of standard therapy? Don't they know I could die?"

Most cancer patients tend to believe that their health professionals know all that needs to be known to treat cancer. A few years ago this was probably true. Today, however, the fact is that discovery of new approaches, drugs, combination chemotherapy "cocktails," and now biological therapies means that no single individual or group can be entirely knowledgeable.

I badgered him, my oncologist relented and called a colleague of his at the Dana-Farber Cancer Institute in Boston to see what protocols might be available. You can imagine our surprise at hearing literally the next day, that a brand-new protocol was being developed to treat low-grade NHL with autologous BMT as the first-line therapy. The enrollment criteria fit me exactly, and within 2 weeks, I was in Boston undergoing preliminary assessment.

Listening to Hear

When I heard about the research protocol, I was naturally thrilled but, at the same time, apprehensive. The Dana-Farber Cancer Institute stood out in my mind as a place where only the sickest cancer patients go and where many do not survive the ordeal of treatment. My NHL was stage IV, diffuse, and nodular, but also indolent. The use of BMT as primary therapy was still an experimental approach, which meant that I was taking a huge chance in the hope that something unproven would work for me. So, like most patients in my position, I tried hard to hear and understand everything that was said to me, and I followed up by reading journals and discussing the issue with trusted friends. As it turned out, at my first visit I apparently fell deaf; I either did not hear what was said or I completely misunderstood.

I was met in Boston by Dr. George Canellos, a world-famous oncologist, clinician, investigator, and scholar. Very early in our conversation, even before he examined me, I recall that he said something like, "Dr. Stabler, I must caution you that we do not take salvage cases on this protocol." That is all I can remember from what must have been more than a 1-hour-long conversation. As it happened, my good friend Tom Cook had come to Boston with me and had sat in on the interview. When the interview was over, Tom and I went to a bar not far from the hospital. I remember saying to him, "Well, this was a waste of time. He doesn't even want to consider me because I am one of those salvage cases!" I was so despondent and forlorn that it actually made Tom laugh. "What do you mean he won't consider you? Didn't you hear what he said later? You are a prime candidate!" Turning to the people at the table next to ours, he said, "This guy just got admitted to Harvard Medical School!" They applauded and offered congratulations.

I clearly had been so anxious and "loaded for bear" that I completely mistook what Dr. Canellos said. I was reacting to my own gloomy predictions of what I thought the doctor "might" say, and then converted all I heard to match my prediction. I know this happens many times in all kinds of caregiver/patient discussions, especially when complex and novel programs are being worked out. My friend Tom was a godsend that day—I needed another pair of ears and another brain to properly appreciate the message I was being given.

The acquired deafness actually reappeared repeatedly throughout the duration of my treatment. During this period, I was not in the best emotional state and, likewise, my ability to listen and comprehend diminished. There were times when I literally could not understand what was being said to me. It helped to have someone from my family present to record and monitor my conversations with staff. I wondered later

". . . my ability to listen and comprehend diminished. There were times when I literally could not understand what was being said to me. It helped to have someone from my family present . . ."

if there were, in fact, some pieces of information about the protocol that I really did not need to hear, such as the mortality rates and complications associated with the treatment. At this juncture, I have come to believe that the patient must be comfortable with allowing some measure of decision-making to be done by others. When a consent form was presented to me, I immediately flipped through the 13 pages and found the place where I had to sign. I knew that there were risks, but I knew also that this protocol treatment was my chance for complete recovery. For me, the goal was clear, and the legal-ethical issues did not matter. In retrospect, it would have been helpful if I had been given a brief précis of the consent form, perhaps only a paragraph to be reviewed when I was more cognizant.

It also might be helpful to have a clinical staff member assigned as an "ombudsperson/translator" for each patient in a protocol. One of the nurses on my health care team informally served in this capacity for me. She explained the course of treatment and the possible side effects, counseled me about what to do when things were going badly, and generally befriended me. For example, I had wanted to read in my room to pass the time. My nurse advocate explained that the effects of chemotherapy and sedatives would cause such cognitive disruption that I would forget what I read almost as soon as I had read it. She suggested I watch lots of videotapes about inane, easy-to-understand subjects such as gardening or travel.

Boy was she right! My cognition was so poor during the 28 days of inpatient therapy that even a simple conversation became disastrous.

A nutritionist once came in and asked me what I liked to eat. I said, "Can you fix this Hickman catheter for me?"

She answered, "No, I can't do that, but I will ask the nurse to come in."

My response was, "Okay, but can you give me more medicine for nausea? I feel a little bilious."

Nothing made any sense to me, and I felt foolish when trying to describe how I felt when asked by my doctors each day. I once answered the question "How are you?" by saying, "Fine, but that Eskimo bar tasted funny last night." When the puzzled doctor said that chocolate was not on my diet, I replied, "Oh, well, maybe I just ate too much mashed potatoes."

My point is that, in varying degrees, medically ill patients lose their critical faculties in response to the stress of illness and the physical demands of treatment. Asking a patient to make decisions, absorb new information, or even join in a discussion may be beyond his or her capacity, regardless of how alert they may appear. Let someone else handle the issues, or wait until the patient is in a better state of mind.

Accepting Help

When diagnosed with cancer, a person assumes the role of "patient" armed only with innate intelligence and practical life experience. I know I was certainly inept when I first stepped into the role of patient. Then I had a chance early encounter with a nurse who taught me what it takes to be successful as a patient in a research protocol.

I was trying very hard not to become violently ill or nauseated by the chemotherapy as I awaited the BMT at the Dana-Farber Cancer Institute. For some reason, I had it in my head that being "in control" at all times was a good thing. I was taking very large doses of cyclophosphamide that left me with this gut-wrenching urge to be sick, but I steadfastly refused to give in. I breathed deeply, I chanted, I hummed, I even tried to whistle—all in an effort to distract myself from the possibility of having to throw up. At one point, I remember standing on my hospital bed with my head thrown back and arms stretched upward as I swayed and babbled in a vain attempt to avoid being sick. As this was happening, the charge nurse came into the room, looked at me in disbelief, and shouted, "What are you trying to do? Get down from there before you pull out your Hickmans!"

Not to be dissuaded, I whined, "But I can't be sick. I haven't been sick this whole past year of chemo."

She rolled her eyes and said, "Listen, don't you know that chemotherapy can't work unless you let it work? Be still, and quit fighting the treatment." With that, she tugged gently on my pajama sleeve and helped me lie sideways. I proceeded to heave.

Things improved markedly during the next few hours. Recalling this small event, I realize that what the nurse said at that moment may not have been entirely accurate from a technical standpoint, but it was what I needed to hear, and it certainly has stayed with me. Sometimes a patient's fighting spirit can get in the way of the healing process. There comes a time to lie back and simply let things "happen." This realization was my first step toward settling into the role of patient.

Round Two

When I was told in 1997 that my disease was beginning to reactivate and that I once again needed treatment, my first instinct was to resist the entire notion. I had had enough. I wanted to give my body a rest. I had been disease-free for several years, and I had lost the self-image

of patient. The horrors of 7 rounds of chemotherapy followed by local and then total-body irradiation together with high-dose cyclophosphamide were indelibly etched on every cell of my body. I decided that this time I would take another route. I had sought out alternative complementary treatments before; this time I hoped that meditation, biofeedback, healing touch, or some other approach would help me jumpstart the self-healing process. The possibilities renewed my optimism; I was energized to move forward.

As I have stated before, when facing hard decisions, my style is to be proactive; that is, to seek out as many other opinions as I can find. So after talking to my wife and my oncologist, I searched for ideas on the Internet, scanned the latest clinical oncology research reports, called the National Cancer Institute information line, and contacted several other NHL patients whom I knew well. For me, seeking information is almost as comforting as actually making a new discovery. The very act of "doing something" makes me feel better and enables me to displace the anxiety that results from facing my own mortality. As a matter of fact, I often tell folks I counsel, "When in doubt, do something!"

So, taking my own advice, I soon came upon a new body of information about monoclonal antibody therapy. What a relief! Someone was actually trying to promote the natural self-healing process rather than beating up cells with chemotherapy whether or not they were delinquent! It seemed intuitively right to actively seek this novel therapy because it so fit my personal preference for doing the least amount of bodily harm, it was relatively easy and painless to administer, and it was just about to be approved by the Food and Drug Administration. A friend had seen something in the newspaper about this new approach and had sent me a clipping with a note saying, in effect, "Why not try this? What have you got to lose?"

Because the treatment had not reached regulatory approval, getting access to information about it took a little work. Monoclonal antibody therapy was certainly not yet in my hospital's formulary. This is where I really had to push to get things going. All the members of my health care team—the doctors, the nurses, and the pharmacists—agreed that such a protocol was a good fit for me, but no one knew where to start, what was involved, and whether the procedure would be covered under my health-insurance policy. Because I worked at the hospital where the treatment would be administered and because I was a health professional, I knew what needed to be done. I remember wondering how laypersons would be able to get information about new treatment options. Would they know the right questions to ask? Or would they expect that their caregivers would always offer the new treatment options?

I found out later that there is sometimes a gap in time between a drug's approval and release for general use and that during this time, literature is developed to educate patients about the new treatment. I would certainly have benefited from reading something that described monoclonal antibody therapy and discussed how it worked, what side effects I might expect, and so on. But my excitement about this potentially lifesaving approach clouded my critical judgment, and I was glad to do anything that promised hope. I respectfully suggest that as the biological efficacy of new therapies is being considered, pharmaceutical companies should team up with patient-advocacy groups to determine what patients need to know about the new drug and to foster the ability of patients to interact with others who have undergone experimental therapy.

After the "Novelty" Wears Off

I have been on 2 novel therapy regimens in the past 9 years: early autologous BMT at the Dana Farber Cancer Institute in 1991 and monoclonal antibody therapy at the University of North Carolina at Chapel Hill in 1998. Both produced the desired outcome—reducing the tumor load and decreasing the physical symptoms associated with NHL. As I look back at my treatment experiences, 3 lessons stand out in my mind.

First, the patient must be informed of the possibility that novel treatment options are available. I cannot stress enough that in my experience, the need to be a self-starter was critical. Information-gathering is the single best first step any patient can take in searching out new and cutting-edge cancer treatments. Knowing how to use the library and the Internet, being willing to pick up the telephone and call major cancer centers, and staying in touch with the American Cancer Society and the National Cancer Institute are all essential actions; however, if the patient is not motivated, these resources may go untapped.

Second, the patient must learn to suspend apprehension when necessary. Cancer patients are frequently and perhaps even chronically anxious because of the health implications they face. But when the possibility of new and therefore relatively untried therapies arises, the first instinct should not always be to delay or disavow the potential value of these treatment options. Being afraid to try new approaches keeps a patient's options limited and may lead to less positive outcomes. In my experience, it might have been helpful if more of my caregivers had actively pushed for the novel approaches rather than being conservative and pushing for the more tried-and-true remedies.

Third, the information vacuum that separates the development of a novel therapy and the dissemination of information about it to patients must be overcome. Because of regulatory requirements, information about new treatment options is curtailed so that only a limited number of centers and their investigators are fully aware of what is available. Moreover, essential patient education materials are usually delayed until after the therapy has been approved and is in general use. For me, this meant that I undertook monoclonal antibody therapy without fully knowing the possible side effects, and more importantly, my medical caregivers were obliged to work with only the bare essentials of treatment strategies. So, I vote for allocating time to develop collateral materials and other resources to properly educate patients and their caregivers about treatment options. In my opinion, a fully informed and prepared patient is more likely to have a complete and enduring treatment response.

Accommodating Illness

I think patients who are approached about entering clinical protocols have the same questions as those being given their initial diagnosis. What will happen to me? Will I get better? Will the treatment make me sicker? Who will take care of me? As I consider the understandable hesitations that many patients have about experimental treatment regimens, I recall what Dr. Maslow postulated about all human needs and how the fulfillment of those needs motivates and propels us through our lives. In his "hierarchy of human needs," Dr. Maslow listed nourishment, biological stability, and a sense of safety as the most fundamental needs and, therefore, those that must be satisfied first. Only when these needs are satisfied, in Maslow's theory, can an individual go on to address the higher-order needs: love and belonging, self-esteem, knowledge and understanding, and actualization (Maslow, 1998). For the patient with cancer, life's needs are arrested at the most fundamental level, and the desire to learn and understand becomes secondary or is overlooked. However, in my experience, the need for knowledge and understanding actually became a major pathway through which I could

"... in my experience, the need for knowledge and understanding actually became a major pathway through which I could begin to help myself feel safer and ultimately more stable. As I learned more, I also became more competent as a patient, and I became more optimistic and confident, which translated into a better quality of life."

begin to help myself feel safer and ultimately more stable. As I learned more, I became more competent as a patient, and I also became more optimistic and confident, which translated into a better quality of life.

So what worked for me was being an active participant in determining my care plan, pursuing new knowledge about my disease, and building survival techniques, all of which helped me maintain a sense of balance. Maslow's hierarchical order of prepotency suggests that individuals passively accept the need-fulfillment for biological stability and for safety. If this is true, then for many cancer patients, their need-fulfillment is always directly correlated with their state of health. Personal initiative focused only on biological survival seems to me to run counter to the urgent need to act in triggering change. For me, the need to know and to understand seems to be a necessary precursor of biological stability and safety, which in turn lead to the opportunity to pursue love, self-esteem, and fulfillment of personal potential. The needs remain the same; their order of

"... what worked for me was being an active participant in determining my care plan, pursuing new knowledge about my disease, and building survival techniques, all of which helped me maintain a sense of balance."

priority changes under the dire circumstances posed by cancer.

Looking Back: How Health Professionals Can Help

Although I am a proponent of proactive patienthood, the health care provider can be a valuable support system for patients beyond providing direct medical care. Particularly when decisions must be made, patients may first seek advice from those care providers with whom they interact routinely. As such, the health care provider must be prepared to be professional and compassionate, and to provide both technical and practical yet unbiased advice.

Providing Information

I remember Dr. Parker telling me at one point, "Brian, no matter what, if things go wrong, we are absolute wizards at finding other options. We'll always be there to try another treatment." Technically correct or not, this is the kind of reassurance patients like to hear because it offers great comfort in uncomfortable times. Although many patients go on to try novel approaches, they must always know that there are lots of old "standby" options also available. Even the bravest tightrope-walkers perform better when they know they have a safety net.

I can say that I would have felt safer knowing that there were, in fact, other options beyond the novel therapies. In fact, I have wondered whether patients who enroll in clinical studies or undertake approved novel therapies ought to have a short course in coping with the special issues associated with those approaches. It need not be lengthy or extensive; it might be presented in a videotape or an audiotape with a booklet. What patients need is simply some-thing to help dispel the many uncertainties they have.

Raising Hope

In my training as a clinical psychologist, I was taught that anxious people fear the future and depressed people mourn the past. As a patient with cancer, I found that these emotional states can easily coexist: we grieve for our lost health and dread what the future may hold.

The patient's first thought is that the diagnosis of cancer presents an automatic "no-win" situation, and in some instances, this assumption may be correct. However, there is always a possibility for hope, and hope can be nurtured through interactions between the patient and the health care providers. What the health care provider says about the possible treatment outcome or overall prognosis does not impress the patient as much as the attitude, demeanor, and approach he or she uses.

Raising hope is something about which many health professionals are wary, because it implies a certainty of sorts. However, in my opinion, imputing optimism is a critical part of the health care provider's role. No one has ever been sued for imputing optimism. I always looked for signs that my nurses or physicians were implying hope through positive words and gestures—an upbeat tone of voice; strong, steady speech; a reassuring smile—without forthrightly declaring it.

Cancer Survival: More Than a Simple Act of Fate

Time has shown me that the 2 novel cancer therapies I undertook were both effective in different ways. Initially, I needed an autologous BMT to literally save my life—to stem the tide of disease and make life possible. Later, when my quality of life became less than optimal, I turned to monoclonal antibody therapy, in the form of Rituxan®. We know more today about cancer therapy than we did 10 years ago, and the growth curve created by this scientific enlightenment has been exponential. The biotechnology behind the treatment of cancer patients has become so elegantly sophisticated that there now seems to me to be an enormous gap between what we do to treat patients and how we care for them during their treatment. Great scientific gains have overshadowed the fact that to optimally reach and extend the best outcomes of therapy, we must pay more attention to the human experience of cancer patients. What I have referred to as "luck," when all the chips are counted, has more to do with the nature of the expert advice, love, encouragement, guidance, role models, trust, and wisdom that I have encountered than simple chance.

Ten years since my diagnosis is the equivalent of 3,650 days, and every single day I depend on the presence of these qualities in my life. I acknowledge them every day, just before I get up and go out to pick up the morning paper.

Acknowledgments

Thanks are due to so many people that I cannot honestly hope to recall them all here. You know who you are, and I hope you will remember what I have said to each of you personally.

My beloved wife Laura deserves special acknowledgment because it is she who always makes things lighter when bleak times come around. My physicians, the late John Parker, Lee Berkowitz, Andrew Greganti, Timothy Smelzer, and Dennis Ellis, have been the best medical partners anyone could hope for. My friends Bill and Jan Bolen, Cliff and Linda Butler, Fred Kiger, Eric and Penny Jensen, Warren and Laura Piver, Ken and Marlene Whitt, Lynn Nye, and Christy and Keith Bowman have been pillars of support and encouragement, each in their own way. I am grateful to Jean Ranc and Dianne Shaw for their friendship and expert editorial assistance.

Special thanks to my nurses Sandra Blackman, Lisa Williams, Pat Decator, Wendy McBride, Liz Ward, Barbara Clark, and Tom Quinn, who expertly blended the best of cutting-edge cancer therapy with their skill and compassionate care, thereby making possible that which might otherwise not have been possible.

Suggested Reading List

Handler, E. 1996. *Time on Fire: A Comedy of Terrors*. New York, NY: Henry Holt & Co.

Maslow, A. 1998. *Toward a Psychology of Being,* 3rd edn. New York, NY: John Wiley & Sons.

McLaurin, T. 1991. *Keeper of the Moon*. New York, NY: W.W. Norton & Company.

Price, R. 1994. *A Whole New Life: An Illness and a Healing*. New York, NY: Athenium.

Remen, R. 1996. *Kitchen Table Wisdom*. New York, NY: Riverhead Books.

Tsongas, P. 1984. *Heading Home*. New York, NY: Alfred P. Knopf.

CHAPTER 16 | Flu-Like Syndrome

Brenda K. Shelton, RN, MS, CCRN, AOCN®

Biotherapy has become known as the fourth cancer treatment modality. Used alone or in combination with other antineoplastic therapies, biotherapy continues to evolve through clinical studies, and its therapeutic and adverse effects are now relatively well defined. The constellation of symptoms known as "flu-like syndrome" (FLS) is the most common adverse effect of treatment with biological agents (Haeuber, 1989; Sergi, 1991; Skalla, 1996). It is reported as a significant adverse effect, affecting at least 20% of the population receiving treatment with 50% to 95% of biotherapy regimens (Haeuber, 1989; Chiron Corporation, 1992; Schering Corporation, 1992; Conrad and Horrell, 1995; American Hospital Formulary

The author wishes to thank and acknowledge Douglas Haeuber, whose work from the first edition of *Biotherapy: A Comprehensive Overview* served as a foundation for this chapter.

Service, 1996; Burke *et al.,* 1996; Rieger, 1996; IDEC Pharmaceuticals Corporation and Genentech, Inc., 1997; Shelton and Turnbough, 1999).

In this chapter, the pathophysiologic mechanisms and the unique patterns of FLS in specific biotherapy regimens are discussed. The instruments and scales used in assessment and toxicity grading are described. Suggestions for manipulation of therapies and specific interventional strategies are provided. Finally, the current status of nursing research regarding the recognition and management of FLS is discussed.

Characteristics and Effects of the Flu-Like Syndrome

FLS refers to a cluster of constitutional signs and symptoms including fever, **chills**, **rigors**, **myalgias**, **arthralgias**, headache, upper-respiratory symptoms (e.g., cough and nasal congestion),

519

malaise, fatigue, and gastrointestinal symptoms (e.g., anorexia, nausea, vomiting, and diarrhea) (Shelton and Turnbough, 1999). Clinical study documentation and drug information sheets for specific biological agents define FLS differently. This text addresses the first 7 symptoms listed previously, because they are relatively unique to treatment with biological agents.

Impact of FLS on Physical and Emotional Well-Being

FLS is often described as a mild yet troublesome toxic effect (Shelton and Turnbough, 1999). Although not life-threatening, FLS can contribute substantially to the debilitation of already compromised patients, and it adversely affects quality of life (Brophy and Sharp, 1991; Sandstrom, 1996). The cytokines released during FLS increase the metabolic rate and disrupt normal homeostatic mechanisms leading to a number of physical manifestations. Fever or rigors increase metabolic rate and deplete energy, affecting the patient's strength and endurance. These physical effects in patients with preexisting health deviations can cause cardiac failure, respiratory compromise, renal insufficiency, or hepatic compromise (Henker *et al.*, 1997; Shaffer, 1997).

For some patients, anticipation of a flu-like episode following every treatment exacts a high emotional response and influences attitudes about continued therapy (Craig *et al.*, 1995). Among health care providers, nurses are most observant of these responses and most committed to addressing the accompanying quality-of-life issues. Therefore, it is important that nurses acquire a thorough understanding of FLS and develop strategies to help patients cope with this adverse effect.

Presenting Symptoms

FLS as a result of biotherapy encompasses a variety of physical symptoms that mimic an episode of influenza. The specific characteristics of each symptom may vary slightly with the biotherapy regimen. The chief characteristics of each symptom and the common clusters are described in the following text.

FEVER

Fever associated with use of biological agents can vary greatly according to regimen and the patient's immune response. Fever patterns are thought to reflect the mechanism of fever production. Persistent fever tends to be more prominent with cytokine therapies (e.g., interferon [IFN], interleukin-2 [IL-2], and tumor necrosis factor [TNF]) that stimulate inflammatory mediators (Haeuber, 1989), whereas intermittent idiosyncratic fever is noted with tumor lysis or hypersensitivity reactions such as with monoclonal antibody (MAB) and immunoconjugate treatments (Haeuber, 1989; Sievers *et al.*, 1997; Ligand Pharmaceuticals, 1999). Patients who have fever related to treatment with biological agents can develop **tachyphylaxis** (i.e., decreasing symptoms with increased exposure) with continuous cytokine therapy; however, this response is rare when fever occurs with MABs (Herzog *et al.*, 1995; Sandstrom, 1996). Fever patterns that are important to identify include severity, rate of rise, timing, and associated symptoms (e.g., rigors). A generalization of specific fever patterns related to biological agents is shown in Table 16.1 (Haeuber, 1989; Conrad and Horrell, 1995; Du and Williams, 1997; IDEC Pharmaceuticals Corporation and Genentech, Inc., 1997; Shelton and Turnbough, 1999).

CHILLS OR RIGORS

Chills or rigors are defined as muscle contractions that usually accompany a rise in the body's temperature (Holtzclaw, 1992; Shaffer, 1997). When the thermoregulatory set point is increased, the body needs to generate heat to change body temperature. The most effective

Table 16.1   Fever patterns that occur with common biological agents

Biological Agent	Fever Severity*	Onset (after administration)	Peak	Duration
CYTOKINES				
IFN-α	Grade 1–2 DD	2–4 hr	4–6 hr	4–8 hr
IFN-β	Grade 1–2 DD	2–4 hr	4–6 hr	4–8 hr
IFN-γ	Grade 2–3 DD	4–8 hr	10–12 hr	18–20 hr
IL-2 (aldesleukin) bolus infusion or injection	Grade 2–3 DD	1–2 hr	4–6 hr	12–24 hr
IL-2 (aldesleukin) continuous infusion	Grade 3–4 DD	2–4 hr	8–12 hr	for 2–3 days after drug is discontinued
TNF bolus infusion	Grade 3–4 DD	1–2 hr	2–4 hr	4–6 hr
TNF continuous infusion	Grade 2–3 DD	2–4 hr	2–6 hr	24–48 hr
TNF IM or SC injection	Grade 1–3 DD	2–4 hr	3–10 hr	20–24 hr
G-CSF (filgrastim)	Grade 1 NDD	2–4 hr	4–6 hr	8–12 hr
GM-CSF (sargramostim)	Grade 2–3 NDD	2–4 hr	4–6 hr	8–12 hr
IL-11 (oprelvekin)	Grade 1 NDD	2–4 hr	4–8 hr	8–12 hr
MONOCLONAL ANTIBODIES				
Trastuzumab (Herceptin®)	Grade 1 NDD	<15 min	1–2 hr	2–4 hr
Rituximab (Rituxan®)	Grade 1 NDD	2–4 hr	4–6 hr	8–12 hr
RETINOIDS				
Tretinoin (Vesanoid®)	Grade 1–2 NDD	4–8 hr	8–12 hr	12–18 hr

(continued)

Table 16.1 *Continued*

Biological Agent	Fever Severity*	Onset (after administration)	Peak	Duration
IMMUNE MODULATORS				
Levamisole	Grade 1–2	8–12 hr	24 hr	48 hr
BCG	Grade 1–3	8–12 hr	12–18 hr	24 hr
FUSION MOLECULES				
Denileukin difitox (Ontak®)	Grade 1 NDD	6–12 hr	12–24 hr	48 hr

*Fever severity definitions based on National Cancer Institute toxicity criteria (see Table 16.4):
  Grade 1 = 37.1°C–38.0°C.
  Grade 2 = 38.1°C–40.0°C.
  Grade 3 = >40°C for <24 hours.
  Grade 4 = >40°C for >24 hours.
BCG, bacillus Calmette Guérin; DD, dose-dependent; G-CSF, granulocyte colony-stimulating factor; GM-CSF, granulocyte-macrophage colony-stimulating factor; hr, hour; IFN, interferon; IL, interleukin; IM, intramuscular; NDD, not dose-dependent; SC, subcutaneous; TNF, tumor necrosis factor.

method of increasing body heat is to increase muscle activity; hence, shivering, shaking, or rigors (Shaffer, 1997; Henker *et al.*, 1997; Henker, 1999). The severity of rigors usually correlates with a wide disparity between body temperature and the new set point or with the rate of rise in temperature (Shaffer, 1997; Henker, 1999). Chills can be so severe as to cause bronchospasms and respiratory compromise (Shelton and Turnbough, 1999).

MYALGIAS

Myalgias are defined as nonlocalized muscle aches accompanied by weakness that may persist despite rest (Shelton and Turnbough, 1999). Patients describe myalgias as affecting their entire body and influencing their motivation to perform activities of daily living. This symptom is most prevalent with the cytokines or multi-lineage growth factors (Shelton and Turnbough,

1999). The most often reported sites of myalgias are large muscle groups such as the shoulders and thighs (Shelton and Turnbough, 1999), although in this author's experience, patients also complain of jaw aches. Myalgias that tend to persist after other FLS symptoms have abated are likely to be preceded by rigors. It is thought that the muscle activity of rigors causes excess physical stress or exercise, producing fatigued and painful muscles (Haeuber, 1989).

ARTHRALGIAS

Pain or aches in joints at rest or during activity is termed arthralgia. This symptom occurs with use of MABs, cytokines, and growth factors to varying degrees; however, it can be confused with the bone pain associated with some growth factors and TNF. The exact mechanism of arthralgias is unclear. In this author's experience, the joints most affected are those required for weight bearing (e.g., wrists, knees, and ankles). Arthralgias tend to persist after other FLS symptoms have abated.

HEADACHE
Headache associated with biological agents is most likely to occur in the frontal area, to be a sharp pain, and to be accompanied by photophobia (Shelton and Turnbough, 1996). Headaches often occur with a rise in temperature and persist as long as the fever, but they rarely occur alone. Headaches may also be global and are then thought to be related to vascular dilation (Haeuber, 1989; Strauman, 1992).

UPPER-RESPIRATORY SYMPTOMS
Nasal congestion, rhinitis, and cough are common flu-like symptoms that are not quite as common with biotherapy, although it may be merely under-reported because of the severity of other symptoms. It is postulated that the nasal symptoms are the result of vasodilation from inflammatory mediators and are more prevalent with cytokine therapy (Haeuber, 1989; Strauman, 1992). Cough may occur when there is post-nasal drainage down the throat, but it also may be reflective of a more serious adverse effect, such as bronchospasm.

Pathophysiology of the Flu-Like Syndrome

The pathophysiology of FLS is similar to that involved in illness-induced fever. During the past decade, advances in understanding the physiology of fever have paralleled research with biological agents. Whereas some gaps remain in the scientific understanding of fever, many aspects of the febrile condition and its associated symptoms are now clear.

Alterations in the Thermoregulatory Set Point

Fever can be defined as a condition in which the thermoregulatory "set point" governing body temperature is raised above the normal level, although autoregulation of temperature is not impaired (Henker *et al.*, 1997; Saper, 1998; Henker, 1999). Core body temperature may or may not be raised to this same level. This condition should be distinguished from hyperthermia (e.g., related to injury to the hypothalamus), in which core temperature is permanently above the set point and autoregulation is impaired (Kluger, 1991; Holtzclaw, 1992; Henker *et al.*, 1997; Henker, 1999).

The thermoregulatory set point is a narrow range of temperatures around 37°C, the optimal temperature for cell metabolism and body function. When body temperature rises above or falls below the set point, signals are sent to initiate appropriate compensatory cooling or warming mechanisms to return body temperature to the set point range. The thermoregulatory set point rises by either a direct effect of the biological agent administered or in response to contact with substances called **pyrogens**.

Action of Pyrogens

There are two basic types of pyrogens: exogenous and endogenous. Exogenous pyrogens are produced outside the body and include bacterial endotoxins, fungi, viruses, neoplastic cells, and antigenic substances such as certain drugs. Although some exogenous pyrogens may directly influence the thermoregulatory set point in the pituitary-hypothalamus axis, their effects are typically mediated via endogenous pyrogens (EPs) (Bligh, 1982; Dascombe, 1986; Henker *et al.*, 1997).

As implied, EPs are synthesized and released by phagocytic cells (e.g., monocytes and tissue macrophages) and secreted in response to contact with antigenic substances such as bacterial endotoxins. IL-1 has long been considered a prime example of an EP, although TNF, IFNs, and IL-6 also meet the clinical criteria of EPs (Kluger, 1991; Bruce and Grove, 1992; Luheshi, 1998). In a study of patients experiencing the paroxysms of chills and fever caused by malaria, Karunaweera (1992) found that serum TNF levels closely paralleled the occurrence of chills and the rise and fall in temperatures preceding these events by 30 to 60 minutes. This parallel supports the hypothesis that TNF is an EP. Some biological agents, such as the IFNs and TNF, are probably themselves EPs and, therefore, initiate symptom patterns similar to those associated with IL-1 (Dinarello, 1988; Kluger, 1991; Cerami, 1992; Kluger, 1992b). Some researchers suggest that variable cytokine combinations may be responsible for altering the thermoregulatory set point and may account for specific fever patterns seen with biological agents (Hirano, 1992; Kluger, 1992b).

Pyrogens travel via the circulatory system to the *organosum lamina terminalis*, an area in the hypothalamic endothelium where there is stimulation of **prostaglandin** E2 (PGE2) production (Coceani and Akarasu, 1998). PGE2 up regulates the temperature set point located in an area of the brain called the *preoptic anterior hypothalamus* (Coceani, 1986; Dinarello, 1988; Bruce and Grove, 1992). Once the thermoregulatory set point is reset, efferent signals are transmitted to activate autonomic and behavioral compensatory mechanisms, causing increased body temperature.

EPs such as PGE2 are known to stimulate pain receptors and increase muscle proteolysis. These two effects may also be causative factors of myalgias commonly associated with FLS (Baracos, 1983; Haeuber, 1989).

Once released into the circulation, pyrogens initiate various other immunostimulatory effects, as shown in Figure 16.1 (Haeuber, 1989;

Bruce and Grove, 1992; Henker *et al.*, 1997; Shaffer, 1997; Zetterstrom *et al.*, 1998; Shelton and Turnbough, 1999).

Stimulation of Inflammatory-Immune Response and Immunostimulatory Effects

The immunostimulatory effects of pyrogens triggered by administration of biological agents cause activation of the body's inflammatory-immune response. Fever, erythema, vasodilation, edema, and generalized aches are the primary effects of the inflammatory-immune response. Complex immunologic processes work together to cause this group of physical effects, and these processes can also explain many of the adverse effects associated with biotherapy. A better understanding of these relationships can be obtained by analyzing the process of fever.

The first phase of fever, known as the chill or cold stage, represents the body's effort to bring core temperatures up to the new, higher set point. Chills are described as shivering accompanied by the sensation of cold and are the forerunner of fever. The muscular contractions that result in shivering serve to generate heat. Muscular activity involved in shivering during the cold phase of fever is also likely to exacerbate myalgias. Simultaneous with shivering, there is vasoconstriction, which conserves heat through decreased skin perfusion. Furthermore, in response to the sensation of cold, patients will dress warmly or huddle under covers in an attempt to conserve heat.

The second phase of fever, termed the hot or plateau stage, occurs when the core temperature reaches or overshoots the new set point. The patient's skin becomes warm and flushed, the basal metabolic rate becomes elevated, and the patient experiences compensatory tachycardia and tachypnea. Headaches, myalgias, and thirst are other common sensations during this phase.

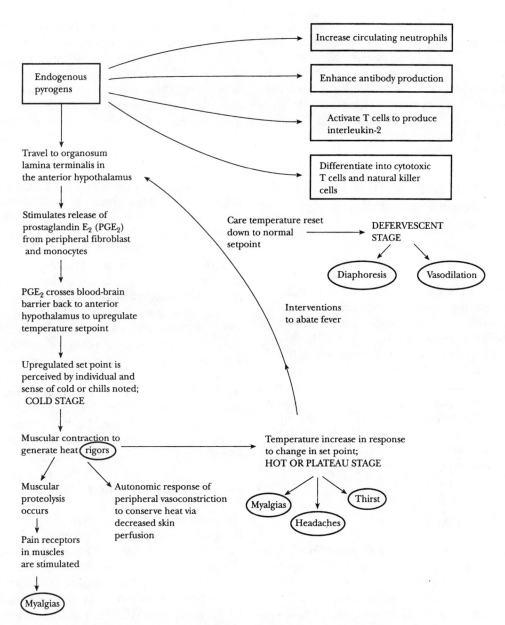

Figure 16.1 Endogenous pyrogens initiate various other immunostimulatory effects

Source: Reprinted with permission from Shelton, B.K., and Turnbough, L. 1999. Flu-like syndrome. In Yarbro, C.H., Frogge, M.H., Goodman, M., and Groenwald, S. (eds). *Cancer Symptom Management*, 2nd edn. Boston, MA: Jones & Bartlett Publishers, Inc., pp. 77–94.

Once the underlying cause of the fever has been treated or antipyretic medications have been administered, the patient enters the defervescent stage. This stage is characterized by diaphoresis, vasodilation, and behavioral indications of excess warmth (Kluger, 1991; Bruce and Grove, 1992; Holtzclaw, 1992; Henker *et al.*, 1997; Shaffer, 1997).

Agent-Specific Patterns of Flu-Like Syndrome Presentation and Severity

It is important for nurses who administer biological agents to be able to recognize the patterns of presentation and severity of FLS that accompany specific biological agents. This knowledge will help nurses determine whether an FLS symptom is a side effect of biotherapy or indication of an infection for which the patient may need treatment. Consideration of agent-specific FLS patterns is also important in establishing the patient education plan, so patients may prepare themselves for the experience that might accompany a particular biotherapy regimen. Table 16.2 is a summary of FLS as seen with common biotherapeutic agents (Shelton and Turnbough, 1999).

Interferons

IFNs tend to cause FLS symptoms that are dose-dependent in occurrence and severity—particularly for the elderly, the very young, or those with concomitant illnesses (Skalla, 1996). IFNs are EPs that directly stimulate PGE2 synthesis, which explains the rapid onset of fever when these agents are administered (Bernheim, 1986; Haeuber, 1989). IFNs also may induce host cells to release IL-1 and TNF, causing a secondary initiation of FLS (Haeuber, 1989). With IFNs, the variations of FLS seen with

specific IFN types are probably caused by the differing immunologic effects of each agent.

IFN-α and IFN-β produce fevers of rapid onset (2 to 4 hours) that typically persist for 4 to 8 hours. These fevers may be preceded by mild chills and accompanied by headache and myalgias. In contrast, IFN-γ causes fevers that tend to peak at 6 to 12 hours and last substantially longer. Upper-respiratory symptoms occur within the first day for most patients, with severity being dose-dependent and variable with individual health tendencies, such as allergies. The symptoms are usually of short duration, lasting a few hours longer than fever (Haeuber, 1989).

The FLS symptom profile may also vary with the route and schedule of IFN administration. Continuous infusion produces less severe effects than intermittent therapy (Haeuber, 1989). Patients who receive IFN-α or IFN-β tend to develop tolerance to FLS with continued administration over time (tachyphylaxis), whereas this does not occur in patients who receive IFN-γ (Haeuber, 1989). In a recent study of bladder-instilled IFN-α, no FLS was noted, supporting the premise that topical cytokine bladder therapy may cause few systemic effects (Portillo *et al.*, 1997).

Hematopoietic Growth Factors

Hematopoietic growth factors (HGFs) have been used with increasing frequency during the past 8 years. Although they are generally associated with few adverse symptoms, FLS has been reported with high doses of **granulocyte-macrophage colony-stimulating factor (GM-CSF)**, oprelvekin (IL-11), and IL-3. Whether HGFs cause FLS depends on where in the hematopoietic sequence they have their effect and which types of cells they stimulate. It appears that most are not innately pyrogenic, but rather cause FLS through indirect pathways (Haeuber, 1989).

Table 16.2 Flu-like syndrome symptoms that occur as a side effect of common biological agents

Medication*	Dose Related Y/N	Headache	Fever	Chills	Arthralgias	Myalgias	Malaise	Nasal Stuffiness
Antithymocyte globulin	N	+	+	+	+	+	+	+
Cytomegalovirus	N	++	+	+	+	+	+	+
Immunoglobulin G			Rate-related	Rate-related		Rate-related		
Erythropoietin	N	+	+	NR	+	UK	NR	NR
Granulocyte colony-stimulating factor (G-CSF)	N	+	Mild	+	+	+	+	NR
Granulocyte-macrophage colony-stimulating factor G	N	++ Mild	++ Mod-Sev	++	++	++ Mod-Sev	++	+
Immunoglobulin	N	+++ Vary	+++ Severe	+	+	+	+	NR
Interferon	Y	++	+++	+++	++	+++ Severe	+++ Severe	+
Interleukin-2	Y	+++ Mild	+++	+++	++	++	+++	+
Interleukin-3	UK	+++	+++ Mild	+++	UK	+	UK	UK
Levamisole	N	+	++	+	+	+	++	NR
All-trans-retinoic acid	Y	+++	+	++	+++	+	NR	UK
Monoclonal antibodies (in general)	N	+	++	+	++	+	NR	NR
Plasma proteins: plasma protein fraction, albumin, plasmanate	N	++	+	+	+	+	+	+
Rituximab	N	++	+++	+++	NR	+	NR	+
Tumor necrosis factor	Y	+++	+++	+++	+	+++	+++	UK
Vaccines: influenza, pneumococcal, measles	N	+	+	+	+	+	+	UK

*Criteria for inclusion were medications that caused ≥3 symptoms of flu-like syndrome.
+, rare; ++, occasional; +++, frequent; UK, unknown; NR, not reported as an adverse effect in product information; Mod, moderate; Sev, severe; Vary, variable severity.

Source: Reprinted with permission from Shelton, B.K., and Turnbough, L. 1999. Flu-like syndrome. In Yarbro, C.H., Frogge, M.H., Goodman, M., and Groenwald, S. (ed). Cancer Symptom Management. 2nd edn, Boston, MA: Jones & Bartlett Publishers, Inc., pp. 77–94.

527

SINGLE-LINEAGE HEMATOPOIETIC GROWTH FACTORS

Erythropoietin, **granulocyte-colony stimulating factor (G-CSF)**, and IL-11 are primarily single-lineage HGFs that affect more mature precursor cells in the erythrocyte lineage, granulocyte lineage, and megakaryocytic lineage, respectively. Cells stimulated by these HGFs tend not to produce cytokines involved in the production of FLS; therefore, it is not surprising that these HGFs are rarely associated with FLS. Erythropoietin has caused FLS in a small number of patients when given by intravenous bolus (Tabbara, 1993; Kulzer et al., 1994). Because G-CSF and IL-11 do have some impact on early multilineage progenitor cells, they may occasionally cause low-grade fever or headache (Kanz et al., 1991; Tepler et al., 1996; Du and Williams, 1997).

MULTILINEAGE HEMATOPOIETIC GROWTH FACTORS

GM-CSF affects both the granulocyte and macrophage/monocyte lineages at higher levels in the hematopoietic sequence of events. Cells in the macrophage/monocyte line are well established as the source of many cytokines involved in fever causation and thus in the symptom pattern of FLS (Kanz, 1991; Grant and Heel, 1992). GM-CSF is generally associated with low-grade fevers (i.e., less than 38°C), although it may cause fevers to rise to 40°C (Haeuber, 1989). Patients who receive GM-CSF may also experience mild chills, transient headaches, and occasionally severe myalgias. These side effects may be more pronounced and more common when the agent is administered intravenously, although they can also appear with subcutaneous administration (Haeuber, 1989; Leonardi et al., 1998).

IL-3, sometimes known as multi-CSF, is a multilineage HGF that promotes the proliferation and differentiation of early multipotential progenitor cells. IL-3 enhances the release of TNF, which may account for its ability to cause FLS (Kanz, 1991; Kurzrock, 1991). Additionally, Gietema et al. (1992) found a dose-dependent increase in serum IL-6 after administration of IL-3, and they suggested that IL-6 may be responsible for the elevated temperatures associated with IL-3 therapy. Adverse effects caused by IL-3 are well characterized and appear to be triggered in the same manner as GM-CSF. Nearly all patients who receive IL-3 experience low-grade fevers accompanied by chills, and at higher dose levels, these side effects have been accompanied by mild headaches (Kurzrock, 1991).

Interleukin-2

IL-2 stimulates the proliferation, differentiation, and activation of T- and B-lymphocytes, natural killer cells, and thymocytes. Both *in vitro* and *in vivo* studies suggest that IL-2 itself is not pyrogenic, but rather induces cells such as T-lymphocytes and macrophages to release IFN-γ and TNF (Michie, 1988; Kintzel and Calis, 1991; Post-White, 1996; Wheeler, 1996). Thus, FLS is caused either directly by these substances or by pathways mediated by other EPs. It has been administered alone and in combination with other biological agents (e.g., IFNs), lymphokine-activated killer (LAK) cells and tumor-infiltrating lymphocytes.

Whether IL-2 is administered alone or in combination with other agents, FLS is a common side effect (Wheeler, 1996). Fever, chills, and rigors sometimes accompanied by myalgias and headache are nearly universal and appear within 2 to 4 hours after initiation of IL-2 therapy (Caliendo et al., 1992; Viele and Moran, 1992). Some FLS symptoms persist for up to 2 months after therapy (Caliendo et al., 1992). With the addition of LAK cells or tumor-infiltrating lymphocytes to IL-2 therapy, mild to severe chills and rigors tend to occur 30 minutes to 4 hours after the first infusion (Caliendo *et al.*, 1992; Viele and Moran, 1992). Although it is difficult to separate the side effects of multi-agent chemobiotherapy regimens from those of treatment with IL-2 alone, there appears to be an additive effect (Margolin *et al.*, 1989; Kintzel and Calis, 1991; Marincola *et al.*, 1995; Taneja *et al.*, 1995). When IL-2 is administered by continuous infusion for several days, FLS symptoms become more intense (Thompson, 1988; Marincola, 1994). Tolerance to FLS symptoms does not appear to develop over successive courses of IL-2 therapy and, in fact, may worsen (Kintzel and Calis, 1991; Caliendo *et al.*, 1993). Thus, the effects of dose, dose interval, rate of infusion, and duration of IL-2 therapy and IL-2-containing regimens on the occurrence and severity of FLS are even more pronounced than with other biological agents.

Monoclonal Antibodies

MABs have been used both diagnostically and therapeutically. Their use is associated with a cluster of FLS symptoms, including chills or rigors, fever, diaphoresis, myalgias, and arthralgias (Baquiran *et al.*, 1996).

With intravenous infusion, 3 distinct side-effect patterns emerge. Events occurring within the first hour of infusion usually indicate hypersensitivity (Haeuber, 1989; Baquiran *et al.*, 1996) or target-cell destruction, and late (i.e., 10-day to 2-week) effects are most likely a serum-sickness reaction (Haeuber, 1989; McKerrow, 1996). Recent reports from studies with rituximab (a MAB targeted toward the CD-20 marker on B-lymphocytes) suggest that FLS appearing within a few hours of MAB administration is probably related to the elimination of circulating target cells (i.e., tumor cells) during the infusion and have compared this effect with the leukocyte-agglutination–in-duced fevers sometimes seen during blood transfusions (Reff *et al.*, 1994). Delayed symptoms seem to be caused by the development of antibodies to MABs (Baquiran *et al.*, 1996). Upper-respiratory symptoms are infusion-related, occurring within 30 minutes to 2 hours of the infusion, and are less frequently observed after the first infusion (Dillman, 1988; Juric *et al.*, 1994; Isaacs *et al.*, 1996; IDEC Pharmaceuticals Corporation and Genentech, Inc., 1997). Infusion-related FLS symptoms may be ameliorated by slowing the infusion rate (IDEC Pharmaceuticals Corporation and Genentech, Inc., 1997).

Tumor Necrosis Factor

TNF, a secretory cytokine of activated monocytes/macrophages and lymphocytes, has a significant role in modulation of both immune and inflammatory responses. In animal studies, Dinarello (1988) observed a biphasic fever curve with TNF administration. The initial rise in temperature is probably caused by a direct effect of TNF on the hypothalamus, as mediated by PGE2; the second temperature spike is related to a subsequent increase in other circulating EPs such as IL-1 (Dinarello, 1988). Stimulation of TNF may also be a primary cause of the development of FLS during treatment with other biological agents.

TNF has been associated with moderately severe FLS. When administered intravenously, rigors occur within 10 to 15 minutes, and a high fever (i.e., 39°C to 40°C) occurs within 1 to 2 hours. When TNF is administered subcutaneously or intramuscularly, adverse effects are somewhat milder and delayed, with temperatures peaking between 2 and 10 hours after injection and remaining elevated for up to 20 hours. With both routes of administration, headaches and myalgias frequently accompany the development of fevers (Aulitzky, *et al.* 1991; Gamm, *et al.* 1991).

Retinoids

All-*trans*-retinoic acid and 9-*cis*-retinoic acid are retinoids licensed for treatment of acute progranulocytic leukemia and Kaposi's sarcoma, respectively. The action of retinoids includes prostaglandin synthesis and activation of IL-2, contributing to FLS associated with these biological agents. Toxicities are dose-related, with the predominant features including headache and arthralgias (Sporn, *et al.* 1994; Qasim *et al.*, 1995; Burke *et al.*, 1996).

Levamisole

Levamisole enhances the clinical activity of immunologically active cells such as monocytes, macrophages, and lymphocytes. The inflammatory-immune physiologic response is evident in the adverse-effect profile. The incidence and severity of fever, chills, headache, myalgias, and arthralgias can vary greatly (Dean, 1996). Grade 4 myalgias and arthralgias have been reported; however, mild FLS is more common. Symptoms usually occur within 12 to 24 hours of the start of treatment and resolve within 2 days after therapy is completed (Qasim *et al.*, 1995).

Immunoconjugates

The newest biotherapeutic agents used in cancer therapy are the cytotoxic fusion proteins that combine MABs or cytokines with cytotoxic agents. The only currently licensed agent in this classification is DAB389IL-2 (denileukin difitox, Ontak®; Ligand Pharmaceuticals). The adverse effects of these proteins are infusion-related and are similar to the effects of MABs

(Sievers *et al.*, 1997; Ligand Pharmaceuticals, 1999).

Assessment and Management of Biotherapy-Induced Flu-Like Syndrome

Assessment

Management of FLS induced by administration of biological agents begins with a thorough assessment of each patient's prior experience with FLS. This analysis includes determination of the timing (i.e., onset, duration, and frequency), setting, location, quality and quantity of the symptoms, associated symptoms, and factors that alleviate or aggravate symptoms. Factors that may exacerbate the severity of FLS (e.g., co-existing illnesses, age, performance status, and nutritional status) should also be evaluated (Sandstrom, 1996). This information will provide baseline data to be used later in judging the effectiveness of interventions and documenting patterns of symptoms.

KEY FACTORS TO BE ASSESSED

Determining the patient's understanding of the cause of the fever is an important factor in the management of FLS. Fletcher and Creten (1986) found that patients and family members were "overly" concerned about the bodily damage that could be caused by fever. In a study conducted in Norway to evaluate the knowledge and attitudes of patients regarding fever, Eskerud *et al.* (1991), found misunderstandings regarding regulation of body temperature to be common. Many of the subjects interviewed in the study thought that moderate fever in both adults and children was life threatening (Eskerud *et al.*, 1991). With regard to cancer, there is an added concern because many patients' initial presentation was fever or FLS, and they may view these symptoms as indicative of disease progression. Thus, it is important to assess the knowledge of the patient and family members regarding the symptoms associated with FLS and to provide information as needed. Reassurance that FLS is an expected side effect and not caused by disease progression can serve to allay fears (Sandstrom, 1996).

Assessment of the distress associated with FLS is an important component of symptom management and will help to identify the meaning of these symptoms to the patient and assist with their management (Rieker *et al.*, 1992). Physical comfort is subjective and is perceived differently by different patients. For example, a temperature of 38°C may be rated as "extremely distressful" by 1 patient but "not distressing at all" by another. The degree of distress caused by FLS may be very important to the decision to treat the adverse effect, because some researchers believe that these manifestations of immune stimulation are best not treated unless they are distressing (Holtzclaw, 1992; Kluger, 1992a).

A final key area that should be assessed in the patient who receives biotherapy is the risk of infection. Although biological agents cause fever and other FLS symptoms, not all fevers are related to therapy. This issue has caused some controversy in the medical literature, especially with respect to HGFs, because they are used to prevent infections in at-risk patients. Vreugdenhil *et al.* (1992) offer a list of criteria for restricting antibiotics in neutropenic patients receiving GM-CSF, given the known propensity of that agent to cause fever and associated symptoms. On the other hand, Khwaja *et al.* (1992) argue that it would be "injudicious" to withhold antibiotic coverage from neutropenic patients receiving GM-CSF. When FLS symptoms appear, it is critical for the nurse to analyze the specific characteristics for conformity with patterns expected from the biological agent administered. The nurse should always maintain a high index of suspicion that a fever may be of infectious etiology (Sergi, 1991).

Throughout the course of therapy, ongoing assessment of the presence and tolerance of FLS is made to determine the success of interventions to lessen side effects and to detect untoward events. Table 16.3 summarizes the most important elements involved in the assessment of the patient experiencing biotherapy-induced FLS (Haeuber, 1989; Sergi, 1991; Conrad and Horrell, 1995; Herzog *et al.*, 1995; Sandstrom, 1996).

TOXICITY GRADING OF FLS

There is little research specifically addressing severity scores for FLS. Some research protocols have developed toxicity scores to use in study reporting (Dillman, 1988; Margolin *et al.*, 1989; Chiron Corporation, 1992; Schering Corporation, 1992; Marincola *et al.*, 1995; American Hospital Formulary Service, 1996; Du and Williams, 1997; IDEC Pharmaceuticals Corporation and Genentech, Inc., 1997), but the specific criteria used to determine toxicity grades 1 through 4 are not available in the scientific literature. This lack of information about toxicity grade has occurred in part because of inconsistencies in the definition of "FLS cluster." The variability of severity for each specific symptom has also made it difficult to develop a severity index that is inclusive of the symptom cluster. The National Cancer Institute toxicity-grading criteria describe toxicity levels for individual symptoms within the group known as FLS (National Cancer Institute, 1988) but does not have toxicity-grading criteria for the syndrome as a whole. The National Cancer Institute toxicity-grading criteria for these symptoms are summarized in Table 16.4.

NURSING ASSESSMENT SCALES

There are only two published nursing assessment scales for FLS (White, 1992; Shelton and

Table 16.3   Key factors in the assessment of the patient experiencing biotherapy-induced FLS

Neurosensory
Headache pain—intensity or character (throbbing or dull ache), timing (continual or exacerbated with exertion), location (usually frontal)
Visual disturbances—blurred vision, diplopia, photophobia
Dizziness/vertigo—position when it occurs, other associated symptoms
Mental status changes
Emotional lability—dysphoria, euphoria
Musculoskeletal
Joint discomfort—at rest or with weight bearing, accompanying swelling, crepitus
Muscle aches—cramping, spasmotic or dull, location, exacerbating factors, alleviating factors
Inability to stand without lower back or leg pain
Degree of shivering
Dermatologic
Increased skin temperature, erythema
Skin dry or moist
Rash characteristics—color, raised or flat, pruritus, distribution
General
Body temperature—fever or subnormal temperature
Sensation of cold—chills, rigors
Laboratory Findings
Increased lactate dehydrogenase with rigors
Increased creatine kinase with rigors
Elevated erythrocyte sedimentation rate
Hyperglycemia
Increased blood urea nitrogen
Increased creatinine
Leukocytosis

Source: Reprinted with permission from Shelton, B.K., and Turnbough, L. 1999. Flu-like syndrome. In Yarbro, C.H., Frogge, M.H., Goodman, M., and Groenwald, S. (eds). *Cancer Symptom Management* 2nd edn. Boston, MA: Jones & Bartlett Publishers, Inc., pp. 77–94. Table 7.4: p. 82.

Turnbough, 1999). White (1992) used a modified National Cancer Institute toxicity-grading scale with an unstructured interview. Shelton and Turnbough (1996) suggest that patients rate the severity of each symptom and the significance of the distress it causes using a specially designed log (Figure 16.2). This quantification of FLS is modeled after existing nausea and vomiting scales but has not been validated through nursing research.

Management

The first issue to consider with regard to the treatment of FLS associated with biotherapy is whether to "manage" the symptoms at all and, if so, under which circumstances. There is a long-standing controversy regarding the potential therapeutic benefits of fever (Kluger *et al.*, 1998; Henker, 1999). Fever has an ancient phylogenetic history suggestive of an important adaptive response that allows the infected host's immune defenses to respond more effectively to pathogens. In a review of the literature regarding the effects of fever on immunologic defenses, Roberts (1991) concluded that elevated temperatures appear to improve T-lymphocyte responses and increase the sensitization and activation of mononuclear leukocytes. Gietema *et al.* (1992) suggest that fever associated with administration of IL-3 may be "interpreted as a sign of increases in host defenses rather than merely as an adverse effect."

Despite the knowledge that fever is an adaptive response to infection, it cannot be assumed that fever enhances the antineoplastic or immunomodulatory aspects of biotherapy (Kluger, 1992a; Shaffer, 1997). Kluger (1992a), in questioning the practice of identifying fever as a side effect of biotherapy and automatically treating it, wrote:

> Since many tumors seem more sensitive to increases in temperature than normal cells are, I suggest that before fever in patients on treat-

Table 16.4   National Cancer Institute's common toxicity grading criteria for flu-like syndrome

Toxicity	Grade				
	1	2	3	4	5
Headache	None	Mild	Moderate or severe but transient	Unrelenting and severe	—
Aching pain (muscle or bone)	None	Mild, transient; does not interfere with casual daily activity	Moderate; interferes with usual daily activity	Severe; interrupts usual daily activity	Intractable
Fever	None	>38.5°C	>39°C	>40°C	—
Chills	None	Mild, transient	Moderate	Severe	Intractable
Malaise	None	25% of time	50% of time	75% of time	100% of time
Fatigue/asthenia	None	25% of time	50% of time	75% of time	100% of time
Anorexia	None	Able to eat normal meals, loss of hunger	Able to eat 2 meals/day with loss of hunger	Able to eat 1 meal/day with loss of hunger	Unable to eat a meal, some nutritional fluids tolerated

Source: National Cancer Institute. 1993. NCI Common Toxicity Criteria, in *Investigator's Handbook*. Bethesda, MD: *National Institutes of Health—National Cancer Institute*, Appendix 12.

ment with biological response modifiers is "treated," careful consideration be given to the possibility that the fever may be helping the patient to rid himself or herself of the tumor.

This consideration argues for a measured response to FLS in biotherapy (Mackowiak and Plaisance, 1998). Holtzclaw (1992), after studying fever in critically ill patients, advocates a "clarification of the therapeutic goal" before implementing a nursing response to fever. Styrt and Sugarman (1990) offer the following indications for the suppression of fever: (1) risk of damage to the central nervous system (CNS); (2) potential for tissue hypoxia and cardiovascular compromise; and (3) comfort of the patient.

The first criteria for fever suppression (i.e.,

risk for CNS damage) is of particular importance for the patient with neurological problems and for pediatric patients at known risk for febrile seizures. Bone marrow transplant patients receiving busulfan also have a lower seizure threshold and may benefit from fever suppression.

Therapeutic suppression of fever in patients at risk for cardiac or pulmonary dysfunction is especially relevant to cancer patients, many of whom are elderly and have co-existing health conditions (Henker, 1999). There is considerable potential to aggravate one of these disorders by the increased basal metabolic rate, tachycardia, and the increased oxygen demand associated with fevers and chills resulting from the administration of biological agents (Henker, 1999). For every increase in temperature of 1°C, it has been estimated that the metabolic rate

Symptom Documentation Log

Patient Name: _____

Instructions Use this chart daily to record the symptoms that you are experiencing. Rate the symptoms according to severity using a scale of 1 to 4 (see below). Under "Interventions," record what you did for relief, and under "Comments," whether or not it helped. Share this log with your nurse or physician each week.

Date	Symp-toms	Rating	Interventions	Comments

Codes for symptoms present

F = Fever

C = Chills

HA = Headache

M = Muscle aches

J = Joint pain

NC = Nasal congestion/cough

Severity rating for symptoms

1 = Able to carry on daily activities normally

2 = Symptoms mildly affect my day

3 = Severe symptoms, but gained relief after intervention

4 = Severe symptoms; no relief gained

Phone Numbers

Nurse: _____ Phone: _____

Physician: _____ Phone: _____

Home-Care Nurse: _____ Phone: _____

Other: _____ Phone: _____

Comments

Patient's Signature: _____ Date: _____

Nurse's Signature: _____ Date: _____

Figure 16.2 This quantification of FLS is modeled after existing nausea and vomiting scales, but has not been validated through nursing research.

Source: Reprinted with permission from Shelton, B.K., and Turnbough, L. 1999. Flu-like syndrome. In Yarbro, C.H., Frogge, M.H., Goodman, M., and Groenwald, S. (eds). *Cancer Symptom Management* 2nd edn. Boston, MA: Jones & Bartlett Publishers, Inc., pp. 77–94.

increases by 10%, with a proportionate increase in tissue-oxygen requirements (Rosenthal and Silverstein, 1988; Bruce and Grove, 1992; Shaffer, 1997). In a study of fever among Gambian children, Stettler *et al.* (1992) calculated that the caloric cost of fever is 11.7% for each 1°C rise in temperature. Holtzclaw (1990) found that strenuous shivering caused by administration of amphotericin-B caused a fall in oxygen saturation from approximately 98% to less than 80%. Dyspnea and labored breathing were also seen in patients that experienced shivering (Holtzclaw, 1990). An added metabolic consideration for cancer patients is that fever appears to stimulate muscle-protein degradation and causes a negative nitrogen balance (Shelton and Turnbough, 1999). This may be important when a person is in a debilitated or malnourished state and receives a biological agent associated with substantial incidence of FLS.

The final consideration outlined by Styrt and Sugarman (1990) is comfort, an issue of prime importance to nurses. There are both psychological and physical components to comfort; however, the relationship of FLS to comfort has not been well studied. Styrt and Sugarman (1990) point out the ambiguity of using antipyretics for the "symptomatic treatment" of fever because some patients do not find the fever uncomfortable. Certainly, some elements of FLS, including myalgias and headaches, may cause patients discomfort. It is possible that the use of antipyretics may cause a cycle of chills and diaphoresis that is ultimately more uncomfortable for the patient than experiencing a moderate fever. Until such issues are scrutinized, assessing the patient's physical comfort and perception of distress as it relates to FLS remains a priority when assessing the need for symptomatic relief.

The management of biotherapy-related adverse effects will depend on a variety of patient factors, protocol requirements, and physician preferences. In most investigative biotherapy regimens, management strategies are strictly regimented to better evaluate the immunologic effects of the agent. Despite concerns about the negative physiologic effects of abrogating FLS, one must always consider the patient's perception and tolerance for these adverse effects and whether symptom management will influence the patient's ability to cope with and continue therapy. Table 16.5 is a review of approaches to the management of biotherapy-related side effect of FLS.

MANIPULATION OF THE TREATMENT

One approach to treating FLS is altering the treatment plan, although this option may be

Table 16.5   Approaches to the management of biotherapy-related flu-like syndrome

Treatment Manipulation
  Dose
  Schedule
  Route
  Rate of administration
Medications
  Prophylactic
  For fever/myalgias: prostaglandin inhibitors, nonsteroidal anti-inflammatory drugs, (ibuprofen, indomethacin), acetaminophen, aspirin
  For chills/rigors: centrally acting agents, meperidine, other narcotics
  For headache: antihistamines, prostaglandin inhibitors
Nursing Measures
  Extremity wraps
  "Bundling"
  Increase ambient temperature
  Hydration
  Relaxation and guided imagery techniques
  Patient/family education, reassurance

limited by the research protocol. The decision to alter the treatment plan rests with the physician, although nurses can have significant input in deciding how to most effectively implement therapy. Thompson *et al.* (1988) examined the toxicity of IL-2 given at different dose levels by either a 24-hour continuous intravenous infusion or 3-hour intravenous bolus infusions. They found that independent of dose, side effects were substantially more severe with continuous infusions. Daily administration of IFN-α or IFN-β is associated with decreasing incidence and severity of symptoms after 7 to 10 days (Haeuber, 1989). With intermittent (1 or 2 times/week) or cyclic (3 or 4 times/week) administration, however, tachyphylaxis may not occur (Quesada, 1986; Skalla, 1996). Decreasing the rate of intravenous administration of MABs also diminishes side effects (Dillman, 1988, IDEC Pharmaceuticals Corporation and Genentech, Inc. 1997).

Nurses involved in the treatment of patients receiving biological agents should be cognizant of the potential for alleviating FLS through manipulation of the route or schedule of the agent. Many clinicians recommend giving IFN or HGF injections at night so that premedication can be taken and patients can hopefully sleep through the worst of the adverse effects (Herzog *et al.*, 1995; Rieger, 1996; Skalla, 1996). Nurses should monitor patients closely for signs that changes in the administration plan have been beneficial.

MEDICATIONS

The administration of supportive medications provides another approach to controlling biotherapy-related side effects. Prostaglandin inhibitors, antipyretic analgesics, and antihistamines may be effective in the control of FLS (Conrad and Horrell, 1995; Herzog *et al.*, 1995; Rieger, 1996; Sandstrom, 1996; Henker, 1999). Prostaglandin inhibitors such as aspirin and nonsteroidal anti-inflammatory agents block

the synthesis of prostaglandins, both at the hypothalamus and in the muscle tissue. Through this mechanism, they may be effective in controlling fever and other symptoms associated with FLS. Antipyretic analgesics such as acetaminophen alleviate fever and reduce the severity of discomfort from myalgias or headache. Antihistamines block mast-cell degranulation, decreasing vasodilation, thereby reducing rhinitis and headache. The vasodilatory effects of FLS and the loss of fluid through diaphoresis necessitates generous fluid-replacement therapy for these patients as well.

To prevent side effects, many clinicians routinely prescribe premedication before biological agents are administered. Other clinicians use medications as infrequently as possible to allow for determination of toxic effects or to avoid a possible adverse effect on the desired biological activity of the agent (Kluger, 1992a). In addition, there is evidence that the elevated temperatures that frequently occur with biotherapy may be intrinsically involved in the biological effect of the agent or may be important in activation of the agent (Dinarello, 1986; Shaffer, 1997). Even medications as seemingly innocuous as ibuprofen and acetaminophen may have adverse effects on the kidneys and liver (Murphy, 1992; Shaffer, 1997). Issacs (1990) examined the use of antipyretics in a university-based tertiary care center and found that administration orders were often written imprecisely and without clear consideration of the therapeutic goal, resulting in sporadic and inconsistent patterns of administration. In caring for patients who receive biotherapy, nurses should approach the use of these medications in a clear, goal-directed manner.

A novel approach to abrogating adverse effects of the cytokine cascade triggered by some biological agents is the use of a new agent that is currently called CNI-1493 (Cytokine Networks, Inc., 1998). In some studies, this agent is combined with IL-2. CNI-1493 appears to block the pro-inflammatory cytokines without affecting IL-2's indirect effect on the tumor (Cytokine Networks, Inc., 1998).

Chills related to the administration of biological agents can be quite uncomfortable. Meperidine is often effective in controlling this particular side effect (Conrad and Horrell, 1995; Herzog *et al.*, 1995; Rieger, 1996; Sandstrom, 1996). Hydromorphone (Herzog *et al.*, 1995; Rieger, 1996; Shelton and Turnbough, 1999), morphine (Haeuber, 1989), and diazepam (Beattie and Smyth, 1988; Haeuber, 1989) have also been used to abrogate chills. Drawing on the experience of using these agents to control rigors, some recommend giving meperidine prophylactically or therapeutically to relieve chills (Spross, 1988). As with antipyretics, the decision to use meperidine should be based on the type of biological agent administered, its association with chills, a thorough assessment of the patient's experience with that agent, and any additional side effects anticipated from the use of meperidine.

NURSING MEASURES

Nursing care for the individual who is experiencing FLS as a result of biotherapy is directed toward determining effective nonpharmacologic means of symptom management. For example, it may be possible to forestall the development of chills by applying warm blankets, encouraging the patient to wear warmer clothes, or increasing the ambient air temperature during and after administration of biotherapy. The body shivers to generate the necessary heat to match the altered thermoregulatory set point. When the body's baseline temperature is warmer, there is less temperature gradient between the core temperature and the hypothalamic set point, allowing temperature elevation without the discomfort and caloric expenditure of shivering.

Abbey *et al.* (1973) and Rutledge and Holtzclaw (1988) evaluated the effect of wrapping the extremities with several layers of terrycloth towels to diminish the shivering response of patients at risk for this side effect. The goal of this intervention is to stop shivering by warming the extremities, where there is an abundance of thermosensory nerve endings involved in the initiation of shivering (Holtzclaw, 1992). Although bundling the patient who is febrile may appear counterproductive, it is important to remember that the fever caused by biological agents is self-limiting and rarely reaches life-threatening levels (Styrt and Sugarman, 1990; Kluger, 1992b; Shaffer, 1997).

PATIENT EDUCATION

Educating patients and families in the management of FLS is a critical intervention. Whereas an understanding of the pathophysiology of FLS may not relieve symptoms, most patients and families will feel more in control of their treatment and their lives with this knowledge. The experience of fever and chills is often frightening; however, patient education can resolve misunderstandings about these symptoms. One patient-education guide has been published by Shelton and Turnbough (1999). It is critical that patients be instructed to report extremely elevated temperatures not being controlled with antipyretics or fevers unrelated to the normal patterns.

Research

The majority of information regarding biotherapy-related FLS symptoms and its management has been generated from clinical trials of biological agents. Because symptom management is an area of professional nursing expertise, it is important that nurses who work with biotherapy patients direct their research skills toward describing the FLS symptom cluster, determining its patterns with the various agents, evaluating tools to quantify symptoms, and organizing clinical studies to develop effective methods of management (Strauman, 1988; Haeuber, 1989; Sandstrom, 1996; Henker, 1999). In addition, studies to determine the distress associated with these symptoms and the impact of symptoms on quality of life should be given high priority (Stetz et al., 1994; Farrell, 1996).

Once symptoms are described and patterns defined, clinical measurement is the next logical step. The severity of fever can be measured by checking the patient's temperature by mouth, rectum, auditory canal, or skin. Headache, myalgias, or arthralgias can be quantified by measuring associated pain. However, measuring chills (i.e., shivering) is more difficult. The two most common methods of measuring chills documented in the literature are electromyographic measurement and observation of shivering stages. There is limited literature about visual measurement systems, and mechanical measurement systems such as palpation of tremors are less well developed. Abbey et al. (1973) developed an ordinal clinical assessment scale based on the work of others that evaluated shivering severity by observing stages of muscle involvement. The scale, which was adapted by Holtzclaw (1993) for use with post operative cardiac patients, assesses shivering as follows:

0 = no visible or palpable shivering
1 = palpable mandibular vibration or electrocardiograph artifact
2 = visible fasciculation of the head or neck
3 = visible fasciculation of the pectorals and trunk
4 = generalized shaking of the entire body, with or without teeth chattering

Toxicity scales utilized in clinical trials to grade severity of symptoms may also be useful in the clinical setting but may not be sufficiently discriminatory for research purposes.

Prevention and control of chills is another important area for nursing research. There are no published accounts of nursing research of biotherapy-related FLS, but there is literature that offers models for how nurses can approach this subject (Abbey, 1973; Morgan, 1990; Caruso et al., 1992). Interventions may be grouped into two major areas: pharmacological measures and physical measures. Perhaps the most applicable example of such research is the work by Holtzclaw (1990) on the use of extremity wraps to control shivering caused by the pyrogenic drug amphotericin B. In her study, Holtzclaw compared the experiences of a control group and a treatment group who had their arms and legs wrapped with towels to insulate the dominant skin thermosensors during a standard amphotericin B infusion. The end points that Holtzclaw compared were the duration and degree of shivering, total meperidine dosage during the amphotericin-B infusion, and myocardial oxygen consumption. This study may be used as a model to determine the effectiveness of interventions that attempt to control shivering as a symptom of biological agent administration.

Summary

The constellation of symptoms known as FLS is a frequent problem for patients who undergo biotherapy, and the identification and management of this adverse effect is within the domain of professional nursing practice. Nurses caring for patients receiving biological agents must continue to evaluate the incidence of FLS and the severity and distress caused by the symptoms, and to actively participate in decisions concerning treatment of FLS. Research in the area of biotherapy-related FLS has remained limited despite the fact that biological agents have been in use for more than a decade. To date, evaluation and management of shivering has been the most thoroughly researched topic related to biotherapy-induced FLS (Holtzclaw, 1993). As part of our mission to enhance quality of life for patients with cancer, nurses must take a more active role in addressing this problematic adverse effect of biotherapy.

References

Abbey, J., Andrews, C., Avigliano, K., *et al.* 1973. A pilot study: The control of shivering during hypothermia by a clinical nursing measure. *Journal of Neurosurgical Nursing* 5(2): 78–88.

American Hospital Formulary Service. 1996. *AHFS 96 Drug Information*. Bethesda, MD: American Society of Hospital Pharmacists, Inc.

Aulitzky, W., Tilg, H., Gastl, G., *et al.* 1991. Recombinant tumour necrosis factor alpha administered subcutaneously or intramuscularly for treatment of advanced malignant disease: A phase I trial. *European Journal of Cancer* 27(4): 462–467.

Baracos, V., Rodemann, H.P., Dinarello, C.A., *et al.* 1983. Stimulation of muscle protein degradation and prostaglandin E2 release by leukocytic pyrogen (interleukin-1). *New England Journal of Medicine* 308: 553–558.

Baquiran, D.C., Dantis, L., and McKerrow, J. 1996. Monoclonal antibodies: Innovations in diagnosis and therapy. *Seminars in Oncology Nursing* 12(2): 130–141.

Beattie, G., and Smyth, J. 1988. Diazepam ablates the constitutional side effects of gamma IFN. *Medical Oncology, Tumor, and Pharmacotherapeutics* 5(2): 129–130.

Bernheim, H. 1986. Is prostaglandin E2 involved in the pathogenesis of fever? Effects of interleukin-1 on the release of prostaglandins. *Yale Journal of Biology and Medicine* 59(2): 151–158.

Bligh, J. 1982. Thermoregulation: Its change during infection with endotoxin-producing microorganisms. In Milton, A. (ed). *Pyretics and Antipyretics*. New York: Springer-Verlag, pp. 5–24.

Brophy, L., and Sharp, E.J. 1992. Physical symptoms of combination biotherapy: A quality of life issue. *Oncology Nursing Forum* 8(suppl): 25–30.

Bruce, J., and Grove, S. 1992. Fever: Pathology and treatment. *Critical Care Nurse* 12(1): 40–49.

Burke, M.B., Wilkes, G.M., and Ingersen, K. (eds). 1996. *Cancer Chemotherapy, A Nursing Process Approach*, 2nd edn. Boston, MA: Jones & Bartlett Publishers, Inc.

Caliendo, G., Joyce, D., and Altmiller, M.C. 1992. Nursing guidelines and discharge planning for patients receiving recombinant interleukin-2. *Seminars in Oncology Nursing* 9(3 suppl 1): 25–31.

Caruso, C., Hadley, B., Shukla, R., *et al.* 1992. Cooling effects and comfort of four cooling blanket temperatures in humans with fever. *Nursing Research* 41(2): 68–72.

Cerami, A. 1992. Inflammatory cytokines. *Clinical Immunology and Immunopathology* 62(1): S3–S10.

Chiron Corporation. 1992. Proleukin® Aldesleukin for injection. Emeryville, CA: Chiron Therapeutics.

Coceani, F., and Akarsu, E.S. 1998. Prostaglandin E2 in the pathogenesis of fever. An update. *Annals of the New York Academy of Sciences* 856: 76–82.

Coceani, F., Bishai, I., Lees, J., *et al.* 1986. Prostaglandin E2 and fever: A continuing debate. *Yale Journal of Biology and Medicine* 59(2): 169–174.

Conrad, K.J., and Horrell, C.J. (eds) 1995. *Biotherapy. Recommendations for Nursing Course Content and Clinical Practicum*. Pittsburgh, PA: Oncology Nursing Press.

Craig, T.J., Moecki, J.K., and Donnelly, A. 1995. Noncompliance with immunotherapy secondary to adverse effects (letter, comments). *Annals of Allergy, Asthma, and Immunology* 75(3): 290.

Cytokine Networks, Inc. 1998. *CNI-1493: A Novel Small Molecule Cytokine Inhibitor*. Seattle, WA: Cytokine Networks Inc.

Dascombe, M. 1986. The pharmacology of fever. *Progress in Neurobiology* 25(4): 327, 373.

Dean, G.E. 1995. Immunomodulator, differentiation agents, and vaccines. In Rieger, P.T. (ed). *Biother-*

apy: A Comprehensive Overview. Boston, MA: Jones and Bartlett Publishers, Inc., pp. 177–192.

Dillman, J.B. 1988. Toxicity of monoclonal antibodies in treatment of cancer. *Seminars in Oncology Nursing* 4: 107–111.

Dinarello, C.A., Cannon, J.G., and Wolff, S.M. 1988. New concepts on the pathogenesis of fever. *Review of Infectious Diseases* 10: 128–189.

Du, X., and Williams, D. 1997. Interleukin 11: Review of molecular, cell biology, and clinical use. *Blood* 89(11): 3897–3908.

Eskerud, J., Hafvedt, B., and Laerum, E. 1991. Fever: Knowledge, perception, and attitudes: Results from a Norwegian population study. *Family Practice* 8(1): 32–36.

Farrell, M. 1996. Nursing opportunities in biotherapy. *Seminars in Oncology Nursing* 12(2): 82–87.

Fletcher, J., and Creten, D. 1986. Perceptions of fever among adults in a family-practice setting. *The Journal of Family Practice* 22(5): 427–430.

Gamm, H., Lindemann, A., Mertelsman, R., *et al.* 1991. Phase I trial of recombinant human tumour necrosis factor alpha in patients with advanced malignancy. *European Journal of Cancer* 27(7): 856–863.

Gietema, J., Postmus, P., Biesma, B., *et al.* 1992. Acute-phase response in patients given rhIL-3 after chemotherapy (letter to the editor). *Lancet* 339: 1616–1617.

Grant, S., and Heel, R. 1992. Recombinant granulocyte-macrophage colony-stimulating factor (GM-CSF): A review of its pharmacological properties and prospective role in the management of myelosuppression. *Drug Evaluation* 43(4): 516–560.

Haeuber, D. 1989. Recent advances in the management of biotherapy-related side effects: Flu-like syndrome. *Oncology Nursing Forum* 16(6) (suppl): 35–41.

Henker, R. 1999. Evidenced-based practice: Fever-related interventions. *American Journal of Critical Care* 8(1): 481–487.

Henker, R., Kramer, D., and Rogers, S. 1997. Fever. *AACN Clinical Issues in Critical Care* 8(3): 351–367.

Herzog, P.J., Lorenzi, V.G., Sandstrom, K.S., *et al.* 1995. Biotherapy. In Gross, J., Johnson, B.L. (eds). *Handbook of Oncology Nursing,* 2nd edn. Boston, MA: Jones & Bartlett Publishers, Inc., pp. 94–122.

Hirano, T. 1992. Interleukin-6 and its relationship to inflammation and disease. *Clinical Immunology and Immunopathology* 62(1): S60–S65.

Holtzclaw, B. 1990. Control of febrile shivering during amphotericin-B therapy. *Oncology Nursing Forum* 17(4): 521–524.

Holtzclaw, B. 1992. The febrile response in critical care: State of the science. *Heart and Lung* 21(5): 482–501.

Holtzclaw, B. 1993. The shivering response. In Fitzpatrick, J., and Stevenson, J. (eds). *Annual Review of Nursing Research* New York: Springer Publishing Co., pp. 31–55.

IDEC Pharmaceuticals Corporation and Genentech, Inc. 1997. *Rituxan® Rituximab (G48097-RO [544]).* San Diego, CA: IDEC Pharmaceuticals Corporation, and South San Francisco, CA: Genentech, Inc.

Issacs, S., Axelrod, P., and Lorber, B. 1990. Antipyretic orders in a university hospital. *The American Journal of Medicine* 88: 31–35.

Isaacs, J.D., Manna, V.K., Rapson, N., *et al.* 1996. CAMPATH-1H in rheumatoid arthritis—An intravenous dose-ranging study. *British Journal of Rheumatology* 35(3): 231–240.

Juric, J.G., Scheinberg, D.A., and Houghton, A.N. 1994. Monoclonal antibody therapy of cancer. In Pinedo, H.M., Longo, D.L., and Chabner, B.A. (eds). *Cancer Chemotherapy and Biological Response Modifiers.* New York, NY: Elsevier, pp. 152–175.

Kanz, L., Lindemann, M., Oster, W., *et al.* 1991. Hematopoietins in clinical oncology. *American Journal of Clinical Oncology* 14(suppl 1): S27–S33.

Karunaweera, N., Grau, G., Gamage, P., *et al.* 1992. Dynamics of fever and serum levels of tumor necrosis factor are closely associated during clinical paroxysms in plasmodium vivax malaria. *Pro-*

ceedings of the National Academy of Sciences USA 89: 3200–3203.

Khwaja, A., Chopra, R., Goldstone, A., et al. 1992. (letter to the editor). Lancet 339: 1617.

Kintzel, P., and Calis, K. 1991. Recombinant interleukin-2: A biological response modifier. Clinical Pharmacy 10: 110–128.

Kluger, M. 1991. Fever: Role of pyrogens and cryogens. Physiological Reviews 71(1): 93–127.

Kluger, M. 1992a. Drugs for childhood fever (letter to the editor). Lancet 339: 70.

Kluger, M. 1992b. Fever revisited. Pediatrics 90(6): 846–850.

Kluger, M.J., Kozak, W., Conn, C.A., et al. 1998. Role of fever in disease. Annals of the New York Academy of Sciences 856: 224–233.

Kulzer, P., Schaefer, R.M., Krahn, R., et al. 1994. Effectiveness and safety of recombinant human erythropoietin (rHuEPO) in the treatment of anemia of chronic renal failure in nondialysis patients. European Multicentre Study Group. International Journal of Artificial Organs 17(4): 195–202.

Kurzrock, R., Talpaz, M., Estrow, Z., et al. 1991. Phase I study of recombinant human interleukin-3 in patients with bone-marrow failure. Journal of Clinical Oncology 9(7): 1241–1250.

Leonardi, V., Danova, M., Fincato, G., et al. 1998. Interleukin-3 in the treatment of chemotherapy-induced thrombocytopenia. Oncology Reports 5(6): 1459–1464.

Ligand Pharmaceuticals, Inc. 1999. Prescribing information for Ontak® (denileukin difitox). San Diego, CA: Ligand Pharamceuticals.

Luheshi, G.N. 1998. Cytokines and fever: Mechanisms and sites of action. Annals of the New York Academy of Sciences 856: 83–89.

Mackowiak, P.A., and Plaisance, K.F. 1998. Benefits and risks of antipyretic therapy. Annals of the New York Academy of Sciences USA 856: 214–223.

Margolin, K., Rayner, A., Hawkins, M., et al. 1989. Interleukin-2 and lymphokine-activated killer-cell therapy of solid tumors: Analysis of toxicity and management guidelines. Journal of Clinical Oncology 7(4): 486–498.

Marincola, F.M. 1994. Biologic Therapy of Cancer Updates: Interleukin-2. Philadelphia, PA: JB Lippincott. pp. 1–16.

Marincola, F.M., White, D.E., Wise, A.P., et al. 1995. Combination therapy with interferon alfa-2a and interleukin-2 for the treatment of metastatic cancer. Journal of Clinical Oncology 13: 1110–1122.

Michie, H., Eberlein, T., Spriggs, D., et al. 1988. Interleukin-2 initiates metabolic responses associated with critical illness in humans. Annals of Surgery 208(4): 493–503.

Murphy, K. 1992. Acetaminophen and ibuprophen: Fever control and overdose. Pediatric Nursing 18(4): 428–431, 433.

National Cancer Institute. 1988. Investigator's Handbook: Cancer Therapy Evaluation Program. Bethesda, MD: National Cancer Institute.

Portillo, J., Martin, B., Hernandez, R., et al. 1997. Results of 43 months' follow-up of a double-blind, randomized clinical trial using intravescial interferon alpha-2b in the prophylaxis of stage pT1 transitional-cell carcinoma of the bladder. Urology 49(2): 187–190.

Post-White, J. 1996. The immune system. Seminars in Oncology Nursing 12(2): 89–96.

Qasim, M., Marlton, P., and Kurzrock, R. 1995. Biological therapy: Hematopoietic growth factors, retinoids, and monoclonal antibodies. In Pazdur, R. (ed). Medical Oncology. A Comprehensive Review, 2nd edn. Huntington, NY: PRR, pp. 587–597.

Quesada, J.R., Talpaz, M., Rios, A., et al. 1986. Clinical toxicity of interferons in cancer patients: A review. Journal of Clinical Oncology 4(2): 234–239.

Reff, M.E., Carner, K., and Chambers, K.S. 1994. Depletion of B cells in vivo by a chimeric mouse human monoclonal antibody to CD20. Blood 83: 435–445.

Rieger, P.T. 1996. Biotherapy. In Burke, M.B., Wilkes, G.M., and Ingersen, K. (eds). Cancer Chemotherapy. A Nursing Process Approach, 2nd edn. Boston, MA: Jones & Bartlett Publishers, Inc., pp. 43–73.

Rieker, P.P., Clark, E.J., and Fogelberg, P.R. 1992. Perceptions of quality of life and quality of care for patients with cancer receiving biological therapy. *Oncology Nursing Forum* 19: 433–440.

Roberts, N. 1991. Impact of temperature elevation on immunologic defenses. *Reviews of Infectious Diseases* 13: 462–472.

Rosenberg, S.A., Yang, J.C., Topalian, S.L., *et al.* 1994. Treatment of 283 consecutive patients with metastatic melanoma or renal-cell cancer using high-dose bolus interleukin-2. *Journal of the American Medical Association* 271: 907–913.

Rosenthal, T.C., and Silverstein, D.A. 1988. Fever: What to do and what not to do. *Postgraduate Medicine* 83(8): 75–84.

Rutledge, D., and Holtzclaw, B. 1988. Amphotericin-B-induced shivering in patients with cancer: A nursing approach. *Heart and Lung* 17(4): 432–440.

Sandstrom, S.K. 1996. Nursing management of patients receiving biological therapy. *Seminars in Oncology Nursing* 12(2): 152–162.

Saper, C.B. 1998. Neurobiological basis of fever. *Annals of the New York Academy of Sciences USA* 856: 90–94.

Schering-Plough Corporation. 1992. *Intron®-A Interferon alfa-2b Patient Guide*. Kenilworth, NJ: Schering-Plough Corporation.

Sergi, J.S. 1991. Issue 1. The physiology of the flu-like syndrome and the cardiopulmonary and renal symptoms associated with BRM therapy. *Biological Response Modifiers, Perspectives for Oncology Nurses*. San Francisco, CA: Professional Healthcare: 4–10.

Shaffer, C. 1997. The chilling truth about fever. *1997 AACN National Teaching Institute Proceedings*. Aliso Viejo, CA: AACN Corp. (audiotape).

Shelton, B.K. 1998. Biotherapy and biotherapeutic agents: Biological response modifiers. In Kuhn, M.A. (ed). *Pharmacotherapeutics: A Nursing Process Approach,* 4th edn. Philadelphia, PA: FA Davis Co., pp. 830–846.

Shelton, B.K., and Turnbough, L. 1999. Flu-like syndrome. In Yarbro, C.H., Frogge, M.H., Goodman, M., and Groenwald, S. (eds). *Cancer Symptom Management* 2nd edn. Boston, MA: Jones & Bartlett Publishers, Inc., pp. 77–94.

Sievers, E.L., Applebaum, F.A., Spielberger, R.T., *et al.* 1997. Selective ablation of acute myeloid leukemia using an anti-CD33 calicheamicin immunoconjugate. *Blood* 10: 504a.

Skalla, K. 1996. The interferons. *Seminars in Oncology Nursing* 12(2): 97–105.

Sporn, M.B., Roberts, A.B., and Goodman, D.S. 1994. *The Retinoids: Biology, Chemistry, and Medicine,* 2nd edn. New York, NY: Raven Press.

Spross, J. 1988. Fever. In Baird, S.B. (ed). *Decision-making in Oncology Nursing*. Philadelphia, PA: BC Decker, pp. 82–83.

Stettler, N., Schutz, Y., Whitehead, R., *et al.* 1992. Effects of malaria and fever on energy metabolism in Gambian children. *Pediatric Research* 31(2): 101–106.

Stetz, K.M., Haberman, M.R., Holcombe, J., *et al.* 1994. Oncology Nursing Society research priorities survey. *Oncology Nursing Forum* 22: 957–964.

Strauman, J.J. 1992. Issue 3. Strategies for managing symptoms: Biological response modifiers. *Perspectives for Oncology Nurses*. San Francisco, CA: Professional Healthcare: 4–10.

Styrt, B., and Sugarman, B. 1990. Antipyresis and fever. *Archives of Internal Medicine* 153: 298–304.

Tabbara, I. 1993. Erythropoietin: Biology and clinical applications. *Archives of Internal Medicine* 153: 298–304.

Taneja, S.S., Pierce, W., Figlin, R., *et al.* 1994. Management of disseminated kidney cancer. *Urologic Clinics of North America* 21: 625–637.

Tepler, I., Elias, L., Smith, J.W., *et al.* 1996. A randomized placebo-controlled trial of recombinant human interleukin-11 in cancer patients with severe thrombocytopenia due to chemotherapy. *Blood* 87(9): 3607–3614.

Thompson, J., Lee, D., Lindgren, C., *et al.* 1988.

Influence of dose and duration of infusion of interleukin-2 on toxicity and immunomodulation. *Journal of Clinical Oncology* 6(4): 669–678.

Viele, C.S., and Moran, T.A. 1993. Nursing management of the nonhospitalized patient receiving recombinant interleukin-2. *Seminars in Oncology Nursing* 9(3 suppl 1): 20–24.

Vlachoyi, Annopoulos, P.G., Tsiferetaki, N., Dimitriou, J., *et al.* 1996. Safety and efficacy of recombinant gamma interferon in the treatment of systemic sclerosis. *Annals of the Rheumatic Diseases* 55(10): 761–768.

Vreugdenhil, G., Preyers, F., Croockewit, S., *et al.* 1992. Fever in neutropenic patients treated with GM-CSF representing enhanced host defense (letter to the editor). *Lancet* 339: 1118–1119.

Wheeler, V.S. 1996. Interleukins: The search for an anticancer therapy. *Seminars in Oncology Nursing* 12(2): 106–114.

White, C.L. 1992. Symptom assessment and management of outpatients receiving biotherapy: The application of a symptom report form. *Seminars in Oncology Nursing* 8(4 suppl 1): 23–28.

Zetterstrom, M., Sundgren-Andersson, A.K., Ostlund, P., *et al.* 1998. Delineation of the proinflammatory cascade in fever induction. *Annals of the New York Academy of Sciences* 856: 48–52.

Clinical Pearls

Assessment

1. Assess for constellation of signs and symptoms associated with the FLS (e.g., headache, malaise, chills). See Table 16.3.
2. Determine the severity or amount of distress the symptom causes the patient and its impact on quality of life:
   1 = Able to carry on daily activities normally
   2 = Symptoms mildly affect their day
   3 = Severe symptoms, but gained relief after intervention
   4 = Severe symptoms, no relief gained
3. Select criteria to grade common symptoms within the FLS:
   - Headache
   - Aching pain
   - Chills
   - Malaise
   - Fatigue/asthenia
   - Anorexia

   See National Cancer Institute toxicity scale (Table 16.4).
4. Ascertain the patient's prior experience with biological agents and FLS, and level of knowledge related to occurrence of symptoms with prescribed therapy.
5. Assess for co-factors that may impact tolerance of symptoms (e.g., age, performance status).
6. Monitor symptoms over course of therapy to determine occurrence, severity, and pattern.
7. Monitor for risk factors that may predispose to infection (e.g., neutropenia).
8. Assess for signs and symptoms associated with adverse effects of FLS on cardiovascular system (e.g., heart rate above 120 beats per minute, irregular beats, respiratory rate more than 24 breaths per minute, and complaints of chest pain).

Management

1. Decide if treatment of adverse effect is warranted (e.g., use of antipyretics):
   - Determine patient's perception of the distress caused by the symptom.
   - Ascertain risk of CNS complications (e.g., seizures, confusion) caused by symptoms.
   - Evaluate risk for hypoxemia or cardiovascular compromise with symptoms.
2. Approaches to management:
   - Manipulate treatment
     - Continuous infusion produces more adverse effects than intermittent therapy.
     - Determine whether tachyphylaxis is likely to occur and whether effects need to be controlled for limited time.
     - Consider giving intermittent doses in the evening.
   - Treat or prevent adverse effects with medications
     - Fever and aches: Premedicate and administer antipyretics about 1 hour prior to anticipated fever and throughout 24 hours after stopping agent. May use acetaminophen, although nonsteroidal anti-inflammatory agents (i.e., prostaglandin inhibitors), such as naprosyn or indomethacin may also be used. Due to the pathophysiologic basis of these symptoms, these agents are also better at managing myalgias, arthralgias, and headache.
     - Rigors: Keeping patient warm at time near anticipated fever spike may prevent chills. Demerol, morphine, dantrolene, and Valium have been used prophylactically and to abrogate chills.
     - Dehydration: Assure intake of adequate fluids and electrolytes.
   - Supportive care
     - Use warm clothing and blankets during chills.
     - Provide emotional support.
     - Assist the patient and family in limiting physical demands during the time of anticipated adverse effects.
     - Develop an individualized system to define the timing and distress produced for each patient by these symptoms.

Patient Education

1. Anticipate and inform patient of the constellation of symptoms typical with each specific therapy regimen.
2. Anticipate and inform patient of the typical onset, peak, and duration of the adverse effects with each specific therapy regimen.
3. Advise patient of strategies to prevent FLS or reduce severity:
   - Anticipate timing and limit activities.
   - Anticipate timing and take prescribed premedications.
4. Teach reportable symptoms:
   - Fever > 39.5° or persisting > 4 hours
   - Confusion
   - Seizures
   - Palpitations

Key References

Dinarello, C.A. 1999. Cytokines as endogenous pyrogens. *The Journal of Infectious Diseases* 179(suppl 2): S294–S304.

Henker, R., Kramer, D., and Rogers, S. 1997. Fever. *AACN Clinical Issues in Critical Care* 8(3): 351–367.

Kluger, M.J., Kozak, W., Conn, C.A., *et al.* 1998. Role of fever in disease. *Annals of the New York Academy of Sciences* 856: 224–233.

Mackowiak, P.A., and Plaisance, K.F. 1998. Benefits and risks of antipyretic therapy. *Annals of the New York Academy of Sciences* 856: 214–223.

Sergi, J.S. 1991. Issue 1. The physiology of the flu-like syndrome and the cardiopulmonary and renal symptoms associated with BRM therapy. *Biological Response Modifiers: Perspectives for Oncology Nurses.* San Francisco, CA: Professional Healthcare: 4–10.

Shelton, B.K., and Turnbough, L. 1999. Flu-like Syndrome. In Yarbro, C.H., Frogge, M.H., Goodman, M., and Groenwald, S. (eds). *Cancer Symptom Management* 2nd edn. Boston, MA: Jones & Bartlett Publishers, Inc., pp. 77–94.

White, C.L. 1992. Symptom assessment and management of outpatients receiving biotherapy: The application of a symptom report form. *Seminars in Oncology Nursing* 8(4 suppl 1): 23–28.

CHAPTER 17 | Fatigue

Grace E. Dean, RN, MSN

Fatigue is probably the only condition that both healthy and ill people experience daily. As a symptom of illness, fatigue is often the first indication of some abnormal process (Epstein, 1995). Patients have learned to accept fatigue as a companion of illness and often do not mention it unless they are asked. When patients voluntarily complain of fatigue, it has become overwhelming or it has begun to severely interfere with their lives.

Fatigue, as a subjective experience, may not be clearly evident when assessing the oncology patient. However, many studies report that fatigue is the most commonly cited symptom in patients with cancer and that some level of

The author wishes to thank and acknowledge the work of Karen Skalla and Paula Trahan Rieger, whose work from the first edition of *Biotherapy: A Comprehensive Overview* served as a foundation for this chapter.

fatigue exists in nearly all patients, especially those actively undergoing treatment with biological agents (Winningham *et al.*, 1994). Fatigue has been documented to be associated with all modes of cancer treatment: chemotherapy, radiation therapy, surgery, and biotherapy.

To characterize the epidemiology of cancer-related fatigue, a telephone survey was conducted with 100,000 randomly selected households in the United States (Vogelzang *et al.*, 1997), and 419 patients with cancer were recruited. These patients provided access to 200 primary caregivers (usually family members) who were also interviewed by telephone. Also included in the survey were 197 of 600 randomly sampled oncologists (unrelated to the patients) who returned a questionnaire regarding perceptions and attitudes concerning fatigue in cancer patients. Seventy-eight percent of the patients reported experiencing fatigue—

defined as a general feeling of debilitating tiredness or loss of energy—during the course of their disease and treatment. Patients reported that fatigue significantly affected their daily routines (32%), and many patients experienced fatigue daily (32%). The caregivers of patients reported observing fatigue in 86% of patients, whereas oncologists perceived that 76% of their patients experienced fatigue. Sixty-one percent of patients reported that their daily lives were more adversely affected by fatigue than by cancer-related pain, whereas only 37% of oncologists perceived this to be the situation. The investigators suggested that these diverse perceptions of fatigue may reflect the fact that fatigue is more prevalent than pain in patients with cancer and that fatigue is tolerated better. Additionally, the authors surmised that the higher emphasis on pain compared with fatigue reflects the significant educational efforts aimed at improving the awareness and management of pain in patients with cancer.

Information regarding fatigue in patients receiving biotherapy for cancer is limited (Piper *et al.*, 1989b). When fatigue is mentioned, it is usually in the context of tolerability to the treatment regimen, and few details are given. Nail and Winningham (1993) suggested that the limited information about the incidence and characteristics of fatigue associated with biotherapy indicates that the prevalence and magnitude of fatigue resulting from biotherapy are more severe than that associated with other cancer treatments. Fatigue related to biotherapy may exceed the patient's level of tolerance to the point that he or she might terminate therapy.

Quesada *et al.* (1986) found that fatigue in patients receiving interferon frequently resulted in job absenteeism, social withdrawal, and a rise in total hours of sleep per day; in extreme cases, it limited patients' ability to participate in some physical activities. The social implications of fatigue, therefore, may be profound. Financial resources may become limited as pa-

tients are forced into disability programs, or worse, out of a job. Patient outcomes may then become compromised due to difficulties in maintaining health insurance, problems gaining access to care, or the financial barriers of pursuing aggressive treatment. A thorough understanding of fatigue, consequently, may lead to initiation of effective interventions that ultimately improve patient outcomes.

Fatigue may have particular significance to some patients. In today's society, it has become increasingly necessary for all eligible family members to be employed. The experience of fatigue may be especially difficult for those who place a special significance on their role as primary breadwinner or caregiver (Davis, 1984). The deterioration in level of functioning may be mildly bothersome to some or intolerable to others, especially for those formerly independent individuals who must now surrender to the "sick role" (Davis, 1984).

The essence of the nursing role is to facilitate self-care in the patient. Nail *et al.* (1991) documented fatigue as the most commonly reported symptom (81%) in a sample of chemotherapy outpatients. They suggested that the continuing trend in oncology for chemotherapy to be delivered on an outpatient basis necessitates a shift in responsibility for control of side effects from nurse to patient. It is imperative that we empower patients to develop the self-care abilities necessary to cope with fatigue. This has been proven to be a challenge because fatigue has been shown to interfere with self-care activities (Davis, 1984; Rhodes *et al.*, 1988).

Despite the serious consequences of this symptom, little is known about the patterns or mechanisms of fatigue in patients treated with chemotherapy and especially in those treated with biological agents. Several problems become evident when examining research related to fatigue. The examination of fatigue in a variety of clinical situations by several disciplines other than nursing has hindered efforts to establish both a universal definition and theory of fatigue. Furthermore, ambiguous literature and a lack of specific tools to measure fatigue have created difficulties in establishing assessment and management guidelines.

This chapter will address the current level of understanding about the clinical nature of fatigue. Definitions of fatigue, its pathophysiology, and its clinical presentation in treatment with biotherapy will be discussed. Research that has guided development of nursing assessment and intervention techniques will be presented. A broad understanding of fatigue as a biotherapy-related problem will facilitate development of effective nursing interventions, which will then help nurses prepare patients to develop self-care abilities and improve the outcomes of their cancer treatment.

Definition of Fatigue

No standard definition for fatigue exists. Whereas scientists in several disciplines have studied fatigue, they have placed their own parameters on the concept and have used their special focus to interpret it. Physiologists have studied the effect of a reduction in performance as a result of fatigue. Pathologists have focused on the pathophysiological aspects of fatigue, such as neuromuscular or metabolic disorders. Psychologists have studied the effect of fatigue on the whole organism, examining its effect on motivation and mental and physical health. Fatigue is often the first indication of physical or mental illness. The fact that fatigue is the seventh most common complaint brought to primary-care physicians lends support to the notion that the lay public uses fatigue as a primary indicator of illness (Epstein, 1995).

Fatigue may be characterized as the disruption of physical, psychological, or spiritual well-being by tiredness or weakness that prevents an individual from functioning at ex-

pected potential. Fatigue has been described using such terms as tiredness, exhaustion, weakness, lack of energy, lack of purpose, sleepiness, and changes in ability to concentrate. Many different factors appear to influence fatigue in cancer patients. Table 17.1 provides a description of theories, frameworks, and models that represent aspects of fatigue experienced by patients with cancer and different philosophical viewpoints about the symptom.

Piper *et al.* (1987) proposed a definition for fatigue from which a conceptual model was developed. The definition for fatigue was later revised to: "In contrast to tiredness, subjective fatigue is perceived as unusual, abnormal, or excessive whole-body tiredness disproportionate to or unrelated to activity or exertion" (Piper, 1993). Piper divides fatigue into two categories: acute and chronic. Acute fatigue is perceived as normal or expected tiredness characterized by localized intermittent symptoms, rapid onset, and short duration. Acute fatigue serves a protective function. Chronic fatigue, in contrast, is perceived as abnormal or excessive generalized tiredness. It is constant or recurrent for at least a month with an insidious onset and cumulative effect. The function of chronic fatigue is unknown. Additional research is needed to further support Piper's definition and model.

Pickard-Holley (1991) defines fatigue as a condition characterized by the subjective feeling of increased discomfort and decreased functional status related to a decrease in energy. Factors involved may be physical, mental, emotional, environmental, physiological, and pathological, with a voluntary component. Fatigue is characterized as a state of increased discomfort and decreased efficiency that may be experienced as tiredness or weakness and that is usually resolved by rest or sleep.

Aistars (1987) defines fatigue as subjective feelings of generalized weariness, weakness, exhaustion, and lack of energy resulting from

Table 17.1   Nursing theories, models, and frameworks

Theory/Model/Framework	Description
Accumulation hypothesis	Suggests that accumulated waste products in the body result in fatigue.
Depletion hypothesis	Suggests that muscular activity is impaired when the supply of substances such as carbohydrates, fats, adenosine triphosphate, and proteins is not available to the muscle. Anemia also can be considered a depletion mechanism.
Biochemical and physiochemical phenomena	Proposes that production, distribution, use, equalization, and movement of substances such as muscle proteins, glucose, electrolytes, and hormones may influence the experience of fatigue.
Central nervous system control	Grandjean (1968) proposes that the central control of fatigue is placed in the balance between two opposing systems: the reticular activating system and the inhibitory system, which is believed to involve the reticular formation, the cerebral cortex, and the brain stem.
Adaptation and energy reserves	Selye (1976) suggests that each person has a certain amount of energy reserve for adaptation and that fatigue occurs when energy is depleted. Selye's hypothesis incorporates ideas from the other hypotheses, but focuses on the person's response to stressors.
Psychobiologic entropy	Proposes to associate activity, fatigue, symptoms, and functional status based on clinical observations that persons who become less active as a result of disease or treatment-related symptoms lose energizing metabolic resources.
Aistars' organizing framework	This framework is based on energy and stress theory and implicates physiologic, psychologic, and situational stressors as contributing to fatigue. Aistars (1987) attempts to explain the difference between tiredness and fatigue within Selye's general adaptation syndrome.
Piper's integrated fatigue model	Piper (1987) suggests that fatigue mechanisms influence signs and symptoms of fatigue. Changes in biological patterns such as host factors, metabolites, energy substrates, disease, and treatment along with psychosocial patterns impact a person's perception and lead to fatigue manifestations. The fatigue manifestations are expressed through the person's behavior.
Attentional fatigue model	Use of attentional theory linked to attentional fatigue. When increased requirements or demands for directed attention exceed available capacity, the person is at risk for attentional fatigue.

Source: Reprinted with permission from Barnett, M. 1997. Fatigue. In Otto, S. (ed). *Oncology Nursing*, 3rd edn. St. Louis, MO: Mosby, p. 670.

prolonged stress that is directly or indirectly attributable to the disease process. Fatigue results from exertion or stress and leads to increased discomfort and decreased efficiency. It causes deterioration of both mental and physical abilities. These commonalities are also expressed by Rhoten (1982). Rhoten's model combines attitude, speech patterns, general appearance, subjective description, concentration, and activity level to reflect the many different aspects encompassed by the word fatigue.

Cognitive change or attentional fatigue has

been identified in patients with chronic, life-threatening illness (Cimprich, 1992). Attentional fatigue occurs when increased demands for directed attention over long periods exceed the available capacity. The observable behavior would be reduced cognitive or mental effectiveness such as memory, concentration, ability to focus, learning, problem-solving, or planning activities (Cimprich, 1992).

Another definition of fatigue is provided by the University of Kansas School of Nursing's Center for Biobehavioral Studies of Fatigue Management (Aaronson *et al.*, 1999). In 1992, they studied fatigue in persons with diabetes, rheumatoid arthritis, and chronic fatigue syndrome, as well as caregivers and healthy individuals. Whereas patients with cancer were not included in their study, much can be learned from their experience with other diagnostic causes of fatigue. The biobehavioral definition of fatigue that guides their research is ". . . the awareness of a decreased capacity for physical and/or mental activity due to an imbalance in the availability, utilization, and/or restoration of resources needed to perform activity" (Aaronson *et al.*, 1999).

Many factors may contribute to both the mechanism and manifestation of fatigue, which hinders attempts to derive a universal definition. This is particularly true for biotherapy-related fatigue. It is often easier, therefore, to understand fatigue as a concept that varies in definition.

Theoretical Frameworks for Fatigue

Fatigue theory is diverse in both focus and philosophy. Historically, the goals of theory development have been to establish theory in healthy populations and then progress toward ill populations. Early studies examining fatigue were performed in order to investigate optimal worker productivity (Grandjean, 1968; Yoshi-take, 1971) and have laid the foundation for current investigations of fatigue in oncology populations.

Grandjean (1968) was one of the pioneers in development of fatigue theory on the physiological level. In studying fatigue in industrial workers, he developed a theory to explain the fatigue produced by "monotonous surroundings." He believed that the activation and inhibition systems of the brain were on opposite ends of a continuum. The reticular activating system (RAS) is responsible for activating an alert state in the organism using sensory afferent stimulation. Pathways exist from the RAS to the cortex that provide a feedback mechanism. Inhibition from the cortex takes two forms: active or passive. Active inhibition results from increased inhibitory impulses from the brain stem, whereas passive inhibition is the result of decreased sensory input or decreased cortical feedback. Depending on which system input predominates, the organism becomes either aroused or fatigued. Grandjean proposed that in monotonous surroundings there is a decrease in both afferent sensory impulses and feedback from the cortex resulting in fatigue.

In keeping with the philosophy of the profession, nursing has focused on development of a holistic theory for fatigue. The most well-known models will be reviewed in this chapter. Although additional research is needed to support these models, they are important to review for their historical significance. Piper *et al.* (1987) proposed a "fatigue framework" (see Figure 17.1). Biological and behavioral factors are modified by the perception of fatigue. Fourteen patterns are thought to influence fatigue: accumulation of metabolites, energy and energy substrate patterns, activity/rest patterns, sleep/wake patterns, disease patterns, treatment patterns, symptom patterns, psychological patterns, oxygenation patterns, regulation/transmission patterns, environmental patterns, social patterns, life events, and unique circadian rhythms and innate host factors.

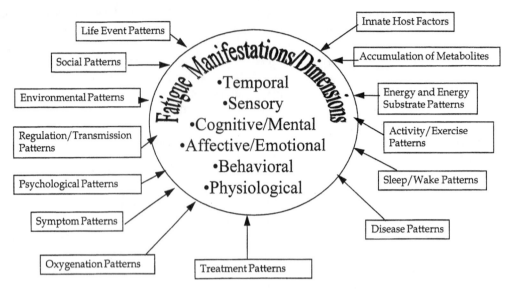

Figure 17.1   Integrated Fatigue Model©

Source: © 1997. Reprinted with permission. Barbrara F. Piper, DNSc, RN, AOCN®, FAAN.

Aistars (1987) utilized the "stress response" as a model for fatigue. The basis for her hypothesis is that prolonged stress causes fatigue. Persons with cancer frequently suffer from extreme stress over a long period of time. Activation of the RAS and sympathetic nervous system as a result of stress results in the prolonged release of stress hormones, which ultimately leads to depletion of energy stores. Consequently, these persons experience a high level of fatigue.

Energy and its relationship to fatigue have been explored by several authors (Mayer *et al.*, 1984; Koeller, 1989) interested in cancer cachexia. Patients receiving interferon often experience significant weight loss and fatigue. This concept must be compared with findings in another study (Kaempfer and Lindsey, 1986), which demonstrated that patients with cancer vary in their energy requirements. Something other than energy requirements alone must be functioning to produce fatigue. Winningham *et al.* (1994) described the Winningham Psychobi-

ological-Entropy (PEH) model for fatigue expanding on the concept of energy requirements and the possible relationship in producing fatigue. In this model, fatigue is defined as an energy deficit, and relational associations between fatigue and disease, treatment, activity, rest, symptom perception, and functional status are proposed (see Figure 17.2). The PEH model uses the energetic approach to determine the optimal balance between restorative rest and restorative activity or exercise. Because the PEH model is directive in terms of conceptual relationships, it provides suggestions for the development of nursing interventions to manage fatigue.

Few nursing models exist that describe fatigue in physiological detail. One model has been proposed; it is based on neurophysiological principles and evaluates the interaction of both central and peripheral components. This model incorporates the peripheral system (muscles and nerves) and central components (psyche/brain and spinal cord) that may influence perception

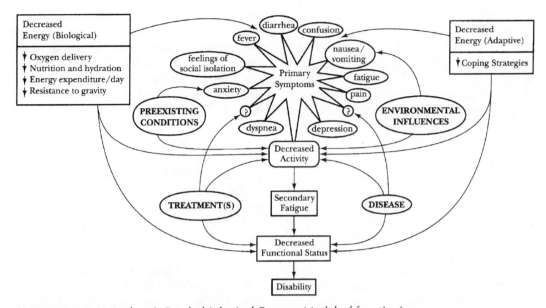

Figure 17.2 Winningham's Psychobiological-Entropy Model of functioning

of fatigue. Impairment of central components causes lack of motivation, impaired spinal cord transmission, and exhaustion or malfunction of brain cells in the hypothalamic region. Damage to the peripheral component can cause impaired peripheral nerve function in transmission at the neuromuscular junction, thereby affecting muscle-fiber activation. Both are hypothesized to play a role in chronic fatigue. The central mechanism may be the key to explaining the extreme fatigue of biotherapy-treated patients (Gibson and Edwards, 1985; Piper *et al.*, 1989a).

The development of clinically based models to examine fatigue and design interventions to manage fatigue offers exciting prospects. Nursing theory is only beginning to identify proposed models for fatigue. To date, these models are concerned with fatigue as a general concept and are not specific to biotherapy-related fatigue. Several researchers studying biotherapy have proposed mechanisms for biotherapy-related fatigue that will be reviewed in the following section.

Presentation and Pathophysiology of Fatigue

Interferon

The two side effects of interferon (IFN) that are the most difficult to manage are fatigue and alterations in the central nervous system. Fatigue is profound at doses equal to or greater than 20 MIU daily. This potentially therapeutic drug was reduced or discontinued in 50% to 100% of patients within 2 to 4 weeks when given in high doses (Quesada *et al.*, 1986). In addition, older patients or those with poor performance status are often more severely affected. Mayer *et al.* (1984) examined IFN-induced weight loss in a phase I clinical trial.

The prevalence of fatigue among patients studied was 70%, making it the most commonly reported side effect of therapy. Another study (Wadler *et al.*, 1989) documented fatigue at interferon doses of 6 to 18 MIU per day as being dose dependent (the higher the dose, the higher the level of fatigue). Fatigue has been reported with IFN-α at doses as low as 2 MIU daily (Gastl *et al.*, 1989). In the same study, fatigue was not reported when IFN was administered at doses of 0.2 to 0.6 MIU daily. A dose-dependent relationship does not become evident until the dose is approximately 2 to 3 MIU daily.

Exacerbation of fatigue becomes apparent when IFN is used in combination with other modalities (Piper *et al.*, 1989b). A study by Wadler *et al.* (1989) demonstrated that with administration of 5-fluorouracil and IFN-α, patients developed fatigue or malaise during the second week of therapy. Daily administration of IFN-α produced more fatigue than intermittent administration. The level of fatigue varied from none to extreme (requiring dose reduction) in the patients participating in the study. Interleukin-2 (IL-2) combined with IFN-α was shown to produce two dose-limiting toxicities: hypotension and chronic fatigue (associated with a decrease in performance status) (Lee *et al.*, 1989). Although fatigue improved between cycles, a decrease of up to 30 points in the Karnofsky Performance Status was seen in patients receiving high doses of IL-2 and IFN.

Quesada *et al.* (1986) and Adams *et al.* (1984) have suggested that IFN-induced fatigue, decreases in appetite, and cognitive-emotional disorders may be caused by central nervous system or frontal lobe neurotoxicity. Postulated causes of this toxic encephalopathy are direct effects of IFN on the frontal lobe or on deeper brain structures. IFN may impede neurotransmitters, cause an alteration of cholinergic balance, or cause the release of other substances that affect frontal lobe functions. Other biological agents cause similar symptoms, thereby enabling this theory to be applied to other biological treatments. The central or peripheral release of substances such as cytokines (e.g., tumor necrosis factor [TNF]) affects sensations of appetite and fatigue. This humoral effect is supported by a study described by Grandjean (1968) where the cerebral spinal fluid of sleep-deprived animals, when injected into other animals, produced fatigue. Repeated administration of biological agents may render fatigue a chronic toxic effect along with weight loss, anorexia, and malaise (Koeller, 1989). Patients diagnosed with chronic fatigue syndrome are also thought to be influenced by a central mechanism triggered by peripheral stimulation (Potempa *et al.*, 1986). Although a central mechanism is postulated to be the cause of fatigue, the pathophysiologic mechanisms remain poorly defined in humans (Lindner *et al.*, 1997).

Davis (1984) was one of the first nurses to conduct research on IFN-induced fatigue. She designed a correlational study to determine the impact of fatigue on the functional status of 16 melanoma patients who received a cumulative dose of INF-α ranging from 100 to 2,000 MIU. Fatigue was measured by the Pearson-Byars Scale (Pearson and Byars, 1956) and the Fatigue Symptom Checklist (Yoshitake, 1969). The impact of fatigue on physical performance status was measured with an adapted Sickness Impact Profile (Gilson *et al.*, 1975). Results from this study suggested a relationship between IFN therapy and fatigue. Specific symptoms related to the fatigue that were reported were walking slower (70%), sleeping more or sitting most of the day (50%), decreased sexual activity (50%), eating less (43%), and engaging in fewer social activities (43%). Positive correlations between fatigue measures and reported symptoms suggested a statistically significant relationship ($p \leq .001$). Statistical significance was also found between fatigue scores and cumulative dose of IFN ($r = .537$; $p = .001$).

There was no relationship between length of therapy and amount of fatigue. Mean dysfunctional scores correlated positively with cumulative IFN dose ($p \leq .005$), especially in sleep and socialization activities. The most common symptoms reported were leg weakness, a need to lie down, difficulty thinking, and impatience.

A study by Rieger (1987) described the changes in fatigue level, functional status, and muscular strength experienced by 30 patients with cancer who received treatment with IFN-α and IFN-γ, alone, together, or in combination with ampligen (an interferon inducer). Fatigue was measured before therapy and at 1 week, and at 1 month of therapy using the Pearson-Byars Scale, and muscle strength was measured at the same time points using the Jamar hand-held dynamometer. Functional quality of life was measured using the Functional-Living Index for Cancer (Schipper et al., 1984). Over time, there was no significant difference demonstrated for fatigue, functional quality of life, or muscle strength. Grip strength decreased significantly only in the group receiving IFN-α alone. Significant negative correlation was found between fatigue scores and quality of life. Complaints of fatigue, as documented in the medical record, increased from approximately 47% at baseline to 74% at the 1-month time point. This suggests that the fatigue measures used were not sufficiently sensitive to adequately measure the fatigue experienced. The limitations of this study include its small sample size and a comparison of groups receiving different types of therapy.

Skalla (1992) examined correlates of fatigue in patients treated with IFN. The purpose of this descriptive study was to investigate the behavioral, physiological, and biochemical factors that might affect subjective ratings of fatigue and simultaneously to question how fatigue might be different in patients with cancer versus healthy populations. This was a pilot study that addressed the feasibility of extending the research to a larger population. The convenience sample consisted of three groups: five medical oncology patients receiving treatment with interferon (group 1), five oncology patients matched to the first group for primary malignancy and stage of disease (group 2), and five healthy subjects matched to the first group for age and sex (group 3). The use of normal controls is unique in the fatigue literature.

The level of fatigue was expected to be highest in the IFN group and negligible in the healthy control group. Correlates of fatigue were classified and examined according to the framework developed by Piper et al. (1987) and included physiological variables, biochemical factors, and behavioral factors. Physiological variables included disease status, disease stage, duration of illness, pain, and performance status. Behavioral variables as measured by the Profile of Mood States (POMS) included mood, social support, marital status, and sleep changes. Many biochemical factors could be measured as potential correlates to fatigue, e.g., medications, liver function tests, and chemistries; however, this study was limited in examining only complete blood count.

The researcher briefly interviewed patients and completed a chart review for pertinent information including performance status, employment, marital status, sex, race, presence of pain, sleep patterns, date of diagnosis, perceived social support, disruption of social activities, current hematological laboratory values, and current cancer therapy. The tool chosen to measure fatigue was a 10-cm visual analogue scale (VAS). Patients were asked to measure both the "amount of fatigue experienced today" and their "usual amount of fatigue." Measures for other variables included a short version of the POMS and a brief questionnaire.

The IFN group scored highest in the categories of fatigue level, pain ratings, duration of illness, and hours of sleep per night. Group 1 had the highest mean score (x) for fatigue (x

= 43.80 mm, sd = 27.76). The score for group 2 was slightly lower (x = 40.20 mm, sd = 25.85), with group 3 experiencing the least amount of fatigue (x = 20.40 mm, sd = 23.13). These differences were not statistically significant and may have been limited by the small sample size. It is important to note that in this study, some level of fatigue was reported in all groups.

Biochemical variables, as measured by the complete blood count, were all lower in the IFN group than in the disease control group. This may have affected the fatigue rating. The effect of IFN-altering hematological values is well documented (Silver *et al.*, 1985; Radin *et al.*, 1989) and was consistent with the findings of this study.

The physiological variables of disease status, duration of illness, performance status, and pain may be difficult to evaluate as separate entities. Most of the cancer patients studied (80%) had metastatic disease. The highest mean duration of illness was found in the IFN group; this may support Aistars' theory that prolonged stress causes fatigue (Aistars, 1987). Performance status, as measured by the Karnofsky scale, was rated at 90 for all of the patients with cancer. These results differ from those of Davis (1984) who found significant differences in performance status among patients receiving IFN. This study also did not find that IFN dose correlated with the level of fatigue as was found in Davis's study at cumulative doses greater than 100 MIU.

The primary limitation of this study was the small sample size. Data collection of fatigue correlates was limited by the documentation of laboratory values in the chart and the sensitivity of the tool used to measure performance status.

The experience of fatigue over time was described in a study of 30 individuals with malignant melanoma receiving treatment with 5 miu/m² of IFN-α three times a week (Dean *et al.*, 1995). Fatigue was measured with the Piper Fatigue Scale (PFS) at baseline and at the end of each 2 weeks of treatment for 2 consecutive months. This resulted in a total of five measurement points over two months of treatment. Reported mean fatigue scores from each PFS subscale and total PFS revealed low baseline fatigue scores that gradually increased until scores peaked at the fourth week of treatment. Mean fatigue scores then declined at week 6 but increased again at week 8. The pattern of fatigue was consistent over time, with the most extreme scores in the affective subscale, followed by the sensory, temporal, total fatigue, and severity subscale scores. The emotional response to fatigue was intense in this sample, whereas the severity scores, which are linked to functional abilities, were least affected. The authors suggested that study results could be used by nurses to help patients prepare for the experience of extreme fatigue.

Interleukin-2

Fatigue is a prevalent side effect in patients receiving IL-2 therapy and is dose and schedule dependent. In general, higher doses of IL-2 and more prolonged therapy will intensify the level of fatigue (Piper *et al.*, 1989b). Other side effects experienced by the patient receiving therapy with IL-2, such as nausea and vomiting, anemia, diarrhea, mental status changes, hypotension, and fever, will increase perceived levels of fatigue. Numerous medications (e.g., antinausea and antipruritic medications) used to control IL-2–related side effects may also contribute to the intensity of fatigue experienced by the patient. Therapy combining IL-2 with other agents known to cause fatigue, such as IFN and chemotherapy, can also result in increased levels of fatigue (Farrell *et al.*, 1990; Janisch, 1990; Siegel and Puri, 1991; Viele and Moran, 1993).

Limited information exists about patterns of fatigue in patients receiving therapy with IL-2.

In reports from clinical trials evaluating the efficacy of IL-2, fatigue is frequently described in association with flu-like symptoms. When described, it is characterized solely as present in a given percentage of patients. When fatigue is frequent and severe (e.g., with IFN- and IL-2–related fatigue), it is often characterized as a dose-limiting toxic effect. In clinical trials, fatigue is generally graded as 1 (none), 2 (mild), 3 (moderate), or 4 (severe). Measures of performance status may also be used to characterize fatigue. Data presented from a phase II clinical trial conducted by the National Biotherapy Study Group that evaluated continuous infusion IL-2 in patients with advanced malignancies reported fatigue as a predominant side effect. Over 90% of patients spent more than 12 hours per day in bed (Sharp, 1993). Fatigue is a common occurrence in patients receiving outpatient administration of IL-2, whether IL-2 is administered by the subcutaneous route or as a bolus or continuous intravenous infusion. The degree of fatigue is dose- and schedule-dependent (Viele and Moran, 1993). Fatigue is often more severe in patients receiving IL-2 therapy than in those receiving IFN. These patients frequently spend the majority of the day in bed and are unable to perform self-care activities. It may take up to 6 to 8 weeks for fatigue to resolve after completion of therapy (Piper *et al.*, 1989b).

Hodges (1992) investigated the pattern of fatigue as measured by the Zubrod scale in patients with metastatic malignant melanoma during their first course of treatment with IL-2 alone or IL-2 in combination with IFN-α. Therapy consisted of a 4-day continuous infusion of IL-2 that started on day 1. In the group receiving IFN (group 2), injections were given on days 1 through 4. All patients were given a break from therapy on days 6 and 7. During the study, this cycle was repeated for 4 weeks for group 1 (IL-2-only) and for 3 weeks for group 2. Each 3- or 4-week cycle constituted

a course of therapy. This study used a retrospective record review to gather data that was grouped by biotherapy treatment. Limitations were secondary analysis of existing data, the use of the Zubrod scale as a measure of fatigue, and a lack of data on analysis of fatigue status between courses of IL-2.

In both groups, the percentage of fatigue increased during treatment, with the highest levels of fatigue occurring on the last full day of treatment. Although slight recovery did occur during the break period each week, Zubrod scores never returned to pretreatment levels. During treatment, approximately 25% of patients in group 1 experienced fatigue severe enough to require assistance with activities of daily living. Patients in group 2 experienced a greater degree of fatigue than those in group 1. No significant relationship between fatigue and the selected toxicity criteria was found for either group during all weeks of treatment; however, anorexia did correlate significantly with the level of fatigue in patients in group 2. Although this study cannot be generalized to all populations, it does provide information on the patterns and level of fatigue experienced by patients receiving therapy with IL-2 and IL-2/IFN-α.

The mechanisms that cause IL-2–related fatigue remain unknown. Both central and peripheral mechanisms may be involved in biotherapy-related fatigue states. It has been hypothesized that the release of cytokines such as TNF may affect the sensations of fatigue and appetite. In patients receiving IL-2 therapy, the release of cytokines such as IFN-γ and TNF combined with the capillary leak syndrome may cause alterations in neuroendocrine secretion, brain electrical activity, and blood-brain barrier permeability (Piper *et al.*, 1989b). It is likely that the significant number of systemic side effects experienced with IL-2 both impact and have a causal role in the development of IL-2–related fatigue.

Tumor Necrosis Factor

Fatigue is also common in patients receiving therapy with TNF, although the patterns of fatigue are not well documented. In the majority of phase I trials evaluating TNF, hypotension is reported as the dose-limiting side effect, although fatigue is occasionally mentioned in this context. Fatigue is reported in approximately 50% to 92% of patients receiving TNF (Moldawer and Figlin, 1988; Alexander and Rosenberg, 1991). The route of administration does not appear to affect the level of fatigue. When TNF is given in combination with other biological agents that are known to cause fatigue, its severity generally increases (Martin, 1991).

The precise mechanism responsible for TNF-related fatigue remains unknown. It is possible that TNF-related fatigue may result from biochemical and morphologic changes in skeletal muscle (St. Pierre et al., 1992). These pathologic changes in muscle would require a patient to exert an additional amount of effort to perform physical activity and maintain body posture, hence resulting in fatigue. It has been hypothesized that the muscle wasting associated with cachexia is mediated by TNF. Although there are experiments linking TNF and skeletal muscle wasting, the precise mechanisms remain unclear. TNF may affect both the synthesis and degradation rate of protein stores in muscle. The ultimate effect probably depends on other variables, including tumor type, tumor status, and the general condition of the patient. Nevertheless, the involvement of muscle in the occurrence of TNF-related fatigue will play a role in determining the level of the patient's self-care abilities or the patient's ability to participate in an exercise program.

Hematopoietic Growth Factors

Fatigue is more consistently reported as a side effect of granulocyte-macrophage colony-stimulating factor (GM-CSF) than with other hematopoietic growth factors. In general GM-CSF–associated fatigue is mild in nature and resolves readily upon cessation of therapy. The ability of GM-CSF to activate monocytes, which in turn leads to the expression of TNF and IL-1, may be the mechanism that causes this fatigue. Fatigue was the most commonly reported side effect in patients with acquired immune deficiency syndrome (AIDS) receiving GM-CSF, although it is difficult to separate the effects of therapy from the underlying effects of the disease (Lynch et al., 1988).

IL-3 is generally well tolerated, but there have been reports of debilitating fatigue following its administration. Reilly and McKeever (1993) reported significant levels of fatigue in patients with aplastic anemia or myelodysplastic syndrome receiving therapy with IL-3 in a phase I/II clinical trial. Patients reported a decreased ability to perform daily activities, decreased job performance, and time lost from work as a result of fatigue. The onset of fatigue occurred 3 hours after receiving IL-3 with a duration up to 8 hours. Owing to this pattern of fatigue, it was recommended that patients receive IL-3 in the evening so that they might sleep through the fatigue episode. The authors report diminished levels of fatigue with this intervention. This abstract does not discuss the tools used to measure fatigue. In addition, symptoms associated with aplastic anemia and myelodysplastic syndrome such as anemia and that may cause fatigue, are not reviewed.

The occurrence of fatigue is uncommon with administration of granulocyte colony-stimulating factor or erythropoietin. Because anemia is known to cause fatigue and to impact the level of fatigue, the administration of erythropoietin to treat anemia may actually decrease fatigue in many patients.

Monoclonal Antibodies

Fatigue is not a side effect commonly associated with the administration of monoclonal antibodies. Malaise is a more common side effect of this treatment and occurs in association with fever, chills, and diaphoresis. This constellation of symptoms occurs most frequently in patients with hematologic malignancies during the removal of circulating target cells and it resolves quickly upon cessation of therapy (Dillman, 1988).

Measurements of Fatigue

A review of the literature on cancer-related fatigue revealed that the majority of fatigue measures in research have been restricted to one-dimensional scales with limited reliability and validity (Irvine et al., 1991; Richardson, 1998). Some of the earliest questionnaires used to measure fatigue were developed by psychologists to evaluate fatigue in healthy workers in industrial settings (Kashiwagi, 1971; Yoshitake, 1971). These same questionnaires were then used on diverse patient populations. The prevalence and intensity of fatigue was the major focus of these and other questionnaires. However, fatigue—like pain—is not only a physical symptom but also a multidimensional concept that has physical, psychological, social, and spiritual aspects.

As a symptom, fatigue requires a precise definition and means of measurement. Symptoms are established as medically legitimate only when they can be isolated conceptually and when their boundaries can be defined and displayed conclusively (Monks, 1989). Questions regarding the validity and legitimacy of symptoms arise when these concrete parameters are not met. Consequently, fatigue has been regarded as a companion symptom to be tolerated or endured as long as the "real diagnosis" is being actively sought.

The presence of fatigue is established based on the subject's reported experience of it. To date, no perfect correlations have been established between physiological fatigue and perception of fatigue; therefore, the subjective report dominates the existence of fatigue (Christensen et al., 1987). Subjectivity implies that the distress from fatigue is difficult to measure by someone other than the individual. The individual is able to communicate the type, intensity, duration, and impact of fatigue on his or her daily activities and describe the experience in ways that others can comprehend. The level of fatigue should be assessed at multiple points in time to understand its pattern.

A variety of tools, reflective of the diversity of definitions for fatigue, exist to measure the phenomenon of fatigue in patients receiving biotherapy. It is measured, with few exceptions, using a modified tool for other aspects of fatigue such as psychological or physical symptom distress rather than as a tool specific for fatigue. Measurements exist that describe either subjective or objective parameters of fatigue. Some measures have been used in a temporal fashion, whereas others capture fatigue at a certain moment in time. Reliability and validity data are beginning to accrue regarding the use of these tools to measure fatigue in cancer populations.

Tools that measure subjective fatigue are VASs, the Pearson-Byars Fatigue Feeling Tone Checklist (Pearson and Byars, 1956); The Fatigue Symptom Checklist (Yoshitake, 1969); various symptom distress scales, original and adapted (McCorkle and Young, 1978); and the POMS (short and long forms) (McNair et al., 1971; Shacham, 1983). Objective parameters have been measured by behavioral indicators such as alterations in general appearance, level of activity, communication patterns, attitudes, and functional performance status.

Physiological indicators to measure fatigue may include changes in levels of neurotransmitters, electromyograms, heart rate, oxygen consumption rate, degree of anemia, temperature, blood glucose, thyroid function, electrolyte levels, and indirect calorimetry. Biochemical indicators used in measuring fatigue are changes in pH, lactate and pyruvate measurements, the proportion of fast twitch to slow twitch fibers (determined by muscle biopsy), and levels of metabolic end products (determined by magnetic resonance spectroscopy).

The two most frequently used tools for measuring fatigue are the VAS and the POMS. The VAS is simple and lends itself easily to clinical practice with end points expressing the two extremes of the fatigue continuum. The POMS is the most reliable and valid tool to date. The original POMS measures various aspects of mood in a 64-item questionnaire. Descriptive adjectives are rated on a scale of 0 (not at all) to 4 (extremely). The adjectives are grouped into six subscales that reflect the emotional dimensions of fatigue: tension-anxiety, depression-dejection, anger-hostility, vigor-activity, fatigue-inertia, and confusion-bewilderment. A shortened version of the POMS was developed by Shacham (1983) with a sample of oncology patients and was designed specifically for use on ill populations. The short version includes 37 items, but retains high correlation scores for mean subscale scores. The shortened POMS has been used by Jamar (1989), Oberst et al. (1991), and Blesch et al. (1991) to study fatigue in patients with cancer. The POMS (both short and long forms) is available through the Educational and Industrial Testing Service, San Diego, CA.

Several questionnaires have been developed to measure fatigue in patients with cancer: the PFS (Piper et al., 1989a), the Multidimensional Fatigue Inventory (MFI) (Smets et al., 1995), The General Fatigue Scale (GFS) (Meek et al., 1997), the Functional Assessment of Cancer Therapy-Fatigue and -Anemia Scales (FACT-F and FACT-An) (Cella, 1997), and the Brief Fatigue Inventory (BFI) (Mendoza et al., 1999). The Rhoten Fatigue Scale was designed to assess postsurgical fatigue and has not been proven reliable and valid for use in cancer populations (Rhoten, 1982).

The PFS was originally developed as a 44-item questionnaire (Piper et al., 1989a). There were 41 visual analogue questions with scores ranging from 0 to 100 and three open-ended questions that addressed perceived cause, relief measures, and additional word descriptors at the end of the PFS. After extensive testing, a factor analysis in a large sample of women with breast cancer was conducted to reduce the number of items without decreasing the instrument's reliability (Piper et al., 1996). The new version of the PFS is composed of four subscales and a total of 22 items: behavioral/severity (six items), affective meaning (five items), sensory (five items), and cognitive/mood (six items). Subscale scores are calculated by adding the scores of all the items within a particular subscale and dividing the sum by the number of items. The total fatigue score is calculated by adding the four subscale scores together and dividing by four. This questionnaire is available with either a visual analogue (0 to 100 mm) or numeric (0 to 10) scale. The PFS has been tested in cancer patients; pregnant women; pre-, peri-, and postmenopausal women; and caregivers of cancer patients. It has excellent reliability and validity estimates in those populations studied. Patients have commented that the 44-item tool was too long and the tool design did not accommodate patients not experiencing fatigue. The new PFS questionnaire can be scored by hand or computer.

The MFI is a 20-item, five-point Likert scale that can be self-administered in about 10 minutes (Smets et al., 1995). This tool includes five dimensions of fatigue—general, physical, mental, reduced motivation, and reduced activity—which have been supported through confirmatory factor analyses (Smets et al., 1996). Psychometric properties have been tested in several patient populations, including patients with cancer receiving radiation therapy, patients with chronic fatigue syndrome, students of medicine and psychology, army recruits, and junior doctors (Smets et al., 1998).

Another tool in the arsenal of fatigue measures is the GFS, a nine-item measure that is scored on a 10-point scale anchored by "no fatigue" and "greatest possible fatigue" (Meek et al., 1997). The items were designed to help ascertain the pattern of cancer-related fatigue through evaluation of the patient's present level of fatigue ("today"), the patient's level of fatigue most days and the high and low levels of fatigue experienced in the past 48 hours and the past month. In addition, the general intensity, distress, and impact of fatigue are assessed.

New measures of fatigue and anemia in the oncology population come from the researchers who developed the Functional Assessment of Cancer Therapy-General (FACT-G), a core instrument that measures the four general domains of quality of life: physical, social/family, emotional, and functional well-being (Cella et al., 1993). The FACT-F is composed of the FACT-G plus a 13-item fatigue subscale. The FACT-An scale is composed of the FACT-F plus seven items that address concerns related to anemia that are distinct from fatigue. This 13-item fatigue subscale was tested on a sample of 50 patients with either solid tumors or hematologic malignancies (Cella et al., 1997). The FACT-F, FACT-An, and the 13-item fatigue subscale were found to successfully discriminate fatigue in patients based on hemoglobin (Hgb) level and Eastern Cooperative Oncology Group (ECOG) performance status. Additionally, when patients were divided into two groups by Hgb levels, the 13-item fatigue subscale was able to distinguish patients with an Hgb level greater than 12 g/dL from those with an Hgb level less than 12 g/dL. Whereas this study demonstrates promise in research on the relationship between subjective fatigue and anemia, it is by no means conclusive and suggests that further research is needed.

An additional tool used to assess fatigue is the Brief Fatigue Inventory (BFI) (Mendoza et al., 1999), a questionnaire developed for the rapid assessment of the severity of fatigue and intended for use in clinical screening and clinical trials. The BFI is a nine-item numerical questionnaire modeled after the Brief Pain Inventory (Cleeland, 1989). Initial testing of the instrument demonstrated an internal consistency coefficient of 0.96. Concurrent validity with the POMS-Fatigue subscale ($r = .88$, $p < .001$) and the fatigue subscale of the FACT ($r = .84$, $p < .001$) were good. Early results of clinical trials assessing the BFI demonstrate that it is a reliable instrument that allows for the rapid assessment of a single dimension of fatigue (severity) in patients with cancer.

Tools such as those described here may be used in conjunction with measurements of physiological parameters to identify patients who may be at risk for or are experiencing significant fatigue while being treated with biological agents. Some tools may be more useful and realistic for the clinical setting, whereas others may be more appropriate for research purposes. For a complete review of tools for the measurement of fatigue, see Piper, 1997.

Assessment and Management of Biotherapy-Related Fatigue

Assessment

A thorough assessment of fatigue in which both subjective and objective data are gathered provides the foundation for management of fatigue. Fatigue should be assessed before therapy to provide baseline information, during therapy to evaluate its severity and determine effectiveness of interventions and after therapy to determine when fatigue is resolved. The criteria for analyzing a symptom (described in Chapter 14) and the theoretical models of fatigue described earlier in this chapter provide a framework for assessing fatigue.

Before therapy, the patient's risk for development of fatigue should be determined. Knowledge of biological agents known to cause the highest levels of fatigue will enable the care team to preplan strategies to combat fatigue. It is important to assess the factors that either predispose the patient to fatigue or influence the level of fatigue experienced (see Figures 17.1 and 17.2) Examples include disease patterns; activity and rest patterns; energy patterns (nutritional intake); sleep and rest patterns; treatment patterns; symptom patterns such as anemia, nausea, and pain; and oxygenation patterns (Piper *et al.*, 1987; McDaniel and Rhodes, 2000). An inventory of the patient's medications may also reveal substances that contribute to or influence fatigue levels (e.g., alcohol, caffeine, narcotics, sedatives, hypnotics, or antihypertensives) (Piper, 1991a).

The patient's perception of fatigue provides subjective data. Important areas to assess include usual patterns of functioning and any changes that have resulted due to treatment; the patient's perception of fatigue, how distressing the symptom of fatigue is (Rhodes and Watson, 1987); and the physical, emotional, and psychological symptoms experienced (Piper *et al.*, 1989a). Physical symptoms may include expressions about whole-body tiredness; feeling "drained," "weary," "listless," or "pooped"; or feeling tired in the eyes, arms, or legs. Emotionally, fatigue may be described as unpleasant or as a lack of motivation. Behaviorally, patients or family members may notice that it takes longer to perform physical activities or that more effort is required. Some activities may no longer be attempted as they are viewed as requiring "too much energy." Mental or cognitive symptoms may include difficulty concentrating or reading or difficulty thinking clearly (Piper, 1993).

In clinical practice, one of the simplest ways to assess fatigue is to have the patient rate the level of fatigue on a scale of 0 to 10, with 0 being "no fatigue" and 10 being "the most

possible fatigue" (Winningham *et al.*, 1994). Having the patient maintain a fatigue diary or journal can yield a significant amount of information about fatigue patterns. Determining temporal levels of fatigue (e.g., when fatigue levels are highest) and which types of factors aggravate and alleviate fatigue will help determine which intervention is needed.

Objective indicators of fatigue include physiological, biochemical, and behavioral factors. In the clinical setting, behavioral factors are the most easily assessed. Examples include performance status (Karnofsky and Zubrod are the most frequently used), physical appearance, and affect (Piper, 1991b).

It is also important to assess social support systems. Patients often need assistance from family or friends during periods of acute or chronic fatigue. The patient with a limited support system may need referrals to obtain other assistance. Evaluation of support from the patient's place of employment should also occur, as work schedules may need to be altered during periods of significant levels of fatigue. Support systems should be reassessed regularly during therapy, because increased role demands can lead to fatigue and strain in caregivers (Jensen and Givens, 1991) and social isolation for the patient and family.

Management Strategies

MEDICATIONS

Few published reports address the use of medications to decrease fatigue in patients receiving biotherapy. Piper (1993) summarizes the few studies that have tested the effects of medications on subjective fatigue; however, none were conducted in patients with cancer. A summary on fatigue in cancer patients by Bruera and MacDonald (1988) reviews the use of methylprednisolone and various amphetamines and their derivatives (e.g., methylphenidate) on patients with cancer and reports varying responses. Anecdotal reports (Quesada *et al.*, 1986) have been written about the use of methylphenidate in patients receiving therapy with IFN-α with varying success rates. The use of medications to alleviate biotherapy-related fatigue remains an area that requires further investigation. When possible, medications that may cause decreased energy and tiredness (e.g., hypnotics and antihistamines) should be eliminated.

MANIPULATION OF TREATMENT

Few published reports exist today, but additional research may begin to delineate the patterns of fatigue associated with different doses of biological agents (e.g., high doses versus low doses), different routes of administration (e.g., subcutaneous, intravenous bolus, or continuous intravenous infusion), and combinations of biological agents. The information may provide a basis for modifying dosing schedules such that equal clinical outcomes are achieved using regimens that cause lower levels of fatigue and less-toxic effects. Because of their role in ongoing assessment of tolerance to therapy, nurses should work collaboratively with physicians to determine dosing schedules that are best tolerated by the patient.

At lower doses, most biological agents tend to cause less fatigue than at higher doses, although this will vary depending on the patient's clinical status. It has been reported that intermittent scheduling (two to three times per week) of IFN is best tolerated and causes less fatigue (Quesada *et al.*, 1986). Others have reported that evening administration of IFN is tolerated better than morning administration and causes less fatigue and fewer side effects (Abrams *et al.*, 1985). A pilot study by Dean *et al.* (1993) evaluated the effect of time of therapy administration (morning vs. evening) on the recurrence of fatigue. Patients with metastatic melanoma were randomized to receive either morning (8 A.M.) or evening (5 P.M.) administration of

IFN-α. Symptom distress was measured by the Symptom Distress Scale (McCorkle and Young, 1978) and the PFS (Piper *et al.*, 1989) before treatment began and every 2 weeks for 2 months. Early results demonstrated less symptom distress with evening administration than with morning administration at the 4-week time point. Although there was no statistical difference in fatigue ratings between the two groups, a plot of mean scores for the morning group showed a trend for the scores to increase over time, whereas scores for the evening group seemed to plateau at 4 weeks.

Stepwise escalation of the dose over time has been reported to assist in achieving higher doses with better tolerance (Talpaz *et al.*, 1997). Patients treated with IFN and IL-2 responded to brief rest periods with resolution of fatigue prior to the next cycle or course of therapy. The optimal dose, route, and schedule is yet to be determined for most biological agents; therefore, future research efforts should focus on regimens that are tolerated with less fatigue and symptom distress while maintaining clinical efficacy.

NURSING MEASURES

Several publications have reviewed clinical interventions for cancer-related fatigue (Aistars, 1987; Rieger, 1988; Brophy and Sharp, 1991; Piper, 1991a, 1991b, 1993; Clark *et al.*, 1992; Skalla and Lacasse, 1992a, 1992b; Clark and Lacasse, 1998; Groopman, 1998; Portenoy *et al.*, 1999; Ream and Richardson, 1999; Winningham and Barton-Burke, 1999; McDaniel and Rhodes, 2000). To date, the majority of clinical interventions used for fatigue in patients with cancer, and specifically for biotherapy-related fatigue, do not have an empirical foundation (Winningham *et al.*, 1994). However, the prevalence of this side effect and its impact on patient's quality of life provide a unique opportunity for nurses to initiate clinical research in this arena. Table 17.2 provides an

Table 17.2 Recommendations for clinical practice regarding cancer-related fatigue

Assessment	Education	Interventions
• Differentiate fatigue from depression. • Evaluate patterns of activity and rest during the day and over time. • Assess for the presence of correctable correlates or contributors to fatigue (e.g., dehydration, anemia, electrolyte imbalance). • Determine the patient's attentional ability. • Monitor the effects of fatigue on perception of quality of life. • Evaluate the efficacy of self-care fatigue interventions on a regular and systematic basis.	• Provide anticipatory guidance regarding the likelihood of experiencing fatigue and of the fatigue patterns associated with particular treatments. • Educate patients and families regarding deleterious effects of prolonged bedrest and too much inactivity. • Educate patients and families about expectancies of fatigue related to disease and treatment.	• Help patients and families identify what fatigue-promoting activities they can modify and how to modify them. • Encourage patients to maintain a journal to identify fatigue patterns. • Establish priorities for safe activities based on usual social role and cultural values. • Encourage activity within individual limitations; make goals realistic by keeping in mind state of disease and treatment regimens. • Suggest individualized environmental or activity changes that may offset fatigue. • Maintain adequate hydration and nutrition. • Promote an adequate balance between activity and rest. • Recommend physical therapy referral for patients with specific neuromusculoskeletal deficits. • Schedule important daily activities during time of least fatigue and eliminate nonessential, unsatisfying activities. • Address the negative impact of psychological and social stressors and how to modify or avoid them.

Source: Adapted with permission from Winningham, M., Nail, L., Burke, M., *et al.* 1994. Fatigue and the cancer experience: The state of the knowledge. *Oncology Nursing Forum* 21(1): 23–36.

overview of recommendations for clinical practice regarding cancer-related fatigue.

A useful analogy for assisting patients in coping with fatigue is to have them think about personal energy stores as a "bank" (Piper, 1991a; Skalla and Lacasse, 1992a). "Deposits" and "withdrawals" are made over time to achieve a balance between activities that are energy-restoring and those that are energy-depleting. Several studies have reported useful activities for managing fatigue (Rhodes *et al.*, 1988; Piper and Dodd, 1991; Robinson and Posner, 1992). In patients receiving therapy with either IL-2 or IFN-α (Robinson and Posner, 1992), self-care interventions identified by patients as helpful included rest or sleep, maintaining their usual routine, or exercising lightly. Patients reported that interventions that helped them reduce fatigue were "helping me with household chores" or "driving me to work." A surprising finding of the study was that only 31% of family members' recommendations and only 46% of nurses's suggestions for alleviating fatigue corresponded with those of the patients. Although the sample size was limited, the results of this study suggest that nurses need to be more adept at assessing fatigue, and both nurses and family members should verify the effectiveness of suggested interventions with the patient.

ENERGY RESTORATION

Numerous interventions have been suggested in the literature to assist patients in replenishing energy stores. Napping and resting are the most frequently used and suggested interventions. Patients may need to take short naps during the day following periods of activity or take a nap prior to a period of planned activity in order to ensure adequate energy levels. However, the majority of patients experiencing biotherapy-related fatigue experience chronic fatigue and should be cautioned to avoid too much rest, as this can negatively impact fatigue levels.

Maintaining normal sleep patterns at night is encouraged.

Despite anorexia being a common problem in patients receiving biotherapy, adequate hydration and nutrition are important in maintaining or restoring energy levels. Fluids are hypothesized to assist with excretion of cell destruction end products that may be associated with fatigue. Adequate energy stores are necessary for optimal muscle functioning. See Chapter 18 for suggestions about enhancing nutritional intake.

Relaxation or diversional activities such as visiting friends, reading, listening to music, watching a movie, or involvement in a hobby may also be energy enhancing. Cimprich (1993) tested an intervention aimed at increasing subjects' participation in activities thought to maintain or restore directed attention. Patients who had undergone surgery were randomly assigned to an intervention of setting aside a minimum of 30 minutes, 3 times a week for restorative activities or a control group of no intervention. Compared with a control group, the experimental group showed higher rates of returning to work and of engaging in newly initiated, purposeful activities. Although not a proven intervention for patients receiving biotherapy, this study provides a basis for future research about strategies to improve patient ability to direct attention and combat mental fatigue.

Management of correlates of fatigue such as anemia, nausea and vomiting, and pain can also enhance energy stores. In theoretical models described earlier in this chapter, these factors are proposed to influence or cause fatigue. Additionally, several qualitative studies recently reported that patients described other symptoms as the cause of their fatigue (Dean *et al.*, 1995; Ferrell *et al.*, 1996). Successful interventions for management of these factors are available, therefore, they should be assessed and treated when present.

Although limited, a research base does exist

for using exercise as an intervention to combat fatigue. Winningham proposed the idea of a fatigue-inertia spiral (Winningham, 1992). Symptoms, such as fatigue, can lead to an actual or perceived need for bed rest and limited activity (hypodynamia). This results in physiologic changes, which in turn lead to lower energetic capacity and heightened feelings of fatigue. The more fatigued a patient feels, the more he or she tends to rest, which leads to more physiologic changes. Over time, this spiral can result in profound decreases in functional status (see Figure 17.3). An individualized endurance exercise training program might serve as the foundation of an effective energy restoring regimen.

Winningham (1983) reported results from a rehabilitation project involving patients with breast cancer who were receiving chemotherapy. Patients placed on the Winningham Aerobic Interval Training (WAIT) protocol for 10 weeks exhibited increases in objective measures of functional capacity and reported increased feelings of internal control as compared with a control group that did not exercise. Sub-

sequent work using the same exercise program documented a decreased perception of fatigue as measured by the POMS fatigue subscale (MacVicar and Winningham, 1986). Mock *et al.* (1994) evaluated a modified version of the rhythmic walking program in patients with breast cancer. This exercise protocol, described in the booklet *Rhythmic Walking: Exercise for People Living with Cancer* (Winningham *et al.*, 1990) is a low-intensity, self-care walking program that is associated with less risk and costs less than the WAIT protocol. In this study, the nonexercise group reported twice the fatigue of the exercise group. Although these studies are not generalizable to biotherapy-related fatigue, they do provide a sound rationale for the use of exercise to diminish sensations of fatigue. Serendipitously, many patients who exercise regularly and are receiving biological agents such as IFN report fewer problems with fatigue.

Mock *et al.* (1997) reported preliminary results on their exercise intervention for management of fatigue and emotional distress during radiation therapy for breast cancer. The experimental intervention involved a brisk, self-paced, 10- to 45-minute walk, four or five times a week. An experimental design was used with a convenience sample of 50 women with stage I/II breast cancer who were randomly assigned to the exercise program or usual care. The exercise group scored significantly higher than the usual-care group on physical functioning, as measured by the differences in pre- and post-test scores on the 12-Minute Walk Test ($p = .01$). Symptom intensity was significantly higher in the usual-care group, especially with respect to fatigue, anxiety, and difficulty sleeping. This study demonstrated that patients with breast cancer receiving radiation therapy may safely acquire physical and psychosocial benefits from a modest exercise program.

Any exercise program should be individualized based on the patient's clinical status. Risk

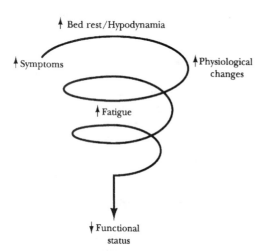

Figure 17.3 The fatigue/inertia spiral

Source: © 1991, 1994. Maryl L. Winningham, RN, PhD, FACSM. Used with express written consent of the author. Graphics by Linda Bishop.

factors such as lytic bone lesions, thrombocytopenia, fever, or neutropenia may be contraindications for an exercise program (Piper, 1991a). Guidelines and precautions for the use of exercise as an intervention have been reported (Winningham, 1991). In addition, St. Pierre *et al.* (1992) cautions that in patients who are cachectic or receiving TNF as therapy, nurses should be concerned that the development of fatigue may involve changes in skeletal muscle protein stores. Physiologic factors may exist that predispose patients with cancer to develop fatigue or to experience an adverse response to exercise.

ENERGY CONSERVATION/UTILIZATION

Other interventions designed to limit or relieve fatigue center on effective utilization of existing energy stores. Environmental modifications, scheduling activities for times when energy levels are at their peak, pacing activities, eliminating nonessential activities, requesting assistance from family members or friends, and using energy-saving equipment to do household chores can be helpful. The nurse can assist patients in coping with fatigue by jointly reviewing their normal day's activities and obligations and making adjustments to fit current energy levels. Frequent follow-up assessments will assist in verifying the effectiveness of these changes. Nurses should also assist with scheduling laboratory tests and diagnostic studies so that patient energy stores are not depleted by repeated trips to the hospital or clinic.

STRESS REDUCTION

The Aistars Organizing Framework (Aistars, 1987), based on energy and stress theory, implies that physiologic, psychologic, and situational stressors contribute to fatigue. By educating patients about effective coping strategies and facilitating their use of existing coping strategies, nurses can help patients decrease stressors. Although not well researched, this may be useful in decreasing fatigue levels. Participation in support groups may also help patients decrease fatigue levels by reducing stress. Depression and anxiety are also related to fatigue; therefore, these symptoms should be watched for and treated when present. Several studies have demonstrated that a patient's perceived ability to manage symptoms correlates with fatigue distress (Pickard-Holley, 1991; Jones, 1993). Patient education on fatigue-management strategies can empower the patient to more effectively cope with therapy (Skalla and Lacasse, 1992b).

PATIENT EDUCATION

Johnson *et al.* (1988) reported that perception of fatigue may be reduced by providing the patient with information that prepares them to view fatigue as an expected part of treatment rather than a sign of disease progression. Other researchers investigating fatigue have also noted the importance of anticipatory guidance and counseling for symptom management (Holland, 1991; Yeager *et al.*, 1993). Teaching should include a definition of fatigue, the symptoms that may be experienced with specific biological agents, and when symptoms are expected to occur. Patients should also be aware of the expected duration of fatigue (e.g., acute or chronic) and should be assured that chronic fatigue does not necessarily signal the recurrence of disease, progression of disease, or lack of response to therapy. Discussing what other individuals have found useful in preventing and eliminating fatigue is helpful. Patients should be instructed to report early signs and symptoms of fatigue so that interventions can be instituted immediately in an attempt to prevent fatigue from worsening (Piper, 1991a; Skalla and Lacasse, 1992a). Reportable signs and symptoms of severe chronic fatigue include spending all day in bed or on a couch, being able to perform only minimal activities of daily living, and decreased ability to concentrate.

Research on Fatigue

Cancer-related fatigue has taken on new importance since this book was first published in 1995. At that time, the Oncology Nursing Society (ONS) had just held its first consensus conference on the state of the knowledge about fatigue (Winningham *et al.*, 1994). The resulting state-of-the-knowledge paper offered suggestions for managing fatigue and outlined critical areas of research for the ONS (see Table 17.2). Important areas for research include developing a research-based definition of fatigue, clarifying concepts related to fatigue (e.g., weakness or tiredness), differentiating acute versus chronic fatigue, determining the mechanisms of fatigue, delineating predictors of fatigue and patterns of fatigue associated with different types of therapy, and testing interventions to alleviate fatigue. These issues are important to research about biotherapy-related fatigue.

The ONS instituted the Fatigue Initiative through Research and Education (FIRE) to focus attention on the much-neglected area of symptom assessment and management. This major initiative, supported by Ortho Biotech, Inc., had three major components: research, professional education, and public education.

One part of the research component of FIRE involved the funding of a 3-year, multi-institutional research project ($500,000) to evaluate the effectiveness of exercise in reducing cancer-related fatigue. Additionally, three instrumentation grants ($50,000) were awarded to support the development and testing of instruments that clinicians can use to assess fatigue in a variety of clinical settings. The Clinical Research Scholars Program, another part of the research component, was initiated to establish a cadre of clinical collaborators, academic-based nursing faculty, and clinical-nurse researchers to move forward with the science and practice of fatigue research.

The professional-education component was officially instituted in 1996 when the ONS conducted a workshop about the state of the knowledge on fatigue. The purpose of the forum was to study, exchange ideas, and utilize new information about cancer-related fatigue. The workshop, which brought together approximately 200 attendees and experts in fatigue research, education, and practice, was designed for both clinicians and staff educators. Workshop attendees had to be nominated by their local ONS chapter president and had to share the information they learned with their local chapter members. Since the workshop, many of the attendees have conducted inservices and workshops on the topic of cancer-related fatigue for their health-care colleagues.

The public-education component of FIRE was initiated in 1998 when ONS launched its first National Cancer Fatigue Awareness Day. The event was sponsored by educational grants from the Oncology Nursing Foundation and Ortho Biotech, Inc. It has become an annual event with the 1999 theme being "Fight Fatigue: It Helps" and the 2000 theme being "Get Energized . . . Conquer Fatigue." Marketing activities, including public service announcements, were developed to get media attention and promotional kits, which included fatigue-assessment scales, and informational and educational literature (English and Spanish), was mailed to potential participants across the United States. Promotional and planning guides are available through the Oncology Nursing Society web site (http://www.ons.org).

Critical review of fatigue literature is problematic. The lack of consistent research tools and theory have created a body of literature that must be carefully reviewed for bias before conclusions can be drawn. As an early pioneer of fatigue research, Grandjean (1968) initially made an important point that must be considered when studying fatigue in patients treated with biological agents. During the assessment of fatigue, the testing process itself is a stress that alerts the organism, which may mask a previous state of fatigue. As a result of this response, tests that measure fatigue may provide results that report lower fatigue levels than were actually experienced. Current investigations (Cimprich, 1992) address "attentional fatigue" as a concept applied to cancer patients. This type of fatigue is another theoretical bias that could be introduced into a study that administers lengthy tools to measure fatigue. Thought must be given to these factors when reviewing the results of any study that investigates fatigue.

One of the earliest studies of fatigue conducted by nurses was a study initiated by Freel and Hart (1977) that examined fatigue in patients with multiple sclerosis. Haylock and Hart (1979) completed a study of fatigue in oncology patients who were receiving radiation therapy. Since then, nurses have documented fatigue in cancer patients receiving biotherapy (Davis, 1984; Mayer et al., 1984; Rieger, 1987; Hodges, 1992; Skalla, 1992) as well as chemotherapy (Jamar, 1989; Blesch et al., 1991; Nail et al., 1991; Pickard-Holley, 1991; Schwartz, 1998; Berger and Farr, 1999), radiation therapy (Oberst et al., 1991; Irvine et al., 1998), and surgery (Rhoten, 1982). An initial review by Irvin et al. (1991) provided a concise overview of the research literature investigating fatigue in patients with cancer. Current research efforts are focused on attempts to characterize the clinical nature of fatigue in patients with cancer.

Few studies have been published that document patterns of fatigue associated with biological agents. Precise mechanisms for fatigue experienced with biological agents have yet to be determined.

St. Pierre et al. (1992) looked at the relationship between fatigue, cachexia, and TNF. Cachexia was found in earlier research (Mayer et al., 1984) to be associated with IFN administration and may play a role in fatigue associated with muscle wasting. St. Pierre and colleagues have expanded this concept to create a cause-effect relationship by proposing a biochemical mechanism that causes changes in skeletal muscle physiology that may affect fatigue. The research by St. Pierre provides critical groundwork in nursing research from a physiologic perspective. It would be useful and relatively easy to include measurements such as albumin and blood pH, in an expanded form of this study, to provide data that may support this type of theory. The data provided by this type of research may also provide physiologic data to support the Piper et al. (1987) theoretical model for fatigue. Questions that address the physiologic relationship between fatigue and other symptoms that contribute to fatigue must be explored.

Investigation of the relationship between fatigue and biological agents could be enhanced in many ways. Due to the subjective nature of fatigue, qualitative research should be combined with quantitative research to steer further research efforts in appropriate directions. Biological agents seem to have a particular dose-relationship with fatigue; studies that examine the physiologic relationship of this phenomenon may yield specific information about the clinical nature of fatigue that could then guide efforts that focus on other treatment modalities. It is important to include healthy control populations in these studies to differentiate the effects of disease and treatment on fatigue. Additional questions may be answered by comparing two patient populations, for example, one receiving IFN for treatment of a malignancy and one receiving IFN for a nonmalignant disease such as hepatitis. Finally, there is a critical need for research that concentrates on the development of tools that adequately measure fatigue. Measures specific for fatigue must be developed that are reliable and valid and that can be easily applied in the clinical setting.

Summary

Fatigue is one of the most commonly occurring side effects in patients undergoing biotherapy.

Therapy with agents such as IFN and IL-2 are known to cause debilitating levels of fatigue that can affect the patient's quality of life. In fact, the severity of fatigue experienced during biotherapy may be dose-limiting; patients may opt to discontinue an otherwise effective cancer therapy because of the negative effects of fatigue. As with many quality-of-life issues, the management of fatigue is typically relegated to the nursing staff; therefore, nurses are in the best position to effect advances in fatigue research.

During the past 10 years, research has emerged that describes the patterns and intensity of biotherapy-related fatigue, but few of the interventions commonly recommended for its management have been evaluated to confirm efficacy or risk (Winningham *et al.*, 1994). Nursing research has only begun to formulate theory that explains the nature of fatigue and to develop tools that adequately measure fatigue. Studies examining the functional aspects of fatigue are needed. Findings from such studies could be used to justify research funding and would provide the groundwork for studies of interventions to alleviate fatigue. As the "state of the knowledge" regarding fatigue continues to progress, empirical interventions for treatment of fatigue should begin to emerge. Nurse researchers will remain at the forefront of these efforts, and nurse clinicians will continue to integrate research into practice and to advocate for management of fatigue in the patients for whom they provide care.

References

Aaronson, L., Teel, C., Cassmeyer, V., *et al.* 1999. Defining and measuring fatigue. *Image: Journal of Nursing Scholarship* 31(1): 45–50.

Abrams, P., McClamrock, E., and Foon, K. 1985. Evening administration of alpha interferon. *New England Journal of Medicine* 312: 443–444.

Adams, F., Quesada, J., and Gutterman, J. 1984. Neuropsychiatric manifestations of human leukocyte interferon therapy in patients with cancer. *Journal of the American Medical Association* 151: 938–941.

Aistars, J. 1987. Fatigue in the cancer patient: A conceptual approach to a clinical problem. *Oncology Nursing Forum* 14(6): 25–30.

Alexander, R., and Rosenberg, S. 1991. Tumor necrosis factor: Clinical applications. In DeVita, V., Hellman, S., Rosenberg, S. (eds). *Biological Therapy of Cancer*. Philadelphia, PA: J.B. Lippincott, pp. 378–392.

Barnett, M. 1997. Fatigue. In Otto, S. (ed). *Oncology Nursing*, 3rd edn. St. Louis, MO: Mosby, p. 670.

Berger, A., and Farr, L. 1999. The influence of daytime inactivity and nighttime restlessness on cancer-related fatigue. *Oncology Nursing Forum* 26(10): 1663–1671.

Blesch, K., Paice, J., Wickman, R., *et al.* 1991. Correlates of fatigue in people with breast or lung cancer. *Oncology Nursing Forum* 18(1): 81–87.

Brophy, L., and Sharp, E. 1991. Physical symptoms of combination biotherapy: A quality-of-life issue. *Oncology Nursing Forum* 18(1 suppl): 25–30.

Bruera, E., and MacDonald, R. 1988. Overwhelming fatigue in advanced cancer. *American Journal of Nursing* 88: 99–100.

Cella, D. 1997. The Functional Assessment of Cancer Therapy-Anemia (FACT-An) scale: A new tool for the assessment of outcomes in cancer anemia and fatigue. *Seminars in Hematology* 34(3 suppl 2): 13–19.

Cella, D., Tulsky, D., Gray, G., *et al.* 1993. The Functional Assessment of Cancer Therapy (FACT) scale: Development and validation of the general measure. *Journal of Clinical Oncology* 11: 570–579.

Christensen, T., Kehlet, H., Vesterberg, K., *et al.* 1987. Fatigue and muscle amino acids during surgical convalescence. *Acta Chirurgica Scandinavica* 153: 567–570.

Cimprich, B. 1993. Development of an intervention

to restore attention in cancer patients. *Cancer Nursing* 16(2): 83–92.

Clark, J., McGee, R., and Preston, R. 1992. Nursing management of responses to the cancer experience. In Clark, J., and McGee, R. (eds). *Oncology Nursing Society Core Curriculum for Oncology Nursing*, 2nd edn. Philadelphia, PA: W.B. Saunders, pp. 67–155.

Clark, P., and Lacasse, C. 1998. Cancer-related fatigue: Clinical practice issues. *Clinical Journal of Oncology Nursing* 2(2): 45–53.

Cleeland, C. 1989. Measurement of pain by subjective report. In Chapman, C., and Loeser, J. (eds). *Issues in Pain Measurement,* vol. 12 of *Advances in Pain Research and Therapy.* New York, NY: Raven Press, pp. 391–403.

Davis, C. 1984. Interferon-induced fatigue (unpublished master's thesis). Yale University, New Haven, CT.

Dean, G., Spears, L., Ferrell, B., *et al.* 1995. Fatigue in patients with cancer receiving interferon alpha. *Cancer Practice* 3(3): 164–172.

Dean, G., Spears, L., Quan, W., *et al.* 1993. Evening administration of interferon-alpha significantly reduces symptom distress in patients with metastatic melanoma. *Society for Biological Therapy 8th Annual Meeting Programs and Abstracts* 82 (abstract).

Dillman, J. 1988. Toxicity of monoclonal antibodies in the treatment of cancer. *Seminars in Oncology Nursing* 4(2): 107–111.

Epstein, K. 1995. The chronically fatigued patient. *Medical Clinics of North America* 79(2): 315–327.

Farrell, M., Gray, P., and Creekmore, S. 1990. Longterm biological therapy using interleukin-2 plus cyclophosphamide as a treatment for patients with melanoma: Nursing responsibilities. *Oncology Nursing Forum* 17(2 suppl): 239 (abstract).

Ferrell, B., Grant, M., Dean, G., *et al.* 1996. "Bone tired": The experience of fatigue and its impact on quality of life. *Oncology Nursing Forum* 23(10): 1539–1547.

Freel, M., and Hart, L. 1977. Fatigue phenomena of multiple-sclerosis patients. Grant no. 5R02-NM-00524-02. Washington, DC: U.S. Department of Health, Education, and Welfare Division of Nursing, p. 118.

Gastl, G., Werter, M., DePauw, B., *et al.* 1989. Comparison of clinical efficacy and toxicity of conventional and optimum biological response modifying doses of interferon alpha in the treatment of hairy-cell leukemia: A retrospective analysis of 39 patients. *Leukemia* 3(6): 453–460.

Gibson, H., and Edwards, R. 1985. Muscular exercise and fatigue. *Sports Medicine* 2(2): 120–132.

Gilson, B., Gilson, J., Bergner, M., *et al.* 1975. The sickness-impact profile: Development of an outcome measure of health care. *American Journal of Health Care* 65(12): 1304–1310.

Grandjean, E. 1968. Fatigue. *American Industrial Hygiene Association Journal* 31: 401–411.

Groopman, J. 1998. Fatigue in cancer and HIV/AIDS. *Oncology (Huntington)* 12(3): 335–344.

Haylock, P., and Hart, L. 1979. Fatigue in patients receiving localized radiation therapy. *Cancer Nursing* 2(6): 461–469.

Hodges, C. 1992. A preliminary study of fatigue in patients receiving IL-2 biotherapy (unpublished master's thesis). The University of Texas Health Science Center School of Nursing, Houston, TX.

Holland, J. 1991. Fatigue in the patient with cancer during the week following a chemotherapy treatment. *Oncology Nursing Forum* 18(2): 54 (abstract).

Irvine, D., Vincent, L., Bubela, N., *et al.* 1991. A critical appraisal of the research literature investigating fatigue in the individual with cancer. *Cancer Nursing* 14(4): 188–199.

Irvine, D., Vincent, L., Graydon, J., *et al.* 1998. Fatigue in women with breast cancer receiving radiation therapy. *Cancer Nursing* 21(2): 127–135.

Jamar, S. 1989. Fatigue in women receiving chemotherapy for ovarian cancer. In Funk, S., Tornquist, E., Champagne, M., Copp, L., and Weise, R. (eds). *Key Aspects of Comfort.* New York: Spring Hill Publishing, pp. 224–233.

Janisch, L. 1990. Nursing management of side effects of interleukin-2 and interferon alfa-2a administered as subcutaneous injections. *Oncology Nursing Forum* 17(2 suppl): 102 (abstract).

Jensen, S., and Givens, B. 1991. Fatigue affecting family caregivers of cancer patients. *Cancer Nursing* 14(4): 181–187.

Johnson, J., Nail, L., Lauver, D., *et al.* 1988. Reducing the negative impact of radiation therapy on functional status. *Cancer* 61: 46–51.

Jones, L. 1993. Correlates of fatigue and related outcomes in individuals with cancer undergoing treatment with chemotherapy (Unpublished doctoral dissertation). State University of New York, Buffalo, NY.

Kaempfer, S., and Lindsey, A. 1986. Energy expenditure in cancer. *Cancer Nursing* 9(4): 194–199.

Kashiwagi, S. 1971. Psychological ratings of human fatigue. *Ergonomics* 14(1): 17–21.

Koeller, J. 1989. Biological response modifiers: The interferon-alpha experience. *American Journal of Hospital Pharmacy* 46(2 suppl): S11–S15.

Lee, K., Talpaz, M., Rothberg, J., *et al.* 1989. Concomitant administration of recombinant human interleukin-2 and recombinant interferon alpha-2a in cancer patients: A Phase I study. *Journal of Clinical Oncology* 7(11): 1726–1732.

Lindner, D., Kalvakolann, D., and Borden, E. 1997. Increasing effectiveness of interferon-α for malignancies. *Seminars in Oncology* 24(3 suppl 9): S9–S99, S9–S104.

Lynch, M., Yanes, L., and Todd, K. 1988. Nursing care of AIDS patients participating in a Phase I/II trial of recombinant human granulocyte-macrophage colony-stimulating factor. *Oncology Nursing Forum* 15: 463–469.

MacVicar, M., and Winningham, M. 1986. Promoting the functional capacity of cancer patients. *Cancer Bulletin* 38: 235–239.

Martin, G. 1991. TNF and IL-2. *Oncology Nursing Forum* 18(2): 307 (abstract).

Maxwell, M. 1984. When the cancer patient becomes anemic. *Cancer Nursing* 7(4): 321–326.

Mayer, D., Hetrick, K., Riggs, C., *et al.* 1984. Weight

loss in patients receiving recombinant leukocyte-A interferon (IFLrA): A brief repost. *Cancer Nursing* 7(1): 53–56.

McCorkle, R., and Young, K. 1978. Development of a symptom distress scale. *Cancer Nursing* 1: 373–378.

McDaniel, R., and Rhodes, V. 2000. Fatigue. In Yarbro, C., Frogge, M., Goodman, M. and Groenwald, S., (eds). *Cancer Nursing: Principles and Practice*, 5th edn. Sudbury, MA: Jones & Bartlett Publishers, Inc., pp. 737–753.

McNair, D., Lorr, M., and Doppelman, F. (eds). 1971. *Manual for the Profile of Mood States*. San Diego, CA: Educational and Industrial Testing Service, pp. 3–29.

Meek, P., Nail, L., and Jones, L. 1997. Internal consistency, reliability, and construct validity of a new measure of cancer-treatment-related fatigue: The general fatigue scale. *Oncology Nursing Forum* 24(2): 334–335 (abstract).

Mendoza, T., Wang, X., Cleeland, C., *et al.* 1999. The rapid assessment of fatigue severity in cancer patients. *Cancer* 85(5): 1186–1196.

Mock, V., Burke, M., Sheehan, P., *et al.* 1994. A nursing rehabilitation program for women with breast cancer receiving adjuvant chemotherapy. *Oncology Nursing Forum* 21(5): 899–907.

Mock, V., Dow, K., Meares, C., *et al.* 1997. Effects of exercise on fatigue, physical functioning, and emotional distress during radiation therapy for breast cancer. *Oncology Nursing Forum* 24(6): 991–1000.

Moldawer, N., and Figlin, R. 1988. Tumor necrosis factor: Current clinical status and implications for nursing management. *Seminars in Oncology Nursing* 4(2): 120–125.

Monks, J. (1989). Experiencing symptoms in chronic illness: Fatigue in multiple sclerosis. *International Disabilities Studies* 11: 78–82.

Nail, L., Jones, L., Greene, D., *et al.* 1991. Use and perceived efficacy of self-care activities in patients receiving chemotherapy. *Oncology Nursing Forum* 18(5): 883–887.

Oberst, M., Chang, A., and McCubbin, M. 1991.

Self-care burden, stress appraisal, and mood among persons receiving radiotherapy. *Cancer Nursing* 14(2): 71–78.

Pearson, R., and Byars, G. 1956. The development and validation of a checklist for measuring subjective fatigue. School of Aviation Medicine, USAF, Randolf AFB, TX (Report No. 56-115).

Pickard-Holley, S. 1991. Fatigue in cancer patients: A descriptive study. *Cancer Nursing* 14: 13–19.

Piper, B. 1991a. Alteration in comfort: Fatigue. In McNally, J., Somerville, E., Miaskowski, C., *et al.* (eds). *Guidelines for Oncology Nursing Practice*, 2nd edn. Philadelphia: W.B. Saunders, pp. 155–162.

Piper, B. 1991b. Alterations in energy: The sensation of fatigue. In Baird, S., McCorkle, R., and Grant, M. (eds). *Cancer Nursing: A Comprehensive Textbook*. Philadelphia: W.B. Saunders, pp. 894–908.

Piper, B. 1993. Fatigue. In Carrieri-Kohlman, V., Lindsey, A., and West, C. (eds). *Pathophysiological Phenomena in Nursing: Human Responses to Illness*, 2nd edn. Philadelphia: W.B. Saunders, pp. 279–302.

Piper, B. 1997. Measuring fatigue. In Frank-Stromborg, M., and Olson, S. (eds). *Instruments for Clinical Health-Care Research,* 2nd edn. Sudbury, MA: Jones & Bartlett Publishers, Inc., pp. 482–496.

Piper, B., Dibble, S., and Dodd, M. 1996. The revised Piper Fatigue Scale: Confirmation of its multidimensionality and reduction in number of items in women with breast cancer. *Oncology Nursing Forum* 23(2): 352 (abstract).

Piper, B., and Dodd, M. 1991. Self-initiated fatigue interventions and their perceived effect. *Oncology Nursing Forum* 18(2): 391 (abstract).

Piper, B., Lindsey, A., and Dodd, M. 1987. Fatigue mechanisms in cancer: Developing nursing theory. *Oncology Nursing Forum* 14: 17–23.

Piper, B., Lindsey, A., Dodd, M., *et al.* 1989a. Development of an instrument to measure the subjective dimension of fatigue. In Funk, S., Tornquist, E., Champagne, M., *et al.* (eds). *Key Aspects of Comfort: Management of Pain, Fatigue, and Nausea*. New York: Springer Publishing Co., pp. 199–208.

Piper, B., Rieger, P., Brophy, L., *et al.* 1989b. Recent advances in the management of biotherapy-related side effects: Fatigue. *Oncology Nursing Forum* 16(suppl 6), 27–34.

Portenoy, R., and Itri, L. 1999. Cancer-related fatigue: Guidelines for evaluation and management. *Oncologist* 4(1): 1–10.

Potempa, K., Lopez, M., Reid, C., and Lawson, L. 1986. Chronic fatigue. *Image* 18: 165–169.

Quesada, J., Talpaz, M., Rios, A., *et al.* 1986. Clinical toxicity of interferons in cancer patients: A review. *Journal of Clinical Oncology* 4(2): 234–243.

Radin, A., Grant, B., Anderson, J., *et al.* 1989. Toxicity of interferon-alpha in the chronic myeloproliferative disorders: Preliminary results of collaborative Phase II trial. *Blood* 74(7 suppl 1): 236a.

Ream, E., and Richardson, A. 1999. From theory to practice: Designing interventions to reduce fatigue in patients with cancer. *Oncology Nursing Forum* 26(8): 1295–1303.

Reilly, L., and McKeever, S. 1993. Fatigue management in the patient treated with the biological response modifier interleukin-3. *Oncology Nursing Forum* 20(2): 218 (abstract).

Rhodes, V., and Watson, P. 1987. Symptom distress—The concept: Past and present. *Seminars in Oncology Nursing* 3: 242–247.

Rhodes, V., Watson P., and Hanson, B. 1988. Patients' descriptions of the influence of tiredness and weakness on self-care abilities. *Cancer Nursing* 11: 186–194.

Rhoten, D. 1982. Fatigue in the postsurgical patient. In Norris, C. (ed). *Concept Clarification in Nursing*. Rockville: Aspen Systems Corporation, pp. 277–295.

Richardson, A. 1998. Measuring fatigue in patients with cancer. *Supportive Care Cancer* 6(2): 94–100.

Richardson, A. 1998. Fatigue in patients receiving

chemotherapy: Patterns of change. *Cancer Nursing* 21(1): 17–30.

Rieger, P. 1987. Interferon-induced fatigue: A study of fatigue measurement. *Sigma Theta Tau International 29th Biennial Convention Book of Proceedings* A163.

Rieger, P. 1988. Management of cancer-related fatigue. *Dimensions in Oncology Nursing* II(3): 5–8.

Robinson, K., and Posner, J. 1992. Patterns of self-care needs and interventions related to biological response modifier therapy: Fatigue as a model. *Seminars in Oncology Nursing* 8(4 suppl 1): 17–22.

Schipper, H., Clinch, C., McMurray, A., *et al.* 1984. Measuring the quality of life of cancer patients: The functional living index—Cancer: Development and validation. *Journal of Clinical Oncology* 2(5): 472–483.

Selye, H. 1976. *The Stress of Life.* New York, NY: McGraw-Hill.

Shacham, S. 1983. A shortened version of the profile of mood states. *Journal of Personal Assessment* 47(3): 305–306.

Sharp, E. 1993. Case management of the hospitalized patient receiving interleukin-2. *Seminars in Oncology Nursing* 9(3 suppl 1): 14–19.

Siegel, J., and Puri, R. 1991. Interleukin-2 toxicity. *Journal of Clinical Oncology* 9: 694–704.

Silver, H., Connors, J., and Salinas, F. 1985. Prospectively randomized toxicity study of high-dose versus low-dose treatment strategies for lymphoblastoid interferon. *Cancer Treatment Reports* 69(7–8): 743–750.

Skalla, K. 1992. Correlates of fatigue in patients treated with interferon: A pilot study (unpublished master's thesis). MGH Institute of Health Professions, Boston, MA.

Skalla, K., and Lacasse, C. 1992a. Fatigue and the patient with cancer: What is it and what can I do about it? *Oncology Nursing Forum* 19: 1540–1541.

Skalla, K., and Lacasse, C. 1992b. Patient education for fatigue. *Oncology Nursing Forum* 19: 1537–1539.

Smets, E., Garssen, B., Bonke, B., and Haes, J. 1995. The Multidimensional Fatigue Inventory (MFI): Psychometric qualitites of an instrument to assess fatigue. *Journal of Psychosomatic Research* 39: 315.

Smets, E., Garssen, B., Cull, A., and Haes, J. 1996. Application of the Multidimensional Fatigue Inventory (MFI-20) in cancer patients receiving radiotherapy. *British Journal of Cancer* 73: 241–245.

St. Pierre, B., Kasper, C., and Lindsey, A. 1992. Fatigue mechanisms in patients with cancer: Effects of tumor necrosis factor and exercise on skeletal muscle. *Oncology Nursing Forum* 19(3): 419–425.

Talpaz, M., Kantarjian, H., O'Brien, S., *et al.* 1997. The M. D. Anderson Cancer Center experience with interferon-alpha therapy in chronic myelogenous leukaemia. *Baillieres Clinical Hematology* 10(2): 291–305.

Viele, C., and Moran, T. 1993. Nursing management of the nonhospitalized patient receiving recombinant interleukin-2. *Seminars in Oncology Nursing* 9(3 suppl 1): 20–24.

Visser, M., and Smets, E. 1998. Fatigue, depression, and quality of life in cancer patients: How are they relatedn. *Support Care Cancer* 6: 101–108.

Vogelzang, N., Breitbart, W., Cella, D., *et al.* 1997. Patient, caregiver, and oncologist perceptions of cancer-related fatigue: Results of a tripart association survey. *Seminars in Hematology* 34(3 suppl 2): 4–12.

Wadler, S., Lyver, A., and Wiernik, P. 1989. Clinical toxicities of the combination of 5-fluorouracil and recombinant interferon-alpha-2a: An unusual toxicity profile. *Oncology Nursing Forum* 16(6 suppl): 12–15.

Winningham, M. 1983. Effects of bicycle ergometry program on functional capacity and feelings of control in women with breast cancer (doctoral dissertation). Ohio State University, Columbus, OH.

they related. *Support Care Cancer* 6: 101–108.

tigue: Implications for people receiving cancer therapy. In Carroll-Johnson, R. (ed). *The Biotherapy of Cancer-V* (monograph). Pittsburgh, PA: Oncology Nursing Press, pp. 16–21.

Winningham, M., and Barton-Burke, M. (eds). 1999. *Fatigue in Cancer: A Multidimensional Approach.* Sudbury, MA: Jones & Bartlett Publishers, Inc.

Winningham, M., Glass, E., and MacVicar, M. 1990. Rhythmic walking: Exercise for people living with cancer. Ohio State University, Arthur G. James Cancer Hospital and Research Institute, Columbus, OH.

Winningham, M., Nail, L., Burke, M., *et al.* 1994. Fatigue and the cancer experience: The state of the knowledge. *Oncology Nursing Forum* 21(1): 23–36.

Yeager, K., Dibble, S., and Dodd, M. 1993. The experience of fatigue among patients receiving chemotherapy. *Oncology Nursing Forum* 20(2): 297 (abstract).

Yoshitake, H. 1971. Relations between the symptoms and the feeling of fatigue. *Ergonomics* 14(1): 175–186.

Yoshitake, H. 1969. Rating the feelings of fatigue. *Journal of Science and Labor* 45(7): 422–432.

Clinical Pearls

Assessment

1. Determine a fatigue-severity rating with "0" being no fatigue and "10" representing the worst possible fatigue. A score greater than 6 would indicate the need for intensive evaluation and management by the health care team.
2. Evaluate the pattern of fatigue (i.e., cancer-related versus activity-related).
3. Review pertinent clinical tests (e.g., laboratory values, vital signs, and x-rays).
4. Note any change in the effect of fatigue (e.g., anxiousness, drowsiness, or depression).

Management

1. Treat any underlying causes of fatigue that are amenable to therapy (e.g., anemia, electrolyte imbalance, malnourishment, depression, or hormonal changes).
2. Teach patients the importance of maintaining a balance between rest/sleep and activity/exercise.
3. Teach patients energy-conservation techniques.
4. Teach patients signs and symptoms that should be reported to the health-care team: tiredness on awakening, reduction in activity level exhibited by decreased functional status, difficulty concentrating (e.g., inability to follow conversations or find the right word in conversation).

Key Resources

Worldwide Web Sites

www.cancerfatigue.org
www.fatiguenet.com
www.oesweb.com (click on CE for fatigue information)
www.oncolink.upenn.edu (scroll down to symptoms)

Books and Book Chapters

McDaniel, R., and Rhodes, V. (2000). Fatigue. In Yarbro, C., Frogge, M., and Goodman, M., and Groenwald, S. (eds). *Cancer Nursing,* 5th edn. Sudbury, MA: Jones & Bartlett Publishers, Inc. pp. 737–753

Winningham, M. 1999. Fatigue. In Yarbro, C., Frogge, M., and Goodman, M. (eds). *Cancer Symptom Management*, 2nd edn. Sudbury, MA: Jones & Bartlett Publishers, Inc., pp. 58–76.

Winningham, M.L., and Barton-Burke, M. (eds). 1999. *Fatigue in Cancer: A Multidimensional Approach*. Sudbury, MA: Jones & Bartlett Publishers, Inc.

Newsletters

Fatigue Forum. Sponsored by Ortho Biotech and produced by Oncology Education Services. Available from Ortho Biotech product representatives and online at the OES web site.

Articles

Aaronson, L., Teel, C., Cassmeyer, V., *et al.* 1999. Defining and measuring fatigue. *Image: Journal of Nursing Scholarship* 31(1): 45–50.

Clark, P., and LaCasse, C. 1998. Cancer-related fatigue: Clinical practice issues. *Clinical Journal of Oncology Nursing* 2(2): 45–53.

Curt, A. 2000. The impact of fatigue on patients with cancer: Overview of FATIGUE 1 and 2. *Oncologist* 5(suppl 2): 9–12.

Mock, V. 1998. Breast cancer and fatigue: Issues for the workplace. *AAOHN Journal* 46(9): 425–431.

Nail, L. 1995. Fatigue and weakness in cancer patients: The symptoms experience. *Seminars in Oncology Nursing* 11(4): 272–278.

Piper, B. 1993. Fatigue. In Carrieri-Kohlman, V., Lindsey, A., and West, C. (eds). *Pathophysiological Phenomena in Nursing: Human Responses to Illness*, 2nd edn. Philadelphia, PA: W.B. Saunders, pp. 279–302.

Ream, E., and Richardson, A. 1999. From theory to practice: Designing interventions to reduce fatigue in patients with cancer. *Oncology Nursing Forum* 26(8): 1295–1303.

Simon, A., and Zittoun, R. 1999. Fatigue in cancer patients. *Current Opinion in Oncology* 11(4): 244–249.

Winningham, M., Nail, L., Burke, M., *et al.* 1994. Fatigue and the cancer experience: The state of the knowledge. *Oncology Nursing Forum* 21(1): 23–36.

CHAPTER 18 | Anorexia as a Side Effect of Biotherapy

Linda Cuaron, RN, MN, AOCN®

Anorexia is a common side effect of biotherapy and one of the most common neurological side effects of biotherapy (Plata-Salaman, 1998). Anorexia is the loss of the desire to eat, leading to reduced food intake (Laviano *et al.*, 1996a). The incidence, expected severity, and treatment of anorexia in the patient who is receiving chemotherapy or radiation therapy has been well described. In contrast, the impact of anorexia and related treatment considerations for the patient receiving biotherapy are only recently in the literature.

In many chronic diseases, including cancer, anorexia contributes to the cachexia syndrome. The word *cachexia* is derived from the Greek words *kakos*, meaning *bad*, and *hexis*, meaning *condition* (Tisdale, 1997a). Cachexia involves muscle-wasting, weight loss, depletion of fat and protein stores, an increase in the amount of body water, and many metabolic changes (Hardin, 1993). This **catabolic** state and its precursor, anorexia, have been hypothesized to derive from the **autocrine**, endocrine, **paracrine**, and **intracrine** actions of cytokines on various receptor sites in the body (Langstein and Norton, 1991; Bartholomew and Hoffman, 1993; Laviano *et al.*, 1996a; Plata-Salaman *et al.*, 1996b; Plata-Salaman, 1998). The idea that cytokines might be involved in processes such as cachexia and anorexia was first considered because individuals with cancer often had the same metabolic alterations as patients with chronic infection. Additionally, cachectin, a factor known to contribute to wasting syndrome, was found to be identical to tumor necrosis factor (TNF).

There is evidence from a large body of animal research that prolonged exposure to cytokines, either as a result of cancer, chronic infections, long-term immune reactions, or therapeutic administration, can induce weight loss, anorexia, and cachexia (Socher *et al.*, 1988; Matthys and Billiau, 1997). Further support comes from research in which tumor-induced cachexia in animals is reversed with administration of anti-IFN-γ or anti-TNF antibodies (Langstein and Norton, 1991). Clinical experience over the years has shown that anorexia is a significant side effect of several biological agents, especially when given at high doses (Plata-Salaman, 1998).

Biotherapy is also used to treat noncancer diseases such as the use of interferon-α (IFN-α) for hepatitis B and C and IFN-β for treatment of relapsing multiple sclerosis. Anorexia may occur as a side effect of biotherapy given for noncancerous diseases or when biotherapy is given as an adjuvant therapy for cancer treatment. It is thought that neurological side effects, including anorexia, are mediated through target sites in both the peripheral nervous system and central nervous system (CNS). Anorexia may also be a part of a constellation of biotherapy-associated side effects that include fatigue, depression, and endocrine-mediated mechanisms (Jones *et al.*, 1998; Lucinio *et al.*, 1998; Valentine *et al.*, 1998).

Anorexia as a side effect of biotherapy is very likely a complex and multifactorial process. Biotherapy, in part, relies on the elements of a competent immune system for its mechanism of action. This chapter describes some of the normal processes that regulate appetite and eating patterns, and the role of nutrients in the maintenance of a healthy immune system. The pathophysiological processes, as well as the conceptual models that describe the numerous factors thought to play a role in the development of anorexia and cachexia as a side effect of biotherapy, are presented. The role of cytokines as direct (i.e., CNS or hypothalamic) or indirect (i.e., serotonergic) mediators of anorexia are described. Gastrointestinal, somatic (e.g., depression, fatigue), and disease-related factors that may influence the occurrence or severity of anorexia are also described.

Presentation of Anorexia

Determining whether anorexia in a patient receiving biotherapy is related to the treatment can pose a complex problem for nurses and physicians because cancer patients often exhibit changes in eating behavior; in fact, changes in normal eating habits may even be the presenting symptom of malignancy (Langstein and Norton, 1991; Laviano *et al.*, 1996b). Data from the Eastern Cooperative Oncology Group show that 50% of oncology patients have some weight loss at the time of their diagnosis (Langstein and Norton, 1991). Additionally, it has been shown that the resting-energy expenditure of patients with cancer is usually increased, but caloric intake is seldom increased (Langstein and Norton, 1991).

Anorexia can interfere with the receipt of adequate treatment, affect the ability to complete the course of therapy, and significantly interfere with quality of life (Laviano *et al.*, 1996b). The severity of anorexia induced by biotherapy depends on the type of biological agent used; the dose, duration, timing, and route of administration; and the disease state and clinical condition of the patient. Anorexia may manifest as the loss of desire to eat or a decrease in food intake, and may be accompanied by other side effects such as nausea, vomiting, taste aversions, constipation, or diarrhea. It can result from alterations in food perception, alterations in taste and smell, early satiety, or delayed gastric emptying.

A complex interaction of psychological, gastrointestinal, metabolic, neuronal, endocrine, and nutritional factors contributes to the regulation of appetite and eating patterns. Since the concept of *homeostasis* was first coined by Walter Cannon in the early 1900s, researchers have been interested in describing the possible factors that contribute to a move away from homeostasis, as is seen in anorexia or cachexia. Rowland *et al.* (1996) conducted a comprehensive review of these factors and prefaced their findings by acknowledging that "... human feeding is extremely complex, and physiological variables form, at best, a crude template on which the many aspects of the behavior are sculpted in an ever-changing way."

The Role of Nutrients in Immune Function

Nutrients, including proteins, carbohydrates, lipids, fluids, vitamins, and minerals, are essential to immune function. Changes in nutrient intake can significantly affect the cells of the immune system and alter the regulation of immunity (Table 18.1). In the malnourished patient, the thymus and lymphoid tissues undergo atrophy, the number of circulating T cells decreases, and there are alterations in cell-mediated immunological functions (Terr *et al.*, 1991). Additionally, natural killer cell–killing ability is decreased, and a depressed response to vaccines is seen (Shronts, 1993). Immunodeficiency in the elderly was studied and found to be associated with a zinc deficiency (Cakman *et al.*, 1997). Additionally, in the elderly, zinc is absorbed at a lower rate than in younger individuals. Some of the immune deficiencies thought to be associated with zinc deficiency are poor wound-healing,

Table 18.1 Nutrients that have a role in immunocompetence

	Nutrient	Immunomodulation
Vitamins	A	Deficiency reduces lymphocyte response to mitogens and antigens.
		Modest doses of β-carotene and retinoids stimulate immune responses.
	B complex (B₆)	Deficiency associated with decreased antibody response and impaired cellular immunity.
	C	Extreme deficiency impairs phagocyte function and cellular immunity.
	D	Deficiency causes anergy in the delayed hypersensitivity skin test.
	E	Deficiency decreases antibody response to T-cell-dependent antigens: effect compounded by selenium deficiency.
Minerals/Trace Elements	Iron	Necessary for optimum neutrophil and lymphocyte function. Free iron necessary for bacterial growth.
	Zinc	Deficiency associated with susceptibility to infection, abnormal cell-mediated immunity, depressed circulating thymic hormones, and altered complement phagocyte function. Excess associated with immunosuppression.
	Copper	Deficiency associated with increased rate of infections, depressed reticuloendothelial system and microbicidal activity of granulocytes, impaired antibody response, and depressed thymic hormone.

(continued)

Table 18.1 *Continued*

	Nutrient	Immunomodulation
Minerals/Trace Elements *(cont.)*	Selenium	Deficiency reduces antibody responses.
	Iodine	Decreased microbicidal activity of neutrophils in hypothyroid patients; improved function followed treatment.
	Manganese	Required for normal antibody synthesis and/or secretion; excess inhibits antibody formation and chemotaxis, and increases susceptibility to pneumococcal infection.
	Magnesium	Deficiency causes thymic hyperplasia, impaired humoral and cell-mediated immunologic responsiveness, depressed immunoglobulins (IgG$_1$, IgG$_2$, IgA).
Other	Calories	Obese individuals have mild impairment of cell-mediated immunity and phagocyte function. Calorie deprivation associated with decreased circulating immune complex levels, decreased anti-DNA antibodies, increased thymocyte proliferation in response to exogenous IL-2, and increased IL-2 production in response to stimulation with mitogens.
	Lipids	
	Omega-6	Essential fatty acid deficiency results in lymphoid atrophy and depressed antibody responses. Excess polyunsaturated fatty acid (linoleic and arachidonic acid) induce atrophy of lymphoid tissue, diminish T-cell immune responsiveness to antigenic stimulation and delayed hypersensitivity; hypercholesterolemia is associated with reduced cell-mediated immunity and phagocyte function.
	Omega-3 (eicosanoids or fish oil)	Form prostaglandins and leukotrienes that play a role in linking the actions of T-suppressor and T-helper cells; lessen immunosuppression associated with burns; improve experimental models of arthritis.
	Protein	Deficiency results in decreased production of labile proteins; e.g., immunoglobulins; depressed cellular immunity including cutaneous hypersensitivity and phagocyte function; quantity and activity of complement is reduced.
	Tyrosine and Phenylalanine	Restriction has been associated with enhancement of cytotoxic immunity in tumor-bearing animals.
	Arginine	Stimulates lymphocyte mitogenesis; suppresses tumor growth.
	Glutamine	Substrate for macrophages and T-lymphocytes.
	Nucleotides (RNA, uracil)	Play a vital role in T lymphocyte-mediated immunity. Deprivation results in increased susceptibility to a bacterial challenge, depressed cutaneous hypersensitivity and response of lymphocytes to mitogens; suppresses cardiac allograft rejection and experimental graft-versus-host disease.

Ig, immunoglobulin; IL, interleukin.

Source: Shronts, E. 1993. Basic concepts of immunology and its application to clinical nutrition. *Nutrition in Clinical Practice* 8(4): 177–183; and American Society of Enteral-Parenteral Nutrition, with permission.

decreased **chemotaxis** by neutrophils and monocytes, and hypoplasia of the lymphoid system. Zinc supplementation may benefit the elderly by reversing immunodeficiency. Additionally, vitamins A, B_6, B_{12}, C, E, and folic acid are involved in synthesis of DNA and proteins, as well as in the maturation of immune cells. Deficiencies in trace elements such as copper, iron, manganese, and selenium generally suppress immune function (Cakman *et al.*, 1997).

The Role of Cytokines in Altering Metabolism

Cytokines have been shown to alter protein, carbohydrate, and lipid metabolism. TNF in-

creases muscle proteolysis, protein oxidation, and hepatic protein synthesis. It also decreases **lipogenesis** and has multiple effects on glucose synthesis and clearance. Other cytokines such as interleukin (IL)-1, IL-6, IFN-γ, and D-Factor (leukemia-inhibitory factor) also affect the metabolism of proteins, carbohydrates, and lipids (Table 18.2) (Laviano *et al.*, 1996b). Cytokines can function as mediators of defense in ways that are essential for processes such as antibody formation, tumor-killing, and T-cell response. The role of cytokines as a mediator of disease is manifested by fever, inflammation, metabolic dysfunction, tissue degradation, anorexia, shock, and death. The interrelationship between nutrition, cytokine production, and biological function during normal and pathologic condi-

Table 18.2   Cytokine-mediated effects on protein, carbohydrate, and lipid metabolism

Cytokine	Metabolism		
	Protein	Carbohydrate	Lipid
TNF	Increased muscle proteolysis Increased protein oxidation Increased hepatic protein synthesis	Increased glycogenolysis Decreased glycogen synthesis Increased glyconeogenesis Increased glucose clearance Increased lactate production	Decreased lipogenesis
IL-1	Increased hepatic protein synthesis	Increased gluconeogenesis Increased glucose clearance	Increased lipolysis Decreased LPL synthesis Increased fatty acids synthesis
IL-6	Increased hepatic protein synthesis		Increased lipolysis Increased fatty acids synthesis
IFN-gamma			Decreased lipogenesis Increased lipolysis Decreased LPL activity
D-Factor (LIF)			Decreased LPL activity

IFN, interferon; IL, interleukin; LIF, leukemia inhibitory factor; LPL, lipoprotein lipase; TNF, tumor necrosis factor.

Source: Laviano, A., Renvyle, T., and Yang, Z. 1996b. From laboratory to bedside: New strategies in the treatment of malnutrition in cancer patients. *Nutrition* 12(2): 112–122, with permission.

tions is demonstrated in Figure 18.1 (Meydani, 1996).

Presentation of Cachexia

Cachexia is a common and potentially debilitating complication of several chronic diseases such as cancer and **acquired immunodeficiency syndrome (AIDS)**. Cachexia, also termed "wasting syndrome," is defined as an unintentional weight loss of more than 10% of total body weight. Depletion of total body weight and metabolically active body-cell mass is related to mortality; when this degree of loss occurs, death is usually imminent. Anorexia, defined as energy input that is consistently less than energy expenditure, is central to cancer-related cachexia.

Maintenance of skeletal and **visceral protein** is essential to survival. In the normal state, when acute fasting occurs, skeletal muscle is catabolized to provide amino acids for **gluconeogenesis**. If chronic fasting occurs, the normal muscle breakdown decreases and the body conserves nitrogen to maintain body mass. This type of conservation does not usually occur in patients who have cancer. What follows is muscle atrophy, myopathy, visceral organ atrophy, hypoalbuminemia, and abnormalities of immune regulation, protein metabolism, and liver-protein synthesis (Langstein and Norton, 1991). The resulting metabolic abnormalities that follow include decreases in body lipid mass, body muscle mass, body glycogen mass, and energy expenditure. Increases are seen in serum-lipid levels, serum-triglyceride levels, total body water, and glucose production (Figure 18.2). The human response to cachexia is characterized by profound weight loss, loss of muscle mass, severe fatigue, weakness, and depression. In some cases, there is an alteration in total functional capacity and debilitating diarrhea.

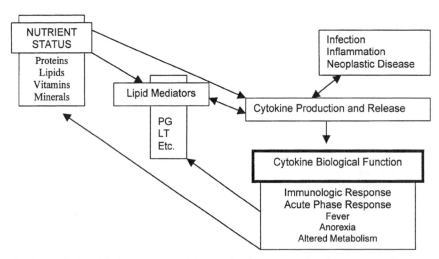

Figure 18.1   Interrelationship between nutrition and infectious and inflammatory diseases mediated by cytokines

Source: Meydani, S. 1996. Effect of (n-3) polyunsaturated fatty acids on cytokine production and their biologic function. *Nutrition* 12(suppl): S8–S14, with permission.

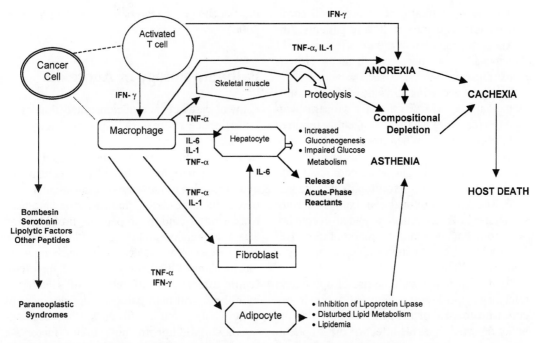

Figure 18.2   Proposed cytokine-mediated mechanism of cancer cachexia

Abbreviations: IFN-γ, interferon-gamma; IL, interleukin; TNF-α, tumor necrosis factor-α.

Source: Langstein, H., and Norton, J. 1991. Mechanisms of cancer cachexia. *Nutrition and Cancer* 5(1): 103–123, with permission.

Occurrence of Anorexia

The occurrence of anorexia in the patient receiving biotherapy will vary depending on the type of therapy; the dose, route, and duration of therapy; and the effects of combined use of chemotherapy, radiation therapy, and surgery (Sandstrom, 1996). Skalla (1996) identified anorexia as a clinical toxic effect of IFN-α and IFN-β when given at high cumulative doses. The occurrence of anorexia with IFN alpha-2a (Roferon®A) varies with the doses used and the disease treated. When IFN alpha-2a was given as treatment for hairy-cell leukemia, anorexia occurred in 43% of patients; likewise, anorexia occurred in 48% of patients treated for chronic myelogenous leukemia and 65% of patients

treated for AIDS-related Kaposi's sarcoma (depending on the schedule). With IFN alpha-con1 (Infergen®) as treatment for hepatitis C, anorexia occurred in 24% (at dose of 9 mcg three times a week) and 21% (at dose of 15 mcg three times a week) of patients. With IFN beta-1a (Avonex®) as treatment for relapsing-remitting multiple sclerosis, anorexia occurred in 7% of patients, but was not reported to occur with the use of IFN beta-1b (Betaseron®). With IFN gamma-1b (Actimmune®) as treatment for chronic granulomatous disease, anorexia occurred as a side effect in 3% of patients (*Physicians' Desk Reference,* 2000).

IL-2 and IL-11 are the only interleukins currently approved by the Food and Drug Administration (FDA). When IL-2 is given as approved by the FDA for treatment of renal-cell carcinoma, anorexia occurs in 20% of patients. Anorexia is not reported as a side effect of IL-11 (Neumega®), a platelet growth factor (*Physicians' Desk Reference, 2000*).

Anorexia occurring as a side effect of monoclonal antibody (MAB) therapy with trastuzumab (Herceptin®) as a single agent is reported in 14% of patients. When trastuzumab is combined with paclitaxel, the occurrence of anorexia reached 24%, but when combined with an anthracycline (i.e., doxorubicin), the rate was 31%. The MAB rituximab (Rituxan®) does not list anorexia as an infusion-related event, but does note that anorexia was reported more frequently in re-treated patients (*Physicians' Desk Reference, 2000*).

As demonstrated with the use of oprelvekin (Neumega®), a low incidence of anorexia occurs with the use of growth factors. Anorexia is not reported as a side effect of the 2 epoetin alfa products approved by the FDA, Procrit® and Epogen®. Anorexia reportedly occurred in 9% of patients treated with the **granulocyte colony-stimulating factor (G-CSF)** filgrastim (Neupogen®); however, the placebo group in the blinded study reported an 11% incidence of anorexia (*Physicians' Desk Reference, 2000*). A rather high incidence of anorexia was reported among patients receiving **granulocyte-macrophage colony-stimulating factor (GM-CSF)** or sargramostim (Leukine®); however, these patients were receiving autologous (54%) and allogeneic (51%) bone-marrow transplant (BMT). Additionally, the patients in the placebo-controlled arm of the studies leading to the regulatory approval of sargramostim reported even higher rates (58% for autologous and 57% for allogeneic BMT of anorexia, which suggests that other factors may have contributed to the anorexia. In a study of sargramostim versus placebo for treatment of acute myelogenous leukemia, anorexia was reported in 13% of patients in the sargramostim group versus 11% in the placebo group (*Physicians' Desk Reference, 2000*).

Pathophysiology of Anorexia

Clinical research has demonstrated that cytokines induce anorexia when administered peripherally or directly into the brain (Plata-Salaman, 1998). In addition to inducing anorexia via peripheral and CNS mechanisms, cytokines also modulate gastrointestinal activities, induce metabolic changes, modulate neurotransmitter and neuropeptide profiles, and affect the endocrine system (Plata-Salaman, 1998). Research that describes the therapeutic mechanisms of biotherapy, as well as the **pleiotropic** effects and side effects of **secondary cytokines**, will help guide the development of effective interventions for the side effect of anorexia. In addition to the cytokine factors, it is also important to consider environmental, metabolic, enzymatic, somatic, and hormonal factors that play a role in regulation of food intake. There also may be other factors that have not yet been elucidated by research that will give us a better understanding of biotherapy-related anorexia and the strategies for managing this side effect (Hellerstein *et al.*, 1989; Fantino and Wieteskas, 1993; Tsujinaka *et al.*, 1996; Hill *et al.*, 1997; Plata-Salaman, 1998).

Central Nervous System Mediators of Anorexia

Research has demonstrated that the major CNS sites involved in anorexia are the lateral hypothalamus (LH), the paraventricular nucleus (PVN), and the ventro-medial hypothalamus (VMH). The VMH may be a satiety center, responsible for the feeling of fullness, whereas the LH is more involved with initiation of feeding and other neuronal activities related to food intake. The VMH and LH are involved in the control of food intake and energy balance via neurons. These neurons sense **endogenous** factors such as glucose levels.

The Role of Cytokines in the Development of Anorexia

CYTOKINE CASCADE

Although there is variability in the exact mechanisms of action and side effects associated with different cytokines, some general principles remain true. A consistent mechanism of action of biotherapy is **immunomodulation**, which often results in the induction of secondary cytokines. Cytokines are essential in regulating the immune response to foreign antigens, pathogens, and virus. Cytokines also have an effect on the regulation of fever and inflammatory responses, and the control of cellular metabolism and nitrogen balance (Karmali, 1996). Cytokine actions are often redundant and they can influence the synthesis of other cytokines, which can lead to a cascade of events in which a second or third cytokine mediates the actions of the original cytokine (Abbas *et al.*, 1991). Because cytokines do not enter cells directly, connection with receptors on the cell membrane via cytokine **ligands** is necessary for signal transduction. Such events may result in the induction of enzymes or secondary messengers, such as cyclic adenosine monophosphate (cAMP), protein kinase C, and phospholipase A, or the synthesis of **prostaglandins** from the precursor **arachidonic acid** (Hellerstein *et al.*, 1989; Abbas *et al.*, 1991).

Administration of certain cytokines induces inflammatory processes and immunological reactions, and stimulates macrophages and other immune cells to synthesize and release other secondary cytokines. Cytokine release is rarely, if ever, a singular event. Cytokines stimulate many other types of cells and generate a cytokine cascade that results in the expression or secretion of other secondary cytokines. TNF-α

induces the expression of IL-1, IL-6, and IL-8. IL-1 induces the expression of IL-2, IL-3, IL-4, IL-6, IL-8, IL-9, and colony-stimulating factors. IFN-α can induce the expression of IL-1, IL-2, IL-6, IL-8, TNF-α, and IFN-γ. There is strong evidence that this cascade plays an important role in the development of anorexia (Terr *et al.*, 1991; Plata-Salaman, 1998).

TUMOR NECROSIS FACTOR AND ANOREXIA

It is well understood that TNF causes anorexia. TNF-α is also known as cachectin and is implicated as contributing to cachexia. TNF mediates acute inflammation and also stimulates mononuclear phagocytes and vascular endothelial cells to secrete IL-1 and IL-6 into the circulation. TNF is also known to cause severe metabolic disturbances such as a fall in glucose concentrations. As shown in experimental studies, long-term systemic administration of TNF causes cachexia. This cachexia is produced in part as a result of anorexia and partly by increased metabolism and lipolysis (Abbas *et al.*, 1991).

Metabolically, TNF increases muscle proteolysis, protein oxidation, and hepatic protein synthesis (Laviano *et al.*, 1996b). Glucagon and TNF act synergistically, resulting in the increased uptake of circulating amino acids by hepatocytes, which then support the increased production of **acute-phase proteins** and the preservation of hepatic mass (Hardin, 1993). In muscle tissue, TNF increases gluconeolysis and lactate production as it decreases glycogen levels. TNF also suppresses lipogenesis. The action of TNF differs depending on its site of production. Anorexia results when TNF is produced in the CNS, and severe cachexia occurs when TNF is secreted peripherally (Laviano *et al.*, 1996b).

TNF is also associated with reduced hepatic albumin synthesis, as seen in inflammatory states (Hardin, 1993). Increased vascular permeability, either as a result of inflammation or the administration of IL-1, also can contribute to hypoalbuminemia. It is important to recognize that cytokines are notorious for acting in both a paracrine and an autocrine manner, and in synergy with each other so that they might exert their effects at serum concentrations that are too low to measure (Matthys and Billiau, 1997). Relatively low concentrations of these cytokines can exert a significant action resulting in anorexia because of their synergistic activity. For example, IFN-γ augments TNF activity, and IL-1 acts synergistically with TNF (Yang *et al.*, 1994). In addition to the synergistic activity of cytokines, clinical evidence has shown that the threshold of cytokine concentrations necessary to induce anorexia is lower than the amount needed to produce fever (Plata-Salaman, 1996b).

Endogenous TNF has a relatively short half-life of approximately 15 minutes. Although structurally unrelated to IL-1 and possessing a different cellular receptor, TNF and IL-1 have overlapping biological activities. Many cells in the immune system (e.g., monocytes, pulmonary and peritoneal macrophages, and hepatic Kupffer cells) and certain cells in the CNS (e.g., astrocytes and microglia) produce TNF-α (Hardin, 1993; Lucinio *et al.*, 1998). Studies have demonstrated that bolus infusions of TNF in humans result in a 30% increase in metabolic rate (Starnes, 1991). TNF exerts systemic effects such as increasing the synthesis of prostaglandins and directly affecting carbohydrate metabolism in muscle cells. This results in the induction of anaerobic glycolysis, as characterized by increased cellular-membrane transport of glucose and depletion of glycogen stores (Hardin, 1993; Tisdale, 1997b). Hypertryglyceridemia also is induced in animals treated with TNF; however, this condition does not seem to be related to cachexia or anorexia (Tisdale, 1997b).

TNF-α contributes to **proteolysis** of the skeletal muscle cell, resulting in **asthenia** and loss of total body mass. TNF-α, IL-6, and IL-1 act on hepatocytes to induce increased gluconeogenesis and impaired glucose metabolism. These cytokines also contribute to the release of acute-phase proteins generating an inflammatory-like condition. TNF-α and IL-1 act on the fibroblasts, which in turn release more IL-6. TNF-α and IFN-γ act on the adipocytes to cause lipidemia, disturbance of lipid metabolism, and inhibition of lipoprotein lipase. These actions add up to the process of anorexia, compositional depletion of the body and asthenia, which ultimately can lead to cachexia and death.

CYTOKINES AS CENTRAL MEDIATORS OF ANOREXIA

Researchers used several animal models to research the effect of cytokines in inducing anorexia, including a **parabiotic** model. In a parabiotic model, the vascular systems of two mice are joined via **anastomosis** so that they share a small portion of each other's circulatory system. In one study, researchers implanted a nonmetastasizing tumor in an animal that had been surgically joined to another animal. These animals shared a small (i.e., 1.5%) amount of their circulatory content. Results of this experiment demonstrated that the nontumor-bearing animal shared the weight loss and decreased food intake of the animal with the tumor. This supported the concept that there is some humoral mediator of anorexia, such as cytokines, that might be present in very small amounts and that might exert a profound effect, resulting in anorexia and weight loss (Norton *et al.*, 1985).

In another study, plasma was collected and pooled from experimental rats who had been implanted with a sarcoma tumor and had become terminally cachectic (Illig *et al.*, 1992). Blood was collected from a group of control animals in the same manner. The collected plasma was then introduced in a blinded fashion to 20 normal rats. Rats who received the plasma collected from the tumor-bearing rats experienced immediate and profound anorexia. The total food intake decreased, and the mean daily nitrogen balance was negative for the rats in the experimental group. This study further supports the idea that cancer-associated anorexia and cachexia is transmissible in plasma and may be mediated by one or more circulating molecules.

Animals treated with IL-1β will ingest the same or a larger quantity of carbohydrate and significantly less protein, whereas fat intake decreases or remains unchanged. Cytokines such as IL-1, TNF-α, and IFN act on the peripheral nervous system, CNS, or both to induce anorexia. This action can be blocked with specific inhibitors (e.g., corticosteroids), anticytokine MABs or **polyclonal** antibodies, or the appropriate cytokine-receptor antagonists (Matthys and Billiau, 1997). Inhibitors such as antipyretics that have been shown to block certain neurological side effects of cytokines, such as fever, are not effective in restoring appetite (Plata-Salaman, 1996a).

EFFECTS OF DIRECT STIMULATION OF THE CNS WITH CYTOKINES

In animal studies, local application of IFN-α to parts of the brain has been shown to cause excitation of glucose-sensitive cells in the VMH. In the same study, cytokines such as IFN-α, IL-1, and TNF caused inhibition of activity in the LH or "hunger center" of the brain (Dafney et al., 1996).

Intracerebral administration of TNF-α and IL-1 in experimental animals produced anorexia (Plata-Salaman et al., 1988). Although fluid intake initially declined as well, it was not a long-term effect as was the suppression of feeding. Equal or greater doses of TNF-α and IL-1 administered peripherally did not have the same degree of effect as the intracerebral method. Although there is not sufficient evidence to state any conclusion related to cytokine-induced anorexia, there is sufficient data

to build a hypothesis for testing. It is known that the release of one cytokine may induce the secondary release of other cytokines. There can be a synergistic effect caused by the administration of more than one cytokine (specifically, IL-1α or IL-1β and TNF). Cytokines can act in both an autocrine and paracrine manner. Certain cytokines, such as IL-1, may be much more potent in suppressing feeding than other cytokines. IL-1β at concentrations generated by disease or pathogens induces short- and long-term anorexia by reducing both meal size and meal duration. At higher pharmacological concentrations, IL-1β also decreases meal frequency. IFN also has been shown to reduce meal size and meal duration, whereas IL-8 appears to reduce only meal size (Plata-Salaman, 1996b).

Depression and Anorexia

Major depression will have an impact on appetite and nutritional status. Depression is a more common manifestation in patients with cancer and chronic illness, with as many as 48% of cancer patients meeting the criteria for diagnosis of a depressive psychiatric disorder—compared to 6% of the general population (Valentine et al., 1998). Biotherapy with agents such as IFN-α and IL-2 may increase the level of depression. Walker et al. (1997) state that patients taking **immunochemotherapy** with IL-2 report higher levels of depressed mood, more confusion, and a greater incidence of appetite impairment and weight loss than patients taking chemotherapy alone. Valentine et al. (1998) report that a single dose of 1.5 MIU of IFN-α results in subjective complaints of memory loss, depression, and lack of initiative. With chronic administration, some patients exhibit symptoms of major depression that include significant decrease in appetite and weight loss. Although these processes are not yet fully understood, there has been recent evidence to suggest that different clinical depressive subsyndromes may be the result of different neuro-chemical and neuroendocrine alterations that affect eating behaviors. For example, patients with melancholic depression tend to exhibit ruminative thinking, agitation, and weight loss, possibly reflecting activation of a stress-response system. In contrast, some patients will experience an "atypical" depression that is manifested by fatigue, lethargy, hypersomnia, and increased appetite. This may be the result of inactivation or lack of responsiveness of the hypothalamic-pituitary-adrenal axis (HPA) (Valentine et al., 1998). Many biological systems are altered when a person experiences major depression. The most prominent alteration is seen in the endocrine system, which includes the HPA, hypothalamic-pituitary-thyroid, and growth hormone axes (Valentine et al., 1998).

The Hypothalamic-Pituitary-Adrenal Axis

The hypothalamus is the best-studied eating-associated CNS site. The amygdala is a part of the brain that is rich in neuropeptides and responds to emotional states. **Catecholaminergic** cells in the brainstem communicate with the hypothalamus to control stress. The hypothalamus secretes corticotropin-releasing hormone (CRH), which stimulates the re-lease of adrenocorticotropin-releasing hormone (ACTH) from the pituitary gland. The release of hormones by this complex network is re-ferred to as the stress response (Post-White, 1996). IFN-α has structural similarities with ACTH and β-endorphin (Valentine et al., 1998). Studies have shown that IFN-α can ei-ther stimulate or inhibit the HPA axis, de-pending on the physiologic concentration (Saphier et al., 1994).

The HPA gland axis responds to cytokine activation with neuroendocrine release when-ever the immune system is activated by disease or cytokine administration. CRH is released from the hypothalamus and ACTH is released from the pituitary gland. Increased levels of glucocorticoids that have been released from the adrenal glands serve to dampen the inflam-matory response and inhibit the synthesis and release of IL-1 and TNF-α. This may be an innate mechanism responsible for preventing over-responsiveness of the immune system (Plata-Salaman, 1996a).

CYTOKINE INFLUENCE ON THE HPA AXIS

Exogenous administration of IFN-α has been shown to stimulate the release of ACTH and cortisol; however, after three weeks, the HPA axis adapts and there is no further ACTH or cortisol-stimulatory response. These patients remain hyper-responsive to CRH (Jones et al., 1998), which results in an abnormally increased release of ACTH and cortisol. This may account for the ongoing anorexia that some patients experience. As a direct or indirect effect of bio-logical therapy, some patients may experience changes in metabolic stimuli such as altered glucose levels, alterations in neurotransmitters and their precursors, hormonal factors, gastro-intestinal and pancreatic factors, and other psy-chobiological factors (Rowland et al., 1996).

The Influence of Tumor on the Development of Anorexia and Cachexia

Figure 18.2 shows the mechanism, suggested by Langstein and Norton, by which tumors might cause cancer cachexia. In addition to cy-tokine activity, certain types of tumor cells se-crete substances that decrease appetite. Oat-cell tumors, for example, secrete bombesin (BBS), a known factor in appetite suppression. As a result of the cell-mediated response of T cells in the presence of an antigen, such as a tumor, IFN-γ is secreted. IFN-γ is a potent activator of the macrophage and the resulting cascade of secondary cytokines, such as TNF-α, IL-6, IL-1, and IFN-γ, has the potential to affect many tissue and organ systems.

The Neurobiology of Food Intake and Anorexia

An area of great interest concerning biotherapy-mediated anorexia involves the effects of central hormones and neurotransmitters on the brain. Substances that are known to have an impact on anorexia include oxytocin, norepinephine, CRH (a 41-amino acid peptide), and serotonin (Rowland et al., 1996). Opioid receptor antagonists such as naloxone reduce food intake initially, but the effects diminish over time (Rowland et al., 1996). Research has linked the activation of oxytocin-containing neurons to both CRH and insulin, suggesting a connection between these factors and the reduction of food intake. Another intriguing area of research in anorexia involves the study of the role of serotonin. Peripheral administration of serotonin decreases food intake. Although peripherally administered serotonin does not readily cross the blood-brain barrier (BBB), peripheral administration of IL-1 has been shown to increase brain tryptophan (TRP) concentrations, which then increase serotonin synthesis. Additionally, the infused IL-1 increases serotonin release. This results in the action of serotonin on neural receptors, which creates a physiologic cascade, whereby the sum of the cytokine and tryptophan availability amplifies the release of serotonin. These findings have led to work by Laviano et al. (1996a) that proposes a serotonergic model for anorexia.

Serotonergic Mechanistic Hypothesis

This serotonergic mechanistic model proposes that peripherally produced IL-1 acts on the tryptophan-plasma pool to facilitate its crossing the BBB. The resulting increase in brain tryptophan levels increases the synthesis of serotonin, which leads to anorexia. Previous descriptions in this chapter and other chapters in this book clearly identify the production of IL-1 as a process of a cytokine cascade that is stimulated by administration of many types of biotherapy.

A study with humans conducted by Cangiano et al. (1994) provided information that showed a close relationship between the level of plasma-free TRP and the development of anorexia. The experimental group included 20 cancer patients in whom tumors were totally resected. Eight of the patients had baseline anorexia. For control purposes, they were sex- and age-matched with six subjects undergoing a noncancer-related surgery. None of the patients in the control group had baseline anorexia, and none developed infection during the study period. At baseline, the plasma-free TRP concentrations in the cancer patients with anorexia were significantly higher than those found in the patients who did not have anorexia. A portion of the patients with cancer who were initially reported to have anorexia experienced a disappearance of it after surgical removal of the tumor. The disappearance of anorexia corresponded to the reduction of plasma-free TRP and a reduction of the plasma-free TRP/large neutral amino acids (LNAA) ratio. The LNAA group includes leucine, valine, isoleucine, tyrosine, phenylanaline, and methione. Conversely, for those patients who continued to experience anorexia after surgery, the plasma-free TRP and the plasma-free TRP/LNAA ratio remained significantly elevated. This important measurement was felt to be confirmation that there was increased TRP crossing the BBB.

This work was further developed into a hypothetical model when, in 1996, researchers from Syracuse University of New York and Rome, Italy, published results of collaborative studies that offered a hypothesis for the serotonergic mechanistic hypothesis of the development of anorexia (Figure 18.3). In this model,

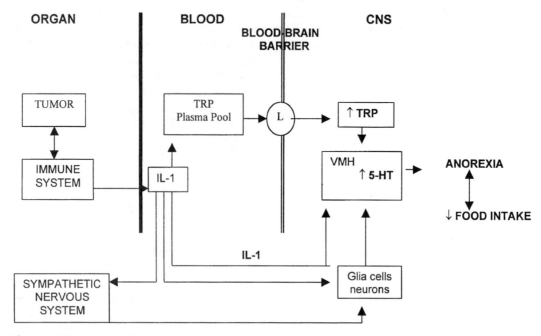

Figure 18.3 Proposed serotonergic model of anorexia. Based on experimental and clinical data, it is likely that cancer-related anorexia is mediated by the peripheral and central interrelationships between cytokines such as IL-1 and the serotonergic system.

Abbreviations: CNS, central nervous system; HT, hydroxytryptamine; IL, interleukin; TRP, tryptophan; VMH, ventromedial nucleus of hypothalamus.

Source: Laviano, A., Renvyle, T., and Yang, Z. 1996b. From laboratory to bedside: New strategies in the treatment of malnutrition in cancer patients. *Nutrition* 12(2): 112–122, with permission.

tumor growth was shown to increase plasma-TRP concentrations, resulting in increases in the brain-tryptophan concentrations. This finding led to the synthesis of hypothalamic serotonin, which was linked to the development of anorexia and a decrease in food intake (Laviano *et al.*, 1996b).

Transport of cytokines from peripheral circulation to the brain may occur across the circumventricular organs, which lack a BBB, or possibly through the BBB. IL-1 also may cause an increase in tryptophan crossing the BBB, thereby increasing serotonin synthesis. IL-1 is able to cross the BBB and enter the VMH, where it modulates neuronal activity via cal-

cium channels (Meguid *et al.*, 1996). There is also a release of cytokines from immune cells within the brain, including brain macrophages, microglia, astrocytes and, during an acute-phase response or inflammatory process, endothelial cells (Plata-Salaman, 1996a). Although there are still many questions regarding the serotonergic mechanistic hypothesis, it is an exciting step toward the understanding of anorexia.

Gastrointestinal Factors Related to Anorexia

The primary natural stimuli responsible for decreasing food intake is satiation or satiety. *Sati-*

ation is defined as the combination of processes that terminate ongoing feeding; *satiety* is the composite of processes that inhibit active food-seeking or between-meal intake. Early animal studies showed that large meals produce longer periods of satiety (Rowland *et al.*, 1996). Later work demonstrated that slow intravenous infusion of metabolizable fuels (e.g., glucose) decreased food intake by increasing the interval between meals (Rowland *et al.*, 1996).

Gastrointestinal factors such as cholecystokinin (CCK) and BBS and pancreatic factors such as insulin, amylin, and glucagon are all endogenous satiety factors. CCK is normally released during and after meals. In experimental settings, CCK has been shown to reduce meal size. Studies have shown that the anorectic effect of peripherally injected CCK is totally eliminated after surgically cutting either the gastric branches or the vagus nerve, suggesting that this compound has a peripheral site of action. Additionally, the CCK molecule is too large to cross the BBB. Recent work has shown that this anorectic effect can be blocked with a selective antagonist. BBS is a gastrointestinal peptide that differs from CCK, in that it probably acts centrally on the brain. Research is underway that is mapping the most likely sites of action of these gastrointestinal factors (Rowland *et al.*, 1996).

Both insulin and amylin are released from pancreatic beta cells after food intake. Although experimental work has shown a role for amylin in decreasing food intake, it is still not known whether amylin will possess actions similar to insulin in mediating food intake and body weight. Glucagon, however, has been well defined as a satiating agent whose primary site of action is the liver (Rowland *et al.*, 1996).

Other circulatory factors that may play a role in satiety-related anorexia via satiety include a large glycoprotein named *satietin* and the protein *leptin*. The synthesis, release, and site of action for satietin is still unknown; however,

central administration of partially purified satietin in research animals has resulted in anorexia. Leptin is a protein thought to be secreted by adipose tissue as a result of reduction in body weight, and may be regulated by insulin. It also may be involved in the mediation of other circulatory factors, but further research will need to be done before significant claims can be made (Rowland *et al.*, 1996). Of note is the fact that the receptor for leptin shows strong similarity to cytokine receptors in the brain, primarily IL-6.

Assessment and Management of Anorexia

Nursing Assessment

Objective measures are important in assessing the presence and degree of anorexia. The criteria used to measure severe weight loss in hospitalized patients may be useful in evaluating weight loss in patients receiving biotherapy. Losses of more than 2% total body weight per week, more than 5% per month, more than 7.5% in three months, and more than 10% in six months are considered severe (Ottery, 1996). The Common Toxicity Criteria is the scale used to grade the severity of nutritional or metabolic toxicity by research groups, as follows: 0 = a loss of 5% or less; 1 = a loss of 5 to 9%; 2 = a loss of 10 to 19.9%; and 3 = a loss of 20% or more during therapy.

PHYSICAL EXAMINATION
The physical examination, including a review of body systems, is key to identifying signs of nutritional problems and is based on the concept that body composition is divided into three compartments: protein, fat, and extracellular mass. Protein consists of somatic protein, made up mostly of skeletal muscle mass and visceral protein, which includes plasma protein, hemo-

globin, several clotting factors, and antibodies. Fat includes subcutaneous, intramuscular, and intra-abdominal fat. Extracellular mass includes extracellular water, circulating protein, and the skeleton. Skeletal muscle mass can be measured by **anthropometric** measurements or **skinfold** measurements. These measurements are useful for determining changes over the long-term rather than the short-term clinical situations.

LABORATORY MEASUREMENTS

Whereas visceral protein cannot be measured directly, it can be estimated by measuring serum albumin, transferrin, fat, and extracellular mass (Ottery, 1996). Assessment of extracellular mass involves evaluation of the patient's hydration status; the presence and extent of edema, including sacral and tibial edema and ascites; unusual fluid loss; and the source of this loss. Laboratory studies add objective data to the subjective information obtained from other tools and aids in assessing the patient's current physical status. Blood chemistries provide information related to energy stores and energy production. Correcting abnormal electrolyte levels is necessary before instituting nutritional support.

Serum albumin is the best single prognostic indicator with which to predict the patient's risk for morbidity and mortality, but it is not a sensitive indicator of acute or short-term changes in nutritional status. Serum transferrin, an iron-transport protein, is more sensitive than albumin to changes in nutritional status, but may be modified by other conditions including hepatitis and liver dysfunction. Prealbumin is useful in assessing the impact of nutritional interventions, but can be altered by stress and infection as well as recent increases in protein intake. Total iron-binding capacity indicates the amount of iron in the blood to which transferrin can bind. Increased levels indicate iron deficiency; lower-than-normal levels indicate ane-

mia. Values can be altered by infections. A complete blood count, including total lymphocyte count, is useful in assessing immune competency but may be altered by acute illness, stress, infection, and drug therapy. Other useful laboratory values include renal- and liver-function studies, glucose as a measure of pancreatic-endocrine function, and skin-test antigens or delayed cutaneous-hypersensitivity testing to gauge systemic-immune function.

STANDARDIZED MEASURE OF ANOREXIA

Ottery (1996) proposes the use of a standardized tool, the Patient-Generated Subjective Global Assessment of Nutrition Status (PG-SGA), to adequately assess the patient's nutritional status. Disease stage, metabolic stress, symptoms, food intake, and functional capacity are assessed with the PG-SGA. Ottery also recommends that anthropomorphic measurements be taken to track loss of muscle and fat, as well as the presence of edema and ascites. Results of this assessment are based on a combination of clinical judgment and subjective data. The medical history and physical examination are the primary sources of the data. The assessment also includes a section for a patient's subjective response to questions about weight change, food intake, symptoms, and functional capacity. The health-care professional completes information on history, metabolic demand, and physical appearance, and then scores the evaluation. This information can then be transferred to an algorithm that directs the plan of action for nutritional intervention. This particular method of assessment provides more complete information because it includes the patient report; a physical examination, including anthropometric measurements; laboratory studies; and a detailed patient history. This tool is described in detail in several oncology nursing resources and may also be obtained from the Society for Nutritional Oncology Adjuvant Therapy (Ottery, 1996).

MEDICAL HISTORY

Assessment of weight loss should include an evaluation for pain, depression, nausea/vomiting, constipation/diarrhea, oral mucosa alterations, food intolerance, and anorexia. When gathering patient-history data, the patient and a family member or caregiver should be interviewed. Open-ended questions allow more complete information to be obtained. Questions should be related to the patient's medical and surgical history, current disease state, current medications, diet, social status, and income history. The assessment should include an evaluation of alcohol and tobacco use, as well as the patient's activity level and functional measurements of muscle strength. The patient's weight history, including current, usual, and ideal weight, should also be obtained.

When collecting medical-history data, all medical diagnoses, surgeries, and other therapeutic interventions should be included. Disease processes that might interfere with the ingestion and absorption of nutrients, which increase metabolic needs or affect the mouth and gastrointestinal tract, should be noted. Symptoms such as stomatitis, dry mouth, and changes in taste and smell have an impact on nutrition and should be assessed. The names of all medical prescriptions, over-the-counter-drugs, and vitamin and mineral supplements; the dose, frequency, and route of administration; and start dates need to be described as well. Performance status as an indicator of energy level and self-care ability is also an important measure.

DIETARY HISTORY

Dietary history and intake is useful in identifying areas where adjustments can be made to increase caloric, protein, and micronutrient intake. Consideration should be given to frequency of eating, the types of foods eaten, and the size of the meals, as well as the patient's food preferences. Questions about food allergies and food intolerances (e.g., lactose) should be included. Social factors such as living alone, eating alone, eating in restaurants, and the ability to shop for and prepare food should be assessed.

Dietary history is best reported through the use of a food diary maintained by the patient for a number of days. It should include an account of the amount of food ingested so that caloric and nutrient intake can be better evaluated. This method is preferred over the 24-hour diet recall because the accuracy of the latter can be affected by poor memory or unusual but temporary changes in the diet.

Management of Anorexia

Early identification of the impact of poor nutrition on health outcomes in the patient experiencing anorexia is an important nursing measure. After a thorough assessment, action should be taken to remedy factors that may contribute to decreased nutrient intake.

INTERVENTIONS TO ENHANCE NUTRIENT INTAKE

The enteral route is the most desired route for nutrient intake for reasons of convenience and the maintenance of normal gut flora, transit, and histology (Cunningham, 1997). Alternative methods such as tube-feeding and intravenous therapy are usually not necessary for patients receiving biotherapy; however, liquid or protein supplements taken orally can be of great value. If recommending the use of commercial supplements, it is important to ensure that they meet the patient's specific needs, particularly regarding the ability to tolerate lactose. Ideally, the supplements will be used between meals to enhance intake rather than as a substitute for meals. Patients receiving biotherapy may report thick and tenacious oral secretions and difficulty tolerating milk or milk-based drinks. An alternative is to create blended supplemental drinks using apple juice as a base, then adding a protein powder and frozen fruit such as bananas.

Patients may report that their appetite is greater earlier in the day, so adjustment of the meal schedule to allow for larger meals at breakfast and lunch should be encouraged. Strategies such as eating small, frequent meals and eating whenever hungry may also be helpful. Food restrictions should be removed if possible (i.e., cardiac-prudent, low-fat diets). Remember that in most cases, treatment is temporary and returning to a preferred diet can occur after therapy is complete. Keep tasty, healthy snacks on hand. Arranging food attractively, creating a pleasant environment for eating, dining with family or friends, or watching a favorite TV program or video while eating may enhance intake. Exercising about half an hour before eating may stimulate the appetite. Eliminate odors that may affect appetite. Other strategies include turning on exhaust fans while cooking and using boiling bags, the microwave, covered pans, or outdoor grills for food preparation. Recognize that favorite foods may no longer seem appealing and should be excluded. Avoid eating in therapy or treatment areas that may generate a recall or aversive stimulus. Patients may report taste changes that interfere with appetite. For those who experience a metallic taste, try switching to plastic utensils. For those who experience a salty taste, try adding a pinch of sugar to the food. Add strong seasonings such as garlic, onion, and ginger, or marinate meat, fish, and chicken to intensify flavors (Keim and Smith, 1996).

Hydration is a crucial part of the diet for patients receiving biotherapy. Water is essential to facilitate digestion, control body temperature, and carry nutrients and waste products through the body. It also cushions joints and internal organs. The role of hydration in maintaining homeostasis will vary depending on the type of biotherapy used. If the side-effect pro-

file of the biotherapy regimen includes fever, diaphoresis, and potential dehydration, adequate hydration and supplemental intravenous (IV) hydration is essential. If the side-effect profile of the biotherapy regimen involves capillary-leak syndrome, the management of the fluid status becomes more challenging because fluids are easily shifted to tissue spaces.

MAINTAINING FLUID BALANCE WITH CAPILLARY-LEAK SYNDROME

With biotherapy using drugs that cause severe capillary-leak syndrome, such as high-dose IL-2, the maintenance of fluid balance and renal perfusion is carefully orchestrated. Some practitioners administer albumin or packed red blood cells (PRBC) if hemoglobin is low, followed by a diuretic. The large molecules of the albumin or PRBC create a greater hydrostatic pressure within the vein, thereby causing the flow of water out of the tissue spaces and back into the blood vessels. At this time, the diuretic is administered, thereby relieving the patient of potentially dangerous edema while perfusing the kidneys.

MAINTAINING FLUID BALANCE WITH DEHYDRATION

For therapies that involve fever-related dehydration such as IFN-α, oral and/or IV hydration is important. Fever can cause extra fluid loss through diaphoresis and rapid breathing. Dehydration is a serious problem. When dehydrated, blood pressure falls and circulation decreases. Be aware of the warning signs of dehydration, including headache, lack of energy, weakness, dizziness, and nausea. These symptoms may be side effects of therapy; however, an intervention that aims to correct dehydration should be considered. Remember that thirst is not always an indicator of need. By the time a person feels thirsty, they have already lost about 1% of the body's water. Plain water is usually better than a sport drink when trying to replace rapid water loss because the sugar and electrolytes in sport drinks slow the absorption of water into the body. However, if trying to enhance caloric intake, use fruit juices or milk. Some patients receiving high-dose regimens may require IV hydration.

PATIENT EDUCATION

Patient education should address the following questions: What is expected of the therapy? What are the potential side effects that may affect eating habits? How can the patient and significant others manage changes in eating habits? What should be reported to the nurse and physician, and when? Providing information and education to the patient and the caregiver can help them make the choices and changes in environmental conditions that promote improved nutrient intake. Referral for consultation with a dietitian, if available, is an appropriate measure. Encourage patients to keep a small notebook with them at all times to note what triggers side effects, remedies that work or do not work, and questions to ask the nurse, nutritionist, or doctor (Keim and Smith, 1996). Patients and family members should be taught to recognize the side effects of the prescribed therapy.

SUPPORTIVE MEDICATIONS

The role of supportive medications in the treatment of anorexia and cachexia for patients receiving biotherapy has not been extensively studied. There are a number of agents that have anticachectic properties and, with further study, may show a benefit for those patients (Table 18.3); however, confident recommendations cannot be made until research demonstrates efficacy in ameliorating side effects without decreasing the therapeutic intent of the biotherapy.

Unlike chemotherapy, biotherapies depend on the pleiotropic effects of the immune system to generate an anticancer effect. Steroids or hormonal medications that have proven effi-

Table 18.3   Anticachectic therapeutic agents, classified according to their mode of action

Agents inhibiting cytokine production
   Corticosteroids
   Pentoxifylline
   Cannabinoids
   N-3 fatty acids
Agents inhibiting cytokine action on target organs
   Specific anticytokine monoclonal antibodies
   Specific cytokine-receptor antagonists
Agents counteracting cytokine-induced
   metabolic abnormalities
   Anabolic steroids
   Growth hormone
   Insulin-like growth factor I
   Megestrol acetate
   Cyproheptadine
   Branched-chain amino acids
   Glutamine
   Arginine
   Nucleotides
Nonspecific agents
   Standard nutritional support (parenteral and
   enteral nutrition)

Source: Adapted from Laviano, A., Renvyle, T., and Yang, Z. 1996b. From laboratory to bedside: New strategies in the treatment of malnutrition in cancer patients. *Nutrition* 12(2): 112–122, with permission.

cacy in improving appetite in patients receiving chemotherapy have not been fully studied in patients receiving biotherapy. Because steroids are known to inhibit certain immunologic activity—specifically, inhibition of antigen presentation by macrophage (Oppenheim, 1997)—they are not commonly used for side-effect management in biotherapy.

Megestrol acetate is a hormonal agent used to increase weight gain in patients with cancer or AIDS. Megestrol acetate was noted to promote weight gain while being used to treat patients with advanced breast cancer. Several studies have demonstrated that megestrol acetate increases appetite and body weight but not lean body mass. In a study by Loprinzi *et al.* (1990) comparing patients with advanced incurable cancer who were given 800 mg of megestrol acetate to a control group, the patients experienced improved appetite ($p = .003$) and food intake ($p = .009$). The megestrol-acetate group also reported significantly less nausea ($p = .001$) and emesis ($p = 0.009$). No significant toxic effects were reported, with the exception of mild edema. Although the patients in this study were receiving many different anti-tumor therapies, it is not clear whether any of the patients were receiving biotherapy. Although this drug has not been studied in patients receiving biotherapy, this is an area that would benefit from research.

Both delta-9-tetrahydrocannabinol (THC) and cannabidiol (CBD) are protein-bound cannabinoids and are major components of marijuana. It is theorized that cannabinoids act via endorphin receptors or by inhibiting prostaglandin synthesis (Laviano *et al.*, 1996b). THC is the major psychoactive element in marijuana, whereas CBD has no evidence of **psychoactivity**. Marijuana components have been utilized in clinical practice as an antiemetic and appetite stimulant as the oral drug Dronabinol®. Watzl *et al.* (1991) conducted studies that showed that both THC and CBD are immunomodulatory and can potentially alter cytokine secretion of human peripheral blood mononuclear cells. These *in vitro* studies and the impact of these findings on the efficacy of biotherapy have not been studied; however, this is an area that warrants more research.

Pentoxifylline, a TNF inhibitor, has been studied for its effect in reducing anorexia. Indeed, in animal models it has been shown to reduce anorexia by reducing TNF-α levels. This effect has been replicated in a small study of patients with cancer (Dezube *et al.*, 1993) and shown to improve the patient's sense of well-being, improve the appetite, and increase weight gain. However, these patients were not

receiving any therapy while enrolled in this study. Pentoxifylline also has been shown, *in vitro*, to be a potent inhibitor of IL-2 and IFN-γ (Thanhauser *et al.*, 1993) and to inhibit cytokine release from microglia (Chao *et al.*, 1992). Again, the concern with patients receiving biotherapy is the degree to which pentoxifylline might inhibit production of TNF-α, IL-2, IFN-γ, or other cytokines that might be providing an antitumor or antiviral effect and whether **downregulation** of any of these cytokines would negatively affect the therapeutic outcome.

Cyproheptadine, an antiserotonergic antihistamine, was thought to have the potential for treating anorexia. Although cyproheptadine has properties that block serotonin, it has failed to demonstrate any efficacy in decreasing anorexia or decreasing weight loss in cancer patients. Kardinal *et al.* (1990) report the results of a 1990 study with 293 patients with cancer. The patients were stratified based on their primary site of disease, the severity of weight loss during the preceding 2 months, and whether they were receiving cisplatin-containing chemotherapy or abdominal radiation therapy. The experimental group in this double-blinded, placebo study received two 4-mg tablets of cyproheptadine three times daily. Doses were modified for toxic effects such as sedation or nausea/vomiting attributable to the study drug. Results of this study demonstrated modest improvement in appetite and less nausea, but no reduction in weight loss. The researchers felt that two factors influenced the meager results. First, in many patients with anorexia, cachexia, or both, any appetite-stimulating effect may be overpowered by the cancer state. Secondly, this intervention might have been "too little, too late" (Kardinal *et al.*, 1990). Further research in this area with other antiserotonergic drugs is needed.

Another drug that has been studied for treatment of anorexia is hydrazine sulfate, which is an inhibitor of gluconeogenesis, a process that is accelerated as a result of increased levels of certain cytokines. One early study of patients with advanced cancer showed that administration of hydrazine sulfate resulted in increases in body weight, improvement in appetite, and increases in caloric intake (Chlebowski et al., 1987). However, these findings could not be supported in larger, randomized, placebo-controlled clinical trials (Loprinzi et al., 1994a and 1994b). Data from these studies also showed either no difference between treatment arms or trends for poorer survival and poorer quality of life. Experts suggest that caution be practiced regarding the use of this drug as an "energizer" for cancer patients, citing the results of studies that failed to demonstrate efficacy and indicated that the drug had a negative impact on quality of life (Herbert, 1994).

Directions for Research

Agents That Inhibit Cytokine Production

Several pharmacological and nutritional factors have been identified as inhibitors of cytokine production and have been investigated for their efficacy in treating anorexia and cachexia in the cancer patient. Anticytokine antibodies, corticosteroids, pentoxifylline, cannabinoids, and n-3 fatty acids or "fish oils" are known to inhibit cytokine production (Laviano et al., 1996a). Of chief importance in looking at agents that inhibit cytokine production is the possible reduction of the therapeutic effect of the administered or the induced secondary cytokines (Matthys and Billiau, 1997).

IL-6 has been implicated in the development of cachexia. Studies with IL-6 **transgenic mice** showed that administration of an anti-mouse IL-6 receptor antibody completely reversed the muscle-wasting that had been induced in these

mice (Tsujinaka et al., 1996). This supports the value of further study using receptor antibodies to block the effects of other secondary cytokines while measuring whether the therapeutic efficacy of the biotherapy is maintained.

Convincing evidence has shown that IL-6 inhibits TNF production in animals, but the results in humans are still conflicting (Laviano et al., 1996a). In addition to suppressing gene transcription of TNF, pentoxyfylline has been shown to reduce the production of other cytokines (Laviano et al., 1996a). Pentoxyfylline has also been shown to block the release of secondary cytokines induced by bacillus Calmette-Guérin (BCG), including TNF, IL-2, and IFN-γ. Of interest in this study was that IL-2–generated lymphocyte-activated killer-cell cytotoxicity was unaffected even when pentoxyfylline was used at the highest concentration (i.e., 200 mcg/mL) (Thanhauser et al., 1993). Others have compared the ability of pentoxyfylline versus dexamethasone to block the release of TNF and have found support for selective efficacy of both substances in vitro (Chao et al., 1992). If this drug is able to block TNF production, it may decrease the severity of cytokine-induced side effects such as anorexia.

N-3 FATTY ACIDS

Epidemiological studies first correlated a lower incidence of cardiovascular and inflammatory disease with the intake of n-3 fatty acids or "fish oils" (Laviano et al., 1996a). Karmali (1996) reviewed the studies of the effects of two components of marine fish oils, eicosapentaenoic acid (EPA) and docosahexaenoic acid (DHA) in relation to cytokines and cachexia therapy. During periods of inflammation, TNF and IL-1 stimulate the production of arachidonic acid metabolites, which are implicated in some of the tissue-damaging actions of these cytokines. Administration of EPA and DHA, in most cases, results in a reduction of arachidonic acid. It is then postulated that if TNF activity is mediated from arachidonic acid metabolism, EPA may serve as an antagonist or inhibitory factor to the cachectic effects of TNF. Human studies have shown a decrease in the production of inflammatory cytokines when moderate to high levels of n-3 fatty acids were taken orally (Meydani and Dinarello, 1993).

Three important considerations associated with the use of n-3 fatty acids include the concentration of fish oil, relationship of EPA to DHA, and intervention to reduce the oxidative stress. Increased free-radical activity has been noted in animals fed diets of the highly oxidizable n-3 fatty acids (Meydani, 1996). Some of the risks associated with free radicals include stroke, emphysema, cataracts, and cancer. Vitamin E is a fat-soluble antioxidant that has been shown to have a membrane-protective effect from the oxidative damage of straight fish oil. This topic presents an opportunity for nursing research to evaluate the effect of balanced supplementation with EPA, DHA, n-3 fatty acids, and vitamin E on the biotherapy-related side effects of anorexia.

Hellerstein *et al.* (1989) induced anorexia in laboratory rats who were treated with rhIL-1β to compare the effects of fish-oil feeding on cytokine and prostaglandin production. They were studying the effects of administration of rhIL-1β and whether a diet of fish oil would decrease anorexia. They found that chronic daily administration of rhIL-1β decreased food intake in the chow-fed and corn-oil-fed rats, but had no effect on fish-oil-fed rats. The researchers felt that the anorexia was mediated by prostaglandins because they could block the acute anorexic effects by pretreating with prostaglandin inhibitor, ibuprofen, at 10 mg/kg IV before injection of rhIL-1β. Acetaminophen did not block the anorexic effects. Fish-oil feeding also decreased IL-1-stimulated prostaglandin E_2 production.

Meydani *et al.* (1993) conducted an *in vivo* study on the effect of dietary n-3 fatty acid intake on cytokine production in 12 healthy women. Each subject received a combination of n-3 fatty acids (i.e., 1.680 g of EPA, 0.720 g of DHA, and 600 mg of other fatty acids) and 6 IU of vitamin E per day. Results showed that n-3 fatty acid administration significantly decreased the production of IL-1β, TNF-α, and IL-6 in the subjects. Other immunologic functions that decreased were the T-cell mediated function, IL-2 production, and **mitogenic** response.

Agents That Counteract Cytokine-Induced Metabolic Changes

Insulin-like growth factor (IGF)-1 (somatomedin-C) stimulates amino-acid uptake and protein synthesis as it inhibits lipolysis. Early research in animal studies has shown promise with continuous subcutaneous infusion of IGF-1 resulting in reduction of muscle protein and lean tissue loss. Careful studies are needed to further evaluate IGF-1, because it has the ability to cause transformation or mitosis in epithelial cells, raising concern that it might promote tumor growth (Laviano *et al.*, 1996b).

Anabolic steroids are known to preserve body protein stores and promote nitrogen retention. There has been little research with this type of therapy, but potential problems include fluid retention and hepatic toxicity.

Branched-chain amino acids (BCAA) are utilized in total parenteral nutrition, which has been shown to improve nitrogen balance, utilization of amino acids, and muscle-protein metabolism, although its use in cancer patients has been controversial. Interest in the possible role of BCAA in cytokine therapy lies in its ability to compete with tryptophan for entry into the CNS. Cangiano *et al.* (1996) conducted a pilot study with cancer patients who were experiencing anorexia. Patients were given BCAA orally, resulting in a decrease in the severity of anorexia and an increase in spontaneous food intake. Large controlled studies are needed to confirm these results.

Summary

In biotherapy, where immunomodulation is often the primary desired mechanism of action, any strategy that decreases that action should be rigorously scrutinized. As our understanding of the processes involved in the development of anorexia grows, we can expect to see more research that explores interventions for this complicated side effect. This is a prime area for nursing research and reports of successful interventions for anorexia. There is no doubt that progress in our ability to improve nutritional status for patients receiving biotherapy is critical to a favorable outcome. More regimens are appearing that utilize biotherapy as a singular intervention or in combination with other interventions. The multiple outcomes of decreasing adverse side effects, maintaining or improving quality of life, and achieving the therapeutic objective are reasonable goals for health-care professionals dealing with biotherapies. Continued research and educational efforts will help us achieve these outcomes.

References

Abbas, A., Lichtman, A., and Pober, J. 1991. Cytokines. In Abbas, A., Lichtman, A., and Pober, J. (eds) *Cellular and Molecular Immunology*. Philadelphia, PA: W. B. Saunders Company, pp. 225–243.

Bartholomew, S., and Hoffman, S. 1993. Effects of peripheral cytokine injection on multiple unit activity in the anterior hypothalamic area of the mouse. *Brain, Behavior and Immunity* 7: 301–316.

Cakman, I., Kirchner, H., and Rink, L. 1997. Zinc supplementation reconstitutes the production of interferon-α by leukocytes from elderly persons. *Journal of Interferon and Cytokine Research* 17: 469–472.

Cangiano, C., Laviano, A., Meguid, M., et al. 1996. Effects of administration of oral branched-chain amino acids on anorexia and caloric intake in cancer patients. *Journal of the National Cancer Institute* 88(8): 550–552.

Cangiano, C., Testa, U., Muscarito, M., et al. 1994. Cytokines, tryptophan, and anorexia in cancer patients before and after surgical tumor ablation. *Anticancer Research* 14: 1451–1456.

Chao, C., Hu, S., Close, K., et al. 1992. Cytokine release from microglia: Differential inhibition by pentoxifylline and dexamethasone. *Journal of Infectious and Diseases* 166: 847–853.

Chlebowski, R., Bulcavage, L., Grosvenor, M., et al. 1987. Hydrazine sulfate in cancer patients with weight loss. *Cancer* 59: 406–410.

Cunningham, R. 1997. *The Anorectic-Cachectic Syndrome in Cancer*. New Brunswick, NJ: The Cancer Institute of New Jersey.

Dafny, N., Prieto-Gomez, B., and Reyes-Vasquez, G. 1996. Effects of interferon on the central nervous system. In Reder, A. (ed). *Interferon Therapy of Multiple Sclerosis*. New York, NY: Marcel Dekker, Inc.

Dezube, B., Sherman, M., Fridovich-Keil, J., et al. 1993. Downregulation of tumor necrosis factor expression by pentoxifylline in cancer patients: A pilot study. *Cancer Immunology and Immunotherapy* 36: 57–60.

Fantino, M., and Wieteska, L. 1993. Evidence for a direct central anorectic effect of tumor necrosis factor-alpha in the rat. *Physiology and Behavior* 53: 477–483.

Hardin, T. 1993. Cytokine mediators of malnutrition: Clinical implications. *Nutrition in Clinical Practice* 8(2): 55–59.

Hellerstein, M., Meydani, S., Meydani, M., et al. 1989. Interleukin-1 induced anorexia in the rat. *Journal of Clinical Investigation* 84: 228–235.

Herbert, V. 1994. Three stakes in hydrazine sulfate's heart, but questionable cancer remedies, like vampires, always rise again (Editorial). *Journal of Clinical Oncology* 12(6): 1107–1108.

Hill, A., Siegel, J., Rounds, J., *et al.* 1997. Metabolic responses to interleukin-1. *Annals of Surgery* 225(3): 246–251.

Illig, K., Maronian, N., and Peacock, J. 1992. Cancer cachexia is transmissible in plasma. *Journal of Surgical Research* 52(4): 353–358.

Jones, T., Wadler, S., and Hupart, K. 1998. Endocrine-mediated mechanisms of fatigue during treatment with interferon-α. *Seminars in Oncology* 25(1 suppl 1): 54–63.

Kardinal, C., Loprinzi, C., Schaid, D., *et al.* 1990. A controlled trial of cyproheptadine in cancer patients with anorexia and/or cachexia. *Cancer* 65: 2657–2662.

Karmali, R. 1996. Historical perspective and potential use of n-3 fatty acids in therapy of cancer cachexia. *Nutrition* 12(1 suppl): S2–S4.

Keim, R., and Smith, G. 1996. *What to Eat Now.* Seattle, WA: Sasquatch Books.

Langstein, H., and Norton, J. 1991. Mechanisms of cancer cachexia. *Nutrition and Cancer* 5(1): 103–123.

Laviano, A., Meguid, M., Yang, Z., *et al.* 1996a. Cracking the riddle of cancer anorexia. *Nutrition* 12(10): 706–710.

Laviano, A., Renvyle, T., and Yang, Z. 1996b. From laboratory to bedside: New strategies in the treatment of malnutrition in cancer patients. *Nutrition* 12(2): 112–122.

Loprinzi, C., Ellison, N., Schid, D., *et al.* 1990. Controlled trial of megestrol acetate for the treatment of cancer anorexia and cachexia. *Journal of the National Cancer Institute* 82(13): 1127–1132.

Loprinzi, C., Goldberg, R., Su, Q., *et al.* 1994b. Placebo-controlled trial of hydrazine sulfate in patients with newly diagnosed non-small-cell lung cancer. *Journal of Clinical Oncology* 12(6): 1126–1129.

Loprinzi, C., Kuross, S., O'Fallon, J., *et al.* 1994a. Randomized placebo-controlled evaluation of hydrazine sulfate in patients with advanced colo-

rectal cancer. *Journal of Clinical Oncology* 12(6): 1121–1125.

Lucinio, J., Kling M., and Hauser, P. 1998. Cytokines and brain function: Relevance to interferon-α induced mood and cognitive changes. *Seminars in Oncology* 25(1 suppl 1): 30–38.

Matthys, P., and Billiau, A. 1997. Cytokines and cachexia. *Nutrition* 13(9): 763–770.

Meguid, M., Yang, Z., and Gleason, J. 1996. The gut-brain brain-gut axis in anorexia: Toward understanding of food intake regulation. *Nutrition* 12(1 suppl): S57–S62.

Meydani, S. 1996. Effect of (n-3) polyunsaturated fatty acids on cytokine production and their biological function. *Nutrition* 12(suppl): S8–S14.

Meydani, S., and Dinarello, C. 1993. Influence of dietary fatty acids on cytokine production and its clinical implications. *Nutrition in Clinical Practice* 8(2): 65–72.

Meydani, S., Endres, S., Woods, M., *et al.* 1991. Oral (n-3) fatty acid supplementation suppresses cytokine production and lymphocyte proliferation: Comparison between young and older women. *Journal of Nutrition* 121: 547–555.

Norton, J., Moley, J., Green, J., *et al.* 1985. Parabiotic transfer of cancer anorexia/cachexia in male rats. *Cancer Research* 45(11): 5547–5552.

Oppenheim, J., and Ruscetti, W. 1997. Cytokines. In Stites, D., Terr, A., and Parslow, T. (eds). *Basic and Clinical Immunology.* Norwalk, CT: Appleton and Lange, pp. 146–168.

Ottery, F. 1996. Definition of standardized nutritional assessment and interventional pathways in oncology. *Nutrition* 12(1 suppl): S15–S19.

Physicians' Desk Reference. 2000. Montvale, NJ: Medical Economics Company.

Plata-Salaman, C. 1996a. Anorexia during acute and chronic disease. *Nutrition* 12(2): 69–78.

Plata-Salaman, C. 1998. Cytokines and anorexia: A brief overview. *Seminars in Oncology* 25(1 suppl 1): 64–72.

Plata-Salaman, C., Oomura, Y., and Kai, Y. 1988. Tumor necrosis factor and interleukin-1β: Suppression of food intake by direct action in the central nervous system. *Brain Research* 448: 106–114.

Plata-Salaman, C., Sonti, G., Borkoski, J., *et al.* 1996b. Anorexia induced by chronic central administration of cytokines at estimated pathophysiological concentrations. *Physiology and Behavior* 60(3): 867–875.

Post-White, J. 1996. Principles of immunology. In McCorkle, R., *et al.* (eds). *Cancer Nursing.* Philadelphia, PA: W. B. Saunders Company, pp. 185–187.

Rowland, N., Morien, A., and Li, B. 1996. The physiology and brain mechanisms of feeding. *Nutrition* 12(9): 626–639.

Sandstrom, S. 1996. Nursing management of patients receiving biological therapy. *Seminars in Oncology Nursing* 12(2): 152–162.

Saphier, D., Roerig, S., and Ito, C., 1994. Inhibition of neural and neuroendocrine activity by alpha-interferon: neuroendocrine, electrophysiological, and biochemical studies in the rat. *Brain, Behavior and Immunology* Mar; 8(1): 37–56.

Shronts, E. 1993. Basic concepts of immunology and its application to clinical nutrition. *Nutrition in Clinical Practice* 8(4): 177–183.

Skalla, K. 1996. The interferons. *Seminars in Oncology Nursing* 12(2): 97–105.

Socher, S., Friedman, A., and Martinez, D. 1988. Recombinant human tumor necrosis factor induces acute reductions in food intake and body weight in mice. *Journal of Experimental Medicine* 167: 1957–1962.

Starnes, H. 1991. Biological effects and possible clinical applications of interleukin-1. *Seminars in Hematology* 28(2 suppl 2): 34–41.

Terr, A., Dubey, D., and Yunis, E. 1991. Physiologic and environmental influences on the immune system. In Stites, D., and Terr, A. (eds). *Basic and Clinical Immunology.* Norwalk, CT: Appleton & Lange, pp. 187–199.

Thanhauser, A., Beiling, N., Bohle, A., *et al.* 1993. Pentoxifylline: A potent inhibitor of IL-2 and IFN-gamma biosynthesis and BCG-induced cytotoxicity. *Immunology* 80: 151–156.

Tisdale, M. 1997a. Biology of cachexia. *Journal of the National Cancer Institute* 89(23): 1763–1773.

Tisdale, M. 1997b. Cancer cachexia: Metabolic alterations and clinical manifestations. *Nutrition* 13(1): 1–7.

Tsujinaka, A., Fujita, J., Ebisui, C., *et al.* 1996. Interleukin-6 receptor antibody inhibits muscle atrophy and modulates proteolytic systems in interleukin-6 transgenic mice. *Journal of Clinical Investigation* 97(1): 244–249.

Valentine, A., Meyers, C., Kling, A., *et al.* 1998. Mood and cognitive side effects of interferon-α therapy. *Seminars in Oncology* 25(1 suppl 1): 39–47.

Walker, L., Walker, M., Heys, S., *et al.* 1997. The psychological and psychiatric effects of rIL-2 therapy: A controlled clinical trial. *Psychooncology* 6(4): 290–301.

Watzl, B., Scuderi, P., and Watson, R. 1991. Marijuana components stimulate human peripheral blood mononuclear cell secretion of interferon-gamma and suppress interleukin-1 alpha in vitro. *International Journal of Immunopharmacology* 13(8): 1091–1097.

Yang, Z., Koseki, M., Meguid, M., *et al.* 1994. Synergistic effect of rhTNF-α and rhIL-1α in inducing anorexia in rats. *American Journal of Physiology* 267(4 pt 2): R1056–R1064.

Key References

Albrecht, J.T., and Canada, T.W. 1996. Cachexia and anorexia in malignancy. *Hematology Oncology Clinics of North America* 10(4): 791–800.

Bloch, A. 2000. Nutrition support in cancer. *Seminars in Oncology Nursing* 16(2): 122–127.

Body, J.J. 1999. The syndrome of anorexia-cachexia. *Current Opinions in Oncology* 11(40): 255–260.

Cunningham, R., and Bell, R. 2000. Nutrition in cancer: An overview. *Seminars in Oncology Nursing* 16(2): 90–98.

Gagno, B., and Bruera, E. 1998. A review of the drug treatment of cachexia associated with cancer. *Drugs* 55(5): 675–688.

Grant, M., and Dravits, K. 2000. Symptoms and their impact on nutrition. *Seminars in Oncology Nursing* 16(2): 113–121.

Grant, M.M., and Rivera, L.M. 1995. Anorexia, cachexia, and dysphagia: The symptom experience. *Seminars in Oncology Nursing* 11(4): 266–271.

Han-Markey, T. 2000. Nutritional considerations in pediatric oncology. *Seminars in Oncology Nursing* 16(2): 146–157.

Nelson, K.A. 2000. The cancer anorexia-cachexia syndrome. *Seminars in Oncology* 27(1): 64–68.

Proceedings of the University of Colorado Cancer Center Conference: Recent Developments and Future Directions in the Research and Management of Anorexia and Cachexia. Cancun, Mexico, October 23–25, 1997. 1998. *Seminars in Oncology* 25(2 suppl 6): 1–122.

Yarbro, C.H., Frogge, M.H., and Goodman, M. (eds). 2000. *Cancer Symptom Management: Patient Self-Care Guides*, 2nd edn. Sudbury, MA: Jones & Bartlett Publishers, Inc.

Yarbro, C.H., Frogge, M.H., and Goodman, M. (eds). 1999. *Cancer Symptom Management*, Part III. Symptoms of Alterations in Nutrition, 2nd edn. Sudbury, MA: Jones & Bartlett Publishers, Inc.

Newsletters

SUPPORTIVE SOLUTIONS

This 4-color quarterly newsletter is made available by the Ambassador 2000 program, a national project for oncology nurses, with funding from the Supportive Care Division of Bristol-Myers Squibb Oncology/Immunology. *Supportive Solutions* discusses the issues related to pain, fatigue, and nutrition for patients with cancer. Distribution is 27,000 and is also available on the Oncology Education Services web site: *http://www.oesweb.com/Publications/*.

CHAPTER 19 | Mental Status Changes Associated with Biotherapy

Christina A. Meyers, PhD, ABPP

Biotherapy is increasingly being used to treat various malignancies and infectious diseases. When cytokines were first introduced, it was hoped that they would not be toxic to the nervous system because (1) they were natural products of the body; (2) it was believed that they did not penetrate the **blood-brain barrier (BBB);** and (3) neurotoxic side effects were not observed in preclinical animal models (Goldstein and Laszlo, 1988). However, clinical trials have since shown that cytokines produce significant toxic effects and that neurological side effects are at times the major dose-limiting side effect (Adams *et al.,* 1984; Denicoff *et al.,* 1987; Lenk *et al.,* 1989).

Although neurotoxic effects are rare after treatment with monoclonal antibodies and hematopoietic growth factors, interferon-alpha (IFN-α), interleukin-2 (IL-2), and tumor necrosis factor (TNF) produce significant acute, subacute, and chronic toxic effects that have considerable impact on patients' quality of life. These agents are now known to cause alterations in cognitive functioning and mood, often in the absence of neurological signs. The alterations in cognitive functioning are usually acute and reversible (Meyers and Scheibel, 1990), but there is growing concern that some cytokines can produce lasting cognitive deficits (Meyers *et al.,* 1991b; Meyers and Abbruzzese, 1992).

Neurotoxic side effects, even when subtle, may impair patients' abilities to function in their usual activities of daily living, impose greater burdens on support systems, lessen the ability to effectively treat other symptoms, and frustrate the attempts of physicians to continue cancer therapy as planned. The side effects are often so distressing that the patient will discontinue an effective treatment. Quantification of the neurotoxic effects associated with biotherapy may aid the development of less toxic but equally efficacious dosing and scheduling and may even guide the development of agents that can protect the nervous system from the toxic effects of immunotherapy. In addition, assessment, counseling, and intervention strategies may be put into place to enhance the patient's quality of life and ability to function.

Biotherapy-associated neurotoxicity is also of interest because it demonstrates an interaction between the immune system and the brain. Many cytokines, via their role in mounting a host response to infection and inflammation, have profound effects on brain activity when introduced into the systemic circulation (Mattson *et al.*, 1983; Farkkila *et al.*, 1984). This suggests that cytokines can communicate information about immune system functioning to the central nervous system (CNS) (Dafny *et al.*, 1985). Thus, increased understanding of the effect of cytokines on brain function may open a window into the neuroimmune interactions that underlie normal cognitive functioning.

The effects of antineoplastic agents on the nervous system are reflected in altered behavior and mood, in addition to peripheral neuropathy and other well-described neurologic syndromes. Cognitive impairments and mood changes, often in the absence of neurological signs, may be seen in patients who are receiving agents that affect CNS function. This chapter describes the assessment of cognitive and emotional changes that result from administration of biotherapy, the patterns of both acute and chronic neurotoxic symptoms that are seen with various biotherapy agents, the mechanisms of these effects, and the interventions that can be put into place to help patients cope with these symptoms.

Assessment of Neurobehavioral Functioning

Distinguishing cognitive impairment from emotional reactions to illness and stress is very important, but the differential diagnosis of neurobehavioral changes is often difficult. A patient who is apathetic, withdrawn, and lacks motivation may be depressed or may be experiencing treatment-related neurotoxicity. Levine *et al.* (1978) reported that 64% of cancer patients with **delirium** (generally from toxic metabolic **encephalopathy**) were misdiagnosed as being depressed. Treatment of depression may be inappropriate in a patient who is experiencing cognitive changes caused by biotherapy. However, biotherapy also can directly cause depression and other psychiatric symptoms; therefore, assessment of mood is also critical (Valentine *et al.*, 1998).

Impairment of neurobehavioral functioning may impair the patient's ability for self-care and ability to follow the therapeutic regimen; it may also necessitate alterations in lifestyle or the need for supervision and special safety measures. Neuropsychological assessment of brain function is often helpful in determining the nature and extent of cognitive impairments that are not detected in routine medical evaluations.

Formal neuropsychological assessment involves the administration of standardized **psychometric tests** that comprehensively evaluate brain function. Table 19.1 is a list of the cognitive domains assessed. This detailed description of intellectual status and personality characteristics allows for rational planning and management. Conferences held with the patient, family members, and health-care team can utilize this knowledge of the patient's capabilities and limitations to help set realistic goals; to determine his or her capacity for independent self-care, including the ability to drive, manage finances, and handle emergencies; and to determine what

Table 19.1 Neuropsychological assessment of cognitive functioning

Intellectual Functions
  Attentional abilities
  Abstract reasoning
  Problem solving

Memory
  Working memory capacity
  Retention of information over time
  Verbal vs. visual memory
  Remote memory

Language
  Naming
  Fluency
  Comprehension
  Reading and writing

Visual Perception
  Scanning
  Discrimination
  Construction

Motor Functions
  Strength
  Motor speed
  Coordination and dexterity

Executive (Frontal Lobe) Functions
  Cognitive flexibility (shifting mental set, multi-
    tasking)
  Motivation
  Social judgment
  Planning
  Learning from experience
  Insight and self-awareness

Mood
  Depression
  Anxiety
  Agitation
  Withdrawal

types of management and compensatory techniques might be most useful.

Of course, not every individual needs or would benefit from an extensive neuropsychological evaluation. The nurse is in an excellent position to assess the patient's mental status and determine whether an extended assessment is warranted. A number of standardized, brief mental status examinations are available, such as the Mini-Mental State Examination (Folstein *et al.,* 1975). This exam includes assessment of orientation (time and place), registration (ability to name objects), attention and calculation, recall (ability to recall the named objects), and language (ability to follow commands and repeat phrases). However, tests of this type only identify patients with severe, global cognitive problems and do not specify the type of disorder. For instance, the performances of demented, nondemented, brain-damaged, and control groups significantly overlap on the Mini-Mental State Examination (Auerbach and Faibish, 1989). The cognitive impairments associated with biotherapy tend to be specific and not global. For the most part, careful evaluation of the patient's general behavior, appearance, ability to maintain a logical conversation, ability to give a concise and accurate history, and ability to paraphrase and comprehend instructions will guide the nurse in evaluating attentiveness, mood, language, and short-term memory (Strub and Black, 1981). Difficulty with this type of evaluation or complaints from patients about difficulties performing their normal work and leisure activities should prompt referral for a more detailed neuropsychological or psychiatric examination, or a combination of these.

Presentation of Mental Status Changes

Mental status changes that result from the neurotoxic effects of cytokines have tremendous potential to impact patients' perceived quality of life. Knowledge of which cytokines are most likely to cause neurotoxic side effects and the ability to recognize the presentation of mental status changes are the first steps toward assisting patients to cope with these effects. This section focuses primarily on cytokines known to cause neurotoxic effects: IFN-α, IL-2, and TNF. Table 19.2 is an overview of these effects. Acute neurotoxicity associated with cytokines resembles "flu-like" symptoms and is reviewed in Chapter 16.

Table 19.2   Neurological side effects associated with biological agents*

Interferon-α
  Confusion
  Depression**
  Hypersomnia
  Difficulty concentrating**
  Memory problems**
  Trouble with calculations
  Slowed thinking**
  Impaired motor coordination**
  Impaired visual-motor skills
  Impaired frontal lobe functioning**
  Paraesthesias

Interleukin-2
  Confusion**
  Hypersomnolence**
  Difficulty concentrating**
  Agitation
  Withdrawal from social contact
  Irritability**
  Depression
  Bizarre dreams
  Paranoia
  Delusions
  Hallucinations

Tumor Necrosis Factor
  Confusion
  Somnolence
  Lethargy

*The occurrence and severity of side effects tend to increase as the dose is increased. Most side effects are readily reversible when therapy is discontinued. However, some may persist or progress when off treatment.

**More frequently seen.

Interferon-α

Within a week of receiving IFN-α therapy, many patients develop temporary deficits in verbal concept formation, visual-motor skills (*i.e.,* the ability to copy drawings), and mental flexibility (Adams *et al.,* 1984). Adams reported that individuals who received IFN-α developed increasing fatigue, lack of spontaneity, and apathy—symptoms similar to those seen in patients whose frontal lobe function is impaired. Iivanainen *et al.* (1985) also reported cognitive impairments in patients with amyotrophic lateral sclerosis who received IFN-α therapy. Their study of five patients revealed a generalized slowing of behavior and deficits in verbal memory, ability to sequence, motor coordination, and visual-motor skills. The symptoms resolved following the discontinuation of treatment. These impairments of motor skills and executive functions were also interpreted as reflecting frontal lobe dysfunction. Intellectual functioning did not appear to decline during treatment, and there were never any impairments in basic language or visual-perceptual skills.

Pavol *et al.* (1995) found that 50% of leukemia patients treated with IFN-α had memory deficits compared with 25% of similar patients not on IFN-α. In addition, significantly more patients on IFN-α had deficits on tests of speed of information processing and executive function.

Electrophysiologic studies support the findings of frontal lobe dysfunction during IFN-α therapy. The abnormalities seen on electroencephalography typically include background slowing with intermittent, very slow waves in the frontal region (Rohatiner *et al.,* 1983;

Smedley *et al.,* 1983; Farkkila *et al.,* 1984; Suter *et al.,* 1984).

MOOD CHANGES

A number of investigators have reported that patients who are receiving IFN-α become depressed (Talpaz *et al.,* 1986; Renault *et al.,* 1987; Pavol *et al.,* 1995), although Adams *et al.* (1984) did not find that depression was a side effect of IFN-α. One study found that more than half of the patients have findings on personality testing reflecting significant depression and agitation (Pavol *et al.,* 1995). Two articles reported on neuropsychiatric symptoms that developed in patients with chronic active hepatitis who were receiving IFN-α. The incidence of overt symptoms ranged from 7% to 17%, most frequently organic personality syndromes, depression, and frank delirium (McDonald *et al.,* 1987; Renault *et al.,* 1987). These side effects usually appeared 1 to 3 months into therapy and improved within 3 to 4 days after decreasing the IFN-α dose. Unfortunately, the reports on emotional symptoms associated with IFN-α therapy relied on interviews and other subjective measures of emotional status. Therefore, some symptoms of depression may not be differentiated from the fatigue-asthenia syndrome that is a common side effect of IFN-α.

Recently, it was reported that the development of mania may also be associated with IFN-α treatment (Strite *et al.,* 1997). However, one study failed to find significant adverse cognitive or mood effects of natural IFN-α, raising the question of a difference between the natural and recombinant products (Mapou *et al.,* 1996). However, this study also used lower doses and a shorter duration of treatment than the other studies cited.

CHRONIC TOXICITY

Many patients who receive IFN-α over a period of months to years complain of difficulties with mood, memory, and clarity of thinking. A retrospective review reported the neuropsychological test profiles of 16 patients with chronic myelogenous leukemia treated with IFN-α for 5 to 86 months (Meyers *et al.,* 1993). These patients had no history of psychiatric or neurologic problems and were well educated (*i.e.,* average of 15 years). They performed in the impaired range on tests of verbal memory, information-processing speed, and ability to shift mental set (*i.e.,* frontal lobe functioning). Personality testing revealed elevations on measures of depression, somatic concern, and denial; in contrast, reasoning skills tended to remain in the normal range. This pattern of slowed thinking, memory difficulty, impaired executive functioning, and mood changes is consistent with the clinical syndrome of **subcortical dementia** (Cummings, 1990). In fact, the types of difficulties that patients on IFN-α experience are very similar to those experienced by patients with multiple sclerosis, a condition that may also be associated with a subcortical dementia.

Interleukin-2

IL-2 also causes alterations in behavior and cognition. In general, as doses are increased, these alterations become more pronounced. In one report, 50% of patients who received IL-2 developed delirium, and more than one third were combative and agitated (Denicoff *et al.,* 1987). These symptoms resolved following discontinuation of treatment. Another study found that mental status changed in 32% of patients with renal cell carcinoma (von der Maase *et al.,* 1991). Many patients who received IL-2 developed depression (Krigel *et al.,* 1988) and tended to withdraw from social contact. Difficulty concentrating or reading (Rieger and Weatherly, 1989) and hypersomnia, in addition to the fatigue-asthenia syndrome, were also seen.

Single photon emission computed tomography (SPECT), which images regional cerebral perfusion, has been used to further quantify the physiologic changes caused by IL-2. In one patient, SPECT revealed diminished blood flow in both frontal lobes in the absence of anatomic abnormalities on a computed tomographic scan (Meyers *et al.,* 1994). The neuropsychological test abnormalities, which also indicated frontal lobe dysfunction, and the regional cerebral blood flow abnormalities resolved one month after treatment was discontinued.

Tumor Necrosis Factor

TNF is a highly neurotoxic agent. In one report, approximately 86% of patients who received TNF developed dose-limiting neurotoxic effects (Lenk *et al.,* 1989). In fact, induction of TNF in the brain may be one of the mechanisms of IL-2 neurotoxicity (Mier *et al.,* 1990). Elevated TNF levels induced by IL-2 administration have been associated with destruction of brain white matter in animal studies (Ellison and Merchant, 1991). The type of cognitive and emotional changes seen in TNF and IL-2 neurotoxicity are similar. Neuropsychological test findings in patients who experience TNF or combination TNF/IL-2 toxic effects have shown mild to moderate deficits of attentional abilities, verbal memory, motor coordination, and ability to shift mental set (*i.e.,* to think flexibly). Intellectual functions, as in the case of IFN-α toxicity, are preserved.

Route Of Administration

The methods of treatment administration and prior treatment with cytokines are factors influencing cytokine neurotoxicity. Intraventricular administration in particular may be associated with more severe neurotoxic side effects, which has limited the use of cytokines in treating leptomeningeal disease. In one study, seven of nine patients (78%) treated with intraventricular

IFN-α for leptomeningeal disease developed severe neurotoxic effects that did not appear to be dose dependent (Meyers *et al.,* 1991a). These patients became increasingly confused and developed expressive speech difficulty, which finally evolved into **mutism** after cumulative IFN-α doses between 14 and 54 MU. The clinical picture was one of a wakeful vegetative state in which the patients could open their eyes to stimulation but would not follow commands and were otherwise completely unresponsive. It took an average of 17 days for the patients to return to their pretreatment levels of function, and two died before recovering. All of the patients who developed this neurotoxic syndrome had previously received whole-brain radiation therapy for leptomeningeal disease, suggesting a synergism between brain irradiation and IFN-α.

A recently completed study using intraventricular IL-2 for leptomeningeal disease revealed less alarming but significant neurotoxicity. Of 20 patients who received neuropsychological testing before and during therapy, 10 (50%) exhibited significant deterioration in cognitive performance (Sherman and Meyers, 2000). The most common problems were memory, frontal lobe executive function, and generalized slowing of behavior—a pattern consistent with frontal-subcortical dysfunction. It is often difficult, however, to sort out the effects of treatment from the effects of progressive disease in these patients.

Irreversible and Delayed Neurotoxicity

There is increasing evidence that cytokine neurotoxicity does not always resolve following the discontinuation of treatment. One study reviewed the neuropsychological evaluations of 46 cancer patients who had received a number of chemotherapeutic and biological agents. These patients were referred for pretreatment assessment before starting a new phase I protocol (Meyers and Abbruzzese, 1992). None of them had a history of neurologic or psychiatric disorder, and all had been off prior therapy for at least 3 weeks. Cognitive deficits were observed in 18% of individuals who had been treated with chemotherapy only but in 53% of patients who had also received cytokines. This finding suggests that treatment with cytokines places certain individuals at greater risk for developing neurobehavioral deficits and that these deficits may persist after treatment is discontinued. Therefore, long-term follow-up of patients treated with biotherapy is warranted.

INTERFERON-α

Studies of IFN-α neurotoxicity already described reported prompt resolution of symptoms when treatment was discontinued, usually within several days to 2 weeks. However, some individuals continue to manifest difficulties with cognition and emotional functioning even years after IFN-α has been discontinued (Meyers et al., 1991b). The impairments of neurobehavioral function, which included memory loss, frontal lobe dysfunction, and outright dementia, could not be attributed to other therapy, changes in disease status, or other medical problems. Although most of the individuals had mild to moderate impairments, a number had very severe cognitive deficits, including progressive dementia, **extrapyramidal motor symptoms,** and florid psychiatric symptoms that necessitated involuntary hospitalization.

INTRAVENTRICULAR INTERLEUKIN-2

Treatment with intraventricular IL-2 may also cause progressive and delayed deterioration of mental functions. Patients rarely survive long after the diagnosis of leptomeningeal disease, but there is a published case report of a woman who was treated successfully with intraventricular IL-2 (Meyers and Yung, 1993). Following the diagnosis of metastatic melanoma to the leptomeninges, she was treated with 9 MU of intraventricular IL-2 over 1 month. She did well following this treatment, with no evidence of tumor recurrence. However, 3 months after her treatment ended, she developed cerebellar signs consisting of a wide-based gait and impaired balance. Neuropsychological testing revealed mild impairments of memory and motor coordination with high-average intellectual ability. Four years after therapy with IL-2, the patient had become exceedingly slow, with significant declines in memory and motor coordination. Intellectual function remained unimpaired. Magnetic resonance imaging revealed lesions in the subcortical white matter. This patient was no longer able to work and was confined to a wheelchair as a result of progressive subcortical dementia.

Pathophysiology of Mental Status Changes

Although the CNS is normally protected by the BBB, the development of cytokine neurotoxicity implies that these substances somehow gain access to the brain. There are several ways that cytokines may bypass this barrier and alter neural activity: (1) by altering vascular permeability, permitting substances normally excluded to enter the brain; (2) by diffusing through circumventricular organs where the BBB is normally leaky; (3) by inducing second messengers and signaling molecules that can cross the barrier; and (4) by transmitting signals to the brain by the vagus nerve or other nerve pathways to the brain (Licinio et al., 1998).

Cerebrovascular Alterations

IL-2 is known to alter cerebrovascular permeability, inducing the so-called capillary leak syndrome, which may allow cytokines and other naturally excluded substances into the brain (Ellison *et al.,* 1987) or cerebrospinal fluid (Saris *et al.,* 1988). Although IL-2 also causes vasogenic edema, the amount of cerebral edema does not appear to correlate with the severity of neurotoxic symptoms (Saris *et al.,* 1989). Changes in vascular permeability may also cause acute focal neurologic events that clinically resemble strokes (Bernard *et al.,* 1990).

IFN-α is an antiangiogenic agent, and its action against tumor blood vessels is one of its therapeutic actions in cancer treatment (Kaban *et al.,* 1999). The use of IFN-α can delay the healing of peripheral ischemic injuries (Cid *et al.,* 1999), but it is unknown whether it can affect cerebral vasculature.

Hypothalamic Actions

There are several lines of evidence suggesting that both IL-2 and IFN-α alter brain activity through actions at circumferential organs associated with the hypothalamus. First, patients who receive cytokines develop fever, anorexia, lethargy, and hypersomnia (Smedley *et al.,* 1983; Sarna *et al.,* 1989), symptoms that are similar to those seen following damage to various areas of the hypothalamus (Anand and Brobeck, 1951; Feldman and Waller, 1962; Ellison *et al.,* 1970; Kupferman, 1981). Second, systemic IFN-α and IL-2 alter electrophysiological activity within the hypothalamus in animal studies. Whereas IFN-α causes neuronal excitability within 5 minutes of systemic administration (Calvet and Gresser, 1979; Dafny, 1983), IL-2 takes somewhat longer to alter neural activity, suggesting that there may be some intermediary steps involved (Bindoni *et al.,* 1988). Systemic administration of TNF also causes an increase in the firing rate of neurons in the circumventricular region of the hypothalamus (Shibata and Blatteis, 1991). Finally, IL-1 has been shown to cause fever and neuroendocrine alterations through an action at the anterior hypothalamus (Tsagarakis *et al.,* 1989).

Areas of the hypothalamus have connections with the brainstem, frontal cortex, and all structures of the limbic system (Berk and Finkelstein, 1982; Issacson, 1982; Carpenter and Sutin, 1983; Villalobos and Ferssiwi, 1987a and 1987b). Thus, it is interesting that the electrophysiological and neuropsychological studies previously cited also suggest brainstem and frontal lobe dysfunction.

Induction of Secondary Cytokines

Interactions among cytokines are complex and include both stimulatory and inhibitory effects. IFN-α administration induces IL-1, IFN-γ, and TNF-α (Licinio *et al.,* 1998). IL-1 has receptors on neurons within the hypothalamus and causes specific alterations in hypothalamic function (Farrar *et al.,* 1987; Breder *et al.,* 1988; Kabiersch *et al.,* 1988). IL-2 also induces production of TNF (Mier *et al.,* 1990), and TNF and IL-1 are synergistically toxic (Waage and Espevik, 1988).

Neuroendocrine Alterations

Neuroendocrine disturbances occur often during cytokine therapy and may have an effect on brain function. Glucocorticoids can cross the BBB (McEwen *et al.,* 1968 and 1986) and have receptors within the CNS (McEwen and Micco, 1980). Glucocorticoid receptors are found within frontal brain regions and neurons of the septo-hippocampal system, a neural network thought to be important for emotion and memory (Gray, 1982; Lynch, 1986; Squire, 1987). In fact, endocrine disturbances are often found in patients with affective disorders (Sachar, 1982). As previously cited, memory and mood alterations are specifically affected by cytokine administration.

Administration of cytokines is known to induce a stress hormone response, elevating cortisol levels (Atkins *et al.,* 1986; Tracey *et al.,*

1987). Corticosterone can potentiate neurotoxic damage within the septo-hippocampal system by enhancing the vulnerability of neurons to other insults; for example, seizure, hypoxia-ischemia, excitatory amino acids, and antimetabolites (Holsboer, 1988; Sapolsky et al., 1988; Stein and Sapolsky, 1988; Masters et al., 1989). These effects have been observed primarily in the hippocampal areas that contain high levels of glucocorticoid receptors (Sapolsky, 1985; Johnson et al., 1989). In addition to inducing stress hormones, cytokines may behave as neuroendocrine hormones themselves. For instance, IFN-α has structural and functional similarities to the adrenocorticotrophic hormone (Blalock and Smith, 1980; Blalock and Stanton, 1980).

Neurotransmitter Alterations

The areas in which IFN has been shown to cause neuronal excitability are also areas with high numbers of opiate receptors (Prieto-Gomez et al., 1983; Dafny et al., 1985). IFN has been shown to have structural similarities to endorphins and to have opiate-like neurotransmitter activity (Blalock and Smith, 1981; Dafny et al., 1983). In fact, many of the effects of IFN can be reversed by the opiate antagonist naloxone. The progressive catatonia observed clinically in patients treated with intraventricular IFN-α are similar to the symptoms seen in animals treated with kappa opiate agonists (Meyers et al., 1991a). This has prompted animal laboratory researchers to determine the opioid-dopamine basis for the behavioral effects of this cytokine.

In one study, rats were trained to discriminate the effects of d-amphetamine from saline. When the rat was given d-amphetamine, it pushed a particular lever for food; when it was given saline, it pushed a different lever. This discrimination response is known to be mediated by the dopamine system. When the dose

of amphetamine was cut in half, the animal responded randomly. However, when the dose of amphetamine was halved and the animal also received IFN-α, it responded just as if it had received the full dose of amphetamine; this is called a *potentiation response* (Ho et al., 1992). Ho et al. also found that the opiate antagonist naloxone suppressed this effect and that morphine had the same effect as IFN-α. Opiate receptor activity subsequently modulates the release of dopamine, which may be a factor in the extrapyramidal motor abnormalities seen in about one third of patients who receive IFN-α. These data suggesting that IFN-α binds to opiate receptors have guided current interventional drug trials against IFN-α toxicity. In fact, the long-acting opiate antagonist naltrexone has shown promise as treatment for the neurocognitive side effects of IFN-α (Valentine et al., 1995).

Nursing Intervention Strategies

Mental status changes that result from biotherapy represent a significant nursing challenge. Unless the symptoms experienced are severe and significantly affect patient function, doses are frequently not altered so that the agent's full therapeutic benefit may be realized. Awareness of common neurotoxic effects related to biotherapy and appropriate interventions will assist the nurse in developing strategies to help patients cope (Sparber and Biller-Sparber, 1993).

One of the greatest interventions that can be provided to patients experiencing the neurotoxic effects of biotherapy is *knowledge*. The potential neurotoxic symptoms of this treatment are frequently not explained to the patient, sometimes because the primary physician does not fully recognize the impact of even subtle symptoms on social and vocational functioning. Not infrequently, patients who experience these symptoms without adequate warning may wonder if they are going "crazy" or will inaccurately attribute their symptoms to other causes. Reassurance that these symptoms are related to therapy can help reduce patient and family anxiety.

In addition, health-care providers may not consider subtle neurobehavioral impairments very important in the context of the disease being treated. However, knowing that treatment-related neurobehavioral changes are common and that they can often be managed with a few compensation techniques can help alleviate the patient's anxiety and improve his or her psychosocial functioning. Even simple techniques such as taking intermittent naps, making lists, and taking special care to plan and organize activities may be all that is necessary to effectively cope with these symptoms.

Baseline assessment of individuals who will be treated with biotherapy agents is critical. It is often difficult to determine whether depression or memory loss are caused by the patient's reaction to his diagnosis or concurrent psychosocial problems or are directly attributable to treatment-related neurotoxicity. The baseline assessment will provide the nurse and health-care team with knowledge about potential risk factors that the patient may bring to the situation (*i.e.,* pre-existing neurobehavioral difficulties related to previous treatment or other neurologic illness, psychosocial stressors, or other medications that can affect mental status) and will help them detect changes in neurobehavioral functioning over time. Because mental status changes associated with biotherapy are often subtle, it is important to request input from the family or significant others. They are often the first to recognize changes in the patient. Ongoing assessment during therapy is paramount. Simple observations such as determining the patient's ability to follow directions, fill out hospital meal menus, answer general orientation questions, and do calculations can provide

significant information regarding neurotoxic side effects (Sparber and Biller-Sparber, 1993).

Baseline and interval assessments of the patient's neurocognitive functioning will also guide the implementation of safety measures and compensation techniques. For instance, a patient with memory problems may inaccurately report the type, frequency, or amount of medication he or she has been taking, leading to subtherapeutic or toxic medication levels. A person with poor motivation and apathy caused by frontal lobe dysfunction may appear depressed or uncompliant and may have difficulty initiating and following through with personal hygiene routines, performing usual work and leisure activities, and so on. For inpatients experiencing side effects such as confusion or hypersomnia, appropriate safety measures, such as fall precautions, should be initiated.

Medical management of neurotoxic symptoms is one area of intervention that may be helpful. Low doses of selective serotonin reuptake inhibitors such as fluoxetene have been found to be effective in reducing psychological symptomatology, whether organically mediated, reactive, or both (Valentine *et al.,* 1998). Tricyclic antidepressants have more adverse side effects, but agents such as amitriptyline may also serve as co-analgesics for the diffuse joint pain and body aches frequently associated with cytokine therapy.

Some groups have advocated prophylactic antidepressant treatment for individuals who are scheduled to receive IFN-α. In the case of very high-dose therapy, such as is used in the treatment of malignant melanoma, prophylactic therapy might be of benefit because the incidence of depression is very high (Miller *et al.,* 1999). However, the incidence of depression in most settings is probably no more than 30%; therefore, prophylactic treatment with antidepressants is unnecessary in at least 70% of patients, exposing them to potential adverse effects with no benefit. At present, there is no good way to predict which patients are likely to experience depression in advance, but aggressive treatment when symptoms occur is usually efficacious.

Development of other agents, many of which are still in the experimental stages, is based on research about the specific mechanisms of action cytokines have on specific neurotransmitter and neuroendocrine systems in the brain. Opiate antagonist therapy in patients complaining of neurotoxic effects of IFN-α has shown promise (Valentine *et al.*, 1995). Approximately 75% of the patients treated so far have had relief from symptoms on this therapy, although some individuals have experienced intolerable side effects.

Research

Although there is a growing understanding of the neurobehavioral deficits experienced by patients who receive biotherapy, much more research is needed in the area of nursing interventions directed toward specific deficits. To date, there are few reports of research pertaining to the mental status changes that occur after biotherapy. Nurses are in a unique position to influence this area because they coordinate inpatient and outpatient care, directly treat patients' symptoms, and function as researchers. It will become increasingly important for nurses and the entire health-care team to develop and implement proactive programs for their patients—including determination of the cost/benefit ratio and efficacy of such programs—to ensure the best quality of life for patients undergoing biotherapy. Interventions designed for patients who are receiving biotherapy will need to include patient education about potential symptoms, psychological support, safety measures, and coordination of adjunct services in neuropsychology, psychiatry, and rehabilitation. Studies that evaluate patterns of neurotox-

icity and associated distress will assist with nursing assessment during therapy.

Future Directions

The use of cytokines will continue to expand as experience with new agents increases and the number of illnesses found to respond to cytokine therapy multiplies. It is increasingly important to consider the long-term impact of these compounds on the social, vocational, and psychological functioning of the individuals being treated. Early detection and some interventions for neurotoxic effects are now feasible, and better intervention strategies are being developed. The potential for progressive brain injury and subsequent disability will need to be considered in developing ancillary treatments to improve the risk/benefit ratio of therapy and to enhance the quality of life of patients who receive biotherapy.

References

Adams, F., Quesada, J., and Gutterman, J. 1984. Neuropsychiatric manifestations of human leukocyte interferon therapy in patients with cancer. *Journal of the American Medical Association* 252: 938–941.

Anand, B., and Brobeck, J. 1951. Hypothalamic control of food intake in rats and cats. *Yale Journal of Biological Medicine* 24: 123.

Atkins, M., Gould, J., Allegretta, M., *et al.* 1986. Phase I evaluation of recombinant interleukin-2 in patients with advanced malignant disease. *Journal of Clinical Oncology* 4: 1380–1391.

Auerbach, V., and Faibish, G. 1989. Mini-mental state examination: Diagnostic limitations. *Journal of Clinical and Experimental Neuropsychology* 11: 75 (abstract).

Berk, M., and Finkelstein, J. 1982. Efferent connections of the lateral hypothalamic area of the rat: An autoradiographic investigation. *Brain Research Bulletin* 8: 511–526.

Bernard, J., Ameriso, S., Kempf, R., *et al.* 1990. Transient focal neurologic deficits complicating interleukin-2 therapy. *Neurology* 40: 154–155.

Bindoni, M., Perciavalle, V., Berretta S., *et al.* 1988. Interleukin-2 modifies the bioelectric activity of some neurosecretory nuclei in the rat hypothalamus. *Brain Research* 462: 10–14.

Blalock, J., and Smith, E. 1980. Human leukocyte interferon: Structural and biological relatedness to adrenocorticotropic hormones and endorphins. *Proceedings of the National Academy of Sciences of the USA* 77: 5972–5974.

Blalock, J., and Smith, E. 1981. Human leukocyte interferon (HuIFN-α): Potent endorphin-like opioid activity. *Biochemistry and Biophysics Research Communication* 101: 472–478.

Blalock, J., and Stanton, J. 1980. Common pathways of interferon and hormonal action. *Nature* 283: 406–408.

Breder, C., Dinarello, C., and Saper, C. 1988. Interleukin-1 immunoreactive innervation of the human hypothalamus. *Science* 240: 321–324.

Calvet, M., and Gresser, I. 1979. Interferon enhances the excitability of cultured neurones. *Nature* 278: 558–560.

Carpenter, M., and Sutin, J. 1983. *Human Neuroanatomy.* Baltimore: Williams & Wilkins.

Cid, M., Hernandez-Rodriguez, J., Robert, J., *et al.* 1999. Interferon-alpha may exacerbate cryoblobulinemia-related ischemic manifestations: An adverse effect potentially related to its antiangiogenic activity. *Arthritis & Rheumatism* 42: 1051–1055.

Cummings, J. 1990. *Subcortical Dementia.* New York: Oxford University Press.

Dafny, N. 1983. Interferon modifies EEG and EEG-like activity recorded from sensory, motor, and limbic-system structures in freely behaving rats. *Neurotoxicology* 4: 235–240.

Dafny, N., Prieto-Gomez, B., and Reyes-Vasquez, C. 1985. Does the immune system communicate with the central nervous system? Interferon modifies central nervous activity. *Journal of Neuroimmunology* 9: 1–12.

Dafny, N., Zielinnski, M., and Reyes-Vasquez, C. 1983. Alteration of morphine withdrawal to naloxone by interferon. *Neuropeptides* 3: 453–463.

Denicoff, K., Rubinow, D., Papa, M., *et al.* 1987. The neuropsychiatric effects of treatment with interleukin-2 and lymphokine-activated killer cells. *Annals of Internal Medicine* 107: 293–300.

Ellison, M., and Merchant, R. 1991. Appearance of cytokine-associated central nervous system myelin damage coincides temporarily with serum tumor necrosis factor induction after recombinant interleukin-2 infusion in rats. *Journal of Neuroimmunology* 33: 245–251.

Ellison, M., Povlishock, J., and Merchant, R. 1987. Blood-brain barrier dysfunction in cats following recombinant interleukin-2 infusion. *Cancer Research* 47: 5765–5770.

Ellison, G., Sorenson, C., and Jacobs, B. 1970. Two feeding syndromes following surgical isolation of the hypothalamus in rats. *Journal of Comparative and Physiological Psychology* 70: 173–188.

Farkkila, M., Iivanainen, M., Roine, R., *et al.* 1984. Neurotoxic and other side effects of high-dose interferon in amyotrophic lateral sclerosis. *Acta Neurologica Scandinavica* 70: 42–46.

Farrar, W., Killian, P., Ruff, M., *et al.* 1987. Visualization and characterization of interleukin-1 receptors in brain. *Journal of Immunology* 139: 459–463.

Feldman, S., and Waller, H. 1962. Dissociation of electrocortical activation and behavioral arousal. *Nature* 196: 1320–1322.

Folstein, M., Folstein, S., and McHugh, P. 1975. "Mini-mental state": A practical method for grading the cognitive state of patients for the clinician. *Journal of Psychiatric Research* 12: 189–198.

Goldstein, D., and Laszlo, J. 1988. The role of interferon in cancer therapy: A current perspective. *CA-A Cancer Journal for Clinicians* 38: 258–277.

Gray, J. 1982. *The Neuropsychology of Anxiety: An Inquiry into the Functions of the Septo-Hippocampal System.* New York: Oxford University Press.

Ho, B., Huo, Y., Lu, J., *et al.* 1992. Opioid-dopaminergic mechanisms in the potentiation of *d*-amphetamine discrimination by interferon-α. *Pharmacology, Biochemistry, and Behavior* 42: 57–60.

Holsboer, F. 1988. Implications of altered limbic-hypothalamic-pituitary-adrenocortical (LHPA)-function for neurobiology of depression. *Acta Psychiatrica Scandinavica* 341(suppl): 72–111.

Iivanainen, M., Laaksonen, R., Niemi, M., *et al.* 1985. Memory and psychomotor impairment following high-dose interferon treatment in amyotrophic lateral sclerosis. *Acta Neurologica Scandinavica* 72: 475–480.

Issacson, R. 1982. *The Limbic System.* New York: Plenum Press.

Johnson, M., Stone, D., Bush, L., *et al.* 1989. Glucocorticoids and 3,4-methylenedioxymethamphetamine (MDMA)-induced neurotoxicity. *European Journal of Pharmacology* 161: 181–188.

Kaban, L., Mulliken, J., Ezekowitz, R., *et al.* 1999. Antiangiogenic therapy of a recurrent giant cell tumor of the mandible with interferon alfa-2a. *Pediatrics* 103: 1145–1149.

Kabiersch, A., Del Rey, A., Honegger, C., *et al.* 1988. Interleukin-1 produces changes in norepinephrine metabolism in the rat brain. *Brain, Behavior, and Immunity* 2: 267–274.

Krigel, R., Padavic-Shaller, K., Rudolph, A., *et al.* 1988. A phase I study of recombinant interleukin-2 plus recombinant beta interferon. *Cancer Research* 48: 3875–3881.

Kupferman, I. 1981. Hypothalamus and limbic system II: Motivation. In Kandel, E., and Schwartz, J. (eds). *Principles of Neural Science.* New York: Elsevier, pp. 450–460.

Lenk, H., Tanneberger, S., Muller, U., *et al.* 1989. Phase II clinical trial of high-dose recombinant human tumor necrosis factor. *Cancer Chemotherapy and Pharmacology* 24: 391–392.

Levine, P., Silberfarb, P., and Kipowski, Z. 1978. Mental disorders in cancer patients: A study of 100 psychiatric referrals. *Cancer* 43: 1385–1391.

Licinio, J., Kling, M., and Hauser, P. 1998. Cytokines and brain function: Relevance to interferon-α-induced mood and cognitive changes. *Seminars in Oncology* 25(suppl 1): 30–38.

Lynch, G. 1986. *Synapses, Circuits, and the Beginnings of Memory.* Cambridge, MA: MIT Press.

Mapou, R., Law, W., Wagner, K., *et al.* 1996. Neuropsychological effects of interferon alpha-n3 treatment on asymptomatic human immunodeficiency virus-1-infected individuals. *Journal of Neuropsychiatry and Clinical Neuroscience* 8: 74–81.

Masters, J., Finch, C., and Sapolsky, R. 1989. Glucocorticoid endangerment of hippocampal neurons does not involve deoxyribonucleic acid cleavage. *Endocrinology* 124: 3083–3088.

Mattson, K., Niiranen, A., Iivanainen, M., *et al.* 1983. Neurotoxicity of interferon. *Cancer Treatment Reports* 67: 958–961.

McDonald, E., Mann, A., and Thomas, H. 1987. Interferons as mediators of psychiatric morbidity: An investigation in a trial of recombinant interferon-alfa in hepatitis B carriers. *Lancet* 2: 1175–1177.

McEwen, B., De Kloet, E., and Rostene, W. 1986. Adrenal steroid receptors and actions in the central nervous system. *Physiological Reviews* 66: 1121–1188.

McEwen, B., and Micco, D. 1980. Toward an understanding of the multiplicity of glucocorticoid actions on brain function and behavior. In De Weid, D., and van Keep, P. (eds). *Hormones and the Brain.* Baltimore: University Park, pp. 11–28.

McEwen, B., Weis, J., and Schwartz, L. 1968. Selective retention of corticosterone by limbic structures in rat brain. *Nature* 220: 911–912.

Meyers, C., and Abbruzzese, J. 1992. Cognitive functioning in cancer patients: Effect of previous treatment. *Neurology* 42: 434–436.

Meyers, C., Mattis, P., Pavol, M., *et al.* 1993. Pattern of neurobehavioral deficits associated with interferon-α neurotoxicity. *Proceedings of the Ameri-*

can *Association for Cancer Research* 34: 218 (abstract).

Meyers, C., Obbens, E., Scheibel, R., *et al.* 1991a. Neurotoxicity of intraventricularly administered alpha interferon for leptomeningeal disease. *Cancer* 68: 88–92.

Meyers, C., and Scheibel, R. 1990. Early detection and diagnosis of neurobehavioral disorders in cancer patients. *Oncology* 4: 115–122.

Meyers, C., Scheibel, R., and Forman, A. 1991b. Persistent neurotoxicity of systemically administered interferon-alpha. *Neurology* 41: 672–676.

Meyers, C., Valentine, A., Wong, F., *et al.* 1994. Reversible neurotoxicity of IL-2 and TNF: Correlation of SPECT with neuropsychological testing. *Journal of Neuropsychiatry and Clinical Neurosciences* 6: 285–288.

Meyers, C., and Yung, W. 1993. Delayed neurotoxicity of intraventricular interleukin-2: A case report. *Journal of Neuro-Oncology* 15: 265–267.

Mier, J., Vachino, G., Lempner, M., *et al.* 1990. Inhibition of interleukin-2-induced tumor necrosis factor release by dexamethasone: Prevention of an acquired neutrophil chemotaxis defect and differential suppression of interleukin-2-associated side effects. *Blood* 76: 1933–1940.

Miller, A., Musselman, D., Penna, S., *et al.* 1999. Pretreatment with the antidepressant paroxetine prevents cytokine-induced depression during IFN-alpha therapy for malignant melanoma. *Neuroimmunomodulation* 6: 237 (abstract).

Pavol, M., Meyers, C., Rexer, J., *et al.* 1995. Pattern of neurobehavioral deficits associated with interferon-alfa therapy for leukemia. *Neurology* 45: 947–950.

Prieto-Gomez, B., Reyes-Vazquez, C., and Dafny, N. 1983. Differential effects of interferon on ventromedial hypothalamus and dorsal hippocampus. *Journal of Neuroscience Research* 10: 273–278.

Rieger, P., and Weatherly, B. 1989. Can your nursing skills meet the challenge of a patient receiving IL-2? *Dimensions in Oncology Nursing* 3: 9.

Renault, P., Hoofnagle, J., Park, Y., *et al.* 1987.

Psychiatric complications of long-term interferon-alfa therapy. *Archives of Internal Medicine* 147: 1577–1580.

Rohatiner, A., Prior, P., Burton, A., *et al.* 1983. Central nervous system toxicity of interferon. *British Journal of Cancer* 47: 419–422.

Sachar, E. 1982. Endocrine abnormalities in depression. In Paykel, E. (ed). *Handbook of Affective Disorders*. New York: Guilford Press, pp. 191–201.

Sapolsky, R. 1985. A mechanism of glucocorticoid toxicity in the hippocampus: Increased neuronal vulnerability to metabolic insults. *Journal of Neuroscience* 5: 1228–1232.

Sapolsky, R., Pacan, D., and Vale, W. 1988. Glucocorticoid toxicity in the hippocampus: *In vitro* demonstration. *Brain Research* 453: 367–371.

Saris, S., Patronas, N., Rosenberg, S., *et al.* 1989. The effect of intravenous interleukin-2 on brain water content. *Journal of Neurosurgery* 71: 169–174.

Saris, S., Rosenberg, S., Friedman, R., *et al.* 1988. Penetration of recombinant interleukin-2 across the blood-cerebrospinal fluid barrier. *Journal of Neurosurgery* 69: 29–34.

Sarna, G., Figlin, R., Pertcheck, M., *et al.* 1989. Systemic administration of recombinant methionyl human interleukin-2 (Ala 125) to cancer patients: Clinical results. *Journal of Biological Response Modifiers* 8: 16–24.

Sherman, A., and Meyers, C. 2000. Pre-treatment cognitive performance predicts survival in patients with leptomeningeal disease. *Journal of the International Neuropsychological Society* [abstract] 6: 200.

Shibata, M., and Blatteis, C. 1991. Human recombinant tumor necrosis factor and interferon affect the activity of neurons in the organum vasculosum laminae terminalis. *Brain Research* 562: 323–326.

Smedley, H., Katrak, M., Sikora, K., *et al.* 1983. Neurological effects of recombinant human interferon. *British Medical Journal* 286: 262–264.

Sparber, A., and Biller-Sparber, K. 1993. Immunotherapy and neuropsychiatric toxicity. *Cancer
Nursing* 16: 188–192.

Squire, L. 1987. *Memory and Brain.* New York:
Oxford University Press.

Stein, B., and Sapolsky, R. 1988. Chemical adrena-
lectomy reduces hippocampal damage induced
by kainic acid. *Brain Research* 473: 175–180.

Strite, D., Valentine, A., and Meyers, C. 1997. Manic
episodes in two patients treated with interferon-
alpha. *Journal of Neuropsychiatry and Clinical
Neurosciences* 9: 273–276.

Strub, R., and Black, F. 1981. *Organic Brain Syndromes.* Philadelphia: F.A. Davis Company.

Suter, C., Westmoreland, B., Sharbrough, F., *et al.*
1984. Electroencephalographic abnormalities in
interferon encephalopathy: A preliminary report.
Mayo Clinic Proceedings 59: 847–850.

Talpaz, M., Kantarjian, H., McCredie, K., *et al.* 1986.
Hematologic remission and cytogenic improvement induced by recombinant human interferon-
alpha in chronic myelogenous leukemia. *New England Journal of Medicine* 314: 1065–1069.

Tracey, K., Lowry, S., Fahey, T., *et al.* 1987.
Cachectin/tumor necrosis factor induces lethal
shock and stress-hormone responses in the dog.
Surgical Gynecology and Obstetrics 164:
415–422.

Tsagarakis, S., Gillies, G., Rees, L., *et al.* 1989.
Interleukin-1 directly stimulates the release of

corticotropin-releasing factor from rat hypothalamus. *Neuroendocrinology* 9: 98–101.

Valentine, A., Meyers, C., Kling, M., *et al.* 1998.
Mood and cognitive side effects of interferon-
α therapy. *Seminars in Oncology* 25(suppl 1):
39–47.

Valentine, A., Meyers, C., and Talpaz, M. 1995.
Treatment of neurotoxic side effects of interferon-
α with naltrexone. *Cancer Investigation* 13:
561–566.

Villalobos, J., and Ferssiwi, A. 1987a. The differential ascending projections from the anterior,
central, and posterior regions of the lateral hypothalamic area: An autoradiographic study. *Neuroscience Letters* 81: 89–94.

Villalobos, J., and Ferssiwi, A. 1987b. The differential descending projections from the anterior, central, and posterior regions of the lateral
hypothalamic area: An autoradiographic study.
Neuroscience Letters 81: 95–99.

von der Maase, H., Geertsen, P., Thatcher, C., *et al.*
1991. Recombinant interleukin-2 in metastatic
renal cell carcinoma: A European multicentre
phase II study. *European Journal of Cancer* 27:
1583–1589.

Waage, A., and Espevik, T. 1988. Interleukin-1 potentiates the lethal effect of tumor necrosis factor
alpha/cachectin in mice. *Journal of Experimental
Medicine* 167: 1987–1992.

Clinical Pearls

Assessment

Baseline assessment of mental status
General behavior
Appearance
Ability to maintain a logical conversation
Ability to provide a concise and logical history
Ability to comprehend instructions
Evaluation for risk factors that may predispose to more severe mental status changes
Pre-existing neurobehavioral problems
History of depression
Psychosocial stressors
Medications that may affect mental status
Periodic assessment during course of therapy
Ability to continue activities of daily living
Assess for signs of slowed thinking, trouble with calculations
Obtain input from family members or significant others

Management Strategies

Determine need for safety measures
Design creative strategies to effectively cope with symptoms (e.g., making list for memory problems, use of calculators, adjustment of job responsibilities)
Determine need for medical management
Determine need for referral for complete neuropsychiatric evaluation

Patient Education

Review with patient prior to initiation of therapy potential for alteration in mental status
Teach reportable signs and symptoms
Inability to function in job, activities of daily living, or leisure activities
Excessive somnolence
Depression

Key References

Baile, W. 1996. Neuropsychiatric disorders in cancer patients. *Current Opinions in Oncology* 8(3): 182–187.

Bender, C., Monti, E., and Kerr, M. 1996. Potential mechanisms of interferon neurotoxicity. *Cancer Practice* 4(1): 35–39.

Depression Guidelines Panel. 1993. *Depression in primary care: Detection, diagnosis and treatment. Quick reference guide for clinicians, Number 5.* Rockville, MD: United States Department of Health and Human Services, Public Health Service, Agency for Health Care Policy and Research (AHCPR Publication No. 93-0552).

Lerner, D., Stoudemire, A., and Rosenstein, D. 1999. Neuropsychiatric toxicity associated with cytokine therapies. *Psychosomatics* 40(5): 428–435.

Lovejoy, N.C., Tabor, D., and Deloney, P. 2000. Cancer-related depression: Part II—Neurologic alterations and evolving approaches to psychopharmacology. *Oncology Nursing Forum* 27(5): 795–808.

Lovejoy, N.C., Tabor, D., Matteis, M., *et al.* 2000. Cancer-related depression: Part I—Neurologic alterations and cognitive-behavioral therapy. *Oncology Nursing Forum* 27(4): 667–678.

McDonald, M., Passik, S., Dugan, W., *et al.* 1999. Nurses' recognition of depression in their patients with cancer. *Oncology Nursing Forum* 26(3): 593–599.

Myers, C.A. 1999. Mood and cognitive disorders in patients receiving cytokine therapy. *Advances in Experimental Medicine and Biology* 461: 75–81.

Myers, C.A. 2000. Neurocognitive dysfunction in cancer patients. *Oncology* (Huntington) 14(1): 75–79.

Pirl, W., and Roth, A. 1999. Diagnosis and treatment of depression in cancer patients. *Oncology (Huntington)* 13(9): 1293–1301.

Sparber, A., and Biller-Sparber, K. 1993. Immunotherapy and neuropsychiatric toxicity. *Cancer Nursing* 16: 188–192.

Trask, P.C., Esper, P., Riba, M., *et al.* 2000. Psychiatric side effects of interferon therapy: Prevalence, proposed mechanisms, and future directions. *Journal of Clinical Oncology* 18(11): 2316–2326.

Valente, S., and Saunders, J. 1997. Diagnosis and treatment of major depression among people with cancer. *Cancer Nursing* 20(3): 168–177.

Valentine, A., Meyers, C., Kling, M., *et al.* 1998. Mood and cognitive side effects of interferon-α therapy. *Seminars in Oncology* 25(suppl 1): 39–47.

CHAPTER 20 | Patient Education

Kimberly A. Rumsey, RN, MSN, OCN®

Patient education is a vital component of the nurse's role in caring for patients who receive biotherapy. It can also be one of the most challenging and rewarding aspects of caring for these patients. Often, the education provided by nurses may prepare patients to receive therapy at home and thereby experience improved quality of life.

Patient education has been defined as "any set of planned, educational activities designed to improve the patient's health behaviors and/ or health status" (Hayward and Kahn, 1995; Lorig, 1996). The ultimate goal of patient education is to help patients and their family members to develop the necessary skills and knowledge for adaptation to the alterations in their health and life style.

In the past several years, there has been an increased emphasis on patient education. Pa-tients today desire information about their health and want to participate in their own care. In 1972, the American Hospital Association first published *A Patient's Bill of Rights* (American Hospital Association, 1992), which listed 12 rights of patients. According to this document, patient education is an integral component of the care a patient should expect from health care providers. Explicit in *A Patient's Bill of Rights* is the right to receive information about diagnosis, prognosis, treatment options, and side effects. Published more recently, *The Cancer Survivors' Bill of Rights* (American Cancer Society, 1995) provides cancer survivors the right to be informed about future problems with insurance coverage and employment. Many state and national agencies require that health care professionals provide patient education. The Joint Commission for the Accreditation of Healthcare Organizations (JCAHO) specifies that "patients receive nursing care based on a documented assessment of their needs," including biophysical, psychosocial, environmental, self-care, educational, and discharge needs (JCAHO, 1999). The Health Care Financing Administration (HCFA) also has specific requirements regarding the education of patients for institutions that participate in Medicare and Medicaid programs (HCFA, 1989). HCFA requirements are updated regularly in the Federal Register, a daily publication that is also available online (*http://www.access.gpo .gov/su_docs*). In addition to JCAHO and HCFA requirements, state nurse practice acts address the role of nursing in patient education, either directly or indirectly. In the *Standards of Oncology Education: Patient/Family and Public* (Oncology Nursing Society, 1995), the Oncology Nursing Society (ONS) states that nurses at the generalist and advanced practice levels are responsible for patient education related to cancer care. More recently, the Oncology Nursing Society published the Patients' Bill of Rights for Quality Cancer Care, which states that all individuals have a right to the availability of and access to education about cancer risks and life-style changes that influence the incidence of cancer, including educational activities that are effective and appropriate for diverse populations (Oncology Nursing Society, 1998). Besides being mandated by state and national organizations, patient education may benefit all who are involved, including patients and family members, health care providers and institutions, and society in general. Today's health care environment requires patients to gain the skills, knowledge, and self-confidence necessary to be able to manage their own disease (Lorig, 1996). Educated consumers are better able to participate in their own care and facilitate early discharge, thereby lowering health care costs.

Obviously, patient education should be a high priority for nurses in direct contact with patients. Although patient education is viewed as a role of the nurse, in reality, more technical or clinical skills often take priority (Faller and Lawrence, 1994). Kruger (1991) surveyed staff nurses, nurse administrators, and nurse educators for their attitudes regarding the role of patient educator and perceptions of personal ability to perform this role. Results indicated that all three groups valued the role of patient educator but did not feel they could perform it satisfactorily. Although some patient education is being successfully conducted, evidence suggests that it is inadequate (Kruger, 1991). Several trends in health care, including early discharge and an increase in the use of ambulatory care facilities and home care, provide new challenges for the nurse implementing the patient education process. One of the major obstacles is lack of preparation of the person assuming the role of patient educator (Close, 1988; Rabel, 1992).

Using the nursing process as a framework, this chapter will describe the process of educating biotherapy patients and their family members. For the purpose of this chapter, use of the term *patient* will also include family members and significant others.

The Process of Patient Education

The role of patient educator can be successfully implemented by the nurse. With planning, the proper tools, and practice, patient education can become a rewarding component of the role of the nurse in all care settings. Systematic patient education results in an increased incidence of adherence to medication regimen, longer persistence of behavior modification, decreased recovery time, and better utilization of health care resources (Hayward and Kahn, 1995). Additional benefits from systematic patient-education programs include decreased liability and improved recruitment and retention of patients (Hayward and Kahn, 1995). A partnership between nurses and patients is necessary for successful patient education. With communication, negotiation, and motivation, nurses and patients are able to work together to progress through the process of patient education. The nursing process provides a familiar and practical framework to follow for teaching patients (Close, 1988; Kaufman, 1989; Redman, 1997).

Assessment

Assessment is a key component in the patient education process and forms the basis for the patient teaching plan. The ability to assess patients' learning needs and styles assists the nurse in providing individual instruction, promoting effective use of resources, identifying specific information that is important to patients, and saving valuable time (Volker, 1991; Lorig, 1996).

The three most important sources of information when assessing the learning needs of patients receiving biotherapy are the patients themselves, the medical record, and other members of the health care team. Formal and informal interviews with patients and family members provide most of the needed information, but a written questionnaire may be helpful and time efficient for the nurse. The medical record provides basic information about health status, including previous learning needs and teaching already completed. Discussions with other members of the health care team enables nurses to expand and validate their assessments (Volker, 1991). Often, biotherapy patients have been in the health care system for a considerable length of time and have developed a wealth of knowledge about their disease and its treatment. Adequate learning needs assessment will identify areas that may need reinforcement, areas that require extensive teaching, and areas that need only review.

A comprehensive learning needs assessment includes assessment of the patient's ability, readiness, and willingness to learn, as well as areas of knowledge deficit.

ABILITY TO LEARN

Assessment of patients' physical and cognitive status provides information about their ability to learn. Patients should be assessed for physiologic barriers to learning, such as sensory impairment (visual, auditory) or impaired motor ability so that adjustments can be made in the teaching plan to overcome these barriers (Phillips, 1999). For example, a patient with visual disturbance may require written materials with large print and extensive verbal instructions. An assessment of the patient's ability to communicate verbally in English is also very important in planning teaching strategies. It may be necessary to schedule a translator in advance or present a non-English version of a video or written material. In addition, literacy level should be assessed. Nurses tend to use many printed materials as adjuncts to one-to-one teaching. A study of American Cancer Society (ACS) patient education literature showed that this material has an average reading level of grade 11.9 (Meade *et al.*, 1992), even though approximately 23 million adults in the United States read at or below a 5th grade level. Sarna and Ganley (1995) studied the readability and content of educational material developed specifically for patients with lung cancer and assessed the materials at a 10th-grade or higher reading level. It has been suggested (Meade, 1992; Sarna and Ganley, 1995; Maynard, 1999) that patient-education materials be developed at a 5th- or 6th-grade reading level to benefit more individuals. Many patients are hesitant to verbalize their difficulty in reading and may try to conceal it. In fact, several studies have found that a patient's reported grade level did not reflect his or her actual reading and comprehension abilities (Cooley *et al.*, 1995; Wilson,

1995). It is imperative that nurses be able to recognize the nonverbal cues to poor reading skills, including poor attention span, little or no interest in the topic, feelings of frustration, and slow reading speed. Patients also may be unable to answer questions regarding the content of the literature or may request that someone else read the literature (Meade *et al.*, 1992). Low literacy levels can sometimes indicate other limitations to learning such as poor organization of thoughts or impaired ability to learn and synthesize new information. Nurses must be careful not to stereotype patients because of low literacy, but to adapt their teaching strategies to meet patients' needs. Furthermore, nurses should always use simple vocabulary and lay terminology during their communications with patients (Redman, 1997).

The learning style of the patient should be assessed to ensure optimal use of teaching time and resources. Patient education is more successful when nurses respond to patients' individual learning styles (Villejo and Meyers, 1991; Phillips, 1999). Numerous learning style theories have been described in the literature, each based on several assumptions. First, each person has a predominant learning style that may be different from that of other people. Second, no one style is superior to another. Third, individuals may process information predominantly by one style, but may also use other styles. It is essential to know patients' preferences prior to initiating the teaching session. The nurse must assess how patients learn best, whether through visual stimuli (reading literature, viewing videos), auditory stimuli (listening to tapes, lectures), or tactile stimuli (handling equipment, return demonstration with critique). Most people prefer a combination of verbal and written stimuli (Hinds *et al.*, 1995) in their education. Information on learning style and patient preferences provides the rationale for the teaching activities and tools that are chosen for the educational endeavor.

To assess learning syle, nurses can simply ask patients how they best learn.

READINESS AND WILLINGNESS TO LEARN

Patients' readiness and willingness to learn are vital components of the learning needs assessment. Patients want health education for 3 reasons: to facilitate active participation in their health care, to prepare them for the future, and to decrease their anxiety (Hinds *et al.*, 1995). Several factors should be assessed that may influence patients' readiness and willingness to learn, including sociocultural background, emotional state, and patient/family goals. Patients should be questioned, in a sensitive manner, about their sociocultural background. Responses should be evaluated in light of current health status and life style (Redman, 1997). For example, a male patient from Saudi Arabia may respond negatively to instruction from female nurses. In this situation, having a male nurse do the teaching may provide a more successful educational session. Religious beliefs about treating illness should be considered. If patients' religious beliefs do not allow administration of blood products, nurses may need to emphasize other measures that can be implemented to ensure the safety of thrombocytopenic patients.

The goals of patients help to determine readiness and willingness to learn. For example, if a patient's goal is to be at home for a child's birthday, the nurse's educational sessions on self-injection of interferon would be well received. Nurses should recognize the goals verbalized by patients and assist them in setting realistic goals within the expectations of the health care system. Agreement on the goals by patients and the health care team should help ensure that they are met.

The emotional state of patients influences their ability, as well as their readiness and willingness, to learn and should be included in the learning needs assessment (Redman, 1997). Common emotions may have a detrimental effect on teaching and may require that sessions be delayed. A small amount of anxiety, for example, is normal and sometimes can increase patients' receptiveness to learning. Too much anxiety, however, can be overwhelming and decrease patients' ability, readiness, and willingness to learn.

KNOWLEDGE DEFICITS

A patient's learning deficits must be assessed during the learning needs assessment. It is vital to assess previous knowledge and experience that may affect current needs. For example, a mother who has been administering insulin subcutaneously to her child should be able to apply the concepts to giving herself subcutaneous interferon. By assessing her previous experience with injections, the nurse can then know to assess the patient's injection technique and to then teach and reinforce accordingly. It is also important to note topics that patients are most concerned about or interested in. If patients are nervous about actually administering the subcutaneous injection, the nurse may want to plan a demonstration/return demonstration of the injection technique before teaching reconstitution and drawing up the medication. Nurses must also consider specific skills needed by family members to adequately care for patients.

A comprehensive learning needs assessment will assist the nurse in formulating a teaching plan that can be agreed upon by all and that will optimally meet the needs of the patient within the constraints imposed by the health care system.

Planning

Once the comprehensive learning needs assessment is complete, the nurse should develop a plan for patient education. All providers have a responsibility to contribute to the care of the patient, including patient education. In addition, there is a need to standardize and organize patient education so that each patient receives essential information. A multidisciplinary teaching plan outlines expected outcomes for the patient, reduces duplication, and improves communication and collaboration among the multidisciplinary team (North et al., 1999). See Table 20.1 for the standardized teaching plan used for biotherapy patients at The University of Texas M. D. Anderson Cancer Center. The plan should be formulated in partnership with the patient and other members of the health care team. Components of the plan include goals and objectives of learning, material to be presented, and teaching strategies to be implemented.

GOALS

The initial step in developing the teaching plan is identifying the goals to be accomplished. Goals give the teaching session direction and act as a guide for evaluation at the completion of the session. For this reason, goals are sometimes referred to as expected outcomes or learning objectives. The goals should directly reflect the learning needs of the patient as determined by the assessment that was previously completed (Redman, 1997; Phillips, 1999).

There are five essential characteristics of an effective goal. First, the goal must be mutually acceptable. Patients should take part in the goal setting (Redman, 1997), or at least verbalize acceptance of the goal, to promote cooperation and compliance. The goal should also be realistic, specifying an outcome that can be accomplished. Sometimes it is helpful to set subgoals that will help move learners toward the overall goal while giving them a feeling of accomplishment. For example, the goal of teaching patients how to perform subcutaneous self-injection could be broken down into several smaller goals, such as reconstitution of medication,

Table 20.1 The University of Texas M. D. Anderson Cancer Center biotherapy patient teaching plan

Team Member	Objective/Expected Outcome	Content	Teaching Method

MD/Fellow/RN	I. Patients will be able to explain, in their own words, basic immune function, as evidenced by:
	• Expressing comprehension of their immune system, how it functions, and the role it plays in their treatment.
	Patients will be able to explain, in their own words, their treatment plan (including frequency of administration and duration) and its rationale, as evidenced by:
	• Expressing understanding of what type of treatment they will have, for how long, and why it is necessary.
		I. Immune Function
		Biotherapy
		A. Definition
		B. Goals of therapy
		  1. Diagnostic
		  2. Therapeutic
		  3. Supportive
		C. Commercial versus investigative use
		  1. Purpose of treatment
		  2. Informed consent
		D. Treatment regimen
		  1. Route of administration
		    a. frequency of administration
		    b. duration of therapy
		  2. Location
		    a. clinic
		    b. station 19
		    c. inpatient
		    d. hometown—referring MD
		  3. When
		    a. scheduled appointments
		    b. follow-up/evaluation
		E. Laboratory and diagnostic tests
		F. Special requirements (e.g., extended hospital admission or need to remain in vicinity for extended period of time)
			Individual instruction:
			• *Understanding the Immune System*, NCI booklet
			• *Biotherapy: A Patient Guide* (The University of Texas, M. D. Anderson Cancer Center)
			• Injection series videotapes (MDA-TV x27287):
			  IM #82-1-92
			  SC #80-1-92
			  Mixing Meds #81-1-92
			• *What are Clinical Trials all About?* NCI booklet
			• Treatment-specific patient information drug card(s)
			• Other applicable print material (refer to Patient Education Clearinghouse listing and Patient/Family Learning Center) and videotapes (refer to Patient Guide for Listings and Numbers)
			• Printed calendar
			• Question/answer period

MD/Fellow/RN

II. Patients will be able to identify potential side effects and appropriate self-management, as evidenced by:

- Verbalizing an understanding of [potential] side effects of their treatment.

II. Side Effects
A. Key areas
1. Incidence
2. Severity
3. Self-management
B. Potential side effects
1. Constitutional symptoms
   a. fever
   b. chills
   c. arthralgia
   d. malaise
   e. flushing
2. Neurological side effects
3. Renal toxicity
4. Hematologic side effects
5. Hepatic side effects
6. Dermatologic side effects
   a. erythema at injection site(s)
   b. itching
   c. rash
   d. dryness
   e. desquamation (dry or wet)
7. GI side effects*
   a. anorexia
   b. weight loss
   c. nausea/vomiting
   d. diarrhea
   e. mucositis
8. Cardiovascular/ pulmonary side effects, e.g., capillary leak syndrome
9. Allergic reactions

Individual instruction:
- Treatment-specific patient information drug card(s)
- Treatment specific videotapes (MDA-TV x27287):
  Introduction to Interferon #832-1-87
  Introduction to Interferon (Spanish) #956-1-90

- *Eating Hints*, NCI Booklet
- *Nausea & Vomiting: What You Can Do* (if applicable, i.e., treatment with IL-2)

- Other applicable print materials (refer to Patient Education Clearinghouse listing) and videos (refer to Patient Guide for listing and numbers)

(continued)

629

Table 20.1 *Continued*

Team Member	Objective/Expected Outcome	Content	Teaching Method
MD/Fellow/RN (cont.)	• Describing in their own words the appropriate management of those side effects.	IIa. Reporting of signs and symptoms A. Reportable signs and symptoms 1. Continuing fever of 40°C 2. Weight gain of 5–10 kg over 1 week 3. Weight loss of 5–10 kg over several weeks 4. Shortness of breath 5. Dizziness 6. Inability to perform ADL 2° fatigue 7. Alteration in mental status 8. Inflammation at injection site 9. Any other unusual signs/symptoms	
	• Identifying who to contact for reportable side effects.	B. Who to contact 1. MDACC a. Clinic staff b. RN/fellow/attending MD c. Station 19—after 5 P.M., weekends, holidays 2. Outside MDACC a. Local MD b. Local hospital	Clinic handout
RN/Pharmacist	III. Patients will be able to self-administer IM/SC injection, as evidenced by: • Accurate return demonstration of drug reconstitution.	III. Self Administration A. Types of equipment 1. Medication 2. Diluent 3. Alcohol swabs	Individual instruction Demonstration/return demonstration

630

Responsible	Objectives	Content Outline	Resources

	• Accurate return demonstration of technique for self-administration of IM/SC injection.
	• Describing in their own words the proper way to store and dispose of the medication and equipment.
		4. Syringes
		5. Needles
		B. Aseptic technique
		  1. Definition
		  2. Parts of equipment that may be handled
		C. Method of reconstitution
		D. Withdrawing liquid from the vial
		  1. Proper dose
		E. Site selection and rotation
		F. Injection techniques
		G. Storage of the medication
		  1. Stability of medication (single/multiple dose vial)
		H. Disposal of equipment at home
			Injection series videotapes (MDA-TV x27287):
			  IM #82-1-92
			  SC #80-1-92
			  Mixing Meds #81-1-92
			
			Patient information cards:
			• Subcutaneous injection
			• Intramuscular injection
			• Drawing up a liquid medication dose preparation instruction sheet

RN/Social Worker	IV. Patients will adjust to their altered life style and cope effectively with psychosocial issues related to their diagnosis and treatment, as evidenced by:
	• Identifying problem/issues in need of follow-up.
	• Identifying appropriate strategies and resources for coping with their diagnosis and/or treatment.
	• Seeking information and assistance.
	• Taking actions to promote coping (i.e., participating in discussion/support group)
		IV. Psychosocial issues
		A. Common problems
		  1. Depression
		  2. Hopelessness
		  3. Decisional conflict
		  4. Financial concerns
		  5. Housing
		  6. Transportation
		B. Support services
		  1. Social work
		  2. Discussion/support groups—hospital & community
		  3. Referrals
		C. How to access community resources
			One-on-one discussion
			
			Referral assistance
			
			Applicable print material (refer to Patient Education Clearinghouse Listing, Patient/Family Learning Center) and videos (refer to Patient Guide for listing and numbers)

(continued)

Table 20.1 *Continued*

Team Member	Objective/Expected Outcome	Content	Teaching Method

MD/Fellow/ RN/Pharmacist	V. Patients will be aware of reimbursement issues common to the biotherapy patient, as evidenced by:
	
	• Verbalizing an understanding of common problems related to reimbursement.
	
	• Having and referring to written material as needed.
	
	• Identifying available resources (educational, financial, etc.) as they relate to biotherapy patients.
		V. Reimbursement Issues
		A. Common problems
		  1. Investigative therapy
		  2. Off-label use
		  3. Cost of therapy
		  4. Lack of insurance coverage for self-administered medications
		B. Support services
		  1. Hospital pharmacy
		  2. Pharmaceutical company
		  3. Reimbursement programs
			One-on-one discussion
			
			Referral/assistance
			
			Applicable print material

*Dietary consult for nutritional problems.

Source: Adapted and reprinted with permission, The University of Texas M. D. Anderson Cancer Center, Department of Patient Education, Houston, Texas. ADL, activities of daily living; IM/SC, intramuscular/subcutaneous; MDACC, M. D. Anderson Cancer Center; MDA-TV, M. D. Anderson television.

drawing up the correct dosage, injection technique, and disposal of the equipment at home. An effective goal must also be measurable and patient centered. The goal should be written clearly in behavioral terms. Well-written goals begin with an action verb (e.g., state, discuss, demonstrate), are limited to one task, and specify a time frame in which the goal should be met. Teaching goals are best if they are written down in a formal document. Written goals help to communicate what is expected to patients and other health care professionals, especially if they are always documented in the same manner and kept in an agreed upon location. In summary, to produce the expected result, goals must be mutually agreed upon by all parties involved; be realistic, measurable, and patient centered; and be written in an identified, consistent location.

CONTENT

Using the information provided by the learning needs assessment, nurses can determine content areas to be included in the teaching plan. The content chosen should reflect the identified learning needs and meet the outlined goals or objectives. In the *Standards of Oncology Education: Patient/Family and Public* (Oncology Nursing Society, 1995), the ONS outlines the knowledge, skills, and attitudes related to the management of human responses to cancer that should be included in patient education. Adams (1991) provides an indepth discussion of the common educational needs of patients across the various phases of cancer care. In prioritizing content, nurses must balance what the patient needs to know with what they want to know. A content outline should be written, beginning with basic ideas and moving toward complex concepts. It is also important to determine which member of the health care team will be responsible for teaching the content. By writing down the content to be taught and indicating the responsible person, nurses can facilitate communication with the patient and other members of the health care team and ensure successful educational endeavors.

Topics to be discussed with patients who are receiving biotherapy include the treatment plan, side effects and management, and self-administration techniques (Rieger and Rumsey, 1992). When discussing the treatment plan, nurses should be sure to include information regarding the goal of the therapy (diagnostic, therapeutic, or supportive), details about the specific treatment protocol (including how, where, and when the agents are to be administered), laboratory and diagnostic tests that are necessary, and any other special requirements of the treatment regimen. Topics that must be covered when educating patients about potential side effects include incidence and severity, self-management, and reportable signs and symptoms. In addition, because many biological agents are given as long-term therapy, it may be necessary for patients to learn to self-administer the treatment.

TEACHING STRATEGIES

The final step in developing the teaching plan is to identify the method of teaching and the specific teaching aids that will be used. Through careful planning, nurses can choose appropriate teaching techniques and adjuncts that will improve the teaching session.

Principles of adult learning should be considered when selecting teaching strategies (Phillips, 1999). According to Knowles (1980), the approach used when teaching adults is so different from that used with children that a new term, **andragogy**, was developed to describe "the art and science of helping adults learn." He puts forth the following four principles that outline the concepts of andragogy:

1. Adults are independent and self-directed learners.
2. The past experiences of adults serve as a resource for learning.

3. Readiness to learn emerges from the need to cope with a developmental task or social role.
4. Adults need to see immediate benefits from learning.

The chosen teaching strategies should not only reflect the learning needs assessment, goals and objectives, and content to be presented, but also should be based on these principles of adult learning, while corresponding to the learning style of the patient or family member. If these factors are all considered when choosing teaching strategies, teaching effectiveness should be improved (Close, 1988).

Several methods are popular for teaching patients. Most patient teaching is done on a one-to-one basis. This provides nurses an opportunity for continuous assessment of the patient and for building a relationship; moreover, the nurse can adapt teaching to individual learning needs. Usually several teaching methods are employed to improve understanding. It is important to decide which content is to be taught via one-to-one teaching and which is to be taught in a group environment. Group teaching is appropriate for groups of patients with similar learning needs. Generally, basic concepts, such as aseptic technique or the technique for drawing up medication, are appropriate for group teaching. There are several advantages to group teaching. Many times, patients who share a common need will become supportive of and learn from each other. Teaching a group of patients will also save time for nurses. More individualized content, such as the exact dosage to draw up, is appropriate for one-to-one presentation with the learner.

Techniques that can be employed for either individuals or a group include lecture, demonstration/return demonstration, and role playing. Lecture, the traditional teaching strategy, is a formal method of teaching. Content that might be appropriate for this technique includes details of the treatment plan and specific goals of therapy. Although lecture is the most frequently used technique, it poses several disadvantages. A lecture is usually given in a classroom setting at a specific time each day. Patients must make adjustments in their schedule to be able to attend. Another drawback is that lecture is a passive form of learning. Because adult learners need to actively participate in their learning, lecture may be inappropriate. Lecture would also be unsuitable for patients who have difficulty understanding or are slow in processing the English language. If lecture is used, it may be helpful to use analogies to clarify or to illustrate a specific point. For example, the analogy of fertilizer on grass can be used to illustrate the effect of colony-stimulating factors on the hematopoietic stem cells. Demonstration/return demonstration can be extremely helpful when teaching a psychomotor skill such as self-injection. With this technique, nurses can demonstrate step-by-step, so that the patient can imitate exactly what the nurse does. Role playing can provide a nonthreatening environment for the patient to act out new behaviors. For example, the nurses may have patients act out a telephone call in which they are reporting signs and symptoms. This will enable the patient to understand what information to have on hand when calling the nurse or physician.

Teaching aids should be incorporated with each of these teaching strategies, because they increase the learner's interest and reinforce learning. Numerous resources are available to assist nurses in educating patients who are receiving biotherapy, including printed material, posters and flip charts, videos, physical models, and computer programs.

Printed material is routinely used for biotherapy patients. Printed materials are helpful for presenting background information and step-by-step procedures. Another advantage is that patients can read the material at their convenience and refer to it if a question arises.

When choosing printed materials, nurses must consider the data obtained in the learning needs assessment. All too often, patients who cannot read are expected to have mastered information provided only in the written material. The written material should be evaluated for literacy level. The more pictures in the printed material, the better patients will retain the information (Meade *et al.*, 1992). For agents approved by the Food and Drug Administration, a good source of written information is the pharmaceutical company that distributes the agent. The American Cancer Society (ACS) and the National Cancer Institute (NCI) have printed materials, some of which are free, for the biotherapy patient. Some major cancer centers have produced materials that are available for a nominal charge (Tables 20.2, 20.3, and 20.4). If an area has a large population of people who do not speak or read English, it may be necessary to translate materials into other languages. Many of the ACS and NCI booklets are already available in Spanish.

Audio-visual aids such as videos have become more widely accepted in the past few years. Videos allow the patient to learn at his

Table 20.2   Educational resources available from pharmaceutical companies

Amgen *www.amgen.com/*
  Books
    Analogy Book
  Pamphlets
    Chemotherapy and Neupogen®
    Neupogen® Reimbursement Guide for the Patient
    Questions and Answers about Therapy with Neupogen® (Filgrastim)
    Patient Guide to Therapy with Neupogen®
  Videos
    Self-Injection Video (English and Spanish)
    Patient Guide to Therapy with Neupogen®
  Other
    Calendar with Laboratory Data
    Neupogen® (Filgrastim) Patient Fact Sheet
    Pediatric Package (includes Sammy Syringe, Marvin's Marvelous Medicine, Your Body, and
      G-CSF pamphlet)
Chiron *www/chiron.com/*
  Videos
    Interleukin-2: Patient Management Strategies (videotape)
    Interleukin-2: Therapy: Information for Patients and Their Families (videotape and booklet)
Genentech BioOncology *www.biooncology.com*
  Audiotape program
    Cancer Survivor's Toolbox™: Building skills that work for you (program to help people with
      cancer and their families to develop skills that can help them meet the challenge of cancer).
      English and Spanish.
  Pamphlets
    Finding Your Way Series (educational series on breast cancer)
      Finding Your Way through the Breast Cancer Diagnostic Process
      Finding Your Way after Breast Cancer Diagnosis

(continued)

Table 20.2 *continued*

Finding Your Way through Metastatic Breast Cancer
Finding Your Way—Clinical Trials: You May Benefit from Joining a Scientific Study
Finding Your Way—Resource Guide: Reaching Out to Breast Cancer Resources
Learning about treatment with Herceptin® therapy
HER2 Protein Overexpression in Metastatic Breast Cancer
Patient-focused reimbursement services; Herceptin®
Stepping Stones Series: Your connection to information and supportive resources
  Living with Cancer
  Non-Hodgkin's Lymphoma: An Introductory Guide
  Making Choices
  Finding Information about NHL
  Showing that You Care
  Questions & Answers about Rituxan® (Rituximab)
Immunex *www.immunex.com/*
Monograph
  The Cells of the Hematopoietic Cascade
  Understanding Your Bone-Marrow Transplant: A Patient's Guide
Videos
  The Cells of the Hematopoietic Cascade
  A Patient's Guide to Self-Injection
  Understanding Your Bone-Marrow Transplant: A Videotape for Patients
Other
  Hematopoiesis Chart
  A Patient Guide to Self-Injection (instruction and site recording chart)
Ortho-Biotech *www.procrit.com*
Audio-cassettes
  Rhu Epo and the Anemia of Cancer and Chemotherapy: Two Sides of an Inpatient Story
  Understanding and Overcoming Fatigue
Books
  Rhu Epo and the Anemia of Cancer and Chemotherapy: Two Sides of an Inpatient Story
  Resource Catalog
Brochures
  Understanding and Overcoming Fatigue
Pamphlets
  Anemia in Cancer: Getting Your Energy Back
  Dimensions of Caring: Understanding and Overcoming Fatigue
Videotapes
  Coping with Fatigue
  Subcutaneous Injection: A Patient's Guide to Correct Injection Technique
Other
  Patient Diary
  Self-Injection Starter Kit
  Subcutaneous Injection: A Patient's Guide to Correct Injection Technique (flip chart)

Table 20.2 *continued*

Roche Laboratories *www.roche.com*
  Pamphlet
    Patient Guide
  Video
    Self-Administration
  Other
    Complete Home Administration Kit
    Medication Travel Cooler
Schering Plough *www.sp-research.com/*
              www.crossingbridges.com/
  Pamphlet
    Taking Control of Your Therapy
  Video
    Self-Injection
  Other
    Patient Information Card
    Patient Kit (home supplies plus brochures on self-administration)

or her convenience and again have the advantage of easy reference if questions should arise. In addition, videos can serve as a stimulus for group discussion, decrease patient anxiety, and improve communication with patients with low literacy levels (Meade, 1996). If a video is not available on a topic that is frequently taught, the nurse may consider producing an original one. Meade (1996) describes a systematic process to produce videos for cancer education and research. It is crucial that nurses remember to evaluate and reinforce information that is learned via video. Videos that cover information regarding specific agents, side effects and management, reimbursement, and injection technique are available from pharmaceutical companies and major cancer centers.

The cost of the videos and special equipment required to view them may be prohibitive for some health care agencies. In this instance, flip charts and posters may prove helpful. Flip charts can be useful when teaching step-by-step procedures such as injection technique. The patient who is learning to reconstitute and draw up the medication can follow along in the flip chart while practicing with the needle and syringe.

Physical models may also prove invaluable when teaching psychomotor skills such as self-injection. Traditionally, patients have practiced injection on oranges and rolled towels. These have served the purpose but are not very lifelike. There are models available that are lifelike and can be actually injected. Other models are available to help patients identify landmarks and choose a proper site for their injection (see Figures 20.1 and 20.2).

The usefulness of computers in today's health care environment is becoming more apparent. Computers can provide individualized information to help patients alter their behavior; help the health care worker assess, prioritize, and track patient needs; and facilitate thorough, accurate communication between the health care worker and patient (Williams *et al.*, 1995). Computer-based patient-education systems can be frequently updated and easily individualized to a patient's specific needs. In addition, the

Table 20.3   Educational resources available from NCI or ACS

National Cancer Institute
1-800-4-CANCER *(www.nci.nih.gov/)*
   Advanced Cancer: Living Each Day
   The Immune System: How It Works
   Managing Interleukin-2 Therapy
   Patient to Patient: Clinical Trials and You
   Taking Time: Support for the People with
      Cancer and the People Who Care About
      Them
   Understanding the Immune System
   What Are Clinical Trials About?
   When Cancer Recurs: Meeting the Challenge
      Again
American Cancer Society
Call your local ACS office *(www.cancer.org/)*
   Pamphlets
      Cancer: Your Job, Insurance, and the Law
      Definitions Book
      Finding New/Better Ways to Control
         Cancer—Getting Involved in Clinical
         Trials
   Videos
      Employment, Insurance, and Cancer Patients
      What Are Clinical Trials About?
   Slide Set
      Cancer: Your Job, Insurance and the Law

Table 20.4   Educational resources available from The University of Texas M. D. Anderson Cancer Center

M. D. Anderson Cancer Center
1-713-792-7128 *(www.mdanderson.org/)*
Biotherapy: A Patient Guide
Cards
• Administration of Subcutaneous Injection
• Disposal Tips for Home Health Care
• Erythropoietin
• Granulocyte Colony-Stimulating Factor
  (G-CSF)
• Human Leukocyte Interferon or
  Lymphoblastoid Interferon (Wellferon)
• Injection Packet
• Interferon
• Intramuscular Injection Instructions
• rGM-CSF (recombinant granulocyte-
  macrophage colony-stimulating factor)
Drug Sheets
• Interleukin-2
• Interleukin-3
• Interleukin-4
• Interleukin-11
• Monoclonal Antibodies (Diagnostic)
• Monoclonal Antibodies (Therapeutic)
• Tumor Necrosis Factor
Videos
• Administration of Intramuscular Injection
• Administration of Subcutaneous Injection
• Coping with Interferon
• Interferon
• Life's Journeys
• Reconstitution of Medication

computerized system provides access to a limitless inventory that would be impossible to store by conventional means (Hayward and Kahn, 1995). The Internet enables health care professionals and patients to obtain the most current information on a range of topics. A major point of concern regarding computer-based patient-education systems is the potential for hardware failure, which would cause instant loss of all information. Additional barriers for many hospitals and clinics include expense (initial costs and upgrades), finding adequate space for a workstation, and the time required to teach staff and patients how to use the new system.

Patient-education software can be classified as noninteractive or interactive. Noninteractive systems compile patient information sheets into an easily manipulable electronic collection that can be printed individually or in sets. They also can be customized, indexed, searched, and updated easily (Hayward and Kahn, 1995). Interactive systems require that the patient interact directly with the computer. With these systems, the computer presents information and

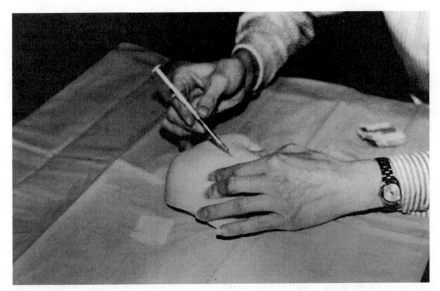

Figure 20.1   Injection model

Source: Reprinted with permission from Rieger, P., and Rumsey, K. 1992. Responding to the educational needs of patients receiving biotherapy. In Carroll-Johnson, R. (ed). *The Biotherapy of Cancer-V* (monograph). Pittsburgh, PA: Oncology Nursing Society and Roche Laboratories, pp. 10–15.

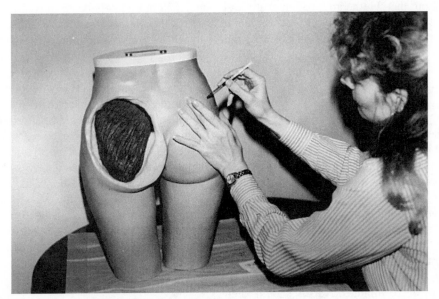

Figure 20.2   Injection model

Source: Reprinted with permission from Rieger, P., and Rumsey, K. 1992. Responding to the educational needs of patients receiving biotherapy. In Caroll-Johnson, R. (ed). *The Biotherapy of Cancer-V* (monograph). Pittsburgh, PA: Oncology Nursing Society and Roche Laboratories, pp. 10–15.

the patient is able to respond to that information. The computer records and responds to the patient's response, providing immediate feedback and additional information. The patient is in control of the educational process, determining the pace and pathway of teaching. He or she may choose to repeat information, seek more detailed information, or proceed.

Many individuals may find computers intimidating; however, patients of all ages, educational backgrounds, and socioeconomic statuses have been satisfied and welcome computer-assisted patient education as a teaching aid (Hayward and Kahn, 1995; Williams *et al.*, 1995). If planning to use computers as a teaching aid, nurses must assess the computer skills of the patient during the learning needs assessment. Even if patients are comfortable with computers, nurses should plan to spend some time orienting patients to the objectives and program.

Because of the amount and complexity of information that biotherapy patients are expected to learn, the nurse should incorporate a variety of teaching strategies and aids into the teaching plan. This will help to provide effective and efficient teaching sessions.

Implementation

Once the plan is complete, it may be implemented. During this stage, nurses must remain creative and flexible in order to accomplish their goals with the materials and time available. If planned well, the implementation should go smoothly.

A frequent obstacle to teaching is time. A definite time must be established with the patient for the teaching session. Most one-to-one teaching sessions are relatively short, usually lasting 10 or 20 minutes. Nurses should keep the patient's schedule and preferences in mind when scheduling teaching time. Some patients may prefer the time period after morning care. Those who do not have evening visitors may prefer that teaching be done during that time. Nurses should also consider when family members are available for sessions. Once the time has been mutually agreed upon, the nurse should make certain that other patient responsibilities will not interfere. Nurses may need to make arrangements so that the needs of other patients are taken care of during that time. One way to accomplish this is to trade time with another nurse. Another way to overcome the obstacle of time is to incorporate teaching into patient care. By explaining site-selection and injection technique while you are performing an injection, the nurse is actually teaching or reinforcing teaching that may have been accomplished with written materials or via video.

During the implementation of the teaching plan, the nurse should promote compliance and give feedback to the patient. If the teaching plan has been mutually agreed upon, compliance will more likely occur. It is also important to limit the amount of new knowledge presented at each session. If too much information is provided the patient may become overloaded and confused, which may lead to noncompliance. Keeping the patient actively involved during the implementation phase will also improve compliance. Patients should be apprised of their progress continually. Positive feedback will enhance self-esteem and motivate patients to continue in their educational endeavors. Any small success should be praised, and difficulties should be corrected gently. Nurses should be honest in their feedback and be aware of their nonverbal communication, as patients are able to judge genuineness.

Evaluation

Evaluation is the final component of the teaching process. Evaluation should be ongoing during the entire teaching process, not just when teaching is complete. Evaluation and documentation are the most frequently omitted steps in the process (Close, 1988). This component assists nurses in evaluating their ability and skill in teaching. It helps give the patients feedback on what they have already learned and may help to motivate them to learn more (Kaufman, 1989). Once the teaching session is over, many nurses consider teaching complete or plan to evaluate learning at a later time. Evaluation should occur at the time of teaching and reevaluation should be performed later as well. In today's climate of liability, accountability, and quality assurance, evaluation and documentation become crucial steps in the process.

Evaluation can be defined as the continuous and systematic review of the patient's progress during and after the teaching session. It not only determines whether the learner learned what was taught but also helps to determine whether the nurse's time was well spent (Kaufman, 1989).

Evaluation should relate back to the original goals that were written for the teaching plan. These goals can be used to judge the effectiveness of the teaching and clarify content and method for evaluation. For example, the patient should respond in a verbal manner if the goal required him or her "to state, verbalize, or describe" the goal of the treatment protocol. A return demonstration without coaching may be required for a psychomotor skill such as self-injection. After evaluating the patient's learning, the nurse might have to revise part or all of the teaching plan and begin again. Nurses should reconsider components of the learning needs assessment, teaching strategies, and aids that were used and barriers to teaching/learning and should make the appropriate changes to the plan.

Evaluation of patient teaching should be incorporated into each clinic or hospital visit.

Nurses should be ready to correct any misconceptions or bad habits that the patient may have developed. Patients who demonstrated successful self-injection 6 months ago may have forgotten the sterile technique or may have begun to take "short cuts" when reconstituting medication. It is imperative that nurses remember to periodically evaluate retention of and compliance with learned material.

Patient education is not complete until the teaching has been documented (Kaufman, 1989). As with the nursing process, "if it was not documented, it was not done." The JCAHO (1999) requires that nursing care data related to patient assessments, nursing diagnoses and/or patient needs, nursing interventions, and patient outcomes are permanently integrated into the medical record. Besides proving that the requirement for patient education from JCAHO and other accrediting agencies has been met, documentation serves several other purposes, including communicating teaching and progress to other members of the health care team and providing a legal record of the teaching that has been completed and the learner's response to the teaching.

Documentation of patient teaching should include several components. All of the learning needs that have been identified should be listed and prioritized with the target date for completion. It is important to indicate whether a family member was present during the teaching or whether the patient was the only one to receive the information. The resources used (such as a standardized teaching plan or standard of care) and teaching aids used (written materials, videos) should also be listed. The outcome of the teaching should be documented. Any unresolved goals must be documented and a follow-up plan should be identified. Nurses may also want to consider having the learner sign a statement saying that the goal was accomplished. A multidisciplinary documentation tool can be useful for communicating to members of the health care team (see Figure 20.3).

Future Directions

A relatively new trend in patient education is the development of patient-learning centers, which enable patients and family members free access to textbooks, lay literature, videos, audiocassettes, models, pamphlets, article files, computer programs, and Internet access. Staff and volunteers are available to help the patient locate information. Some centers may also provide support groups, classes and skills labs for learning necessary skills, cancer-prevention programs, and periodic cancer screenings. These resource centers provide medical information to patients and their families to facilitate informed decision making (Eddleman and Warren, 1994; Kantz et al., 1998). During these times of health care reform, it has become even more important that patients receive adequate and appropriate patient education to be able to care for themselves at home. As our population grows older and lives longer, health care professionals will encounter with greater frequency barriers to learning such as vision and auditory impairment, negative life experiences, and chronic diseases. Nurses in particular will have to improve their assessment and teaching skills (Mooney, 2000; Treacy and Mayer, 2000). As our methods of early detection and treatment of cancer continue to improve, the numbers of cancer patients and cancer survivors will increase. Health care professionals will need to consider the needs of this population and provide more information on survivorship issues. Nurses will have to become astute not only at knowing if patients are receiving accurate and appropriate information but also at detecting sensory overload (Close, 1988). The needs of the minority population will continue to grow. Members of the health care team will become more sensitive to their cultural differences and will find better ways of communicating with this population. More people will have problems with literacy. Teaching aids will need to become increasingly more visual and auditory. Research is needed on the use of teaching technologies, such as computer-based patient education and home video (Mooney, 2000), that will be implemented to meet the educational needs of the individual. The health care system will be different from what it is today. Changes in the system will influence the methods and content taught to patients and family members, as well as the time frame in which the teaching/learning is to be accomplished.

Nurses will have to examine their own values and attitudes about their role as patient educators over the next few years. They must demonstrate the value they place on education of the patient by advertising their role in patient education through publication in lay journals, prioritizing patient education over non-nursing activities, and implementing research on the economic, physiologic, social, and psychological benefits of patient education (Close, 1988). In these times of health care reform, nurses must be clear about and must publicize who they are and what they do that benefits the patient to ensure themselves an appropriate role in a new health care system.

As cancer care moves to the ambulatory-care setting and away from inpatient care, cancer patients and their family members are expected to assume tremendous responsibility for recovery, treatment, and follow-up care at home. Similarly, health care professionals face an enormous challenge if, during their brief contacts with patients and family members, they are to provide the understanding of treatment and the skills needed to implement the regimen at home (Mooney, 2000; Treacy and Mayer, 2000). The health care team must identify, agree upon, and implement the components of a comprehensive education program efficiently and

THE UNIVERSITY OF TEXAS
MD ANDERSON
CANCER CENTER

**INTERDISCIPLINARY PATIENT
TEACHING RECORD**

PATIENT IDENTIFICATION

DATE & INITIALS	INCLUDE: learning needs, teaching tools, comments, identity of learner and learner's signature (optional)	Content Area	Barriers to Teaching	Plan	Method	Outcomes	Resolved: Date & Initials

INITIALS	NAME & TITLE	INITIALS	NAME & TITLE	INITIALS	NAME & TITLE

TEAM MEMBERS: ☐ APN   ☐ Case Mgr   ☐ Chaplain   ☐ Diagnostic Imaging   ☐ LVN   ☐ MD   ☐ OT   ☐ PT   ☐ RD   ☐ RN
☐ RPh   ☐ RT   ☐ RTT   ☐ SP   ☐ SW   ☐ Translator   ☐ Other _____

CONTENT AREA

1. Illness/Disease
2. Diagnostic Procedures
3. Treatment Plan
4. Medications
5. Medical Equipment
6. Nutrition/Diet
7. Potential Food/Drug Interaction
8. Personal Hygiene
9. Rehabilitation Techniques
10. Available Community Resources
11. When/How to Obtain Further Treatment
12. Continuation of Care at Home or Health Care Facility
13. Other*

BARRIERS TO TEACHING

N = No
Yes, barriers exist, Indicate barrier:

A = Acuity of Illness	**F** = Financial Implication	**R** = Religion
C = Culture	**H** = Hearing	**S** = Sight
CL = Cognitive Limitations	**L** = Language	**O** = Other*
D = Desire and Motivation	**LI** = Literacy	
E = Emotional	**M** = Mobility	

PLAN

S = Standard
TP = Teaching Plan
CP = Clinical Path
O = Other*

METHOD

C = Class
E = Explanation
V = Video
P = Printed Material
D = Demonstration
O = Other*

OUTCOMES

AP = Applied Knowledge
V = Verbalized Understanding
D = Demonstrates Skills
N = No Evidence of Learning*
NP = Needs Practice*
NR = Needs Reinforcement*
O = Other*

*Requires Comments

INTERDISCIPLINARY PATIENT TEACHING RECORD - File under Allied Health   602091/5205 7/99

Figure 20.3   Teaching Record

Source: Reprinted with permission from The University of Texas M. D. Anderson Cancer Center.

effectively if patients and their families are to follow complex self-care regimens, manage pain and side effects, and cope with the emotional issues that often accompany the diagnosis and treatment of cancer. We are in the midst of an information revolution that will profoundly impact oncology practice (Ambinder, 2000). Oncology nurses will continue to be at the forefront as we assist our patients in understanding an ever expanding body of knowledge and how it impacts their care.

References

Adams, M. 1991. Information and education across the phases of cancer care. *Seminars in Oncology Nursing* 7(2): 105–111.

Ambinder, E.P. 2000. Oncology and the information age. In Bast, R., Kufe, D., Pollock, R., Weichselbaum, R., Holland, J., Frei, E. (eds). *Cancer Medicine*, 5th edn. Hamilton, Ontario: B.C. Decker Inc., pp. 2454–2468.

American Cancer Society. 1995. The *Cancer Survivor's Bill of Rights*. Atlanta, GA: American Cancer Society.

American Hospital Association. 1992. *A Patient's Bill of Rights*. Chicago, IL: American Hospital Association.

Close, A. 1988. Patient education: A literature review. *Journal of Advanced Nursing* 13(2): 203–213.

Cooley, M., Moriarty, H., Berger, M., *et al.* 1995. Patient literacy and the readability of written cancer educational materials. *Oncology Nursing Forum* 22(9): 1345–1351.

Eddleman, J., and Warren, C. 1994. Cancer resource center: A setting for patient empowerment. *Cancer Practice* 2(5): 371–378.

Faller, N., and Lawrence, K. 1994. Patient education: Patient willingness versus nursing skill. *Ostomy, Wound Management* 40(7): 32–34, 36, 38.

Hayward, R., and Kahn, G. 1995. Patient education. In Osherhoff, J. (ed). *Patients, Information, and Communication*. Philadelphia, PA: American College of Physicians, pp. 93–109.

Health Care Financing Administration (HCFA). 1989. Code of Federal Regulations, *Federal Register* 53(116): 22506–22513.

Hinds, C., Streater, A., and Mood, D. 1995. Functions and preferred methods of receiving information related to radiotherapy: Perceptions of patients with cancer. *Cancer Nursing* 18(5): 374–384.

Joint Commission on Accreditation of Healthcare Organizations (JCAHO). 1999. *Comprehensive Accreditation Manual for Hospitals*. Oakbrook Terrace, IL: Joint Commission.

Kants, B., Wandel, J., Fladger, A., *et al.* 1998. Developing patient and family education services: Innovations for the changing health care environment. *Journal of Nursing Administration* 28(2): 11–18.

Kaufman, M. 1989. ABC's of patient education. *Advancing Clinical Care* 4(3): 26–28.

Knowles, M. 1980. *The Modern Practice of Adult Education: From Pedagogy to Andragogy*. New York, NY: Cambridge, The Adult Co.

Kruger, S. 1991. The patient educator role in nursing. *Applied Nursing Research* 4(1): 19–24.

Lorig, K. 1996. *Patient Education: A Practical Approach*. Thousand Oaks, CA: Sage Publications.

Maynard, A.M. 1999. Preparing readable patient-education handouts. *Journal for Nurses in Staff Development* 15(1): 11–18.

Meade, C. 1996. Producing videotapes for cancer education: Methods and examples. *Oncology Nursing Forum* 19(1): 51–55.

Mooney, K.H. 2000. Oncology nursing education: Peril and opportunities in the new century. *Seminars in Oncology Nursing* 16(1): 25–34.

North, M., Harbin, C., and Clark, K. 1999. A patient-education MAP: An integrated, collaborative approach for rehabilitation. *Rehabilitation Nursing* 24(1): 13–18.

Oncology Nursing Society. 1998. *Patients' Bill of Rights for Quality Cancer Care*. Pittsburgh, PA: Oncology Nursing Press.

Oncology Nursing Society. 1995. *Standards of Oncology Education: Patient/Family and Public.* Pittsburgh, PA: Oncology Nursing Press.

Phillips, L.D. 1999. Patient education: Understanding the process to maximize time and outcomes. *Journal of Intravenous Nursing* 22(1): 19–35.

Redman, B.K. 1997. *The Practice of Patient Education.* St. Louis, MO: Mosby Yearbook.

Rieger, P.T., and Rumsey, K.A. 1992. Responding to the educational needs of patients receiving biotherapy. In Carroll-Johnson, R. (ed). *The Biotherapy of Cancer* (monograph). Pittsburgh, PA: Oncology Nursing Society and Roche Laboratories, pp. 10–15.

Sarna, L., and Ganley, B. 1995. A survey of lung-cancer patient-education materials. *Oncology Nursing Forum* 22(10): 1545–1550.

Treacy, J.T., and Mayer, D.K. 2000. Perspectives on cancer patient education. *Seminars in Oncology Nursing* 16(1): 47–56.

Villejo, L., and Meyers, C. 1991. Brain function, learning styles, and cancer-patient education. *Seminars in Oncology Nursing* 7(2): 97–104.

Volker, D. 1991. Needs assessment and resource identification. *Oncology Nursing Forum* 18(1): 119–123.

Wilson, F. 1995. Measuring patients' ability to read and comprehend: A first step in patient education. *Nursing Connections* 8(4): 17–25.

Williams, R., Boyles, M., and Johnson, R. 1995. Patient use of a computer for prevention in primary-care practice. *Patient Education and Counseling* 25(3): 283–292.

Key Resources

American Cancer Society
http://www.cancer.org

American Society of Clinical Oncology
http://www.asco.org

Cancer Care, Inc.
http://cancercare.org

Cancereducation.com
http://www.cancereducation.com

Cancer Facts
http://www.cancerfacts.com

Cancer Information Network
http://www.cancernetwork.com

Cancer News on the Net
http://cancernews.com

CancerSource.Com
http://cancersource.com

Cancer Survivors Toolkit
http://www.cansearch.org/programs/toolbox

John Hopkins Cancer Center
http://www.hopkinscancercenter.org

Dr. Koop's Web Site
http://www.drkoop.com

MEDLINE*plus*
http://medlineplus.gov/

Memorial Sloan Kettering Cancer Center
http://www.mskcc.org

National Cancer Institute
http://www.nci.nih.gov/

Oncology Nursing Society—Patient Information and Education Resource (PIER)
http://www.ons.org

Patient Advocacy Foundation
http://www.patientadvocate.org/

Roswell Park Cancer Institute
http://www.roswellpark.org

University of Pennsylvania
http://www.oncolink.upenn.edu

The University of Texas M.D. Anderson Cancer Center
http://www.mdanderson.org

CHAPTER 21

The Role of Disease Management in Reimbursement for Biotherapy

Alma Yvette DeJesus, RN, MSN, AOCN®

In the last decade, tremendous progress has been made in the development and use of biotherapy as treatment for cancer. Recent advances in molecular biology and genetic engineering have been instrumental in facilitating the identification, formulation, and availability of biological agents for both investigational and therapeutic usage. In the past, health services were provided without significant concern about the costs involved. In today's world of shrinking resources and cost-containment, the health-care professional must try to balance these restraints against the continuing evolution of innovative therapies and technology, such as biotherapy, that are often considered costly.

The author wishes to thank and acknowledge Mary McCabe, whose work from the first edition of *Biotherapy: A Comprehensive Overview* served as the foundation for this chapter.

Reimbursement has been challenging when using biotherapy agents for several reasons. At first, when biotherapy agents were being evaluated in clinical research trials for efficacy in the treatment of or as supportive therapy for cancer, there were many third-party payers who would not support any treatment that was part of research efforts. Once research supported the efficacy of using biological agents and regulatory approval was received, denial of reimbursement related to use in a clinical trial became less problematic.

The vast majority of biotherapy is administered in the outpatient setting. Therefore, how much the patient's insurance will pay for therapy often depends on whether the policy covers prescription or self-administered drugs. For example, the exclusion by Medicare of prescription drugs necessitates that patients on this program receive biological agents such as

647

hematopoietic growth factors in the physician's office. At the other extreme, health maintenance organizations (HMOs) may mandate that patients self-administer biological agents, even though they may not reimburse for patient education. The challenge of obtaining insurance coverage for biotherapy represents one of numerous obstacles in providing and identifying new cancer treatments and ensuring quality patient care.

Disease management is a systematic approach to patient care in which coordination of medical services is extended across the entire health-care delivery system (Harris, 1996). Health-care systems have utilized disease-management concepts for many years; however, in recent years, there has been a shift in focus. Traditionally, health-care systems focused on discrete episodes of care. The current focus is on providing high-quality care across a continuum, considering all phases rather than specific episodes. Increased use of biotherapy has presented the opportunity to develop new disease-management strategies for improving patient outcomes, health-care delivery, practice patterns, and resource utilization that incorporate the expanding armamentarium of biological agents. Applying a disease-management approach when using biotherapy to treat patients with cancer represents innovative evidence-based medicine. Biotherapy can be integrated into clinical pathways—considered one of several disease-management tools—to provide quality oncology care and as a strategy for managing costs.

In this chapter, reimbursement issues related to cancer care using biotherapy are thoroughly reviewed. Disease management and how it may be used as a tool to integrate biotherapy into the delivery of cancer care also is discussed. There are many challenges today with the changing health-care system, and those challenges often seem even greater when dealing with a life-threatening disease such as cancer.

The oncology nurse has the opportunity to advocate on behalf of the patient when decisions concerning provision of cancer care in a managed-care environment are made and, through political activism, to impact health-care financing at the state and national levels.

The Impact of Health-Care Financing on Biotherapy

Since the mid-1980s, when interferon (IFN)-α gained Food and Drug Administration (FDA) approval, researchers and oncologists have recognized the safety and efficacy of biological agents in treating cancer and other diseases. Many biological agents, such as erythropoietin, granulocyte colony-stimulating factor (G-CSF), granulocyte-macrophage colony-stimulating factor (GM-CSF), and interleukin (IL)-2, received regulatory approval in the 1990s and are considered important drugs for use in the management of cancer. Biological agents are now available for a variety of clinical indications (see Table 1.6, Chapter 1). In addition, many promisingnew biological agents— including multiple ILs, stem-cell factor, antisense compounds, and retinoids—are currently under investigation.

Along with advances in biotherapy are many economic and socioeconomic issues regarding the high cost of health care. The nation's total spending for health care is projected to increase from $1.0 trillion in 1996 to $2.1 trillion in 2007, which represents an average annual increase of 6.8%. It has been estimated that cancer will become one of the top five diseases with respect to treatment cost. The total cost of cancer care in the United States today is estimated at $107 billion, which includes $37 billion in direct medical costs, $11 billion in productivity loss, and $59 billion in mortality cost (American Cancer Society, 2000). Treatment of breast, lung, and prostate cancers accounts for more than half of the direct medical costs. At the start of the 20th century, cancer was the eighth-leading cause of death in this country; today, unfortunately, it is the second. An estimated 1,220,100 new cases of cancer will be diagnosed in the year 2000 (American Cancer Society, 2000).

Recent developments and increased use of biotherapy as a major component of cancer therapy have had a significant impact on health-care expenditures. In fact, a portion of the $37 billion in direct medical costs represents treatment with biological agents and the technology employed to produce them. To provide quality patient care in a cost-conscious environment, the health-care team is discovering that it must be knowledgeable about the financial impact of cancer care, including costs associated with biotherapy and how to most effectively integrate its use into the clinical management of patients. A new approach used increasingly to assist these efforts is disease-management programs, which guide the health-care team in focusing on quality care, while simultaneously considering resource consumption.

Reimbursement Issues

Daily reports in both the lay press and professional journals outline the financial challenges that the health-care industry faces as it attempts to stabilize expenditures. The health-care system has been operating at a growth rate higher than that of any other industry; costs have simply risen beyond the sustainability of a social and political system. Employers, third-party payers, and governments have all initiated attempts to control the dollars used for provision of health-care services (Porter-O'Grady, 1998). Economic considerations have become an integral part of legislative proposals regarding health-care planning, clinical research, and patient care. Initial comprehensive efforts at ap-

propriate resource consumption began with the federal government's introduction of the Medicare prospective payment system (PPS), which categorizes patient admissions into diagnostic-related groups (DRG). "Like-type" patients were placed into groupings that would determine hospital reimbursement. The industry quickly moved from a fee-for-service reimbursement system to one of fixed-sum reimbursement. Suddenly, there were limits placed on reimbursement for each service provided. For the first time, both the health-care system and providers had to learn to control expenditures. Although the DRG system was first mandated for Medicare, it was ultimately adopted by many states for the Medicaid program as well.

In the 1980s, managed-care organizations (MCOs) began to emerge. Market forces began to prevail, with extremely competitive insurance rates being negotiated between payers and providers. In the managed-care system, the provider is a gatekeeper, or manager, of the client's health. It was hoped that this philosophy would encourage a "wellness" orientation to health care versus the current "illness" orientation. The managed-care company or the provider assumes some degree of financial responsibility for the care that is given. In capitated contracts, the provider or system is paid a set amount of money per patient life to provide care for the patient; this can also be related to specialty practices such as oncology care. Physician practices began to see a decrease in income, either through negotiated discount rates or capitated risks contracts (Pulcini and Mahoney, 1998). In markets with a heavy penetration of managed care, such as California, an increasing trend has been toward capitated contracts. Many practices have begun to experience financial difficulties, or even bankruptcy, especially when high-cost oncology drugs are included within the capitated rate.

These efforts resulted in an increasing shift

of care to the ambulatory setting. A significant amount of cancer care is now given in ambulatory practice settings such as university- or community-hospital–based centers, HMOs, physician group or private practices, federal health systems, and freestanding centers. In 1998, the Health Care Financing Administration (HCFA) released a proposed rule for ambulatory payment classifications (APCs) in an attempt to develop a PPS for the hospital outpatient setting. (This regulation does not affect inpatient care or services delivered in the physician office setting.) When the proposed rules were released, concern spread throughout the cancer community because the HCFA had suggested that chemotherapy drugs be placed in one of four categories, ranging in reimbursement from approximately $50 to slightly more than $200. Analysis by the Association of Community Cancer Centers (ACCC) and the Lewin Group, an independent research firm, indicated that the losses of such a proposal would have been profound and may have caused cancer service lines to be shut down. Moreover, the proposal did not include any reimbursement for supportive-care drugs, a category in which hematopoietic growth factors were included.

During the commentary period, the oncology community deluged the HCFA and Congress with letters and calls protesting the proposed rule. In 1999, the Omnibus Budget Reconciliation Act was signed by President Clinton that, in part, addressed APCs. Instead of four categories for all drugs, the bill instructs HCFA to pay for drugs at either the APC or 95% of the average wholesale price, whichever is higher. The bill also mandated that HCFA update APCs annually to ensure their cost relevance and accuracy. HCFA released the final rule in April 2000; it was available on the HCFA web site (*http:// www.HCFA.gov/regs/hopps/default.htm*) and was also published in the *Federal Register* on April 7, 2000. Comments on the final ruling were due by June 6, 2000. As this book goes

to press, the Secretary of the Department of Health and Human Services and the Administrator of the HCFA made announcements encouraging Medicare intermediaries to reimburse hospitals and physicians treating Medicare patients according to a drug pricing survey conducted by the Department of Justice (DOJ). The HCFA "hopes" to encourage this change by October 1, 2000. The DOJ survey includes 16 commonly used chemotherapy and supportive drugs. Analysis of reimbursement at this level by the ACCC indicates significant underreimbursement to providers of cancer care, generating significant losses. Once again, the oncology community has deluged Congress and the HCFA with letters and calls. As of July 2000, the issue remained unresolved (*http:// www.assoc-cancer-ctr.org*). The oncology community will continue to monitor APCs as they become integrated in the reimbursement system for oncology care.

The economic focus of clinical decision-making now plays a role in all aspects of health care, including recommending an appropriate level of care based on the care setting, providing clinical justification for the care being rendered, and determining whether the recommended intervention is considered evidence-based practice. These issues are equally important with regard to the use of biological agents in oncology care.

There are several reasons why reimbursement strongly affects the use of cancer therapies. First, biotherapy often involves an agent that is investigational or that may be combined with another technology, such as bone-marrow transplant in solid tumors. Insurance policies govern reimbursement; therefore, if the selected therapy is investigational, the cost burden may be transferred to the patient, who then may have to pass up what could be a successful treatment option. This creates a cost burden on patients and the fear of not being able to receive treatment for their cancer. Second, some standard oncology practices involve the use of approved drugs in treatment regimens or patient populations not specified on the FDA-approved drug label. Third, biotherapy is relatively costly. These three issues represent the primary reimbursement challenges for clinicians and patients seeking the treatment opportunities offered by biological agents and other investigational cancer therapies.

Effects of Reimbursement on Clinical Trials

Cancer is a serious, life-threatening disease for which therapy is not always curative and is sometimes toxic. As research continues to explore new methods of treating this life-threatening disease, there is increasing emphasis on providing quality patient care throughout the continuum and maintaining quality of life for patients. Therefore, clinical investigation is an important element of cancer care, and investigational therapy represents a measurable process for patients for whom no standard therapy is applicable. Many biological agents are still investigational or, once approved, remain under investigation in combination with other agents or for additional indications. Investigational protocols offer patients access to the newest therapy in the confines of scientific evaluation.

By definition, a drug or biological agent is listed as investigational when the FDA has not approved the drug in any form for use in medical treatment. The evaluation of such agents must be conducted as a formal, peer-reviewed clinical trial. The distinction between scientifically valid clinical research and the nonevidence-based, nonresearch use of investigational therapy is an important one. It is vital that the patient understands the treatment and treatment outcome when an agent is used for a nonapproved indication outside the confines of a clinical trial. Furthermore, such use adds no scientific or valid knowledge to the identifica-

tion and evaluation of new cancer therapies. It ultimately does not contribute to achieving overall quality patient care.

In a clinical trial of an investigational cancer agent, knowledge is accumulated in a step-wise fashion in which the continued evaluation is dependent on specific results or assumptions. The scientific process can be seen as a twofold event: induction (learning from experience) and deduction (confirming what is learned) (Sheiner, 1997). Clinical trials are conducted in three distinct phases. In a phase I study, the goal is to identify the maximum safe dose of the new agent. In a phase II study, the efficacy of the drug is evaluated using outcome measures, such as tumor response. In phase III studies, a randomized comparison of the investigational and standard treatments is done. The results from a phase III study provide scientific evidence that the new therapy is better than the already existing best-known therapy. Once these studies are completed, additional clinical trials and FDA approvals may follow.

Despite the fact that cancer treatment given in the context of a scientifically valid, peer-reviewed clinical trial represents care, many insurers are reluctant to cover such therapy. In fact, investigational therapies are likely to be specifically excluded from the contract language in an insurance policy. GM-CSF, G-CSF, and IL-2, for example, could never have been evaluated in clinical trials without insurance support to cover the treatment costs. The reason for this was related to the high costs of investigational therapies without having an understanding of the outcomes of the care following the treatment. The National Cancer Institute (NCI) and other professional oncology organizations (i.e., National Coalition of Cancer Research, Oncology Nursing Society [ONS], American Society of Clinical Oncology) are supportive of legislation that encourages insurance companies and government-sponsored health-care plans to provide benefits that cover clinical-trial participation. Caregivers (e.g., physicians and nurses) can encourage insurance companies to reimburse for treatment costs incurred during clinical trials by providing evidence-based literature describing the treatment plan. This material can be reviewed by the company's medical director, who decides whether to cover treatment costs; this information is usually provided in a "Letter of Medical Necessity."

The technological explosion that occurred in medicine in the last 10 years, which enabled clinicians to incorporate biotherapy as a major component of cancer therapy, would not have occurred without the benefit of the clinical-trial process. Recently, the American Society of Clinical Oncology, which represents 14,000 cancer specialists, requested that insurance companies nationwide follow suit with those in New Jersey, where patients are reimbursed for the cost of participating in cancer clinical trials (Pear, 1999). If insurance companies in other states adopt this policy, access to new, promising, and otherwise unavailable therapies would be enhanced. Some federal organizations have followed the lead of the New Jersey insurance companies. The NCI has addressed the issue of reimbursement by negotiating agreements in principle and practice with agencies such as Medicare and the American Association of Health Plans. The agreement is to cover the cost of patient care provided through clinical trials sponsored by the National Institutes of Health. If these efforts continue, reimbursement challenges will decrease. As of June 2000 in the 106th Congress, several bills that would mandate coverage for clinical trials in both government and private insurance plans remained under discussion. On June 7, 2000, President William Clinton issued an executive order from the White House announcing that Medicare would pay for patient care and treatment costs for patients enrolled in clinical trials. This landmark measure was hailed as a significant step in ensuring the highest quality of care and treatment for American seniors.

State legislation that mandates coverage of patient-care costs for specific cancer clinical trials has been introduced and passed in Maryland, Rhode Island, and Georgia, and is under consideration in several other states (National Cancer Institute, 1998). At the federal level, a similar mandate was proposed as part of the Patient's Bill of Rights Act of 1998 (Patient's Bill of Rights, 1998). As of July 2000, each house of Congress passed a patient's bill of rights. These two bills were in conference committee to formulate a single piece of legislation that would then be sent back to each house for consideration.

The obstacles impeding reimbursement for investigational therapy or for drugs used for off-label indications have the potential to significantly influence the amount of clinical cancer research and care that is delivered. Historically, a coalition of payers has supported the research and the patient-care components of clinical trials (Friedman and McCabe, 1992), including the federal government, the pharmaceutical industry, third-party insurers, and private institutions such as universities. The coalition has been changing for a number of years as agencies and institutions struggle to limit health-care expenditures. Payer groups today, for example, are more open to granting reimbursement for care given through clinical trials when a "Letter of Medical Necessity" is provided for their review. This increase in support will contribute to the future of cancer research, which is an essential and well-established health-care priority.

The health-care team is encouraged to become fully knowledgeable about the clinical, financial, and patient outcomes of investigational treatments such as biotherapy so it can lend support in addressing reimbursement issues. Refusal to reimburse for peer-reviewed, scientifically valid clinical trials, such as those sponsored by the NCI, limits the research that can be done, thereby slowing the development of new therapies (Pear, 1993). Investigators at the University of Chicago documented the incidences in which reimbursement issues caused delayed completion or early closure of studies of biological agents such as IL-2 (Vogelzang and Richards, 1989).

Reimbursement restrictions also have the potential to impact how medical research is conducted. The reimbursement structure for clinical research varies with each sponsor. The costs of conducting clinical research are categorized as direct and indirect. It is important to be able to distinguish the costs of care involved with clinical research compared to standard care. Several studies recently demonstrated that clinical-trial costs may be less than standard-care costs. At the May 2000 meeting of the American Society of Clinical Oncology, findings from two studies revealed that the cost of treating patients enrolled in clinical trials may be less than the cost of treating similar patients who receive standard care. A multicenter pilot study conducted by the American Association of Cancer Institutes (AACI) and a single-center study conducted at Memorial Sloan-Kettering Cancer Center found numerical but not statistically significant savings. The AACI study entitled "A Multicenter Study of the Costs of Enrolling Cancer Patients on Phase II Clinical Trials" involved 35 protocol patients who were matched for age, gender, tumor type, stage, and treatment period with an equal number of controls. Data on charges were collected for 6 months following enrollment. Comparison of total charges for the two cohorts indicated a savings of almost 11% for the trial group (i.e., $57,524 compared with $63,721). The Memorial Sloan-Kettering study was entitled "Clinical Trial Costs Are Similar to and May Be Less than Standard Care and Inpatient Charges at an Academic Center and Are Similar to Major, Minor, and Non-Teaching Hospitals." The study evaluated 77 patients enrolled in phase II or III clinical trials who were matched with 77 similar patients undergoing standard care. All were Medicare-eligible patients and had primary tumors of the colon, rectum, prostate,

lung, breast, cervix, or ovary. Using a New York State database of health-care charges, the investigators found that 6 months of combined inpatient and outpatient care cost $6,280 (17%) less for the trial population than for the patients receiving standard care. The cost difference was statistically significant only in association with lung cancer because a greater part of treatment was provided on an outpatient basis. Similar studies conducted at the Mayo Clinic and elsewhere during the last 10 years have generally concluded that the treatment of patients in clinical trials is only 5% to 10% more costly than standard care, which is not statistically significant (ACCC website, accessed June 1, 2000).

Disease-management tools such as practice guidelines and clinical pathways outline the plan of care and the associated costs to treat a certain cancer, which enables the institution to measure outcomes and manage the cost to deliver care. One way to encourage insurance companies to reimburse patients for the costs of participating in clinical research is to incorporate cost-effectiveness and cost-benefit analyses in the trial design. If these issues are identified prior to beginning the research protocol, decisions can be made to determine additional funds that are needed to conduct it. Understanding the costs of care allows the health-care team to become more sensitive to the costs of hospitalization, treatments, and medications. This, in turn, may allow the health-care team to manage, as well as determine, other options to conduct research in a cost-conscious manner.

Insurance Coverage of "Off-Label" Use of Approved Drugs

Continuous efforts to improve cancer care have led to off-label use of some drugs. "Off-label" refers to the use of a drug in ways not indicated on the FDA-approved drug label. Amendments to the Federal Food, Drug and Cosmetics Act passed in 1962 charged the FDA with evaluating the effectiveness and safety of all new drugs, but did not grant the FDA the authority to restrict a physician's use of an oncology drug once it has been approved. The *FDA Drug Bulletin* of April 1982 states, "The FDA Act does not limit the manner in which a physician may use an approved drug. Once a product has been approved for marketing, a physician may prescribe it for use in treatment regimens or patient populations that are not specified on approved labeling" (FDA, 1982). This publication also stated that off-label use of a drug might be appropriate and rational in certain circumstances, for example, the application of a drug therapy that has been extensively reported in the medical literature.

Medicare guidelines permit wider therapeutic use of oncology drugs than that indicated on approved labeling, provided the therapy is "medically reasonable and necessary" (U.S. Department of Health and Human Services, 1987). It is difficult to measure "medically reasonable and necessary"; however, this value might be quantifiable with tools such as practice guidelines, clinical pathways, and outcome measures. Using disease-management tools "medically reasonable and necessary" could have quantifiable measures, which should focus on outcomes such as tumor response, quality of life, patient satisfaction, and appropriate resource consumption. This information should be collected about all biological agents in any health-care setting. The goal is to confirm the benefits of biotherapy as a cancer treatment.

The ACCC first documented the extent to which off-label use of oncology drugs constitutes standard care in clinical oncology in 1988. In a national survey of oncologists, the ACCC determined that 46% of chemotherapy drugs are used in off-label treatment (Mortenson, 1988). The survey demonstrated that a majority of cancer treatments are established after the initial

marketing of the specific agents (Moertel, 1991).

A random survey of oncologists who were members of the American Society of Clinical Oncology found that off-label drug usage was widespread (U.S. General Accounting Office, 1991). One third (33.2%) of the more than 5,000 documented administrations of cancer drugs were for off-label indications. More significantly, for more than half (56.0%) of the patients treated, at least one drug in their treatment regimen was prescribed for off-label use. In general, the rate of off-label use reported in the study was higher in those cases in which there was no agreement on the best therapy. In addition, the rate of off-label drug use as palliative treatment was almost twice that of off-label drug use with curative intent. In the treatment of colorectal cancer, more than 50% of patients were treated with at least one drug off-label. In the treatment of lung cancer, all patients were treated with at least one drug off-label (U.S. General Accounting Office, 1991).

In an effort to curb rising health-care costs, insurance companies are increasingly restrictive in granting coverage for off-label use of oncology drugs because they consider this inappropriate without scientific support for efficacy. Until the U.S. General Accounting Office (GAO) survey was undertaken, however, only anecdotal reports of such limited coverage of off-label use existed. The GAO study was able to assess the extent of reimbursement denials and the effect of those denials on the treatment of cancer patients. Approximately half of the respondents reported that a third-party payer had denied reimbursement for the cost of a drug when it was used for an off-label indication. Three of four oncologists who reported reimbursement denials for off-label use of a drug stated that the rate of denials had increased in recent years. Study results also showed that the policies of third-party payers resulted in 8% to 11% of oncologists altering their preferred course of treatment for difficult-to-treat diseases such as metastatic colon cancer, non-small-cell lung cancer, and malignant melanoma (Laetz and Silberman, 1991).

IFN-α, which was approved by the FDA in 1986 for use in treating hairy-cell leukemia and AIDS-related Kaposi's sarcoma, was the biological agent that brought attention to insurance companies' denials to cover off-label drug use. This occurred because IFN is expensive, because it is often administered by the patient or in an outpatient setting, and because insurers were initially reluctant to accept data supporting off-label indications (Huber, 1988). As more biological agents received regulatory approval, denial of payment for off-label use became less problematic. The value of some biological agents, such as the CSFs, has been quantified because they provide outcomes such as decreases in the use of antibiotics related to neutropenic fever, the duration of neutropenia following chemotherapy, and the length of hospital stay due to infection. Practice guidelines developed by the National Comprehensive Cancer Network, the American Society of Clinical Oncology, and other well-known organizations indicate when CSFs are clinically indicated (see related discussion in Chapter 7). Evidence-based literature was used in developing these practice guidelines to ensure that appropriate indications were identified. Evidence-based medical practice is another essential component of disease management. If the health-care system continues to improve and report collectively on patient outcomes associated with the delivery of care, reimbursement challenges should decrease because payers will have a better understanding of the outcomes they are financially supporting. Many states have attempted to pass legislation that requires insurers to reimburse for new uses of drugs that are listed in three major drug reference books; more than a dozen states have been successful.

Reimbursement in the Setting of Managed Care

The use of biotherapy in cancer care is often perceived as costly, although studies are beginning to evaluate the cost-effectiveness of some biological agents, such as epoetin-alfa versus standard care (e.g., the use of transfusions) (Meadowcroft *et al.*, 1998). The majority of oncology care provided today is within the framework of some type of cost-containment system; therefore, a discussion of managed care and how it relates to reimbursement for patients receiving biotherapy is important. Managed care has many economic and policy implications for individuals receiving oncology care. Under managed care, the financing and delivery of health care is integrated through contractual relationships among purchasers, insurers, and providers. Common features of managed-care systems are provision of care to a specific patient population, provision of care by a select group of providers, limitations on benefits to enrollees who use providers outside the system, and prior authorization requirements to access a limited number of specialists. The goal of a managed-care system is to provide quality health care in a cost-efficient manner (Simmons and Goforth, 1997).

Generally, managed care encompasses several organizations. Health-care purchasers such as government agencies, Medicare, Medicaid, labor unions, and employers contract with benefit providers to offer coverage to enrollees. The providers or MCOs are categorized by the degree of control, accountability, and financial risks. Some MCOs only require precertification of elective admissions and case management of catastrophic illness such as cancer. In contrast, HMOs provide both health-care financing and delivery, may own their own hospitals and clinics, and employ salaried physicians who are authorized to see only plan enrollees. Finally, the other available option is the preferred provider organization (PPO), which allows enrollees to choose from a network of hospitals and physicians. PPOs offer discounted fees for service; however, enrollees may seek care outside the network at a higher cost (Simmons and Goforth, 1997).

Typically, to reduce overall medical costs, MCOs use capitated contracts, which allocate a fixed amount of funds per month to cover the medical expenses of each plan enrollee. This fee is given to the provider on a monthly basis and is applied to any care needed by an enrollee. Some cancer-care centers and networks are beginning to test special capitation rates for the total care of cancer patients, specifically a subcapitation for disease-specific medical care, in which the primary caregiver is the cancer team. The cancer team assumes responsibility and financial risk for the care (Wermeling *et al.*, 1997). When negotiating such contracts, whether to include the costs of antineoplastic agents and supportive-care drugs is an extremely important consideration owing to their high costs. Many oncology practices are going bankrupt after entering into capitated arrangements that include coverage of antineoplastic drugs.

The trend for the new millennium is to shift control of Medicare and Medicaid from the government to local and regional HMOs for the management of their respective populations. Many states already have Medicare pilot programs with voluntary enrollment; currently, 3.4 million people are enrolled in Medicare risk plans. It is estimated that by the year 2006, voluntary enrollment will increase to 10 million people. Medicaid enrollment in managed-care programs increased from 2.7 million to 11.6 million between 1991 and 1996 (Gelinas and Fountain, 1997). However, as of July 2000 many insurers have begun to drop their Medicare HMO plans, citing financial losses as the rationale (Schramm, 2000).

As MCOs become larger and gain leverage

in the health-care industry, there will be greater price demands and performance concessions from oncologists and cancer-care centers. Many questions arise regarding how this trend will affect cancer care; for example: Will managed care limit access to research or clinical trials? Will managed care limit referrals to specialists? Will managed care limit access to aggressive treatments (e.g., biotherapy or bone-marrow transplantation), palliative care, psychosocial support, or hospice facilities?

Managed care often places restrictions on where patients can receive their care. For example, patients may have to obtain prechemotherapy labwork or X-rays across town from their oncologists. Patients with complex cases (e.g., rare tumors or multiple cancers) may not be able to access care at larger, comprehensive cancer-care centers; in some instances, managed care may even restrict referral to oncology specialists. Depending on the patient's plan, deductible expenses (up to 20% of charges) and co-pays can reach large sums, given the high costs of treating cancer. The oncology nurse is increasingly challenged to provide cancer care within the constraints of the current health-care financing system and to serve as a patient advocate while doing so.

Reimbursement in the Setting of Federal Programs

Aged and disabled individuals are covered by the Medicare program, which provides for a variety of services such as hospital insurance and related medical insurance for eligible persons 65 and older. The Medicare program also covers disabled persons under 65 who have been entitled to Social Security benefits for at least 24 consecutive months. Another group of individuals that the Medicare program covers is individuals under age 65 with chronic renal disease who are currently insured by or entitled to Social Security benefits. Regarding reimbursement issues, the Medicare program is divided into two parts: Part A and Part B.

Part A of the program deals with hospital insurance charges, including coverage for charges of inpatient hospital stays, transfers from the hospital to extended-care facilities, and discharge to home-health-care charges. Understanding the coverage provided by Medicare Part A assists health-care professionals in facilitating the selected treatment plan appropriate for the patient. Part B of the program deals with voluntary medical insurance activities and all outpatient-care issues. This part of the program provides protection against the cost of the physician services, hospital outpatient services, home-health care, and other health services such as physical and occupational therapy. Specific rules and regulations pertain to items that will and will not be covered under Part B. One of the major limitations of Medicare is that the cost of prescription drugs (i.e., oral and injectable drugs) is not covered. The majority of biological agents are administered on an outpatient basis by injection and, therefore, are impacted by this regulation. During the 106th Congress, there has been significant debate on how to include the costs of prescription drugs in Medicare benefits. As this book goes to press, the debate is unresolved. Certain home-health services will be covered only if the patient is considered homebound. Although it can represent a significant challenge, knowing and understanding the rules and regulations of state and federal programs is essential for the health-care team to facilitate quality patient care. Differences are known to exist across the country on the types of services covered by Medicare. Although this information is readily available on a variety of Internet sites, it may be difficult to locate precise answers to patients' questions. When using biotherapy for an individual covered by Medicare, it would be of value to determine which issues need to be addressed to provide the best care in a safe environment

with the least cost burden on the patient. Many patients have a second policy that may cover prescriptions or deductibles incurred.

Disease Management

Because reimbursement issues continue to create barriers, there is a growing interest in measuring outcomes of cancer care. Outcome measures are essential for guiding informed health-care decisions and determining what type of financial support will be needed to provide care. According to Schlenker (1996), outcomes should be measured because (1) payers want information about results of the care delivered; (2) outcomes are an integral part of accreditation; (3) consumers have a right to know what to expect from a treatment; (4) regulatory agencies want information about outcomes; and (5) the outcome is the basic reason for providing care. Measuring outcomes is another essential component of disease management. There are several ways to measure outcomes using investigational protocols and disease-management tools, such as **practice guidelines** and **clinical pathways**.

Disease management is a concept created to ensure delivery of quality patient care and to support outcome research while focusing on resource utilization. A major goal of disease management is to reduce variations in practice and increase efficiency. Disease-management programs are based on evidence-based medical practice and focus on clinical, functional, cognitive, and financial outcomes. A disease-management program can be implemented to coordinate oncology services across the continuum of care so that the care is integrated and patient-focused, thereby optimizing those clinical, functional, cognitive, and financial outcomes.

With the challenges and changes in the health-care setting in the past decade, health-care professionals recognize the need to better understand patient care while focusing on outcomes. This better understanding should concentrate on issues such as efficacy and efficiency. The disease-management concept can be applied in many health-care settings. Academic and tertiary-care referral centers are viewed as two of the most-challenged settings with regard to changes occurring in health-care delivery because the academic influence on institutions is viewed as more costly than its influence on community-based care (Morris, 1996). There is limited evidence showing that outcomes in academic facilities represent better planning and delivery of care compared with that in community-based settings.

In any setting, a disease-management program could be used to establish measurable outcomes of patient care. Five essential tools are needed to implement a disease-management program: practice guidelines, clinical pathways (i.e., care protocols), a case-management system, outcomes analysis, and patient education.

A practice guideline may be defined as a systematically developed flow chart that helps practitioners and patients make decisions about appropriate health care for specific clinical indications, such as breast cancer (Figure 21.1). A guideline is an overview of what is done when caring for patients across the continuum—from the evaluation phase through surveillance and possible recurrence. Guidelines are developed using results of evidenced-based medical practice and are often set up as algorithms with decision-branching points based on results of disease staging, tests, or treatments.

A clinical pathway is a multidisciplinary approach to a plan of care that specifies how to carry out certain treatments or procedures within the practice guideline for a specific clinical indication (Figure 21.2). For example, if treating a woman with early breast cancer, a simple mastectomy followed by radiation may be the treatment of choice. The clinical pathway

for a simple mastectomy outlines the major interventions that will take place during the plan of care. The pathway defines the period in which the plan of care will be achieved. The pathway is composed of various categories of care, including assessment, treatments, medications, diagnostic tests, performance status, teaching, psychosocial support, and discharge planning. The clinical pathway represents evidence-based medicine that reflects "best practice." (See Appendix A.)

Case management involves the coordination of health and financial matters during and between episodes of care for optimal clinical and financial outcomes. This process focuses on the individual patient during an episode of care. A team of health-care professionals manages a specific caseload of patients. A case manager coordinates care during the continuum, and should be able to identify the needs and resources of the patient during his or her care.

Outcomes analysis is the end result of a certain action or intervention. Outcomes are measurable changes in health status that can be attributed to a prior or concurrent treatment. The outcomes of care may have a long- or short-term effect and may be favorable or not favorable (Donabedian, 1985). Outcomes may be divided into the following three categories:

- Clinical outcomes represent the patient's physiological outcomes and can be subdivided into cognitive, functional, and psychosocial outcomes.
- Satisfaction outcomes represent the patient's perception of the care rendered from the process as well as the structural perspectives.
- Financial outcomes represent the cost of the care received.

Outcomes are seen as the product following a patient's interaction with the health-care system.

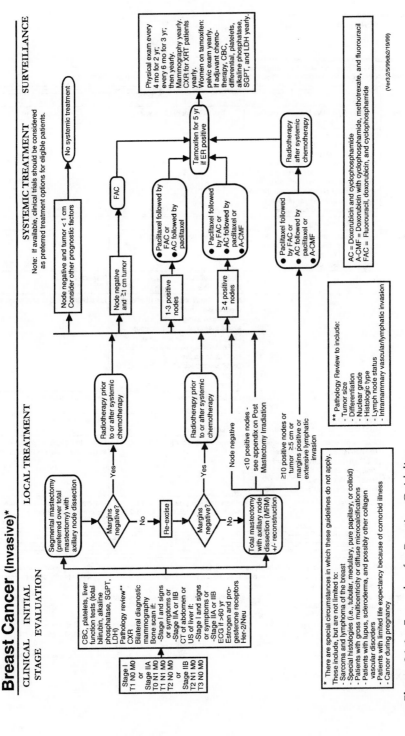

Figure 21.1 Example of a Practice Guideline

This practice guideline was created by the National Comprehensive Cancer Network and modified by The University of Texas M. D. Anderson Cancer Center for our own patient population. The core development team at M. D. Anderson working on this practice guideline included Dr. S. Eva Singletary, Dr. Eric A. Strom, and Dr. Richard Theriault.

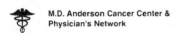

M.D. Anderson Cancer Center &
Physician's Network

Pathway:BrS3 Partial(Seg)Mastectomy with Ax Node Dissection; Possible SLN Biopsy
THIS PATH IS A GENERAL GUIDELINE: CARE IS REVISED TO MEET THE INDIVIDUAL PATIENT'S NEEDS BASED ON MEDICAL NECESSITY.

Date			
Category of Care	Pre-Operative Visit (Internal Evaluation)	Day of Surgery (Outpatient)	Post-Op Day #1
Assessment / Eval	Obtain consent. Schedule pre-op lymphoscintigraphy with Nuclear Medicine. If SLN biopsy, schedule isotope injection with Nuclear Medicine. If localization needed, schedule isotope injection with mammogram or ultrasound and Nuclear Medicine. Verify insurance authorization.		
Consult	Surgery Scheduling		
Diagnostic Test	Pre-op tests (completed within 30 days), if abnormal MDA evaluation Dx Bilateral Mammogram review Review outside pathology	Repeat abnormal pre-op tests	
Treatment		Drain to suction Incision care	Inspect incision
Medication		Ancef 1 Gm IV x 1 pre-op (if allergic, Cleocin 900mg IV x 1) Phenergan 25mg IV q6h prn, N/V MSO4 2-4mg IV q2-3h prn, pain Lortab 5mg po q3h prn, pain Tylenol 650mg po q4h prn MOM 30cc po prn D5 1/2NS 1000cc with 20 mEq KCl @ 100cc/hr Heparin lock when tolerating po	Lortab 5mg po q3h prn, pain
Performance Status / Activity		Out of bed to chair	Return to pre-op status
Nutrition	Diet as tolerated NPO after midnight prior to surgery	NPO until awake Diet as tolerated	Diet as tolerated
Teaching / Psychosoc	Assess pt for barriers to learning Provide educational materials Pre/Post-op teaching & wound drain/cath care Reach to Recovery Interactive video: CHOICES (optional)	Reach to Recovery (notify)	Reach to Recovery (verify) Pt demonstrates wound/cath care
Discharge Planning	Review discharge needs	Meds/supplies prepared for pt discharge : Lortab 5 mg #20, 1-2 po q4-6h prn	Discharge instructions reviewed Return appt scheduled

Outcome Criteria	Discharge Criteria: patient afebrile; catheter drainage <200cc/8h; pain controlled with oral medications; incision without redness/drainage; patient returns to pre-op status; no N/V, tolerates diet; patient/family demonstrates ability to manage wound/catheter care.
Followup Criteria	Non-Invasive Breast Cancer: Return appt. every year with a diagnostic mammogram. Invasive Breast Cancer: Six month appt.: mammogram of treated breast only. Years 1-2: Return appt. q4mo x 2 yr, with yearly mammogram and CXR if received radiotherapy. Years 3-5: Return appt. q6mo x 3 yr, with yearly mammogram and CXR if received radiotherapy. >5 years: Yearly exam with mammogram and CXR if received radiotherapy.

Figure 21.2   Example of a Clinical Pathway

Patient education is one of the most essential components of health-care delivery. It is important for patients to know what to expect from a treatment experience. Educating the patient and family members about the plan of care can significantly impact the outcome of care over a period of time. Patient-education materials should provide information that describes the activities and procedures that will be performed during a set period. The patient-education materials should be designed to encourage patient and family involvement in health-care decisions and practices, as appropriate.

The concept of disease management is based on a trilogy of factors that Donabedian (1980) identified as key to patient care: structure, process, and outcome, defined as follows:

- Structure refers to all of the relatively stable attributes, both material and organizational, of the setting in which care is provided.
- Process is what physicians and other practitioners do for patients. It demonstrates how skillfully they deliver care and focuses on the outcome.
- Outcome is the change in health status, for better or for worse, that can be attributed to the care being provided, such as the care delineated in a pathway.

In an effort to evaluate quality care, the emphasis must be shifted from structures to processes to outcomes within the continuum of care. This shift can be translated as having the right things, to doing things right, to having the right things happen (Mitchell *et al.*, 1998). All three concepts are essential for a successful disease-management program. However, certain challenges are involved in achieving process and outcomes that must be addressed.

Process is what is done "to" or "for" patients; for example, if a patient is receiving biotherapy for treatment of cancer, the clinical pathway will outline that care. The pathway consists of steps that should be taken to maximize the potential for a good outcome, and it should represent the established care procedure(s) as documented in the medical literature. The pathway is an example of evidence-based medical practice and can be seen as the vehicle or the baseline of established care that guides health-care teams in caring for patients receiving biotherapy. Pathways should describe the standard of care for all patients receiving biotherapy. It must be remembered, however, that pathways are only a guideline to care, and that care must be provided as clinically appropriate and necessary on a patient-by-patient basis.

According to the Institute of Medicine, *quality* is defined as "the degree to which health services for individuals and populations increase the likelihood of desired outcomes and are consistent with current professional knowledge" (Institute of Medicine, 1990). Outcomes have been discussed for at least several decades. It is a challenge in any health-care setting to define, measure, and analyze patient-care outcomes. In the academic setting, where patient care is usually developed—new and on the "cutting edge"—the associated costs of patient care are high. However, it is an even greater challenge to demonstrate that the outcomes can be measured in any health-care setting. For this reason, it is essential to establish a consistent methodology in the evaluation of patient care by using the guidelines and pathways. The use of these disease-management tools leads to reproducibility and value of patient care.

Strategies for Obtaining Reimbursement

Although the reimbursement debate is taking place within state and national forums, the effect of restricted reimbursement is felt directly by patients seeking treatment and by the health-care professionals providing care. For oncology nurses, reimbursement challenges are encountered daily. In today's world, care can no longer be provided without questions that relate to costs and the types of service a patient's insurance—be it government or private—will cover. It is the nurse's responsibility to be informed when interacting with patients seeking information about reimbursement for a recommended therapy. First, it is important to have accurate information about the reimbursement potential of the therapy. Next, it is essential to know the process involved in working with insurers. In the hospital setting, this may mean helping patients understand how to negotiate their insurance coverage or working with case managers to secure the needed care. For nurses in the outpatient setting, this often involves direct communication with insurance companies. Several tactics are effective, as follows:

- Assemble packets of appropriate data (i.e., published literature demonstrating treatment efficacy) to be reviewed by the insurance company's medical director.
- Update records about important institutional studies being conducted.
- Provide data that demonstrate the standards of excellence of clinical investigators and ongoing clinical trials.
- Utilize the assistance of pharmaceutical-company reimbursement services available to provide support in securing reimbursement for patients (Table 21.1).
- Accurately and thoroughly identify costs and use the appropriate Clinical Procedural Terminology (CPT) coding.
- Educate third-party payers about new therapies and the rationale for any specialized requirements, such as monitoring, laboratory tests, or equipment.

In addition to institutionally based reimbursement efforts, nurses can pursue individual and professional activities that address the need to provide economically efficient care. The following patient-care issues should be considered:

- Economic issues when designing equipment and treatment strategies
- Potential self-care options for the patient
- Discharge planning strategies that minimize hospital stays and provide for continuity of care at home
- Development of an institutional model that balances cost and quality in clinical care, such as a disease-management program using practice guidelines and clinical pathways

Nurses should view patient education about the financial issues of treatment as part of the informed-consent process. In some clinical trials, such as bone-marrow transplant studies, insurance coverage is an eligibility requirement. Patients generally assume that their insurance covers such therapy and are frequently shocked to discover that it is not necessarily the case. Table 21.2 summarizes strategies that may assist nurses in negotiating the reimbursement maze.

To truly effect change, nurses must work collaboratively with other providers of oncology care and professional associations to enact health-care reform at the governmental level. There are numerous misperceptions on the part of the public and legislators regarding charges for care in clinical practice. Price markups on drug costs represent an excellent example of the current deficiencies in the reimbursement system. These markups are often portrayed as an attempt to reap huge profits at the expense of payers and patients and therefore, are targeted in cost-cutting efforts. In reality, it is difficult to bill for many of the services provided to patients. Many services, such as education about symptom management and vital psychosocial interventions, are performed by the

Table 21.1   Pharmaceutical-company–sponsored reimbursement services

Company	Programs	Biological Agents	Telephone
Amgen (Thousand Oaks, CA)	• Reimbursement Hotline • Reimbursement Assistance Program (Safety Net®)	• G-CSF (Neupogen®) • Erythropoietin (Epogen®) (dialysis indication only) • IFN-α (Infergen®)	1-800-272-9376 1-800-272-9376 1-888-508-8088
Chiron Corporation (Emeryville, CA)	Reimbursement Hotline	IL-2 (Proleukin®)	1-800-775-7533
Genentech (South San Francisco, CA)	Genentech Reimbursement Information Program	Trastuzumab (Herceptin®) Rituximab (Rituxan®)	1-800-879-4747 or 1-800-TRY-GRIP
Genetics Institute, Inc. (Cambridge, MA)	BENEFIX Reimbursement and Information Program	IL-11 or oprelvekin (Neumega®)	1-888-638-6342 or 1-888-NEUMEGA
Hoffmann-La Roche, Inc. (Nutley, NJ)	Oncoline™ (Hepatitis) Cost-Assistance Program	• Interferon-alfa-2a (Roferon®-A) • Tretinoin (Vesanoid®)	1-800-443-6676 1-800-227-7448
Immunex Corporation (Seattle, WA)	Reimbursement-Support Program	• GM-CSF (Leukine®) • Etanercept (Enbrel®)	1-800-321-4669 1-800-282-7704
Ligand Pharmaceuticals (San Diego, CA)	Reimbursement Assistance	Denileukin Diftitox (ONTAK®)	1-877-654-4263
Ortho Biotech (Raritan, NJ)	• ProCrit® Cost-Sharing Program • Procritline® Financial Assistance Program (FAP)	Erythropoietin (Procrit®)	1-800-553-3851
Schering Corporation (Kenilworth, NJ)	Schering's Commitment to Care, Financial Assistance Programs: • Drug Assistance • Patient Assistance • Indigent Patient	Interferon alfa-2b (Intron®)	1-800-521-7157

Abbreviations: G-CSF, granulocyte colony-stimulating factor; GM-CSF, granulocyte-macrophage colony-stimulating factor; IFN-α, interferon-alpha; IL, interleukin.

nurse. Therefore, it is important and necessary for nurses to be involved in specific reimbursement cases as patient advocates, as well as in national groups working toward reimburse-ment-policy solutions. As health-care reform activities begin to address oncology-reimbursement issues, the direction of the discussion and the development of solutions should involve

Table 21.2   Nursing strategies for assisting patients with reimbursement issues

1. Be informed.
   - Have accurate information regarding the therapy, including knowledge of supportive literature.
   - Be familiar with information sources.
2. Know the process of working with insurers.
   - Develop a working relationship with third-party payers (e.g., case managers, medical directors).
   - Document the benefits and scientific basis for the treatment planned.
3. Assist patients with financial issues as part of the informed-consent process.
   - Educate patients about financial responsibility for specific aspects of treatment.
   - When relevant, inform patients of reimbursement issues involving off-label use of drugs and investigational therapy.
   - Facilitate and promote strategies for reimbursement.
   - Access pharmaceutical-company–reimbursement information services and indigent-patient programs.
4. Develop cost-effective care plans.
   - Include economic considerations in clinical decision-making for equipment and treatment strategies.
   - Develop an institutional model that balances cost and quality in clinical care.
5. Get involved.
   - Participate in professional organizations involved in setting national reimbursement standards in oncology.

nurses. Oncology nurses should join with them as active participants in educating and influencing legislators and health-care-provider groups. There are several options for nurses to participate in the effort to impact policy. Start with the issues that are most frustrating in daily practice. Are there currently bills before Congress that relate to this issue? If so, nurses should write or call their Senator and Representatives to voice their concerns and why they think the proposed bill would either help or hinder resolution of the problem. If there is no pending legislation, a potential solution can be suggested. The collective voice of many nurses supporting or opposing a particular bill can make a difference, as evidenced by the success of the original APC proposal.

Being part of a professional organization such as the ONS is another way to become aware of issues and to participate in efforts to impact health-care policy. ONS has many resources to assist in developing such skills (see Key Resources). Nurses have the power to help their patients and impact quality cancer care if they only choose to use it.

Conclusion

There is evidence to suggest that the U.S. health-care system is reforming in certain ways; however, the problems of oncology reimbursement are not easy to resolve. It is hoped, however, that as health-care-reform programs are proposed, designed, and implemented, the commitment to providing the most effective cancer therapies will continue to be a national health-care priority. It is important that ethical, scientific research questions continue to be addressed and that patients continue to receive care of the highest quality, which should be mutual goals of all groups involved in health care.

The new Information Age will continue to make patients better consumers of health care today. This will in turn force hospitals, insurance carriers, and MCOs to simultaneously focus on quality patient care and efficient and appropriate resource consumption. Health-care systems must keep up the pace while providing consumers with the best quality care in the most cost-effective manner. Health-care providers play a major role in this changing health-care environment. The challenge is to quantify the outcomes of care that are delivered by using disease-management tools such as practice guidelines and clinical pathways. Use of these tools would facilitate measures to ensure and/ or improve quality care, as measured by patient outcomes. Collecting outcomes provides quantifiable information by using a systematic disease-management approach and would further contribute to the evidence-based literature.

References

American Cancer Society. 2000. *Cancer Facts and Figures 2000*. Atlanta, GA: American Cancer Society.

American Society of Clinical Oncology. 1993. *Reimbursement Position Statements* (fact sheet). Washington, DC: ASCO, Government Relations Office.

Association of Community Cancer Centers. 1991. *Cancer treatments your insurance should cover* (pamphlet). Rockville, MD: ACCC.

Donabedian, A. 1980. *Explorations in Quality Assessment and Monitoring*, Vol. 1. Ann Arbor, MI: Health Administration Press, pp. 79–85.

Donabedian, A. 1985. *The Methods and Findings of Quality Assessment and Monitoring: An Illustrated Analysis*, Vol. 3. Ann Arbor, MI: Health Administration Press, p. 256.

Food and Drug Administration. 1982. Use of approved drugs for unlabeled indications. *FDA Drug Bulletin* 12: 4–5.

Friedman, M., and McCabe, M. 1992. Assigning care costs associated with therapeutic oncology research: A modest proposal. *Journal of the National Cancer Institute* 84(10): 760–763.

Gelinas, M.A., and Fountain, M. 1997. Management of cancer services: Trends and opportunities. *Cancer Management* 2(5): 6–15.

Harris, J.M. 1996. Disease management: New wine in new bottles? *Annals of Internal Medicine*, 124: 838–842.

Huber, S. 1988. Reimbursement issues with interferon therapies. *Seminars in Oncology* 15(5): 54–57.

Institute of Medicine. 1990. *Medicare: A Strategy for Quality Assurance*, Vol. 1. Washington, DC: Institute of Medicine, pp. 19–44.

Laetz, T., and Silberman, G. 1991. Reimbursement policies constrain the practice of oncology. *Journal of the American Medical Association* 266(21): 2996–2999.

McCabe, M. 1992. Reimbursement of biotherapy: Present status, future directions: Perspective of the hospital-based oncology nurse. *Seminars in Oncology Nursing* 8(4): 3–7.

Meadowcroft, A.M., Gilbert, C.J., Maravich-May, D., *et al.* 1998. Cost of managing anemia with and without prophylactic epoetin-alfa therapy in breast-cancer patients receiving combination chemotherapy. *American Journal of Health System Pharmacy* 55(18): 1898–1902.

Mitchell, P.H., Ferketich, S., and Jennings, B.M. 1998. Quality health outcomes model. *Image Journal of Nursing Scholarship* 30(1): 43–46.

Moertel, C. 1991. Off-label drug use for cancer therapy and national health-care priorities. *Journal of the American Medical Association* 266(21): 3031–3032.

Morris, M. 1996. Disease-management program at an academic medical center. *Best Practices and Benchmarking in Healthcare* 1(3): 1–8.

Mortenson, L. 1988. Audit indicates half of chemotherapy uses lack FDA approval. *Journal of Cancer Program Management* 3(2): 21–25.

National Cancer Institute: State Cancer Legislative Database Program. 1998. Bethesda, MD.

Pear, R. 1993. Health-care costs up sharply again, posing a new threat. *The New York Times*, January 5: Section A, p. 1, column 6.

Pear, R. 1999. Managed-care plans agree to help pay the costs of their members in clinical trials. *The New York Times*, February 9: Section A, p. 21, column 1.

Patient's Bill of Rights Act of 1998, H.R. 3605/ S.1890, Sec. 106. *Coverage for individuals participating in approved clinical trials.* Washington, DC, March 31, 1998.

Porter-O'Grady, T. 1998. Contemporary issues in the workplace: A glimpse over the horizon into the new age of health care. In Mason, D.J., and Leavitt, J.K. (eds). *Policy and Politics in Nursing and Health Care*, 3rd edn. Philadelphia, PA: W.B. Saunders, pp. 261–279.

Pulcini, J., and Mahoney, D. 1998. Health-care financing. In Mason, D.J., and Leavitt, J.K. (eds). *Policy and Politics in Nursing and Health Care*, 3rd edn. Philadelphia, PA: W.B. Saunders, pp. 80–99.

Schlenker, R.E. 1996. Outcomes across the care continuum: Home-health care. Presented at the AAN Conference of Outcome Measures and Care Delivery Systems, Washington, DC.

Schramm, S.L. 2000. Developing tools for better medical management of Medicare populations. *Managed Care Interface* 13(1): 43–47.

Sheiner, L.B. 1997. Learning versus Confirming in Clinical Drug Development. *Clin Phamacol Ther* 61(3): 275–291.

Simmons, W.J., and Goforth, L. 1997. The impact of managed care on cancer care review and recommendations. *Cancer Practice* 5(2): 111–117.

U.S. Dept. of Health & Human Services. 1987. *Medicare Carriers Manual*, Part 3—Claims Process, Coverage, and Limitations, HCFA-Pub 14-3, Transmittal No. 1204. Washington, DC, August, pp. 2–25.

U.S. General Accounting Office. 1991. Off-label drugs: Reimbursement policies constrain physicians in their choice of cancer therapies. Washington, DC: Publication PEMD 91-14.

Vogelzang, N., and Richards, J. 1989. Third-party reimbursement issues during a Phase I trial of interleukin-2. *Journal of the National Cancer Institute* 81(7): 544–545.

Wermeling, D.P., Piecoro, L.T., and Foster, T.S. 1997. Financial impact of clinical research on a health system. *American Journal of Health-System Pharmacy* 54(15): 1742–1751.

Young, J. 1993. Southern state enacts off-label drug legislation. *Oncology Issues* 8(2): 6.

Young, J. 1993. States acting on off-label legislation. *Oncology Issues* 8(1): 8.

Key Resources

Web Sites

Association of Community Cancer Centers Web Site
  http://www.assoc-cancer-ctrs.org.acccII.html
Oncology Nursing Society—Capitol Hill Updates.
  http://www.ons.org

Books and Book Chapters

Britt, T., Schraeder, C., and Shelton, P. (eds). 1998. *Managed Care and Capitation: Issues in Nursing.* Washington, DC: American Nurses Publishing, Pub #9803MC.

Mason, D.J., and Leavitt, J.K. (eds). 1998. *Policy and Politics in Nursing and Health Care,* 3rd edn. Philadelphia, PA: W.B. Saunders.

Oncology Nursing Society. 1998. *Health Policy Toolkit.* Pittsburgh, PA: Oncology Nursing Press.

Raber, M., and Bailes, J. 2000. Clinical oncology in a changing health care environment. In Bast, R.C., Kufe, D.W., Pollock, R.E., Weichselbaum, R.R., Holland, J.F., and Frei, E. (eds). *Cancer Medicine,* 5th edn. Hamilton, Ontario: B.C. Decker, Inc., pp. 1035–1038.

Weeks, J. 2000. Outcomes assessment. In Bast, R.C., Kufe, D.W., Pollock, R.E., Weichselbaum, R.R., Holland, J.F., and Frei, E. (eds). *Cancer Medicine,* 5th edn. Hamilton, Ontario: B.C. Decker, Inc., pp. 1039–1044.

Articles

Bloche, M.G. 2000. Fidelity and deceit at the bedside. *Journal of the American Medical Association* 283(14): 1881–1884.

Ellrodt, G., Cook, D., Lee, J., *et al.* 1997. Evidence-based disease management. *Journal of the American Medical Association* 278(20): 1687–1692.

Epstein, R.S., and Sherwood, L.M. 1996. From outcomes research to disease management: A guide for the perplexed. *Annals of Internal Medicine* 124: 832–837.

Haylock, P.J. 2000. Healthy Policy and Legislation: Impact on cancer nursing and care. *Seminars in Oncology Nursing* 16(1): 76–84.

Lieberman, A., and Rotarius, T. 1999. Managed care evolution—where did it come from and where is it going? *Health Care Management* 18(2): 50–57.

Selis, S. 2000. Will defined contribution catch on? *healthcarebusiness* March/April 2000: 26, 28, 71.

CHAPTER 22 | The Future of Cancer Therapy

Paula Trahan Rieger, RN, MSN, CS, AOCN®, FAAN

Introduction

What part will biotherapy play in the cancer-treatment armamentarium of the future? Will biotherapy be remembered as a historical event, a bright meteor of the 1980s and 1990s? Or will it assume prominence as a full-fledged fourth modality of cancer therapy, used both as a single mode of treatment and in combination with other cancer-therapy modalities in a variety of both hematological and solid tumors?

Two attempts have been made to establish immunotherapy, the forerunner of biotherapy, in cancer therapeutics. First, in the early 1900s, Coley's toxins, crude bacterial extracts, were given subcutaneously and intralesionally to patients with sarcoma and other tumors. At that time, those extracts were the only known systemic treatment for cancer (Balkwill, 1989). In the 1970s, the bacillus Calmette-Guérin (BCG) vaccine, the *Corynebacterium parvum* vaccine, and other nonspecific immunomodulators were used with some success in the treatment of melanoma and other cancers; however, they were not consistently effective in clinical trials (Oldham, 1998a).

Although the success of an immunological approach to the treatment of cancer is regarded optimistically, the unfortunate fact is that most patients are not cured by this approach. A number of explanations have been proposed to account for the failure of a strictly immunological approach to cancer treatment. One is that the tumor antigens or HLA antigens expressed on the tumor cell are not sufficient in quantity to trigger an effective immune response. Another explanation is that the tumor lacks co-stimulatory molecules that are

669

critical for eliciting a T-cell response. T lymphocytes from patients with cancer may have defects in signalling molecules important in generating immune responses. A third explanation is that tumors may express molecules that suppress the immune response (Hershey, 1999). The extent to which these proposed mechanisms of resistance to immune rejection of tumors can be overcome by therapeutic interventions has yet to be fully explored. Potential approaches include blocking immunosuppressive molecules through the use of monoclonal antibodies (MABs) targeted toward inhibitory factors or using recombinant soluble receptors to neutralize the inhibitory factors. Using molecules such as chemokines to attract immune cells to the tumor site is another option. Hence, a strict focus on stimulating the immune system to fight cancer remains an active area of focus. As our understanding of the immune system and its interaction with cancer has improved, newer strategies have emerged that target immune responses. There has been a resurgence of interest in the use of vaccines for the treatment of cancer. New approaches include the use of vaccines in association with the appropriate co-stimulatory molecules (see Chapter 10).

Immunotherapy no longer aptly describes the modern use of biological substances in medicine; hence, the birth of the term "biotherapy." According to Oldham (1998a), biotherapy is not immunotherapy revisited but rather a new therapy. Major technological improvements have provided a sound foundation for the development of biotherapy into a useful form of cancer treatment.

Individuals who are optimistic about the future of biotherapy say that several key events have contributed to the development of current biological agents. The first important achievement was progress in **molecular biology** and the development of genetic engineering. The ability to identify specific genes responsible for immunologically active molecules such as cytokines has led to the use of recombinant technology to produce these molecules. Recombinant proteins are specific products that are more purified than previously used nonspecific immunostimulants such as BCG. This technology has also provided large quantities of these immunological proteins, which has permitted broadscale testing of these agents in cancer therapy. Numerous biological molecules (e.g., interferons [IFNs], interleukins [ILs], and hematopoietic growth factors) now have regulatory approval for use in the treatment of cancer and other diseases.

A second key event was development of the hybridoma technique, the fusing of an immortal cell to an antibody-producing cell, which yielded very specific antibodies directed at a desired tumor target. These antibodies, known as MABs, have found wide application in diagnostic use and continue to be explored for therapeutic use both alone (i.e., naked) or in conjugate form (e.g., with immunotoxins) and in other new chimeric forms.

A third event was the ability to culture and expand in number clonally activated lymphocytes, lymphokine-activated killer cells, or tumor-infiltrating lymphocytes (TILs) and return them in large numbers to the patient. This technology has been investigated in combination with existing therapies and currently forms the basis for gene transduction of TILs with cytokine genes, such as tumor necrosis factor (TNF), as a means to augment the TIL's tumoricidal capabilities (Hoffman et al., 2000).

Finally, technological advances in instrumentation, computer capabilities, molecular biology, and assay methods have enabled investigators to precisely determine the nature of existing molecules (Oldham, 1998a) and to develop new molecules. Some of these advances have allowed investigators to determine specific nucleotide sequences using an automated method. One example of this novel technology is the polymerase chain reaction technique, which has become an essential tool in gene research, enabling technicians to copy and describe gene sequences. *In vitro* evolution is a new, important laboratory method to evolve molecules with desired properties. The emerging field of directed molecular evolution is a process by which novel genes are generated for commercial use. For example, companies such as Maxygen (Santa Clara, CA) have developed proprietary technologies, known as MolecularBreeding™, that brings together advances in molecular biology and classical breeding while capitalizing on the large amount of genetic information being generated by the genomics industry. The objective is to develop multiple products in a broad range of industries, including agriculture, chemicals, and protein pharmaceuticals. A single gene or multiple genes are cleaved into fragments and recombined, creating a population of novel gene sequences. The novel genes created by the DNA-shuffling process are then selected for one or more desired characteristics. This selection process yields a population of genes that becomes the starting point for the next cycle of recombination. This process is repeated until genes expressing the desired properties are identified. The hope is that the new genes can manufacture proteins that are much better at certain tasks than nature's originals. One biological agent targeted by Maxygen is IFN. The goal, in effect, is to produce IFNs that are more effective against viruses than those produced naturally. In the future, this technique may provide for tremendous variability in tailored biological molecules (Maxygen, 2000).

Because of these technological advances and other continuing discoveries, new possibilities exist for the steady progress of biotherapy in the coming years. Chemotherapy remains the primary systemic modality used for cancer treatment. Although effective in treating nu-

merous malignancies, the major problem associated with chemotherapy is its nonspecificity (Hellman, 1998). Both malignant and nonmalignant cells are affected by chemotherapy, often resulting in serious adverse effects. Breakthroughs in understanding the transformation of a normal cell into a malignant cell and the identification and refinement of biological proteins have led to the ability to more selectively target the tumor for therapy. As knowledge in these areas continues to grow and as molecular biology becomes increasingly sophisticated, the ability to identify the underlying "defect" in a given malignancy and then "correct it" will become a reality.

The explosion of knowledge about cancer genetics and the molecular basis of neoplasia in the past two decades have begun to change the basic management of cancer as a disease. It is hoped that these advances will ultimately translate into improved patient survival or even cancer prevention (Cannistra, 1997). The discovery of genes that become altered or mutated during the process of carcinogenesis will provide new clues and insights into how to determine individual risk for developing cancer, will provide prognostic indicators for those who develop cancer, and will generate new modalities for the treatment of cancer. Much of the knowledge gained has resulted from work related to the Human Genome Project initiated in 1990. The ultimate goal of this project is to generate information, tools, and molecular approaches that will increase our understanding of both normal and abnormal gene structure and function. It is anticipated that the sequencing of all three billion base pairs of human DNA will be completed by the end of 2003 (Collins *et al.*, 1998). In June 2000, The Human Genome Project public consortium announced that it had assembled a working draft of the sequence of the human genome. This draft contains overlapping fragments that cover approximately 90% of the genome, thus some gaps and ambiguities remain. The next step will be the integration of new technologies and the wealth of information generated into the clinical management of diseases, including cancer (Collins and Jenkins, 1997).

This chapter will review developing areas of biotherapy that represent opportunities for the continued advancement of cancer treatment. The ongoing discovery of novel biological proteins such as ILs, as well as the production of genetically engineered molecules, will be reviewed and methods for increasing the therapeutic index of drugs through innovative dosing and delivery will be examined. The next step in the future of cancer care is molecular oncology. The remainder of this chapter will discuss the integration of genetic information into three major areas of cancer management: risk management and cancer prevention, diagnosis and prognosis assessment, and treatment. As a prerequisite to understanding these advances in cancer care, oncology nurses must first have a solid foundation in cell biology, genetics, and the molecular basis of cancer (see Chapter 3). Specific clinical examples will be used to illustrate current and future incorporation of this knowledge into the management of cancer.

Discovery of New Agents

Progress with established treatment strategies and the introduction of new approaches in biotherapy continue at rapid rates. Discoveries of new biological proteins, such as IL-18, that may have therapeutic benefit have steadily added to the armamentarium available for investigation in clinical trials (Lebel-Binay *et al.*, 2000). Furthermore, the melding of molecular biology and immunology has led to the creation of a variety of novel biological agents through the use of recombinant DNA technology to genetically engineer proteins such as fusion toxins (Foss *et al.*, 1998).

New Developments in Interleukins

The discovery and evaluation of cytokines continue to be active areas of research. Newly discovered molecules are assigned successive IL numbers as their gene sequences are described. Not all ILs are studied in cancer clinical trials because their primary function may not appear applicable to cancer therapy. An example of such a cytokine is IL-5.

ILs are being evaluated for use as hematopoietic growth factors and as anticancer agents. Currently, IL-1, IL-3, and IL-6 are being investigated in clinical trials for their potential role as hematopoietic growth factors (Dinarello, 1998; Maslak and Nimer, 1998; Mangi and Newland, 1999). This field is progressing rapidly, and ILs have potential use as supportive therapy in combination with high-dose chemotherapy, radiation therapy, and bone-marrow transplant or as supportive therapy in diseases such as myelodysplastic syndrome, in which inadequate production of blood cell lines is seen.

A second area of IL development focuses on ILs as anticancer agents. Clinical investigation of IL-2, for example, led to its approval by the Food and Drug Administration (FDA) in 1992 for treatment of renal-cell cancer. Both IL-6 and IL-12 have shown preclinical evidence of potential use as anticancer agents and remain under investigation for efficacy in the treatment of cancer (Golab and Zagozdzon, 1999). ILs utilized as single tumoricidal agents may have limited clinical application until their biology and multiple functions that overlap with other ILs are better understood. It is more likely that the combination of these agents and other forms of therapy, such as chemotherapy, may provide the most effective tumoricidal therapy (Bukowski, 2000) (see Chapter 4).

Chemokines

Chemokines belong to a large family of chemo attractant molecules involved in the directed migration of immune cells. They are small, inducible, secreted, chemotactic cytokines that make up the largest mammalian cytokine superfamily (Devalaraja and Richmond, 1999). They achieve their cellular effect by direct interaction with cell-surface receptors. Chemokine receptors comprise a family of seven transmembrane domain G protein–coupled receptors differentially expressed in diverse cell types. Pharmacological analysis of chemokine receptors is at an early stage of development. Biological activity of chemokines is finely controlled by the varied display, binding affinity, and/or signal-transducing mechanisms of receptors. A receptor nomenclature system, ratified by the International Union of Pharmacology, has helped to facilitate clear communication in this area (Murphy *et al.*, 2000).

Chemokines appear to be involved in a variety of proinflammatory and autoimmune diseases, which makes them and their receptors very attractive therapeutic targets. Biological activities have been most clearly defined in leukocytes, where chemokines coordinate development, differentiation, anatomic distribution, trafficking, and effector functions, thereby regulating innate and adaptive immune responses. Chemokines are known to be beneficial in wound healing, hematopoiesis, the clearance of infectious organisms, lymphocyte development, and homeostasis. Dysregulation is associated with chronic inflammatory conditions such as arthritis (Devalaraja and Richmond, 1999). More than 50 chemokines were identified as of July 2000; they are classified into four subgroups designated CXC (e.g., IL-8), CC (e.g., regulated upon activation normal T-cell expressed and secreted [RANTES]), C (e.g., lymphoactin), and CX_3C (e.g., fractalkine).

Improved understanding of chemokine biology may lead to therapeutic indications. IL-8 has angiogenic activity that is believed to account for its tumor-growth–promoting effect. Other chemokines such as IP-10 have angiostatic effects and, therefore, suppress tumor growth. In the future, the effects of chemokines on tumors must be carefully characterized so that the appropriate therapeutic use can ensue (i.e., the use of antagonists to those chemokines with tumor-promoting effects) (Oppenheim *et al.*, 1997). Tumors use multiple means to blunt and circumvent immunotherapeutic approaches. By learning to identify and counteract downregulatory mechanisms and utilizing immunostimulants to maximum effectiveness, the therapeutic potential of biotherapy may be fully realized.

Advances in Dosing, Delivery, and Development of Drugs

In Chapter 4, issues surrounding dosing and scheduling of biological agents were reviewed. Once the appropriate dose for a given biological agent in a specific situation is identified, how can this dose be delivered? Several novel methods, including regional perfusion therapy, the use of lipid vesicles as novel drug–delivery systems, combination therapies, and MAB immunoconjugate therapy, are currently being investigated. The ultimate goal is to increase the concentration of drug at the tumor site without systemic toxicity.

Liposomes as Novel Drug–Delivery Systems

Liposomes are lipid vesicles composed of single or multiple concentric phospholipid bilayers. These vesicles are formed spontaneously when an aqueous solution is added to a dried lipid film (Bangham *et al.*, 1974). Over the past decade, the potential use of liposomes as drug carriers has been recognized. Their unique ability to encapsulate both **hydrophilic** and **hydrophobic** drugs has led to numerous investigations evaluating their use in the administration of antimicrobial agents (Lopez-Berestein, 1987), antifungal agents (Lopez-Berestein et al., 1989), chemotherapeutic agents (Lautersztain et al., 1986), and biological agents. The primary objective in using liposomes as drug carriers is to enhance the therapeutic index of the drug. This can be accomplished by maintaining or amplifying the therapeutic activity of a drug, decreasing toxicity, or both. Liposomes are appealing as drug carriers because they are easy to prepare, they are biodegradable, and they lack toxicity. The fact that liposomes naturally target organs rich in reticuloendothelial cells (e.g., liver, spleen, and bone marrow) provides further opportunity for investigation (Lopez-Berestein, 1985; Leyland-Jones, 1993).

Liposomes can function as sustained-release systems for drugs, and the rate of release can be manipulated. Benefit can be gained from the substantial changes in pharmacokinetics that often accompany the association of drugs with liposomes. New formulations of liposomes, sterically stabilized with substances like surface-grafted polyethylene glycol (PEG), have circulating half-lives in humans of up to 2 days. These long circulation times allow for the concentration of liposomal drugs in regions of increased vascular permeability, such as solid tumors, and decreased delivery of drug to normal tissues. Alterations of the biodistribution of drugs, when they are liposome associated, generally lead to significant overall decreases in drug toxicity but can also increase toxicity in some tissues. The use of targeting ligands to increase the selectivity of delivery of liposomal drugs to target tissues is currently under development. An understanding of how liposome association can alter drug properties can lead to their rational development in the treatment of many diseases (Allen, 1998).

Because liposomes are rapidly cleared from the circulation by the reticuloendothelial system (phagocytic cells primarily located in the liver and spleen) (Fidler, 1992), liposomes are potentially useful as delivery agents for immunomodulators that increase the tumoricidal activity of monocytes and macrophages. One such immunomodulator, muramyl dipeptide (MDP), is a component of bacterial cell walls that is capable of activating an immune response. However, it has an extremely short half-life in the bloodstream (Fidler, 1992), thus limiting its clinical usefulness. The agent MTP-PE is a synthetic analogue of MDP that has been investigated in clinical phase I studies to evaluate its toxicity and potential efficacy as an anticancer agent. The trials involved parenteral administration of liposomal MTP-PE for 1 hour twice weekly for 4 to 9 weeks. Patients experienced moderate toxic effects, primarily chills, fever, nausea and vomiting, fatigue, and hypertension. Toxic effects were most severe after the first dose, but were not cumulative (Murray et al., 1989, Creaven et al., 1990). The maximum tolerated dose was 6 mg/m^2, and the optimal biological dose to produce activation of blood monocytes was 2 to 4 mg/m^2. Only one patient with a renal-cell cancer had an objective response to treatment with MTP-PE. Therefore, liposomal MTP-PE can target and activate cytotoxic properties of monocytes and macrophages and is generally well tolerated.

Kleinerman et al. (1995) evaluated the use of liposomal MTP-PE in patients with osteosarcoma. Osteosarcoma appears to be an ideal disease in which to employ liposomal MTP-PE as an additional adjuvant to current chemotherapy regimens. The lung is the most frequent site of metastases, and pulmonary micrometastases are considered to be present in the majority of patients at diagnosis. Approximately 40% of patients with osteosarcoma develop pulmonary metastases despite the administration of adjuvant chemotherapy. A nationwide randomized phase III trial is under way in newly diagnosed osteosarcoma patients in conjunction with the Children's Cancer Study Group and the Pediatric Oncology Group (Kleinerman *et al.*, 1995).

Several liposomal drug preparations have received regulatory approval. Daunorubicin citrate liposome (DaunoXome®, NeXstar Pharmaceuticals, Inc., San Dimas, CA) has regulatory approval for the treatment of acquired immune deficiency syndrome-related Kaposi's sarcoma. This approach is also being evaluated in the treatment of cancers such as leukemias and lymphoma (Cortes *et al.*, 1999). Long-circulating formulations of liposomes containing lipid derivatives of PEG, sterically stabilized liposomes (SLs), have now been coupled to MABs at the PEG termini of these liposomes. MAB-targeted SLs (immunoliposomes [SILs]) containing entrapped anticancer drugs are predicted to be useful in the treatment of hematological malignancies such as B-cell lymphomas or multiple myeloma, in which the target cells are present in the vasculature.

Lopez de Mendes *et al.* (1999) evaluated single doses (3 mg/kg) of doxorubicin-SIL (anti-CD19) administered intravenously. This formulation resulted in a significantly improved therapeutic benefit, including some long-term survivors. From their results, these investigators inferred that targeted anti-CD19 liposomes containing the anticancer drug doxorubicin may be selectively cytotoxic for B cells and may be useful in the selective elimination of circulating malignant B cells *in vivo*. Three lipid amphotericin-B preparations have now been approved by the FDA for the treatment of fungal infections (Rust and Jameson, 1998).

Polymer Conjugates

Polymer conjugation may also be used to alter the biodistribution, elimination, and rate of metabolism of covalently bound drugs. The field has evolved in two primary directions: (1) conjugation of biologically active protein drugs to improve efficacy and reduce toxicity and (2) rational design of polymer-drug conjugates to facilitate controlled release and targeting of conventional low-molecular-weight chemical entities, particularly cytotoxic agents. PEG has been the most widely used polymer for protein conjugation. Conjugates are comprised of three parts: the protein, a linker, and the polymer. PEG conjugates have been developed with the IFNs, IL-2, and hematopoietic growth factors. It is hoped that conjugation will allow for prolonged half-times, a reduction of immunogenicity, and improved solubility of the drug (Duncan and Spreafico, 1994). Clinical trials have evaluated the use of pegylated compounds (Johnston *et al.*, 2000); however, as of June 2000, none had received regulatory approval.

Combination Therapies

The development of biological agents in many ways parallels that of chemotherapy. After the efficacy of a single agent has been established, greater response rates may be achieved by combining this agent with others in a variety of schedules. As reviewed in Chapter 4, combination therapy can have several goals. An agent such as a hematopoietic growth factor can be used to decrease the toxicity of another treatment modality, such as chemotherapy or radiation therapy. An example is the use of granulocyte colony-stimulating factor to abrogate toxic hematologic effects following treatment with high-dose, myelosuppressive chemotherapy. Another goal would be to combine biological agents with each other or with chemotherapy to achieve a synergistic or additive therapeutic effect. The research conducted to date has only begun to solve the problem of finding the optimal dose and schedule of biological agents to maximize the potential antitumor effects of each agent while not increasing toxicity to the patient. Not all of these potential combinations will prove valuable, but they may offer insights into newer, more effective combinations.

Pharmacogenomics

Pharmacogenomics is an emerging scientific discipline that examines the genetic basis for individual variations in response to therapeutics. Genetic polymorphisms are a major cause of individual differences in drug response. Genotyping allows determination of individual DNA sequence differences for a particular trait. Therefore, rapid and accurate detection of genetic polymorphisms has great potential for application to drug development, animal toxicity studies, improvement of human clinical trials, and post-market monitoring surveillance for drug efficacy and toxicity (Shi *et al.*, 1999). Clinical pharmacogenomics promises to increase the safety and efficacy of drug prescription; decrease the incidence of adverse drug reactions; help improve public health; and presage in an era of personalized, predictive, and prophylactic medicine (Hess and Cooper, 1999). Genetic polymorphisms in drug-metabolizing enzymes, transporters, receptors, and other drug targets have been linked to inter individual differences in the efficacy and toxicity of many medications. Pharmacogenomic studies are rapidly elucidating the inherited nature of these differences in drug disposition and effects, thereby enhancing drug discovery and providing a stronger scientific basis for optimizing drug therapy on the basis of each patient's genetic constitution (Evans and Relling, 1999). Clinical pharmacogenomics stands to become the basis for the new millennium's practice of medicine and to have a profound impact on the clinical practice.

Drug Design

In conventional drug discovery, the pharmaceutical industry has historically relied on dis-covering drug leads by screening and sifting through vast inventories of naturally occurring and man-made chemicals in search of previously undiscovered substances with the desired biological activity. This approach has become increasingly unsatisfactory because it is costly and inefficient, and the discovery of new compounds has continued to decline. Given the emergence of new technologies, the idea of designing drugs no longer remains far-fetched.

Nearly every drug molecule works through structural interaction with a target or receptor molecule or protein that plays key roles in all biological processes. In the most common model for this interaction, the drug molecule inserts itself into a functionally important indentation of its target protein, like a key in a lock. The molecule then binds there and either induces or, more commonly, inhibits the protein's normal function. This universal drug-target scheme suggests a powerful alternative approach to drug discovery. If it were possible to identify, in advance, the appropriate protein target for a given therapeutic need, and if enough were known about the distinguishing structure of that target protein, it ought to be feasible to design the structure of an ideal drug to interact with it. This approach offers the promise of eliminating much of the inefficiency of conventional drug discovery (Kuhlmann, 1999; Agouron, 2000; Schreiber, 2000).

New Developments in Genetically Engineered Molecules

The creation of novel molecules through genetic engineering or through the linking of toxic substances to biological agents, specifically to MABs, will continue to further the introduction of new biological agents and cancer therapies. One of the greatest assets of certain biological agents is the ability to selectively target therapy to the tumor cell. This represents a major advance in the treatment of cancer compared with nonselective therapies such as chemotherapy. Numerous avenues exist by which this goal may be achieved. MAB immunoconjugates represent one avenue and remains an active area of focus (see Chapter 8 and Chapter 9.). However, one of the problems with this approach is that whatever substance has been attached to the MAB may dissociate. To solve this problem, an area of focus has been the use of genetically engineered molecules. Fusion proteins, molecules designed with parts of 2 molecules but produced as 1 complete protein, solve this problem. As the use of recombinant proteins for the treatment of disease continues, the use of novel fusion proteins will continue to progress (Russell and Clarke, 1999).

Denileukin Difitox

One example of a fusion protein is the DAB_{486} IL-2 molecule, in which the native binding domain of diphtheria toxin has been replaced with human IL-2 (Figure 22.1). The resulting diphtheria toxin-related cytokine fusion protein binds to its respective receptor, in this instance IL-2, and is internalized by receptor-mediated endocytosis and then efficiently eliminates the target cell. This molecule has been investigated as a treatment for a variety of hematologic malignancies (Cobb *et al.*, 1991; Foss *et al.*, 1998). To date, administration of the diphtheria toxin–based fusion proteins targeted toward the high-affinity IL-2 receptor have been found to be safe, well tolerated, and capable of inducing remission in refractory hematologic malignan-

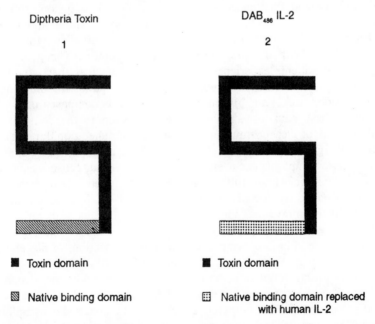

Figure 22.1   Interleukin-2 (IL-2) fusion toxin. DAB_{486} IL-2 is a genetically engineered ligand toxin created by replacing the binding domain of diphtheria toxin with sequences for human IL-2

Source: Reprinted with permission from Cobb, P., LeMaistre, C., and Jackson, L. 1991. Clinical evaluation of immunotoxins. *Cancer Bulletin* 43(3): 233–239. Copyright 1991 Medical Arts Publishing Foundation; Houston, Texas.

cies. In February 1999, denileukin difitox (Ontak®; Ligand Pharmaceuticals, San Diego, CA) received regulatory approval for the treatment of patients with persistent or recurrent cutaneous T-cell lymphoma whose malignant cells express the CD25 component of the IL-2 receptor. A randomized, double-blind study was conducted to evaluate doses of 9 or 18 mcg/kg/day given as an intravenous infusion over at least 15 minutes in 71 patients with recurrent or persistent cutaneous T-cell lymphoma. Patients received a median of 6 courses of therapy with denileukin difitox. More than 60% of the patients entered had stage Ib or more advanced stage disease. Overall, 30% of patients treated with denileukin difitox experienced an objective tumor response (e.g., 50% reduction in tumor burden that was sustained for 6 weeks). Seven patients achieved a complete response, and 14 patients achieved a partial response (Olsen *et al.*, 1998; Ligand Pharmaceuticals, 1999).

The administration of denileukin difitox is associated with toxicity. With the first dose, approximately 70% of patients experience an acute hypersensitivity–type reaction characterized by hypotension, back pain, dyspnea, vasodilation, rash, chest pain or tightness, tachycardia, dysphagia or laryngismus, syncope, and, rarely, allergic reaction or anaphylaxis (1% each). These symptoms occur either during the infusion or within 24 hours following it. Symptoms are managed by decreasing the rate of infusion and by the intravenous administration of antihistamines, corticosteroids, and, occasionally, epinephrine. Flu-like symptoms were experienced by up to 91% of patients within several hours to days after infusion of denileukin difitox. These symptoms were generally mild and responded well to antipyretics and/or antiemetics. A vascular-leak–type syndrome also occurred in some patients and was characterized by 2 or more of the following symptoms: hypotension, edema, hypoalbumi-

nemia, or a combination of these. The onset of these symptoms is generally delayed, occurring within the first 2 weeks of infusion. Research continues to evaluate the role of denileukin difitox in other hematologic malignancies such as lymphoma (LeMaistre *et al.*, 1998) and other diseases such as psoriasis (Bagel *et al.*, 1998). Only modest clinical improvement has been seen with its use in rheumatoid arthritis (Dinant and Dijkmans, 1999).

Etanercept

A second fusion protein has also received regulatory approval. Etanercept (Enbrel®; Immunex Corp., Seattle, WA) was approved in November 1998 for the treatment of moderately to severely active rheumatoid arthritis in patients who have had an inadequate response to one or more disease modifying anti-rheumatic drugs (DMARDs). This fusion protein, classified as an immunoadhesin, combines the structural features of antibodies with high-affinity cell-surface receptors. The goal is to inhibit the activity of factors that would normally bind to the receptors in the body. Etanercept (TNFR:Fc) is composed of 2 soluble TNF receptors fused to the constant fragment of a human immune globulin (Fc). It selectively binds TNF, an important cytokine in the cascade of reactions that cause the inflammatory processes of rheumatoid arthritis (Jarvis and Faulds, 1999). In a multicenter, double-blind trial, 180 patients with refractory rheumatoid arthritis were randomly assigned to receive subcutaneous injections of placebo or 1 of 3 doses of TNFR:Fc (0.25, 2, or 16 mg/m^2 body-surface area) twice weekly for 3 months (Moreland, 1998). The clinical response was measured by changes in composite symptoms of arthritis defined according to American College of Rheumatology (ACR) criteria. Treatment with TNFR:Fc led to significant reductions in disease activity, and the therapeutic effects of TNFR:Fc were dose related. At 3 months, 75% of the patients in the group assigned to 16 mg/m^2 TNFR:Fc had improvement of 20% or more in symptoms, compared with 14% of patients in the placebo group ($p < .001$). In the group assigned to the 16 mg/m^2 dose, the mean percent reduction in the number of tender or swollen joints at 3 months was 61%, compared with 25% in the placebo group ($p < .001$). The most common adverse events were mild injection-site reactions and mild upper-respiratory-tract symptoms. There were no dose-limiting toxic effects, and no antibodies to TNFR:Fc were detected in serum samples. The authors concluded that in this 3-month trial, TNFR:Fc was safe, well tolerated, and associated with improvement in the inflammatory symptoms of rheumatoid arthritis.

Additional studies evaluated TNFR:Fc in combination with methotrexate. A randomized study by Weinblatt *et al.* (1999) evaluated the addition of etanercept or methotrexate in 89 patients with persistently active rheumatoid arthritis. In a 24-week, double-blind randomized trial, patients were assigned to receive either TNFR:Fc plus methotrexate or placebo plus methotrexate. The addition of TNFR:Fc to methotrexate resulted in a rapid and sustained improvement. Seventy-one percent of patients met the ACR 20 criteria and 39% met the ACR 50 criteria (i.e., 20% and 50% improvement, respectively) in number of swollen joints, plus reduction in at least 3 of the following: pain, patient self-assessment of disease status, patient self-assessment of disability, physician's global assessment of disease status, or reduction in acute-phase reactants. The authors concluded that the combination was safe and well tolerated and provided significantly greater clinical benefit than methotrexate alone. Issues that remain to be answered with respect to the use of TNFR:Fc in patients with rheumatoid arthritis are (1) when, in the course of therapy, should the drug be used and (2) whether there are ways to predict which patients will best respond. A new era in the treatment of autoimmune disease has begun in which agents that specifically target a part of the pathophysiology of the disease are utilized (O'Dell, 1999).

Bifunctional Monoclonal Antibodies

Another example of using genetically engineered molecules to treat tumors is the use of bifunctional, or bispecific, MABs. Bispecific antibodies have 2 different specific antigen-binding sites, one on each arm of the antibody molecule (Cao and Suresh, 1998). This approach has immense potential in biological and immunological fields, with applications ranging from immunohistochemistry, immunoassays, radio-immunodiagnosis, radioimmunotherapy, and biological therapy. For example, antibodies have been designed in which one arm of the antibody binds to the tumor and the second arm binds to a drug, toxin, or effector cell. For use in immunohistochemistry, one arm can be designed to bind to a particular tissue and the other to peroxidase. Clinical trials are actively investigating the use of bispecific MABs in patients with cancer. For example, 15 patients with refractory Hodgkin's disease were treated in a phase I/II dose-escalation trial with the natural-killer-cell–activating bispecific MAB HRS-3/A9, which is directed against the Fc gamma–receptor III (CD16 antigen) and the Hodgkin's-associated CD30 antigen. Eight patients developed human anti-mouse immunoglobulin antibodies, and 5 patients showed an allergic reaction after attempted retreatment. One complete and one partial remission (lasting 6 and 3 months, respectively), 2 minor responses (lasting 1 and 15 months), stable disease in 2 patients (one each for 2 and 17 months), and 1 mixed response were achieved. There was no clearcut dose-side effect or dose-response correlation. The investigators felt further clinical trials with this novel immunotherapeutic approach were warranted; however, they emphasized the necessity to reduce the immunogenicity of the murine bispecific antibodies (Hartmann *et al.*, 1998).

Receptor-Based Therapy

Another approach to cancer treatment capitalizes on the natural biology of the tumor. Receptors expressed on the surface of tumor cells may serve as potential targets for therapy; therefore, receptor-based therapy will remain an active area of research. Clinical trials evaluating the use of receptor-based therapy are being pursued actively by researchers as new targets are discovered and molecules developed. Human epithelial tumors frequently express high levels of epidermal growth factor (EGF) receptor and of its **ligand**, transforming growth factor-alpha (TGF-α). It has been suggested that an autocrine pathway constituted by the EGF receptor and TGF-α may have an important role in human tumors (Derynck *et al.*, 1987). In some tumors, expression of high levels of the EGF receptor and its ligand TGF-α are associated with a poor prognosis. The use of MABs that block the binding of TGF-α or activation of the EGF receptor may inhibit proliferation of tumor cells expressing this receptor. This approach was reviewed in Chapter 9. As the understanding of this family of receptors and its ligands progresses, new targets for therapeutic intervention in cancer, such as signal-blocking, will ensue (Wells, 1999).

A naturally occurring IL-1–receptor antagonist was discovered in 1985. This protein binds to the IL-1 receptor with an affinity similar to IL-1, but does not have **agonist** activity when coupled to that receptor (Dinarello, 1998). Clinical trials are in progress evaluating its use in modulating the deleterious effects of IL-1 in diseases such as rheumatoid arthritis (Maini and Taylor, 2000).

New Developments in Understanding the Biology of Cancer

Multiple events are involved in the initiation, promotion, and expression of a malignancy. Cancer is a genetic disease, one that is characterized by genetic instability and long-term uncontrolled growth of cells. For a cell to function normally, control of growth, differentiation, and programmed cell death must be evident. These complex processes involve a cascade of cellular events and proteins that are encoded by DNA. Alteration in the DNA through mutations, deletions, or translocations result in aberrations that have been well documented to affect cell growth, differentiation, and programmed cell death. These disruptions and the resulting abnormally functioning proteins result in the disease recognized as cancer. The discovery of genes that become altered or mutated during the process of carcinogenesis will provide new clues and insights into how to determine individual risk for developing cancer, will provide prognostic indicators for those who develop cancer, and will generate new modalities for the treatment of cancer.

Identification of individuals who carry an increased risk of developing certain types of cancer and an understanding of the risk factors associated with the development and the causes of cancer are necessary to maximize cancer prevention strategies. To design the most effective cancer prevention interventions, one must relate these interventions to the principles of carcinogenesis. The oncology professional of the future must focus on the "therapy" of cancer at all stages, starting with the first initiated cell and dysplasia, not solely invasive and metastatic cancer (Alberts, 1999). Tremendous opportunities will exist to integrate the current understanding of the biology of cancer into new strategies for earlier intervention in its prevention (Figure 22.2).

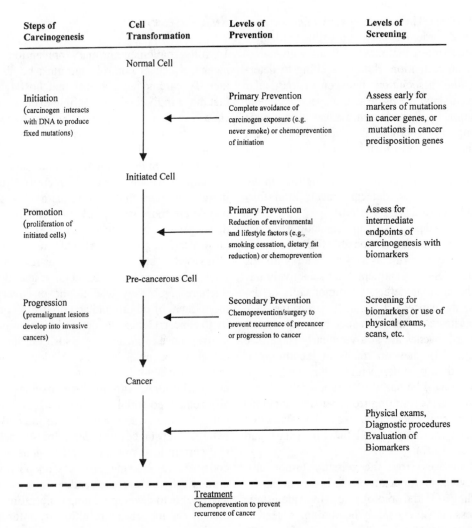

Steps of Carcinogenesis	Cell Transformation	Levels of Prevention	Levels of Screening
	Normal Cell		
Initiation (carcinogen interacts with DNA to produce fixed mutations)		Primary Prevention Complete avoidance of carcinogen exposure (e.g. never smoke) or chemoprevention of initiation	Assess early for markers of mutations in cancer genes, or mutations in cancer predisposition genes
	Initiated Cell		
Promotion (proliferation of initiated cells)		Primary Prevention Reduction of environmental and lifestyle factors (e.g., smoking cessation, dietary fat reduction) or chemoprevention	Assess for intermediate endpoints of carcinogenesis with biomarkers
	Pre-cancerous Cell		
Progression (premalignant lesions develop into invasive cancers)		Secondary Prevention Chemoprevention/surgery to prevent recurrence of precancer or progression to cancer	Screening for biomarkers or use of physical exams, scans, etc.
	Cancer		
			Physical exams, Diagnostic procedures Evaluation of Biomarkers

Treatment
Chemoprevention to prevent
recurrence of cancer

Figure 22.2   An alternative view of cancer prevention

Source: Reprinted with permission from Rieger, P.T. (in press). The impact of genetic information in the management of cancer. In Calzone, C.A., Jenkins, J., Masny, A., and Strauss Tranin, A. (eds). *Recommendations for Cancer Genetics Nursing Practice and Education.* Pittsburgh, PA: Oncology Nursing Press.

The manner in which cancer is screened for will also be dramatically altered in the future. Imagine that long before tumors arise, a test could detect biological clues about tissue injury by specific cancer-causing agents or the impending evolution of precancerous changes. Circulating tumor markers, biological substances either produced by the tumor or released by the host in response to the tumor, have long been used to monitor the efficacy of treatment

(Bosl, 1995). The emerging view of cancer as a genetic disorder has made it possible to identify genetic markers that may associate with malignant transformation. Studies seeking to determine the association between a particular environmental exposure and a specific genetic alteration associated with a given tumor type are ongoing. The hope is that, in the future, it will be possible to identify individuals at risk for the development of cancer before it occurs, as compared with current screening that, in the majority of cases, detects cancers after they have developed (Israel, 1996).

Continued progress in understanding the molecular mechanisms responsible for carcinogenesis and cancer metastases is leading to the development of treatments that selectively target the cellular defects of tumor cells or decrease the cancer cell's ability to survive once it metastasizes. Although such molecular treatment approaches are at a very early stage (see Chapter 13), they do represent the future of cancer therapy. Increasingly, therapeutic approaches will be based on targeting the abnormal processes resulting from genetic mutations and reasserting normal checks and balances that translate into normal cell function (Stass and Mixson, 1997).

Metastases from the primary tumor ultimately cause the death of the host. An understanding of the biology of the metastatic process, however, is only beginning. Researchers have begun to define the process of metastasis and subsequent invasion and to characterize this process into sequential steps. Elucidation of the cellular processes and interactions responsible for each step will provide future avenues for impeding these processes. Potential antimetastasis therapies include prevention of tumor invasion, antiadhesive therapy, modulation of tumor vascularization, anticoagulation therapy, and genetic manipulation (Narod, 1998; Fidler, 1999).

Risk Assessment

To fully implement primary prevention as a means of cancer control, one must be able to identify carcinogenic agents and host factors that make individuals susceptible to developing cancer. In the future, the ability to more specifically determine an individual's risk for developing a particular type of cancer (i.e., low, moderate, or high risk) will become reality. For example, a growing area is the identification of individual traits that may explain why some people are more susceptible than others to the development of cancers after exposure to known carcinogens such as cigarette smoke and ultraviolet light (upper- and lower-respiratory-tract cancers and skin cancers, respectively). Such research may lead to the discovery of biomarkers of inborn and acquired susceptibility to cancer. Genes that determine an individual's response to a carcinogen also fall into this category. Examples include variations in genes that encode a family of enzymes known as cytochrome P450. As a group, these enzymes generally render potential carcinogens harmless by detoxifying a wide range of both internal and external substances. Epidemiologists believe that certain forms of the *CYP1A1* gene, which codes for an enzyme that acts on polycyclic aromatic hydrocarbons, render smokers more susceptible to developing lung cancer. Environmental carcinogenesis resulting from tobacco-smoke exposure is a complex process that can involve activation of procarcinogens that lead to adduct formation and subsequent failure of DNA repair, which should normally remove these adducts. Studies have begun to demonstrate that DNA-repair capacity influences risk for lung cancer among individuals (Amos *et al.*, 1999). It is hoped that advances in molecular epidemiology will refine estimates of cancer risk by considering variations in innate and acquired susceptibility within populations. In reality, however, because of the complex nature of the events leading to the development of cancer, it is reasonable to assume that more than one single event or characteristic will be related to an increased risk for developing cancer (Perera, 1996; Perera, 2000).

Approximately 5% to 10% of all cancers have recognizable familial clusterings. Hereditary mutations, in conjunction with acquired mutations, play a fundamental role in the development of these cancers. These inherited mutations place individuals at a heightened risk for the development of cancer and have important implications for the prevention and detection of cancer. More than 50 types of cancer have demonstrated a familial clustering indicative of inherited predisposition, including colorectal, breast, and ovarian cancer; melanoma; and medullary thyroid cancer (Fraser *et al.*, 1997; Collins, 1999; Rieger, 2000). The recent discovery of genes associated with some of these hereditary cancers has translated into the ability to test for the presence of these genes in individuals, which is known as predisposition genetic testing. Predisposition genetic testing, which represents one of the newest strategies for identifying individuals at increased risk, has limited clinical application at this time. Although technology is rapidly moving forward, a gap exists between our ability to identify those individuals who carry an increased risk and our acquisition of knowledge of the appropriate approaches to reduce the associated mortality and morbidity. The management of hereditary cancer syndromes represents an important focus of future research in the prevention of cancer and hopefully will provide information relevant to the prevention of sporadic forms of cancer.

Chemoprevention

An emerging approach to the management of cancer is strategies designed to prevent the development of cancers. The use of pharmacologic agents that will arrest or reverse the multistage process of cancer development is known as chemoprevention (Greenwald, 1996; Anonymous, 1999). As more is understood about the nature of carcinogenesis, the ability to intervene at the earliest stages is rapidly becoming possible. Recognition that dysplastic lesions (e.g., oral leukoplakia) are biologically significant is a paradigm shift that can lead to the design of effective prevention measures. In addition, study of the intrinsic biological mechanisms that may prevent these lesions from becoming invasive and metastatic can also offer insight into the design of new, effective therapeutic strategies (Sporn and Lippmann, 1997).

Over the last 10 to 15 years, there have been numerous trials to evaluate the effectiveness of various agents in the chemoprevention of cancer. Conceptually, chemoprevention agents may be classified into two basic categories: agents that prevent initiation of the carcinogenic process (i.e., "blocking" agents) and those that prevent further promotion or progression of lesions that have already been established (i.e., "suppressing" agents). In reality, the distinction between these categories is often artificial. The major categories of agents used in the chemoprevention of cancer include the following (Greenwald *et al.*, 1995; Swan and Ford, 1997):

- Retinoids, natural and synthetic analogues of vitamin A
- Estrogen response modifiers (e.g., tamoxifen and raloxifene)
- Deltanoids, natural and synthetic analogues of vitamin D
- Androgen analogues (e.g., finasteride [Proscar])
- Agents that alter ovulation (e.g., oral contraceptives)

- Agents that suppress cell proliferation (e.g., difluoromethylornithine)
- Nonsteroidal anti-inflammatory drugs (e.g., aspirin, ibuprofen, sulindac)
- Agents that protect cells from oxidative stress (e.g., vitamin E)
- Agents that block carcinogens from binding to DNA (e.g., oltipraz and acetylcysteine)

Randomized trials have evaluated the use of chemopreventive agents in the following areas: prevention of solid tumors such as breast, prostate, lung, and colorectal cancers in people at increased risk; reversal of premalignant conditions such as cervical dysplasia, premalignant skin lesions, and oral premalignancies; and prevention of second primary cancers in patients who have had head and neck, lung, or bladder cancers (Sporn and Lippmann, 1997; Swan and Ford, 1997). The Breast Cancer Prevention Trial sponsored by the National Cancer Institute–funded National Surgical Adjuvant Breast and Bowel Project was designed to evaluate the ability of tamoxifen to decrease breast-cancer incidence in women at high risk for developing the disease. The trial was started in 1992 and reached full accrual in 1997. Eligibility for the trial was based on risk for developing breast cancer and was determined by both family history and nongenetic risk factors such as age of menarche, parity, and history of breast biopsies. In April 1998, preliminary results from this trial demonstrated a 49% decreased incidence of breast cancer in women taking tamoxifen versus those taking placebo (Fisher *et al.*, 1998). In 1999, tamoxifen received regulatory approval for the chemoprevention of breast cancer in women with increased risk for developing the disease. The Prostate Cancer Prevention Trial is an intergroup effort in the United States managed by the Southwest Oncology Group in collaboration with the Eastern Cooperative Oncology Group and the Cancer and Leukemia Group B. This 10-year study will achieve its primary end point in October 2004. At the start of the study, 18,882 men over 55 years of age with normal digital rectal examinations and serum prostate-specific antigen levels of less than or equal to 3.0 ng/ml were randomized to take finasteride (5 mg/day) or placebo (1 tablet/day). Newer generation trials will evaluate the use of vitamin E and selenium in the chemoprevention of prostate cancer (Nelson *et al.*, 1999). In December 1999, celecoxib (Celebrex; Searle, Chicago, IL, and Pfizer, New York, NY) received regulatory approval for use in patients with familial adenomatous polyposis to reduce the number of colorectal polyps.

Detection

Through early detection of precancerous lesions or localized and thus manageable cancers, the ability to cure or slow the progress of disease, to prevent complications, to limit disability, and to enhance quality of life would all be maximized (Frank-Stromberg, 1997). Efforts have been made to identify biomarkers that would serve to identify cancer predisposition or the detection of early, premalignant lesions before the development of invasive malignancy. It is anticipated that in the near future, tests will detect biological clues of tissue injury by specific cancer-causing agents or the impending evolution of precancerous changes. A variety of new tumor markers will be discovered that will aid clinicians in the detection of cancer at the earliest possible stage. Lysophosphatidic acid (LPA), a bioactive phosopholipid, is being evaluated as a potential marker to screen for breast and ovarian cancers. (Eder *et al*, 2000).

Studies seeking to determine the association between a particular environmental exposure and a specific genetic alteration associated with a given tumor type are ongoing. For example, new assays based on polymerase chain reaction amplification of genetic material, a sort of molecular photocopier, and sequence-specific

DNA probes can be used to identify oncogene activation and/or loss of tumor-suppressor genes in premalignant lesions or body fluids (Raj *et al.*, 1998). Cells obtained from colonic washing in individuals with adenomatous polyps have been used in assays to detect a mutated *ras* gene. Other studies have utilized stool specimens to detect the presence of K-*ras* mutations as a screening tool for colorectal cancer. Similar studies using sputum and bladder washings in the early detection of head and neck, lung, and bladder cancer have shown promising results. For optimal screening of high-risk populations, assays that use blood and body fluids are desirable because these substances are more readily available than tissue. Protein-based markers are potentially powerful because they are amenable to simple blood tests (e.g., prostate-specific antigen for prostate cancer and CA-125 for ovarian cancer).

It is now becoming possible to assay for oncogene products, tumor-derived growth factors, and genetic alterations in exfoliated cells. The hope is that, in the future, it will be possible to identify individuals at risk for the development of cancer before it occurs, as compared with current screening that, in the majority of cases, detects cancers after they have developed (Israel, 1996). Successful integration of molecular methods for the detection and diagnosis of cancer will require understanding of the accuracy of the marker, technological aspects with regard to the assay used to test for the marker, and the accessibility of material needed to assay for the marker. Once markers are identified, the precise cutoff for accurate detection of clinical disease will need to be determined. Identified molecular changes may not necessarily progress to cancer. Only prospective testing in patients at risk of cancer will empirically identify the critical threshold for accurate detection of the smallest tumors (Cairns and Sidransky, 1999).

This information is also anticipated to have application as a prognostic indicator. A future is envisioned in which oncologists will have the technological tools and information to evaluate a tumor cell, much like a detective dusts for fingerprints. A "molecular fingerprint" of the tumor will be available that can provide clues as to whether a tumor is likely to grow fast or slow or to metastasize and, if so, to where. This type of information will have tremendous implications in how initial therapy for cancer is developed (Kustka, 1998). Some tests are already in clinical use. Matritech NMP22® is a quantitative microplate enzyme immunoassay that can identify bladder cancer patients who are at risk for rapid recurrence or occult disease. The test is performed on a single voided urine sample and is twice as sensitive as urine cytology. The test may ultimately prove useful in identifying those patients who may benefit from more or less aggressive management. NMP22 is a nuclear matrix protein found in human epithelial cells. The majority of patients with bladder cancer release large quantities of NMP22 into their urine (Matritech, 2000).

The Oncor INFOMR™ HER-2/*neu* test has regulatory approval to identify the presence or absence of increased copies of the HER-2/*neu* gene in women with breast cancer. This prognostic indicator is being evaluated for effectiveness in determining whether a breast cancer is likely to return (Press *et al.*, 1997; Oncor, 2000).

Protein-chip technology gives researchers a means of rapid, differential protein-expression analysis to find novel protein disease markers or analyze the effect of drug treatments using biological samples such as serum, urine, or tissue extracts. Ciphergen (Palo Alto, CA) has developed the ProteinChip System to provide this service. At the 1999 meeting of the American Association for Cancer Research, a group from the National Cancer Institute presented a paper on the use of this system. This new technology will ultimately allow for the characterization of proteins associated with specific forms of cancer, from benign to preinvasive to invasive carcinoma, and may reveal potential diagnostic markers to monitor carcinogenic-disease progression as well as potential targets for therapeutic drugs (Paweletz *et al.*, 1999; Ciphergen, 2000).

Treatment

CONTROL OF ABERRANT GENE EXPRESSION

Antisense Therapy

Cancer results from the "turning on" of certain genes and the "turning off" of others. The ability to synthesize natural **oligodeoxynucleotides** (ODNs) through automation presents the possibility of selectively modifying the activity of any given gene. Antisense RNA and DNA are small synthetic ODN chains (oligos) that bind with specific messenger RNAs and can turn off the gene. The principle of this therapy, therefore, involves interference in the process by which the cell expresses its genetic information. The information transfer from DNA to RNA (known as **transcription**) and from RNA to protein (known as **translation**) is disrupted. Theoretically, one could design an antisense oligo to block the function of a proto-oncogene. Although this approach remains at a very early stage, the ability may one day exist to treat certain cancers with antisense oligos that affect genes involved in the formation and progression of tumors and in the metastasis to and invasion of other organs.

Preliminary results of several clinical studies have demonstrated the safety and, to some extent, the efficacy of antisense ODNs in patients with malignant diseases. Clinical response was observed in some patients suffering from ovarian cancer who were treated with antisense targeted against the gene encoding for protein kinase C-α. Some hematological diseases treated with antisense oligos targeted against the *bcr/abl* and the *bcl2 m*RNAs have shown promising clinical response (Kronenwett and Haas, 1998). Antisense therapy has been useful in the treatment of cardiovascular disorders including restenosis after angioplasty, vascular bypass graft occlusion, and transplant coronary vasculopathy. Antisense ODNs also have shown promise as antiviral agents (Galderisi *et al.*, 1999). Key problems to overcome with the application of antisense agents remain cellular uptake and compartmentalization, specificity, and undesired digestion of these ODNs by extracellular and intracellular enzymes (Bennett, 1998).

Triplex Therapy

The triplex approach, known as such because the oligomer winds around the double-stranded helix of DNA to form a triple-stranded helix, blocks transcription. Triplex therapy has not yet entered clinical trials. Before this approach can move from concept to reality, several important constraints must be overcome. Current studies are focusing on solving such problems as induction of binding between the oligonucleotide and the DNA, specificity of binding of the oligonucleotide to the target DNA, stability of the triplex once binding occurs, and specificity (i.e., delivery to tumor but not to normal cells) (Askari and McDonnell, 1996; Chan and Glazer, 1997).

Transcription Factors

Another approach to controlling gene expression would be the use of molecules that suppress inappropriate transcription. These molecules would do so by binding to activator or coactivator proteins and preventing them from attaching to promoter or enhancer regions of DNA and initiating creation of inappropriate RNA transcripts. Currently, the majority of research in this area is focused on identifying and cataloguing transcription factors, but it will soon turn to the development of treatments that act on transcription factors involved in the misexpression of specific proteins (Papavassiliou, 1998).

Ribozymes

Ribozymes provide another approach to blocking translation. This approach is based on the principle that specific RNA structures have the ability to function as enzymes. These RNA enzymes can split RNA. The insertion into cells of genes that code for selected ribozymes could result in the elimination of unwanted RNA strands and, therefore, block the manufacture of unwanted proteins. Ongoing preclinical studies in this area are targeting transcripts for the *bcr-abl* fusion gene, the H-*ras* mutant gene, and aberrant *p53* (James and Gibson, 1998; Macpherson *et al.*, 1999).

CONTROL OF METASTASES

Antiangiogenic Drugs

Tumor neovascularization is established through secretion of angiogenic molecules. The process of angiogenesis consists of a series of interactive events: quiescent endothelial cells are stimulated by angiogenic factors to degrade the underlying basement membrane, to migrate within the interstitial matrix, to proliferate, and to organize themselves into tubular structures that become mature blood vessels. During angiogenesis, the endothelial cells undergo functional changes and show molecular features that are different from those of normal, quiescent endothelium. In normal physiology (e.g., wound healing), this process is finely regulated. Stimulatory and inhibitory factors are in balance, and, simply put, the body knows when to quit. In cancer, this regulatory process is out of balance, and things do not know when to quit. These differences can be exploited to selectively target tumor endothelium and to prevent neovessel formation. Therefore, it appears plausible that inhibition of this process could be a potential anticancer therapy (Fidler, 1999; Folkman, 2000).

Several methods exist for inhibition of pathological angiogenesis. One involves blocking the expression or production of angiogenic factors (e.g., vascular endothelial growth factor and basic fibroblast growth factor) or neutralizing their activity. A second is blocking capillary endothelial cells from responding to angiogenic factors. Natural angiogenesis inhibitors, such as angiostatin, are associated with tumors whereas others, such as platelet factor 4 and IFN-α, are not. Endostatin is a specific inhibitor of endothelial-cell proliferation, migration, and angiogenesis. Clinical studies evaluating several classes of antiangiogenic factors are now in progress to the point where a remarkably diverse group of more than 24 such drugs is currently undergoing evaluation in phase I, II, or III clinical trials (Kerbel, 2000; Libutti and Pluda, 2000).

An example of an angioinhibin is TNP-470, an analogue of fumagillin, an antibiotic derived from the fungus *Aspergillus fumigatus fresenius*. This compound has demonstrated potent inhibition of endothelial-cell growth (Kusaka *et al.*, 1991). Phase I trials evaluating its use in a variety of advanced malignancies are now in progress. Clinical trials of endostatin began in 1999. The drug currently is being tested in phase I clinical trials through Dana-Farber Partners Cancer Care (Boston, MA), The University of Texas M. D. Anderson Cancer Center (Houston, TX), and the University of Wisconsin (Madison, WI). Preliminary data presented at the National Cancer Institute's semiannual phase I progress meeting showed encouraging results regarding the safety of the drug and indicated potential effects of endostatin in cancer patients suffering from progressive disease. Full results will not be available until thorough analysis of data and completion of clinical studies (EntreMed, 2000; Oncology News Today, 2000).

Metalloproteinases

A key characteristic of malignancy is the ability of tumor cells to cross physiologic boundaries and invade normal tissues. Another approach to inhibiting metastasis is to administer inhibitors of proteolytic enzymes (known as matrix metalloproteinases [MMPs]) that cancer cells use to degrade extracellular matrices (i.e., to invade adjacent tissues). Local production of MMPs is implicated in supporting tumor growth, invasion, and angiogenesis. The MMPs are a family of zinc-dependent enzymes that have been divided into five subgroups: collagenases, gelatinases, stromelysins, membrane-type MMPs, and others. Synthetic MMP inhibitors are a new class of investigational therapeutic agents under active investigation to potentially arrest tumor growth, invasion, and metastasis by inhibiting angiogenesis and the degradation of healthy tissue matrix (Nelson *et al.*, 2000).

Several MMP inhibitors are currently in clinical trials. Marimastat (BB-2516) (British Biotech, Inc., Annapolis, MD) is the first MMP inhibitor to enter clinical trials. It is currently under phase III study in combination with chemotherapy in the treatment of small-cell lung cancer and pancreatic and gastric carcinoma (Jones *et al.*, 1999). Phase III clinical trials are under way to evaluate the MMP inhibitor prinomastat (AG3340; Agouron Pharmaceuticals, La Jolla, CA) in combination with the anticancer drugs paclitaxel and carboplatin for the treatment of advanced non-small-cell lung cancer and with mitoxantrone and prednisone for the treatment of hormone-refractory prostate cancer (Shalinsky *et al.*, 1999).

CONTROL OF THE CELL CYCLE

The multistage process of carcinogenesis involves the progressive acquisition of mutations and epigenetic abnormalities in the expression of multiple genes that have highly diverse functions. An important group of these genes is involved in cell-cycle control. Normal cell-cycle progression relies on the cell's ability to translate extracellular signals such as mitogenic stimuli and intact extracellular matrices to efficiently replicate DNA and divide. Normal mechanisms regulating the progression of cells

through the cell cycle include cyclin kinase inhibition; the G_1 restriction point and the retinoblastoma protein (pRb) pathway; accuracy of DNA replication and DNA repair; the G_2 to M transition; apoptosis and the *p53* pathway; proteolytic, in particular ubiquitin-dependent, mechanisms involved in the initiation of DNA synthesis in the separation of sister chromatids; and the telophase to G_0/G_1 transition. Cancer cells evolve in part by overriding normal cell-cycle regulation (McDonald and El-Deiry, 2000).

Many molecular approaches to controlling cellular proliferation revolve around *p53* function. Mutations in *p53* itself have been documented to occur in more than 60% of all cancers (Levine, 1997); *p53* has been denoted as "the guardian" of the genome. When the cell's DNA is damaged, the usual breakdown of p53 ceases and concentrations of p53 begin to build. If the DNA damage is substantial, the cell essentially gives up on the idea of repairing itself and commits suicide. With this choice, *p53* turns on the synthesis of proteins that commit the cell to self-destruction (or apoptosis). If the damage is less severe, then p53 switches on the synthesis of other proteins that, in turn, block the cyclins so that the cell cycle is frozen in place. The cell then has time to repair the damaged DNA before it starts to divide again. If *p53* becomes mutated, as in cancer, it allows for an increase in DNA damage within the cell as well as numerical and structural alterations in chromosomes. Potential therapeutic strategies include development of drugs that mimic the inhibitory effects of p53 protein on cell division; insertion, through gene therapy, of a functional, normal *p53* gene into cells; or use of antisense oligomers to block expression of mutated *p53* (Chang *et al.*, 1995; McCormick, 1999; Tzatsos and Papavassiliou, 1999).

Another important group of molecules include the cyclin-dependent kinases (Cdks). Their function mainly consists of phosphorylating the pRb family of proteins to direct the cell toward a series of events that end in generating two sister cells from one mother cell. The eukaryotic cell cycle is regulated by the periodic synthesis and destruction of cyclins that associate with and activate Cdks. Inhibitors of Cdks, such as p21 and p16, also play important roles in cell-cycle control coordinating internal and external signals and by impeding proliferation at several key checkpoints. Understanding how these proteins interact to regulate the cell cycle has become increasingly important to researchers and clinicians with the discovery that many of the genes that encode cell-cycle regulatory activities are targets for alterations that underlie the development of cancer (Sellers and Kaelin, 1997).

CELL SIGNALING

One strategy impacting cellular proliferation would be to interfere with growth-regulatory signals from the cell surface to the nucleus that regulate cell-cycle progression and proliferation. One potential target is the ras oncoprotein. The normal *ras* genes are critical regulators of numerous physiologic processes. The ras protein serves as a key intermediate in signal-transduction pathways that mediate proliferative and other types of signals, largely from upstream of receptor tyrosine kinases (binding of a growth factor to its receptor) to a downstream cascade of protein kinases. When mutated, the ras protein becomes "locked" in its active state, and continual signals for growth are sent to the nucleus. *Ras* mutations are particularly prevalent in gastrointestinal malignancies such as colorectal and pancreatic cancers.

Farnesylation is a process necessary for biological activation of the ras protein. The protein becomes anchored to the cytoplasmic side of the cell plasma membrane by posttranslational farnesylation of a cysteine residue to a select site on the ras protein. The enzyme that recognizes and farnesylates ras is known as

ras farnesyltransferase (FT). Novel anticancer compounds are being designed that would inhibit the function of the mutated ras protein by interfering at different stages of this process (Qian *et al.*, 1997; Rowinsky, 1999). The goal is to render the ras protein inactive and unable to send signals for growth to the nucleus.

SCH66336 is one of the first FT inhibitors to undergo clinical testing. Adjei *et al.* (2000) recently reported a phase I trial to assess the maximum tolerated dose, toxicities, and biological effectiveness of SCH66336 in inhibiting FT *in vivo*. Twenty patients with solid tumors received 92 courses of escalating SCH66336 doses given orally twice a day (b.i.d.) for 7 days every 3 weeks. Gastrointestinal toxicity (i.e., nausea, vomiting, and diarrhea) and fatigue were dose-limiting at 400 mg of SCH66336 b.i.d. Moderate reversible renal insufficiency, secondary to dehydration from gastrointestinal toxicity, was also seen. Inhibition of prelamin A farnesylation in buccal mucosa cells of patients treated with SCH66336 was demonstrated, confirming that SCH66336 inhibits protein farnesylation *in vivo*. One partial response was observed in a patient with previously treated metastatic non-small-cell lung cancer, who remained on study for 14 months. This study not only established the dose for future testing on this schedule (i.e., 350 mg b.i.d.) but also provides the first evidence of successful inhibition of FT in the clinical setting and the first hint of clinical activity for this class of agents (Adjei *et al.*, 2000).

Additional molecules are being studied that are important in the process of signal transduction, and compounds are being designed to inhibit their activity. Potential targets include inhibitors of tyrosine kinases (Klohs *et al.*, 1997) and protein kinase C. Small molecular inhibitors of the EGF receptor, platelet-derived growth factor receptors (i.e., flk-1/KDR and flt-1), fibroblast growth factor receptor, and src family of tyrosine kinases are under development, with a focused effort to discover tyrosine kinase inhibitors with increased potency, increased selectivity, better pharmacokinetics, and decreased toxicity. Some EGF receptor tyrosine kinases are now in or are about to enter clinical trials as potential anticancer agents. Tyrosine kinases continue to remain an extremely attractive target for the design of potent and selective inhibitors that will represent an important new class of therapeutic agents for a variety of diseases for which current therapy is still insufficient. Potent and selective inhibitors of receptors involved in neovascularization such as fibroblast growth factor receptor, Flk-1, or Flt-1 are less prevalent in the literature, and the discovery of tyrosine kinase inhibitors that can inhibit neovascularization remains a fertile area for drug discovery (Klohs et al., 1997).

One inhibitor of protein kinase C being evaluated is bryostatin 1, a macrocyclic lactone. A phase I study in patients with relapsed non-Hodgkin's lymphoma or chronic lymphocytic leukemia evaluated the maximum-tolerated dose, major toxicities, and possible antitumor activity of bryostatin 1. Generalized myalgia was the dose-limiting toxicity. Eleven of 29 patients achieved stable disease for 2 to 19 months. Future studies will define the precise activity of bryostatin 1 in subsets of patients with lymphoproliferative malignancies and its efficacy in combination with other agents (Varterasian et al., 1998). In a follow-up phase II trial in patients with lymphoma or chronic lymphocytic leukemia, Varterasian et al. (2000) administered bryostatin 1 by a 72-hour continuous infusion every 2 weeks at a dose of 120 mcg/m² per course. In 25 patients, the administration of bryostatin alone resulted in one complete remission and one partial remission. Patients whose disease progressed while receiving bryostatin 1 were eligible to participate in a feasibility study of vincristine administered by bolus intravenous injection immediately

after the completion of the bryostatin 1 infusion. The authors concluded that the addition of vincristine at a dose of 2 mg was feasible and that further study is warranted.

Su101 is a tyrosine kinase inhibitor that interferes with signal transduction by inhibiting platelet-derived growth factor receptor–mediated tyrosine phosphorylation, DNA synthesis, cell-cycle progression, and cellular proliferation. A phase I study in patients with solid tumors by Eckhardt et al. (1999) concluded that Su101 was well tolerated when given as a 24-hour continuous infusion at doses up to 443 mg/m²/week for 4 consecutive weeks every 6 weeks. Further dose escalation was precluded by infusate volume constraints; however, biologically relevant doses were obtained. The authors stated that optimal clinical development of this agent will require the use of novel trial designs and strategies, that is involvement of patients with malignancies in which aberrant cellular proliferation is primarily mediated by platelet-derived growth factor–dependent pathways (Eckhardt et al., 1999; Hudes, 1999).

CELL SENESCENCE

Normal human cells have a limited life span in culture, which is called the Hayflick limit. Cancer cells are known to be immortal; that is, they do not die as normal cells do. Recent studies have indicated that telomere shortening is one of the important meters utilized by cells to determine the Hayflick limit and that activation of a mechanism to maintain telomere length is essential for cells to become immortal. Normal human cells undergo a finite number of cell divisions and ultimately enter a nondividing state called replicative senescence. The proposed mechanism for this "molecular clock" that triggers senescence is telomere shortening. It is generally believed that cells must have a means to maintain telomeres to progress to malignancy. Most cancers do this by activating an enzyme called telomerase, which adds telomeric repeats to the telomere ends. Recently, expression of this enzyme has been shown to extend the life span of cells. Recent and future advances in the telomerase field may lead to better diagnostic and treatment protocols for many different cancer types. The development of anti-telomerase therapies will be an active area of investigation. However, certain critical questions must be answered before this strategy can be applied: Which normal cells manufacture telomerase? What is the importance of telomerase to those cells? Cells may have other mechanisms that compensate forthe loss of telomerase, and such "telomere-salvaging pathways," which could negate anti-telomerase therapies, have to be identified (Burger *et al.*, 1997; Shay, 1997; Klingelhutz, 1999). Such discoveries may be facilitated by recent regulatory approval of the TRAPeze® ELISA telomerase-detection kit (Intergen Company, Purchase, NY), a rapid enzyme-linked immunosorbent assay used to detect telomerase activity in cell or tissue extracts that may have implications for cancer diagnosis and prognostics (Hirose *et al.*, 1997; Anonymous, 1998; Bodnar *et al.*, 1998; Intergen Company Website, 2000).

A second mechanism of cell death is that of apoptosis. In this process, cells that have become superfluous or disordered will self-destruct. For example, cells that have incurred significant genetic damage generally initiate this process of "cell suicide" so that the genetic damage is not perpetuated. Apoptosis is a process distinct from necrotic cell death, which occurs when a cell is severely injured. Swelling is a defining feature of necrosis. In apoptosis, very different changes are seen. First, there is no swelling; instead, the dying cell shrinks and pulls away from its neighbors. The nucleus is dramatically changed, with chromatin condensing into one or more distinct blobs near the nuclear envelope. Apoptotic cells are then ingested by scavenger cells that reside in all tissues. Cells that are not consumed come apart and divide into a number of apoptotic bodies that contain pieces of the nucleus. Cancer cells neglect to sacrifice themselves on cue; that is, they seem unable to die. In many tumors, genetic damage apparently fails to induce apoptosis because the cells have inactivated genes involved in the apoptotic process (e.g., *p53* or *bcl-2*).

Finally, it is now well documented that most cytotoxic anticancer agents induce apoptosis, raising the intriguing possibility that defects in apoptotic programs contribute to treatment failure. This expanding body of knowledge related to apoptosis and cancer has allowed for the development of therapeutic strategies aimed at restoring apoptosis in cancer cells. Examples are blocking *bcl-2* expression with antisense oligonucleotides and introducing apoptosis inducers such as wild-type *p53* into cells via liposomes or viral vectors (Duke *et al.*, 1996; Lotem and Sachs, 1996; Shiff and Rigas, 1997; Lowe and Lin, 2000).

Biological Agents in Other Diseases

As an understanding of the pathophysiology of a variety of disease states such as autoimmune diseases, sepsis, and organ rejection following transplantation has unfolded, so have novel therapies emerged in the treatments of these conditions. The administration of biological agents or strategies to suppress the effects of proinflammatory cytokines represents an examples of such strategies. The use of MABs in the treatment of organ rejection or rheumatoid arthritis was described in Chapter 9 and represents a prime example of such therapies.

The biological therapy of sepsis provides another example. The role of IL-1 as a mediator during severe bacterial infection or septic shock has been supported by numerous studies (see Chapter 6). Clinical trials with experimental immunotherapeutic agents (e.g., MABs targeted toward the IL-1 receptor) for severe sepsis and septic shock have been largely unsuccessful, despite seemingly convincing preclinical evidence of significant benefits of these antisepsis therapies. Lessons learned from past failures should provide insights into the design and implementation of successful clinical trials for new antisepsis agents in the future (Maini and Taylor, 2000).

Wound healing is a complex process that, in most cases, leads to complete healing of the wound. The three phases of wound-healing have been described as the inflammatory phase, which begins immediately and lasts for 2 to 5 days; the proliferation phase, which lasts from 2 days to 3 weeks; and the remodeling phase, which can last as long as 2 years (Stadelmann *et al.*, 1998). In some patients, impediments to effective wound healing exist, such as in diabetics or those with venous leg ulcers. Application of the pathophysiology of wounds and the role of growth factors in all three phases of this process have led to the novel new treatments to improve wound healing.

Platelet-derived growth factor can now be produced by recombinant-DNA technology. Becaplermin gel (Regranex®, Ortho McNeil Pharmaceutical, Raritan, NJ) has now received regulatory approval for the treatment of lower-extremity diabetic neuropathic ulcers that extend into the subcutaneous tissue or beyond and have an adequate blood supply. Clinical trials have demonstrated its effectiveness in conjunction with good ulcer-care practice in complete healing of diabetic ulcers (Smiell *et al.*, 1999). In the future, several growth factors may be used in combination to treat chronic ulcers (Kunimoto, 1999).

Conclusion

Advances in molecular biology have essentially made the human genome available as a source of potentially therapeutic biological agents (Oldham, 1998b; Russell and Clarke, 1999). Constant discovery of new agents and the refinement of molecules through genetic-engineering techniques will continue to provide new therapeutic avenues. The "molecularization of medicine" has led to a more thorough understanding of the molecular basis of disease and disease pathogenesis. This has led in turn to the development of recombinant proteins, derived from nature's medicine chest, for the treatment of disease. Within this context, a more complete understanding of the biology of cancer will lead to increasingly selective therapy and ultimately to repair of underlying cellular defects. Gene therapy is one aspect of this potential that continues to grow, with the number of new strategies and protocols increasing at an exponential rate.

Yet, despite this promising growth, there are reasons for concern about the future of these therapies. One of the primary concerns is that of costs for development and the dilemma of who will pay these costs. What roles should the government, pharmaceutical companies, and the consumer play in realizing the usefulness of this new technology?

Another concern is the time-consuming product-development process (see Chapter 4). Oldham (1998b) pointed out the need to develop a new paradigm for the development and licensing of new biological agents. He argued that because biotherapy works through the body's physiologic mechanisms and cellular receptors in a manner that is different from that of chemotherapeutic agents, different evaluative methods are required. Biological agents such as IFN, believed in the 1970s to be the "magic bullet" for curing cancer, are now beginning to be used in a more rational manner. For example, after 2 decades of clinical research, there now appears to be a better understanding of IFN's effects and of how to combine IFN with other treatment modalities for an improved therapeutic outcome. The cost of discovering these optimal therapeutic strategies for other biological agents could be prohibitive unless new methods for development of biotherapy are created. In the future, there may be more potentially valuable biological agents than means to develop them into approved treatments, so priorities will have to be determined. Finding a balance among the cost of development, the potential treatment value of an agent, and the needs of the patient will be the challenge in the next decade.

The future of clinical cancer research as a viable entity must be ensured. The bridge to the new millennium requires a strong clinical-research infrastructure, built by attracting the brightest and most energetic physician/scientists to the field of cancer research and by maintaining adequate funding. In conjunction with the translation of basic science research into clinical practice ("bench to bedside"), the flow of knowledge from the bedside to the bench must also occur. Attention to infrastructure is a must to realize effective cancer control (Freireich, 1997).

The next 20 years will represent one of the most exciting eras in the management of cancer as the secrets of its causes are unlocked. The ability to determine the cellular defect for a given cancer and then to design effective therapy may one day become reality. Biotherapy has the potential to be a part of this revolution. Nurses caring for patients receiving biotherapy will be continually challenged to remain abreast of changes in a rapidly expanding field and to chart new territory in developing strategies of care for these patients through clinical practice and research.

References

Adjei, A., Erlichman, C., Davis, J., *et al.* 2000. Phase I trial of the farnesyltransferase inhibitor SCH66336: Evidence for biological and clinical activity. *Cancer Research* 60(7): 1871–1877.

Agouron Pharmaceuticals. 2000. Available at *http//www.agouron.com.* Accessed June 1, 2000.

Alberts, D. 1999. A unifying vision of cancer therapy for the 21st century. *Journal of Clinical Oncology* 17(11 suppl): 13–21.

Allen, T. 1998. Liposomal drug formulations: Rationale for development and what we can expect for the future. *Drugs* 56: 747–756.

Amos, C., Xu, W., and Spitz, M. 1999. Is there a genetic basis for lung cancer susceptibility? *Recent Results in Cancer Research* 151: 3–12.

Anonymous. 1999. Prevention of cancer in the next millennium: Report of the Chemoprevention Working Group to the American Association for Cancer Research. *Cancer Research* 59: 4743–4758.

Askari, F., and McDonnell, W. 1996. Antisense-oligonucleotide therapy. *New England Journal of Medicine* 334: 316–318.

Bagel, J., Garland, W., Breneman, D., *et al.* 1998. Administration of DAB389IL-2 to patients with recalcitrant psoriasis: A double-blind, phase II multicenter trial. *Journal of the American Academy of Dermatology* 38: 938–944.

Balkwill, F. 1989. Cytokines in Cancer Therapy. New York, NY: Oxford University Press.

Bangham, A., Hill, M., and Miller, N. 1974. Preparation and use of liposomes as models of biological membranes. In Korn, E. (ed). *Methods in Membrane Biology.* New York, NY: Plenum Publishing Corporation, vol. 1, pp. 1–68.

Bennett, C. 1998. Antisense oligonucleotides: Is the glass half full or half empty? *Biochemical Pharmacology* 55: 9–19.

Bodnar, A.G., Ouellette, M., Frolkis, M., *et al.* 1998. Extension of life span by introduction of telomerase into normal human cells. *Science* 279 (5349): 349–352.

Bosl, G. 1995. Circulating tumor markers. In MacDonald, J., Haller, D., and Mayer, R. (eds). *Manual of Oncologic Therapeutics.* Philadelphia, PA: J.B. Lippincott, pp. 49–54.

Bukowski, R. 2000. Cytokine combinations: Therapeutic use in patients with advanced renal-cell carcinoma. *Seminars in Oncology* 27: 204–212.

Burger, A., Bibby, M., and Double, J. 1997. Telomerase activity in normal and malignant mammalian tissues: Feasibility of telomerase as a target for cancer chemotherapy. *British Journal of Cancer* 75: 516–522.

Cairns, P., and Sidransky, D. 1999. Molecular methods for the diagnosis of cancer. *Biochimica et Biophysica Acta* 1423(2): C11–C18.

Cannistra, S. 1997. "Cancer defeated": Not if, but when—Introducing the Biology of Neoplasia series. *Journal of Clinical Oncology* 15: 3297–3298.

Cao, Y., and Suresh, M. 1998. Bispecific antibodies as novel bioconjugates. *Bioconjugate Chemistry* 9: 635–644.

Chan, P., and Glazer, P. 1997. Triplex DNA: Fundamentals, advances, and potential applications for gene therapy. *Journal of Molecular Medicine* 75: 267–282.

Chang, F., Syrjanen, S., and Syrjanen, K. 1995. Implications of the *p53* tumor-suppressor gene in clinical oncology. *Journal of Clinical Oncology* 13: 1009–1022.

Ciphergen. 2000. Available at *http://www.ciphergen.com.* Accessed June 1, 2000.

Cobb, P., LeMaistre, C., and Jackson, L. 1991. Clinical evaluation of immunotoxins. *Cancer Bulletin* 43(3): 233–239.

Collins, F., and Jenkins, J. 1997. Implications of the Human Genome Project for the nursing profession. In Lashley, F. (ed). *The Genetic Revolution: Implications for Nursing.* Washington, DC: American Academy of Nursing, pp. 9–13.

Collins, F. 1999. The Human Genome Project and the future of medicine. *Annals of the New York Academy of Sciences* 882: 42–55 (discussion, pp. 56–65).

Collins, F., Patrino, A., Jordan, E., et al. 1998. New goals for the Human Genome Project 1998–2003. *Science* 282: 682–689.

Cortes, J., O'Brien, S., Estey, E., et al. 1999. Phase I study of liposomal daunorubicin in patients with acute leukemia. *Investigational New Drugs* 17(1): 81–97.

Creaven, P., Cowens, J., Brenner, D., et al. 1990. Initial clinical trial of the macrophage activator muramyl tripeptide-phosphatidylethanolamine encapsulated in liposomes in patients with advanced cancer. *Journal of Biological Response Modifiers* 9(5): 429–498.

Derynck, R., Goeddel, D., Ullrich, A., et al. 1987. Synthesis of messenger RNAs for transforming growth factors α and β and the epidermal growth factor receptor by human tumors. *Cancer Research* 47: 707–712.

Devalaraja, M., and Richmond, A. 1999. Multiple chemotactic factors: Fine control or redundancy? *Trends in Pharmacological Sciences* 20: 151–156.

Dinant, H., and Dijkmans, B. 1999. New therapeutic targets for rheumatoid arthritis. *Pharmacy World and Science* 21: 49–59.

Dinarello, C. 1998. Interleukin-1, interleukin-1 receptors and interleukin-1 receptor antagonist. *International Reviews of Immunology* 16: 457–499.

Duke, R., Ojcius, D., and Young, J. 1996. Cell suicide in health and disease. *Scientific American* 275: 80–87.

Duncan, R., and Spreafico, F. 1994. Polymer conjugates: Pharmacokinetic considerations for design and development. *Clinical Pharmacokinetics* 27(4): 290–306.

Eckhardt, S., Rizzo, J., Sweeney, K., et al. 1999. Phase I and pharmacologic study of the tyrosine-kinase inhibitor SU101 in patients with advanced solid tumors. *Journal of Clinical Oncology* 17(4): 1095–1104.

Eder, A.M., Sasaqawa, T., MGO, M., et al. 2000. Constitutive and lysophosphatidic acid (LPA)-induced LPA production: Role of Phospholipase D and phospholipase A2. *Clinical Cancer Research* 6(6): 2482–2491.

EntreMed. 2000. Available at *http//www.entremed.com.* Accessed June 1, 2000.

Evans, W., and Relling, M. 1999. Pharmacogenomics: Translating functional genomics into rational therapeutics. *Science* 286: 487–491.

Fidler, I. 1992. Therapy of disseminated melanoma

by liposome-activated macrophages. *World Journal of Surgery* 16: 270–276.

Fidler, I. 1999. Critical determinants of cancer metastasis: Rationale for therapy. *Cancer Chemotherapy and Pharmacology* 43(suppl): S3–S10.

Fisher, B., Costantino, J., Wickerham, D., *et al.* 1998. Tamoxifen for prevention of breast cancer: Report of the National Surgical Adjuvant Breast and Bowel Project P-1 Study. *Journal of the National Cancer Institute* 90: 1371–1388.

Folkman, J. 2000. Tumor angiogenesis. In Bast, R., Kufe, D., Pollock, R., Weischelbaum, R., Holland, J., and Frei, E. (eds). *Cancer Medicine*, 5th edn. Hamilton, Ontario: B. C. Decker, Inc., pp. 132–152.

Foss, F., Saleh, M., and Krueger, J., *et al.* 1998. Diphtheria toxin fusion proteins. *Current Topics in Microbiology and Immunology* 234: 63–81.

Frank-Stromberg, M. 1997. Cancer screening and early detection. In Varricchio, C., Pierce, M., Walker, C., *et al.* (eds). *A Cancer Source Book for Nurses*. Atlanta, GA: American Cancer Society, pp. 43–55.

Fraser, M., Calzone, K., and Goldstein, A. 1997. Familial cancers: Evolving challenges for nursing practice. In Hubbard, S.M., Goodman, M., and Knobf, M.T. (eds). *Oncology Nursing Updates*. Cedar Knolls, NJ: Lippincott-Raven Healthcare, 4(3): 1–18.

Freireich, E. 1997. The future of clinical cancer research in the next millennium. *Clinical Cancer Research* 3: 2563–2570.

Galderisi, U., Cascino, A., and Giordano, A. 1999. Antisense oligonucleotides as therapeutic agents. *Journal of Cellular Physiology* 181: 251–257.

Golab, J., and Zagozdzon, R. 1999. Antitumor effects of interleukin-12 in preclinical and early clinical studies (review). *International Journal of Molecular Medicine* 3: 537–544.

Greenwald, P. 1996. Chemoprevention of cancer. *Scientific American* 275: 96–99.

Greenwald, P., Kelloff, G., and Burch-Whitman, C. 1995. Chemoprevention. *CA: A Cancer Journal for Clinicians* 45: 31–49.

Hartmann, F., Renner, C., and Jung, W. 1998. Anti-CD16/CD30 bispecific antibodies as possible treatment for refractory Hodgkin's disease. *Leukemia and Lymphoma* 31: 385–392.

Hellman, S. 1998. The first century of cancer chemotherapy (editorial). *Journal of Clinical Oncology* 16(7): 2295–2296.

Hershey, P. 1999. Impediments to successful immunotherapy. *Pharmacology & Therapeutics* 81(2): 111–119.

Hess, P., and Cooper, D. 1999. Impact of pharmacogenomics on the clinical laboratory. *Molecular Diagnosis* 4: 289–298.

Hirose, M., Abe-Hashimoto, J., Ogura, K., *et al.* 1997. A rapid, useful and quantitative method to measure telomerase activity by hybridization protection assay connected with a telomeric repeat amplification protocol. *Journal of Cancer Research and Clinical Oncology* 123: 337–344.

Hoffman, D., Gitlitz, B., Belldegrun, A., *et al.* 2000. Adoptive cellular therapy. *Seminars in Oncology* 27: 221–233.

Hudes, G. 1999. Signaling inhibitors in the clinic: New agents and new challenges (editorial). *Journal of Clinical Oncology* 17(4): 1093–1094.

Intergen Company. 2000. Available at *http://www.intergenco.com/locations.html*. Accessed June 1, 2000.

Israel, M. 1996. Molecular genetics in the management of patients with cancer. In Bishop, M., and Weinberg, R. (eds). *Scientific American Molecular Oncology*. New York, NY: Scientific American, Inc., pp. 205–237.

James, H., and Gibson, I. 1998. The therapeutic potential of ribozymes. *Blood* 91: 371–382.

Jarvis, B., and Faulds, D. 1999. Etanercept: A review of its use in rheumatoid arthritis. *Drugs* 57: 945–966.

Johnston, E., Crawford, J., Blackwell, S., *et al.* 2000. Randomized, dose-escalation study of SD/01 compared with daily filgrastim in patients receiving chemotherapy. *Journal of Clinical Oncology* 18(13): 2522–2528.

Jones, L., Ghaneh, P., Humphreys, M., *et al.* 1999. The matrix metalloproteinases and their inhibitors in the treatment of pancreatic cancer. *Annals of the New York Academy of Sciences* 880: 288–307.

Kerbel, R. 2000. Tumor angiogenesis: Past, present and the near future. *Carcinogenesis* 21(3): 505–515.

Kleinerman, E., Gano, J., Johnston, D., *et al.* 1995. Efficacy of liposomal muramyl tripeptide (CGP 19835A) in the treatment of relapsed osteosarcoma. *American Journal of Clinical Oncology* 18: 93–99.

Klingelhutz, A. 1999. The roles of telomeres and telomerase in cellular immortalization and the development of cancer. *Anticancer Research* 19: 4823–4830.

Klohs, W., Fry, D., and Kraker, A. 1997. Inhibitors of tyrosine kinase. *Current Opinion in Oncology* 9: 562–568.

Kronenwett, R., and Haas, R. 1998. Antisense strategies for the treatment of hematological malignancies and solid tumors. *Annals of Hematology* 77: 1–12.

Kuhlmann, J. 1999. Alternative strategies in drug development: Clinical pharmacological aspects. *International Journal of Clinical Pharmacology and Therapeutics* 37: 575–583.

Kunimoto, B. 1999. Growth factors in wound healing: The next great innovation? *Ostomy Wound Management* 45(8): 56–64.

Kusaka, M., Sudo, K., Fujita, T., *et al.* 1991. Potent antiangiogenic action of AGM-1470: Comparison to the fumafillin parent. *Biochemistry and Biophysics Research Communication* 174: 1070–1076.

Kustka, B. 1998. Molecular diagnostics takes one small step forward. *Journal of the National Cancer Institute* 90(8): 564–565.

Lautersztain, J., Perez-Soler, R., Khokhar, A., *et al.* 1986. Pharmacokinetics and tissue distribution of liposome-encapsulated *cis*-bis-*N*-decycliminodi-acetato-1,2-diaminocyclohexane-platinum (II). *Cancer Chemotherapy and Pharmacology* 18: 93–97.

Lebel-Binay, S., Berger, A., Zinzindohoue, F., *et al.* 2000. Interleukin-18: Biological properties and clinical implications. *European Cytokine Network* 11(1): 15–26.

LeMaistre, C., Saleh, M., Kuzel, T., *et al.* 1998. Phase I trial of a ligand fusion-protein (DAB389IL-2) in lymphomas expressing the receptor for interleukin-2. *Blood* 91: 399–405.

Levine, A. 1997. *p53*, the cellular gatekeeper for growth and division. *Cell* 88: 323–331.

Leyland-Jones, B. 1993. Targeted drug delivery. *Seminars in Oncology* 20: 12–17.

Libutti, S., and Pluda, J. 2000. Antiangiogenesis: Clinical applications. In Rosenberg, S.A. (ed). *Principles and Practice of the Biologic Therapy of Cancer*, 3rd edn. Philadelphia, PA: Lippincott, Williams, and Wilkins, pp. 844–863.

Ligand Pharmaceuticals. 1999. Ontak® package insert. San Diego, CA: Ligand Pharmaceuticals.

Lopes de Menezes, D., Pilarski, L., and Allen, T. 1999. *In vitro* and *in vivo* targeting of immunoliposomal doxorubicin to human B-cell lymphoma. *Cancer Research* 58(15): 3320–3330.

Lopez-Berestein, G. 1985. Prospects for liposomes as a novel-drug delivery system. *Cancer Bulletin* 37(4): 203–206.

Lopez-Berestein, G. 1987. Liposomes as carriers of antimicrobial agents. *Antimicrobial Agents and Chemotherapy* 31(5): 675–678.

Lopez-Berestein, G., Bodey, G., Fainstein, V., *et al.* 1989. Treatment of systemic fungal infections with liposomal amphotericin B. *Archives of Internal Medicine* 149: 2533–2536.

Lotem, J., and Sachs, L. 1996. Control of apoptosis in hematopoiesis and leukemia by cytokines, tumor suppressors, and oncogenes. *Leukemia* 10: 925–931.

Lowe, S., and Lin, A. 2000. Apoptosis in cancer. *Carcinogenesis* 21: 485–495.

Macpherson, J., Ely, J., Sun, L., *et al.* 1999. Ribozymes in gene therapy of HIV-1. *Frontiers in Bioscience* 4: D497–505.

Maini, R., and Taylor, P. 2000. Anti-cytokine therapy for rheumatoid arthritis. *Annual Review of Medicine* 51: 207–229.

Mangi, M., and Newland, A. 1999. Interleukin-3 in hematology and oncology: Current state of knowledge and future directions. *Cytokines, Cellular & Molecular Therapy* 5: 87–95.

Maslak, P., and Nimer, S. 1998. The efficacy of IL-3, SCF, IL-6, and IL-11 in treating thrombocytopenia. *Seminars in Hematology* 35: 253–260.

Matritech. 2000. Available at *http://www.matritech. com.* Accessed June 1, 2000.

Maxygen. 2000. Available at *http://www.maxygen.- com.* Accessed June 1, 2000.

McCormick, F. 1999. Cancer therapy based on *p53*. *Cancer Journal from Scientific American* 5: 139–144.

McDonald, E., and El-Deiry, W. 2000. Cell cycle control as a basis for cancer drug development (review). *International Journal of Oncology* 16(5): 871–886.

Moreland, L. 1998. Soluble tumor necrosis factor receptor (p75) fusion protein (ENBREL) as a therapy for rheumatoid arthritis. *Rheumatic Diseases Clinics of North America* 24: 579–591.

Murphy, P., Baggiolini, M., Charo, I., *et al.* 2000. International union of pharmacology. XXII. Nomenclature for chemokine receptors. *Pharmacological Reviews* 52: 145–176.

Murray, J. 1991. Current clinical applications of monoclonal antibodies. *Cancer Bulletin* 43(2): 152–162.

Murray, J., Kleinerman, E., Tatom, J., *et al.* 1989. Phase I trial of liposomal muramyl tripeptide phosphatidylethanolamine in cancer patients. *Journal of Clinical Oncology* 7(12): 1915–1925.

Narod, S. 1998. Cancer genetics '98: Host susceptibility to cancer progression. *American Journal of Human Genetics* 63: 1–5.

Nelson, A., Fingleton, B., Rothenberg, M., *et al.*

2000. Matrix metalloproteinases: Biological activity and clinical implications. *Journal of Clinical Oncology* 18(5): 1135–1149.

Nelson, M., Porterfield, B., Jacobs, E., *et al.* 1999. Selenium and prostate cancer prevention. *Seminars in Urologic Oncology* 17: 91–96.

O'Dell, J. 1999. Anticytokine therapy—A new era in the treatment of rheumatoid arthritis? *New England Journal of Medicine* 340: 310–312.

Oldham, R. 1998a. Cancer biotherapy: General principles. In Oldham, R. (ed). *Principles of Cancer Biotherapy*, 3rd edn. Dordrecht, The Netherlands: Kluwer Academic Publishers, pp. 1–15.

Oldham, R. 1998b. Speculations for 2000 and beyond. In Oldham, R. (ed). *Principles of Cancer Biotherapy*, 3rd edn. Dordrecht, The Netherlands: Kluwer Academic Publishers, pp. 493–497.

Olsen, E., Duvic, M., Martin, A., *et al.* 1998. Pivotal phase III trial of two dose levels of DAB_{389} IL-2 (Ontak®) for the treatment of cutaneous T-cell lymphoma (CTCL) (abstract). *Journal of Investigative Dermatology* 11: 678.

Oncology News Today. Low-dose endostatin therapy discussed. Available at *http://www. cancernetwork. com.* Accessed June 1, 2000.

Oncor. 2000. Available at *http://www.oncor.com.* Accessed June 1, 2000.

Oppenheim, J., Murphy, W., Chertox, O., *et al.* 1997. Prospects for cytokine and chemokine biotherapy. *Clinical Cancer Research* 3: 2682–2686.

Papavassiliou, A. 1998. Transcription-factor-modulating agents: Precision and selectivity in drug design. *Molecular Medicine Today* 4: 358–366.

Paweletz, C., Ornstein, D., Gillespie, J., *et al.* 1999. A novel, proteomic approach to monitor carcinogenic disease progression using surface-enhanced desorption ionization spectroscopy (SELDI) of laser capture microdissection (LCM)-derived cells from cancer tissue (abstract). *Proceedings of the American Association of Cancer Research* 40: Abstract #2717.

Perera, F. 1996. Uncovering new clues to cancer risk. *Scientific American* 274: 54–62.

Perera, F. 2000. Molecular epidemiology: On the path to prevention? *Journal of the National Cancer Institute* 92: 602–612.

Press, M., Bernstein, L., Thomas, P., *et al.* 1997. HER-2/*neu* gene amplification characterized by fluorescence *in situ* hybridization: Poor prognosis in node-negative breast carcinomas. *Journal of Clinical Oncology* 15(8): 2894–2904.

Qian, Y., Sebti, S., and Hamilton, A. 1997. Farnesyl-transferase as a target for anticancer drug design. *Biopolymers* 43: 25–41.

Raj, G., Moreno, J., and Gomella, L. 1998. Utilization of polymerase chain-reaction technology in the detection of solid tumors. *Cancer* 82: 1419–1442.

Rieger, P.T. 2000. Counseling on genetic risk for cancer. In Yarbro, C., Hansen-Frogge, M., Goodman, M., *et al.* (eds). *Cancer Nursing: Principles and Practice*, 5th edn. Sudbury, MA: Jones & Bartlett Publishers, Inc., pp. 189–213.

Rieger, P.T. (in press). The impact of genetic information in the management of cancer. In Calzone, K.A., Jenkins, J., Masny, A., and Strauss-Tranin, A. *Recommendations for Cancer Genetics in Nursing Practice and Education.* Pittsburgh, PA: Oncology Nursing Press.

Rowinsky, E., Windle, J., and Von Hoff, D. 1999. Ras protein farnesyltransferase: A strategic target for anticancer therapeutic development. Biology of neoplasia series. *Journal of Clinical Oncology* 17(11): 3631–3652.

Russell, C., and Clarke, L. 1999. Recombinant proteins for genetic disease. *Clinical Genetics* 55: 389–394.

Rust, D., and Jameson, G. 1998. The novel lipid delivery system of amphotericin B: Drug profile and relevance to clinical practice. *Oncology Nursing Forum* 25(1): 35–48.

Schreiber, S. 2000. Target-oriented and diversity-oriented organic synthesis in drug discovery. *Science* 287(5460): 1964–1969.

Sellers, W., and Kaelin, W. 1997. Role of the retinoblastoma protein in the pathogenesis of human cancer. *Journal of Clinical Oncology* 15: 3301–3312.

Shalinsky, D., Brekken, J., Zou, H., *et al.* 1999. Broad antitumor and antiangiogenic activities of AG3340, a potent and selective MMP inhibitor undergoing advanced oncology clinical trials. *Annals of the New York Academy of Sciences* 878: 236–270.

Shay, J.W. 1997. Telomerase in human development and cancer. *Journal of Cell Physiology* 173(2): 266–270.

Shi, M., Bleavins, M., and de la Iglesia, F. 1999. Technologies for detecting genetic polymorphisms in pharmacogenomics. *Molecular Diagnostics* 4: 343–351.

Shiff, S., and Rigas, B. 1997. Nonsteroidal anti-inflammatory drugs and colorectal cancer: Evolving concepts of their chemopreventive actions. *Gastroenterology* 113: 1992–1998.

Smiell, J., Wieman, T., Steed, D., *et al.* 1999. Efficacy and safety of becaplermin (recombinant human platelet-derived growth factor-BB) in patients with nonhealing, lower-extremity diabetic ulcers: A combined analysis of four randomized studies. *Wound Repair and Regeneration* 7: 335–346.

Sporn, M., and Lippmann, S. 1997. Chemoprevention of cancer. In Holland, J., Bast, R., Morton, D., *et al.* (eds). *Cancer Medicine*, vol. 4. Baltimore, MD: Williams & Wilkins, pp. 495–508.

Stadelmann, W., Digenis, A., and Tobin, G. 1998. Impediments to wound-healing. *American Journal of Surgery* 176: 39S–47S.

Stass, S., and Mixson, J. 1997. Oncogenes and tumor suppressor genes: Therapeutic implications. *Clinical Cancer Research* 3: 2687–2695.

Swan, D., and Ford, B. 1997. Chemoprevention of cancer: Review of the literature. *Oncology Nursing Forum* 24: 719–727.

Tzatsos, A., and Papavassiliou, A. 1999. Molecular "rehabilitation" by rational drug targeting: The challenge of p53 in cancer treatment. *Anticancer Research* 19: 4353–4356.

Varterasian, M., Mohammad, R., Eilender, D., *et al.* 1998. Phase I study of bryostatin 1 in patients with relapsed non-Hodgkin's lymphoma and chronic lymphocytic leukemia. *Journal of Clinical Oncology* 16(1): 56–62.

Varterasian, M., Mohammad, R., Shurafa, M., *et al.* 2000. Phase II trial of bryostatin 1 in patients with relapsed low-grade non-Hodgkin's lymphoma and chronic lymphocytic leukemia. *Clinical Cancer Research* 6(3): 825–828.

Weinblatt, M., Kremer, J., Bankhurst, A., *et al.* 1999. A trial of etanercept, a recombinant tumor necrosis factor receptor:Fc fusion protein, in patients with rheumatoid arthritis receiving methotrexate (see comments). *New England Journal of Medicine* 340: 253–259.

Wells, A. 1999. EGF receptor. *International Journal of Biochemistry and Cell Biology* 31: 637–643.

Key References

Alberts, D. 1999. A unifying vision of cancer therapy for the 21st century. *Journal of Clinical Oncology* 17(11 suppl): 13–21.

Bast, R.C., Kufe, D.W., Pollock, R.E., Weichselbaum, R.R., Holland, J.F., and Frei, E. (eds). 2000. *Cancer Medicine*, 5th edn. Hamilton, Ontario: B.C. Decker, Inc.

Cannistra, S. 1997. "Cancer defeated": Not if, but when—Introducing the Biology of Neoplasia series. *Journal of Clinical Oncology* 15: 3297–3298.

Collins, F., and Jenkins, J. 1997. Implications of the human genome project for the nursing profession. In Lashley, F. (ed). *The Genetic Revolution: Implications for Nursing*. Washington, DC: American Academy of Nursing, pp. 9–13.

Collins, F. 1999. The human genome project and the future of medicine. *Annals of the New York Academy of Sciences* 882: 42–55 (discussion, pp. 56–65).

Collins, F., Patrino, A., Jordan, E., et al. 1998. New goals for the Human Genome Project 1998–2003. *Science* 282: 682–689.

Johnston, E., Crawford, J., Blackwell, S., et al. 2000. Randomized, Dose-Escalation Study of SD/01 Compared With Daily Filgrastim in Patients Receiving Chemotherapy. *Journal of Clinical Oncology* 18(13): 2522–2528.

Meyerson, M. 2000. Role of Telomerase in Normal and Cancer Cells. *Journal of Clinical Oncology* 18(13): 2626–2634.

Oldham, R. 1998. Speculations for 2000 and beyond. In Oldham, R. (ed). *Principles of Cancer Biotherapy*, 3rd edn. Dordrecht, The Netherlands: Kluwer Academic Publishers, pp. 493–497.

Rosenberg, S.A. (ed). 2000. *Principles and Practice of the Biologic Therapy of Cancer*, 3rd edn. Philadelphia, PA: Lippincott Williams and Wilkins.

Seminara, D. (ed). 1999. Innovative Study Designs and Analytic Approaches to the Genetic Epidemiology of Cancer. *Journal of the National Cancer Institute Monographs*, Number 26. Oxford, England: Oxford University Press.

Talpaz, M., Sawyers, C., Kantarjian, H., et al. 2000. Activity of an ABL specific tyrosine kinase inhibitor in patients with BCR-ABL positive acute leukemias, including chronic myelogenous leukemia in blast crisis. *Proceedings of the American Society of Clinical Oncology* 19: abstract #6.

Yarbro, C.H. (ed). 2000. Cancer nursing in the 21st century. *Seminars in Oncology Nursing* 16(1): 1–84.

Zajtchuk, R. 1999. New technologies in medicine: Biotechnology and nanotechnology. *Disease-a-Month* 45(11): 451–495.

APPENDIX A

Biotherapy Care Pathway Advocate Health Care

Patient's Name: _____

Date of Admission: _____ 　　　　　Attending Physician: _____

Components	Day 1	Day 2	Day 3	Day 4	Day 5	Outcomes Day 6/Discharge
Date						
Outcomes	☐ Pt's temperature returns to baseline prior to each IL-2 dose ☐ Pt's weight remains within 3 lbs of baseline ☐ Pt ambulates without dizziness	☐ Pt's temperature returns to baseline prior to each IL-2 dose ☐ Pt's weight remains within 3 lbs of baseline ☐ Pt ambulates without dizziness	☐ Pt's temperature returns to baseline prior to each IL-2 dose ☐ Pt's weight remains within 3 lbs of baseline ☐ Pt ambulates without dizziness ☐ Pt's lungs remain clear to auscultation ☐ Pt remains orientated to person, time & place ☐ Pt drinks 6 to 8 glasses of fluids without emesis	☐ Pt's temperature returns to baseline prior to each IL-2 dose ☐ Pt's weight remains within 3 lbs of baseline ☐ Pt ambulates without dizziness ☐ Pt's lungs remain clear to auscultation ☐ Pt remains orientated to person, time & place ☐ Pt drinks 6 to 8 glasses of fluids without emesis	☐ Pt's temperature returns to baseline prior to each IL-2 dose ☐ Pt's weight remains within 3 lbs of baseline ☐ Pt ambulates without dizziness ☐ Pt's lungs remain clear to auscultation ☐ Pt remains orientated to person, time & place ☐ Pt drinks 6 to 8 glasses of fluids without emesis	☐ Pt is afebrile ☐ Pt is orientated to person, time & place ☐ Pt/so given written instructions of when to call MD/RN with a phone number
Assessment/ Monitoring	☐ Weight daily _____ ☐ Intake & Output ☐ Assess lung sounds, mental status & vital signs prior to each IL-2 dose. Notify MD if: • symptomatic hypotension occurs • temperature doesn't return to baseline prior to each IL-2 dose • crackles heard in lungs • change in mental status	☐ Weight _____ (if weight > 3 lbs over baseline, notify MD) ☐ Intake & Output ☐ Assess lung sounds, mental status & vital signs prior to each IL-2 dose. Notify MD if: • symptomatic hypotension occurs • temperature doesn't return to baseline prior to each IL-2 dose • crackles heard in lungs • change in mental status	☐ Weight _____ (if weight > 3 lbs over baseline, notify MD) ☐ Intake & Output ☐ Assess lung sounds, mental status & vital signs prior to each IL-2 dose. Notify MD if: • symptomatic hypotension occurs • temperature doesn't return to baseline prior to each IL-2 dose • crackles heard in lungs • change in mental status ☐ Increase temperature assessment to q4h if neutropenic	☐ Weight _____ (if weight > 3 lbs over baseline, notify MD) ☐ Intake & Output ☐ Assess lung sounds, mental status & vital signs prior to each IL-2 dose. Notify MD if: • symptomatic hypotension occurs • temperature doesn't return to baseline prior to each IL-2 dose • crackles heard in lungs • change in mental status ☐ Assess temperature q4h (if neutropenic)	☐ Weight _____ (if weight > 3 lbs over baseline, notify MD) ☐ Intake & Output ☐ Assess lung sounds, mental status & vital signs prior to each IL-2 dose. Notify MD if: • symptomatic hypotension occurs • temperature doesn't return to baseline prior to each IL-2 dose • crackles heard in lungs • change in mental status ☐ Assess temperature q4h (if neutropenic)	☐ Weight _____ (if weight > 3 lbs over baseline, notify MD)

702

Tests	□ CBC-baseline □ Chemistry profile-7, LDH and Liver profile	□ CBC □ If ANC < 500 institute neutropenic precautions □ If platelets < 10,000 transfuse □ Chemistry profile-7 and liver profile □ If creatinine > 4.3 hold IL-2/IFN-α □ If SGOT > 153, SGPT > 204, or total bili > 4.5, hold IL-2/IFN-α □ If K, Mg or phosphorus are low replace IVPB per MD order	□ CBC □ If ANC < 500 institute neutropenic precautions □ If platelets < 10,000 transfuse □ Chemistry profile-7 and liver profile □ If creatinine > 4.3 hold IL-2/IFN-α □ If SGOT > 153, SGPT > 204, or total bili > 4.5, hold IL-2/IFN-α □ If K, Mg or phosphorus are low replace IVPB per MD order
Functional/ Rehabilitation	□ Patient ambulates in hallways TID	□ Patient ambulates in hallways TID □ If dizziness or hypotension present ambulate with assistance only	□ Patient ambulates in hallways TID □ If dizziness or hypotension present ambulate with assistance only □ Refer pt for PT if appropriate to maintain activity status	□ Patient ambulates in hallways TID □ If dizziness or hypotension present ambulate with assistance only	□ Patient able to ambulate independently without dizziness
Nutrition	□ Diet as tolerated	□ Push salty fluids with calories (juice, Gatorade, lemonade, pop)	□ Push salty fluids with calories (juice, Gatorade, lemonade, pop)	□ Push salty fluids with calories (juice, Gatorade, lemonade, pop)	□ Patient is able to drink fluids (6–8 glasses per day) and is not vomiting

(continued)

Patient's Name: _____

Date of Admission: _____

Attending Physician: _____

Components	Day 1	Day 2	Day 3	Day 4	Day 5	Outcomes Day 6/Discharge
Date						
Medications	☐ IL-2 IVPB q8hours ☐ IFN-α sq at 16:30 ☐ Famotidine daily ☐ Heplock IV line when not in use (use IV fluid sparingly) NO STEROIDS NO Antihypertensives NO PRBCs unless medically emergent	☐ IL-2 IVPB q8hours ☐ IFN-α sq at 16:30 ☐ Famotidine daily NO STEROIDS NO Antihypertensives NO PRBCs unless medically emergent ☐ Obtain order to start fluids for symptomatic hypotension and/or oliguria 500cc NS IV bolus or 1000cc NS over 24 hours per MD order	☐ IL-2 IVPB q8hours ☐ IFN-α sq at 16:30 ☐ Famotidine daily ☐ Cipro BID NO STEROIDS NO Antihypertensives NO PRBCs unless medically emergent ☐ Obtain order to start fluids for symptomatic hypotension and/or oliguria 500cc NS IV bolus or 1000cc NS over 24 hours per MD order	☐ IL-2 IVPB q8hours ☐ IFN-α sq at 16:30 ☐ Famotidine daily ☐ Cipro BID NO STEROIDS NO Antihypertensives NO PRBCs unless medically emergent ☐ Obtain order to start fluids for symptomatic hypotension and/or oliguria 500cc NS IV bolus or 1000cc NS over 24 hours per MD order	☐ IL-2 IVPB q8hours ☐ IFN-α sq at 16:30 ☐ Famotidine daily ☐ Cipro BID NO STEROIDS NO Antihypertensives NO PRBCs unless medically emergent ☐ Obtain order to start fluids for symptomatic hypotension and/or oliguria 500cc NS IV bolus or 1000cc NS over 24 hours per MD order	☐ Pt is discharged with oral antibiotic prescription if ANC < 1000
Treatments	☐ Insert PICC ☐ K-thermia PRN chills/fever	☐ PICC line care ☐ K-thermia PRN chills/fever	☐ PICC line care ☐ K-thermia PRN chills/fever	☐ PICC line care ☐ K-thermia PRN chills/fever	☐ PICC line care ☐ K-thermia PRN chills/fever	
Teaching	☐ Instruct patient/so on side effects of medications and self management strategies using: ☐ Drug cards ☐ Videos (IL-2 & IFN-α) ☐ Biotherapy Patient Guide booklet ☐ Instruct pt/so in sc self injection techniques	☐ Continue pt/so instructions on medications ☐ Demonstrate to pt/so sc self injection ☐ Instruct pt/so on care of PICC line, if line will be left in place, postdischarge ☐ Instruct pt/so on care of PICC line, if line will be left in place, postdischarge	☐ Continue patient/so instructions on medications ☐ Have pt/so return demo of sc injection (have pt/so give 16:30 IFN-α) ☐ Instruct pt/so on care of PICC line, if line will be left in place, postdischarge	☐ Continue patient/so instructions on medications ☐ Have pt/so return demo of sc injection (have pt/so give 16:30 IFN-α) ☐ Instruct pt/so on care of PICC line, if line will be left in place, postdischarge	☐ Continue patient/so instructions on medications ☐ Instruct pt/so on care of PICC line, if line will be left in place, postdischarge	☐ Pt/so state names of medications, correct dose and route, possible side effects and self-management strategies for all medications patient will take at home ☐ Pt/so demonstrates ability to perform sc injection of biologic medication if appropriate ☐ Pt/so demonstrates ability to care for PICC line if appropriate

Spiritual/ Psychosocial/ Discharge Planning	□ Advanced directive in chart Y N □ Assessment by care coordinator, social worker and/or pastoral care □ Care Manager to arrange for outpatient biologic therapy as indicated □ Begin planning for discharge	□ Continue discharge planning	□ Continue discharge planning	□ Refer pt/so to social worker/pastoral care as appropriate □ Continue discharge planning	□ Advise pt/so about community services available such as support groups □ Continue discharge planning	□ Pt/so given written information of community resources available to them D/C plans in place: □ Pt has prescriptions □ Pt has in writing date & time of next MD/RN appointment
Initials	AM _____ PM _____ NOC _____	AM _____ PM _____ NOC _____	AM _____ PM _____ NOC _____	AM _____ PM _____ NOC _____	AM _____ PM _____ NOC _____	AM _____ PM _____ NOC _____

Abbreviations: ANC, absolute neutrophil count; BID, twice a day; bili, bilirubin; CBC, complete blood count; D/C, discharge; h, hour; IFN-α, interferon-alpha; IFN, interferon; IL, interleukin; IL-2, interleukin-2; IV, intravenously; IVPB, intravenous piggyback; K, potassium; LDH, lactate dehydrogenase; MD, medical doctor; Mg, magnesium; NS, normal saline; NOC, night shift; PICC, peripherally inserted central catheter; PRBC, packed red blood cell; PRN, as required; Pt, patient; PT, physical therapy; q, every; RN, Registered nurse; so, significant other; sc, subcutaneously; SGOT, serum glutamic–oxalacetic transaminase; SGPT, serum glutamic pyruvic transaminase; TID, three times a day.

APPENDIX B | Quick Summary Pages

INTERLEUKINS

Quick Summary Page

Agent: Interleukin-2, aldesleukin (Proleukin®)
Manufacturer: Chiron Corporation
Emeryville, CA

Aldesleukin, a human recombinant interleukin-2 (IL-2) product, is a highly purified protein produced by recombinant DNA technology. Aldesleukin possesses the biological activity of human native IL-2.

Website: *http://www.chiron.com/*

First approved by the FDA in May 1992.

Regulatory Approvals

Disease	*Dosing*
Metastatic renal-cell carcinoma	Two 5-day treatment cycles separated by a rest period of 9 days: 600,000 IU/kg administered every 8 hours by a 15-minute IV infusion for a total of 14 doses. Patients treated with this schedule received a median of 20 doses because of toxicity.

Metastatic melanoma   Two 5-day treatment cycles separated by a rest period of 9 days: 600,000 IU/kg administered every 8 hours by a 15-minute IV infusion for a total of 14 doses. Patients treated with this schedule received a median of 18 doses because of toxicity.

Pharmacokinetics

Elimination: Metabolized in the kidneys, with little or no bioactive protein excreted in the urine. High plasma concentration occurs following short IV infusion, with a half-life of 13 minutes. Following subcutaneous administration, peak levels are achieved in 5 hours.

Setting

Hospital, for regulatory approved doses.

Many patients currently receive aldesleukin in the ambulatory setting when receiving low to moderate dosing schedules.

Diagnostic/Laboratory Tests

The following clinical evaluations are recommended for all patients prior to beginning treatment and then daily during drug administration for the regulatory approved dose.

Standard hematologic test, including CBC, differential, and platelet counts; blood chemistries, including electrolytes, renal, and hepatic function test; chest x-rays.

All patients should have baseline pulmonary function test with arterial blood gases and evaluation of cardiac function using a stress thallium study.

Daily monitoring during therapy should include vital signs with orthostatic blood pressure measurement, weight, and clinical pulmonary assessment.

Administration

Vial Sizes:

22×10^6 IU/vial (18 million IU [1.1 mg] per mL when reconstituted)

Single-use vials, discard unused portion.

Reconstitute with 1.2 mL sterile water for injection by directing diluent against the side of the vial to avoid excess foaming.

Swirl gently to mix. Do not shake.

Dilute the reconstituted aldesleukin dose in 50 mL of 5% dextrose injection and infuse over 15 minutes. ***Do not use in-line filters when administering aldesleukin.***

Caution: Avoid reconstitution or dilution with bacteriostatic water for injection or 0.9% Sodium Chloride Injection because of increased aggregation. Dilution with albumin can alter the pharmacology of aldesleukin. *Do not mix with other drugs.*

Storage/Stability: Store in a refrigerator at 2° to 8°C.

Administer within 48 hours of reconstitution. Bring to room temperature before administration to the patient.

Storage During Travel

Protect from extremes in temperature. Do not leave medication in the car or trunk. When traveling by airplane, take vials on board in passenger cabin so that medication will not be exposed to temperature extremes in the baggage compartment. Vials should be transported in a cooler, near but not touching ice packs. Do not use dry ice as it may freeze the vials.

General Precautions (see package insert for details)

- Monitor for capillary leak syndrome (CLS). Following administration of aldesleukin, CLS begins immediately and results from the extravasation of plasma proteins and fluid into the extravascular space and loss of vascular tone. The CLS may be associated with cardiac arrhythmias, angina, MI, respiratory insufficiency requiring intubation, GI bleeding or infarction, renal insufficiency, and mental status changes.
- Early administration of dopamine (1 to 5 mcg/kg/min) to patients manifesting CLS, before the onset of hypotension, can help maintain organ perfusion, particularly to the kidney, thereby preserving urine output.
- Aldesleukin may exacerbate autoimmune disease.
- Patients with significant cardiac, pulmonary, renal, hepatic, or CNS impairment should be excluded from therapy with high-dose aldesleukin.
- In high-dose therapy, all patients with an indwelling central line should receive antibiotic prophylaxis effective against gram-positive organisms. Aldesleukin administration is associated with impaired neutrophil function (chemotaxis), with an increased risk for infection including sepsis and bacterial endocarditis.
- **Avoid concurrent use of glucocorticoids as they may reduce the anti-tumor effectiveness of aldesleukin.**
- Antihypertensives may potentiate the hypotension seen with aldesleukin.
- See package insert for clinical guidelines for holding or interrupting a dose or discontinuation of therapy. Organ systems most often involved include cardiovascular, pulmonary, renal, CNS, GI, and hepatic.
- The use of premedication with acetaminophen and/or nonsteroidal anti-inflammatory agents is commonly used to control the flu-like symptoms.

Resources for Patients

Website: *www.chiron.com*

> See *For the patient*. Includes sections on disease overview, disease treatments, patient resources, and educational resources.
> *Interleukin-2: Information for Patients and Their Families.* 1997. Write to Attn: Interleukin-2 Therapy Medicalliance, Inc., 5565 Sterett Place, Ste. 200, Columbia, MD 21044-9590.
> Video: *Interleukin-2 Therapy: Information for Patients and Their Families.* Available through American Medical Communications, Houston, TX (713) 590-1475.
> *National Kidney Association Interleukin-2 and Biologic Therapy.*

Resources for Professionals

Chiron Professional Services Department
To request specific product information and educational materials

Open Monday through Friday, 6 A.M. to 5 P.M. PST

To contact, please call 1-800-CHIRON-8, selection #2 (within the United States)

Reimbursement Hotline: 1-800-775-7533

Proleukin® inpatient management guidelines

Proleukin® outpatient management guidelines

Reprint: *Seminars in Oncology Nursing.* Management of patients receiving interleukin-2 therapy, 9(3 Suppl 1): 1–35, August 1993.

Physicians and Nurses, Guidelines for Proleukin® (aldesleukin) therapy

Biotherapy: Considerations for Oncology Nurses

CE accredited newsletter

Published by Scientific Frontiers, Inc.

1105 Taylorsville Road

P.O. Box 827

Washington Crossing, PA 18977

Provided as a professional service by Chiron.

Monograph on IL-2 produced by Chiron: Rieger, P.T. (ed). 1998. Interleukin-2: A paradigm for developing nursing strategies for patient management. Beachwood, OH: Pro ED Communications, Inc.

INTERFERONS

Quick Summary Page

Agent: Interferon-alfa-2a (Roferon®-A)
Manufacturer: Roche Laboratories
Nutley, NJ

Roferon® is a highly purified protein, biosynthetic human interferon produced by recombinant DNA technology using genetically engineered *Escherichia coli (E. coli)* bacterium.

Website: *http://www.roche.com*

First approved by the FDA in 1986.

Regulatory Approvals

Disease	*Dosing*
Hairy-cell leukemia	Induction: 3 MIU daily SC or IM injection for 16–24 weeks Maintenance: 3 MIU three times per week (TIW)
Kaposi's sarcoma	Induction: 36 MIU daily IM or SC injection for 10–12 weeks (Gradual dose escalation starting from 3 MIU to 9 MIU to 18 MIU, then to 36 MIU, may help decrease initial toxicity) Maintenance: 3 MIU three times per week (TIW)
Chronic myelogenous leukemia (CML)	9 MIU daily by SC or IM injection (Gradual dose escalation starting from 3 MIU for three days to 6 MIU for three days to 9 MIU may help decrease initial toxicity)
Hepatitis C	3 MIU administered SC or IM injection for 12 months (48 to 52 weeks), three times per week (TIW) New Dosage Regimen: An induction regimen of 6 MIU three times a week for 12 weeks followed by the standard regimen given for an additional 12 to 36 weeks (approved 11/99)

Pharmacokinetics

Absorption: Maximum serum concentration for IM or SC injection occurs 3.8 and 7.3 hours, respectively, after administration. After IV use, concentrations peak at the end of the infusion.

Half life: Elimination half-lives are approximately 3.7 to 8.5 hours (mean 5.1 hours).

Metabolism/Excretion: It is believed that proteolytic degradation occurs in the kidney where most of the drug is catabolized.

Setting

Primarily ambulatory

Diagnostic/Laboratory Tests

Hematologic survey, routine blood chemistries including liver function studies, assay for presence of hepatitis virus (with hepatitis).

Administration

Vial Sizes:

Single-use injectable solution 3 MIU per mL, 6 MIU per mL, 9 MIU per mL, 36 MIU per mL

Single-use prefilled syringes (for SC injections only) 3 MIU per 0.5 mL; 6 MIU per 0.5 mL; 9 MIU per 0.5 mL

Multidose injectable solution 9 MIU; 18 MIU (use within 30 days once vial is entered)

Store in the refrigerator 2° to 8°C.
Do not freeze. Do not shake.

Storage During Travel

Protect from extremes in temperature. Do not leave medication in the car or trunk. When traveling by airplane, take vials on board in passenger cabin so that medication will not be exposed to temperature extremes in the baggage compartment. Vials should be transported in a cooler, near but not touching ice packs. Do not use dry ice as it may freeze the vials.

General Precautions (see package insert for details)

• Should not be used in patients with a history of severe psychiatric disorders, and therapy should be discontinued in patients developing severe depression, suicidal ideation, or other severe psychiatric disorders. Should be used with caution in patients with a history of cardiac disease or debilitating medical conditions such as pulmonary disease or diabetes mellitus prone to develop ketoacidosis; in patients with abnormally low peripheral blood cell counts; in patients who are receiving agents known to cause myelosuppression; and in patients with a history of endocrine disorders. Exacerbation of autoimmune disease has been reported. Monitor renal and hepatic function.

Resources for Patients

The new Roferon®-A HCV Patient Support System is designed to educate patients about the side effects of therapy with Roferon®-A. The kit contains an educational brochure and a Spanish- and English-language video; a booklet with "Frequently Asked Questions about Hepatitis C"; and a workbook/diary so that patients can monitor their responses to therapy.

PATH (Partners Allied in the Treatment of Hepatitis) Compliance Kit can be obtained by calling 1-800-527-6243 or directly through local product sales representative.

Resources for Professionals

1-800-776-3376

Can request information on product use, adverse drug reactions, safety issues, product complaint line, and medical needs program.*

---

*M.D. must submit request for application for a patient with financial need for covering drug expenses.

Can request a videotape, booklet, and personal care kit (e.g., syringes, cooler) specific to Roferon®-A and suitable for patients or professionals.

Product Information Line
1-800-526-6367

Quick Summary Page

Agent: Interferon-alfa-2b, recombinant (Intron® A)
          Manufacturer: Schering Corporation
               Kenilworth, NJ

Intron® A is a highly purified protein, biosynthetic human interferon produced by recombinant DNA technology using genetically engineered *Escherichia coli (E. coli)* bacterium.

Websites: **For information on current research:**
          http://www.sp-research.com
          For corporate information:
          http://www.schering-plough.com

First approved by the FDA in 1986.

Regulatory Approvals

Disease	*Dosing*
Hairy-cell leukemia	2 MIU/m² SC or IM injection three times per week (TIW) for up to 6 months
Kaposi's sarcoma	30 MIU/m² SC or IM injection three times per week (TIW)
Hepatitis B	30–35 MIU/week SC or IM daily as either 5 MIU daily or 10 MIU three times per week for 16 weeks Pediatric: 3 MIU/m² three times per week (TIW) for the first week followed by dose escalation to 6 MIU/m² (maximum 10 MIU TIW) administered SC for 16–24 weeks
Hepatitis C	3 MIU SC or IM injection three times per week (TIW) for 16 weeks depending on response, for 18–24 months
Condyloma acuminata	10 MIU/1.0 cc inject 0.1 cc per lesion three times per week for three weeks
Melanoma	Induction: 20 MIU/m² IV 5 days/week for 4 weeks (Place appropriate dose of reconstituted IFN into a 100 mL bag of 0.9% sodium-chloride injection, USP. Infuse over 20 minutes) Maintenance: 10 MIU/m² SC or IM injection three times per week (TIW) for 48 weeks
Follicular lymphoma	5 MIU SC injection three times per week for up to 18 months in conjunction with an anthracycline-containing chemotherapy regimen

Pharmacokinetics

Absorption: Maximum serum concentration for IM or SC injection occurs 3–12 hours after administration. After IV use, concentrations peak at the end of the infusion.

Half-life: Elimination half-lives are approximately 2–3 hours.

Metabolism/Excretion: It is believed that proteolytic degradation occurs in the kidney where most of the drug is catabolized.

Setting

Primarily ambulatory

Diagnostic/Laboratory Tests

Hematologic survey, routine blood chemistries including liver function studies (especially important during induction phase for malignant melanoma), assay for presence of hepatitis virus (with hepatitis).

Administration

Vial Sizes:

Solution:

Single-use injectable solution 3 MIU per 0.5 mL; Pak-3 (six 3 MIU vials, syringes, and alcohol)
Single-use injectable solution 5 MIU per 0.5 mL; Pak-5 (six 5 MIU vials, syringes, and alcohol)
Single-use injectable solution 10 MIU per 1.0 mL; Pak-10 (six 10 MIU vials, syringes, and alcohol)

Multidose injectable solution 18 MIU; 25 MIU (use within 30 days once vial is entered)
3 MIU multidose pen (6 doses × 3 MIU/0.2 mL)
5 MIU multidose pen (6 doses × 5 MIU/0.2 mL)
10 MIU multidose pen (6 doses × 10 MIU/0.2 mL)

Sterile Powder:

Sterile powder with diluent 3 MIU; Pak-3 (six 3 MIU vials, six syringes of diluent)
Sterile powder with diluent 5 MIU, 10 MIU, 18 MIU, 25 MIU, 50 MIU
Swirl gently to mix. *Do not shake.*

Combinations

For use in the treatment of hepatitis C:
Rebetron™ 1200/Pak-3 Combination therapy
   84 Rebetol® 200-mg capsules
   Intron® A 3 MIU pack (6 vials of 3 MIU/0.5 mL)
Rebetron™ 1000/Pak-3 Combination therapy
   70 Rebetol® 200-mg capsules
   Intron® A 3 MIU pack (6 vials of 3 MIU/0.5 mL)
Rebetron™ 600/Pak-3 Combination therapy
   42 Rebetol® 200-mg capsules
   Intron® A 3 MIU pack (6 vials of 3 MIU/0.5 mL)
Rebetron™ 1200/MDV
   84 Rebetol® 200-mg capsules
   Intron® A 18 MIU pack (6 doses of 3 MIU/0.5 mL)

Rebetron™ 1000/MDV
    70 Rebetol® 200-mg capsules
    Intron® A 18 MIU pack (6 doses of 3 MIU/0.5 mL)
Rebetron™ 600/MDV
    42 Rebetol® 200-mg capsules
    Intron® A 18 MIU pack (6 doses of 3 MIU/0.5 mL)
Rebetron™ 1200/3 MIU pen
    84 Rebetol® 200-mg capsules
    Intron® A 3 MIU multidose pen (6 doses × 3 MIU/0.2 mL)
Rebetron™ 1000/3 MIU pen
    70 Rebetol® 200-mg capsules
    Intron® A 3 MIU multidose pen (6 doses × 3 MIU/0.2 mL)
Rebetron™ 600/3 MIU pen
    42 Rebetol® 200-mg capsules
    Intron® A 3 MIU multidose pen (6 doses × 3 MIU/0.2 mL)

Store in the refrigerator 2° to 8°C.
Do not freeze.

Storage During Travel

Protect from extremes in temperature. Do not leave medication in the car or trunk. When traveling by airplane, take vials on board in passenger cabin so that medication will not be exposed to temperature extremes in the baggage compartment. Vials should be transported in a cooler, near but not touching ice packs. Do not use dry ice as it may freeze the vials.

General Precautions (see package insert for details)

- Should not be used in patients with a history of severe psychiatric disorders, and therapy should be discontinued in patients developing severe depression, suicidal ideation, or other severe psychiatric disorders. Should be used with caution in patients with a history of cardiac disease or debilitating medical conditions such as pulmonary disease or diabetes mellitus prone to develop ketoacidosis; in patients with abnormally low peripheral blood cell counts; in patients who are receiving agents known to cause myelosuppression; and patients with a history of endocrine disorders. Exacerbation of autoimmune disease has been reported. Monitor renal and hepatic function.

Resources for Patients

Package insert available for patients.
    Crossing Bridges: Your Link to a World of Support and Caring (pamphlet)
    Crossing Bridges is a voluntary therapy compliance program available at no cost to malignant melanoma patients on INTRON® A. Designed to supplement the advice of oncologists and their nurses, the program provides patients with up-to-date medical information regarding their treatment, as well as resources to manage their treatment challenges and side effects such as depression, fatigue, nausea, and loss of appetite. The program is a research study for malignant melanoma patients who are prescribed INTRON® A.

Be in Charge: A Program to Help You Get Through Intron® A Therapy
Commitment to Care Program: assistance and reimbursement program for indigent patients
Interferon Information Sheet
Cancer Care Brochure
Melanoma Fact/Fiction Card
Patient Guide for Melanoma
Side Effects Card
Website: *http://www.melanoma.com*

Resources for Professionals

Drug Information Service (1-800-526-4099)
Monday–Friday 9 A.M. to 4 P.M. EST
    Provides literature search and general product information.

Patient Care Consultant Program
    Provides nurses with specialty backgrounds for consultation and education to nurses working in doctors' offices.

Quick Summary Page

Agent: Interferon alfacon-1 (Infergen®)
            Manufacturer: Amgen, Inc.
                        Thousand Oaks, CA

Infergen® is a recombinant non-naturally occurring type-1 interferon. The 166-amino acid sequence of Interferon alfacon-1 was derived by scanning the sequences of several natural IFN-α subtypes and assigning the most frequently observed amino acid in each corresponding position. Four additional amino-acid changes were made to facilitate the molecular construction, and a corresponding synthetic DNA sequence was constructed using chemical synthesis methodology. IFN alfacon-1 is produced in *E. coli* cells that have been genetically altered by insertion of a synthetically constructed sequence that codes for IFN alfacon-1.

Website: *http://www.amgen.com*

Regulatory Approvals

Disease	*Dosing*
Chronic hepatitis C virus infection	9 mcg SC injection three times per week (TIW) for 24 weeks. At least 48 hours should elapse between doses.
	Expanded Indication: Subsequent treatment of HCV-infected patients who have tolerated an initial course of interferon therapy with 15 mcg of Interferon alfacon-1 for 24 weeks (approved 12/99).

Setting
Primarily ambulatory

Diagnostic/Laboratory Tests
Hematologic survey, routine blood chemistries including liver function studies, assay for presence of hepatitis virus (with hepatitis), triglycerides, thyroid functions.

Administration
Vial Sizes:
> Single-dose, preservative-free vials 9 mcg per 0.3 mL (dispensing pacs of 6 vials) or 15 mcg per 0.5 mL (dispensing pacs of 6 vials)
> Single-dose, preservative-free prefilled syringes 9 mcg/0.3 mL (dispensing pacs of 6 prefilled syringes)
> Single-dose, preservative-free prefilled syringes 15 mcg/0.5 mL (dispensing pacs of 6 prefilled syringes)
> Use only one dose per vial; do not reenter the vial. Discard unused portions. Do not save unused drug for later administration.

Store in the refrigerator 2° to 8°C.
Do not freeze. Do not shake. Do not expose to direct sunlight.

Storage During Travel
Protect from extremes in temperature. Do not leave medication in the car or trunk. When traveling by airplane, take vials on board in passenger cabin so that medication will not be exposed to temperature extremes in the baggage compartment. Vials should be transported in a cooler, near but not touching ice packs. Do not use dry ice as it may freeze the vials.

General Precautions (see package insert for details)
- Should not be used in patients with a history of severe psychiatric disorders, and therapy should be discontinued in patients developing severe depression, suicidal ideation, or other severe psychiatric disorders. Should be used with caution in patients with a history of cardiac disease; in patients with abnormally low peripheral blood cell counts who are receiving agents known to cause myelosuppression; and in patients with a history of endocrine disorders. Exacerbation of autoimmune disease has been reported. Monitor renal and hepatic function.

Resources for Patients
> *Patient Center*® accessed through the website. Includes a therapy guide, called *Infergen and You,* for patients taking Infergen®, and the quarterly newsletter, *Living Well,* for patients with chronic hepatitis C.
> *Safety Net*® *Program*: Patient-assistance program to help medically indigent patients with chronic hepatitis C. Accessed via the COMPASS™ Support Line at 1-888-508-8088. Ask to speak with a reimbursement specialist. Open 7 days per week/24 hours per day.

Resources for Professionals

Infergen® Fact Sheet

Infergen® Prescribing Information

Resource guide for treatment with Infergen®, a link to continuing education programs for pharmacists offered by the University of Wisconsin, and *Hepatitis Care Views*, a quarterly newsletter for hepatology nurses and health-care professionals.

Hep in Cite (Hepatitis C Information & Support): Newsletter found under professionals resources on website, targeted toward helping patients to live with and manage hepatitis C.

Quick Summary Page

Agent: Interferon alfa-n3, human leukocyte derived (Alferon® N)
Manufacturer: Interferon Sciences, Inc.
New Brunswick, NJ

Alferon® N is a sterile aqueous formulation of purified, natural, human IFN-α protein for use by injection. It is manufactured from pooled units of human leukocytes induced by incomplete infection with a murine virus (Sendai virus) to produce interferon alfa-n3.

Website: *http://www.interferonsciences.com/*

First approved by the FDA in 1989.

Regulatory Approvals

Disease	*Dosing*
Condyloma acuminata	Intralesional injection 250,000 IU/wart 2×/week for up to 8 weeks. Inject into the base of each wart, preferably using a 30-gauge needle.

Pharmacokinetics

In a study of intralesional use of interferon alfa-n3 injection for the treatment of condylomata acuminata, plasma concentrations were below the detection limit of the assay.

Setting

Physician's office or ambulatory clinic

Diagnostic/Laboratory Tests

In patients with condyloma acuminata, decreased white blood cell counts were seen approximately 11% of the time.

Administration

Vial Sizes:
5 MIU/1.0 mL vials

Store in refrigerator 2° to 8°C.
Do not freeze. Do not shake.

Storage During Travel

Protect from extremes in temperature. Do not leave medication in the car or trunk. When traveling by airplane, take vials on board in passenger cabin so that medication will not be exposed to temperature extremes in the baggage compartment. Vials should be transported in a cooler, near but not touching ice packs. Do not use dry ice as it may freeze the vials.

General Precautions (see package insert for details)

- Contraindicated in patients with hypersensitivity to human IFN-α or any component of the product, patients who have anaphylactic sensitivity to mouse immunoglobulin, egg protein, or neomycin. Use with caution in patients with debilitating medical conditions because of the flu-like symptoms. Caution fertile women to use effective contraception during use.

Resources for Patients

Patient Assistance Program (1-888-Alferon)
Request patient-specific product information on-line or by calling 1-888-Alferon.

Resources for Professionals

The ALFERON Access Program® consists of three components:
Distribution Services: a centralized distributor for wholesalers, home-care agencies, pharmacies, hospitals, and physician offices.
Clinical and Product Information Services: where clinicians and patients can learn more about Alferon® N Injection.
Reimbursement Information Services: offers assistance with reimbursement issues.
1-888-ALFERON. The ALFERON Access Program® is staffed from 8 A.M. to 7 P.M. EST. For additional information about the program, you can fax questions to 1-888-FAXXAFN.

Quick Summary Page

Agent: Interferon beta-1a, recombinant (Avonex®)
Manufacturer: Biogen
Cambridge, MA

Avonex® is a purified, sterile, lyophilized protein products produced by recombinant DNA technology and formulated for use by injection. It is produced by mammalian cells (i.e., Chinese hamster ovary cells) into which the human IFN-β gene has been introduced. The amino-acid sequence of interferon beta-1a is identical to that of natural human IFN-β. The mechanism of action by which it exerts its actions in multiple sclerosis (MS) are not clearly understood.

Website: *http://www.biogen.com/*

First approved by the FDA in May 1996.

Regulatory Approvals

Disease	*Dosing*
Multiple sclerosis (relapsing/remitting)	30 mcg IM once per week

Pharmacokinetics

Peak serum concentrations occurred between 1 to 8 hours, with an elimination half-life of 8 to 10 hours, depending on the route of administration (SC or IM).

Setting

Primarily ambulatory

Diagnostic/Laboratory Tests

Hemoglobin, complete and differential WBC counts, platelet counts and blood chemistries, including liver function tests. Recommended prior to initiation of therapy and at periodic intervals thereafter.

Administration

Vials Sizes:

Powder for injection, lyophilized 33 mcg (6.6 MIU). Preservative-free/single-use vial

Reconstitute with provided diluent 1.1 mL and swirl gently to dissolve.

AVONEX® is available in the following package configurations: Package

(Administration Pack) containing four Administration Dose Packs (each containing one vial of AVONEX®, one 10-mL (10 cc) diluent vial, two alcohol wipes, one 3-cc syringe, one Micro Pin® vial access pin, one needle, and one adhesive bandage).

Store in the refrigerator 2° to 8°C. If unavailable, may be stored at room temperature for up to 30 days. Following reconstitution, use as soon as possible (within 6 hours or less).

Do not freeze. Do not shake. Do not expose to high temperatures.

Storage During Travel

Protect from extremes in temperature. Do not leave medication in the car or trunk. When traveling by airplane, take vials on board in passenger cabin so that medication will not be exposed to temperature extremes in the baggage compartment. Vials should be transported in a cooler, near but not touching ice packs. Do not use dry ice as it may freeze the vials.

General Precautions (see package insert for details)

- Contraindicated in patients with known hypersensitivity to natural or recombinant IFN-β, albumin human, or any other component of the formulations. Use with caution in patients with depression or history of depression, preexisting seizure disorders, and debilitating conditions such as cardiac conditions.

Resources for Patients

Training Materials: patients first receive AVONEX® Patient Instruction Materials, including a video cassette and a manual that describe the appropriate ways to store AVONEX®, prepare for injections, and administer the drug. To order AVONEX® Patient Instruction Materials, call 1-800-456-2255.

The Avonex Alliance

The Avonex Alliance was developed by Biogen as an ongoing, comprehensive support program to help people with relapsing MS, their care partners, and health care professionals working together to help manage MS with AVONEX® (Interferon beta-1a).

Patient support program website: *http://www.avonex.com/patientsupp/*

Includes information on getting started, determining insurance coverage, obtaining AVONEX®, free injection training (Avonex Administration Training Program, an Interim HealthCare service), and the AVONEX® support line.

Resources for Professionals

The Avonex Support Line

A toll-free Avonex Support Line provides product information, reimbursement counseling, and information about Biogen's optional distribution and training programs. The number is 1-800-456-2255 and is available Monday through Friday, 8:30 A.M. to 8 P.M. EST.

Biogen's Special Distribution Options

In addition to offering AVONEX® through traditional retail channels, Biogen has established two special distribution options that provide direct billing of patients' health plans (referred to as "assignment of benefits") so that patients can avoid having to pay for the drug upfront and then filing claims for reimbursement. The Avonex Pharmacy Network, a service of Olsten Health Services, provides assignment of benefits for patients wishing to pick up AVONEX® at a local pharmacy. Avonex Direct Delivery, a service of Nova Factor, provides assignment of benefits for patients preferring the convenience of direct shipment to their home or workplace.

Quick Summary Page

Agent: Interferon beta-1b, recombinant (Betaseron®)
    Manufacturer: Chiron Corporation
        Emeryville, CA
    Distributor: Berlex
        Richmond, CA

Betaseron® is a purified, sterile, lyophilized protein product produced by recombinant DNA technology and formulated for use by injection. It is produced by bacterial fermentation of a strain of *E. coli* that bears a genetically engineered plasmid containing the gene for human IFN-β_{ser17}. The native gene is altered in a way that substitutes serine for cysteine at position 17. Interferon beta-1b is a highly purified protein with 165 amino acids. The mechanism of action by which it exerts its actions in multiple sclerosis (MS) is not clearly understood.

Websites: *http://www.berlex.com/*
    http://www.betaseron.com/

First approved by the FDA in July 1993.

Regulatory Approvals

Disease	*Dosing*
Multiple sclerosis (relapsing/remitting)	0.25 mg (8 MIU) SC every other day, evidence of efficacy after 2 years is not known.

Pharmocokinetics

Peak serum concentrations occurred between 1 to 8 hours, with an elimination half-life of 8 to 10 hours, depending on the route of administration (SC or IM). With IV administration, half-life values range from 8 minutes to 4 hours.

Setting

Primarily ambulatory

Diagnostic/Laboratory Tests

Hemoglobin, complete and differential WBC counts, platelet counts and blood chemistries, including liver function tests. Recommended prior to initiation of therapy and at periodic intervals thereafter.

Administration

Vials Sizes:

Powder for injection, lyophilized 0.3 mg (9.6 MIU). Preservative-free single-use vial. Discard unused portions. Reconstitute with provided diluent 1.2 mL and swirl gently to dissolve. Use within 3 hours of reconstitution.

Store in the refrigerator 2° to 8° C.
Do not freeze. Do not shake.

Storage During Travel

Protect from extremes in temperature. Do not leave medication in the car or trunk. When traveling by airplane, take vials on board in passenger cabin so that medication will not be exposed to temperature extremes in the baggage compartment. Vials should be transported in a cooler, near but not touching ice packs. Do not use dry ice as it may freeze the vials.

General Precautions (see package insert for details)

- Contraindicated in patients with known hypersensitivity to natural or recombinant IFN-β, albumin human, or any other component of the formulations. Use with caution in patients with depression or history of depression, preexisting seizure disorders, and debilitating conditions such as cardiac conditions.
- Injection site necrosis (ISN) has been reported in 5% of patients in controlled clinical trials. Typically, ISN occurs within the first 4 months of therapy, although post-marketing reports have been received of ISN occurring over 1 year after initiation of therapy. Necrosis may occur at single or multiple injection sites. The necrotic lesions are typically 3 cm or less in diameter, but larger areas have been reported. While necrosis has commonly extended only to subcutaneous fat, there are also reports of necrosis extending to and including fascia overlaying muscle. In some lesions where biopsy results are available, vasculitis has been reported. For some lesions, debridement and, infrequently, skin grafting has been required. Other injection site reactions occurred in 85% of

patients in the controlled MS trial, at one or more times during therapy. There was redness, pain, swelling, and discoloration. In general, these were transient and did not require discontinuation of therapy.

Resources for Patients

A patient information sheet is provided with the product and is available on the website.

Betaseron® patient handbook

Patient Assistance Program 1-800-788-1467

MS Pathways Program: offers comprehensive patient programs, including resource center, brochures *Caring for a Loved One with MS* and *MS Management Gets Personal*, peer support groups, newsletter *Messages*, reimbursement options, Betaseron® starter kit (personal journal, videotape on learning to use Betaseron®, administration supplies, patient guide *Your Guide to Starting Therapy with Betaseron*, and information regarding financial assistance).

Access these resources by calling 800-788-1467.

Resources for Professionals

Website: *http://www.betaseron.com/healthpro/*

Health Professionals' Forum is a dynamic section designed for health professionals, such as physicians, nurses, nurse practitioners, and pharmacists, who are involved in the care and treatment of patients with multiple sclerosis. In this section, Continuing Medical Education (CME) and other educational programs are offered to aid such caregivers in their professional development and in their care of MS patients.

The Betaseron® Training Program

The Betaseron® Training Program provides a registered nurse to conduct a personalized training session on the administration of Betaseron® to all patients referred by their physician. In addition to the initial training session, the program includes 3 follow-up telephone calls to answer questions that the patient or caregiver may have and to encourage compliance with Betaseron® therapy. Physicians can refer patients to this program by calling 800-788-1467.

Berlex Professional Services Department 1-888-BERLEX4 (1-888-237-5394) between 8 A.M. and 5 P.M. PST.

Option 1:   To report adverse events.
Option 2:   Questions regarding the use of Betaseron® therapy.
Option 3:   Questions regarding the use of Fludara.
Option 4:   Questions regarding other products.

To report adverse events due to Betaseron® therapy, call 888-237-5394.

Online MS Resource Library to order copies of recently published MS-related articles.

Quick Summary Page

Agent: Interferon gamma-1b, recombinant (Actimmune®)
Manufacturer: InterMune Pharmaceuticals, Inc.
3294 West Bayshore Road
Palo Alto, CA 94303

Actimmune® is a single-chain polypeptide containing 140 amino acids. It is produced by fermentation of a genetically engineered *Escherichia coli* bacterium containing the DNA that encodes for the human protein IFN-γ.

Websites: *http://www.actimmune.com*
http://intermune.com

First approved by the FDA in December 1990.
Approved for osteopetrosis in February 2000.

Regulatory Approvals

Disease	*Dosing*
Chronic granulomatous disease	50 mcg/m² (1.0 MIU/m²) for patients whose BSA is > 0.5 m² and 1.5 mcg/kg/dose for patients whose BSA is ≤ 0.5 m². Administer SC three times per week (TIW). (To decrease frequency and severity of infections)
Osteopetrosis	50 mcg/m² (1.0 MIU/m²) for patients whose BSA is > 0.5 m² and 1.5 mcg/kg/dose for patients whose BSA is ≤ 0.5 m². Administer SC three times per week (TIW).

Pharmocokinetics
The mean elimination after IV administration was 38 mintues. After IM and SC dosing, the mean half-life was approximately 3 and 6 hours, respectively.

Setting
Primarily ambulatory

Diagnostic/Laboratory Tests
In addition to tests normally required for monitoring patients with chronic granulomatous disease, or osteopetrosis, it is recommended that prior to initiation of therapy and every 3 months during treatment that hematologic tests, including complete blood counts, differential and platelet counts, blood chemistries including renal and liver function tests, and urinalysis, be done.

Administration
Vial Sizes:
  100 mcg/0.5 mL single-dose vials. Stable for a maximum of 12 hours at room temperature. Single-dose vial; discard unused portion.

Store in the refrigerator 2° to 8°C.
Do not freeze. Do not shake.

Storage During Travel
Protect from extremes in temperature. Do not leave medication in the car or trunk. When traveling by airplane, take vials on board in passenger cabin so that medication will not be exposed to temperature extremes in the baggage compartment. Vials should be transported in a cooler, near but not touching ice packs. Do not use dry ice as it may freeze the vials.

General Precautions (see package insert for details)
Contraindicated in patients with known hypersensitivity to natural or recombinant IFN-γ, *E. coli* derived products, or any other component of the formulations. Use with caution in patients with depression or history of depression, preexisting seizure disorders, and debilitating conditions such as cardiac conditions. Exercise caution when administering interferon gamma in combination with other potentially myelosuppressive agents.

Resources for Patients
  See website: *www.actimmune.com*
  Information on reimbursement assistance program and patient assistance program: 800-577-9112

Resources for Professionals
  See website: *www.actimmune.com*

MONOCLONAL ANTIBODIES

Quick Summary Page

Agent: Trastuzumab (Herceptin®)
                    Manufacturer: Genentech, Inc.
                                    South San Francisco, CA

Herceptin® (Trastuzumab) is a recombinant DNA-derived humanized monoclonal antibody that selectively binds with high affinity to the extracellular domain of the human epidermal growth factor receptor 2 protein, HER2. The antibody is an IgG_1 kappa that contains human framework regions with the complementarity-determining regions of a murine antibody (4D5) that binds to HER2. The humanized antibody against HER2 is produced by a mammalian cell (i.e., Chinese hamster ovary [CHO]) suspension. Herceptin is a sterile, white to pale yellow, preservative-free lyophilized powder for intravenous (IV) administration.

Website: *http://www.gene.com*

First approved by the FDA in September 1998.

Regulatory Approvals

Disease—Metastatic Breast Cancer

Herceptin® (Trastuzumab) as a single agent is indicated for the treatment of patients with metastatic breast cancer whose tumors overexpress the HER2 (human epidermal growth factor receptor 2) protein and who have received one or more chemotherapy regimens for their metastatic disease. Herceptin® in combination with paclitaxel is indicated for treatment of patients with metastatic breast cancer whose tumors overexpress the HER2 protein and who have not received chemotherapy for their metastatic disease. Herceptin® should only be used in patients whose tumors have HER2 protein overexpression.

Dose

Initial loading dose 4 mg/kg administered as a 90-minute infusion

Weekly maintenance dose of 2 mg/kg administered as a 30-minute infusion

In 25% to 30% of women with metastatic breast cancer, there is a genetic alteration in the HER2 gene that produces an increased amount of the growth factor receptor protein on the tumor-cell surface. This HER2 protein overexpression is believed to be associated with more aggressive disease. HER2 protein overexpression is determined by immunohistochemical testing. Patients should contact their physician to discuss testing for HER2 overexpression.

Pharmacokinetics

In studies using a loading dose of 4 mg/kg followed by a weekly maintenance dose of 2 mg/kg, a mean half-life of 5.8 days (range = 1 to 32 days) was observed. Between weeks 16 and 32, trastuzumab serum concentrations reached a steady-state with mean trough and peak concentrations of approximately 79 and 123 microgram/mL, respectively.

Setting
May be given in the ambulatory setting.

Diagnostic/Laboratory
As clinically indicated.

Administration
Vial Sizes:

Each vial contains 440 mg of Herceptin® as a lyophilized, sterile powder. Each carton contains one vial of 440-mg Herceptin®; one 30-mL vial of Bacteriostatic Water for Injection, USP, 1.1% benzyl alcohol.

Each vial should be reconstituted with the diluent supplied to yield a multidose solution containing 21 mg/mL trastuzumab. May be used for 28 days following reconstitution when stored properly. The trastuzumab solution should be added to a 250-mL bag of 0.9% sodium chloride, USP. **Dextrose (5%) solution should not be used.** Gently invert the bag to mix the solution.

Stability/Storage:
Vials of Herceptin® are stable at 2° to 8°C prior to reconstitution.

Storage During Travel
Protect from extremes in temperature. Do not leave medication in the car or trunk. When traveling by airplane, take vials on board in passenger cabin so that medication will not be exposed to temperature extremes in the baggage compartment. Vials should be transported in a cooler, near but not touching ice packs. Do not use dry ice as it may freeze the vials.

General Precautions (see package insert for details)
No known contraindications.

Warnings
- **Cardiotoxicity:** Signs and symptoms of cardiac dysfunction, such as dyspnea, increased cough, paroxysmal nocturnal dyspnea, peripheral edema, S_3 gallop, or reduced ejection fraction, have been observed in patients treated with Herceptin®. Congestive heart failure associated with Herceptin® therapy may be severe and has been associated with disabling cardiac failure, death, and mural thrombosis leading to stroke. The clinical status of patients in the trials who developed congestive heart failure were classified for severity using the New York Heart Association classification system (I–IV, where IV is the most severe level of cardiac failure).
- Candidates for treatment with Herceptin® should undergo thorough baseline cardiac assessment including history and physical exam and one or more of the following: EKG, echocardiogram, and MUGA scan. There are no data regarding the most appropriate method of evaluation for the identification of patients at risk for developing cardiotoxicity. Monitoring may not identify all patients who will develop cardiac dysfunction.
- *Extreme caution* should be exercised in treating patients with pre-existing cardiac dysfunction.
- *Patients* receiving Herceptin® should undergo frequent monitoring for deteriorating cardiac function. The probability of cardiac dysfunction was highest in patients who received Herceptin® concurrently

with anthracyclines. The data suggest that advanced age may increase the probability of cardiac dysfunction. Pre-existing cardiac disease or prior cardiotoxic therapy (e.g., anthracycline or radiation therapy to the chest) may decrease the ability to tolerate Herceptin® therapy; however, the data are not adequate to evaluate the correlation between Herceptin®-induced cardiotoxicity and these factors.

- Discontinuation of Herceptin® therapy should be strongly considered in patients who develop clinically significant congestive heart failure. In the clinical trials, most patients with cardiac dysfunction responded to appropriate medical therapy often including discontinuation of Herceptin®. The safety of continuation or resumption of Herceptin® in patients who have previously experienced cardiac toxicity has not been studied. There are insufficient data regarding discontinuation of Herceptin® therapy in patients with asymptomatic decreases in ejection fraction; such patients should be closely monitored for evidence of clinical deterioration.
- Hypersensitivity reactions, including fatal anaphylaxis.
- Infusion reactions, including some with a fatal outcome.
- Pulmonary events, including adult respiratory distress syndrome and death.
- While the serious adverse events related to anaphylaxis and pulmonary events were observed in clinical trials, some of the events reported in the postmarketing setting were more severe. Additionally, the following observations have not been previously reported: adult respiratory distress syndrome, anaphylaxis, and death within 24 hours of a Herceptin® infusion.
- Serious adverse events of greater severity than previously reported include: urticara, bronchospasm, angioedema, hypotension, dyspnea, wheezing, pleural effusions, pulmonary infiltrates, noncardiogenic pulmonary edema, and pulmonary insufficiency and hypoxia requiring supplemental oxygen or ventilatory support.
- Most patients with fatal events had significant pre-existing pulmonary compromise secondary to instrinsic lung disease and/or malignant pulmonary involvement. Because it appears that patients with significant pre-existing pulmonary compromise may be at greater risk, these patients should be treated with *extreme caution*. Patients experiencing any of the severe infusion-associated symptoms such as anaphylaxis or adult respiratory distress syndrome should have the Herceptin® infusion discontinued and appropriate medical therapy administered.

Precautions

- General: Herceptin® (trastuzumab) therapy should be used with caution in patients with known hypersensitivity to trastuzumab, Chinese Hamster Ovary cell proteins, or any component of this product.
- Drug Interactions: There have been no formal drug interaction studies performed with Herceptin® in humans.

Adverse Reactions

- Infusion-Associated Symptoms: During the first infusion with Herceptin®, a symptom complex most commonly consisting of chills and/or fever was observed in about 40% of patients. The symptoms were usually mild to moderate in severity and were treated with acetaminophen, diphenhydramine, and meperidine (with or without reduction in the rate of Herceptin infusion). Herceptin® discontinuation was infrequent. Other signs and/or symptoms may include nausea, vomiting, pain (in some cases at tumor sites), rigors, headache, dizziness, dyspnea, hypotension, rash, and asthenia. The symptoms occurred infrequently with subsequent Herceptin® infusions.

Do Not Administer as an IV Push or Bolus

- It is advisable to keep emergency drugs (e.g., epinephrine, antihistamines, corticosteroids) readily available at the bedside for immediate use in the event of a reaction during administration.

Resources for Patients

Website: *http://www.herceptin.com/*

Patient Perspective: Online information on therapy with Herceptin®, monoclonal antibodies, patient stories, and patient materials.

Patient Assistance Program
Single Point of Contact (SPOC^SM)
1-888-249-4918
6 A.M. to 5 P.M. PST

Patient Education Booklets:
  Finding Your Way—Information for Women with Breast Cancer
  Finding Your Way through the Breast Cancer Diagnostic Process
  Finding Your Way after Breast Cancer Diagnosis
  Finding Your Way through Metastatic Breast Cancer
  Finding Your Way™ *Clinical Trials: You May Benefit from Joining a Scientific Study*
  Finding Your Way™ *Resource Guide: Reaching out to Breast Cancer Resources* (coming 2000)
  Learning about Treatment with Herceptin Therapy

Website: *http://www.her2status.com*

Website developed and maintained by F. Hoffmann-La Roche Ltd. for patients and professionals with information on breast cancer and HER2 status.

Resources for Professionals

Website: *http://www.biooncology.com/*

Oncology Resource Center: information on monoclonal antibodies, slides that may be downloaded, patient teaching/counseling information, upcoming meetings

Finding Your Way—Information for Women with Breast Cancer

Folder with materials to order patient education booklets for educating women about breast cancer and to increase awareness of the biology of breast cancer, molecular testing, and new treatment options. Call 1-800-818-9188 to order.

  Consult product sales representative regarding the availability of monographs on the use of Herceptin® in patients with breast cancer.
  Herceptin® (Trastuzumab): Targeted biologic therapy for patients with HER2 protein overexpressing metastatic breast cancer Lecture notes and slide set.
  Herceptin® (Trastuzumab): A Mini Slide Kit for Healthcare Professionals. Genentech, Inc., 1999.
  Uninsured Patient Assistance Program
  1-800-879-4747

Quick Summary Page

Agent: Rituximab (Rituxan®)
Jointly marketed: IDEC, San Diego, CA
Genentech, South San Francisco, CA

Rituximab is a genetically engineered chimeric murine/human monoclonal antibody directed against the CD20 antigen found on the surface of normal and malignant B lymhocytes. This antigen is expressed on >90% of B-cell non-Hodgkin's lymphomas (NHL) but is not found on hematopoietic stem cells, pro-B cells, normal plasma cells, or other normal tissues. The constant portion (Fc) of rituximab recruits immune effector functions to mediate B-cell lysis.

Websites: *http://www.gene.com*
http://www.rituxan.com

First received approval by the FDA in November 1997.

Regulatory Approvals

Disease	*Dosing*
Non-Hodgkin's lymphoma, relapsed or refractory low-grade or follicullar, CD20 positive, B-cell non-Hodgkin's lymphoma	375 mg/m^2 given as an IV to patients with infusion weekly for four doses.
	First Infusion: Initiate infusion at 50 mg/hour; if tolerated, escalate rate in 50-mg/hour increments every 30 minutes to a maximum of 400 mg/hour.
	Subsequent Infusions: Initiate at 100 mg/hour; escalate rate in 100-mg/hour increments every 30 minutes to a maximum of 400 mg/hour as tolerated.

Pharmocokinetics

Administration of Rituximab results in a rapid and sustained depletion of circulating and tissue-based B-cells. Mean serum half-life was 59.8 hours after the first infusion and 174 hours after the fourth infusion. The wide range seen in half-lives may reflect variable tumor burden among patients as peak and trough serum levels are inversely correlated with baseline values for the number of circulating CD20 positive B-cells and measures of disease burden.

Setting

Primarily ambulatory

Diagnostic/Laboratory

Obtain complete blood counts and platelet counts at regular intervals during Rituximab therapy and more frequently in patients who develop cytopenias.

Administration

Vial Sizes:

10 mg/mL, preservative-free, in 10- and 50-mL single-use vials

Storage/Stability:

Vials are stable at 2 to 8°C. Protect vials from direct sunlight. Stable at room temperature for 12 hours.

Storage During Travel

Protect from extremes in temperature. Do not leave medication in the car or trunk. When traveling by airplane, take vials on board in passenger cabin so that medication will not be exposed to temperature extremes in the baggage compartment. Vials should be transported in a cooler, near but not touching ice packs. Do not use dry ice as it may freeze the vials.

General Precautions (see package insert for details)

- Type I hypersensitivity or anaphylactic reactions to murine proteins or to any component of this product are rare, but may occur.
- Emergency drugs (e.g., epinephrine, antihistamines, corticosteroids) should be readily available at the bedside for immediate use in the event of a reaction during administration.
- Rituximab-induced B-cell depletion occurred in 70–80% of patients and was associated with decreased serum immunoglobulins in a minority of patients. The incidence of infection does not appear to be increased.
- **Do not administer by IV push or as an IV bolus. Hypersensitivity reactions may occur.**
- Consider premedication with acetaminophen and diphenhydramine before each infusion of Rituximab. This may attenuate the infusion-related events. Because of the potential for hypotension, consideration should be given to holding hypertensive medication 12 hours prior to the infusion.
- Administer infusion at a rate of 50 mg/hour. If hypersensitivity or infusion-related events do not occur, escalate the infusion rate in 50 mg/hour-increments every 30 minutes to a maximum of 400 mg/hour.
- Subsequent infusions can be initiated at a rate of 100 mg/hour and increased by 100 mg/hr to a maximum of 400 mg/hour.
- **Do not mix or dilute Rituximab with other drugs. May be mixed for infusion with either 0.9% sodium chloride or 5% dextrose in water.**

Warnings

- Tumor lysis syndrome may occur, especially in patients with high numbers of circulating malignant cells.
- For severe allergic reactions (e.g., bronchospasm, hypotension, and angioedema), the infusion should be interrupted and resumed at a 50% reduction in rate once symptoms have completely resolved. Treatment of symptoms with diphenhydramine and acetaminophen is recommended; additional treatment with bronchodilators or IV saline may be indicated.
- Infusion-related complex symptoms consisting of fever and chills/rigors occurred in the majority of patients during the first Rituximab infusion. Other infusion-related symptoms included nausea, urticaria, fatigue, headache, pruritus, bronchospasm, dyspnea, sensation of tongue or throat swelling, rhinitis, vomiting, hypotension, flushing, and pain at the disease sites. These reactions generally occurred within 30 minutes to 2 hours of beginning the first infusion, and resolved with slowing or interruption of the infusion and with supportive care (e.g., IV saline, diphenhydramine, and acetaminophen).

Resources for Patients

Genentech Assistance Program provides medication for medically indigent patients.
1-800-879-4747

Website: *http://www.rituxan.com/patient*

Stepping Stones a series of educational materials for people living with non-Hodgkin's lymphoma. *Stepping Stones* is a program to help patients learn more—not just about Rituxan®—and non-Hodgkin's lymphoma (NHL)—but also about how to live better with cancer and cancer treatment. *Stepping Stones* consists of a patient-to-patient video and a series of short, easy-to-read brochures. Additional elements are planned for future years.

Video: *Person to Person*

Brochures: Questions and Answers About Rituxan® (rituximab)
Making Choices: Understanding Your Treatment Alternatives for Non-Hodgkin's Lymphoma
Living with Cancer: Learning to Take Care of Yourself
Showing That You Care: How You Can Help if Someone You Know Has Cancer
Finding Information About NHL: Learning to Live with Non-Hodgkin's Lymphoma

Brochures available online or may be ordered through the product sales representative.

Resources for Professionals
Medical Information Line
1-800-821-8590

Education Materials
Rituxan® Administration Video
Rituxan® Administration Resource Kit (includes dosing, mixing, and administration guidelines and charts, question-and-answer pamphlet, and tear-out patient information sheet).
Non-Hodgkin's Lymphoma Classification Wall Chart
Non-Hodgkin's Lymphoma Classification Pocket Pamphlet
See *Stepping Stones* under Resources for Patients

Website: *http://www.rituxan.com/professional*

Online prescribing information:
Dosing and Administration Guide
Dosage and Infusion Rate Finder
Reference Sheets for Patients
Dosage and Administration Video and Slides

Suggested Readings
Patient Education and Counseling

Website: *http://www.biooncology.com/*

Oncology Resource Center: information on monoclonal antibodies, slides that may be downloaded, patient teaching/counseling information, upcoming meetings
Uninsured Patient Assistance Program
1-800-879-4747

Quick Summary Page

Agent: Gemtuzumab ozogamicin (Mylotarg™)
Marketed by: Wyeth Ayerst Laboratories
Philadelphia, PA
Developed by: Wyeth Ayerst and Celltech Group

Mylotarg™ is the first targeted chemotherapy agent using monoclonal antibody technology. A potent anti-tumor antibiotic, calicheamicin is combined with an antibody that binds to the CD33 antigen, a glycoprotein commonly found on leukemic cells. The antibody portion of Mylotarg™ binds to the CD33 antigen found on the surface of leukemic myeloblasts and immature normal cell of myelomonocytic lineage, but not on normal hematopoietic stem cells. The anti-CD33 antibody portion of Mylotarg™ binds with the CD33 antigen resulting in the formation of a complex that is internalized. Upon internalization, the calicheamicin derivative is released inside the lysosomes of the myeloid cell, resulting in DNA strand breaks and cell death.

Mylotarg™ is a humanized monoclonal antibody and is the first drug specifically approved to treat patients with relapsed AML.

Website: *www.ahp.com*

FDA approval May 2000.

Regulatory Approvals

Disease

AML *(CD33 positive)* in patients 60 years or older who have relapsed for the first time and are poor candidates for cytotoxic therapy.

Dosing

9 mg/m², as a 2-hour IV infusion with prophylactic medication of diphenhydramine 50 mg PO and acetaminophen 650–1000 mg PO one hour prior to Mylotarg™ administration, repeating the acetaminophen × 2 doses at 4-hour intervals posttreatment with Mylotarg™.

Recommended treatment is a total of 2 doses of Mylotarg™ with 14 days between doses.

Pharmocokinetics

Half-life: Elimination half-lives of total and unconjugated calicheamicin is about 45 and 100 hours, respectively. Following the second dose of Mylotarg™, the total half-life was increased to about 60 hours.

Metabolism/excretion: Metabolic studies indicate hydrolytic release of the calicheamicin derivative from Mylotarg™. After *in vitro* incubation metabolites were found in human liver microsomes and cytosol. Metabolic studies characterizing the possible isozymes involved in the metabolic pathway of Mylotarg™ have not been performed.

Setting

Primarily ambulatory under the supervision of a physician who is experienced in the use of the cancer chemotherapeutic agents.

Diagnostic/Laboratory Tests

Electrolytes, hepatic function studies, complete blood counts (CBCs) and platelet counts should be monitored during Mylotarg™ therapy. Mylotarg™ is not known to interfere with any routine diagnostic tests.

Administration

Mylotarg™ is a sterile, white, preservative-free lyophilized powder containing 5 mg of drug conjugate in a 20-mL amber vial. *Do not administer as an intravenous push or bolus.*

Storage

Store at 2 to 25°C (36 to 77°F). *The drug product is light sensitive and must be protected from direct and indirect sunlight and unshielded fluorescent light during the preparation and administration of the infusion.*

General Precautions (see package insert for details)

The use of Mylotarg™ is contraindicated in patients with a known hypersensitivity to gemtuzumab ozogamicin or any of its components. Mylotarg™ may cause fetal harm when administered to pregnant women.

Warnings (see package insert or online information for details)

Severe myleosuppression occurs in all patients given the recommended dose of Mylotarg™. Careful hematologic monitoring is required and systemic infections should be treated.

Mylotarg™ can also produce a postinfusion symptom complex of fever and chills, and less commonly hypotension and dyspnea. Prophylactic medications should be given as described above and two additional posttreatment doses, one every four hours. *Vital signs should be monitored during the infusion and for four hours following the infusion.*

Patients receiving Mylotarg™ also experienced infection, bleeding, and mucositis.

Abnormalities of liver function were transient and generally reversible.

Resources for Patients

Complete product information in package insert

Resources for Professionals

Complete product information in package insert
Lists of scientific publications are available on the website.

Quick Summary Page

Agent: Infliximab (Remicade®)
Developed and Marketed by: Centocor, Inc.
Malvern, PA

Through a merger completed on October 6, 1999, Centocor became a wholly owned subsidiary of Johnson & Johnson, worldwide manufacturer of health care products.

Infliximab is the first of a new class of therapeutic agents used in the treatment of Crohn's disease. Infliximab is a chimeric (human/murine) monoclonal antibody that works by inhibiting activity of tumor necrosis factor alpha (TNF-α), which is a mediator of inflammation. It is composed of human constant and murine variable regions. Infliximab is produced by a recombinant cell line cultured by continuous perfusion and is purified by a series of steps that includes measures to inactivate and remove viruses.

Website *http://www.centocor.com/remicade/*

FDA approval August 1998.

Regulatory Approvals

Crohn's disease

Treatment of moderately to severely active Crohn's disease for the reduction of the signs and symptoms, in patients who have an inadequate response to conventional therapy. The safety and efficacy of therapy continued beyond a single dose have not been established.

Treatment of patients with fistulizing Crohn's disease for the reduction in the number of draining enterocutaneous fistula(s). The safety and efficacy of therapy continued beyond 3 doses have not been studied.

Rheumatoid Arthritis

For reduction in signs and symptoms of rheumatoid arthritis in patients who have had an inadequate response to methotrexate. (Approved 11/99)

Dosing

The recommended dose of Infliximab is 5 mg/kg given as a single intravenous infusion for treatment of moderately to severely active Crohn's disease in patients who have had an inadequate response to conventional therapy.

In patients with fistulizing disease, an initial 5 mg/kg dose should be followed with additional 5 mg/kg doses at 2 and 6 weeks after the first infusion.

Dosing

The recommended dose of Infliximab is 3 mg/kg given as an intravenous infusion followed with additional 3 mg/kg doses at 2 and 6 weeks after the first infusion, and every 8 weeks thereafter. Should be given in combination with methotrexate.

Pharmacokinetics

Half-life

Infliximab has a prolonged terminal half-life and is predominantly distributed within the vascular compartment. A single infusion of the recommended dose of 5 mg/kg resulted in a median Cmax of 118 mcg/mL, a median Vd equal to 3.0 liters and a terminal half-life of 9.5 days.

Corticosteroid use significantly increased the Vd of Infliximab from 2.8 to 3.3 liters (a 17% increase, possibly secondary to corticosteroid-mediated changes in electrolyte balance and fluid retention). No evidence of accumulation was observed after repeated dosing in patients with fistulizing disease given 5 mg/kg Infliximab at weeks 0, 2, and 6, or in patients with moderate or severe Crohn's disease retreated with 4 infusions of 10 mg/kg Infliximab at 8-week intervals.

Metabolism/Excretion

Not specified.

Setting
Primarily ambulatory under the supervision of a physician.

Diagnostic/Laboratory Tests
As clinically indicated.

Administration
Vial Sizes:
Infliximab (Remicade®) lyophilized concentrate for injection is supplied in individually boxed single-use vials in the following strength: 100 mg infliximab in a 20-mL vial.

Remicade® vials do not contain antibacterial preservatives. Therefore, the vials after reconstitution should be used immediately, not re-entered or stored. The diluent to be used for reconstitution is 10 mL of sterile water for injection, USP. The total dose of the reconstituted product must be further diluted to 250 mL with 0.9% sodium chloride injection, USP. The infusion concentration should range between 0.4 mg/mL and 4 mg/mL. The Remicade® infusion should begin within 3 hours of preparation.

Studies have indicated that reconstituted Remicade® and diluted Remicade® infusion solution are incompatible with plasticized PVC (polyvinylchloride) equipment or devices. Diluted Remicade® solutions should be prepared only in glass infusion bottles or polypropylene or polyolefin infusion bags and administered through polyethylene-lined administration sets.

Storage
Store the lyophilized product under refrigeration at 2 to 8°C (36 to 46°F). Do not freeze. Do not use beyond the expiration date. This product contains no preservative.

General Precautions (see package insert for details)
Contraindications
Infliximab should not be administered to patients with known hypersensitivity to any murine proteins or other component of the product.

Warnings
Hypersensitivity
Infliximab has been associated with hypersensitivity reactions that differ in their time of onset. In some cases, urticaria, dyspnea, and/or hypotension have occurred during infusion or within 2 hours of Infliximab infusion. In other cases, when patients were retreated with Infliximab following a 2- to 4-year period without Infliximab treatment, fever, rash, headache, sore throat, myalgias, polyarthralgias, hand and facial edema and/or dysphagia were observed 3–12 days following infusion.

Infliximab should be discontinued for severe reactions. Medications for the treatment of hypersensitivity reactions (e.g., acetaminophen, antihistamines, corticosteroids, and/or epinephrine) should be available for immediate use in the event of a reaction.

Autoimmunity
Anti-TNFα therapy may result in the formation of autoimmune antibodies and, rarely, in the development of a lupus-like syndrome. If a patient develops symptoms suggestive of a lupus-

like syndrome following treatment with Infliximab and is positive for antibodies against double-stranded DNA, treatment should be discontinued.

Precautions
Immunosuppression
TNFα mediates inflammation and modulates cellular immune response; therefore, the possibility exists for anti-TNFα therapies, including Infliximab, to affect normal immune responses.

Malignancy/Infection
Patients with long duration of Crohn's disease and chronic exposure to immunosuppressant therapies are more prone to develop lymphomas and infections.
Human Antichimeric Antibody (HACA) Development
134 of the 199 Crohn's disease patients treated with Infliximab were evaluated for HACA; 18 (13%) were HACA-positive (the majority at low titer, 1:20). Patients who were HACA-positive were more likely to experience an infusion reaction.

Resources for Patients
Complete product information in package insert

Resources for Professionals
Complete product information in package insert

Website: *http://centocor.com/remicade*

Quick Summary Page

Agent: Daclizumab (Zenapax®)
          Manufacturer: Roche Laboratories
                    Nutley, NJ

Website: *http://www.rocheusa.com/*

Approved December 11, 1997

Daclizumab is an immunosuppressive, humanized IgG1 monoclonal antibody produced by recombinant DNA technology that binds specifically to the alpha subunit (Tac subunit) of the human high-affinity interleukin-2 receptor that is expressed on the surface of activated lymphocytes. Daclizumab is a composite of human (90%) and murine (10%) antibody sequences. It functions as an IL-2 receptor antagonist by inhibiting the binding of IL-2 to its receptor. Daclizumab inhibits IL-2-mediated activation of lymphocytes, a critical pathway in the cellular immune response involved in allograft rejection.

Regulatory Approvals

Disease

Organ rejection, prophylaxis: Prophylaxis of acute organ rejection in patients receiving renal transplants. It is used as part of an immunosuppressive regimen that includes cyclosporine and corticosteroids.

Dosing

1 mg/kg IV as a bolus infusion over 15 minutes. The standard course of therapy is for five doses. The first dose should be given 24 hours prior to transplantation. Give the four remaining doses at intervals of 14 days.

Pharmocokinetics

In vitro and *in vivo* data suggest that serum levels of 5 to 10 mcg/mL are necessary for saturation of the Tac subunit of the IL-2 receptors to block the responses of activated T-lymphocytes.

Setting

Ambulatory or inpatient

Diagnostic/Laboratory

As clinically indicated

Administration

Vial Sizes:

25 mg/5 mL preservative-free; in single use vials

Preparation:

Mix the calculated volume of daclizumab with 50 mL of sterile 0.9% sodium chloride solution and administer via a peripheral or central vein over a 15-minute period. When mixing the solution, gently invert the bag to avoid foaming.

Do not shake.

The product contains no antimicrobial preservative or bacteriostatic agents. Once the solution is prepared, administer IV within 4 hours. May be held longer, refrigerated at 2 to 8°C for 24 hours. If not used within 24 hours, discard.

Storage/Stability:

Vials are stable at 2 to 8°C. Protect vials from direct sunlight. Stable at room temperature for 4 hours.

General Precautions (see package insert for details)

Emergency drugs (e.g., epinephrine, antihistamines, corticosteroids) should be readily available at the bedside for immediate use in the event of an allergic reaction during administration. Reactions have not been observed but may occur during the administration of proteins.

The incidence and types of adverse events were similar in both placebo-treated and daclizumab-treated patients (all received cyclosporine and corticosteroids) in the preliminary clinical trials. GI disorders were the most commonly reported effects.

Do not infuse or add any other drug substances simultaneously through the same intravenous line.

Daclimuzab is not for direct injection.

Resources for Patients
See linked website, *The Transplant Patient Partnering Program,* provided as an educational resource by Roche Pharmaceuticals.

Website: *http://www.tppp.net*

Resources for Professionals
Website: *http://www.rocheusa.com/programs/contacts.html*

1-800-526-0625

Quick Summary Page

Agent: Muromonab-CD3 (Orthoclone OKT®3)
Manufacturer: Ortho Biotech
Raritan, NJ

Muromonab-CD3 is a murine monoclonal antibody to the T3 (CD3) antigen of human T-cell that functions as an immunosuppressant first approved by the FDA in 1986. The antibody is a biochemically purified IgG_{2a} immunoglobulin. It reverses graft rejection probably by blocking the T-cell function, which plays a major role in acute allograft rejection.

Website: *http://www.jnj.com*

Regulatory Approvals

Disease	*Dosing*
Organ rejection: Treatment of acute organ rejection in patients receiving renal transplants	5 mg/day for 10 to 14 days. Begin treatment once acute renal rejection is diagnosed.
Cardiac/hepatic allograft rejection: Treatment of steroid-resistant acute allograft rejection	5 mg/day for 10 to 14 days. Begin treatment when it is determined that a rejection has not been reversed by an adequate course of corticosteroid therapy.

Pharmocokinetics
In vitro and *in vivo* data suggest that serum levels > than 0.8 mcg/mL block the function of cytotoxic T cells.

Setting
Hospital or ambulatory treatment center

Diagnostic/Laboratory
Monitor the following tests prior to and during therapy:
BUN, serum creatinine, hepatic transaminases, alkaline phosphatase, bilirubin, CBC with differential and platelets

Chest x-ray within 24 hours before initiating treatment, which should be free of any evidence of heart failure or fluid overload

Quantitative T-lymphocyte surface phenotyping

Testing for human-mouse antibody titers is strongly recommended; a titer of 1:1,000 is a contraindication for use

Administration

Vial Sizes:

5 mg/5 mL.

Administer as an IV bolus in <1 minute.

Do not give by IV infusion or in conjunction with other drug solutions.

Preparation:

Draw solution into a syringe through a low protein-binding 0.2- or 0.22-micrometer filter.

Muromonab-CD3 is for IV use only.

Do not add or infuse with other drugs simultaneously through the same IV line. If the same IV line is used for sequential infusion of several different drugs, flush with saline before and after infusion of muromonab-CD3.

Storage/Stability:

Refrigerate at 2 to 8°C.

Do not freeze or shake.

General Precautions (see package insert for details)

Cytokine release syndrome: The majority of patients experience fever and chills, headache, tremor, nausea/vomiting, diarrhea, abdominal pain, malaise, muscle/joint ache and pains, and generalized weakness with the first few doses. This is attributed to the release of cytokines by activated lymphocytes or monocytes. The syndrome typically begins 30 to 60 minutes following administration of a dose and may persist for several hours.

Cytokine release syndrome may be prevented or minimized by pretreatment with 8 mg/kg of methylprednisolone given 1 to 4 hours prior to administration of the first dose of muromonab-CD3 and by closely following recommendations for dosage and treatment duration.

If hypersensitivity reaction is suspected, discontinue the drug immediately and do not resume therapy or re-expose the patient to muromonab-CD3. Serious acute hypersensitivity reactions may require emergency treatment with epinephrine and other resuscitative measures.

Serious and occasionally fatal, immediate (usually within 10 minutes) hypersensitivity (anaphylactic) reactions have occurred. Manifestations of anaphylaxis may appear similar to manifestations of the CRS.

Patients more at risk for serious complications from CRS may include those with unstable angina; recent MI or symptomatic ischemic heart disease; heart failure of any etiology; pulmonary edema of any etiology; any form of chronic obstructive pulmonary disease; intravascular volume overload or depletion of any etiology; cerebrovascular disease; patients with advanced symptomatic vascular disease or neuropathy; history of seizures; septic shock.

Make efforts to correct or stabilize background conditions prior to initiation of therapy.

Emergency drugs (e.g., epinephrine, antihistamines, corticosteroids) should be readily available at the bedside for immediate use in the event of an allergic reaction during administration.

Patients should be monitored closely at the initiation of the infusion.

Drug Interactions:

Do not use with indomethacin because encephalopathy and other CNS effects have occurred with concurrent use.

Once opened, use the ampule immediately because there is no bacteriostatic agent present; discard any unused portion.

Advise patients to seek medical attention at the first sign of skin rash, urticaria, rapid heartbeat, difficulty in swallowing and breathing, or any swelling that may suggest angioedema or other allergic reaction.

Resources for Patients
Website: *http://www.jnj.com*

Resources for Professionals
See product sales representative.

Quick Summary Page

Agent: Basiliximab (Simulect®)
Distributor: Novartis Pharmaceuticals Corporation
East Hanover, NJ 07936

Simulect® is a chimeric monoclonal antibody, produced by recombinant DNA technology. It is a glycoprotein obtained from fermentation of an established mouse myeloma cell line genetically engineered to express plasmids encoding the RFT5 antibody that binds selectively to the IL-2R alpha. While in circulation, Simulect impairs the response of the immune system to antigenic challenges.

Website: *www.us.novartis.com*

FDA approval: May 13, 1998.

Regulatory Approvals

Disease

Prophylaxis of acute organ rejection in patients receiving renal transplant when used as part of an immunosuppressive regimen that includes cyclosporine and corticosteroids.

Dosing

Adult: Two doses of 20 mg each. The first dose given within 2 hours prior to transplantation surgery. The second dose should be given four days after transplantation.

Pediatric Use: Two doses of 12 mg/m², up to a total in each dose of 20 mg, using the same schedule as for adult use.

Pharmacokinetics

Absorption: Peak serum concentration following IV infusion of 20 mg over 30 minutes is 7.1 ± 5.1 mg/L. The extent and degree of distribution to various body compartments has not been fully studied.

Half-life: Terminal half-life is 7.2 ± 3.2 days.

Metabolism/Excretion: Complete and consistent binding to IL-2R alpha is maintained as long as serum Simulect® levels exceed 0.2 mcg/mL. *In vitro* studies using human tissues indicate that Simulect® binds only to lymphocytes.

Setting
Inpatient in a facility equipped and staffed with adequate laboratory and supportive medical resources.

Diagnostic/Laboratory Tests
As clinically indicated.

Administration
For intravenous use.

Vial Sizes:
Supplied in a single-use glass vial containing 20 mg of basiliximab. Preparation includes adding 5 mL of sterile water for injection, USP to the vial containing basiliximab. Shake the vial gently to dissolve the powder. The reconstituted solution should be diluted to a volume of 50 mL with normal saline or 5% dextrose for infusion. When mixing, gently invert the bag to avoid foaming.

Do not shake.

Storage:
Reconstituted basiliximab should be used immediately. If not used immediately, store at 2 to 8°C for 24 hours or at room temperature for 4 hours. Discard the reconstituted solution if not used within 24 hours.

General Precautions (see package insert for details)
The use of Simulect® is contraindicated in patients with a known hypersensitivity to basiliximab or other components of the product. Simulect® should be administered under qualified medical supervision. Anaphylactoid reactions following the administration of Simulect® have not been observed, but can occur following the administration of proteins. Medications for the treatment of severe hypersensitivity reactions should be available for immediate use. Simulect® does not appear to add to the background of adverse events seen in organ transplantation. The most frequently reported adverse events were gastrointestinal disorders.

Resources for Patients
Website: *www.us.novartis.com*

1-888-NOW-NOVA (toll free), Monday through Friday, 8:30 A.M. to 5 P.M. EST.

Resources for Professionals
Novartis Pharmaceuticals Corporation
59 Route 10
East Hanover, NJ 07936
973-781-8300

1-888-NOW-NOVA (toll free), Monday through Friday, 8:30 A.M. to 5 P.M. EST.
Rx Pharmaceuticals Media Relations
Telephone: 973-781-5486
Fax: 973-781-7828

HEMATOPOIETIC GROWTH FACTORS

Quick Summary Page

Agent: Oprelvekin (Neumega®)
  Manufacturer: Genetics Institute, Inc.
    Cambridge, Massachusetts
    Subsidiary of American Home Products

Oprelvekin, the active ingredient in Neumega®, is produced in *E. coli* by recombinant DNA methods. The protein is nonglycosylated. Oprelvekin (interleukin-11) is a thrombopoietic growth factor that directly stimulates the proliferation of hematopoietic stem cells and megakaryocyte progenitor cells and includes megakaryocyte maturation, resulting in increased platelet production.

Websites: *http://www.genetics.com/*
  http://www.neumega.com/

First received regulatory approval in November 1997.

Regulatory Approvals

Disease/Condition

Neumega® is indicated for the prevention of severe thrombocytopenia and the reduction of the need for platelet transfusions following myelosuppressive chemotherapy in patients with nonmyeloid malignancies who are at high risk of severe thrombocytopenia.

Dosing

50 mcg/kg once daily started by subcutaneous injection 6 to 24 hours following chemotherapy until post-nadir platelet count is greater than or equal to 50,000 cells/mcL.

Pharmacokinetics

Peak serum levels following subcutaneous injection of 50 mcg/kg occurred at 3.2 hours post-injection. Terminal half-life was approximately 7 hours.
Elimination: Primarily in the kidney, molecule is metabolized prior to excretion.

Setting

Ambulatory

Diagnostic/Laboratory Tests

Complete blood count including platelet count prior to chemotherapy and at regular intervals during oprelvekin therapy. Monitor platelet counts during the time of the expected nadir and until adequate recovery has occurred. Continue dosing until post-nadir platelet count is 50,000 cells/mcL.

Administration

Vial Sizes:

Neumega® is available for subcutaneous administration in single-use vials containing 5 mg of oprelvekin as a sterile, lyophilized powder. When reconstituted with 1 mL of sterile water for injection, USP, the resulting solution has a pH of 7.0 and a concentration of 5 mg/mL. Direct diluent against the side of the vial and swirl contents gently. Avoid excessive or vigorous agitations. Use within 3 hours of reconstitution.

Do not reenter or reuse the single-use vials. Discard any unused portion.

Stability/Storage:
Store in a refrigerator at 2 to 8°C.

Do not freeze.

Storage During Travel
Protect from extremes in temperature. Do not leave medication in the car or trunk. When traveling by airplane, take vials on board in passenger cabin so that medication will not be exposed to temperature extremes in the baggage compartment. Vials should be transported in a cooler, near but not touching ice packs. Do not use dry ice as it may freeze the vials.

General Precautions (see package insert for details)
- Hypersensitivity to oprelvekin or any component of the product.
- Oprelvekin is known to cause fluid retention; use with caution in patients with clinically evident congestive heart failure (CHF) and patients who may be susceptible to developing CHF.
- Monitor preexisting fluid collections, such as pleural effusions, pericardial effusions, or ascites. Consider drainage if medically indicated.
- Monitor fluid balance and institute appropriate medical management as required.
- **Capillary leak syndrome has not been observed.**
- Adverse events associated with Neumega® were mild to moderate in severity, associated with fluid retention, and were reversible after discontinuation of dosing. The most common adverse events associated with Neumega treatment included peripheral edema, dyspnea, tachycardia, and conjunctival redness.

Resources for Patients
Neumega® Access Program, a program available to uninsured and underinsured patients based on financial status.
1-888-NEUMEGA
Patient Treatment Diary

Resources for Professionals
Website: *http://www.neumega.com*
Complete Prescribing Information
Product Press Releases
Slide Library (new selections of slides available every month)
Interactive Case Studies

Quick Summary Page

Agent: Filgrastim (Neupogen®)
Manufacturer: Amgen, Inc.
Thousand Oaks, CA

Filgrastim is a human granulocyte colony-stimulating factor (G-CSF) produced by recombinant DNA technology. Filgrastim is produced by *E. coli* bacteria inserted with the human G-CSF gene. As a natural body protein, G-CSF regulates the production of neutrophils within the bone marrow.

Website: *http://www.amgen.com/*

First received FDA approval in February 1991.

Regulatory Approvals

Disease/Condition	*Dosing*
In patients with cancer, following myeloablative chemotherapy to reduce the incidence of infection in patients with nonmyeloid malignancies.	5 mcg/kg/day given daily for up to two weeks by either SC injection, IV bolus infusion, or by continuous SC or IV infusion. Administer no earlier than 24 hours following chemotherapy, or in the time frame of 24 hours before administration of chemotherapy.
Patients with acute myeloid leukemia receiving induction or consolidation chemotherapy to reduce the time to neutrophil recovery.	5 mcg/kg/day given daily for up to two weeks by either SC injection, IV bolus infusion, or by continuous SC or IV infusion. Administer no earlier than 24 hours following chemotherapy, or in the time frame of 24 hours before administration of chemotherapy or until ANC reaches 10,000 cells/mm^3.
Bone-marrow transplant: To reduce the duration of neutropenia and neutropenia-related clinical sequelae in patients with nonmyeloid malignancies undergoing myeloablative chemotherapy followed by BMT.	10 mcg/kg/day given as an IV infusion of 4 or 24 hours or as a continuous 24 hour SC infusion. Administer at least 24 hours following chemotherapy or BMT infusion. Titrate dose by response (see package insert for details).
Peripheral Blood Progenitor Cell (PBPC) Collection: For the mobilization of hematopoietic progenitor cells into the peripheral blood for leukapheresis collection.	10 mcg/kg/day SC, either as a bolus or continuous infusion. It is recommended that filgrastim be given for at least four days before the first leukapheresis and continued till the last.
Severe Chronic Neutropenia (SCN): To reduce the incidence and duration of sequelae of neutropenia.	Congenital: 6 mcg/kg twice daily SC every day Idiopathic or cyclic: 5 mcg/kg as a single SC injection daily. Adjust dose based on patient's clinical course as well as ANC.

Pharmacokinetics

Peak serum levels following subcutaneous injection occurred within 2 to 8 hours following dosing, with longer time corresponding with higher doses. The elimination half-life is approximately 3.5 hours.

Setting

Ambulatory

Diagnostic/Laboratory Tests

Complete blood count including differential and platelet count prior to chemotherapy and at regular intervals (twice per week post-chemotherapy; three times per week post-BMT) during filgrastim therapy. Monitoring during the time of recovery of neutrophils is important to avoid leukocytosis. An initial rise in the neutrophil count is expected. It is important to continue dosing until the post-nadir neutrophil count is 10,000 cells/mm³.

Administration

Vial Sizes:

Neupogen® is available for subcutaneous administration in single-use vials containing 300 mcg/mL or 480 mcg/1.6 mL of liquid.

The vials are preservative-free. Do not reenter or reuse the vials. Discard any unused portion.

Neupogen® may be diluted in 5% dextrose solution for IV administration. *Do not dilute with saline at any time; product may precipitate.*

At concentrations between 5 and 15 mcg/mL, filgrastim should be protected from adsorption to plastic materials by the addition of albumin (human) to a final concentration of 2 mg/mL.

Admixture Incompatibilities: Amphotericin B; cefonicid; cefoperazone; cefotaxime; cefoxitin; ceftizoxime; clindamycin; dactinomycin; etoposide; fluorouracil; furosemide; heparin; mannitor; metronidazole; methylprednisolone; mezlocillin; mitomycin; prochlorperazine; piperacillin; thiotepa.

Stability/Storage:

Store in a refrigerator at 2 to 8°C.

Do not freeze.

Storage During Travel

Protect from extremes in temperature. Do not leave medication in the car or trunk. When traveling by airplane, take vials on board in passenger cabin so that medication will not be exposed to temperature extremes in the baggage compartment. Vials should be transported in a cooler, near but not touching ice packs. Do not use dry ice as it may freeze the vials.

General Precautions (see package insert for details)

Hypersensitivity to filgrastim, *E. coli* derived proteins, or any component of the product. Adverse events associated with Neupogen® were mild. The majority of adverse experiences in clinical trials were associated with the underlying malignancy or cytotoxic chemotherapy. The most common adverse event associated with Neupogen® treatment included medullary bone pain. Other effects seen occasionally include decreased platelet count; however, counts will generally remain within normal limits.

Resources for Patients

Educational materials may be ordered online at *http://www.amgen.com* under patient resources. Materials include the following:

Video: *What I Wish I Knew*—Features six women who offer hope and help in dealing with breast cancer.

Starting Over: How stem-cell support helps rebuild your immune system after high-dose chemotherapy. A video guide for patients and caregivers.

Brochure: *Patient to Patient: Sharing our Experiences with Chemotherapy. Stem-cell support. Making delivery of your high-dose chemotherapy possible.*

Managing Career and Cancer. What You Need to Know.

Brochures available for downloading from the website in English or Spanish:

Neupogen® (filgrastim): Part of the Good News About Today's Chemotherapy, information about a particular side effect of chemotherapy, a low white blood-cell count, and how one drug, Neupogen®, helps to manage it.

The Most Important Part of Your Treatment Is You. The more you know about cancer, the more you can participate in its treatment. Learn about where to find sources of information and what questions to ask of your doctor.

The First Step in Chemotherapy Is Overcoming Your Fear, information about medicines that are available to manage side effects of chemotherapy and help you lead a more active life.

Journal: *Your personal daily journal*—includes space for addresses and medical information, and recordkeeping.

Online programs patients may register for:

In Your Shoes™—An interactive program for patients with breast cancer that allows them to view actual case studies of people who have gone through chemotherapy for breast cancer.

Amgen Cancer and Chemotherapy Education Support System (ACCESS), a free information and support resource for women with breast cancer.

Resources for Professionals

Website: *http://www.amgen.com*

Project ChemoInsight™: A data collection tool that may help oncology health-care professionals improve chemotherapy outcomes.

Communication Skills Evaluation

Product and Treatment Information

Professional Services Department
1-800-772-6436 (1-800-77-AMGEN)

Safety Net™: Program for patients who are medically indigent. Call 1-800-272-9376.

Amgen Clinical Support Specialist™: Available for consultation or to provide programs related to the use of hematopoietic growth factors and patient management. Access by contacting Amgen product sales representative.

Professional Speakers Bureau

Quick Summary Page

Agent: Epoetin-alfa (ProCrit®)
     Manufacturer: Amgen Inc.
            Thousand Oaks, CA
     Distributed by: Ortho Biotech
            Raritan, NJ

PROCRIT® is a genetically engineered version of the body's natural hormone, erythropoietin. Produced primarily in the kidneys, erythropoietin stimulates the division and differentiation of committed erythroid progenitors in the bone marrow. Epoetin-alfa is manufactured by recombinant DNA technology; the gene for human erythropoietin is inserted into mammalian cells. The recombinant product contains the identical amino-acid sequence of natural erythropoietin.

Through a product-licensing agreement, Johnson & Johnson acquired the rights to develop and market recombinant human erythropoietin. In the United States, Ortho Biotech (Ortho Biotech was established in 1990 by Johnson & Johnson as the first biotechnology subsidiary of a major health-care company) markets recombinant human erythropoietin, manufactured by Amgen, Inc., under the tradename ProCrit® (epoetin alfa). Janssen/Cilag, a Johnson & Johnson company, markets this product internationally under the tradename Eprex® for a variety of indications, including CRF patients receiving dialysis treatment.

Website: *www.procrit.com*

First received FDA approval in 1989 for chronic renal failure.

Regulatory Approval

Disease/Condition	*Dosing*
Approved for the treatment of anemia in patients with chronic renal failure	50–100 U/kg 3×/week by intravenous infusion until target hemoglobin is reached
Approved for the treatment of anemia in AZT-treated HIV-infected patients (Epo level ≥ 500 mU/mL)	100 U/kg 3×/week SC injection or by intravenous infusion for 8 weeks as a starting dose.

Approved for the treatment of anemia in cancer patients on chemotherapy	150 U/kg 3×/week SC or by intravenous infusion until target hemoglobin is reached.
	Alternate schedule: Some institutions have tried an alternate schedule of 40,000 U SC q week. If after 4 weeks Hgb level has not increased more than 1 g/dL from baseline, dose may be increased to 60,000 U weekly.
Reduction of allogeneic blood transfusions in surgery patients (elective, non-vascular, noncardiac surgery)	300 U/kg/day SC for 10 days prior to surgery, the day of surgery, and 4 days after surgery.
	Alternate schedule: 600 U/kg SC q week (21, 14, and 7 days before surgery and on the day of surgery).

Pharmacokinetics

Circulating half-life is 4 to 13 hours in patients with CRF following IV administration. Peak serum levels are achieved from 5 to 24 hours after SC administration in patients with CRF, and decline slowly thereafter.

Setting

Primarily ambulatory

Diagnostic/Laboratory Tests

At baseline, perform CBC with differential and platelet count and repeat at regular intervals as clinically determined.

Determine hematocrit twice weekly (CRF) and once weekly (HIV-infected patients and patients with cancer) until stabilized, then at regular intervals.

- Because of the time required for erythropoiesis and the red-cell half-life, allow a minimum of 4 weeks to determine initial responsiveness. Following a dosage adjustment, allow 2 to 6 weeks to determine effectiveness.
- See package insert for full instructions for dosage adjustments.

Suggested target hematocrit range is 30% to 36%.

If hematocrit increases too rapidly (> 4 points in a 2-week period), dosage should be decreased.

Prior to and during therapy, monitor patient's iron status by measurement of serum ferritin (should be at least 100 ng/mL) and transferrin saturation (should be at least 20%). Patients may require supplementation with ferrous sulfate to achieve full therapeutic benefit of epoetin-alfa.

In HIV-infected patients and patients with cancer on chemotherapy, at baseline an erythropoietin (Epo) level will assist in determining those patients who are most likely to respond to therapy. In HIV-infected patients, those with an initial Epo level ≥500 mU/mL are less likely to respond. In patients with cancer, those with an initial Epo level ≥200 mU/mL are generally not recommended to receive therapy.

Reasons to consider for delayed or diminished response: functional iron deficiency; underlying infectious, inflammatory or malignant processes; occult blood loss; underlying hematologic diseases; vitamin deficiencies (folic acid or B_{12}); hemolysis, aluminum intoxication; osteitis fibrosa cystica; and increase zidovudine dosage.

Administration
Vial Sizes:

Single-use vials of injectable solution with no preservative 2,000 U/mL; 3,000 U/mL; 4,000 U/mL; 10,000 U/mL; 40,000 mU/mL

Multidose vials of injectable solution with preservative 10,000 U/mL in 2-mL vials; 20,000 U/mL in 1-mL vial. Do not shake vials because prolonged shaking may denature the glycoprotein, rendering it inactive.

Do not reuse or reenter single-use vials. Discard unused portion.
Multidose vials: Discard 21 days after initial entry.

Compatibility: Do not give in conjunction with other drug solutions.

Stability/Storage:
Store in a refrigerator at 2 to 8°C.

Do not freeze.

Storage During Travel

Protect from extremes in temperature. Do not leave medication in the car or trunk. When traveling by airplane, take vials on board in passenger cabin so that medication will not be exposed to temperature extremes in the baggage compartment. Vials should be transported in a cooler, near but not touching ice packs. Do not use dry ice as it may freeze the vials.

General Precautions (see package insert for details)

The use of epoetin-alfa is contraindicated in patients with uncontrolled hypertension; hypersensitivity to mammalian cell-derived products or human albumin. Not intended as a substitute for emergency transfusion in severe anemia. In general, epoetin-alfa is well tolerated. In the CRF population, the most common side effects observed were hypertension and headache. Monitor blood pressure at baseline and at regular intervals.

Resources for Patients

Website: *http://www.procrit.com*
             http://www.4Anemia.com

A consumer-friendly site with the basics on anemia, treatment options, news, and research developments.

Strength for Living™   *http://www.procrit.com/*
An educational program designed to help women with cancer cope with serious side effects of chemotherapy, such as anemia.

Strength for Caring™ Program
Ortho Biotech is proud to offer Strength for Caring™, an educational program designed to teach family members the skills they need to care for a loved one with cancer.

To locate programs in your area, call 1-888-ICARE80

Surviving Patients Inspire through Resources, Information, and Treatment tips (The SPIRIT Project): A program founded in 1981 by CHEMOcare, to provide support to people undergoing treatment for cancer and to their families. The SPIRIT project is a gift from cancer survivors designed to help patients rekindle their spirits. Printed brochure available from product sales representative, or call 1-800-55-CHEMO.

Brochure: *When I Started Chemotherapy I was Tired All the Time* may be ordered or viewed online.

Resources for Professionals

Customer Service: Open 8:15 A.M. to 4:30 P.M. EST
(800) 325-7504
Reimbursement Hotline: (800) 553-3851
Fax Number: (908) 526-6457

The Importance of Treating Anemia in HIV Patients
Website: *http://www.thebody.com/*
(An AIDS and HIV information resource)

Professional Speakers Bureau (contact product representative)

Dimensions of Caring
8:30 A.M. to 5 P.M. EST
1-800-984-7337

Oncology Nurse Educators
Available for consultation and programs
Check with product sales representative for availability of monographs on anemia and treatment of cancer-related anemia.

Quick Summary Page

Agent: Epoetin-alfa (Epogen®)
Manufacturer & Distributor: Amgen, Inc.
Thousand Oaks, CA

Epogen® is a genetically engineered version of the body's natural hormone, erythropoietin. Produced primarily in the kidneys, erythropoietin stimulates the division and differentiation of committed erythroid progenitors in the bone marrow. Epoetin-alfa is manufactured by recombinant DNA technology; the gene for human erythropoietin is inserted into mammalian cells. The recombinant product contains the identical amino-acid sequence of natural erythropoietin.

Website: *http://www.amgen.com*

First received FDA approval in 1989.

Regulatory Approvals

Disease/Conditions	*Dosing*
Approved for the treatment of anemia in patients with chronic renal failure (CRF)	50–100 U/kg 3×/week by intravenous infusion until target hemoglobin is reached

In 1999, epoetinalfa received approval for use in the treatment of anemia in pediatric patients with CRF.

Starting dose in the pediatric patient is 50 μ/kg TIW; IV or SC.

Approved for the treatment of anemia in AZT-treated HIV-infected patients (Epo level ≥500 mU/mL)

100 U/kg 3×/week SC injection or by intravenous infusion for 8 weeks as a starting dose

Approved for the treatment of anemia in cancer patients on chemotherapy

150 U/kg 3×/week SC or by intravenous infusion until target hemoglobin is reached.

Alternate schedule: Some institutions have tried an alternate schedule of 40,000 U SC q week. If after 4 weeks Hgb level has not increased more than 1 g/dL from baseline, dose may be increased to 60,000 U weekly.

Reduction of allogeneic blood transfusions in surgery patients (elective, nonvascular, noncardiac surgery)

300 U/kg/day SC for 10 days prior to surgery, the day of surgery, and 4 days after surgery.

Alternate schedule: 600 U/kg SC q week (21, 14, and 7 days before surgery and on the day of surgery).

Pharmacokinetics

Circulating half-life is 4 to 13 hours in patients with CRF following IV administration. Peak serum levels are achieved from 5 to 24 hours after SC administration in patients with CRF, and decline slowly thereafter.

Setting

Primarily ambulatory

Diagnostic/Laboratory Tests

At baseline, perform CBC with differential and platelet count and repeat at regular intervals as clinically determined.

Determine hematocrit twice weekly (CRF), then at regular intervals.

- Because of the time required for erythropoiesis and the red-cell half-life, allow a minimum of four weeks to determine initial responsiveness. Following a dosage adjustment, allow two to six weeks to determine effectiveness.
- See package insert for full instructions for dosage adjustments.

Suggested target hematocrit range is 30% to 36%.

If hematocrit increases too rapidly (> 4 points in a two-week period), dosage should be decreased. Prior to and during therapy, monitor patient's iron status by measurement of serum ferritin (should be at least 100 ng/mL) and transferrin saturation (should be at least 20%). Patients may require supplementation with ferrous sulfate to achieve full therapeutic benefit of epoetin-alfa.

Reasons to consider for delayed or diminished response: functional iron deficiency; underlying infectious, inflammatory, or malignant processes; occult blood loss; underlying hematologic diseases; vitamin deficiencies (folic acid or B_{12}); hemolysis, aluminum intoxication; osteitis fibrosa cystica; and increase zidovudine dosage.

Administration
Vial Sizes:

Single-use vials of injectable solution with no preservative 2,000 U/mL; 3,000 U/mL; 4,000 U/mL; 10,000 U/mL; 40,000 U/mL.

Multidose vials of injectable solution with preservative 10,000 U/mL in 2-mL vials; 20,000 U/mL in 1-mL vials

Do not shake vials because prolonged shaking may denature the glycoprotein, rendering it inactive. *Do not reuse or reenter single-use vials. Discard unused portion.*

Multidose vials: Discard 21 days after initial entry.

Compatibility: Do not give in conjunction with other drug solutions.

Stability/Storage:

Store in a refrigerator at 2 to 8°C.

Do not freeze.

Storage During Travel

Protect from extremes in temperature. Do not leave medication in the car or trunk. When traveling by airplane, take vials on board in passenger cabin so that medication will not be exposed to temperature extremes in the baggage compartment. Vials should be transported in a cooler, near but not touching ice packs. Do not use dry ice as it may freeze the vials.

General Precautions (see package insert for details)

The use of epoetin-alfa is contraindicated in patients with uncontrolled hypertension; hypersensitivity to mammalian cell-derived products or the human albumin. Not intended as a substitute for emergency transfusion in severe anemia. In general, epoetin-alfa is well tolerated. In the CRF population, the most common side effects observed were hypertension and headache. On rare occasions, patients experienced seizures in the context of increased blood pressure and increased hematocrit. Monitor blood pressure at baseline and at regular intervals.

Resources for Patients

Online: About Epogen® (epoetin-alfa)
    Epogen® FAQ (most frequently asked questions)
Patient resources: links to organizations that have established websites related to particular diseases.
Patient Assistance Program 1-800-272-9376
Safety Net Program (for Medically Indigent Patients on Dialysis)

Resources for Professionals

Epogen® FAQ (most frequently asked questions)
Epogen® backgrounder
Epogen® prescribing information
Epogen® News

Patient Assistance Program 1-800-272-9376
Open Monday through Friday 9 A.M. to 5 P.M. EST

Kidney Disease Resources

Quick Summary Page

Agent: Sargramostim (recombinant human granulocyte-macrophage colony-stimulating factor [GM-CSF]) (Leukine®)
           Manufacturer: Immunex
                   Seattle, WA

Sargramostim is a recombinant human GM-CSF produced by recombinant DNA technology in a yeast (*S. cerevisiae*) expression system.

Website: *http://www.immunex.com/*

First approved by FDA in March of 1991.

Regulatory Approvals

Disease	*Dosing*
Neutrophil recovery following induction chemotherapy in acute myelogenous leukemia	The recommended dose is 250 mcg/m²/day administered intravenously over a 4-hour period starting approximately on day 11 or 4 days following the completion of induction chemotherapy, if the Day 10 bone marrow is hypoplastic with <5% blasts.
	If a second cycle of induction chemotherapy is necessary, Leukine® should be administered approximately 4 days after the completion of chemotherapy if the bone marrow is hypoplastic with <5% blasts. Leukine® should be continued until an ANC >1,500/mm³ for 3 consecutive days or a maximum of 42 days. Leukine® should be discontinued immediately if leukemic regrowth occurs. If a severe adverse reaction occurs, the dose can be reduced by 50% or temporarily discontinued until the reaction abates.
Mobilization of peripheral blood progenitor cells (PBPC)	The recommended dose is 250 mcg/m²/day administered IV over 24 hours or SC once daily. Dosing should continue at the same dose through the period of PBPC collection. The optimal schedule for PBPC collection has not been established. If WBC > 50,000 cells/mm³, the Leukine® dose should be reduced by 50%. If adequate numbers of progenitor cells are not collected, other mobilization therapy should be considered.
Post-peripheral blood progenitor cell transplantation	The recommended dose is 250 mcg/m²/day administered IV over 24 hours or SC once daily beginning immediately following infusion of progenitor cells and continuing until an ANC >1,500/ mm³ for 3 consecutive days is attained.
Myeloid reconstitution after autologous or allogeneic bone-marrow transplantation	The recommended dose is 250 mcg/m²/day administered IV over a 2-hour period beginning 2 to 4 hours after bone-marrow infusion, and not less than 24 hours after the last dose of chemotherapy or radiotherapy. Patients should not receive Leukine® until the post-

marrow infusion ANC is less than 500 cells/mm³. Leukine® should be continued until an ANC >1,500/mm³ for 3 consecutive days is attained. If a severe adverse reaction occurs, the dose can be reduced by 50% or temporarily discontinued until the reaction abates. Leukine® should be discontinued immediately if blast cells appear or disease progression occurs.

Bone-marrow transplantation failure or engraftment delay — The recommended dose is 250 mcg/m²/day for 14 days as a 2-hour IV infusion. The dose can be repeated after 7 days off therapy if engraftment has not occurred. If engraftment still has not occurred, a third course of 500 mcg/m²/day for 14 days may be tried after another 7 days off therapy. If there is still no improvement, it is unlikely that further dose escalation will be beneficial. If a severe adverse reaction occurs, the dose can be reduced by 50% or temporarily discontinued until the reaction abates. Leukine® should be discontinued immediately if blast cells appear or disease progression occurs.

Pharmacokinetics

At doses of 250 mcg/m² given by SC injection, serum levels peaked in approximately 3 hours. Metabolism of sargramostim has not been well established.

Setting

Primarily ambulatory

Diagnostic/Laboratory Tests

To avoid potential complications of excessive leukocytosis (WBC > 50,000 cells/mm³ or ANC > 20,000 cells/mm³), a CBC with differential is recommended twice per week during Leukine® therapy. Leukine® treatment should be interrupted or the dose reduced by 50% if the ANC exceeds 20,000 cells/mm³. Biweekly monitoring of renal and hepatic function in patients with renal or hepatic dysfunction prior to initiation of treatment is recommended. Carefully monitor body weight and hydration status during administration.

Administration

Vial Sizes:

Leukine® liquid is a preserved (1.1% benzyl alcohol), sterile, injectable solution: 500 mcg/mL.
Cartons of 5 multiple-dose vials of liquid 500-mcg/mL Leukine®
Lyophilized Leukine® is a sterile, white, preservative-free, lyophilized powder: 250- or 500-mcg vials
Cartons of 5 vials of lyophilized 250-mcg Leukine®
Cartons of 5 vials of lyophilized 500-mcg Leukine®
Both Leukine® Liquid and reconstituted lyophilized Leukine® are suitable for SC injection and IV infusion

Preparation of Leukine®

Lyophilized Leukine® requires reconstitution with 1 mL Sterile Water for Injection, USP or 1 mL Bacteriostatic Water for Injection, USP. The Leukine® Liquid injectable and the reconstituted lyophilized Leukine® solutions are clear, colorless, isotonic solutions. The contents of vials reconstituted with different diluents should not be mixed together.

Sterile Water for Injection, USP (without preservative): Leukine® vials contain no antibacterial preservative; therefore, solutions prepared with Sterile Water for Injection, USP, should be administered as soon as possible, and within 6 hours following reconstitution and/or dilution for IV infusion. The vial should not be reentered or reused. Do not save any unused portion for administration more than 6 hours following reconstitution.

Bacteriostatic Water for Injection, USP (0.9% benzyl alcohol): Reconstituted solutions prepared with Bacteriostatic Water for Injection, USP (0.9% benzyl alcohol) may be stored up to 20 days at 2 to 8°C prior to use. Discard reconstituted solution after 20 days. Previously reconstituted solutions mixed with freshly reconstituted solutions must be administered within 6 hours following mixing. Preparations containing benzyl alcohol (including Leukine® Liquid and lyophilized Leukine® reconstituted with Bacteriostatic Water for Injection) should not be used in neonates (see WARNINGS).

Once the vial has been entered, Leukine® liquid may be stored for up to 20 days at 2 to 8°C. Discard any remaining solution after 20 days.

During reconstitution, the diluent should be directed at the side of the vial and the contents gently swirled to avoid foaming during dissolution. Avoid excessive or vigorous agitation; do not shake.

Leukine® should be used for SC injection without further dilution.

Dilution for IV infusion should be performed in 0.9% Sodium Chloride Injection, USP. If the final concentration of Leukine® is below 10 mcg/mL, Albumin (Human) at a final concentration of 0.1% should be added to the saline prior to addition of Leukine® to prevent adsorption to the components of the drug-delivery system. To obtain a final concentration of 0.1% Albumin (Human), add 1 mg Albumin (Human) per 1 mL 0.9% Sodium Chloride Injection, USP (e.g., use 1 mL 5% Albumin [Human] in 50 mL 0.9% Sodium Chloride Injection, USP).

An in-line membrane filter should not be used for intravenous infusion of Leukine®.

Storage/Stability:

Store Leukine® Liquid and reconstituted lyophilized Leukine® solutions under refrigeration at 2 to 8°C.

Do not freeze.

In the absence of compatibility and stability information, no other medication should be added to infusion solutions containing Leukine®. Use only 0.9% Sodium Chloride Injection, USP, to prepare IV infusion solutions.

Storage During Travel

Protect from extremes in temperature. Do not leave medication in the car or trunk. When traveling by airplane, take vials on board in passenger cabin so that medication will not be exposed to temperature extremes in the baggage compartment. Vials should be transported in a cooler, near but not touching ice packs. Do not use dry ice as it may freeze the vials.

General Precautions (see package insert for details)

- Do not use in patients with excessive leukemic myeloid blast in the bone marrow or peripheral blood ≥ (10%); known hypersensitivity to GM-CSF, yeast-derived products, or any component of the product; simultaneous administration with cytotoxic chemotherapy or radiotherapy, or administration 24 hours preceding or following chemotherapy or radiotherapy.
- Use with caution in patients with preexisting cardiac disease as occasional transient supraventricular arrhythmias have occurred.
- Occasional sequestration of granulocytes in the pulmonary circulation has occurred following a sargramostim infusion, resulting in dyspnea. Monitor patients for any respiratory distress during infusion, especially those patients with preexisting lung disease.
- In patients with preexisting pleural and pericardial effusions, administration of sargramostim may aggravate fluid retention; use with caution in preexisting fluid retention, pulmonary infiltrates, or congestive heart failure.
- Benzyl alcohol as a preservative has been associated with a fatal "gasping syndrome" in premature infants.
- First-dose effects: A syndrome with respiratory distress, hypoxia, flushing, hypotension, syncope or tachycardia has occurred rarely following the first use. These signs have resolved with symptomatic treatment and usually do not recur with subsequent doses in the same cycle of treatment.
- The most common adverse events were fever, asthenia, headache, bone pain, chills, and myalgia. These systemic events were generally mild or moderate, and were usually presented or reversed by the administration of analgesics and antipyretics such as acetaminophen.

Resources for Patients

Patient Information Leukine® (sargramostim)
Chemotherapy and You: a booklet about chemotherapy and the older patient.
Website: *http://www.immunex.com/*

Resources for Professionals

Website: *http://www.immunex.com*
Customer Service and Professional Services
(800) IMMUNEX (800-466-8639)
Reimbursement Hotline
(1-800-321-4669)

FUSION PROTEINS

Quick Summary Page

Agent: Etanercept (Enbrel®)
                   Manufacturer: Immunex Corporation
                                   Seattle, WA
                   Marketed by: Immunex and Wyeth-Ayerst Laboratories

Enbrel® is a dimeric fusion protein consisting of the extracellular ligand-binding portion of the human 75 kilodalton tumor necrosis factor receptor linked to the Fc portion of human IgG1. It is produced by recombinant DNA technology in a Chinese hamster ovary mammalian cell expression system.

Website: *www.enbrel.com*

First approved by the FDA on November 2, 1998.

Regulatory Approvals

Disease	*Dosing*
Rheumatoid arthritis patients who have had an inadequate response to one or more diseases modifying antirheumatic (DMARDs).	25 mg twice weekly SC injection, 72 to 96 hours apart
Expanded indication: Reducing the signs and symptoms and delaying structural damage in patients with moderately to severely active rheumatoid arthritis, including those who have not previously failed treatment with a DMARD.	
Polyarticular-course juvenile rheumatoid arthritis in patients who have had an inadequate response to DMARDs (Approved May 28, 1999)	0.4 mg/kg (up to a maximum 25-mg dose) twice weekly SC injection, 72 to 96 hours apart

Pharmacokinetics

> *Absorption:* Maximum serum concentration of 1.2 mcg/mL and time of 72 hours following SC injection of 25 mg of Enbrel®.
> *Half-life:* Median half-life of 115 hours (range 98 to 300 hours) with a clearance of 89 mL/hr.
> *Metabolism/Excretion:* Renal/hepatic. No formal studies conducted to examine the effects of renal or hepatic impairment.

Setting

Primarily ambulatory with the first dose of Enbrel® administered under medical supervision.

Diagnostic/Laboratory Tests

As clinically indicated.

Administration

Vial Sizes:

> Single-use vial of Enbrel® contains 25 mg etanercept, 40 mg mannitol, 10 mg sucrose, and 1.2 mg tromethamine. Supplied in a carton containing four dose trays. Each dose tray contains one

25-mg single-use vial of etanercept, one 1-mL syringe of sterile Bacteriostatic water for injection (USP, containing 0.9% benzyl alcohol), one plunger, and two alcohol swabs.

Injection sites should be rotated.

Store in the refrigerator at 2 to 8°C. *Enbrel® not used within 6 hours of reconstitution should be discarded.*

Do not freeze. Do not vigorously shake.

Storage During Travel

Protect from extremes in temperature. Do not leave medication in the car or trunk. When traveling by airplane, take vials on board in passenger cabin so that medication will not be exposed to temperature extremes in the baggage compartment. Vials should be transported in a cooler, near but not touching ice packs. Do not use dry ice as it may freeze the vials.

General Precautions (see package insert for details)

In post-marketing reports, serious infection/sepsis with fatalities have been reported. Many of these events occurred in patients with underlying diseases that, along with their rheumatoid arthritis, may predispose them to infections. Patients who develop a new infection while on Enbrel® should be monitored carefully. Therapy with Enbrel® should be discontinued immediately in the presence of a severe infection or sepsis. Enbrel® should not be used in patients with active infections, including chronic or localized infections. Caution should be observed when considering the use of Enbrel® in patients with a history of recurring infections or with conditions such as advanced or poorly controlled diabetes.

Live vaccines should not be given concurrently with Enbrel®. Approximately one third of patients developed site reactions that were mild to moderate and did not require discontinuation of therapy. Treatment may result in the formation of autoimmune antibodies.

Resources for Patients

The Dosing System: A resource for patients using Enbrel®, available through your Wyeth-Ayerst Representative

Enliven: Support for patients starting on Enbrel®, available through your Wyeth-Ayerst Representative

Reimbursement Support Line for Enbrel®: Assistance with issues related to insurance coverage and reimbursement. 1-800-282-7704, 8:30 A.M. to 5:30 P.M., EST, Monday through Friday.

Website: *www.enbrel.com*

Resources for Professionals

The Teaching System for the Health Care Professional: A comprehensive office training and education program available through your Wyeth-Ayerst Representative.

Reimbursement Support Line for Enbrel®: Learn more about your patient's insurance overage. 1-800-282-7704, 8:30 A.M. to 5:30 P.M. EST, Monday through Friday.

Website: *www.enbrel.com/physician/patprograms.htm* or 1-888-4ENBREL (436-2735)

Quick Summary Page

Agent: Denileukin diftitox (ONTAK®)
  Manufacturer: Seragen, Inc.
      Hopkinton, MA
   Distributor: Ligand Pharmaceuticals
      San Diego, CA

ONTAK® is a recombinant DNA-derived cytotoxic protein composed of the amino-acid sequences for diphtheria toxin fragments A and B followed by the sequences for interleukin-2 and is produced in an *E. coli* expression system. It is a fusion protein designed to direct the cytocidal action of diphtheria toxin to cells that express the IL-2 receptor.

Website: *www.ligand.com*

FDA approval on February 2, 1999.

Regulatory Approvals

Disease	*Dosing*
Persistent or recurrent cutaneous T-cell lymphoma in patients whose malignant cells express the CD25 component of the IL-2 receptor.	9 or 18 mcg/kg/day, given IV for five consecutive days every 21 days. Infused over at least 15 minutes.

Pharmacokinetics

  Absorption: Variable but proportional to the dose.

  Half-life: Two-compartment behavior with a distribution phase half-life of 2 to 5 minutes and a terminal phase half-life of 70 to 80 minutes.

  Metabolism/Excretion: Renal/hepatic, metabolized by proteolytic degradation. Excreted material shown to be less than 25% of the total injected dose.

Setting

Hospital or facility equipped with IV epinephrine, corticosteroids, antihistamines, and resuscitative equipment and staffed for cardiopulmonary resuscitation.

Diagnostic/Laboratory Tests

  Prior to administration, the patient's malignant cells should be tested for CD25 expression. CBC, blood chemistry with liver and renal function, and serum albumin should be done prior to initiation of ONTAK® and weekly during therapy.

  Because 83% of study patients experienced hypoalbuminemia, serum albumin levels should be monitored prior to the start of each treatment course. ONTAK® administration should be delayed until serum albumin levels are at least 3.0 g/dL.

Administration

Vial Sizes:

  150 mcg/mL sterile, frozen solution (300 mcg in 2 mL) in a sterile, single-use vial, six vials in a package. Store frozen at or below −10°C.

Special Handling
- Must be brought to room temperature, up to 25°C (77°F), before preparation of the dose.
- Vial may be thawed in the refrigerator at 2 to 8°C for not more than 24 hours or at room temperature for 1 to 2 hours.
- ONTAK® *must not be heated.*
- Mix by gentle swirling. *Do not vigorously shake.*
- After thawing, a haze may be visible. Haze should clear when the solution is at room temperature.
- Solution must not be used unless the solution is clear, colorless, and without visible particulate matter.
- ONTAK® *must not be refrozen.*
- Prepare and hold ONTAK® in plastic syringes or soft IV bags. *Do not use a glass container.*
- The concentration of ONTAK® must be at least 15 mcg/mL during all steps in the preparation of the solution for IV infusion. **For each 1 mL of ONTAK® from the vial(s), no more than 9 mL of sterile saline without preservative should then be added to the IV bag.**
- Should be infused over at least 15 minutes.
- **Should not be administered as a bolus injection.**
- Do not mix with other drugs.
- **Do not administer through an in-line filter.**
- Prepared solutions should be administered within 6 hours.
- Unused portions of ONTAK® should be discarded immediately.

General Precautions (see package insert for details)

Contraindicated for use in patients with a known hypersensitivity to denileukin diftitox or any of its components: diphtheria toxin, IL-2, or excipients.

Patients should be monitored for infection because patients with CTCL have a predisposition to cutaneous infection. Immune impairment may result from the binding of denileukin diftitox to activated lymphocytes and macrophages that can lead to cell death.

Flu-like syndrome is common (91% of patients) and occurs within several hours to days after ONTAK® infusion. Symptoms are usually mild to moderate and respond to antipyretics and/or antiemetics.

Warnings:

Acute hypersensitivity reactions reported in 69% of patients during or within 24 hours of ONTAK® infusion. Symptoms included one or more of the following: hypotension, back pain, dyspnea, vasodilatation, rash, chest pain/tightness, tachycardia, dysphagia, syncope, allergic reaction, or anaphylaxis. Management consists of interruption or a decrease in the rate of infusion. *Antihistamines, corticosteroids, epinephrine, and resuscitative equipment should be readily available and also may need to be administered.*

Vascular leak syndrome characterized by two or more of the following three symptoms (hypotension, edema, and hypoalbuminemia) reported in 27% of patients. Special caution should be observed in patients with preexisting cardiovascular disease.

Resources for Patients

Complete product information at *www.ligand.com*

Resources for Professionals

Complete product information at *www.ligand.com*

Testing service for assay of CD25 on skin biopsy samples is available. For information: 1-800-964-5836.

Lists of scientific publications are available on the website.

Ligand Pharmaceuticals: 1-858-550-7500

Reimbursement Assistance Program: 1-877-654-4263

RETINOIDS

Quick Summary Page

Agent: Bexarotene (Targretin®)
Manufacturer: R. P. Scherer
St. Petersburg, FL
Distributor: Ligand Pharmaceuticals
San Diego, CA

Bexarotene is a member of a subclass of retinoids that selectively activate retinoid X receptors. Once activated, these receptors function as transcription factors that regulate the expression of genes that control cellular differentiation and proliferation. Bexarotene inhibits the growth *in vitro* of some tumor cell lines and also induces tumor regression *in vivo* in some animal models.

Website: *www.ligand.com*

First approved by the FDA in December 1999.

Regulatory Approvals

Disease	*Dosing*
Advanced and early stage cutaneous T-cell lymphoma (CTCL), refractory to at least one prior systemic therapy	300 mg/m²/day PO; if no response after eight weeks or more, the dose can be increased to 400 mg/m²/day with careful monitoring. **Should be taken with a meal.**

Pharmacokinetics

Absorption: Variable, dependent on the fat content of the meal, being higher following a fat-containing meal versus a glucose solution. The therapeutic maximum is about 2 hours.

Half-life: Terminal half-life of about 7 hours.

Metabolism/Excretion: Metabolites have been identified in plasma but the relative contribution to the efficacy and safety of Targretin® is unknown. Bexarotene is thought to be eliminated primarily through the hepatobiliary system.

Setting

Primarily ambulatory

Diagnostic/Laboratory Tests

Blood lipid testing should be performed prior to the initiation of Targretin®. Fasting triglycerides should be normal or normalized before therapy with Targretin® begins. Weekly blood lipid testing is recommended due to the fact that hyperlipidemia usually occurs within the first two to four weeks of therapy.

WBC with differential and baseline thyroid function tests should be obtained prior to the initiation of treatment and periodically during therapy with Targretin®. Liver function tests should be obtained prior to treatment and then carefully monitored at one, two, and four weeks; if stable, monitoring then can be done periodically thereafter.

Administration

Targretin® capsules are supplied as 75-mg off-white, oblong, soft gelatin capsules, imprinted with Targretin®, in high-density polyethylene bottles with child-resistant closures.

Safety and efficacy information is based on administration with food. It is therefore recommended that Targretin® be administered with food.

Storage/Stability:

Store at 2 to 25°C. Avoid exposure to high temperatures and humidity after the bottle is opened. Protect from light.

General Precautions (see package insert for details)

Advise patient to avoid pregnancy.

The use of Targretin® is contraindicated in patients with a known hypersensitivity to bexarotene or other components of the product. Targretin® must not be administered to pregnant women or to women who intend to become pregnant. If a woman becomes pregnant while taking Targretin®, treatment must be stopped immediately and counseling initiated due to the high risk of fetal harm.

Warnings (see package insert or online information for details)

Targretin® induces major lipid abnormalities in most patients. These abnormalities must be monitored and treated during long-term therapy. The effects on triglycerides, high-density lipoprotein cholesterol, and total cholesterol are reversible with the discontinuation of therapy, and could generally be minimized by a reduction in the dose of Targretin®.

Pancreatitis may occur and patients with CTCL who have risk factors for pancreatitis should (for the most part) not be treated with Targretin®.

Liver-function abnormalities, hepatic insufficiency, thyroid axis alterations, and leukopenia also have been reported in patients treated with Targretin®.

Patients should be advised to limit vitamin A supplements to avoid potential additive toxic effects.

Patients should be advised to minimize sun exposure as retinoids are associated with photosensitivity.

Resources for Patients

Complete product information at *www.ligand.com*

Resources for Professionals

Complete product information at *www.ligand.com*
Lists of scientific publications are available on the website.
Ligand Pharmaceuticals: 858-550-7500

Quick Summary Page

Agent: Tretinoin (Vesanoid®)
Manufacturer: Roche Laboratories
Nutley, NJ

Tretinoin is all-trans-retinoic acid, a derivative of vitamin A.

Website: *http://www.rocheusa.com/*

First approved by the FDA in November 1995.

Regulatory Approvals

Disease	*Dose*
Induction of remission in patients with acute promyelocytic leukemia	45 mg/m^2/day taken orally in two evenly divided doses until complete remission is documented

All patients should receive standard consolidation and/or maintenance chemotherapy for acute promyelocytic leukemia after completion of induction therapy with tretinoin, unless otherwise contraindicated. Maintain supportive care appropriate for acute promyelocytic leukemia patients during tretinoin therapy.

Setting
Primarily ambulatory

Pharmacokinetics
Following oral administration, peak concentration occurs in 1 to 2 hours.
Metabolism: Cytochrome p450 (CYP) enzymes have been implicated in the oxidative metabolism of tretinoin.
Excretion: Tretinoin is excreted in the urine and the feces.
Interactions: Because tretinoin is metabolized by the hepatic CYP system, there is a potential for alteration of pharmacokinetics in patients administered concomitant medications that are also inducers or inhibitors of this system.

Diagnostic/Laboratory Tests/Monitoring
- Blood: Frequently monitor patient's hematologic profile, coagulation profile, and triglyceride and cholesterol levels. Closely observe patients for signs of leukocytosis.
- Liver Function: Carefully and frequently monitor liver-function test results during therapy.
- Respiratory Function: Closely observe patient for signs of respiratory compromise.
- Pregnancy Test: Within one week before start of therapy, collect blood or urine for a pregnancy test with a sensitivity of at least 50 m IU/L. Delay therapy, if possible, until a negative result from test is obtained. When a delay is not possible, place patient on two reliable forms of contraception. Repeat pregnancy testing monthly throughout therapy.

Absorption of the retinoids is shown to be enhanced when taken with food.

Drug should be given under supervision of a physician experienced in management of acute leukemia and in a facility with laboratory and supportive services sufficient to monitor drug tolerance and protect and maintain a patient compromised by side effects related to administration of the drug, including respiratory compromise.

Administration
Capsules, 10 mg

Storage During Travel
Protect from extremes in temperature. Do not leave medication in the car or trunk. When traveling by airplane, take vials on board in passenger cabin so that medication will not be exposed to temperature extremes in the baggage compartment.

General Precautions (see package insert for details)
- **Advise patient to avoid pregnancy.**
- Instruct patient to use two reliable contraceptive methods simultaneously during therapy and for 1 month following discontinuation.
- Contraception must be used even when there is a history of infertility or menopause, unless a hysterectomy has been performed.
- Confirm diagnosis by detection of t(15;17) genetic marker by cytogenetic studies or other molecular diagnostic techniques. Efficacy of other disease subtypes to tretinoin has not been demonstrated.
- Drug is contraindicated in patients with a known hypersensitivity to retinoids.
- Approximately 25% of APL patients treated with tretinoin have experienced a syndrome called the retinoic acid-APL (RA-APL) syndrome characterized by fever, dyspnea, weight gain, radiographic pulmonary infiltrates, and pleural or pericardial effusions. Generally occurs during the first month of treatment.

Resources for Patients
Consult product sales representative for availability.

Resources for Professionals
Website: *http://www.rocheusa.com*
  Consult product sales representative for availability.
  Product Information Line: 1-800-526-6367

IMMUNOMODULATORS

Quick Summary Page

Agent: ImmuCyst®/TheraCys® (bacillus of Calmette and Guérin [BCG])
Manufacturer: Pasteur Merieux Connaught
Website: *http://www.connaught.com/*

Agent: TICE BCG (BCG vaccine) (OncoTICE®)
Manufacturer: Organon
Website: *http://www.akzonobel.com/*

BCG is a freeze-dried suspension of an attenuated strain of *Mycobacterium bovis* (Bacillus Calmette and Guérin) used in the nonspecific active therapy of carcinoma *in situ* of the urinary bladder. TheraCys® is BCG live and comes from a strain developed at the Pasteur Institute.

Regulatory Approval

Disease
ImmuCyst®/TheraCys®
Primary and relapsed carcinoma *in situ* of the urinary bladder with or without papillary tumors and following failure to respond to other treatment regimens. Drug is used to eliminate residual tumor cells and to reduce the frequency of tumor recurrence.

New Indication: The prophylaxis of primary and recurrent Ta and/or T1 papillary tumors following transurethral resection (TURB) (approved 11/99).

TICE BCG: Primary treatment of carcinoma *in situ* of the bladder in the absence of an associated invasive cancer without papillary tumors or with papillary tumors after transurethral resection, and as primary or secondary treatment for patients with medical contraindications to radical surgery.

Dosing
Induction: 81 mg intravesically under aseptic conditions once weekly for 6 weeks beginning 7–14 days after biopsy or transurethral resection if this procedure is done.

Maintenance Therapy
One treatment given 3, 6, 12, 18, and 24 months following the initial treatment.

One vial (50 mg) given intravesically per catheter once a week for six weeks. Schedule may be repeated if tumor remission is not achieved or if deemed clinically necessary. Thereafter, administer one dose at approximately monthly intervals at least 6 to 12 months.

Setting
Primarily ambulatory

Diagnostic/Laboratory Tests
Urinalysis

Administration
Vial Sizes:
 TheraCys®: 81 mg (1.05 billion ± 0.87 billion colony-forming units after reconstitution) 5% MSG.
  Preservative-free, in single-dose vials with two vials of diluent (3 and 50 mL)
 TICE BCG: 50 mg (1 to 8 × 10^8 CFU) lactose, preservative-free in 2-mL ampules

BCG is instilled directly into the bladder.

Storage/Stability:
Keep BCG and any accompanying diluent refrigerated between 2 to 8°C. At no time should the freeze-dried or reconstituted BCG be exposed to sunlight, direct or indirect. Keep exposure to artificial light to a minimum.

Induction Therapy
• Insert a urethral catheter into the bladder aseptically, drain bladder, and then instill 53 mL of suspension slowly by gravity; withdraw catheter.
• Patient should lie for 15 minutes each in prone and supine positions and also on each side.
• The patient is then allowed to be up, but retains suspension for another 60 minutes, for a total of 2 hours.
• All patients may not be able to retain suspension for 2 hours. Patients may void in less time, if needed.
• At the end of 2 hours, patient should void in a seated position for safety reasons. Disinfect urine voided for 6 hours after instillation with an equal volume of undiluted household bleach and allow to stand for 15 minutes before flushing.

Most local reactions occur following the third intravesicular administration; symptoms usually begin 2 to 4 hours after instillation and persist for 24 to 72 hours. Systemic reactions usually last for one to three days after each intravesicular instillation. Irritative bladder symptoms can be managed symptomatically with phenazopyridine, propantheline, and acetaminophen.
• If bladder catheterization has been associated with bleeding or possible false passage, do not administer drug, and delay retreatment by at least 1 week. Thereafter, resume treatment as if no interruption has occurred.

Storage During Travel
Protect from extremes in temperature. Do not leave medication in the car or trunk. When traveling by airplane, take vials on board in passenger cabin so that medication will not be exposed to temperature extremes in the baggage compartment. Vials should be transported in a cooler, near but not touching ice packs. Do not use dry ice because it may freeze the vials.

General Precautions (see package insert for details)
• Persons handling BCG should be masked, gloved, and gowned and should have no immunological deficiencies. *BCG should be treated as infectious material.*
• Carefully monitor urinary status for evidence of hematuria, urinary frequency, dysuria, and bacterial urinary-tract infection. If there is an increase in patient's existing symptoms, if symptoms persist, or if any symptoms develop, evaluate patient and manage for urinary-tract infection or BCG toxicity.

- Instruct patient to maintain adequate hydration.
- Treatment is contraindicated in patients on immunosuppressive therapy or with compromised immune systems.
- Treatment is contraindicated in presence of urinary-tract infection; use may result in risk of disseminated BCG infection or an increased severity of bladder irritation.
- Monitor closely for signs of systemic BCG infection. If systemic BCG infection is suspected (fever > 39°C or persistent fever > 38°C, severe malaise), consult an infectious-disease specialist and initiate fast-acting antituberculous therapy (BCG systemic infections are rarely evidenced by positive cultures).
- Intravesicular treatment with BCG could complicate future interpretations of skin-test reactions to tuberculin in diagnosis of suspected mycobacterial infections; determine patient's reactivity to tuberculin before administration of BCG.
- Instruct patients to report blood in urine, fever and chills, frequent urge to urinate, increased frequency of urination, increased tiredness or fatigue, joint pain, nausea and vomiting, painful urination, cough (rare), and skin rash (rare), to the health care team.

APPENDIX C | **Plans of Care for Patients Receiving Biological Agents**

Plans of care for patients receiving biological agents

Outcome	Assessment	Interventions	
		Therapeutic	**Educational**
Diagnosis: Knowledge deficit related to treatment with a biological agent*			
• Patient/significant other will verbalize expected side effects of agent and reportable signs and symptoms • Patient/significant other will demonstrate self-administration of agent if indicated	• Assess knowledge of side effects • Assess ability of patient/ significant other to be responsible for self-administration		• Instruct patient/significant other of expected side effects and reportable signs and symptoms • Instruct patient/significant other in reconstitution of agent • Instruct patient/significant other in IM or SC injection technique • Instruct patient/significant other in management of portable infusion pump
Diagnosis: Altered comfort related to chills (commonly occurs prior to fever)			
• Patient/significant other will demonstrate self-care behaviors for management of chills • Patient reports acceptable control of chills	• Assess severity and duration of chills and document • Monitor vital signs frequently and report changes to physician	• Keep patient warm • Avoid icy fluids • Medicate with meperidine 25 to 50 mg IVPB or sublingual Dilaudid as ordered • Antipyretics as ordered	• Instruct patient/significant other in self-management of chills • Instruct patient regarding duration (generally 30 to 60°)

Diagnosis: Fever 101° to 104° (38.4°–40.0°C)

• Patient/significant other will demonstrate self-care behaviors for management of fever • Patient reports acceptable control of temperature	• Monitor temperature frequently every one to four hours for hospitalized patients or with first course of therapy to establish patterns • Assess for complaints of tachycardia, chest pain, or shortness of breath and report to physician • Assess need for work up of potentially infectious episode for fevers unrelated to expected patterns or in neutropenic patients • Report to physician fevers >104°F despite antipyretics or other control measures	• Encourage p.o. fluids • Medicate with antipyretic as ordered • For temperature >103° despite antipyretic, consider —tepid sponge bath or shower —ice packs to temperature-control area —hypothermia blanket, if indicated	• Instruct patient/significant other to monitor temperature • As therapy continues, teach family to monitor temperature pattern in response to medication Report unusual spikes to health-care team • Instruct patient/significant other in self-management of fever • Instruct patient/significant other to report to physician if fever does not resolve after therapeutic measures

Diagnosis: Fatigue related to treatment with biological agents

• Patient maintains independence in activities of daily living and/or uses measures to prevent further immobility	• Assess effect of fatigue on activities of daily living • Assess usual patterns of sleep and rest • Assess for signs and symptoms associated with fatigue • Assess for cofactors that may influence fatigue (anemia, poor nutritional intake, etc.)	• Encourage patient to arrange most strenuous activities according to peak energy levels • Encourage patient to seek assistance with activities of daily living as necessary • Encourage patient to maintain mobility —ambulatory patient: mild exercise; e.g., walking as tolerated —bedridden patient: turn every 2 hours; active/passive range of motion	• Teach patient/significant other about fatigue as an expected side effect of biotherapy and self-management measures to prevent sequelae • Consider energy as a finite resource. How does patient want to "spend" it?

(continued)

Plans of care for patients receiving biological agents *(continued)*

Outcome	Assessment	Interventions	
		Therapeutic	**Educational**
		• Encourage patient to take short naps as required to increase energy levels • Treat cofactors that may contribute to fatigue as appropriate —use epoetin alfa for anemia —institute pain control measures • Evaluate need for use of assistive devices (e.g., walker, cane) to conserve energy stores • Institute measures to assure adequate intake of calories, proteins, and fluids	

Diagnosis: Potential for injury related to allergic reaction (primarily seen with murine monoclonal antibodies)

Outcome	Assessment	Interventions	
		Therapeutic	**Educational**
• Patient will immediately report signs and symptoms of anaphylaxis, hives, or itching	• Prior to administration, review prior allergic episodes to include —agent thought to be responsible —description of the episode (reaction to agent) • During administration, assess for —shortness of breath, wheezing —sneezing, coughing —local or generalized urticaria and/or erythema, itching	• Administer test dose if ordered • Ensure that emergency equipment is available • Ensure that emergency drugs (epinephrine, diphenhydramine, hydrocortisone) are available • Stop infusion immediately for signs of severe allergic reactions (e.g., hypotension, angioedema, shortness of breath) —increase IV fluids	• Teach patient to report: —pain or tightness in chest —dyspnea —inability to speak —generalized itching —symptoms of uneasiness, agitation, warmth, dizziness —desire to urinate or defecate

—notify physician
—institute orders as received

—hypotension
—tachycardia
—cyanosis
—unconsciousness
—emesis and/or diarrhea

Diagnosis: Pain related to myalgias, arthralgias, headaches

- Patient/significant other will demonstrate self-care behaviors for the management of myalgias and headaches
- Patient reports acceptable control of pain

- Assess need for analgesia
  —onset/duration of pain
  —intensity of pain

- Acetaminophen 650 mg po q three to four hours as ordered
- Apply moist heat to aching areas, cool for headache
- Consider use of NSAIDs or stronger analgesics as required
- For headache: adjust environment (quiet, dark room)
- Consider use of massage, reflexology by trained personnel

- Instruct patient/significant other in self-management of myalgias, arthralgias, and headaches

Diagnosis: Pruritis (primarily seen with IL-2)

- Patient identifies/demonstrates measures to control pruritus
- Patient reports acceptable control of pruritus

- Assess pruritis
  —onset/duration
  —characteristics
  —factors that relieve/aggravate the condition
  —treatment used previously
- Assess for signs of skin breakdown

- Water-based lotion and/or cream to affected area p.r.n.
- Use colloidal oatmeal baths in bathwater (tepid water instead of hot)
- Consider use of room humidifier
- Administer medications (e.g., antihistamines) as ordered; may need aggressive around-the-clock administration
- Encourage use of distraction (relaxation techniques, reading, needlework, etc.)
- Soft, cotton clothing

- Teach signs/symptoms of skin changes to report
- Discuss measures to promote skin hydration
- Teach measures to prevent further skin irritation
- Teach relaxation techniques as necessary
- Teach patient to substitute rub, pressure, or vibration for scratching (e.g., rub arms with lotion)

(continued)

Plans of care for patients receiving biological agents *(continued)*

Interventions

Outcome	Assessment	Therapeutic	Educational

Diagnosis: Altered skin integrity related to treatment with biological agents (patients on IL-2 may experience dry desquamation)

Outcome	Assessment	Therapeutic	Educational
• Patient/significant other will verbalize understanding of factors that may cause alteration in skin integrity • Skin integrity will be maintained • Patient/significant other will demonstrate behaviors to maintain skin integrity	• Observe skin daily for any breaks, discoloration, or redness • Observe injection sites for any changes • Observe IV sites for phlebitis, signs of infection (especially in patients on IL-2)	• Turn bedfast patient every two hours • Rotate injection sites for IM/SC agents • Apply moist heat to any inflamed areas • Apply water-based lotion and/or cream to entire body two to three times a day for dry desquamation • Consider use of room humidifier for dryness	• Instruct patient/significant other in individual measures for maintenance of skin integrity • Instruct patient/significant other in causative factors

Diagnosis: Altered thought processes related to treatment with biological agents (e.g., confusion, slowed mentation, somnolence)

Outcome	Assessment	Therapeutic	Educational
• Patient/significant other will verbalize understanding of factors that may cause alteration in thought processes • Patient/significant other will recognize changes in thinking or behavior • Patient will maintain reality orientation	• Assess mental status prior to therapy • Assess mental status each shift or clinic visit and when indicated • Assess amount of pre-medication and/or analgesics patient is receiving	• Orient to time and place if necessary • Allow verbalization of feelings • Refer to mental health professional if indicated • Report changes in mental status to physician • Initiate safety measures if indicated • Evaluate need for instituting therapy with antidepressants • Work with patient/family to develop strategies to compensate for deficit (e.g., lists for memory problems, alarms as reminders)	• Instruct patient/significant other how biological agent may cause alteration in thought process • Inform patient/significant other that this side effect is temporary and generally resolves when therapy is stopped

Diagnosis: Altered nutritional status, less than body requirements related to anorexia, mucositis, nausea, vomiting

- Patient will maintain adequate nutritional status
- Patient/significant other will verbalize understanding of nutritional needs
- Patient/significant other will demonstrate measures to increase nutritional intake

- Weigh patient regularly and record
- Initiate a calorie count if indicated to assess intake
- Assess biochemical measures of nutrition
  —albumin
  —transferrin
  —nitrogen balance

- Provide appetizing food consistent with patient preference
- Provide high-calorie, low-bulk foods
- Use nutritional supplements
- Refer to dietitian for consultation
- Try small, frequent meals
- Try cold foods if patient is sensitive to food odors
- Give antiemetics as ordered In some cases, around-the-clock administration may be necessary
- Discuss with health care team the need for tube feedings, IVH if nutritional status becomes severely compromised
- Consider use of appetite stimulants (e.g., megestrol acetate) if no contraindication
- Institute oral hygiene measures

- Instruct patient/significant other in measures to provide adequate nutrition

(continued)

Plans of care for patients receiving biological agents (*continued*)

| | | Interventions | |
Outcome	Assessment	Therapeutic	Educational
Diagnosis: Altered oral mucous membranes related to treatment with biological agents			

• Patient recognizes and reports changes in mucous membranes
• Patient demonstrates knowledge of oral hygiene protocol
	• Perform oral exam to include:
	  —palate
	  —gingiva
	  —dorsum of tongue
	  —undersurface of tongue
	  —floor of mouth
	  —buccal mucosa
	  —oral pharynx
	  —inner surface of lips
	• Assess normal oral hygiene routine
		• Encourage patient to perform oral hygiene after meals and at bedtime
		• Begin use of salt and soda mouth rinses every two hours and prn
		• Provide lubricant for lips
		• Encourage use of soft tooth brush
		• Consider oral irrigations prn to hydrate mouth and for comfort
		• Avoid use of agents that further dry the oral mucosa
		• Alter diet (e.g., avoid foods such as potato chips) if oral mucosa is inflamed
			• Explain rationale for prophylactic oral hygiene protocol
			• Teach proper oral hygiene protocol
			• Teach signs and symptoms to report to nurse/physician

Diagnosis: Diarrhea related to treatment with biological agents			
• Patient/significant other identifies measures to correct or control diarrhea	• Abdominal assessment every eight hours and prn** • Monitor intake and output every eight hours** • Monitor stools for frequency, volume, consistency and document • Assess perineal/perianal region for skin status • Assess electrolyte balance as indicated, signs of dehydration	• Administer IV fluid as ordered • Encourage adequate p.o. fluid intake • Administer medications that control diarrhea as ordered • Encourage hygiene measures. May consider use of sitz bath and/or barrier creams • Suggest low-residue dietary modifications	• Teach complications of diarrhea (e.g., fluid and electrolyte imbalance, skin breakdown) and prevention measures • Teach signs and symptoms to report

Diagnosis: Altered tissue perfusion related to treatment with biological agents (primarily seen with IL–2)

• Patients will maintain adequate blood pressure	• Assess
	  —orthostatic vital signs every one to four hours
	  —daily weights
	  —intake and output every eight hours***
	• Assess respiratory and cardiovascular system every eight hours or clinic visit for
	  —increased heart rate
	  —decreased blood pressure
	  —complaints of dizziness
	  —complaints of shortness of breath
	  —rales
	• Assess for fluid shifts as evidenced by
	  —peripheral edema
	  —ascites
	  —rales
	  —weight gain
	  —decreased urine output
	• Assess renal function (e.g., BUN, creatinine)
		• Administer IV fluids, colloids, and vasopressors as ordered
		• Institute comfort measures as necessary
		• Institute safety measures:
		  —ambulate with assistance
		  —rise from lying to sitting position slowly
		• Encourage p.o. fluid intake
			• Teach patient/significant other about hypotension as expected side effect of biotherapy and temporary nature of side effect
			• Teach patient/significant other to monitor for side effects while at home (daily weight, temperature t.i.d., etc.) and notify physician of any changes or problems
			• Teach patient/significant other to recognize these signs and symptoms:
			  —peripheral edema
			  —shortness of breath
			  —decreased urinary output
			  —weight gain of 5 pounds
			• Teach patient to rise from lying position slowly

(continued)

Plans of care for patients receiving biological agents (co...

Outcome	Assessment	Therap...
Diagnosis: Altered coping related to changes in disease status and/or new therapy		
• Patient recognizes potential/ actual stressors and facilitates own coping strategies	• Assess patient's perception of stressors and beliefs about the causes • Assess patient's past use of coping strategies • Evaluate patient's ability to problem solve	• Encourage patient to verbalize thoughts and feelings about changes in disease status and new therapy • Identify available resources for support and encourage participation (e.g., American Cancer Society, support groups, chaplain, etc.)	• Teach relaxation te... • Teach problem-solving techniques

* See complete patient teaching plan in Chapter 20.
** For hospitalized patients.
*** For ambulatory patients, assess for oliguria.
Source: Adapted and reprinted with permission from Rumsey, K. A., and P. T. Rieger (eds). Biological Response Modifiers: A self-instructional manual for health professionals. 1992. Chicago: Precept Press.
Abbreviations: IM, intramuscular; IV, intravenous; IVH, intravenous hyperalimentation; IVPB, intravenous piggyback; NSAIDs, non-steroidal antinflamatory drugs; PO, by mouth; prn, as required; q, every; sc, subcutaneous; tid, three times daily.

APPENDIX D | Normograms for Determination of Body Surface Area

Normograms for Determination of Body Surface Area from Height and Weight (Adults)*

Height	Body surface area	Weight

```
Height                              Body surface area          Weight

cm 200 ─┬─ 79 in                        2.80 m²        kg 150 ─┬─ 330 lb
          78                            2.70              145    320
   195                                                    140    310
          77                           2.60               135    300
          76                                              130    290
   190    75                           2.60                      290
          74                           2.50               125    280
   185    73                                                     270
          72                           2.40               120    260
   180    71                           2.30               115    250
          70                                              110    240
   175    69                           2.20               105    230
          68                                              100    220
   170    67                           2.10
          66                                               95    210
   165    65                           2.00
          64                           1.95                90    200
   160    63                           1.90
          62                           1.85                85    190
   155    61                           1.80
          60                           1.75                80    180
   150    59                           1.70
          58                           1.65                75    170
   145    57                           1.60
          56                           1.55                70    160
   140    55                           1.50                       150
          54                           1.45                65
   135    53                           1.40                       140
          52                           1.35                60
   130    51                           1.30                       130
          50
   125    49                           1.25                55    120
          48                           1.20
   120    47                           1.15                50    110
          46                                                      105
   115    45                           1.10                45    100
          44                           1.05                       95
   110    43                           1.00                40     90
          42                                                      85
   105    41                           0.95                35     80
                                                                 75
          40                           0.90
cm 100 ─┴─ 39 in                       0.86 m²        kg 30 ─┴─ 66 lb
                                                                 70
```

* From the formula of DuBois and DuBois. *Arch. Micrn. Med.* 17.863 (1916): $S = W^{0.696} \times H^{0.726} \times 71.84$, or $\log S = \log W \times 0.425 + \log H \times 0.725 + 1.8564$ (S = body surface in square centimeters; W = weight in kilograms; H = height in centimeters). The body surface area is the point of intersection on the middle scale when a straight line joins the height and weight scales (e.g., Patient A weighs 109 kg and is 171 cm tall; the patient's BSA [m²] is 2.2).

Source: Hubbard, S.M., and C.A. Seipp. 1982. Administration of cancer treatments: Practical guide for physicians and oncology nurses. In Devita, V.T., Jr., Hellman, S., and Rosenberg, S.A. (eds) *Cancer Principles and Practices of Oncology.* Philadelphia: Lippincott, 1985.

GLOSSARY

Absorption The rate at which a drug leaves the site of administration and the extent to which this occurs.

Acquired Immune-Deficiency Syndrome (AIDS) A disease caused by the HIV retrovirus that slowly undermines the immune system by destroying helper T cells.

Active specific immunity (ASI) Usually long-lasting immunity that is acquired through production of specific antibodies within the organism that are targeted to the presence of antigens.

Acute-phase proteins Molecules that increase in concentration during infection, e.g., C-reactive protein.

Adaptive immunity Immunity generated in response to a specific antigen. Hallmarks are memory and specificity.

ADCC Antibody-dependent cell-mediated cytotoxicity. A phenomenon in which target cells, coated with antibody, are destroyed by specialized killer cells that bear receptors for the Fc portion of the coating antibody. These receptors allow the killer cells to bind to the antibody-coated target.

Additive The relationship between 2 or more components such that their combined effect is the algebraic sum of their combined effects.

Adenovirus A virus containing DNA as its genetic material.

Adoptive cellular therapy Therapy that involves the transfer to the tumor-bearing host of immune cells with antitumor activity.

Adoptive transfer The transfer of immune cells or serum from one specifically immunized person to another. The goal is to transfer immunity to the nonimmunized person.

Agonist   A drug capable of combining with receptors to initiate drug actions.

Alleles   Variants of genes at a locus.

Alloantigens   Molecules that distinguish one individual from another individual of the same species. An example is the ABO blood type molecule.

Allogeneic   Involving, derived from, or being individuals of the same species but that are distinct antigenically.

Anabolic steroid   Any of a group of usually synthetic hormones that increase constructive metabolism. They are sometimes abused by athletes in training to temporarily increase the size of their muscles.

Anamnestic   "Memory response." A powerful antibody response (of secondary immune response type) following what is assumed to be initial exposure to an antigen.

Anastomosis   A communication between or coalescence of blood vessels.

Andragogy   The art and science of helping adults to learn.

Anergy   A condition in which the body fails to react to an injected allergen or antigen.

Aneuploidy   Presence of unusual numbers of chromosomes.

Angiogenesis   The formation of new microvessels from parent microvessels.

Anhedonia   Absence of pleasure from acts that would ordinarily be pleasurable.

Antagonistic   A substance that neutralizes or impedes the action or effect of another.

Anthelmintic   Of or pertaining to a substance capable of destroying or eliminating parasitic worms.

Anthropometric   The study of human body measurements especially on a comparative basis.

Antiangiogenic   Inhibition of the development of new blood vessels.

Antibody   A protein whose function it is to bind antigen.

Antigen   Any substance that, as a result of coming in contact with appropriate tissues, induces a state of sensitivity. Traditionally, an antigen is thought of as something "foreign" that, when introduced to the immune system, will generate an immune response. Antigens are also molecules that react with antibodies or primed T cells regardless of their ability to generate a response (e.g., histocompatibility antigens, differentiation antigens).

Antigen processing/presenting cells   Non-lymphocyte cells that carry antigen and present it to lymphocytes, resulting in induction of an immune response.

Antigenic determinant   The particular chemical group of a molecule that determines immunological specificity (dominant epitope clusters). This is the part that binds directly with the immunoglobulin or T-cell receptor.

Antigen modulation   The process by which the surface antigen on the cell is internalized or shed into the circulation after binding with antibody.

Anti-idiotype   An antibody targeted to the idiotype found on antibodies.

Antiproliferative   To inhibit the growth of a particular cell.

Apoptosis   Programmed cell death, a genetically controlled process to eliminate old or damaged cells.

Arachidonic acid   A liquid unsaturated fatty acid that occurs in most animal fats, is a precursor of prostaglandins, and is considered essential in animal nutrition.

Arthralgias   Joint pain.

Area under the curve (AUC)   The area under a pharmacology curve that defines the exposure of the target cell to a drug.

Asthenia   Lack or loss of strength, debility.

Attenuate   To lessen the amount, force, or magnitude; weaken.

Autocrine   Binding and activation of a cell by a substance produced by the same cell.

Autoimmunity   A state in which the immune system reacts against self antigens.

Autologous   Derived from the same individual.

B lymphocyte (B cell)   Lymphocytes derived from the bone marrow that develop into plasma cells and are responsible for the production of antibodies.

Bacillus Calmette-Guérin (BCG)   Strain of tubercle bacilli that causes tuberculosis in humans. Attenuated strain is often used as a vaccination against tuberculosis or as a means to nonspecifically stimulate the immune system.

Basophil   A white blood cell with basophilic granules that is similar in function to a mast cell.

Biological response modifiers (BRMs)   Agents or approaches that modify the relationship between tumor and host by modifying the host's biologic response to tumor cells with a resultant therapeutic effect.

Biotherapy   The use of agents derived from biological sources or of agents that affect biological responses.

Biotransformation   Enzymatic alteration of a drug.

Blood-brain barrier   The ability of brain capillaries to restrict the diffusion of substances from the blood supply into the brain because of their unique structure. Brain capillaries have no pores and are tightly wrapped in a sheath of astrocytes.

Bystander effect   Antitumor effect, or cell kill, of cancer cells adjacent to those treated. Generally seen with radiation or transduced cells in gene therapy.

C1q   One of the serum proteins involved in the immune response, the first component of complement.

Capsid   The layer of protein enveloping a virion.

Carcinogenesis   The transformation of normal cells into malignant cells.

Case management   The coordination of health and financial matters during and between episodes of care to achieve optimal clinical and financial outcomes.

Catabolic   Relating to catabolism (i.e., destructive metabolism involving the release of energy and resulting in the breakdown of complex materials within the organism).

Catalysis   The effect that a catalyst exerts on a chemical reaction.

Catalyst   A substance that accelerates a chemical reaction but is not consumed or changed during the reaction.

Catecholaminergic   Involving, liberating, or mediated by catecholamines.

Cationic   Positively charged. An ion that in solution is attracted to the negative electrode.

CD4+ cells   Subset of T cells that function as helper cells, promoting the proliferation, maturation, and immunological function of other cell types.

CD8+ cells   Cytotoxic T cell subset that has the ability to kill cells with foreign macromolecules on their surface.

Cell cycle   The sequence of events required for growth and division of a cell.

Cell-mediated immunity   Immunity mediated by cells, primarily lymphocytes.

Chemoimmunoconjugate   Linking of a drug to an antibody; usually an antineoplastic drug such as doxorubicin or methotrexate.

Chemokine   Chemokines belong to a large family of chemoattractant molecules involved in the directed migration of immune cells.

Chemotaxis   Directional movement by immune cells in response to an inflammatory mediator.

Chills   A sensation of cold.

Chimeric   Composed of parts of different origin.

Chromosome   A structural unit within DNA. A chromosome is composed of genes and transmits hereditary information, normally 46 in man.

Class I MHC   Major histocompatability proteins whose role is to display fragments of proteins originating inside the cell.

Class II MHC   Major histocompatibility proteins whose role is to display fragments of proteins from digested microorganisms.

Clearance   A measure of the speed at which a drug leaves the system.

Clinical pathway   A multidisciplinary approach to a plan of care that specifies how to carry out certain treatments or procedures within the practice guideline for a specific clinical indication.

Colony assays   Analysis of cells produced from a single cell cultivated on special medium.

Complement   A series of serum proteins involved in the mediation of immune reactions. The complement cascade is triggered classically by the interaction of antibody with specific antigen.

Complementarity-determining regions   The hypervariable region of the antibody that binds to an antigen.

Conjugate   The process of attaching a drug, toxin, or radioactive substance to a biological molecule such as an antibody.

Costimulation   Stimulation of the immune response by more than one signal.

Cytogenetics   The study of cytology in relation to genetics.

Cytokines   A generic term for proteins released by cells on contact with a specific anti-gen that serve as messengers between cells. Cytokines effect the growth and differentiation of white blood cells and regulate immune and inflammatory responses.

Cytokine cascade   Network of interactions that occur through mutual cytokine induction; through transmodulation of cell-surface receptors; and by synergistic, additive, or antagonistic interactions that affect the function of a target cell.

Cytoplasm   Gelatinous substance inside the cell.

Cytotoxic   Detrimental to or destruction of cells.

Cytotoxic T cell   Effector T-lymphocyte subset that directly lyses target cells.

Delirium   A type of organic mental disturbance characterized by confusion, decreased ability to attend and process information, and occasional hallucinations or delusions. Agitation is a common feature. This state generally develops over a short period, fluctuates during the day, and is usually reversible when the underlying etiology is corrected. Delirium is often caused by metabolic disturbance or medication effects. This disturbance also is referred to as an acute confusional state and is one of the conditions included under the term encephalopathy.

Deoxyribonucleic acid (DNA)   The type of nucleic acid found principally in the nucleus of animal and vegetable cells. The repository of hereditary characteristics (genetic information). A large, double-helix molecule that controls protein synthesis within a cell.

Differentiation   The process of cell development and maturation. Results in ability to perform specialized functions for a particular cell type.

Differentiation antigens   Antigens (proteins) expressed during different stages of development. For example, different cell-surface antigens are expressed on T cells as they mature.

Disease management A systematic approach to patient care in which coordination of medical services is extended across the entire health care delivery system.

Distribution Movement of a drug from the site of administration to the site of action.

Downregulate Decreased expression of receptors or cell-surface proteins.

Dyscrasia Diseases affecting blood cells or platelets.

Effector A small molecule that binds to a protein and thereby alters the activity of that molecule.

Effector cell A cell that becomes active in response to stimulation.

Encapsulated The surrounding of one substance or compound with a thin coat of another.

Encephalopathy A term used to describe a number of organic mental disturbances, including delirium and post-traumatic confusional states. They are distinguished from more gradual, progressive dementias by their relatively abrupt onset. Depending upon the specific entity, an encephalopathy may be reversible (i.e., toxic-metabolic encephalopathy) or permanent (i.e., severe anoxia).

Endocrine An action that occurs when a substance is secreted by a cell and binds to distant cells in the body.

Endocytosis Internalization of substances from the extracellular environment through the formation of vesicles formed from the plasma membrane.

Endogenous Originating or produced within an organism.

Endotoxin A complex phospholipid-polysaccharide macromolecule that forms part of the cell wall of a variety of gram negative bacteria.

Eosinophil A white blood cell or other granulocyte with cytoplasmic inclusions that stains readily with eosin. A hallmark of acute and chronic allergic responses. Eosinophil levels are also elevated with administration of interleukin-2.

Episomal Related to a genetic determinant (as the DNA of some bacteriophages) that can replicate either autonomously in bacterial cytoplasm or as an integral part of their chromosomes.

Erythropoietin (Epo) Hematopoietic growth factor produced in response to decreased oxygen in the blood circulating through the kidneys; stimulates erythroblast differentiation and recruits immature progenitors.

Esterified Having been converted to an ester. An ester, as defined in organic chemistry, is a compound formed by the combination of an organic acid with an alcohol.

Eukaryotic Descriptor for an organism composed of one or more cells containing visibly evident nuclei and organelles.

Exogenous Originating or produced outside of the body.

Extrapyramidal motor symptoms A symptom constellation that may include rigidity, tremor, slowness of movement, poor coordination, and difficulty maintaining balance. These symptoms are due to dysfunction of subcortical brain regions.

FAB Fragment of antibody containing the antigen-binding site generated by cleavage of the antibody with the enzyme papain, which cuts at the hinge region.

Fc Fragment of antibody without antigen-binding sites generated by cleavage with papain. The Fc fragment contains the C terminal domains of the heavy immunoglobulin chains.

Fc receptor Protein on the surface of immune cells that recognizes the Fc region of an antibody once it has bound an antigen.

FDA Food and Drug Administration.

Feeder layers Semisolid medium used for clonal assays that contain medium, accessory cells, cell extracts, or medium conditioned by tissues.

Flow cytometry   A technique for identifying and sorting cells and their components (as DNA) by staining with a fluorescent dye and detecting the fluorescence usually by laser beam illumination.

Fibroblast   A cell present in the connective tissue that is capable of forming collagen fibers.

FISH   Fluorescent in situ hybridization, using a fluorescent tagged probe to see a molecule of DNA or RNA in its natural location.

Freund's complete adjuvant   A vehicle used to increase antigenicity. A water-in-oil emulsion of antigen, to which killed mycobacterium are added.

Gene   A sequence of nucleotide base pairs within the DNA structure. Contains the genetic code for producing specific proteins.

Gene expression   The process of protein synthesis.

Gene therapy   The insertion of a gene into a patient's cells to reverse an acquired gene defect or to add a new function to the cell.

Genetics   The branch of science concerned with heredity.

Genome   Total genetic information carried by a cell or organism.

Genotype   The makeup of DNA: the description of an organism at the genetic level.

G_0   The phase of the cell cycle when cells are said to be resting or non-dividing.

G_1   The phase of the cell cycle that is sensitive to effects of transcription factors that presumably act on the synthesis of DNA.

Gluconeogenesis   The formation of glucose within the animal body especially by the liver and kidney from precursors other than carbohydrates using amino acids from proteins, glycerol from fats, or lactate produced by muscle during anaerobic glycolysis; also called glyconeogenesis

Graft-versus-host disease   Reaction of a graft rich in immunologically competent cells against the tissue of a genetically nonidentical recipient.

Granulocyte colony-stimulating factor (G-CSF)   Hematopoietic growth factor that stimulates neutrophil production and maturation and enhances the function of mature neutrophils.

Granulocyte-macrophage colony-stimulating factor (GM-CSF)   Hematopoietic growth factor that preferentially supports neutrophil, eosinophil, and macrophage development and interacts with early progenitors; inhibits neutrophil migration.

Growth fraction   The proportion of cells in active proliferation.

HACA   Human anti-chimeric antibody. The immune response generated by the infusion of a chimeric antibody into an immunocompetent individual. The response is targeted to the mouse portion of the antibody.

HAHA   Human anti-human antibody. The immune response generated by the infusion of a human antibody into an immunocompetent individual.

HAMA   Human anti-mouse antibody. The immune response generated by the infusion of a murine antibody into an immunocompetent individual.

Haplotype   "Half of a genotype," refers to the complete set of MHC loci inherited from one parent.

Hapten   An incomplete or partial antigen, incapable of causing antibody production alone but capable of binding to antibody.

Haptenated   An abbreviated form.

Helper/inducer T cell (T_h)   A subset of T lymphocytes (CD4) whose presence is required by B cells for normal antibody production.

Hematopoietic   Pertaining or relating to the formation of blood cells.

Hematopoietic growth factor (HGF) A family of glycosylated proteins that interact with specific cell-surface receptors to regulate the reproduction, maturation, and functional activity of blood cells.

Hematopoietic stem cell An unspecialized cell in the bone marrow that gives rise to differentiated blood cells.

Heterogeneity The wide variability in cell properties within a cancer.

Histiocyte A macrophage, especially a nonmotile macrophage, of extravascular tissues and especially connective tissue.

Histologic examination The examination of stained sections of tissue under the microscope.

Human leukocyte antigen (HLA) complex A complex group of antigens that define human tissue histocompatibility.

Humoral immunity Immunity mediated by the cell-free portion of the blood primarily by antibodies.

Hybridoma A hybrid cell that results from the fusion of an antibody-secreting cell with a malignant cell. The progeny secrete antibody without stimulation and proliferate continuously both *in vivo* and *in vitro*.

Hydrolytic enzymes An enzyme that breaks down a molecule into its constituent parts with incorporation of the elements of water.

Hydrophilic "Water loving." The tendency to attract and hold water.

Hydrophobic "Water hating," the tendency to repel water.

Hyperchromatism Dark staining.

Idiotype The combined antigenic determinants (idiotypes) found on antibodies of an individual that are directed at a particular antigen. Such antigenic determinants are found only in the variable region.

Immune surveillance The concept that immunological mechanisms "recognize" and remove malignant cells as they arise.

Immunization The creation of immunity usually against a particular disease with the goal of making the organism immune to subsequent attack by a particular pathogen.

Immunochemotherapy The combination of immunotherapy and chemotherapy.

Immunoconjugate A generic term to describe the linking of a toxic substance, such as chemotherapy or plant or bacterial toxins, to a cell-binding substance (often a monoclonal antibody).

Immunogenic "Antigenic;" having the properties of an antigen. An immunogen is a molecule capable of inducing an immune response.

Immunoglobulin Protein molecules composed of four polypeptide chains that function as antibodies. There are five classes of immunoglobulins: IgG, M, A, D, and E.

Immunomodulation Alteration of immune responses through inhibition or stimulation.

Immunophenotyping The observed immunological characteristics of an organ or cell.

Immunoregulation Having the biological property of regulating immune responses.

Immunotoxin Monoclonal antibody with a toxin molecule (e.g., diphtheria toxin) attached.

Immunotherapy The use of therapy that stimulates the immune system as its mechanism of action.

INDA Investigational new drug application.

Innate immunity Nonspecific immunity that does not involve the specific recognition of antigen.

Intracrine Secreted within.

Invasion The spread of a tumor into adjacent tissues.

Interleukin Literally, "between leukocytes." This term refers to the signaling and communication that occur between cells in the immune system.

Interleukin-3 (IL-3) Hematopoietic growth factor that causes stem cells to differentiate into granulocytes, macrophages, megakaryocytes, erythrocytes, and lymphocytes.

Isotype Any of the categories of antibodies determined by their physicochemical properties (such as molecular weight) and antigenic characteristics.

Killer-cell inhibitory receptors (KIRs) A family of receptors expressed by natural killer cells. These receptors recognize the class I proteins that are part of the major histocompatibility complex.

Large granular lymphocytes Cells that, after exposure to mediators such as IL-2, can efficiently kill targets that are natural-killer insensitive.

Lectins Protein mitogens.

Leukocyte A white blood cell.

Leukotriene Any of a group of eicosanoids that are generated in basophils, most cells, macrophages, and human lung tissue by lipoxygenase-catalyzed oxygenation. Leukotrienes participate in allergic responses (such as bronchoconstriction in asthma).

Ligand Something that binds, especially molecules that bind to cells or other molecules.

Lipogenesis Formation of fat in the living body especially when excessive or abnormal.

Liposomes A spherical particle of lipid substance suspended in an aqueous medium within a tissue.

Locus The position on the chromosome where the gene is positioned.

Lymph node Any of the rounded masses of lymphoid tissue that are surrounded by a capsule of connective tissue, are distributed along the lymphatic vessels, and contain numerous lymphocytes that filter the flow of lymph passing through the node. Sometimes called a "lymph gland."

Lymphocytes Cells that originate from stem cells and differentiate in lymphoid tissue (as of the thymus or bone marrow) and are the typical cellular elements of lymph. They constitute 20% to 30% of the white blood cells of normal human blood.

Lymphokines Protein molecules secreted by lymphocytes that serve as messengers between cells of the immune system.

Lymphokine activated killer (LAK) cells Peripheral blood lymphocytes capable of lysing a variety of tumor cell lines after exposure to IL-2.

Lysis Destruction of cells, bacteria, and other structures by a specific agent.

Macrophage A phagocytic tissue cell of the mononuclear phagocyte system that may be fixed or freely motile. It is derived from a monocyte and functions in the protection of the body against infection and noxious substances.

Macrophage colony-stimulating factor (M-CSF) Hematopoietic growth factor that activates monocytes prompting macrophage production, and stimulates enhanced cytotoxicity against fungi.

Major histocompatibility complex (MHC) The collection of genes coding for cell-surface compatibility antigens.

Malaise A feeling of general discomfort; often the first indication of infection or disease.

Margination A process that occurs during early phases of inflammation, when leukocytes adhere to the endothelial cells lining blood vessel walls.

Marker Characteristic or factor by which a cell or molecule can be recognized or identified.

Mast cell Specialized immune cell responsible for the secretion of histamine.

Meiosis The process of cell division that results in the production of gametes, each containing one half the normal number of chromosomes.

Memory cell A long-lived lymphocyte that

carries the antibody or receptor for a specific antigen after a first exposure to the antigen and that remains in a less than mature state until stimulated by a second exposure to the antigen at which time it mounts a more effective immune response than a cell that has not been exposed previously.

Memory response The capacity of the immune system to respond much faster and more powerfully to subsequent antigen exposure than the first time.

Metastasis The spread of cancer cells from the primary site to a distant site.

Methanol extraction residue of BCG (MER-BCG) MER, a cell wall fraction of BCG, has been reported to exhibit immunomodulating properties. It has been used as an adjuvant of immunotherapy in cancer patients.

MHC restriction Recognition of foreign antigen only in conjunction with class I MHC antigens.

Mitogen A molecule that can induce nonspecific division and activation of lymphocytes.

Mitosis The process of cell division that results in the production of two daughter cells.

Mitotic index The proportion of cells in a given tissue that are in mitosis at any given time.

Modulate When antigens expressed on the surface of a cell change; that is, they may be shed into the bloodstream or internalized within the cell and no longer expressed on the surface.

Molecular biology Knowledge of how the cell expresses its information from DNA to RNA to protein.

Monoclonal antibody Literally an antibody from a single clone. A clone is the progeny of a single cell. The antibody is homogeneous.

Monocyte A large white blood cell that is formed in the bone marrow, enters the blood, and migrates into the connective tissue where it differentiates into a macrophage.

Monokines Regulatory proteins produced by monocytes.

Mononuclear phagocyte system A system of cells comprising all free and fixed macrophages together with their ancestral cells including monocytes and their precursors in the bone marrow.

Mucosal-associated lymphoid tissue (MALT) A specialized group of lymphoid tissues found in mucosal areas such as the gut or bronchus.

Multipotential colony-stimulating factor (multi-CSF) Another name for interleukin-3.

Mutism The absence of speech in a conscious person who does not have a primary disturbance of language (aphasia) or of motor function (paralysis of voice musculature).

Myalgias Muscle aches.

Myc protein A transcription factor involved in regulation of cell division.

Natural killer (NK) cells Lymphocytes (non B or T) that kill a range of tumor cell targets without antigen specificity. Sometimes known as "large granular lymphocytes."

NDA New drug application.

Neurotropic Having an affinity for or localizing selectively in nerve tissue

Neutrophil Immune cell, mostly found in blood, that ingests and destroys invading microorganisms.

Nucleotide Any compound containing a heterocyclic compund bound to a phosphorylate sugar by an N-glycosyl link.

Nucleus The central structure within a cell that houses the genetic code.

Nude mouse Hairless mouse with congenital absence of the thymus, hence; thymus-dependent areas are depleted of T lymphocytes.

Null cells Lymphocytes that lack both T- or B-cell markers.

OBD Optimal biological dose; may be defined as the minimum dose at which biological activity is maximally stimulated.

2′-5′ oligoadenylate synthetase   A protein that can be induced by IFN, which, when activated, inhibits protein synthesis.

Oligodeoxynucleotides (ODNs)   Short segments of deoxyribonucleic acid (DNA) synthesized primarily in an automatic synthesizer or "gene machine."

Oncofetal   Products that are normally present during embryonic and fetal development but that are either not present or present at very low levels in normal adult tissue. Examples include carcinoembryonic antigen (CEA) and alpha-fetal protein (AFP).

Oncogene   An altered version of a normal-cell gene (proto-oncogene) that can cause cancer.

Organelles   Small organs within a cell.

Outcomes analysis   The end result of a certain action or intervention.

Oxidative phosphorylation   Formation of high energy phosphoric bonds via biochemical process.

Oxidized   Combined with oxygen. The process includes a loss of electrons and a resultant increase in positive valence.

p53 gene   A tumor-suppressor gene that controls the cell cycle transition from the G_1 phase to the S phase.

Parabiotic   Descriptor for the anatomical and physiological union of two organisms either natural (as in Siamese twins) or artificially produced

Paracrine   Binding of a substance and activation of nearby cells.

Passive antibody therapy   Administration of serum-containing antibody.

Perforins   Molecules involved in the destruction of cells. They cause donut-shaped holes to form in the cell membrane, allowing cellular contents to leak out.

Peripheral tolerance   The death of immune cells in the periphery (i.e., circulation or lymphatic system) to reduce the pool of memory cells to a level sufficient to sustain immunologic memory and avoid beneficial immune reactions from becoming harmful.

Phagocytes   Cells that engulf and consume foreign material such as microorganisms and debris.

Phagocytosis   The process of ingestion of microbes, other cells, and foreign particles by phagocytes. Neutrophils and macrophages function as phagocytes.

Phagosome   An intracellular vesicle in a phagocyte formed by invagination of the cell membrane during phagocytosis. It contains phagocytized material. Digestion generally occurs by lysosomal enzymes.

Pharmacodynamics   Defined simply, what the drug does to the body.

Pharmacokinetics   Defined simply, what the body does to a drug.

Phenotype   The observed characteristics of an organism that result from interaction of genes and the environment.

Philadelphia chromosome (Ph¹)   An abnormal chromosome formed as a result of translocation between arms of chromosome 9 and 22. Found in patients diagnosed with chronic myelogenous leukemia.

Phosphorylation   To cause (on organic compound) to take up or combine with phosphoric acid or a phosphorus-containing group.

Photoisomer   One of two or more forms of a compound exhibiting optical isomerism. Compounds that contain the same number of atoms of the same elements but differ in structural arrangement and properties.

Phylogenetic   The description of the evolution of a genetically related set of organisms.

Piloerection   Erection of the hair.

Plasma cell   A lymphocyte that is a mature antibody-secreting B cell.

Plasma concentration   The amount of both free and bound drug in the plasma.

Plasma membrane   Membrane that forms the outer covering of a cell.

Plasmid   A genetic particle physically separate from the chromosome of the host cell that can stably function and replicate. Also called a "para gene."

Pleiotropic   Characterized by the production of multiple effects.

Pleomorphism   Variation in size and shape.

Pluripotent stem cells (PPSC)   An uncommitted cell that produces two daughter cells, one that enters a differentiation pathway and another that returns to a resting pool of cells.

Polyclonal   Proteins from more than a single clone of cells.

Polymerase chain reaction (PCR)   A technique to amplify the specific genes that codes for the variable region of the mouse antibody. The two strands of DNA are separated and the separated strands serve as a template for a complementary strand of DNA. Repetitions of the process can result in more than two million copies of the desired gene in a matter of hours.

PPD   Purified protein derivative. Substance used in intradermal test for tuberculosis.

Practice guideline   A systematically developed flow chart that helps practitioners and patients make decisions about appropriate health care for specific clinical indications, such as colon cancer.

Precursors   Immature forms of blood cells.

Prodrug   A drug that can be converted to a toxic metabolite when metabolized.

Professional antigen-presenting cell (APC)   A group of cells that have the ability to educate T, B, and NK cells to the specific antigens. The most adept of these cells are a closely related family termed dendritic cells (DC).

Progenitors   Earliest committed cells in each lineage.

Promoter   A DNA sequence at which RNA polymerase binds and initiates transcription.

Prostaglandin   Any of various oxygenated unsaturated cyclic fatty acids of animals that have a variety of hormone-like actions.

Protein kinase   An enzyme that switches other enzymes on or off by attaching a phosphate group to them.

Proteolysis   The hydrolysis of proteins or peptides with formation of simpler and soluble products (as in digestion).

Proto-oncogenes   A gene present in the normal genome that appears to have a role in regulation of normal cell growth that is converted into an oncogene through somatic mutation.

Pseudopod   A temporary process put forth for the purpose of locomotion

Psychoactivity   Activity that affects the mind or behavior.

Psychometric testing   The administration of standardized psychological tests with known validity and reliability.

p-value or alpha level   The level of probability that the obtained results are a result of chance alone. Generally .05 alpha level means that generalizing to the real world or in repeating the study you should find these same differences 95 out of 100 times, thus it is unlikely that the differences are due to chance.

Pyrogen   An agent that causes a rise in temperature.

Racemic   The state of being optically inactive and separable into two other substances of the same chemical composition as the original substance, one of which is dextrorotatory and the other levorotatory.

Radioimmunoconjugate   A monoclonal antibody combined with a radionuclide. These conjugates may be used for either diagnostic or therapeutic purposes depending on the radionuclide and the amount of radiation.

RAID (radioimmunodetection) External imaging to disclose foci of increased radioactivity after injection of radioactive antibodies.

Recombinant Genetically engineered; may refer to a whole organism or a single product.

Recombinant DNA Genetically engineered DNA. Often involves the insertion of a gene coding for a specific protein into an expression system such as a bacterium to produce biologically active proteins such as interferon.

Redundance Repetition.

Reticulocyte Immature red blood cells that are larger than mature erythrocytes yet nonnucleated. They circulate in the blood for 1 to 2 days while maturing.

Retinoids Synthetic or naturally occurring analogs of vitamin A.

Retrovirus A virus from the family retroviridae. These viruses possess the enzyme RNA dependent DNA polymerase (reverse transcriptase).

Reverse-transcription polymerase chain reaction (RT-PCR) The process of making cDNA (complementary DNA) using an RNA template and then amplifying copies of the cDNA through PCR techniques.

Ribonucleic acid (RNA) A large molecule consisting of ribonucleoside residues attached to the 3′ hydroxyl of one nucleoside to the 5′ hydroxyl of the next nucleoside by phosphates.

Rigors A feeling of cold with shivering and pallor, accompanied by an elevation of temperature.

Secondary cytokines Cytokines that are induced following the administration or secretion of another cytokine. For example, interleukin-1 stimulates T cells to produce interleukin-2.

SIDs (shared anti-idiotypes) Anti-idiotype antibodies that share an idiotypic determining site with another anti-idiotype.

Signal transduction A process of transmitting information (signal) received on the cell surface to the cell's inner structures and nucleus.

Skinfold A fold of skin formed by pinching or compressing the skin and subcutaneous layers especially in order to estimate the amount of body fat.

Somatic mutation Mutation that occurs in cells other than germline cells.

Stem cell factor (SCF) Hematopoietic growth factor that works at the earliest level of commitment and possibly effects the PPSC.

Subcortical dementia A clinical syndrome characterized by behavioral slowing, loss of memory, frontal lobe dysfunction, and mood and personality changes. Cortical functions such as speech and language tend to be preserved. This syndrome can be due to dysfunction of subcortical brain regions or of the connections between the subcortical and frontal lobe regions. Typical examples of subcortical dementia are Parkinson's disease and Huntington's disease.

Super antigens Antigens that are capable of activating large subsets of T cells.

Suppressor T cell A subset of T lymphocytes responsible for suppression of the immune response.

Synergistic The coordinated action of two or more substances such that the combined action is greater than that of each acting separately.

Syngeneic Genetically identical especially with respect to antigens or immunological reactions.

T$_h$1 A subset of T-helper cells that secrete cytokines that help defend the body against viral or bacterial invasion. Cytokines secreted include IL-2, IFN-γ, and TNF.

T$_h$2 A subset of T helper cells that secretes cytokines that assist in protection from parasitic and mucosal infections. Cytokines secreted include IL-4, IL-5, and IL-10.

T-cell receptor (TCR)   Molecule (as a protein) on the cell surface of the T cell that has an affinity for a specific antigen.

Tachyphylaxis   A progressive decrease in response following repetitive administration of a physiologically or pharmacologically active substance.

T cell   Type of immune system cell responsible for cell-mediated immunity and which makes T-cell receptors instead of antibodies.

Telomerase   An enzyme that allows a cell to replicate indefinitely by replacing telomere length.

Telomere   The ends of chromosomes. Each time a cell replicates, the telomeres shorten, which leads to cell senescence and cell death.

Thymocyte   A cell of the thymus, especially a thymic lymphocyte.

Titers   The standard of strength of a volumetric test solution. The assay value of an unknown measure by volumetric means.

Tolerance   The capacity of the body to endure or become less responsive to a substance.

Tolergens   Molecules that induce a state of immunologic unresponsiveness.

Transcription   The first step in protein synthesis. An RNA molecule or copy of the information within DNA is made within the nucleus. Information transfer from DNA to RNA.

Transduction   Transfer of genetic material from one cell to another by viral infection.

Transformation   A permanent genetic change induced in a cell following incorporation of new DNA.

Transgene   A newly introduced gene.

Transgenic mice   Having chromosomes into which one or more heterologous genes have been incorporated either artificially or naturally.

Translation   The second step of protein syn-

thesis. Information from mRNA is used to make the new protein within the cytoplasmic structures. Information transfer from RNA to protein.

Translocation   Transposition of two segments between nonhomologous chromosomes as a result of abnormal breakage.

Trophoblast   The cell layer that covers the blastocyst and supplies nutrition to the embryo. It erodes the uterine mucosa and forms a cavity that facilitates implantation. These cells do not enter into the formation of the embryo itself.

Tumor-associated antigens   Antigens expressed to a greater degree on tumor cells than on normal cells. There are four basic types: oncofetal, unique, antigens from unrelated tissue, and antigens from the same tissue.

Tumor-infiltrating lymphocytes (TILs)   Lymphocytes obtained from tumor specimens.

Tumor-suppressor gene   A gene that inhibits growth. Loss of function can lead to cell transformation and malignancy.

Tumor volume-doubling time   The time taken for a tumor mass to double its volume of cells.

Ultraviolet light   Invisible radiation of higher energy than visible light.

Unconjugated   A monoclonal antibody with nothing (e.g., toxin or chemotherapy) attached to it. Another term would be a "naked" antibody.

Upregulate   Increased expression of receptors or cell-surface proteins.

Vacuole   A clear space in the substance of a cell that can surround a foreign body and serve as a temporary stomach for the digestion of the body.

Vector   The vehicle that carries a gene into the target cell, getting it through the cell wall into the nucleus and then the chromosome. A "carrier" that is used to introduce foreign genetic material into a host.

Visceral protein   Protein related to an internal organ of the body.

Virion   A virus particle.

Virus   Subcellular parasite with genes of DNA or RNA. Replicates inside the host cell, upon which it relies for energy and protein synthesis. In addition, it has an extracellular form in which the virus genes are contained inside a protective coat.

Wild-type   A phenotype, genotype, or gene that predominates in a natural population of organisms.

Xenograft   A graft transferred from an animal of one species to an animal of another.

INDEX

Note: Page numbers followed by f indicate figures; those followed by t indicate tables.